PSC

First Edition

Patient Self-Care

Helping patients make therapeutic choices

PUBLISHED BY:
Canadian Pharmacists Association
Ottawa, Ontario, Canada

President:	Ron Elliott, BScPharm, FASCP
Executive Director:	Jeff Poston, PhD, MRPharmS
Senior Director, Publications:	Leesa D. Bruce
Editor-in-Chief:	Carol Repchinsky, BSP
Managing Editor:	Christine LeBlanc, B Journalism
Clinical Editors:	Barbara Jovaisas, BSc(Pharm)
	Karen Leahey, BScPhm
	Cynthia Way, BScPharm
Manager, Publication Technology:	Darquise Leblanc
Design and Production:	Lucienne Prévost
Desktop Publishers:	Kathleen Régimbald
	Bob Heathorn

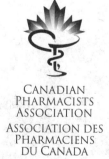

CANADIAN
PHARMACISTS
ASSOCIATION
ASSOCIATION DES
PHARMACIENS
DU CANADA

The editors gratefully acknowledge the assistance of Frances Hachborn, Lili Loorand-Stiver, Robin McIntosh and Louise Welbanks.

Published by:
Canadian Pharmacists Association
1785 Alta Vista Drive
Ottawa, ON K1G 3Y6
Canada

Tel.: (613) 523-7877
Fax: (613) 523-0445

Cover design by:
Ozayr S. Saloojee, Co-Principal,
Blue Pooch Design/Build

Illustrations by:
Lianne Friesen

Index by:
Dianne Baxter,
The Text Therapist

Printed in Canada by:
Webcom Limited

Canadian cataloguing in publication data
Main entry under title: Patient Self-Care

Previously published under title Nonprescription Drug Reference for Health Professionals (NDR).

1. Drugs, nonprescription 2. Self-care, patient
I. Repchinsky, Carol, 1951-
II. LeBlanc, Christine, 1973-
III. Canadian Pharmacists Association

ISBN 10894402-03-0

Table of Contents

Patient Self-Care. Helping Patients Make Therapeutic Choices

Editorial Board

Authors

Dr. John Bachynsky, PhD
University of Alberta, Faculty of Pharmacy &
  Pharmaceutical Sciences
Edmonton, AB

Denis Bélanger, BScPhm
Ottawa Valley Regional Drug Information
  Service
Ottawa, ON

Marie Berry, BScPharm, BA, LLB
Vimy Park Pharmacy
Winnipeg, MB

Carole Beveridge, BScPhm, RNCP
Beveridge & Brown Pharmacy
Cambridge, ON

Michelle Bourassa, BPharm, MSc, DMD
Dentist, private practice, Québec City
Chargée de cours, Faculté de Médecine
  Dentaire, Université Laval
Hospital pharmacist, Trois-Rivières
Québec, QC

Janie Bowles-Jordan, BScPhm
Marchese Pharmacy
Ancaster, ON

Thomas E. R. Brown, PharmD
Sunnybrook & Womens College Health
  Sciences Centre
Toronto, ON

Christinne Campbell, BScPhm
Sunnybrook & Womens College Health
  Sciences Centre
Toronto, ON

**Patricia Carruthers-Czyzewski, BScPhm,
  MSc (Pharmacology)**
Sintera Inc., Health Care Consulting
Ottawa, ON

Shelita Dattani, BSc(Pharm), PharmD
Pharmacy Department,
Queensway-Carleton Hospital
Nepean, ON

Lisa Dolovich, PharmD
Assistant Professor, Faculty of Pharmacy,
  University of Toronto
Assistant Professor, Department of Family
  Medicine, McMaster University
Scientist, Centre for Evaluation of Medicines
Pharmacotherapy Specialist, St. Joseph's
  Healthcare
Hamilton, ON

Barbara Farrell, BScPhm, PharmD
Clinical Research Coordinator
Pharmacy Department
SCO Health Service
Ottawa, ON

Antonietta Forrester, BScPhm
Marchese Pharmacy
Hamilton, ON

Anne M. Friesen, BSc(Pharm), MSc
Pharmacy Department, Seven Oaks Hospital
Winnipeg, MB

Ken Gellatly, OD
Downtown Vision Care
Calgary, AB

L. Maria Gutschi, BScPharm, PharmD
Canadian Forces Medical Group, Department
  of National Defence
Ottawa, ON

Shirley Heschuk, BScPharm, MSc
Faculty of Pharmacy & Pharmaceutical Sciences,
  University of Alberta
Edmonton, AB

Maryann Hopkins, BSP, CDE
The Ottawa Hospital, Riverside Campus
Nepean, ON

Sandra Knowles, BScPhm
Sunnybrook & Womens College Health
  Sciences Centre
Drug Information Centre
Toronto, ON

Debora Kwan, BScPhm, MSc
Pharmacy Department,
Toronto Rehabilitation Institute
Toronto, ON

Roger Larouche, BScPharm
Pharmacie Larouche
Hull, QC

Peter Loewen, BSc(Pharm), PharmD
Pharmacy Department,
UBC Hospital
Vancouver, BC

Lily Lum, BScPharm
Drug Information Pharmacist
Ontario Pharmacists' Association
Drug Information and Research Centre
Don Mills, ON

Mary E. MacCara, PharmD
College of Pharmacy
Dalhousie University
Halifax, NS

Anne Mallin, BScPhm
Manager of Pharmacy Services
Dufferin-Caledon Healthcare Corporation
Orangeville, ON

Penny F. Miller, BSc(Pharm), MA
Senior Instructor, Faculty of Pharmaceutical
  Sciences
Clinical Pharmacist, Department of Family
  Practice, Faculty of Medicine
University of British Columbia
Vancouver, BC

Helen Ng, BScPhm
GlaxoSmithKline
Mississauga, ON

Christine Papoushek, PharmD
Clinical Pharmacy Specialist
Toronto Western Hospital
Toronto, ON

Jennifer Peddlesden, BScPharm, IBCLC
Pharmacist, International Board Certified
  Lactation Consultant
La Leche League Canada Leader
Chestermere, AB

**Laura-Lynn Pollock, BSc(Pharm), RPh,
  NARTC, Dip AC**
Pharmacist/Health Educator
Victoria, BC

Barry Power, BScPhm, PharmD
Director, Practice Development
Canadian Pharmacists Association
Ottawa, ON

Ric M. Procyshyn, PharmD, PhD
Riverview Hospital
Port Coquitlam, BC

Lalitha Raman-Wilms, PharmD, FCSHP
Faculty of Pharmacy, University of Toronto
Toronto, ON

Melanie Rantucci, MScPhm PhD
MJR Pharmacy Communications and Research
Mississauga, ON

Hélène Roy, BPharm, MSc
Pharmacy Department,
Hôpital Ste-Justine
Montreal, QC

Yvonne Shevchuk, BSP, PharmD, FCSHP
Professor of Pharmacy
College of Pharmacy
Saskatoon, SK

Debra Sibbald, BScPhm, MA
  (Adult Education)
Faculty of Pharmacy, University of Toronto
Toronto, ON

Dr. Jeff Taylor, PhD
University of Saskatchewan, College of
  Pharmacy & Nutrition
Saskatoon, SK

Peter Thomson, BSc(Pharm), PharmD
Pharmaceutical Care Coordinator
Medicine and Family Medicine Programs
Winnipeg Regional Health Authority
Assistant Professor, Faculty of Pharmacy
University of Manitoba
Winnipeg, MB

Dorothy Tscheng, BScPhm
Drug Information Pharmacist
Ontario Pharmacists' Association
Drug Information and Research Centre
Don Mills, ON

Régis Vaillancourt, BPharm, PharmD
Clinical Pharmacy Advisor, Canadian Forces
  Health Services
Deputy Chief of Staff – Medical Policy
Pharmacy Policy and Standards
Patient Care Pharmacist
University of Ottawa Heart Institute
Pharmacie Larouche, Hull
Ottawa, ON

Janet Webb, BScPharm, MSc
British Columbia Drug and Poison Information
  Centre
Vancouver, BC

David Wing, BSP, MS
Script Pharmacy
Calgary, AB

Deanne Wong, BScPhm
Pharmacist
Toronto, ON

Irene Worthington, BScPhm
Sunnybrook & Womens College/Health
Sciences Centre
Toronto, ON

Dale Wright, BSP, MSc, MDE
DEW Consulting
Calgary, AB

Practitioner Review Board

List of Illustrations

Glossary of Abbreviated Terms

5HT	5-hydroxytryptamine
AAP	American Academy of Pediatrics
ABG	arterial blood gases
AC	before meals
ACE	angiotensin-converting enzyme
ACEI	angiotensin-converting enzyme inhibitors
ADA	American Dental Association
ADHD	attention deficit hyperactivity disorder
ADL	activities of daily living; aids to daily living
ADR	adverse drug reaction
AFB	acid fast bacilli
AGEP	acute generalized exanthematous pustulosis
AHCPR	Agency for Health Care Policy and Research
AIDS	acquired immunodeficiency syndrome
ALP	alkaline phosphatase
ALS	amyotrophic lateral sclerosis
ALT	alanine transaminase
AMS	acute mountain sickness
ANA	antinuclear antibody
ANC	acid neutralizing capacity
Anti HBe	antibody to HBeAg
Anti HCV	antibody to HCV
AOM	acute otitis media
APSAC	anisoylated plasminogen streptokinase activator complex
aPTT	activated partial thromboplastin time
ARDS	acute respiratory distress syndrome
ASA	acetylsalicylic acid
ASOT	antistreptolysin-o titer
AST	aspartate transaminase
AUA	American Urological Association
BAC	benzalkonium chloride
BAL	bronchoalveolar lavage
BCG	bacillus Calmette-Guérin
BDZ	benzodiazepine
BFHI	Baby-Friendly Hospital Initiative
BID	two times per day
BM	bowel movement
BMD	bone mineral density
BMI	body mass index
BMR	basal metabolic rate
BP	blood pressure
BPH	benign prostatic hyperplasia
BSS	bismuth subsalicylate
C&S	culture and sensitivity
CABG	coronary artery bypass graft
CAD	coronary artery disease
CAM	complementary and alternative medicine
cAMP	cyclic adenosine monophosphate
CBC	complete blood count
CBT	cognitive behavioral therapy
CCB	calcium channel blocker
CCES	Canadian Centre for Ethics in Sport
CDA	Canadian Diabetes Association; Canadian Dental Association
CFGHE	*Canada's Food Guide to Healthy Eating*
cfu/L	colony-forming units/litre
cGMP	cyclic guanosine monophosphate
CHD	coronary heart disease
CHF	congestive heart failure
CI	contraindication
CK	creatine kinase
ClCr	creatinine clearance
CMV	cytomegalovirus
CNS	central nervous system
COPD	chronic obstructive pulmonary disease
CPAP	continuous positive airway pressure
CPhIS	Canadian Pharmacist Intervention Study
CPK	creatine phosphokinase
CRP	C-reactive protein
CSF	cerebrospinal fluid
CT	computed tomography
CTD	connective tissue diseases
CV	cardiovascular
CVA	cerebrovascular accident
CVD	cardiovascular disease
CVP	central venous pressure
CXR	chest x-ray

CYP 2D6	cytochrome P450 2D6		FDA	Food and Drug Administration (USA)
d	day		FEV	forced expiratory volume
DCCT	Diabetes Control and Complications Trial		FHTG	familial hypertriglyceridemia
DEET	diethyltoluamide		FIP	International Pharmaceutical Federation (France)
DEXA	dual energy x-ray absorptiometry		FSH	follicle-stimulating hormone
DHA	dihydroxyacetone		GABHS	group A beta-hemolytic streptococcus
DHE	dihydroergotamine		GAD	generalized anxiety disorder
DHEA	dehydroepiandrosterone		GalU	galactose units
DHT	dihydrotestosterone		GER	gastroesophageal reflux
DI	drug interaction		GERD	gastroesophageal reflux disease
DIC	disseminated intravascular coagulation		GGT	gamma glutamyl transpeptidase
DKA	diabetic ketoacidosis		GI	gastrointestinal
DM	dextromethorphan; diabetes mellitus		GnRH	gonadotropin-releasing hormone
			GPC	giant papillary conjunctivitis
DO	Doctor of Osteopathy		GTN	nitroglycerin
DRE	digital rectal examination		GTT	glucose tolerance test
DSM-IV	*Diagnostic and Statistical Manual of Mental Disorders*, 4th edition		GU	genitourinary
			HACE	high-altitude cerebral edema
DTs	delirium tremens		HAPE	high-altitude pulmonary edema
DU	duodenal ulcer		HAV	hepatitis A virus
DVT	deep vein thrombosis		HBeAg	hepatitis Be antigen
E3G	estrone-3-glucuronide		HBIG	hepatitis B immune globulin
EAC	external auditory canal		HBsAg	hepatitis B surface antigen
EC	emergency contraception		HBV	hepatitis B virus
ECF	extracellular fluid		HCV	hepatitis C virus
ECG	electrocardiogram		HDL-C	high-density lipoprotein cholesterol
ECL	enterochromaffin-like		HDV	hepatitis D (delta) virus
ECP	emergency contraceptive pills		HEMA	hydroxyethyl methacrylate
ECT	electroconvulsive therapy		HEPA	high efficiency particulate air filter
ED	erectile dysfunction			
EDTA	Ethylenediaminetetraacetic acid		hFH	heterozygous familial hypercholesterolemia
EE	ethinyl estradiol			
EGD	esophagogastroduodenoscopy		Hgb	hemoglobin
EHT	endoscopic hemostatic therapy		HH	hiatus hernia
ELISA	enzyme-linked immunosorbent assay		HIV	human immunodeficiency virus
			HLA	human leukocyte antigen
ENT	ear, nose and throat		HPN	high-potency neuroleptic
ERCP	endoscopic retrograde cholangiopancreatography		HPO	hypothalamic-pituitary-ovian
			HPV	human papilloma virus
ESR	erythrocyte sedimentation rate		H_2RA	H_2-receptor antagonist
ESRD	end stage renal disease		HRQOL	health-related quality of life
ETEC	Enterotoxinogenic Escherichia coli		HRT	hormone replacement therapy
ETS	environmental tobacco smoke		HS	bedtime
FAE	fetal alcohol effects		HSG	hysterosalpingogram
FAS	fetal alcohol syndrome		HSV	herpes simplex virus
FCC	Food Chemical Codex		HTN	hypertension
FCH	familial combined hyperlipidemia			

IBCLC	International Board Certified Lactation Consultants
IBD	inflammatory bowel disease
IBS	irritable bowel syndrome
IBW	ideal body weight
ICF	intracellular fluid
ICU	intensive care unit
IFNa	interferon alfa
IHD	ischemic heart disease
IL-1	interleukin-1
IM	intramuscular
INR	International Normalized Ratio
IOP	intraocular pressure
ISA	intrinsic sympathomimetic activity
ISDN	isosorbide dinitrate
IU	international unit
IUCD	intrauterine contraceptive device
IUD	intrauterine device
IV	intravenous
IVIG	intravenous immune globulins
IVP	intravenous pyelogram
J	joule
JVP	jugular venous pressure
KSC	keratonconjunctivitis sicca
LADA	latent autoimmune disease in adults
LBBB	left bundle branch block
LCD	liquor carbonis detergens
LDH	lactic dehydrogenase
LDL-C	low-density lipoprotein cholesterol
LES	lower esophageal sphincter
LFT	liver function test
LH	luteinizing hormone
LLQ	left lower quadrant
LMWH	low-molecular-weight heparins
LP	lumbar puncture
LPN	low-potency neuroleptic
LRTI	lower respiratory tract infection
MAC	mycobacterium avium complex
MAO	monoamine oxidase
MAOI	monoamine oxidase inhibitor
MCV	mean corpuscular volume
MDI	metered-dose inhaler
MDS	myelodysplastic syndrome
MI	myocardial infarction
MMI	methimazole
MMSE	mini-mental state examination
MODY	maturity onset diabetes of the young

MOFS	multiple organ failure syndrome
MOH	medication-overuse headache
MRA	magnetic resonance angiography
MRI	magnetic resonance imaging
MS	motion sickness; multiple sclerosis
MSG	monosodium glutamate
MSK	musculoskeletal
MTP	metatarsophalangeal (foot joint)
NAPRA	National Association of Pharmacy Regulatory Authorities
NDSAC	National Drug Scheduling Advisory Committee
NE	norepinephrine
NEC	necrotizing enterocolitis
NG	nasogastric
NIH	National Institute of Health
NPT	nocturnal penile tumescence
NRT	nicotine replacement therapy
NS	normal saline
NSAIDs	nonsteroidal antiinflammatory drugs
NTD	neural tube defects
NUD	nonulcer dyspepsia (a.k.a. functional dyspepsia)
NYHA	New York Heart Association
N&V	nausea and vomiting
OA	osteoarthritis
OANV	opioid-associated nausea and vomiting
OC	oral contraceptive
OCD	obsessive-compulsive disorder
OCP	oral contraceptive pill
OE	otitis externa
ORS	oral rehydration solution
ORT	oral rehydration therapy
OTC	over-the-counter
PANV	pregnancy-associated nausea and vomiting
PASI	psoriasis area and severity index
PC	after meals
PCNV	postchemotherapy nausea and vomiting
PCP	*Pneumocystis carinii* pneumonia; phencyclidine
PCR	polymerase chain reaction
PD	panic disorder
PDA	panic disorder with agoraphobia
PE	pulmonary embolism
PEEP	positive end-expiratory pressure

PEF	peak expiratory flow
PEFR	peak expiratory flow rates
PFAPA	Pharyngitis and Adenitis syndrome
PFT	pulmonary function test
PG	prostaglandin
PG inhibitors	prostaglandin synthetase inhibitors
PGE1	prostaglandin E1
PID	pelvic inflammatory disease
PKU	phenylketonuria
PMDD	premenstrual dysphoric disorder
PMMA	polymethylmethacrylate
PMN	polymorphonucleocyte
PMS	premenstrual syndrome
PO	by mouth
PONV	postoperative nausea and vomiting
PPD	purified protein derivative (of tuberculin)
PPI	proton pump inhibitors
PR	rectally
PRN	when necessary
PRP	primary Raynaud's phenomenon; planned replacement program (contact lenses)
PSA	prostate specific antigen
PSC	Pheromone Sciences Corp.
PT	prothrombin time
PTCA	percutaneous transluminal coronary angioplasty
PTH	parathyroid hormone
PTSD	post-traumatic stress disorder
PTT	partial thromboplastin time
PTU	propylthiouracil
PUD	peptic ulcer disease
PUVA	psoralen-ultraviolet light (treatment)
PVD	peripheral vascular disease
QHS	each bedtime
QID	four times per day
RAU	recurrent aphthous ulcers
RBC	red blood cell
RE	retinol equivalents
REM	rapid eye movement
RGP	rigid gas permeable
RICE	rest, ice, compression, elevation
RIMA	reversible inhibitors of monoamine oxidase A
RLQ	right lower quadrant

RNA	ribonucleic acid
RNI	recommended nutrient intake
RP	Raynaud's phenomenon
rtPA	recombinant tissue plasminogen activator (alteplase)
RUQ	right upper quadrant
SAC	seasonal allergic conjunctivitis
SAD	seasonal affective disorder
SAH	subarachnoid hemorrhage
SAMe	S-adenosyl-L-methionine
SBT	serum bactericidal titer
SC	subcutaneous
SD	standard deviation
SHARP	swelling, heat, ache, redness, pu (signs of infection)
SIADH	syndrome of inappropriate antidiuretic hormone
SIDS	sudden infant death syndrome
SJS	Stevens-Johnson syndrome
SK	streptokinase
SL	sublingual
SLE	systemic lupus erythematosus
SLR	straight leg raise
SLS	sodium lauryl sulfate
SMBG	self-monitored blood glucose
SNRI	serotonin and norepinephrine reuptake inhibitor
SOGC	Society of Obstetricians and Gynaecologists of Canada
SPF	sun protection factor
SR	sustained release
SRP	secondary Raynaud's phenomenon
SSRI	selective serotonin reuptake inhibitor
SSSS	staphylococcal scalded skin syndrome
STD	sexually transmitted disease
SVT	supraventricular tachycardia
TBSA	total body surface area
TCA	tricyclic antidepressant
TD	tardive dyskinesia
TEN	toxic epidermal necrolysis
TENS	transcutaneous electrical nerve stimulation
TIA	transient ischemic attack
TIBC	total iron binding capacity
TID	three times per day
TIPS	transjugular intrahepatic portosystemic shunt

TLESR	transient lower esophageal sphincter relaxations
TM	tympanic membrane
TMT	tympanic membrane thermometers
TNF	tumor necrosis factor
TOPS	Take Off Pounds Sensibly®
TPN	total parenteral nutrition
TSH	thyroid-stimulating hormone
TSS	toxic shock syndrome
TTH	tension-type headache
TTKG	transtubular K concentration gradient
TUIP	transurethral incision of the prostate
TURP	transurethral resection of the prostate
UBT	urea breath test
UGIB	upper gastrointestinal bleeding
UK	urokinase
USP	United States Pharmacopoeia
UTI	urinary tract infection
UVA	ultraviolet-A
UVB	ultraviolet-B
UVC	ultraviolet-C
VAS	vasoactive substances
VDRL	Venereal Disease Research Laboratories
VF	ventricular fibrillation
VLCD	very-low calorie diet
VLDL	very low-density lipoprotein
VMO	vastus medialis obliquus
VMS	vasomotor symptoms
VON	Victorian Order of Nurses
VSC	volatile sulfur compounds
VSST	visual sexual stimulation tests
VT	ventricular tachycardia
VTE	venous thromboembolism
WBC	white blood cell
WC	waist circumference
WHO	World Health Organization
WOCN	wound ostomy and continence nurse

List of Patient Information Pages

Please photocopy and distribute
theses pages to your clients.

Foreword

The pharmacists' and other health professionals' ever-growing need for information on helping people take care of their own health was first identified by CPhA in 1980 and is even larger now. More drugs and more potent drugs are available to the self-medicating consumer. Herbals are more available and more popular. Consumers continue to claim more responsibility for their own health. Even more, the health care system is demanding that people take care of themselves because it is presumed to be less expensive for the health care system.

As the name of this book implies, patients have become the centre of health care. Every chapter *of Patient Self-Care. Helping Patients Make Therapeutic Choices* begins with patient assessment and goals of therapy. Selection of nonprescription medications is an essential component but so are lifestyle management and prevention strategies. How to provide advice to patients and monitor their therapy for each self-care condition concludes each chapter. In addition, there are invaluable appendices containing practical information for practitioners of ambulatory care.

The Communicating with Patients section is as important as the therapeutic sections. It guides us in how to assess and talk to patients. Don't skip it because you already know it all. I guarantee everyone will learn from (and enjoy) Chapters 2 through 5.

Patient Self-Care. is the third generation of the Canadian Pharmacists Association's publications to guide practitioners making decisions about patient self-care. The original Canadian Self-Medication published in 1980 and again in 1984 evolved into *Self-Medication* (1988 and 1992) and then *Nonprescription Drug Reference for Health Professionals* in 1996. Those books were successful and enduring, satisfying the needs of pharmacists, pharmacy students and other health professionals.

A book like *Patient Self-Care* comes to be published because of the commitment of 7 accomplished editorial board members, 43 expert authors and the staff at CPhA, in particular the publications department headed by Leesa Bruce. I would especially like to recognize our dedicated team: managing editor, Christine LeBlanc; clinical editors, Barbara Jovaisas, Karen Leahey and Cynthia Way; administrative assistant, Sheryl Neilson; and our skilled and artistic production group, Lucienne Prévost, Kathleen Régimbald, Bob Heathorn and Darquise Leblanc.

Carol Repchinsky

How to Use *Patient Self-Care*

The first edition of *Patient Self-Care. Helping Patients Make Therapeutic Choices* contains 65 chapters and 11 appendices. Following the Communicating with Patients section, the book is organized according to body systems.

Each chapter is organized in a similar manner: Pathophysiology, Patient Assessment, Goals of Therapy, Nonpharmacologic Therapy, Pharmacologic Therapy (with emphasis on nonprescription products and brief mention of prescription therapy) and Monitoring of Therapy. Prevention is also addressed when appropriate. An algorithm for Patient Assessment guides users to appropriate referrals to health care professionals.

Pharmacologic Therapy is presented in table format. Products are usually addressed in generic terms. To locate a particular product by brand name, the reader is directed to the Comparative Product Tables in the current edition of *Compendium of Self-Care Products*, published annually by the Canadian Pharmacists Association.

Herbals are included in the discussion of nonprescription therapy if appropriate. An appendix on Complementary and Alternative Medicine provides general information.

Appendices are located within the section to which they relate (e.g., Special Diets in the Nutrition section). If an appendix is more general such as Home Testing, it is included in the final General Appendices section.

Patient Information sheets on self-care conditions follow each chapter and are intended to be photocopied for patients. A list of all Patient Information topics precedes the Foreword to this book.

A Suggested Reading list accompanies each chapter to supplement such headings as Pathophysiology. The entire text is referenced; the reference list follows the Suggested Readings.

The photograph section is located in the centre of the book.

Description and Limitations of Information

Patient Self-Care contains selected information representing the opinions and experience of individual authors. The authors, editors and publishers have tried to ensure the accuracy of the information at the time of publication. Users of *Patient Self-Care* should be aware that the text may contain information, statements and dosages for drugs different from those approved by the Therapeutic Products Directorate, Health Canada. The manufacturers' approval has not been requested for such information. Users are advised that the information presented in *Patient Self-Care* is not intended to be all inclusive. Consequently, health care professionals are encouraged to seek additional and confirmatory information to meet their practice requirements and standards as well as the information needs of the patient.

Introduction Section Highlights

Chapter 1: **Patient Self-Care and Nonprescription Drugs in Health Care**

Self-care and self-medication
Economics of self-care
Safety of self-medication
Medication usage patterns
Product labeling
Regulations
Global perspectives
Canadian drug schedules
Professional control of pharmacist-only products
The role of the pharmacist in self-care
Sources of health care advice

Introduction

Patient Self-Care and Nonprescription Drugs in Health Care

John Bachynsky, PhD and Jeff Taylor, PhD

Minor illnesses and symptoms are by far the most common health problems. More people suffer with colds and headaches than with diabetes and hypertension. Because minor illness and nonprescription drug use is so common, the formal health care system often neglects them.

Economics may be a reason for this neglect. In 2001, Canadian health care expenditures in the private and public sectors exceeded $100 billion.[1] Nonprescription medications account for only a small percentage of this figure. However, nonprescription therapy is a crucial part of any health care system. Understanding minor illness and how consumers use nonprescription medication becomes more important as growing numbers of increasingly potent prescription products are reclassified to nonprescription status. Insight will also be needed as patient traffic involving minor ailments is attempted to be redirected away from doctors' offices and emergency rooms.

At times, the importance of nonprescription medicines may not be fully appreciated even by pharmacists.[2] When questions generated by patients are tracked, their importance becomes evident. A significant percentage of the questions pharmacists receive involve symptoms amenable to self-care (Table 1).[3-5] A report of pharmacist – patient interactions (3743 questions) found the most frequently asked question (19%) was for a recommendation for a nonprescription product.[6] In comparison, requests for renewing prescriptions accounted for only 11.9%.

The majority of nonprescription products are purchased in pharmacies. The self-care products industry in Canada generated approximately $2.9 billion in sales in 1999, of which $2.3 billion was nonprescription drugs and $600 million was natural health products.[7] The top sales categories for 2000 were internal analgesics ($265 million), cough and cold remedies ($257 million), vitamins ($121 million), antihistamines ($90 million), upset stomach remedies ($87 million) and herbal remedies ($77 million).[8] Worldwide sales of nonprescription medicines were about $40 billion in 1999.[9]

Self-Care and Self-Medication

People experiencing symptoms of minor illness may choose to ignore them, use a home remedy, take a medicine or seek professional help. The course chosen will depend on many factors, including past experience with the symptoms and the degree to which they interfere with normal activities.[10-12] Most sufferers tend not to seek professional care.[13]

Table 1: **Inventory of Questions Received by Community Pharmacists**

Questions	Ried et al.[5]	Kirking et al.[4]	Lawrence/Linn[3]
Total number of questions received over study period	1880	1133	2580
Percentage of questions of a "professional" nature	25%	22%	17%
Percentage of "professional" questions involving OTCs	57%	39%	58%

Lay-initiated treatment can include nonpharmacologic measures such as getting rest, exercise, increasing fluid intake, dietary changes, cold packs and attempts at reducing life's stresses.

When professional intervention is not involved, the actions constitute self-care, a group of behaviors that represent the majority of health-related activities. **Self-care** can broadly be considered as all things that people do to protect, maintain or improve their own health.

While always an integral part of patient care, self-care has enjoyed a renaissance over the past few decades. In England, Wilkie writes that "How-to" books on minor illness have documented lay expertise in health care and date back to *Domestic Medicine* (1769), the *Poor Man's Medicine Chest* (1791) and *The Family Physician* (1870).[14] This body of knowledge, however, started to wane in importance in lay circles. Near the end of the 1800s, there was massive growth in the advertising and use of patent medicines, creating a pattern of product use that lasted until the appearance of modern medicines. The growth in medical knowledge and the expectations from the medical profession in the mid-1900s encouraged people to consult their doctor, not only for serious illnesses, but also for minor complaints which would previously have been treated at home. A professional view began to solidify that, in light of medicine's spectacular advances, self-care was unnecessary, even undesirable. Health care professionals are now gradually accepting the concept that patients must take charge of their health and the value of self-care.

Self-medication is a component of self-care. A product available for self-medication purposes is "one that the average consumer can use to treat minor, self-limiting illnesses without the intervention of a prescribing, dispensing or monitoring health professional with relative assurance of its safety and effectiveness."[15] The US Food and Drug Administration (FDA) states that while a physician is a required intermediary between manufacturer and patient when prescription drugs are involved, consumers must rely on their own judgment when using nonprescription products.[16] Manufacturers are required to give consumers enough information to allow appropriate use with a minimum of risk.

Economics of Self-care

Professional acceptance of self-care practices has been slow, but is now part of the reform of the health care system. This coincides with the continuing shift from hospital and medical care to self-treatment, community services and the prevention of disease.

Appropriate use of self-care is rational, efficient and effective therapy. Accordingly, governments have been promoting self-care behaviors to reduce the economic burden on the formal system. In Ontario, an initiative to reduce patient visits to physicians for the common cold was evaluated because $200 million a year was being spent on such visits unnecessarily.[17] In British Columbia, the HealthGuide Program utilizes a guidebook of self-care advice and 24-hour telephone access to nurses to foster less costly interventions.[18] This should also free physician time for more serious conditions.

Pharmacist expertise with minor illness has been demonstrated in an innovative program in England, the Care at the Chemist program, which was established in a general medical practice.[19] Patients appearing at the clinic to see a doctor for minor ailments are instead offered a consultation with a pharmacist. If the patient accepts, a referral form is faxed to a program pharmacy of their choice. The program was implemented in part to reduce clinic case load.

The goal of the Canadian Pharmacist Intervention Study (CPhIS) was to determine the value of pharmacist involvement in minor illness.[20] Participating pharmacists were asked to record all instances where advice was given on nonprescription products over a two-week period. Accounting for under-reporting, then extending the figures to a national level, Canadian pharmacies would have made nearly 50,000 interventions each business day or over 15 million interventions during the year (1993). Using $44 to represent the cost savings per intervention (including prescription cost, physician and dispensing fees), and assuming half of these individuals would have otherwise consulted a physician, an estimated $265.6 million per year would have been saved.

Moving prescription products to nonprescription status, where appropriate, can be safe and cost effective.[21,22] It was estimated in 1994 that switching nonsedating antihistamines back to prescription status in Ontario would cost the province approximately

$11.6 million. This figure represents mainly the costs of physician visits and pharmacy dispensing fees. Another $4.4 million could be added for consumers' time in obtaining prescriptions.[23]

Safety of Self-medication

The minor conditions that typically bother Canadians are listed in Table 2. When people get headaches or start to sniffle, they must make a decision. Should they tough it out? Do they have medicine at home? Are symptoms serious enough to see a doctor, or will asking a friend or parent suffice? Perhaps they will even ignore the symptoms out of fear of a more serious underlying condition. Previous experience with the symptoms will play a role in whatever is decided.

People often choose to use nonprescription products for minor ailments. When purchasing them in a pharmacy, they will also decide whether or not to ask for advice in selecting a product. Familiarity with the products and past experience with pharmacists are important factors in making these decisions.

Appropriate self-medication has two facets — selecting the best product for a given condition (appropriate selection) and using it correctly once purchased (appropriate use). Hundreds of products are available to consumers; dozens may be available for just one indication. Choosing the most appropriate product can be a daunting task, and has become even more challenging with the increase in product line extensions.[25,26] It is understandable, therefore, that pharmacists believe consumers are not comfortable with the selection process. A majority of Canadian pharmacists reported that, if left to themselves, people will often buy inappropriate medication.[27] Pharmacists

have also expressed concern that the public may not consider nonprescription drugs to be "medicines."[28,29]

The safety of self-medication by consumers is the subject of debate. Studies have attempted to quantify user behavior during self-medication[30-34] and how patients interpret common symptoms.[35-39] Karpinski conducted 2000 interviews in 1981 to gather information on self-medication practices.[40] Thirty-three cases of misuse (4.5%) over 731 opportunities were discovered. Misuse was defined as any use which exceeded the dosage recommended on the label or for a condition not listed.

Researchers found that 7.2% of encounters in California pharmacies had the potential for people to purchase the wrong medication.[41] This value was determined by assuming that the 4.3% of consumers advised not to purchase a product, and the 2.9% who were referred to their physician, would have selected needless and/or inappropriate medication.

In Canada, the effect of a pharmacist's advice on patient outcomes involving cold products has been examined.[42] The outcomes of pharmacist interventions were compared to no intervention during product selection. Patients who were counseled tended to know more about certain aspects of their drug therapy, but medications were basically being used appropriately by both groups.

While there are examples that cause concern, available information suggests a reasonable ability on the part of the public to self-medicate. Experience with prescription to OTC switches also seems to indicate a general pattern of safe use.[43-45] Pharmacists therefore have a balancing act to perform — being aware of patient need for information, but at the same time not becoming too paternalistic and impinging on patient freedom to choose medication.

Medication Usage Patterns

Most people have used nonprescription products at sometime. Pharmaceutical industry figures indicate the number of products used by a sample of Canadians over a one-year period was none (10%), one to two (42%), three to five (41%), six or more (7%).[2] Agents used were headache/pain relievers (77% of the sample), cough/cold products (42%), vitamins (28%), upset stomach remedies (26%) and analgesic rubs (19%).

Table 2: **Top 10 Minor Ailments in Canada***[24]

1. Headache (76%)	6. Indigestion (20%)
2. Cough/Cold (70%)	7. Arthritis (16%)
3. Sore throat (47%)	8. Insomnia (14%)
4. Muscle aches/Pains (38%)	9. Menstrual cramps (13%)
5. Sinus congestion (37%)	10. Allergy/Hay fever (12%)

Based on percentage of Canadians who said they suffered from the symptom or ailment during the past 12 months.

Trends indicate there has been a considerable increase in the use of herbals and natural products. The Slone Epidemiology Unit of Boston University surveyed the use of all medications in the ambulatory adult US population in 1998-99.[46] Fourteen percent had taken at least one herbal or natural product in the preceding week. The most common reason for use was "health/good for you" (16%), the same reason given by 35% of those who took vitamins.

Attempts have been made to determine the various factors that might influence nonprescription drug use (beyond simply having the symptoms).[47-50] Women use more products than men. The influence of age on total products used is less clear. Age does influence the type of products used, however, with young people using more acne products and the elderly using more laxatives.

A survey by the Nonprescription Drug Manufacturers Association of Canada created a profile of the average consumer.[24] Women again reported greater use of nonprescription products. The association's observation was that women use more products simply because they recognize a larger number of conditions as treatable. Young adults tend to use a wide range of products on an infrequent basis. The elderly have lower consumption rates overall, but are heavier users of a limited number of products. It was suggested that seniors may be more inclined to seek professional care for symptoms.

Product Labeling

Nonprescription drug products are safe and effective when used as directed. However, because of changing patterns of drug use, the potential for adverse reactions and misuse is increasing.[51] This possibility has increased in part because more medications are now available without a prescription.

Product labels and inserts contain information for safe and effective product use. Safe use requires that the information is actually read. A Health Canada survey found that a majority (62%) of respondents always read package information before purchasing a nonprescription drug product.[52] Only 13% replied that they seldom or never bothered to do so. Data generated by the pharmaceutical industry tend to be more positive on this aspect.[2,53] Historically, leaflets and package information were written in technical language while small package sizes with small print could be difficult for patients to read.[52,54] Regulatory agencies now insist that the information be provided in a way that consumers understand.

Are pharmacists convinced of the value of package information? Only 36% of pharmacists surveyed in one study felt package information helps people make responsible choices. In the same report, 72% of consumers felt it was helpful.[27]

Regulations

Global Perspectives

Nonprescription medications are regulated in all countries. Differences exist, however, among the drugs that are classified as nonprescription and the nature of the restrictions on their sale. France and Sweden, for example, are purported to allow minimal (or no) public access to nonprescription medication outside of pharmacies.[55] In one Australian state, pharmacists are required to speak with the patient every time a pharmacist-class (behind-the-counter) drug is sold. In France, the Netherlands, and Switzerland, pharmacists need merely be physically present on the premises as transactions occur.[56] In England, pharmacists are advised to use structured counseling protocols when discussing OTC medicines with the public.[57,58]

There is the least amount of pharmacy control in the United States; a nonprescription product may be sold from any retail outlet. However, many drugs available without prescription in other parts of the world require prescriptions in the US. The pharmacist profession in the US has lobbied for years to obtain a pharmacist-only category of drug distribution (the so-called "third category") with little success.[55] Supporters state that such a move would better ensure public safety as more agents are switched to nonprescription status. There is also a worry that the sale of potent agents is increasingly in the hands of unskilled retailers. Opponents of the category argue that it goes against free-market principles and that stringent labeling requirements ensure public safety.

In the United States the shift of products from prescription to nonprescription status is increasing. Of specific interest is that the original products identified for a shift were those to treat episodic or acute symptoms. Now, there is greater interest in shifting products for chronic conditions to help low income families afford medication (they have no health insurance with physician access and little income for prescription medication) and to encourage compliance for silent health risks such as hypertension. A review of many potential products for switch, including antimicrobials and statins, has indicated a need for caution in proceeding with the switch due to the open nature of marketing in the US.[59]

Canadian Drug Schedules

In 1991, Health Canada initiated steps to change the Canadian drug distribution system. The main thrust was to harmonize the 10 provincial systems already in place, enabling firms to advertise nationally and allow the public to purchase products under similar conditions in each province. Previously, significant differences existed across jurisdictions — a product sold in three provinces could have had three different conditions of sale. The new legislation called for a prescriptive schedule, sale by pharmacists only (behind-the-counter; no public access) and a category where no sales restrictions applied (unscheduled). Pharmacists argued there should be one more category — pharmacy-only sale.

The National Association of Pharmacy Regulatory Authorities (NAPRA) has now endorsed a proposal for a national drug scheduling model. Drug scheduling is guided by an advisory committee, the National Drug Scheduling Advisory Committee (NDSAC). As of 2002, consistent schedules and harmonization of the national drug schedule model have largely become a reality (Table 3).

Table 3: **Canadian Drug Schedules**

Schedule I	Drugs that require a prescription as a condition of sale.
Schedule II	Drugs that are available only from a pharmacist and without a prescription. There is no opportunity for patient self-selection.
Schedule III	Drugs that are available without a prescription from the self-selection area of a pharmacy, which is operated under the direct supervision of a pharmacist.
Unscheduled	Drugs not listed in Schedules I, II, or III that may be sold from any retail outlet.

When NDSAC considers the placement of a drug, it uses a series of factors for each schedule against which it makes an assessment. The factors differ across schedules and are based on differing degrees of counseling/supervision necessary to encourage appropriate use. Progressively less professional control is required in moving from Schedule I to Unscheduled.

The review process uses a cascading principle whereby a drug is first assessed using the factors for Schedule I (prescription). Should sufficient factors apply, the drug remains in this schedule. If not, the drug is assessed against the factors for Schedule II. A factor in schedule II is as follows: *the initial need for a drug is normally identified by the practitioner, while chronic, recurrent or subsequent use requires monitoring by the pharmacist.* If the agent fails to meet the stipulations of this schedule, it is subsequently assessed against the factors in Schedule III (pharmacy-only). A Schedule III example is: *the drug is a new ingredient for self-medication and the availability of the pharmacist to provide advice can promote appropriate use.* Should the drug not meet the factors for any schedule, it becomes unscheduled (sale allowed in any retail outlet). The usual impetus for considering a change in drug status is a manufacturer's submission prompting one.

Professional Control of Pharmacist-only Products

When a patient *describes* symptoms to a pharmacist, the course of action to be taken is clear — the patient and symptoms will be assessed and a recommendation made. Most requests for a pharmacist-only product, however, occur as a result of a product request at the counter specifically *by name.* Symptoms may not even be mentioned. When a patient directly asks for a Schedule II product, to what extent should pharmacists assess the purchase? Responsibilities under these circumstances are not clear.

Product requests by name can be problematic.[60-65] British pharmacists have stated that detailed questioning may not be necessary when consumers request specific products and may even be counterproductive in terms of customer satisfaction.[60] A similar position is that pharmacists must be readily available to advise pharmacy customers, but do not necessarily have to be involved in every straightforward request for a medicine.[66] One research team found that when products were requested by name, questions posed by pharmacy staff to assess product appropriateness were received with confusion, even hostility and belligerence.[67] Other reports have examined consumer receptiveness to increases in questioning.[68-72]

Pharmacists face a professional dilemma in this area. Many customers request medicines they have used before. Under these circumstances, questioning from a pharmacist may be perceived as interference or interrogation. Conversely, the sale of medicines without professional input could impact on patient care and may weaken the argument for restricting them to behind-the-counter status. Pharmacists and pharmacy organizations continue to wrestle with this issue. In recognition of the problem, the International Pharmaceutical Federation (FIP) stated:[73]

> When a non-prescription medicine is requested by name, the pharmacist should not assume that the inquirer has adequate knowledge of the medicinal product. In all cases the person should be asked if any other medication is being taken and if the medicine has been used previously before deciding whether the medicine requested is appropriate for supply or whether it is necessary to ask additional questions before deciding on the advice to be given.

The Role of the Pharmacist in Self-Care

Advising consumers on self-care is one of the pharmacist's main responsibilities. Duties are outlined in the standards of pharmacy practice, including those of NAPRA. In general, when requested or deemed appropriate, a pharmacist will assess the patient's situation and then consider one of three recommendations: provide assurance that drug therapy is unnecessary; suggest treatment with nondrug measures or a nonprescription drug, or both; or refer the patient to appropriate medical personnel. Pharmacists also have a role in postmarketing surveillance.[74]

A tremendous number of consultations take place every year especially in the areas of cough/cold/allergy, dermatology, gastrointestinal, vitamins/nutrition and analgesics.[75-78] Canadian data are available on estimates of consumer contact with pharmacists. The 1984 Upjohn Study found that 42% of consumers had consulted a pharmacist when treating a minor complaint.[79] In another, a majority (58%) of respondents stated they either always or often consult with a pharmacist before buying a product.[52] Twenty-two per cent said they seldom or never do. A third survey found that 35% claimed at least one consultation with a pharmacist over the previous year; 65% indicated no such interaction had taken place.[2] It was felt that the lack of consultation may simply be due to limited product use or a stable pattern of use.

The above information has limited usefulness because it is based on estimations made by pharmacists and consumers. Pharmacists keeping activity diaries improves the accuracy of study results. Over a five-month period in British Columbia, pharmacists in 56 pharmacies were involved in 3480 interventions involving nonprescription products.[80] On a national scale, CPhIS provided data from 524 pharmacies.[20] Pharmacist records indicated requests for advice on minor illness an average of 2.8 times a day (range 0 to 36), although significant under-reporting was possible.

When consumers are actually observed making purchases in pharmacies, most transactions occur without a pharmacist's assistance. Product sales were tracked in a random sample of 40 pharmacies in Ireland.[81] A total of 632 medicines were purchased during the study period, of which 22.3% were sold with advice. In Australian pharmacies, 27.5% of transactions involved advice following symptom presentation.[76] A small Canadian study observed 860 consumers in one city making purchases, and of these, 11.6% received advice when selecting a product.[82] The highest rate of interaction involved single-entity antihistamines, while one of the lower rates was for analgesics.

The amount of time pharmacists spend with each person is often limited. The public may have little desire to engage in extended conversations regarding minor concerns. In Canada, an average of 90 seconds was observed for a consultation regarding decongestant agents.[42] The advisory role in this instance, however, was carried out by the researcher and may not represent the norm. In another Canadian report involving similar products, the average time that 48 people spent in consultation with pharmacists was 45 seconds each.[83] The minimum was five seconds, with a maximum of just over three minutes. Australian researchers determined that the majority (63.3%) of transactions took 30 to 90 seconds.[76] In England, the mean length for consultations was 96 seconds.[84]

Consultations on behalf of children (130 seconds) were significantly longer than those concerning adults (85 seconds).

When consumers do receive advice on selecting a product, it generally occurs because the consumer initiates the interaction. The public appears to readily accept any recommendation made by pharmacists.[85-88]

Sources of Health Care Advice

Physicians and pharmacists are often the first sources considered for information on nonprescription products and minor illness.[89-95] Some consumers are more apt to consult pharmacists about nonprescription products, but physicians for prescription medicines.[96-98]

Pharmacists have not always finished first or second, however.[99,100] During interviews with American consumers in 2000 households, friends were listed first, advertisements second and physicians third, while pharmacists placed fourth.[101] Pharmacists have been cited as infrequent sources for information among elderly patients.[102] When parents are seeking advice for their children, pharmacists have ranked as the fourth-most important source,[103] but also as high as second.[104]

The Internet is becoming an important source of information. However, pharmacists have an advantage over most sources of nonprescription product-related information because they are knowledgeable experts and can provide immediate input at the time of the purchase. They can also help patients find suitable Internet sites for information on minor illness and nonprescription therapy.

All aspects of self-care and self-medication will continue to be powerful forces in the health care professions and society. Governments are encouraging, or at least are not opposing, this trend. The decline of trust in the traditional health care system and the public's attempt to take more control over its health provide pharmacists with an opportunity to become a more important member of the health care system.

In Canada, there is widespread use of nonprescription medicines for the prevention and treatment of various ailments. Their low cost and effectiveness will likely result in greater use over the next few years, exposing users to more drug-related risk. To reduce this risk as much as possible, pharmacists will be required to meet the changing educational and monitoring needs of the public. In doing so, they will continue to justify their role as the main provider of medicines for self-care.

Suggested Readings

Bissell P, Ward P, Noyce P. Variation within community pharmacy: 1. Responding to requests for over-the-counter medicines. *J Soc Admin Pharm* 1997; 14:1-15.

Community Pharmacists and Self-Medication: Results of a National Survey of Community Pharmacists' Attitudes. Toronto: ABM Research; 1992.

Coons S, McGhan W. The role of drugs in self-care. *J Drug Issues* 1988;18:175-83.

Decima Research. *Attitudes, Perceptions and Behavior Relating to Ethical Medicines: Research Report to the Department of National Health and Welfare.* Ottawa: Minister of Supply and Services Canada; 1990.

Hassell K, Rogers A, Noyce P. Community pharmacy as a primary health and self-care resource: a framework for understanding pharmacy utilization. *Health Soc Care Comm* 2000;8(1):40-49.

Loh E, Waruszynski B, Poston J. Cost savings associated with community pharmacist interventions in Canada: a preliminary economic evaluation of the CPhIS data. *Can Pharm J* 1996;129(1):43-7,52-5.

Nichol M, McCombs J, Johnson K et al. The effects of consultation on over-the-counter medication purchasing decisions. *Med Care* 1992;30:989-1003.

Tully M, Hassell K, Noyce P. Advice-giving in community pharmacies in the UK. *J Health Serv Res Policy* 1997;2(1):38-50.

References

1. Canadian Institute for Health Information. *Total Health Care Spending Surpasses $100 Billion*, Press Release 19 December 2001. Available at www.cihi.ca/medrls/18dec 2001.shtml
2. *Consumer Usage and Attitude Study: Volume I.* Canadian Facts, Toronto: 1991.
3. Lawrence G, Linn L. Requests made in community pharmacies: implications for curriculum. *Am J Pharm Educ* 1978;42:310-13.
4. Kirking D, Maksym C, Neterer P et al. Evaluation of questions received by community pharmacists. *Drug Info J* 1986; 20:69-76.

5. Ried L, Angaran D, Neveaux J. What patients want to know from pharmacists: suggestions for pharmacy education. *Am J Pharm Educ* 1986;50:235-39.

6. DeSimone E, Peterson C, Carlstedt B. Pharmacist – patient interaction and patient expectations. *Am J Pharm Educ* 1977;41:167-71.

7. *Canada's Self-Care Products Industry.* Ottawa: Nonprescription Drug Manufacturers Association of Canada; April 2001.

8. Ghent N. The top 10 OTC categories. *Pharm Post* 2001; Mar:25.

9. Anonymous. OTC sales top $40 bn. *Pharm J* 2000;265:225.

10. Smith M, Knapp D. The ill person. In: Smith M, Knapp D., eds. *Pharmacy, Drugs and Medical Care.* Baltimore: Williams and Wilkins; 1987:15-36.

11. Hedvall M-B. *The Process of Self-Care Decision Making.* Helsingfors: Swedish School of Economics and Business Administration; 1994.

12. Hassell K, Noyce P, Rogers A, Harris J, Wilkinson J. A pathway to the GP: the pharmaceutical 'consultation' as a first port of call in primary health care. *Fam Pract* 1997;14: 498-502.

13. Dean K. Lay care in illness. *Soc Sci Med* 1986;22:275-84.

14. Wilkie P. Modern views of self-medication: What do consumers and patients want from their nonprescription medicines? *Swiss Pharma* 1994;16(11-S):27-9.

15. *The Distribution of Self-Medication Products in Canada.* Ottawa: Nonprescription Drug Manufacturers Association of Canada; 1990.

16. Alsobrook H. An overview of liability for OTC drugs. *Drug Info J* 1992;26:317-28.

17. Vingilis E, Brown U, Koeppen R et al. *Evaluation of the Ministry of Health's Cold Self-Care Public Education Project.* London, ON: Health Intelligence Unit, Faculty of Medicine, University of Western Ontario; 1994.

18. Anonymous. *B.C.'s Health Action Plan.* British Columbia Ministry of Health; 2001.

19. Whittington Z, Hassell K, Noyce P et al. Unravelling consultations for minor ailments. *Pharm J* 2000;265:R8.

20. Loh E, Waruszynski B, Poston J. Cost savings associated with community pharmacist interventions in Canada: a preliminary economic evaluation of the CPhIS data. *Can Pharm J* 1996;129(1):43-7,52-5.

21. Oster G, Huse D, Delea T et al. the risks and benefits of an Rx-to-OTC switch: the case of over-the-counter H$_2$-blockers. *Med Care* 1990;28:834-52.

22. Oster G, Delea T, Huse D et al. The benefits and risks of over-the-counter availability of nicotine polacrilex ("Nicotine Gum"). *Med Care* 1996;34:389-402.

23. Anderson M, Bolton C, Morgan S, Tremblett K. *The Economics of Self-Medication. Queen's Health Policy.* Kingston: Queen's University; 1995.

24. NDMAC Consumer Profile: The Nonprescription Drug User. Ottawa: Nonprescription Drug Manufacturers Association of Canada; 1997.

25. Anonymous. Product knowledge key to selling line extensions. *Pharm News* 1995;Aug (suppl):S5.

26. Anonymous. Confusion over OTC product lines. *Am Pharm* 1994;NS34(12):5.

27. *Community Pharmacists and Self-Medication: Results of a National Survey of Community Pharmacists' Attitudes.* Toronto: ABM Research; 1992.

28. Sharpe T, Smith M, Barbre A. Medicine use among the rural elderly. *J Health Soc Behav* 1985;26:113-27.

29. Williams R. Protecting patients from themselves: self-medication – the pharmacy perspective. *J Pharm Mkt Mgt* 1986; 1(2):109-16.

30. Skinner D. Consumer use of nonprescription drugs. *Can Pharm J* 1985;118(4):206-14.

31. Conn V. Self-management of over-the-counter medications by older adults. *Public Health Nurs* 1992;9(1):29-36.

32. Segall A. A community survey of self-medication activities. *Med Care* 1990;28:301-10.

33. Mount J. Quantity and appropriateness of nonprescribed drug use in a high risk elderly population: prevalence and correlates. *J Soc Admin Pharm* 1991;8:25-32.

34. Paxton R, Chapple P. Misuse of over-the-counter medicines: a survey in one English county. *Pharm J* 1996;256: 313-5.

35. Jones R, Wiese H, Moore R, Haley J. On the perceived meaning of symptoms. *Med Care* 1981;19:710-17.

36. Stoller E, Forster L, Pollow R, Tisdale W. Lay evaluation of symptoms by older people: an assessment of potential risk. *Health Educ Q* 1993;20:505-22.

37. Green K. Student knowledge of appropriate responses to symptoms of illness. *Health Values* 1990;14(2):32-7.

38. Verbrugge L, Ascione F. Exploring the iceberg: common symptoms and how people care for them. *Med Care* 1987;25:539-69.

39. Bell H, McElnay J, Hughes C. Societal perspectives on the role of the community pharmacist and community-based pharmaceutical services. *J Soc Admin Pharm* 2000;17: 119-28.

40. Karpinski K. *National Non-Prescription Drug Survey.* Ottawa: Proprietary Association of Canada; 1985.

41. Nichol M, McCombs J, Boghossian T, Johnson K. The impact of patient counseling on over-the-counter drug purchasing behavior. *J Soc Admin Pharm* 1992;9:11-20.

42. Rantucci M, Segal H. Over-the-counter medication: outcome and effectiveness of patient counselling. *J Soc Admin Pharm* 1986;3:81-91.

43. Kristensen K. Report from Denmark. *Lancet* 1992;339:418.

44. Altherr W. Around the world with new ingredients. *Swiss Pharma* 1994;16(11-S):35-7.

45. Smith F, Martin C. Reclassification of drugs from prescription-only to pharmacy medicines: patterns of use. *J Soc Admin Pharm* 1999;16(1):2-12.

46. Kaufman DW, Kelly JP, Rosenberg L et al. Recent patterns of medication use in the ambulatory adult population of the United States. The Slone Survey. *JAMA* 2002;287:337-344.

47. Stuart B, Grana J. Are prescribed and over-the-counter medicines economic substitutes? *Med Care* 1995;33:487-501.

48. Benrimoj S, Chua S. Predictors of nonprescription medication use. *J Pharm Mkt Mgt* 1990;5(1):3-27.

49. Juergens J, Smith M, Sharpe T. Determinants of OTC drug use in elderly. *J Ger Drug Ther* 1986;1(1):31-46.

50. Northcott H, Bachynsky J. Concurrent utilization of chiropractic, prescription medicines, nonprescription medicines and alternative health care. *Soc Sci Med* 1993;37:431-5.

51. Proposed rules. *Fed Reg* 1997;62(39):9023-62.

52. *Attitudes, Perceptions and Behaviour Relating to Ethical Medicines: A Research Report to the Department of National Health and Welfare.* Ottawa: Drugs Directorate, Health Protection Branch; 1990.

53. Nonprescription Drug Manufacturers Association of Canada. Improving label comprehension. March 1999. Available at: http://www.ndmac.ca. Accessed January 13, 2002.

54. Cheung A. Visual acuity in reading nonprescription drug labels. *Can Pharm J* 1995;127(10):47-50.

55. Gore M, Thomas J. Nonprescription informational services in pharmacies and alternative stores: implications for a third class of drugs. *J Soc Admin Pharm* 1995;12:86-99.

56. *Nonprescription Drugs: Value of a Pharmacist-Controlled Class has Yet to be Demonstrated.* Washington: United States General Accounting Office; 1995.

57. Anonymous. Medicine sales to need written protocols and staff training. *Pharm J* 1994;253:89.

58. Phillips S, Temple D. Writing a protocol. *Pharm J* 1994; 253:570.

59. Reynolds T. Switching from prescription to over the counter. *Ann Int Med* 2002;136:177-178.

60. Anonymous. Missed professional and commercial opportunities, says POM to P group. *Pharm J* 1996;257:205.

61. Almond M. Convenience, constraints and confidence. *Pharm J* 1996;257:548.

62. Jones I. OTC or OTT? – A provocative view. *Pharm J* 1996; 257:268.

63. Anonymous. A national audit. *Pharm J* 1997;258:611.

64. Anonymous. Pharmacists ignore professional guidelines, claims radio programme. *Pharm J* 1996;256:9.

65. Anonymous. Status of drug information. *Pharm J* 1996; 256:665.

66. Anonymous. CA criticism "confusing", says President. *Pharm J* 1994;252:768.

67. Hassell K, Harris J, Rogers A et al. *The Role and Contribution of Pharmacy in Primary Care.* Manchester: National Primary Care Research and Development Centre; 1996.

68. Anonymous. A question of Catch 22. *Chem Drug* 1994;242 (Oct 29):710-711.

69. Krska J, Kennedy E. An audit of responding to symptoms in community pharmacy. *Int J Pharm Pract* 1996;4:129-135.

70. *Consumer Experiences and Attitudes to Buying OTC Medicines in Pharmacy Following the Introduction of the New Protocols.* London: National Opinion Polls Health Monitor Survey; 1995.

71. John D, Evans S. Residents' views and experiences of pharmacy questioning and advice relating to non-prescription medicine purchases. *Int J Pharm Pract* 1997;5:85-90.

72. John D, Evans S. South-east Wales community pharmacists' views on the new medicines sales protocol. *Pharm J* 1996;256:626-628.

73. Anonymous. FIP adopts policy on self-care and self-medication. *Pharm J* 1996;257:373-374.

74. Sinclair H, Bond C, Hannaford P. Pharmacovigilance of over-the-counter products based in community pharmacy: A feasible option? *Pharmacoepidemiol Drug Safety* 1999;8: 479-91.

75. Smith F, Salkind M. Presentation of clinical symptoms to community pharmacists in London. *J Soc Admin Pharm* 1990;7:221-24.

76. Stewart K, Garde T, Benrimoj S. Over-the-counter medication sales in community pharmacy: A. Direct product requests and symptom presentation. *Aust J Pharm* 1985;66: 979-82.

77. Hardisty B. Do assistants take the pharmacists' role in counter-prescribing? *Chem Drug* 1982;218:804-5,808.

78. Marklund B, Karlsson G, Bengtsson C. The advisory services of the pharmacies as an activity of its own and as part of a collaboration with the primary health care services. *J Soc Admin Pharm* 1990;7:111-16.

79. Ryan S. Canadian Pharmacy Services Study: Is the public ready for this? Don Mills, ON: Upjohn Company; 1984.

80. Kerr-Eng S, Stratton T. Nonprescription drug counselling. *Can Pharm J* 1993;126(9):464.

81. Fisher C, Corrigan O, Henman M. A study of community pharmacy practice: 3. Non-prescribed medicines sales and counselling. *J Soc Admin Pharm* 1991;8:69-75.

82. Taylor J, Suveges L. Frequency of consumer-pharmacist interaction during the selection of non-prescription medications. *Can Pharm J* 1994;127(7):27-30.

83. Taylor J, Suveges L. Timing the selection process during the purchase of cough, cold and allergic rhinitis products. *Can Pharm J* 1991;124(11):507,510-11,526.

84. Smith F. A study of the advisory and health promotion activity of community pharmacists. *Health Educ J* 1992;51: 68-71.

85. Anonymous. "I recommend" survey. *Am Drug* 1995;212 (Jul):19-22,25.

86. Anonymous. 93% of consumers report that they purchase OTC products recommended by the RPh. *Pharm Times* 1984;Dec:77.

87. Anonymous. Consumers very satisfied with pharmacist's advice. *Pharm Today* 1991;Sept 13:1.

88. Gannon K. Patients content with OTC information from RPhs. *Drug Topics* 1990;134 (Mar 19):26,28.

89. Cosler L, Schulz R, Baldwin H, Cohen S. Consumer preference for personal drug information source: relationship to perceived importance of drug class. *Drug Intell Clin Pharm* 1986;20:138-42.

90. Stewart K, Garde T, Benrimoj S. Over-the-counter medication sales in community pharmacy: B. Consumer aspects. *Aust J Pharm* 1986;67:270-74.

91. Branstad J-O, Kamil I, Lilja J, Sjoblom M. When topical hydrocortisone became an OTC drug in Sweden – a study of the users and their information sources. *Soc Sci Med* 1994;39:207-12.

92. Harris J. Is the pharmacist a credible source of health information? *Pharm J* 1984;233:143-44.

93. Hoffman C. Canadian Pharmacy Services Study: What your customers think of you! Don Mills, ON: Upjohn Company, 1988.

94. Middleton H. Survey says: good news, bad news for pharmacy. *Pharm Post* 1998;Dec:10.

95. *The AltiMed CFP Report on Pharmacy Services.* AltiMed Pharmaceutical Company; 1997.

96. Rantucci M, Segal H. Public awareness: an assessment of the public response to a display illustrating community pharmacists' roles and services. *Can Pharm J* 1984;117(6): 272-75.

97. Stratton T, Stewart E. The role of the community pharmacist in providing drug and health information: a pilot survey among the public, physicians, and pharmacists. *J Pharm Mkt Mgt* 1991;5(4):3-25.

98. Anderson-Harper H, Scoggin J, Cady P. Pilot study – an investigation of the sources and satisfaction of medication information provided to the elderly. *J Clin Pharm Ther* 1991;16:139-44.

99. Hargie O, Morrow N, Woodman C. Consumer perceptions of and attitudes to community pharmacy services. *Pharm J* 1992;249:688-91.

100. *Self-Medication and the Pharmacist*. Brussels: The European Proprietary Medicines Manufacturers' Association; June 1993;7-43.

101. Gannon K. Where your patients get their information on OTCs. *Drug Topics*, 1990;134(Feb 19):32,34.

102. Smith M, Sharpe T. A study of pharmacists' involvement in drug use by the elderly. *Drug Intell Clin Pharm* 1984;18: 525-29.

103. Bryant B, Mason H. Nonprescription drug use among hospitalized pediatric patients. *Am J Hosp Pharm* 1983;40: 1669-73.

104. Walker R. Supply of OTC medicines for children. *Pharm J* 1983;230:404-9.

Communicating with Patients
Section Highlights

Chapter 2: **Effective Patient Interactions**

What to say when assessing patients
Questioning appropriately
Appropriate language level
Listening effectively
Nonverbal communication
Responding effectively
What to say when counseling patients
Speaking skills
Verbal and nonverbal skills during telephone conversations
What to say at follow-up
Tips for special situations

Chapter 3: **Facilitating Behavior Change**

The transtheoretical model of behavior change
Identifying the stages of change
Characteristics of the process of change
Steps to facilitating behavior change
Developing a plan to facilitate behavior change

Chapter 4: **Preventive Health Care and Lifestyle Management**

Risk factors
Assessment of lifestyle management
Nutrition
Physical activity
Immunization
Smoking cessation
Alcohol
Folic acid in pregnancy
Injury prevention
Strategies to improve lifestyle management and promote health
Counseling for health behavior change
Monitoring for lifestyle changes

Chapter 5: **Triage and Assessment of the Self-medicating Consumer**

What is triage?
Patient assessment
Red flags for referral for more intensive/urgent care

Effective Patient Interactions

Barbara Farrell, BScPhm, PharmD

Effective patient interaction has two major components — how the interaction is organized and how well the pharmacist uses communication skills. The effective use of communication skills is maximized by the use of an organized approach by the pharmacist. An efficient interaction with a patient enables the pharmacist to assess, triage, and if necessary, assist with product selection and provide counseling and follow-up. Use of verbal and nonverbal communication skills at each stage of the interaction ensures that a full description of the presenting complaint and associated symptoms, as well as other relevant information, is gathered from the patient.

There are three major components of an organized approach: assessment and triage, counseling, follow-up.

The "how" and "what" of communication are addressed for each component in this chapter. Most of the "how" of communication skills are covered in the Assessment and Triage section with skills specific to counseling and follow-up found in the next two sections. The "what" of the organized approach lists the types of questions to be asked or topics to be discussed at each stage.

Throughout the interaction, the participants (the pharmacist and the patient) alternate between the roles of "sender" and "receiver" of the message. As a sender, the pharmacist has the responsibility of ensuring that they are transmitting the message clearly, in language understood by the patient and in an environment that is conducive to clear transmission. As a receiver, the pharmacist has the responsibility of listening to what is being transmitted and providing feedback as to whether the message was understood.

Assessment and Triage

The primary purposes of this stage of the interaction with a patient are to determine the nature of the patient's concern or symptom, and evaluate its amenability to self-treatment or need for referral to a physician. Although the pharmacist acts as both a "sender" and "receiver" of messages at this stage, the emphasis is on receipt of messages from the patient. This is also the point at which the pharmacist begins to build the patient's trust.

How
- Introduce yourself
- Find out briefly what the patient needs
- Explain how you can help
- Ensure comfort and privacy if necessary
- Proceed with questioning and basic physical assessment (if required) for assessment and triage

Examples of statements and questions that can be used at each stage are listed in Figure 1.

Use good communication skills. This will help you send messages in a manner that can be understood by the patient and will help you to understand the messages that you receive. Both verbal and nonverbal communication skills are important and should reflect one another. Good verbal communication skills and poor or distracting nonverbal skills send conflicting messages, and the patient may lose confidence in the pharmacist. The reverse is also true.

Verbal communication skills include the ability to question appropriately (Table 1), speak in language that the patient can understand (Table 2), listen effectively (Table 3) and respond using empathy (Table 4).

Figure 1: **What to Say When Assessing Patients**

Introduce yourself
e.g., name, profession

Find out briefly what the patient needs
e.g., "How can I help you?" "What brings you in today?"
(Better than "Can I help you?" which is closed-ended and could prompt "No")

Explain how you can help
e.g., "I may be able to help you feel better. I'll need to ask you a few questions about how you're feeling
to make sure it is something one of these products could help."

Ensure comfort and privacy
e.g., provide tissue, offer water, offer chair, ask if would like to talk in more private area,
ask if needs medication now (e.g., nitroglycerin)

Proceed with questioning for assessment and triage
- Begin with open-ended question to gather lots of information (e.g., "Tell me about your headache.")
- Move to more closed-ended questions to gather focused information about the following:
  "red flags" (Chapter 5)
  duration, onset, frequency, location
  severity
  associated symptoms
  things that make the symptom worse
  things that make the symptom better
  effect on activities of daily living
  medications already tried
- Conduct appropriate basic physical assessment (i.e., inspection, palpation) if required.
- Determine if drugs or certain medical conditions are causing the symptoms.
  (Don't worry if you need to look something up. The patient will appreciate your thoroughness.)
- Avoid counseling or providing information until you have gathered all the information to make a full
  assessment.

Referral (as soon as red flag raised)
e.g., "From what you've described, I think it would be best to see your doctor about this."
Challenge: if referral to the physician is not accepted by the patient, use concern and empathy,
offer to call ahead or send a note — for example, "I'm really concerned about how you're feeling and
I think it's important that your doctor see you as soon as possible. If you like, I can fax them
a note to let them know what we've already discussed and medications you've tried."

Counseling

Table 1: **Question Appropriately**

Use open-ended questions	Use closed-ended questions	Avoid
• When you need to gather symptom information that is uppermost in the patient's mind • When you need to begin a line of questioning • When you want to determine the patient's understanding, level of sophistication of their assessment of the problem and what level of vocabulary would be appropriate for you to use • To convey a willingness to listen • To promote rapport and trust Examples: • Describe... (the feeling to me) • Explain... (how the pain feels) • Tell me about... (the heartburn) • How... (does the headache feel?) • What... (brings you in today?)	• When you want a yes, no or number response • When you want to gather specific, focused information about the nature of the symptoms and treatment • When you need to gather information quickly • When you need to keep a talkative patient focused Examples: • Do you... (have any discharge?) • Have you... (ever had this before?) • Will you... (be able to take this every four hours?) • How many times... (do you wake up during the night?)	• Using only open-ended questions (will make the discussion much longer and unfocused) • Using only closed-ended questions (will prevent discussion from moving to details of which you are unaware, may create passivity) • Asking several questions in succession • Asking leading or biased questions • Asking questions that start with "why" (can seem judgmental and cause defensiveness) • Using slang or medical terminology Examples: • Is the pain mostly in your stomach or is it more like heartburn? What does is feel like? Do you usually get it after you eat? • There isn't any blood in your stool, is there?

Table 2: **Speak at an Appropriate Language Level**[1]

Use:	Not:	Use:	Not:
A lot of phlegm	Productive	Digestive system	Gastrointestinal
High blood pressure	Hypertension	Lower	Decrease
Pain killer	Analgesic	Raise	Increase or elevate
Cough suppressant	Antitussive	Condition	Diagnosis
Shooting pain	Radiating pain	How bad	Severity
Bum	Rectum	On the skin	Topically

Table 3: **Listen Effectively**

You are listening when you:	You are not listening when you:
• Encourage talking (e.g., hm, yes, go on) • Wait during silence (allows the patient a chance to think and react) • Repeat (so you're having difficulty sleeping) • Reflect (why do you think that) • Explore (could you say a bit more about that) • Summarize accurately • Ask questions • Paraphrase	• Are in a hurry (looking at watch) • Interrupt • Change subject for no apparent reason • Ask a question twice • Don't ask any questions at all • Are talking • Don't allow the patient a chance to finish speaking • Lecture • Cut off expressions of feeling • Give advice prematurely

Nonverbal communication transmits more than half of the message that the patient sends and receives. These skills must be practiced when the pharmacist both is speaking to the patient and listening to the patient. Techniques to optimize nonverbal communication are outlined in Table 5.

Counseling

The main purposes of this stage of interaction are to assist with product selection and provide counseling that will enable the patient to gain the most benefit from the product. Again, the pharmacist acts as both "sender" and "receiver" of messages, but with more emphasis on sending messages to the patient. To ensure counseling is effective, pharmacists need to pay attention to transmitting their message clearly and explicitly.

How
- Establish goals
- Help with product selection
- Provide information
- Test for understanding
- Close

Examples of statements and questions that can be used at each stage are listed in Figure 2.

Use communication skills. The same skills highlighted in the Assessment and Triage section apply.

Additional verbal skills that are useful to the counseling component of the interaction include the rate, volume, tone and pitch of speech. These are outlined in Table 6.

The nonverbal skills used in counseling are the same as those used in assessment and triage. You may need to use additional nonverbal skills to indicate the closure of the interaction. Examples are standing up (if sitting), changing stance, shaking hands and sometimes packing up papers or putting pen and paper away.

Table 4: **Respond Effectively***

Use empathy	Avoid automatically giving the following responses until you understand what the patient is feeling
• Make an effort to understand how the patient is feeling**; respond to that feeling • Some of what the patient tells you involves their feelings about it; be sensitive to those feelings	• Judgmental or critical responses (e.g., "Oh, you shouldn't be doing that") • Advising/recommending responses • Reassuring responses (you'll be fine) • Generalizing responses (everybody feels that way) • Distracting responses (changing the subject)

*Some responses will be factual but always consider why the patient raised the point or asked the question.
**You can learn a lot about a patient's feelings by observing their nonverbal behavior: do they look sad? frustrated? angry? weak or sick? worried? in pain?

Table 5: **Nonverbal Communication**

Do	Don't
• Smile • Demonstrate genuine interest and concern • Maintain eye contact; look directly at patient's face at least 60-70% of the time • Use appropriate body language (show interest and concern in your facial expression, maintain appropriate distance from the patient, keep your body posture open, lean forward) • Sit or squat if the patient is sitting, stand if the patient is standing • Have a neat and clean appearance	• Look down or away repeatedly • Look at other objects repeatedly • Cross your arms or your legs • Use distracting gestures • Tilt to one side • Slouch • Stare • Get so close that you are in the patient's "personal space" • Have barriers between you and the patient (desk, counter)

Figure 2: **What to Say When Counseling Patients**

Establish goals
- Find out what the patient's expectation of treatment is (cure? symptom relief?); discuss reasonable expectations
- Find out time frame of expectations; explain reasonable time frame

Help with product selection
- Find out what has or has not worked in the past (useful to ask first because patient may have a product in mind when they begin speaking with you)
- Determine preferences (considering side effects, convenience, cost, beliefs, values, etc.)
- Ask about other drugs and medical conditions that might impact on choice
- If more than one product, explain advantages and disadvantages

Provide information
- Emphasize important points and give reasons
- Provide definite and explicit instructions, including duration of therapy
- Ensure your words cannot be misunderstood
- Consider using written information

Test for understanding
- Ask for feedback (e.g., I want to make sure I explained everything well. Can you tell me the most important points to remember?)
- Ask for demonstration (if applicable)
- Check for signs of understanding (e.g., nodding, saying "hm," "yes," not looking confused or distracted)
- Ask if there are questions
- Clarify misunderstandings

Close
- Summarize important points acknowledging the patient's initial concerns and reiterating key counseling advice
- Explain any required monitoring and follow-up that should be done either by patient or you
- Arrange time and date of follow-up call if necessary
- End graciously

Challenge: Closing an interview with a patient who continues to talk once the product is selected and counseling is provided: try the nonverbal techniques listed above; try a closed-ended question like "Do you have any further questions?"

Follow-up

Use follow-up to determine if the patient's goals were achieved with the plan selected and that no red flag has arisen that would require physician referral. Follow-up is similar in format to a combination of both the assessment/triage phase and the counseling phase. Ideally, it's best if the same person can provide the follow-up as this is the person with whom the patient has developed a relationship.

How
- Introduce yourself
- Explain purpose of follow-up
- Assess response

- Advise if necessary
- Close

Examples of statements and questions that can be used at each stage are listed in Figure 3.

Use good communication skills. A major difference between this type of interaction and the assessment/triage and counseling interactions is that this discussion often takes place by telephone (Table 7).

Since neither you nor the patient will be able to read each other's nonverbal cues as well, particular attention must be paid to clear verbal communication. These are outlined in Table 7.

Patient Self-Care (PSC), 2002

Table 6: **Speaking Skills**

Do	Don't
• Slow down; resist the temptation to "download" information quickly (e.g., learn to pause when there are periods or natural commas in your sentences) • Speak loudly enough so the patient can hear you • Speak in a friendly tone • Raise and lower the pitch of your voice appropriately (lower at the end of sentences, lower if patient is hard of hearing) • Use precise language (e.g., "with an 8 oz glass of water," not "with plenty of water"; "one hour before a meal," not "on an empty stomach") • Write when verbal is not sufficient	• Increase the rate of speech (tempting when you have a lot of information to provide) • Speak so loudly that others in the pharmacy can also hear you (have another staff member tell you if your conversation was heard) • Speak in a condescending or patronizing manner • Speak in a monotonous voice pitch (boring) • Raise your pitch at the end of a sentence (sounds like you are questioning yourself) • Hand out preprinted written information without also providing verbal counseling

Table 7: **Verbal Skills to Use Over the Telephone**

Do	Don't
• Start with a friendly greeting • Speak more slowly than you would face to face • Enunciate clearly • Let the patient know you need to stop talking if you need to pause to write something down or think	• Hold the receiver too far away from your mouth • Use a cell phone or speaker phone (can be difficult to hear on the other end)

Table 8: **Nonverbal Skills to Use During Telephone Conversations**

Do	Don't
• Be prepared • Give your full attention to the phone call • Smile to help ensure your voice carries a friendly tone • Listen carefully to the tone of the patient's voice and their speech in order to determine concerns or misunderstanding	• Put the patient on hold • Be interrupted • Have background noise (e.g., voices, music, ringing telephones) • Be overheard by other people

The nonverbal messages that you send will confirm your real interest and concern for the patient. They will also make it easier for both of you to hear each other. Techniques for optimizing nonverbal communication during telephone conversations are outlined in Table 8.

Tips for Special Situations
The talkative patient who gets off topic:
• Minimize your contribution to the "off topic."
• Acknowledge but continue returning to the questioning or counseling; if possible, try to link the therapy discussion to the "off topic" (e.g., patient starts talking about husband's death 10 years ago; ask "Is that when your stomach problems started?" then focus discussion back on today's presenting complaint).
• Try referring back to the discussion about the presenting complaint and introducing a closed-ended question (e.g., "A few minutes ago, you said that you were having trouble sleeping; have you had this problem before?"), then continue with the line of questioning.

The angry patient:
• Acknowledge anger.

Figure 3: **What to Say at Follow-up**

Introduce yourself and ensure you are recognized as the caller
e.g., "Hello Mr/s. ____, it's Bob, the pharmacist at City Drugstore."

Explain purpose of follow-up
e.g., "We spoke on Thursday about your_____, and I'm calling to see if the medication
you purchased has helped."
Do not apologize for calling!

Assess response
• Start with an open-ended question (e.g., "How has the medication worked for you?")
• Check for red flags (e.g., "Am I correct in thinking that you've had the problem now for two weeks
and that the medication has not helped?")
• Check for adverse effects (e.g., "Have you had any stomach upset with the medication?")

Advise if necessary
• May need to provide further counseling or suggest referral to physician

Close
• Summarize
• Explain any necessary follow-up
• Arrange time and date of follow-up if necessary
• Ask if any further questions, then end graciously
• Allow the patient to hang up first

• Let the patient vent their anger.
• Stay calm.
• Lower your voice, speak slowly and maintain eye contact.
• If you are at fault, agree (agreeing often diffuses anger).
• Avoid defensiveness (which can aggravate the situation).

The depressed/upset/crying patient:
• Offer privacy, tissues, time alone.
• Offer to call someone.
• Ask "Is it something you want to talk about?"

The patient who doesn't want to see their doctor:
• Explain your reasons for concern; be assertive (e.g., "When diarrhea goes on longer than two weeks, it's important to see a doctor because they can tell if there are any serious problems").

The patient who doesn't want to take your OTC advice:
• Determine preferences before recommending a product.

• Explain advantages and disadvantages in terms of patient's medications and medical conditions.

The patient with hearing impairment:
• Ask if the patient can hear you.
• Ask if better to speak to one side.
• Face the patient so they can read your lips.
• Speak more slowly, enunciate clearly and lower your tone of voice to make it easier for the patient to differentiate words.
• Increase your volume of speech but don't shout.
• Use short, simple sentences.
• Keep in mind that your facial expression, body posture and gesture are as important as lip movements for the patient to understand what you are saying.

The patient with vision impairment:
• Tell the patient what you are doing and if there is anyone else present (e.g., a student).
• If writing information, use large print and pastel-colored paper rather than white.

The patient with cognitive impairment:
- Speak slowly.
- Allow time for patient to answer questions.
- Write information down.

The noncommunicative patient:
- Wait during silence so the patient can respond.
- Ask open-ended questions.

The patient with a potentially embarrassing complaint:
- Offer privacy.
- Use closed-ended questions for assessment (e.g., "Do you have any discharge? Is it clear or white?") *not* "Tell me about the discharge."

The elderly patient:
- Slow down your rate of speech.
- Decrease the amount of information given at one time.

The patient with speech impairment:
- Speak slowly.
- Face the patient.
- Let the patient finish speaking.
- Provide writing pads.
- Learn simple sign language if used by the patient.

The patient who does not speak your language:
- Speak slowly and simply.
- Use an interpreter (e.g., caregiver).

The aphasic patient (patients who have perhaps suffered a stroke and have a decreased ability to understand what others are saying and to express themselves):
- Do not shout.

- Avoid complex conversations.
- Be patient.
- Help patient select words by offering a few choices.
- Talk to caregiver.

The caregiver:
- Provide written information for the patient.
- Follow up by telephone (if possible) with the patient.

Suggested Readings

Berger B. Managing the angry patient. *US Pharm* 1999;24(5):78.

Berger B. Building effective relationships with your patients. *US Pharm* 1998;23(8):52.

Dolovich L, Hudson A. Collecting the evidence. *Pharm Pract* 1997;13(5):68.

Janke KK. Developing call-backs to enhance pharmaceutical care. *Can Pharm J* 1995;128(9):17.

Rantucci M. Communicating with a patient with literacy or developmental disabilities. *Pharm Pract* 1998;14(6):21.

Rantucci M. Counselling on nonprescription medications. *Pharm Pract* 1997;13(3):23.

Tindall W, Beardsley R, Kimberlin C. *Communication Skills in Pharmacy Practice: a Practical Guide for Students and Practitioners*. 3rd ed. Philadephia: Lea & Febiger; 1996

References

Rantucci M. *Pharmacists Talking with Patients: a Guide to Patient Counseling*. Baltimore: Williams & Wilkins; 1997.

Chapter 3

Facilitating Behavior Change

Lisa Dolovich, PharmD

Changing one's behavior is the culmination of a complex set of thoughts, beliefs, motivations and actions. Maintaining a new behavior over time requires continued motivation, engagement and interest. Each individual is ultimately responsible for their own health. Health care professionals cannot dictate behavior; they can only help facilitate positive behaviors that would improve a person's health and well-being.

Effectively managing a medical condition almost always requires some type of short- or long-term behavior change. This change could be to adhere to a medication regimen, exercise regularly, decrease dietary fat or salt, reduce body weight, stop smoking, or monitor blood pressure or blood glucose.

It is vital that health care professionals understand how to facilitate behavior change so that people can be as successful as possible in initiating change and maintaining changes that are made. The transtheoretical model of behavior change provides a framework that can help health care professionals individualize their approaches to the needs of the patient.

The Transtheoretical Model of Behavior Change

The transtheoretical model of behavior change is based on an extensive review of leading theories of psychotherapy and behavior change.[1-3] It is called "transtheoretical" because it integrates many major theories of intervention in the psychotherapy and behavior change fields.

The model is an integrative framework for understanding how individuals and populations move towards initiating and maintaining health behavior change. The model deals with intentional behavior change, that is, when individuals are intending to change their own behavior or others are intending to help them change.[4] It has been tested in multiple studies, mainly in patients who had at-risk problem behaviors such as smoking, poor diet and lack of exercise.

This theory encompasses and integrates five core components (Figure 1):
1. Stages of change
2. Processes of change
3. Decisional balance
4. Self-efficacy
5. Temptation

The best chance for successful movement through the stages of change incorporates aspects from all of these core constructs. Each of these constructs will be explained in the next sections.

Stages of Change
There are six stages of change: precontemplation; contemplation; preparation; action; maintenance; termination.[1]

Precontemplation
People who are in this stage of change are not intending to take any action to change their behavior in the foreseeable future (i.e., within the next six months). They are generally uninformed or underinformed about the consequences of their behavior.[1] They may be reluctant or resistant to change. They may have tried to change but became discouraged because they did not succeed.[1]

Contemplation
People in this stage are intending to change, at least within the next six months.[1] They are aware that there is a need for change and are open to information

---

Figure 1: **The Transtheoretical Model of Behavior Change**[1-3]

PRECONTEMPLATION → CONTEMPLATION → PREPARATION → ACTION → MAINTENANCE → TERMINATION

Consciousness-raising

Dramatic relief

    Environmental re-evaluation

    Self-re-evaluation

        Social liberation

        Self-liberation

          Helping relationship

           Contingency management

           Counterconditioning

           Stimulus control

Con > Pro	**Con = Pro**	**Pro ≥ Con**	**Pro > Con**
↓ Confidence	Slightly ↑ confidence	↑ Confidence	Performance
↑ Temptations			Mastery confidence
			↓ Temptations

Pros = benefits; Cons = disadvantages

---

and education. They recognize the benefits (pros) of changing but are also very much aware of the disadvantages (cons). These opposing beliefs can prevent someone from moving on to the next stage. People in this stage are generally not ready for traditional action-oriented programs.[1]

Preparation
People who are in this stage are intending to take action in the immediate future, usually measured as in the next month.[1] They are beginning to set goals and prepare emotionally for change. They are the most open to change.

Action
People in this stage of change have actually engaged in new behaviors within the past six months.[1] They are carrying out plans, dealing with negative forces and developing a fledgling confidence that they can continue with their new behavior. But they may also experience guilt, failure, limits to personal freedom.[5]

Since a person's action is observable, the overall concept of behavior change has often been equated with action, so it is useful to recognize that the action stage is only one of the six stages of change.[1]

Maintenance
People in the maintenance stage have been engaged in the new behavior for at least six months. They are working to prevent relapse. This stage can last anywhere from six months to five years.[1]

Termination
This stage of change includes people who have completely integrated a new behavior into their lifestyle.[1] The new behavior is now a usual action. They are certain they will not return to their old behavior.

Patient Assessment to Identify Stages of Change
An assessment plan to identify what stage of change a person is in for a particular behavior is shown in Figure 2.

Figure 2: **Identifying the Stages of Change**[1,2,5,6]

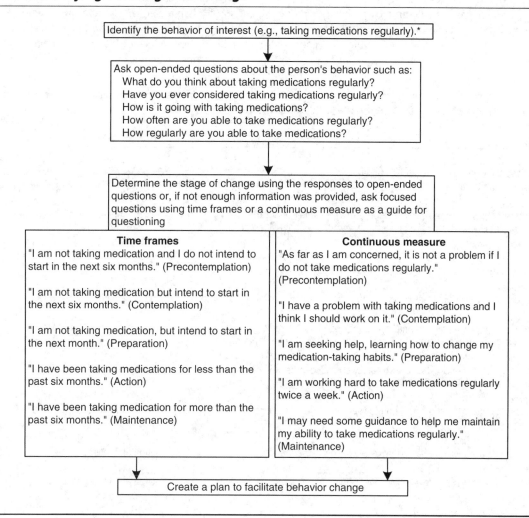

Other behaviors could be exercising regularly, decreasing dietary fat or salt, reducing body weight, stopping smoking, or monitoring blood pressure or blood glucose.

Processes of Change

The processes of change are the covert and overt actions that people use to progress through the stages of change.[1] Different processes of change should be applied at different stages to help people move from stage to stage. This concept is an extremely useful one to consider when developing intervention programs.[1] The processes are listed, defined and matched to the stages of change in Table 1. Health care professionals who recognize the need for a change to occur, and

then design an intervention to help the person go through the specific process of change, will help them achieve success.

Decisional Balance

Decisional balance encompasses the weighing of the pros and cons of behavior change by an individual who is thinking about changing. When lists of pros and cons generated by participants in studies were assessed it was found that the cons were higher than pros of changing for people in precontemplation stage, and the pros were higher than cons for people in the action stage.[2] It has also been shown that the pros must increase twice as much as the cons decrease for a person to move from precontemplation to action.[7] Therefore, a health care professional doing a patient assessment should recognize what a person's decisional balance is likely to be (depending on their stage of change) to help determine whether the predicted balance of a person's particular pros and cons have been detected. Interventions need to target reducing cons or increasing pros accordingly.

Table 1: **Characteristics of the Processes of Change**[1,5]

Process	Applicable stages
Consciousness-raising Gaining and thinking about the causes, consequences and cures for a particular health behavior	Precontemplation and contemplation
Dramatic relief Experiencing or expressing feelings in response to information about the hazards of not changing, and then recovering from this emotional response	Precontemplation and contemplation
Environmental re-evaluation Assessing the differences in one's social environment compared to without a particular behavior (e.g., the effect of smoking on others)	Precontemplation and contemplation
Self-re-evaluation Evaluating one's attitudes and self-image compared to without a particular behavior	Contemplation
Social liberation Recognizing, taking advantage of and supporting social opportunities that help others in the environment with a similar condition to change behaviors	Contemplation and preparation
Self-liberation Realizing that people are capable of successfully engaging in healthy behaviors if they make a commitment to do so	Preparation
Helping relationships The existence of meaningful others who provide support for one's efforts to change	Preparation, action and maintenance
Reinforcement management Rewarding oneself or being rewarded by others for healthy behaviors	Action and maintenance
Counterconditioning Developing and engaging in new behaviors to substitute for old, unhealthy ones	Action and maintenance
Stimulus control Removing cues that trigger relapses in behaviors and adding cues to facilitate healthy ones	Action and maintenance

Table 2: **Steps to Facilitating Behavior Change**

1. Complete an initial general patient assessment (medical and medication history).
2. Identify at-risk behaviors.
3. Identify stages of change for each behavior (Figure 1).
4. Determine individual's priorities for change (focus on only one issue at a time).
5. Ensure these priorities are consistent with urgent health needs based on health consequences.
6. Complete a focused patient assessment for the targeted behavior including the patient's particular history, personal circumstances and personality.
7. Create appropriate strategies that are matched to the stage the patient is in and their individual circumstances.
8. Monitor progress to facilitate movement through stages, respond to relapses and determine if the termination stage occurs.

Table 3: **Stages of Change and Health Care Professional Assessment and Strategies for Intervention**[1,5]

Stage	Characteristics	Example questions to ask for "taking medications"	Strategies to use to create a plan to facilitate behavior change
Precontemplation	Not intending to change within next six mos; discouraged, uninformed, underinformed, has not tried anything; cons outweigh pros; low self-efficacy; temptations are high	What do you see are the benefits of taking medications? What have people said to you about your medical condition? Would you like to read more about the benefits? What pressures do you have to take medications? What kind of help could you get to help you take your medications?	• Educate to raise their consciousness. • Create some uncertainty so people begin to question whether their current behavior patterns are the best ones. • Provide personalized information regarding benefits and risks. • Give information about helpful services available when patient is ready. • Identify barriers to change (e.g., what knowledge gaps or errors exist, what environmental or social issues exist?). • Focus on increasing awareness of the pros of changing. • Do not cheerlead, use persuasive strategies, be argumentative, suggest or expect change, or let information overload occur. • Do not use action-oriented strategies.
Contemplation	Intending to try something within six mos; open to information, education; slightly higher self-efficacy than precontemplations; temptations are high; pros and cons are about equal	What is not so easy about taking your medications? How can I help? Who would help you to take your medications? How would taking your medications help your health? What is one small thing you could do to help you take your medications?	• Help person accept ownership of the problem. • Help identify advantages and try to soften the effect of the disadvantages. • Use a pros versus cons approach and try to eliminate cons (e.g., money, memory aids). • Identify barriers and temptations (self-and environmental evaluations). • Help bolster self-confidence. • Help identify their own and other's attitudes towards new versus old behavior. • Encourage them to talk to you again when they are ready to begin taking their medications. • Do not use action-oriented strategies.
Preparation	Ready to engage in behavior(s) in the next month; beginning to set goals and get emotionally ready for change; pros and cons are about equal or pros are greater than cons	Have you decided if you are going to start medications? When is that? Have you told your doctor you are going to continue on the medications? Have you thought about how you are going to change your schedule to make medication taking easier?	• Help a person commit to a course of action (e.g., suggest a date they start, tell them to tell other people they are starting, contract to make the change, set objective and realistic goals). • Announce course of action to others. • Identify and involve supportive others in the plan for change. • Provide frequent encouragement. • Increase awareness of social policies that support their new behavior (e.g., smoking ban, Canada's Food Guide). • Engage in action-focused education program.

(cont'd)

Table 3: **Stages of Change and Health Care Professional Assessment and Strategies for Intervention**[1,5] *(cont'd)*

Stage	Characteristics	Example questions to ask for "taking medications"	Strategies to use to create a plan to facilitate behavior change
Action	Actually trying to change behavior; improved self-efficacy; pros outweigh cons; temptations are low	How have you had to rearrange your life so that you can take your medications more easily? Who has been helping you stick to your plan? How have you been feeling about how to manage taking your medication?	• Reinforce successes to increase self-efficacy. • Assist with stimulus control (reminders, conduct encouraging follow-up calls). • Support their use of helping relationships. • Highlight decreasing the cons. • Recognize and quickly address faltering behavior change (e.g., frequent monitoring, work to problem-solve unanticipated issues).
Maintenance	Has been engaged in new behaviors for at least six months; working to prevent relapse; self-efficacy is high, temptations are low; taking responsibility for actions	How is taking your medications going? What do you think has been the most helpful thing you did to achieve success? (Reinforce this) Have there been any difficulties with taking your medications over the last while?	• Reinforcement of successes (notes, measurement of results, updates on benefits of activity). • Assist with stimulus control (reminders, conduct encouraging follow-up calls). • Suggest additional behaviors that can add to current success. • Suggest alterations that remove cues that trigger relapses. • Recognize relapses as part of process and assist with getting back on track.
Termination	Zero temptation and 100% self-efficacy; will not return to old habits	How is taking your medications going?	• Recognize that regular health care professional facilitation is no longer required.

Self-efficacy

Self-efficacy is the situation-specific confidence that people have about their ability to cope with high-risk situations without relapsing to their unhealthy or high-risk habit.[1,8] The cognitive beliefs a person has about their self-efficacy influence their activities, motivations, persistence, thought patterns and emotional responses to difficult situations.[8-10] Self-efficacy is low in the initial stage of change and progressively increases as people move through the stages.

Temptation

Temptation is the intensity of urges to engage in a specific habit when in the midst of difficult situations. Common tempting situations that can create difficulties in undertaking or maintaining behavior change include positive social situations, emotional distress and cravings.[1]

Developing a Plan to Facilitate Behavior Change

Once a person's at-risk behavior and stage of change have been identified, a plan to facilitate a person's behavior change can be developed and implemented (Table 2). People do not skip stages. Instead, success occurs when there is movement along the continuum of change.[4] Few people are in the preparation stage for more than one behavior at a time, so it is more helpful to identify the highest priority issue and work on only this behavior. A study examining those who have at-risk behaviors (e.g., smokers) found the distribution to be the following: precontemplation (40%), contemplation (40%), and preparation (20%).[1] A group of arthritis patients who were assessed for their willingness to adopt self-management strategies included 44% of people in the precontemplation stage and 11% of people in the contemplation stage.[11] Given that most people are not in the preparation or action stage for many at-risk behaviors, those who are intending to change will not be helped by conventional action-oriented approaches. Various strategies specific to each stage of change are provided in Table 3.

Suggested Readings

Berger BA, Suchanek Hudmon K. Readiness for change: implications for patient care. *J Am Pharm Assoc* 1997;NS37:321-329.

Prochaska JO, Johnson S, Lee P. The transtheoretical model of behavior change. In: Schron EB et al, eds. *The Handbook of Health Behavior Change.* 2nd ed. New York, NY: Springer Publishing Company; 1998: 59-84.

References

1. Prochaska JO, Johnson S, Lee P. The transtheoretical model of behavior change. In: Schron EB et al, eds. *The Handbook of Health Behavior Chang*e. 2nd ed. New York, NY: Springer Publishing Company; 1998:59-84.
2. Prochaska JO, Velicer WF, Rossi JS et al. Stages of change and decisional balance for 12 problem behaviors. *Health Psychol* 1994;13:39-46.
3. Prochaska JO, DiClemente CC. Transtheoretical therapy: toward a more integrative model of change. *Psychother Theory Res Pract* 1982;19:276-288.
4. Prochaska JO, DiClemente CC, Velicer WF, Rossi JS. Criticisms and concerns of the transtheoretical model in light of recent research. *Br J Addiction* 1992;87:825-835.
5. Berger BA, Suchanek Hudmon K. Readiness for change: implications for patient care. *J Am Pharm Assoc* 1997;NS37: 321-329.
6. Jones H, Edwards L, Belton A, Ledermann B. *Helping People with Diabetes Change.* Lifescan Education Institute; 1998; 1-29.
7. Prochaska JO. Strong and weak principles for progressing from precontemplation to action on the basis of twelve problem behaviors. *Health Psychol* 1994;13:47-51.
8. Bandura A. Self-efficacy: toward a unifying theory of behavior change. *Psychol Rev* 1977;84:191-215.
9. Bandura A. Human agency in social cognitive theory. *Am Psychol* 1989;44:1175-1184.
10. Bandura A. *Social Foundations of Thought and Action.* Englewood Cliffs, NJ: Prentice Hall; 1986.
11. Keefe FJ, Lefebvre JC, Kerns RD et al. Understanding the adoption of arthritis self-management: stages of change profiles among arthritis patients. *Pain* 2000;87:303-313.

Chapter 4

Preventive Health Care and Lifestyle Management

L. Maria Gutschi, BScPharm, PharmD

Prevalence of Risk Factors for Mortality in Canada

Infectious diseases were the major cause of death in North America in 1900. Due to the success of public health, medicine, drugs and perhaps as importantly, increased affluence, this is no longer the case. The major causes of death in Canada at the beginning of the 21st century are:[1]

- Cardiovascular diseases including stroke
- Cancer
- Respiratory diseases including influenza and pneumonia
- Accidental death and suicide

It is estimated that 50% of these causes are linked to lifestyle behaviors, specifically tobacco use, a sedentary lifestyle, unhealthy diet, alcohol use and risky sexual practices related to HIV/AIDS.[2]

Obesity

Obesity is increasing worldwide, reaching epidemic rates in industrialized countries.[3] Current surveys reveal that approximately 50% of the Canadian population is overweight and 16% are obese.[1,3] Obesity rates in children are also climbing,[4] resulting in a disturbing scenario for future health care. Being overweight or obese increases the risk of morbidity from hypertension, dyslipidemia, type 2 diabetes, coronary heart disease, stroke, gallbladder disease, osteoarthritis, sleep apnea and respiratory problems. Less well-known is that obesity is associated with cancers such as esophageal, colon, prostate, endometrial and breast.[5] Furthermore, obesity is also an independent risk factor for all-cause mortality.[6]

Overweight is defined by the World Health Organization (WHO) as a body mass index (BMI) > 25 and *obesity* as a BMI > 30 measured as kg/(height in cm^2). *Morbid obesity* is defined as a BMI > 35. However, the use of BMI does not apply to people over 65 or to conditioned athletes.[6] *Visceral adiposity* assessed by the waist-hip ratio (> 1.0 for males, > 0.85 for females) may be a better indicator for increased risk for cardiovascular disease, diabetes and impaired functioning; patients at high risk have an absolute waist measurement of > 40 inches (102 cm) for males and > 35 inches (88 cm) for females.[3,7]

Folic Acid Deficiency and Pregnancy

The incidence of neural tube defects (NTDs), such as anencephaly and spina bifida, was 7.5 per 10 000 total births in 1997.[8] A family history, history of a previous birth of a baby with an NTD, certain ethnic groups, and folic acid deficiency increase the risk of having a fetus with an NTD.[8] Fortification of flour, pasta and cornmeal with folic acid, mandatory since 1998, is estimated to have increased folate consumption; however, total intakes are still expected to be below the recommended requirements of at least 0.4 mg daily.[8] Supplementation should begin two to three months prior to conception and continue through the first trimester to be effective in reducing NTDs. Folic acid supplementation is also beneficial in reducing the risk of other common congenital anomalies such as limb, some heart, urinary tract and orofacial cleft defects.[8] This poses challenges, as many pregnancies are unplanned. Despite knowledge of folic acid supplementation, only 26.3% of women attending a genetics clinic took folic acid with optimal timing.[9]

Physical Activity

Unfortunately, 57% of the Canadian population is inactive.[1]

Regular exercise benefits health by increasing longevity and reducing morbidity and mortality for coronary heart disease (CHD), hypertension, obesity, diabetes and osteoporosis.[10] Exercise also improves mood and mental outlook, reduces stress and may be beneficial in depression.[11] Regular exercise was identified as a major component of health promotion and disease prevention in the 1990s.[10,12-14] If the sedentary became more active, a 35% reduction in excess CHD could be achieved.[12] The benefits of exercise extend to individuals regardless of body weight and physical activity has benefits even if there is no weight loss.[10,11,15-17] Exercise is beneficial even if the participant is older. Exercise in youth provides no benefit if sedentary as an adult.[16] Furthermore, the risk reduction with moderate exercise compares favorably with coronary artery disease (CAD) risk factors such as smoking, hypertension and high cholesterol levels. Most importantly, the least fit have the most to gain.[16,17]

Infectious Diseases

Influenza and pneumonia cause significant morbidity and mortality in patients with chronic medical conditions, particularly the elderly.[18-22] It is estimated that 8000 Canadians die annually due to these vaccine-preventable diseases.[22] Vaccination is the most effective method for preventing or attenuating influenza, yet only 20 to 40% of adults and children with chronic diseases receive the vaccine on an annual basis.[19] Invasive pneumococcal disease, which includes pneumonia, meningitis and bacteremia, is a vaccine-preventable bacterial disease and accounts for approximately 4500 cases per year in Canada.[22] Pneumococcal vaccination confers benefit in addition to influenza vaccination[18,20] but its uptake has been lower.[23]

Smoking

Smoking directly or indirectly contributes to 21% of all deaths in Canada.[24] The direct health care costs were $3 billion in 1993.[25] Although smoking rates overall have remained at about 30% over the last decade, most alarming is the increase in youth smoking, especially adolescent females.[1,24,25] A recommendation from a health care professional is one of the most important ways of influencing a patient to consider

quitting.[25,26] Since it is estimated that most smokers start smoking as teenagers,[24-27] strategies to prevent smoking are as important as getting patients to quit.

Alcohol

Surveys show that 9% of the population admits to drinking more than the recommended maximal weekly limit.[1] Alcohol contributes to the risk of esophageal, colon, breast and hepatic cancer as well as hepatic and pancreatic disease.[28] Patients who consume large amounts (> seven drinks at a time) episodically are more at risk of adverse effects such as accidental injury and violence.[29] Alcohol use during pregnancy is associated with fetal alcohol syndrome (FAS) and fetal alcohol effects (FAEs).[30]

The regular intake of alcohol is associated with both benefits and risks.[29] Low to moderate doses of alcohol are beneficial for reducing the risk of CHD,[28,29] stroke[31] and the development of heart failure after an MI in older adults.[32] Low doses of alcohol in younger populations are unlikely to have benefit.[29] Cardiovascular benefits can be obtained from one standard drink (45 mL spirits, 150 mL table wine, 360 mL beer) every two days. However, alcohol intake has negative consequences for patients with hypertension[33] and triglyceridemia. The potential benefits of low-dose alcohol must be balanced against the risk that there is no amount of alcohol that is without adverse effects.[28]

Injury Prevention and Drug Poisoning

Injuries are the leading cause of death in children, accounting for 63% of all deaths in Canadians aged 1 to 24 years, due mostly to motor vehicle accidents.[34] However, poisoning is a preventable injury. The death rate from poisonings has fallen from 2.0 in 100,000 in 1958 to 0.5 in 100,000 in 1978 due to the use of child-resistant containers. Parents' knowledge of the phone number of the nearest poison control centre also reduces childhood poisonings.[35]

Goals of Disease Prevention

- Improve quality of life by alleviating symptoms and reducing drug requirements
- Lower risk of developing cardiovascular disease, diabetes, respiratory diseases, vaccine-preventable infections and some cancers

- Prevent death due to accidents
- Decrease risk of NTDs
- Prevent FAS and FAEs

Patient Assessment

Patients can be assessed for lifestyle management and disease prevention, either as primary prevention or as secondary prevention, to maintain, reverse or prevent disease as illustrated in Figure 1.

Who can Benefit From Health Promotion and Disease Prevention?

Medications can be cues to identify patients who may benefit from disease prevention strategies as outlined in Table 1. Every patient or client who visits a pharmacy is a candidate for health promotion. Approaches to care of children and youth are addressed in other references.[35-39]

Strategies to Improve Lifestyle Management and Promote Health (Table 2)

Weight Loss

Health gains such as decreased drug requirements, or prevention of diseases such as diabetes and hypertension, can be achieved with a 5 to 10% reduction in weight (in many patients this represents 5 to 10 kg).[3,6,40,43] Emphasize eating whole foods and reducing processed foods, which tend to be high in fat and salt. A planned diet with a moderate caloric deficit (500 to 1000 kcal), decreased dietary fat to < 30% of total intake, regular physical activity and behavioral modification is the most successful strategy for weight loss and weight maintenance.[3] A low fat diet may not lead to weight loss if there is no associated decrease in total caloric intake. Excess intake of carbohydrates with a high glycemic index (sugars, potatoes, white rice) may also have deleterious effects on lipid parameters.[41] During weight loss, attention should be paid to maintaining an adequate intake of vitamins and minerals, and in women, maintenance of recommended calcium intake is important in those at high risk of osteoporosis. A supplement may be necessary.[6]

Folic Acid in Pregnancy

Counsel all women of childbearing age on a yearly basis regarding the use of folic acid 0.4 mg every day to prevent NTDs. One method to accomplish this is to ensure all women obtaining contraception are informed of the benefits of folic acid and suggest a supplement.

Physical Activity

Pharmacists can promote regular moderate physical activity to all patients and especially to patients with chronic diseases. Perform an assessment of risk (Table 2) before recommending an exercise regimen. Refer patients with known cardiac, pulmonary or metabolic disorders or who have signs and symptoms suggestive of these disorders to a physician. Vigorous activity is not required. Moderate physical activity such as brisk walking (defined as 5 to 6 km/h or 3 to 4 mph), cycling or noncompetitive swimming is sufficient to reduce the risk of cardiovascular mortality and infers many other benefits. Weight loss should not be the only or even the primary goal for patients who start regular exercise. Success should be evaluated according to improvements in chronic disease factors or symptoms and by adopting healthy lifestyle habits, not by weight loss alone.[10]

Immunization

Research shows that pharmacists can effectively identify people who are eligible for vaccination and increase the number who get vaccinated.[22,23,44] Pharmacists can promote vaccination in adults who are in high-risk categories during the influenza season and refer them to either their family physician, local health clinic or pharmacist-initiated clinics. Encouraging pneumococcal vaccination, however, can be done at any time.

Smoking Cessation

Pharmacists can impact smoking rates[27] but most pharmacists do not regularly ask their patients if they smoke.[45] Promote smoking cessation by ascertaining the smoking status of patients and documenting this in the patient's profile.

Alcohol

Since alcohol can potentiate the effects of many medications, pharmacists must emphasize low to moderate drinking. Patients who abstain from alcohol

Figure 1: **Assessment of Lifestyle Management**

What is the patient's current lifestyle?
Current weight and height? (calculate BMI)
What exercise does the patient do regularly? (What activities,
how much, how often?)
Is the patient a smoker? (How many packs per day? For how long?
Ever tried to quit?)
How much alcohol does the patient drink? (How much, how often?)
What does the patient eat?

↓

Does the patient have a **diagnosis** of CVD (HTN,
dyslipidemia, CAD, PVD, stroke), cancer, diabetes, respiratory
diseases, renal failure or depression?

↓

Does the patient have **signs** of the above conditions?
Look for overweight, foot infection, shortness of breath, depressed affect;
ask about blood pressure, neuropathy

↓

Does the patient have **symptoms** of the above conditions?
Ask about chest pain, shortness of breath, exercise capacity, interest in daily activities

↓

Does the patient have **abnormal laboratory values** related to the above conditions?
Ask or obtain information about cholesterol, blood glucose, serum creatinine

↓

How is the patient currently managing these conditions, signs, symptoms
or abnormal laboratory values?

↓

Is the patient pregnant or thinking of becoming pregnant?

↓

What is the patient's immunization history?
Has the patient had previous pneumonia or influenza episodes?

↓

What is the relevant family history (e.g., CVD, cancer)?

↓

Does the patient keep medications out of reach of children or grandchildren and in
childproof containers?

↓

What is the patient's quality of life and functional status?

↓

Determine areas of disease and lifestyle management where prevention could help
reduce risk and improve health for this patient

↓

Assess patient's knowledge of folic acid supplementation, smoking cessation, exercise,
diet, weight loss strategies, importance of reducing alcohol intake, medication safety
strategies, immunization benefits

↓

Assess patient's motivation and readiness to change (Chapter 3)

↓

Prioritize lifestyle and prevention measures to identify what the patient will work on first

↓

Create a plan that includes:
• Reviewing the benefits of implementing lifestyle and prevention measures
• Recommending specific strategies for change (Table 2)
  Self-monitoring plan for the patient to use
  Follow-up and monitoring plan for your use (Table 3)
  Referral to an appropriate health care professional as required

---

BMI = body mass index; CVD = cardiovascular disease; HTN = hypertension; CAD = coronary artery disease; PVD = peripheral vascular disease.

Table 1: **Drugs as Cues for Lifestyle Modification**

Drugs	Disease prevention strategy
Oral contraceptives	Folic acid supplementation Abstinence from alcohol if pregnancy contemplated Smoking cessation
ACEIs, oral hypoglycemics, insulin, beta-blockers, calcium channel blockers, diuretics, nitrates, antiplatelet agents, other cardiac drugs	Smoking cessation if required Exercise guidelines Nutrition guidelines Influenza, pneumococcal vaccination Education on alcohol
Antibiotic therapy for pneumonia, COPD exacerbation	Influenza, pneumococcal vaccination Smoking cessation if required
Corticosteroid inhalers and anti-asthma medications	Influenza, pneumococcal vaccination Smoking cessation if required
Drugs to avoid with alcohol (e.g., antidepressants, narcotics, benzodiazepines)	Promotion of abstinence during drug use Education about low-moderate alcohol consumption
Immunosuppressive agents including chronic corticosteroid use, antimetabolites, interferon, anemia therapy, HIV therapy	Influenza and possibly pneumococcal vaccination
Antipsychotic medications	Exercise guidelines Nutrition guidelines Smoking cessation if required
Most drugs used on a chronic basis	Exercise guidelines Smoking cessation if required

COPD = chronic obstructive pulmonary disease

should not be encouraged to start drinking for its cardiovascular benefits, as there are other options and they may have a reason for abstinence. Inform all pregnant women of the risks of alcohol consumption and FAS. Emphasize abstinence in this population.[28]

Injury Prevention and Drug Poisoning

Ensure that parents of young children know the telephone number of their poison control centre and are aware of the risks of household injury. Needle exchange programs to prevent the transmission of HIV/AIDS and hepatitis B as well as proper waste disposal of excess medications are other disease prevention strategies that can be promoted.

Counseling for Health Behavior Change

Many health care professionals try to get patients to change behavior, "to lose weight, exercise, stop smoking, get cholesterol checked," but it may seem the time and energy required are wasted. Studies show however, that brief, effective interventions are successful[42] and that patients are very interested in preventive care.[46] Patients are responsible for making choices but health care professionals are responsible for the clarity and accuracy of the information presented.

- Be specific and detailed, with an endpoint and a time frame.
- Define small achievable goals.
- Personalize the lifestyle changes.
- Write the goals and changes down in front of the patient.
- Use a handout as an adjunct to a personalized lifestyle recommendation.
- Be as educated as possible about choices and options.
- Be authoritative and not authoritarian.
- Include plans for self-monitoring and reinforcement.

Table 2: **Disease Prevention and Health Promotion for Adults**

Disease prevention	Recommendations	Expected benefits	Onset of benefit	Cautions	Comments
Exercise[10-12,15-17]	150 min moderately intense exercise/wk • 30 min walk at moderate rate (6 km/h) 5 x/wk • May be divided into 10 min segments • Resistance training (climbing stairs, push-ups) and stretching (Tai-Chi, dance) also valuable	↓ all mortality causes ↓ risk of development of disease and type 2 DM ↓ risk of stroke ↓ risk of obesity Improved mental outlook ↓ stress ↑ balance and energy Prevents progressive functional incapacity. Slows progression of osteoporosis.	3-4 wks for lipid values 4-6 wks for mental outlook and mild depression 10 yrs for all-cause mortality Benefits lost if exercise not continued; cannot be "stored up"	Consult physician for: • Uncontrolled HTN (SBP > 150 mm Hg) • Uncontrolled DM • History of CAD • Chest pain on exertion or at rest • Shortness of breath on exertion • Functional disability • Dizziness causing loss of balance • Any loss of consciousness	Discourage vigorous exercise in otherwise sedentary adults. Walking suggested as costs are low and no training required. 10 min sessions accumulated throughout the day is as effective as a single 30 min session. Total energy expenditure is most important.
Nutrition[3,5-7,40,41]	Diet high in vegetables and fruit (5-10 servings), fibre and whole grains, low in saturated fats, rich in omega-3 fatty acids Caloric intake matched to energy expenditure	↓ risk of some cancers (colon, esophageal) ↓ risk of developing CAD ↓ risk of developing type 2 DM ↓ risk of stroke	3-4 wks for lipid values 1-5 yrs for CAD, DM, stroke	Clinical nutritionist or other professional with specialized nutritional expertise for patients with DM, dyslipidemia and CAD. Anorexia and terminal illness contraindications for weight loss. Patients with unstable medical or mental illnesses should be temporarily excluded from weight loss programs.	Healthy nutrition and exercise are more important than weight loss alone. Weight loss indicated if BMI > 25 and comorbidity (DM, HTN, sleep apnea) or abdominal obesity.
Smoking cessation[24-27]	Abstinence	↓ risk of cancer ↓ risk of CV disease including stroke ↓ risk of osteoporosis ↓ risk of lung diseases	6 mos for improvement in respiratory symptoms. 3 yrs for risk reduction of CVD 10 yrs results in risk reduction of cancer to similar to that of non-smokers	None	Address concern for increase in weight as absolute risk of smoking is greater than absolute risk of obesity.

(cont'd)

Table 2: **Disease Prevention and Health Promotion for Adults** (cont'd)

Disease prevention	Recommendations	Expected benefits	Onset of benefit	Cautions	Comments
Alcohol[28-33,42]	Low-moderate alcohol consumption • ≤ 9 standard drinks/wk for females • ≤ 14 standard drinks/wk for males Abstinence if pregnant Abstinence while driving a motor vehicle or boat	↓ risk of CVD achieved with consumption of approximately 1 drink every other day	5-10 yrs for benefit of CVD in older patients (> 50 yrs) Younger patients unlikely to benefit	Consumption outside low risk guidelines associated with • Increased risk of cancer (esophageal, liver, colon, breast) • Increased risk of hypertension • Impaired social functioning Consult physician if problem drinking identified.	Patients with triglyceridemia may be sensitive to ethanol intake.
Immunizations[18,23]	Influenza vaccination for: • > 65 yrs of age • Chronic heart and lung disease • Cancer • Diabetes • Renal disease • Immunosuppression • HIV Pneumococcal vaccination as above plus • Asplenia, sickle cell disease • Chronic CSF leak Tetanus booster every 10 yrs	↓ mortality due to influenza or pneumonia ↓ risk of hospitalization due to these diseases in patients > 65 yrs ↓ morbidity and mortality from tetanus	2 wks; requires yearly vaccination for influenza vaccination 2-3 wks onset to > 10 yrs for pneumococcal vaccination 2-3 wk onset to 10 yr for tetanus	Contraindications to vaccination • Egg allergy for influenza vaccination • Previous pneumococcal vaccination Address concerns regarding common vaccination myths.	Pneumococcal vaccination usually given only once. Recommend acetaminophen prophylactically to prevent fever and myalgias. Influenza vaccination also recommended for patients capable of transmitting influenza to those at high risk. Vaccination is also recommended for pregnant women in high-risk groups.

Injury prevention[34-36]	Parental knowledge of poison control centre Child-resistant medication containers Needle exchange programs. Condom use Seatbelt use	↓ mortality and morbidity from accidents and accidental exposure to drugs and poisons ↓ transmission of HIV, hepatitis B	Immediate	None
Folic acid supplementation[8,9]	All women of child-bearing age should ↑ consumption of folic acid to at least 0.4 mg per day. With history of NTDs, requirements are higher.	↓ incidence of NTDs by 40-60%	Through first trimester where risk is greatest	Should be taken at least 1 mo prior to conception as many pregnancies are unplanned or patient is unaware during the critical period.

DM = diabetes mellitus; HTN = hypertension; SBP = systolic blood pressure; CAD = coronary artery disease; BMI = body mass index; CVD = cardiovascular disease; CSF = cerebrospinal fluid; NTDs = neural tube defects.

Table 3: Monitoring Disease Prevention and Health Promotion

Lifestyle change	Monitoring	Endpoint	Actions
Weight loss and nutrition	**Patient:** weight weekly while on diet, looser clothing, increased mobility, decreased drug requirements **Pharmacist/Physician:** after 3-6 mos	Decrease in 5-10% of body weight over 6 mos	If ineffective, refer to physician and/or a formal weight management program and/or dietitian. If effective, exercise also recommended to prevent weight regain.
Exercise	**Patient:** daily using activity logs, increased stamina and energy **Pharmacist/Physician:** after 3-6 mos	30 min continuous exercise of moderate intensity: walking at 6 km/h or 4 mph pace.	Start with 10 min per day, slowly increasing by 10 min, every 8-10 wks in elderly or sedentary patients. If ineffective, refer to physician or to community resources.
Smoking	See Chapter 11.	See Chapter 11.	See Chapter 11.
Alcohol	**Patient:** weekly intake **Pharmacist/Physician:** after 3-6 mos	Alcohol intake within low-moderate guidelines. Improved blood pressure control.	If ineffective, counsel to stage of change (see Chapter 3). If problem drinking (impaired social functioning), refer to physician.
Folic acid	**Patient:** daily intake. **Pharmacist/Physician:** after 1 mo at next refill of oral contraceptives; then yearly	Daily intake of supplement containing 0.4 mg folic acid.	If ineffective, explain importance and counsel to stage of change (see Chapter 3).
Immunization	**Patient:** at next physician visit during the fall for influenza, at any time for pneumococcal, tetanus. **Pharmacist:** at 3 mos	Immunization with influenza and/or pneumococcal vaccine and/or tetanus.	If ineffective, record in patient profile for recommendation the following year. Assess and address reasons for nonvaccination, counsel to stage of change.
Injury prevention	**Patient:** Poison Control Centre number beside phone, secured medications especially iron-containing products, analgesics, antidepressants, household cleaning supplies. **Pharmacist:** at next refill or after 3 mos	Knowledge of Poison Control Centre number and medications, supplies causing high risk. Proper medication waste disposal.	If ineffective, explain importance and counsel according to stage of change (see Chapter 3).

Monitoring the Patient for Lifestyle Changes

Self-monitoring is important for lifestyle change. Table 3 provides a framework that requires individualization. The pharmacist should provide reinforcement with written plans and logs for self-monitoring, as this has been found to be useful especially for nutrition and exercise recommendations.[12] Further community and governmental resources may be suggested to patients.

What can pharmacists do to help their patients stay healthy? Opportunities should be sought by pharmacists to promote lifestyle changes as the majority of patients will not seek out the pharmacist for health advice, but respond to suggestions well.[47] Surveys of British Columbia and Quebec pharmacists demonstrated pharmacists were able and willing to provide more health-promoting activities but did so mostly in relation to dispensing or selling of medications.[47-49] An area set aside in pharmacies to promote health lifestyle changes should be encouraged. Pamphlets and booklets from various organizations and support groups are freely available. It may be sensible to select one or two interventions and deliver them consistently to meet the goals of both patients and other health care providers. Education on disease prevention should be a way of thinking; in this manner pharmacists may realize their potential for health promotion[46-49] to improve and maintain the health of Canadians.

Suggested Readings

Blenkinsopp A, Panton R, Anderson C. *Health Promotion for Pharmacists*. 2nd ed. Oxford: Oxford University Press; 2000.

Canadian Task Force on Development of The Healthy Heart Kit. *The Healthy Heart Kit: Helping Your Patients Reduce their Risk*, Ottawa, February 1999. Available at: http://www.healthyheartkit.com.

Canadian Task Force on Preventive Health Care. *The Canadian Guide to Clinical Preventive Health Care*. Ottawa: Ministry of Supply and Services; 1994. Available at: http://www.hc-sc.gc.ca/hppb/health-care/pubs/clinical_preventive/index.html.

Lalonde M. *A New Perspective on the Health of Canadians*. Ottawa: Ministry of Supply and Services Canada; 1981. Available at: http://www.hc-sc.gc. ca/hppb/healthpromotiondevelopment/pdf/perspective.pdf.

World Health Organization. *Obesity: Preventing and Managing the Global Epidemic. Report of a WHO Consultation on Obesity*. Geneva; 1997. Executive summary available at: http://www.who.int/ncd/cvd/obesityreport.pdf.

References

1. *Selected Health Indicators. Appendix B. Towards a Healthy Future: Second Report on the Health of Canadians*. Ottawa: Health Canada. Available at: http://www.hc-sc.gc.ca/hppb/phdd/report/stat/eng/index.html. Accessed April 4, 2001.

2. McGinnis JM, Foege WH. Actual causes of death in the United States. *JAMA* 1993;270:2207-12.

3. Lau DCW. Call for action: preventing and managing the expansive and expensive obesity epidemic. *CMAJ* 1999;160:503-5. Available at: http://www.cma.ca/cmaj/vol-160/issue-4/0503.htm. Accessed April 17, 2001.

4. Andersen RE. The spread of the childhood obesity epidemic. *CMAJ* 2000;163:1461-2. Available at: http://www.cma.ca/cmaj/vol-163/issue-11/1461.htm. Accessed April 17, 2001.

5. Josefson D. Obesity and inactivity fuel global cancer epidemic. *BMJ* 2001;322:945. Available at: http://www.bmj.com/cgi/content/full/322/7292/945. Accessed April 17, 2001.

6. Douketis JD, Attia J. Periodic health examination, 1999 update: 1. Detection, prevention and treatment of obesity. *CMAJ* 1999;160(4):513-25. Available at: http://www.cma.ca/cmaj/vol-160/issue-4/0513.htm. Accessed April 17, 2001.

7. National Heart Lung and Blood Institute. *Clinical Guidelines on the Identification, Evaluation, and Treatment of Overweight and Obesity in Adults—The Evidence Report*. Bethesda, MD: National Institutes of Health; June 1998.

8. Van Allen MI, McCourt C, Lee NS. *Preconception health: folic acid for the primary prevention of neural tube defects. A resource document for health professionals*, 2002. Ottawa, Ontario: Minister of Public Works and Government Services Canada, 2002 (Cat Number H39-607/2002E). Available at: http://www.hc-sc.gc.ca/english/folicacid/report/. Accessed April 1, 2002.

9. Dawson LE, Pham B, Hunter AGW. Low rate of adequate folic acid supplementation in well-educated women of high socioeconomic status attending a genetics clinic. *CMAJ* 2001;164(8):1149-1150. Available at: http://www.cma.ca/cmaj/vol-164/issue-8/1149.asp. Accessed April 17, 2001.

10. Fentem PH. ABC of sports medicine: benefits of exercise in health and disease. *BMJ* 1994;308:1291-1295. Available at: http://www.bmj.com/cgi/content/full/308/6939/1291. Accessed April 30, 2001.

11. Lawlor DA, Hopker SW. The effectiveness of exercise as an intervention in the management of depression: systematic review and meta-regression analysis of randomized controlled trials. *BMJ* 2001;322:763-70. Available at: http://www.bmj.com/cgi/content/full/322/7289/763. Accessed April 30, 2001.

12. US Preventive Services Task Force. Section II. Counseling to Promote Physical Activity. In: *Guidelines from Clinical Preventive Services*, 1996.

13. Health Canada: *What Determines Health? Towards a Healthy Future: Second Report on the Health of Canadians.* Available at: http://www.hc-sc.gc.ca/hppb/phdd/report/toward/eng/report.html. Accessed April 4, 2001.

14. *Healthy People 2010. The National Health Promotion and Disease Prevention Objectives.* US Department of Health and Human Services. Available at: http://web.health.gov/healthypeople/publications. Accessed May 2, 2001.

15. Cléroux J, Feldman RD, Petrella RJ. Lifestyle modifications to prevent and control hypertension. 4. Recommendations on physical exercise training. *CMAJ* 1999:160(9 suppl):S21-S28. Available at: http://www.cma.ca/cmaj/vol-161/issue-12/hypertension/index.htm. Accessed April 10, 2001.

16. Kavanagh T. Exercise in the primary prevention of coronary artery disease. *Can J Cardiol* 2001;17(2):115-161.

17. Leermakers EA, Dunn AL, Blair SN. Exercise management of obesity. *Med Clin North Am* 2000;84(2):419-40.

18. Christenson B, Lundbergh P, Hedlund J, Örtqvist Å. Effects of a large-scale intervention with influenza and 23-valent pneumococcal vaccines in adults aged 65 years or older: a prospective study. *Lancet* 2001;357:1008-11.

19. National Advisory Committee on Immunization. Statement on Influenza Vaccination for the 2000-2001 Season. *Can Commun Dis Rep* 26 (ACS-2): June 2000.

20. Nuroti PJ, Butler JC, Breiman RF. Prevention of pneumococcal disease: recommendations of the Advisory Committee on Immunization Practices. *MMWR* 26: (RR-8); 1997.

21. National Vaccine Advisory Committee. Adult immunization programs in non-traditional settings: quality standards and guidance for program evaluation. *MMWR* 49: (RR-1);2000.

22. Health Canada. Influenza and pneumonia. In *Respiratory Diseases in Canada.* Ottawa; 2001. Available at: http://www.hc-sc.gc.ca/pphb-dgspsp/.

23. Gutschi LM, Vaillancourt R, Holmes M et al. Effect of pharmacist interventions on pneumococcal and influenza vaccination rates. A seamless care approach. *Can Pharm J* 1998;131(8):32-38.

24. *Heart Diseases and Stroke in Canada. 6. Risk Factors for Cardiovascular Disease.* Available at: http://www.hc-sc.gc.ca/hpb/lcdc/bcrdd/hdsc97/s06_e.html. Accessed April 17, 2001.

25. Canadian Paediatric Society. Role of the physician in smoking. *Paediatr Child Health* 2001;6(2):89-95.

26. Kottke TE, Battista RN, DeFriese GH et al. Attributes of successful smoking cessation interventions in medical practice. *JAMA* 1988;259:2883-9.

27. American Society of Health-System Pharmacists. ASHP Therapeutic Position Statement of Smoking Cessation. *Am J Health-Syst Pharm* 1999;56:460-466.

28. Bondy S, Rehm J, Ashely M et al. Low-risk drinking guidelines: the scientific evidence. *Can J Public Health* 1999;90(4):264-70.

29. Addiction Research Foundation of Ontario and the Canadian Centre on Substance Abuse. Appendix 1-Moderate drinking and health. *CMAJ* 1994;151(6):821-824.

30. Canadian Pediatric Society. Prevention of fetal alcohol syndrome (FAS) and fetal alcohol effects (FAE) in Canada. *Paediatr Child Health* 1997;2(2):143-5.

31. Berger K, Ajani UA, Kase C et al. Light-to-moderate alcohol consumption and the risk of stroke among U.S. male physicians. *N Engl J Med* 1999;341:1557-64.

32. Abramson JL, Williams SA, Krumholz HM et al. Moderate alcohol consumption and risk of heart failure among older persons. *JAMA* 2001;285(15):1971-7.

33. Campbell NRC, Ashley MJ, Carruthers SG et al. Lifestyle modifications to prevent and control hypertension. 3. Recommendations on alcohol consumption. *CMAJ* 1999;160 (9 suppl):S13-20. Available at: http://www.cma.ca/cmaj/vol-161/issue-12/hypertension/index.htm. Accessed April 10, 2001.

34. Canadian Task Force on Preventative Care. Chapter 28: *Prevention of Household and Recreational Injuries in Children (<15 Years of Age).* Ottawa: Minister of Supply and Services Canada; 1994.

35. McGuigan MA. Common culprits in childhood poisoning: epidemiology, treatment and parental advice for prevention. *Pediatr Drugs* 1999;1(4):313-24.

36. Canadian Task Force on the Periodic Health Examination. The Canadian Guide to Clinical Preventive Health Care. Ottawa: Minister of Supply and Services Canada; 1994. Available at: http://www.hc-sc.gc.ca/hppb/healthcare/pubs/clinical_preventive/index.html. Accessed May 1, 2001.

37. The Canadian Guide to Clinical Preventive Health Care. Pediatric Preventative Care. Available at: http://www.hc-sc.gc.ca/hppb/healthcare/pubs/clinical_preventive/sec2e.htm. Accessed May 1, 2001.

38. Elster AB. Integrating comprehensive adolescent preventive services into routine medicine care. Rationale and approaches. *Pediatr Clin North Am* 1997;44(6):1365-77.

39. American Academy of Pediatrics. Recommendations for pediatric preventive health care: Committee on Practice and Ambulatory Medicine. *Pediatrics* 1995;96:373-4.

40. Leiter LA, Abbott D, Campbell NRC et al. Lifestyle modifications to prevent and control hypertension. 2. Recommendations on obesity and weight loss. *CMAJ* 1999;160(9 suppl):S7-12. Available at: http://www.cma.ca/cmaj/vol-161/issue-12/hypertension/index.htm. Accessed April 10, 2001.

41. Stone NJ, Kushner R. Effects of dietary modification and treatment of obesity: emphasis on improving vascular outcomes. *Med Clin North Am* 2000;84(1):95-122.

42. Barnes HN, Samet JH. Brief interventions with substance-abusing patients. *Med Clin North Am* 1997;81:867-879.

43. Tuomilehto J, Lindström J, Eriksson JG et al. Prevention of type 2 diabetes mellitus by changes in lifestyle among subjects with impaired glucose tolerance. *N Engl J Med* 2001; 344:1343-50.

44. Grabenstein JD. Pharmacists as vaccine advocates: roles in community pharmacies, nursing homes, and hospitals. *Vaccine* 1998;16(18):1705-10.

45. Williams DM, Newsom JF, Brock TP. An evaluation of smoking cessation-related activities by pharmacists. *J Am Pharm Assoc* 2000;40:366-70.

46. Cogswell B, Eggert M. People want doctors to give more preventative care: a qualitative study of healthcare consumers. *Arch Fam Med* 1993;2:611-619.

47. Paluk ED, Stratton RP, Eni GO. Community pharmacists' participation in health education and disease prevention activities. *Can J Public Health* 1994;85:389-92.

48. O'Laughlin J, Masson, P, Déry V et al. The role of community pharmacists in health education and disease prevention: a survey of their interests and needs in relation to cardiovascular disease. *Prev Med* 1999;28:324-31.

49. Kotecki JE, Elanjian SI, Torabi MR. Health promotion beliefs and practices among pharmacists. *J Am Pharm Assoc* 2000; 40:773-9.

Preventive Health Care and Lifestyle Management—Patient Information

- Be active. Engage in moderate activity such as walking for at least 30 minutes five times a week. This can be divided up into 10-minute sessions throughout the day.
    - Obtain a copy of *Canada's Physical Activity Guide to Healthy Active Living*: 1-888-334-9769 or www.paguide.com
    - Use an activity record to keep track of what you do every day – see the attached example.
- Eat sensibly. Eat 5 to 10 servings a day of fruit and vegetables. Increase fibre by eating oatmeal, barley, brown rice, whole wheat and dried beans, peas and lentils. Cut down on fat in cooking and what you add to food. Cut back on meat and choose poultry or fish. Avoid high-fat desserts, snack foods and processed foods. Cut down on calories and portions if you have been told to lose weight.
    - Obtain a copy of *Canada's Food Guide to Healthy Eating* from Health Canada at www.hc-sc.ca/nutrition
    - Use a food record to keep track of what you eat – see the attached example.
- Stop smoking. If you don't smoke, don't start. Talk to your physician or pharmacist about quitting and the options open to you.
- If you drink alcohol, drink in moderation. Don't drink and drive a motor vehicle or a boat. Don't drink if you are pregnant.
    - No more than two standard drinks a day for men
    - No more than one standard drink a day for women
    - Standard drink is: 1.5 oz (45 mL) hard liquor or spirits, 5 oz (150 mL) wine, 12 oz (360 mL) beer
- Get the flu shot every year. Get vaccinated against pneumococcal pneumonia.
    - Discuss vaccination with your physician at your next visit or contact your public health unit (see your blue pages).
    - More information is available at www.canadian-health-network.ca/html/faq/chntopiccategory_13e.html
- If you are contemplating pregnancy, ask your pharmacist about taking folic acid 0.4 mg each day.
- Know the nearest Poison Control Centre phone number. Store medications, cleaning supplies and other toxic substances out of the reach of children.
- Return unused medications to the pharmacy for proper disposal.

My next visit to my doctor is _____

- Supplement, date, directions _____

    _____

    _____

- Poison Control Centre number _____
- Pharmacy name _____

    _____

Physical Activity Log					
Date	**Goal activity**	**Actual**	**Time spent**	**Level of exertion**	**Comments**

Total active time this week:

Average time per day:

Food Record					
Time	**Food**	**Amount**	**Hunger scale (none, little, moderate, very, starved)**	**Time taken to eat**	**Where and what you were doing**

Chapter 5

Triage and Assessment of the Self-medicating Consumer

Barry Power, BScPhm, PharmD

Nonprescription medications are widely accessed by the public using self-selection. However, consultation with a health professional will assist the consumer in selecting an appropriate product or in identifying conditions that may require more intensive medical care. The challenge for the busy health care provider is to quickly determine the seriousness of the condition for which treatment is being sought, and to identify appropriate nonprescription products that can be used for self-treatment. The tools the health care worker uses to make these decisions are triage and patient assessment.

What is Triage?

Triage is the process of quickly determining the presenting complaint of a patient and determining the urgency of the situation. When responding to the self-medicating patient, a pharmacist is able to assess presenting symptoms to determine the most appropriate action:

- Referring for medical assessment
- Recommending treatment with nonpharmacologic therapy or nonprescription medication
- Reassuring patient that no treatment is necessary at this time

In busy locations, it may be necessary to deal with a more seriously ill patient ahead of another, regardless of the order in which they present. This "queue jumping" is based on the severity of the health condition being experienced by each of the patients.

Triage also identifies patients who need more intensive medical care and a referral to an appropriate provider.

Triage is carried out by assessing the patient through discussion of their complaint and by physical assessment, when appropriate. For example, a health care provider may need to inspect a rash to be able to make an appropriate recommendation. Some patients may not be able to explain what their condition looks like, but may be able to show it. Warts, athlete's foot and minor cuts and burns are easily inspected. Efficient, clear communication is the key to successful triage.

Patient Assessment (Figure 1)

A systematic approach by the health care professional will result in consistent and comprehensive patient assessments.

During any interaction, the health care provider assesses a patient by obtaining a history and, if needed, doing a physical exam (mainly inspection and palpation) or obtaining laboratory or diagnostic measurement. Thorough assessment is essential before recommending a nonprescription product, to identify patients who require additional care, and who have special needs requiring careful product selection.

First steps:

- Determine *why* the patient is seeking your help or looking for a nonprescription product.
- Ask the patient to explain to you, in their own words, the condition, symptom or problem that they wish to treat.

Determine the urgency of situation:

- Enquire about red flags indicating the need for more intensive medical attention (Table 1).

Figure 1: **Patient Triage and Assessment**

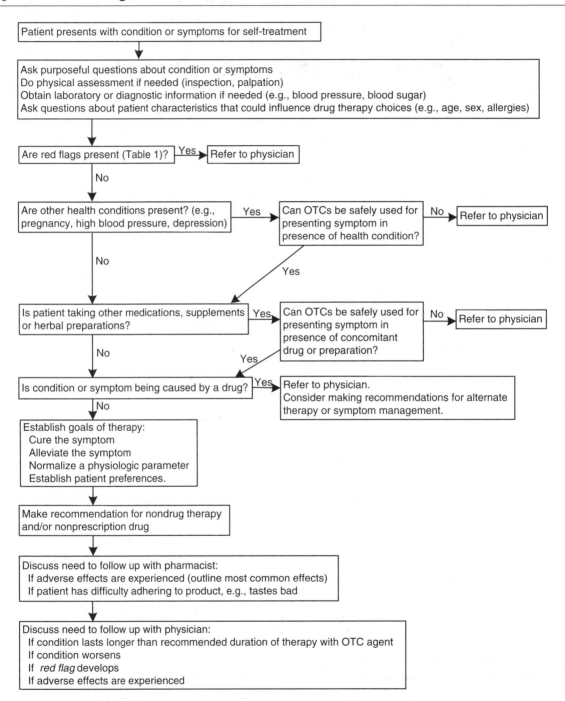

Table 1: **Red Flags for Referral for More Intensive/Urgent Care***

Red flag	Significance of red flag
Change in level of consciousness or change in senses (vision, hearing, taste)	Infection, concussion, stroke, hypoglycemia
Fever in infants	Infection, meningitis
Fever not responding to appropriate measures	Infection
Fever, vomiting, headache, confusion, difficulty bending neck	May indicate meningitis
Sign of infection or inflammation (pus, swelling, fever, redness, tenderness, heat)	Systemic antibiotics or antiinflammatories may be needed
Persistent bleeding	Assess need for hospitalization; may indicate clotting abnormalities
Spontaneous bleeding/bruising	May indicate clotting or blood disorder requiring investigation
Bleeding from any orifice	May indicate more serious internal injuries
Severe pain ("Worst pain I've ever had.")	Possible precursor of cerebral aneurysm
Risk of dehydration, especially in infants/children and the elderly (e.g., vomiting, diarrhea)	Hospitalization or more intensive screening may be required
Pain on urination	May indicate infection
Increasing urinary frequency	May indicate poor glucose control or infection
Discolored urine or feces (rule out drug causes)	May indicate internal bleeding
Increasing breathlessness	May require immediate treatment
Chest pain	May indicate cardiac problems
Paralysis of face, arms, legs; difficulty speaking	Transient ischemic attack, stroke
Yellowing of skin and/or eyes	Jaundice or liver damage
Contraindications to specific nonprescription medications	More intensive medical observations needed

List should not be considered exhaustive.

- Determine the presence of other health conditions potentially impacting on product selection or requiring more intensive medical care (e.g., ulcer, hypertension, asthma).
- Ask women about the possibility of pregnancy.
- Does the patient require treatment immediately (e.g., for vomiting or pain), or can treatment be started at any time (e.g., treatment for warts)?

Assess the situation:
- Much of the information a health care practitioner needs to recommend the use of a nonprescription product will develop from a discussion with the patient.
- It is important to have a complete description of the condition (Figure 1).
- It may be necessary to inspect (e.g., observe a potentially infected cut), measure (e.g., body temperature) or palpate (e.g., ankle swelling) to be able to assess a patient's condition.

Establish the patient's goals:
- Tailor product selection to meet the patient's expectations, where possible. For example, "curing" a cold is not possible, but relief of symptoms is.

- Educating the patient may be needed to set realistic goals.

Select product and counsel:
- Determine appropriate product(s) for condition in question.
- Provide patient with a choice if possible.
- Counsel patient on use, adverse effects, onset of action.
- Provide guidelines for follow-up with physician if necessary (e.g., "If your cold does not clear up in five days, or if it is becoming worse, talk to your doctor.").

Follow-up:
- For some cases, follow-up is important. For example, a parent seeking a rehydration fluid should be contacted in 24 hours to determine if the child is displaying signs of dehydration.
- Follow-up may not be possible in many cases.
- Professional judgment should be used in determining cases for follow-up.
- Documentation will allow for more effective follow-up and continuity of care.

Suggested Readings

Dolovich L, Hudson A. Collecting the evidence. *Pharm Pract* 1997;13(5):68-77.

Longe RL, Calbert JC. *Physical Assessment. A Guide for Evaluating Drug Therapy.* Vancouver, Washington: Applied Therapeutics; 1994.

Central Nervous System Conditions
Section Highlights

Chapter 6: **Insomnia**

Chapter 7: **Depression**

Chapter 8: **Headache**
>
> Clinical features of tension-type headache, migraine and cluster headache
> Red flags for serious headache
> Drug-induced headache
> Medication-overuse headache
> Nonprescription medications for acute therapy of tension-type and migraine
>   headaches
> Nonprescription medications for prophylaxis of migraine headaches

Chapter 9: **Fever**
>
> Methods of measuring body temperature
> Normal pediatric temperature ranges associated with measurement
>   techniques
> Fever in cardiovascular or pulmonary disorders
> Fever in the elderly
> Fever in pregnancy
> Fever phobia

Chapter 10: **Heat-related Disorders**
>
> Heat edema
> Heat cramps
> Heat syncope
> Heat exhaustion
> Heat stroke

Chapter 11: **Nicotine Addiction**
>
> Health risks associated with smoking
> Behavioral modification programs
> Acupuncture and other alternative therapies
> Nicotine replacement therapy

Insomnia

Régis Vaillancourt, BPharm, PharmD

Pathophysiology

Normal sleep involves four to six cycles divided between rapid eye movement (REM) and non-REM. Non-REM sleep consists of four stages and is associated with eye movement and low muscle tone. Stage 1 sleep represents a transition between wakefulness and sleep, and lasts 0.5 to 7 minutes. Stage 2 is a light stage of sleep and comprises up to 50% of sleep time. Stages 3 and 4 (called delta sleep) are characterized by deep, restorative sleep. A decrease in stages 3 and 4 is associated with poor sleep quality. REM sleep is associated with a high level of neuronal activity and dreaming. *REM rebound* occurs upon abrupt discontinuation of agents that suppress REM sleep, such as benzodiazepines or tricyclic antidepressants.[1] This may result in vivid and frightening dreams.

Insomnia is characterized by one or more of the following: difficulty initiating sleep (taking > 30 minutes to fall asleep), change in sleep quality (not having a satisfying sleep), decrease in sleep quantity (not enough sleep) and/or difficulty in maintaining sleep continuity (broken sleep or early morning awakening).[2,3] Insomnia may also present with daytime symptoms such as impaired alertness, fatigue, mood changes (e.g., depression, irritability), diminished concentration, memory difficulty and/or inability to perform complex tasks. Poor sleep is associated with an increased risk of traffic accidents, depression, alcohol abuse, mortality, absenteeism, health care utilization, social disability and a decrease in the quality of life.[4,5]

Insomnia is usually a symptom of another condition.

Table 1 classifies insomnia according to duration of symptoms and lists conditions that may be associated with it.

A Canadian survey indicates that 10.5% of adults experienced an "inability to sleep/insomnia" in a

Table 1: **Types of Insomnia**[1,3,5]

Type	Duration	Possible causes
Acute		
Transient	2-3 days	Acute emotional or physical discomfort (life stress, acute illness, hospitalization, jet lag, environmental disturbance such as noise, light and temperature).
Short term	≤ 3 wks	Acute stressor, usually related to work or family life (death or illness of a loved one, loss of job).
Chronic	> 3 wks	Mood disorders, anxiety disorders, chronic pain, difficulty breathing (asthma, COPD, loud snoring and/or gasping, choking or stopping breathing during sleep (sleep apnea), gastroesophageal reflux disease, hormonal changes associated with pregnancy, perimenopause and menopause, drug and alcohol abuse and dependency, restless legs syndrome, periodic limb movement disorders, circadian rhythm sleep disorders (e.g., shift worker), Parkinson's disease, Alzheimer's disease or some drugs.

COPD = chronic obstructive pulmonary disease

12-month period; of these, 47.3% claimed to have suffered for the whole or part of the year.[6] Insomnia ranked ninth among the most commonly experienced minor ailments.[6] According to the survey, 26.9% of patients suffering from insomnia took an OTC either alone or in combination with prescription, herbal or homeopathic products to manage their insomnia. OTC remedies alone were used by 14.1% of patients.

Populations at risk of insomnia are women, individuals of lower socioeconomic status, patients with chronic medical and psychiatric disorders, and patients with a first-degree relative with insomnia.[7,8] Elderly patients often experience frequent awakenings and increased difficulty in falling asleep again. Their sleep may be shortened even if more time is spent in bed.[7] Younger patients often have more difficulty falling asleep.

Goals of Therapy[3,8,9]

- Prevent symptoms associated with poor sleep such as daytime drowsiness and impairment
- Promote a sound and satisfying sleep (sleep quality, quantity, continuity and initiation)
- Prevent the progression from transient to chronic insomnia
- Prevent dependence on drug therapy
- Reinstate a normal sleep pattern without medication

Patient Assessment

An assessment plan for patients suffering from insomnia is illustrated in Figure 1.

Children less than 12 years of age should not receive nonprescription products to manage insomnia, but should be referred to a physician for complete medical assessment.[10]

Nonpharmacologic Therapy[3,8,9,11-13]

General *sleep hygiene* measures involve health practice and environmental influences relating to sleep. However, they may not be sufficient to manage patients with chronic insomnia.[8,12]
- Establish regular bedtimes and wake-up times.
- Discontinue caffeine four to six hours before bedtime and minimize total daily intake.

- Avoid nicotine near bedtime and upon awakening at night.
- Avoid using alcohol to facilitate sleep onset (alcohol may cause awakening later in the night).
- Avoid eating heavy meals before going to bed, or going to bed hungry.
- Avoid poor sleep environments; minimize noise, light or extreme temperature.
- Exercise regularly. Regular exercise in the late afternoon may deepen sleep; vigorous exercise within three to four hours before bedtime may interfere with sleep.
- Minimize drinking fluids before going to bed to decrease the number of awakenings to void.

Stimulus control is based on the concept that sleep is a conditioned response to temporal (bedtime) and environmental cues. Instructions are aimed at avoiding sleep-incompatible behaviors and regulating the sleep–wake cycle. Stimulus control instructions are the following:
- Go to bed only when sleepy.
- Use the bedroom only for sleep and sex.
- If unable to sleep after 15 to 20 minutes, get out of bed and go to another room to read in a dimly lit environment (avoid watching TV as it radiates a full spectrum of light that may have an arousing effect) and return only when feeling sleepy again.
- Get up at the same time in the morning regardless of sleep duration the previous night.
- Avoid napping during the day.

Pharmacists are unlikely to implement the following forms of nonpharmacologic therapy as they require specialized patient follow-up.

The normal reaction to insomnia is trying to increase the time spent in bed to provide more sleep opportunity, usually resulting in fragmented and poor quality sleep. *Sleep restriction* consists of controlling the amount of time spent in bed but increasing the percentage of time asleep. For example, a patient who sleeps for only six hours but stays in bed for eight hours per night would be asked to decrease the time in bed to six hours. This would be accomplished by changing the bedtime while maintaining wake-up time to maintain a good sleep-wake cycle. The mild state of intentional sleep deprivation promotes more rapid sleep onset and more efficient sleep. The allowable time in bed is gradually lengthened by 15 to 30 minutes as sleep efficiency increases.

Figure 1: **Assessment of Patients with Insomnia**[1,3,6-8]

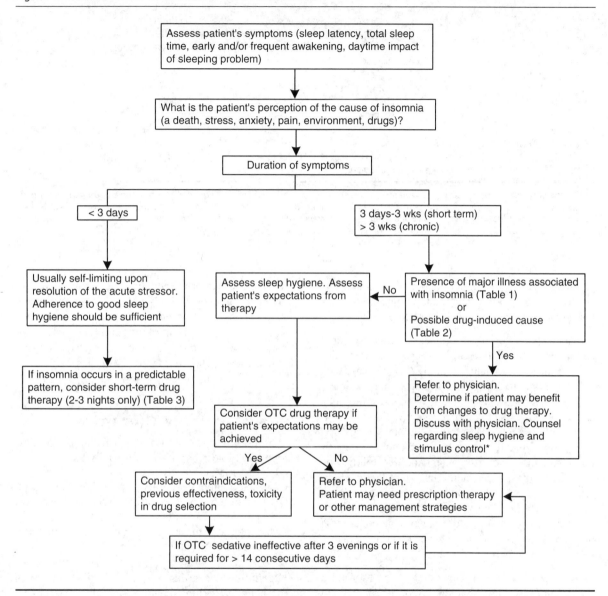

While awaiting a physician visit, recommend maintenance of a sleep diary indicating the usual bedtime, time of arising, the timing and quantity of meals, use of alcohol, exercise, medications and descriptions of the duration and quality of sleep. This may serve as a baseline for assessment of future treatment effects. (See Patient Information.)

Relaxation Strategies

Relaxation procedures and biofeedback focus on somatic arousal, whereas attention-focusing procedures target cognitive arousal. This therapy is aimed either at reducing cognitive arousal, such as intrusive thoughts and racing mind, or at physiologic arousal such as muscle tension.

Cognitive behavioral therapy consists of identifying dysfunctional beliefs and attitudes about sleep and

Table 2: **Drugs Associated with Insomnia**[*,2,9,11]

Alcohol	Corticosteroids	Methylphenidate
Amantadine	Daunorubicin	Nicotine
Amphetamines	Decongestants	Oral contraceptives
Anticholinergics	Diuretics	Pentostatin
Appetite suppressants	Goserelin	Phenytoin
Beta$_2$-agonists	HMG CoA reductase inhibitors	Progesterone[†]
Beta-blockers	Interferon alpha	Quinidine
Bupropion	Leuprolide	Reserpine
Caffeine (in OTCs)	Levodopa	Selective serotonin reuptake inhibitors
Calcium channel blockers	LSD	Selegiline
Clonidine	Medroxyprogesterone	Theophylline
Cocaine	Mefloquine	Thyroid hormone

*The pharmacodynamic mechanisms involved in the occurrence of drug-induced insomnia are penetration of the blood-brain barrier (e.g., lipophilicity), direct effect on the central nervous system (e.g., either stimulant, sedative or drug withdrawal); mental disturbances causing insomnia (e.g., depression or anxiety); and aggravation or occurrence of a medical condition that disturbs sleep (e.g., enuresis, nocturia, sleep apnea, restless legs syndrome, painful erection, gastric irritation).
†Micronized progesterone may cause sedation (See Chapter 52).

replacing them with a more adaptive substitute. It is aimed at creating a new attitude to minimize anticipatory anxiety and arousal, which interfere with sleep.

In patients with chronic insomnia, nonpharmacologic therapy is expected to decrease sleep onset latency by 43%, from a mean latency of 64.3 ± 23.2 minutes before therapy to 36.6 ± 15.8 minutes after the intervention.[12] Similarly, the amount of time awake after sleep onset is expected to decrease by 46.4%, from a mean of 70.3 ± 31.3 minutes before therapy to 37.6 ± 15.7 minutes after the intervention.[9] Clinical improvements have been maintained at follow-ups averaging six months. Stimulus control and sleep restriction appear to be the most effective single therapies. These therapies are compatible with each other and can be combined.[12] Sleep hygiene alone is not as effective as the other forms of nonpharmacologic therapy in chronic insomnia.[12]

The following therapies have shown some promise but require more investigation. *Exercise:* Four 30- to 40-minute endurance training sessions (low impact aerobics, brisk walk) per week, in an elderly population, for a period of 16 weeks, resulted in a significant improvement in sleep quality, decreased sleep latency and increased sleep duration.[13] *Bright light therapy* consisting of bright light exposure (> 4000 lux) from 9 pm to 11 pm every night during a 12-day period, followed by maintenance therapy with bright light exposure twice a week from 9 pm to 11 pm, resulted

in significant improvement in sleep quality and in daytime cognitive functioning.[7] *Low energy emission therapy* consists of an electrically conducting mouthpiece delivering an amplitude-modulated electromagnetic field.[7] Limited data in elderly patients have shown some promise. *Acupuncture* has been used with good results in many cases.[7]

Pharmacologic Therapy[11]

Nonprescription medications for insomnia are described in Table 3. Principles of therapy are:
• Use the lowest effective dose.
• Use intermittent dosing (two to four times weekly).
• Use short term, no longer than 14 consecutive days with an OTC therapy.
• Discontinue medication gradually if used long term.
• Be alert to rebound insomnia.

Alternative Therapies

The herbal **valerian** is included in Table 3 because it is available as a Health Canada approved product and has been assigned a DIN number. **Kava** may promote sleep but there are no long-term studies.[23] Use of kava is not recommended because of several reports of hepatotoxicity. **Chamomile (German), eleuthero (Siberian Ginseng), passion flower, reishi** and **St. John's wort** are other herbals used for insomnia for which there is insufficient evidence to recommend use.

Table 3: Nonprescription Drug Therapy of Insomnia[11]

Drug	Effective dose	Expected clinical benefit	Half-life	Onset of action	Side effects	Comments
Diphenhydramine*[14-17]	12.5-50 mg 30-60 min before bedtime[†] Optimal dose = 50 mg	Subjective improvement in sleep onset, night awakening, duration and quality of sleep	2.4-9.3 h	60-180 min	Morning drowsiness (10-15%). Dizziness (8%). Grogginess (10-19%). Anticholinergic side effects (e.g., delirium, urinary retention). May lower seizure threshold.	Contraindicated in patients suffering from glaucoma, benign prostatic hypertrophy, heart disease, constipation, dry mouth and dry eyes. Dimenhydrinate contains 50-55% diphenhydramine. Anticholinergic effects of concern in the elderly. Drug of choice, especially in patients who experience difficulty falling asleep.
Doxylamine[18]	25 mg	Improvement in sleep onset, night awakening, duration and quality of sleep	10 h prolonged to 15.5 h in elderly men[19]	60-120 min	Feeling tired in the morning (29%), hangover feeling in the morning (3%), feeling drugged (6%). Anticholinergic side effects are rare. May lower seizure threshold.	Less well studied than diphenhydramine; prolonged half-life may explain side effect profile.
Valerian[20]	400-900 mg 30 to 60 min before bedtime	Decreased sleep latency and subjective improvement in sleep quality	Unknown	Unknown	Morning hangover (dose 900 mg). A few cases of hepatotoxicity are reported. One case report of severe withdrawal syndrome after high dose long term.[21] Not recommended in pregnancy.	More likely to be effective in patients who have not received previous therapy. Preparations may differ in effectiveness depending on the age of the extract, species used or growing conditions.[22] Limited data available.

*Despite the efficacy of diphenhydramine, benzodiazepines are considered to be more efficacious.[10]
[†]Slight dose-dependent increase in the hypnotic effect at doses ≤ 50 mg, especially in hypnotic-naïve patients; flat dose response in doses > 50 mg.[16]

Melatonin is a neurohormone synthesized from tryptophan. Naturally occurring melatonin is believed to be involved in the regulation of circadian rhythms and the initiation of sleep.[24] Doses of 0.3 to 1 mg for a few nights before retiring may be effective for insomnia, decreasing sleep latency and variably affecting total sleep time and overall sleep quality. However, evidence for its use in insomnia is weak. Melatonin is effective in preventing or reducing jetlag.[25] Fatigue, headache, dizziness, irritability and abdominal cramps are possible side effects. In doses of 300 mg per day, it may inhibit ovarian function and should be avoided by women trying to conceive. Melatonin is not available in Canada.

Prescription medications that are used to manage insomnia can be divided into four groups.

- The **barbiturates** such as secobarbital and pentobarbital have fallen out of favor due to significant side effects, rapid development of tolerance and dependence, and fatalities with overdose.
- **Benzodiazepines** are commonly used to manage insomnia in view of their efficacy and low toxicity.[1] When compared to placebo, benzodiazepines decrease sleep latency by about 11.7 minutes and increase sleep duration by about 48.4 minutes.[26]
- Sedating **antidepressants** such as amitriptyline and trazodone are also used to manage insomnia. Trazodone is used often in patients experiencing insomnia associated with serotonin reuptake antidepressants.
- Others: **Chloral hydrate** is an older hypnotic that has fallen out of favor, as tolerance develops rapidly. **Zopiclone** is an intermediate-acting hypnotic agent with a half-life of 3.5 to 6.5 hours. It has similar effects to benzodiazepines although potential for dependence may be less. **Zaleplon** is a novel agent with a short half-life of 0.9 to 1.1 hours, resulting in a low incidence of next-morning hangover. This agent is useful for inducing sleep as opposed to increasing sleep duration.

Monitoring of Therapy

Table 4 provides a framework for a monitoring plan, which should be individualized.

Advice for the Patient

Counsel patients who choose drug therapy regarding:
- Sleep hygiene and stimulus control (see Non-pharmacologic Therapy)
- Instructions not to drive or operate machinery while under the influence of the medication
- Instructions not to combine drug therapy with alcohol
- Expected results of drug therapy and management of side effects (Table 4)

Resource Tips

Sleep/Wake Disorders Canada
3080 Yonge Street, Suite 5055, Toronto, ON M4N 3N1
Tel.: (416) 483-9654 or 1-800-387-9253
Fax: (416) 483-7081 http://www.swdca.org
Internet-based information on sleep disorders: http://www. sleepnet.com

Suggested Readings

Asplund R. Sleep disorders in the elderly. *Drugs & Aging* 1999;14(2):91-103.

Holbrook AM, Crowther R, Lotter A, Cheng C, King D. The diagnosis and management of insomnia in clinical practice: a practical evidence-based approach. *CMAJ* 2000;162(2):216-20.

Kupfer DJ, Reynolds CF. Management of insomnia. *N Engl J Med* 1997;336:341-46.

National Center on Sleep Disorders Research, National Heart, Lung, and Blood Institute, National Institute of Health. Insomnia: assessment and management in primary care. *Sleep* 1999;22(suppl 2):s402-8.

Novak M, Shapiro CM. Drug-induced sleep disturbances, focus on nonpsychotropic medications. *Drug Safety* 1997;16(2):133-49.

Wagner J, Wagner ML, Hening WA. Beyond benzodiazepines: alternative pharmacologic agents for the treatment of insomnia. *Ann Pharmacother* 1998;32: 680-91.

References

1. Wagner J, Wagner ML, Hening WA. Beyond benzodiazepines: alternative pharmacologic agents for the treatment of insomnia. *Ann Pharmacother* 1998;32:680-91.

Table 4: **Monitoring Therapy for Insomnia**

Symptoms	Monitoring	Endpoint of therapy[1,3,7-9]	Actions
Inability to fall asleep, frequent nocturnal awakening, early morning awakening, and/or overall quality of sleep.	**Patient:** daily while on drug therapy **Pharmacist:** after 3 and 14 days of therapy or next pharmacy visit	Decrease in sleep latency of ≤ 30 min, decrease in or no nocturnal awakening, duration of sleep of 5-7 h per night[25] and/or improved subjective sleep quality with 3 nights of therapy.	If ineffective after 3 evenings of therapy and treatment still required, refer to a physician. If drug therapy is required for more than 14 consecutive days, **refer** to a physician.
Morning drowsiness, grogginess and/or dizziness. Elderly are more at risk.	**Patient or family member:** daily **Pharmacist:** after 3 and 14 days of therapy or next pharmacy visit	Minimal/acceptable morning drowsiness, grogginess and/or dizziness throughout therapy	Decrease the dose by 50%. If still a problem after dosage adjustment and therapy still required, **refer** to a physician. If symptoms relate to a lack of efficacy see above.
Constipation. Elderly are more at risk.	**Patient:** every 3 days **Pharmacist:** within 1 week or next pharmacy visit	Minimal constipation throughout therapy	Increase dietary fibre, water intake and exercise. If therapy is still indicated and the patient required laxatives **refer** to a physician.
Confusion. Elderly are more at risk.	**Family:** daily **Pharmacist:** within 1 wk of next pharmacy visit	No confusion throughout therapy	Discontinue therapy immediately and **refer** to a physician.
Adherence to good sleep hygiene, stimulus control practice.	**Pharmacist:** after 3 and 14 days of therapy or next pharmacy visit	Continuous good sleep hygiene practice required throughout therapy to ensure long-term therapeutic outcomes are achieved.	If drug therapy is required for more than 14 consecutive days, **refer** to a physician.

2. Novak M, Shapiro CM. Drug-induced sleep disturbances, focus on nonpsychotropic medications. *Drug Safety* 1997; 16(2):133-49.

3. National Center on Sleep Disorders Research, National Heart, Lung, and Blood Institute, National Institute of Health. Insomnia: assessment and management in primary care. *Sleep* 1999;22(suppl 2):s402-8.

4. Zammit GK, Weiner J, Damato N, Sillup GP, McMillan CA. Quality of life in people with insomnia. *Sleep* 1999;22 (suppl 2):S379-85.

5. Stoller MK. Economic effects of insomnia. *Clin Ther* 1994;16: 873-97.

6. NDMAC/ACNielsen. *Health Vision '98.* Ottawa. May 1998.

7. Asplund R. Sleep disorders in the elderly. *Drugs & Aging* 1999;14(2):91-103.

8. Kupfer DJ, Reynolds CF. Management of insomnia. *N Engl J Med* 1997;336:341-6.

9. Therapeutics Initiative. To sleep or not to sleep: here are your questions. *Therapeut Lett* 1995;11.

10. Pray WS. OTC products: age limits for safe use. *US Pharmacist* 1999;24(7):14-22.

11. Maczaj M. Pharmacological treatment of insomnia. *Drugs* 1993;45(1):44-55.

12. Morin CM, Culbert JP, Schwartz SM. Nonpharmacological interventions for insomnia: a meta-analysis of treatment efficacy. *Am J Psychiatry* 1994;151:1172-80.

13. King AC, Oman RF, Brassington GS, Bliwise DL, Haskell WL. Moderate-intensity exercise and self rated quality of sleep in older adults, a randomized controlled trial. *JAMA* 1997;277: 32-7.

14. Rickels K, Morris RJ, Newman H, Rosenfeld H, Weinstock R. Diphenhydramine in insomniac family practice patients: a double-blind study. *J Clin Pharmacol* 1983;23(5-6):234-42.

15. Kudo Y, Kurihara M. Clinical evaluation of diphenhydramine hydrochloride for the treatment of insomnia in psychiatric patients: a double-blind study. *J Clin Pharmacol* 1990;30 (11):1041-8.

16. Sunshine A, Zighelboim I, Laska E. Hypnotic activity of diphenhydramine, methapyrilene, and placebo. *J Clin Pharmacol* 1978;18(8-9):425-31.

17. Teutsch G, Mahler DL, Brown CR, Forrest WH, James KE, Brown BW. Hypnotic efficacy of diphenhydramine, methapyrilene and pentobarbital. *Clin Pharmacol Ther* 1975; 17:195-201.

18. Smith GM, Smith PH. Effects of doxylamine and acetaminophen on postoperative sleep. *Clin Pharmacol Ther* 1985;37:549-57.

19. Friedman H, Greenblatt DJ, Scavone JM et al. Clearance of the antihistamine doxylamine. Reduced in elderly men but not in elderly women. *Clin Pharmacokinet* 1989;16(5):312-6.

20. Plushner SL. Valerian: valeriana officinalis. *Am J Health-Syst Pharm* 2000;57:328,333,335.

21. Garges HP, Varia I, Doraiswamy PM. Cardiac complications and delirium associated with valerian root withdrawal. *JAMA* 1998;280:1566-7.

22. Houghton PJ. The scientific basis for the reputed activity of valerian. *J Pharm Pharmacol* 1999;51(5):505-12.

23. Pepping J. Kava: Piper methysticum. *Am J Health-Syst Pharm* 1999;56:957-58,960.

24. Pepping J. Melatonin. *Am J Health-Syst Pharm* 1999;56:2520-7.

25. Herxheimer A, Petrie KJ. Melatonin for preventing and treating jet lag (Cochrane Review). In: *The Cochrane Library*, Issue I. Oxford: Update Software; 2001.

26. Holbrook AM, Crowther R, Lotter A, Cheng C, King D. The diagnosis and management of insomnia in clinical practice: a practical evidence-based approach. *CMAJ* 2000;162(2):216-20.

Insomnia—Patient Information

To help you sleep better:
- Have regular bedtimes and wake-up times.
- Develop a bedtime ritual to relax before going to bed.
- Go to bed only when sleepy; sleep as much as possible to feel refreshed.
- Use the bedroom only for sleep and sex.
- Regular exercise in the late afternoon may help you sleep; brisk exercise within three to four hours before bedtime may interfere with sleep.
- Do not drink coffee, tea or cola four to six hours before bedtime, and minimize total daily intake.
- Minimize drinking fluids before going to bed to decrease the number of awakenings to void.
- If you cannot sleep after 15 to 20 minutes, get out of bed and go into another room to read in a dimly lit environment (avoid watching TV as the bright light may have an arousing effect) and return only when feeling sleepy again.

- Avoid smoking near bedtime and upon awakening at night.
- Avoid using alcohol to help you fall asleep (alcohol may cause awakening later in the night).
- Avoid eating heavy meals before going to bed or going to bed hungry.
- Avoid poor sleep environments; minimize noise, light, or too cold or too warm temperatures.
- Avoid watching the clock.
- Avoid napping during the day.

If you are given a sleeping pill by your pharmacist:
- Do not drive or operate machinery while under the influence of the medication.
- Do not take with alcohol.
- You may need to see a doctor if:
  —It is not working after three evenings, or
  —You need the medication for more than 14 days in a row, or
  —You feel confused, dizzy or drowsy in the morning.

If you think you need to see a doctor, prepare a **sleep diary** while you are waiting for the appointment. This will help your doctor find the best treatment for you. The diary should include:

Date				
Bedtime				
Rise time				
Time to fall asleep				
Number of awakenings				
Total sleep time				
Number of alcoholic drinks/Time				
Exercise type/Time				
Medication taken				
Quality of sleep 5- very good; 4- good; 3- fair; 2- poor; 1- very poor				
Daytime symptoms: impaired alertness, fatigue, irritability, diminished concentration, other				

Adapted with permission from National Center on Sleep Disorders Research, National Heart, Lung, and Blood Institute, National Institute of Health. Insomnia: assessment and management in primary care. *Sleep* 1999;22(suppl 2):s402-8.

Chapter 7

Depression

Ric M. Procyshyn, PharmD, PhD

Depressive disorders are often referred to as affective disorders. However, the pathology is one of mood reflecting the sustained internal emotional state, rather than one of affect or the external expression of emotional content. Table 1 describes the three depressive disorders with a differential diagnosis.

Pathophysiology

Although the exact cause of depression is not known, the contributors are likely a combination of genetic, psychosocial and biologic factors. The first major biologic theory concerning the etiology of depression proposed that depression was due to insufficient concentrations of monoamine neurotransmitters.[2] These neurotransmitters include noradrenaline, serotonin and dopamine. The evidence for this hypothesis was both observational and circumstantial. That is, it was noted that drugs capable of depleting neurotransmitters

induced depression, whereas the classical antidepressants (tricyclic antidepressants and monoamine oxidase inhibitors [MAOIs]) that increased neurotransmitter levels were effective in treating the symptoms of depression. Thus the prevailing wisdom of the day proposed that individuals with "low" levels of neurotransmitters, for whatever reason (drugs, stress or disease process), would be prone to the symptoms of depression. The classical antidepressants increased levels of neurotransmitters in the synapse by blocking presynaptic reuptake of neurotransmitters (the tricyclic agents), or by preventing the metabolic degradation of neurotransmitters by inhibiting MAOIs.

The monoamine neurotransmitters represent only one of many biological factors believed to play a role in depression. Other factors include neuroendocrine and neuroimmune regulation, sleep abnormalities and aberrant neuronal circuits.[3-7] Various disease states

Table 1: **Classification and Differential Diagnosis of Depressive Disorders**[1]

Disorder	Diagnostic features	Differential diagnosis
Major depressive disorder	Characterized by one or more major depressive episodes (i.e., at least 2 wks of depressed mood or loss of interest accompanied by at least four additional symptoms of depression).	• Substance-induced mood disorder • Mood disorder due to a general medical condition • Dysthymic disorder • Schizoaffective disorder
Dysthymic disorder	Characterized by at least 2 yrs of depressed mood for more days than not, accompanied by additional depressive symptoms that do not meet criteria for a major depressive episode.	• Substance-induced mood disorder • Mood disorder due to a general medical condition • Major depressive disorder
Depressive disorder not otherwise specified	Depressive features that do not meet criteria for major depressive disorder, dysthymic disorder, adjustment disorder with depressed mood, or adjustment disorder with mixed anxiety and depressed mood.	

(Table 2) and medications (Table 3) are also known to be associated with depression.

The lifetime risk for major depressive disorder varies from 10 to 25% for women and from 5 to 12% for men.[9-11] The prevalence rates for major depressive disorder appear to be unrelated to ethnicity, education, income or marital status.[12] The risk of major depressive disorder is 1.5 to 3 times greater among those who have a first-degree biologic relative with depression than among the general population. The risk of recurrence in an individual who has experienced one previous depressive episode is 60%. This increases to 70 and 90% if two or three episodes, respectively, of major depression have occurred.[1]

Goals of Therapy

- Relieve symptoms of depression
- Prevent recurrence
- Prevent suicide

Patient Assessment

An assessment plan for patients suffering from depression is illustrated in Figure 1. Refer patients meeting the criteria for either major depression or dysthymic disorder to a physician. Due to the association between depression and suicide, an assessment of risk factors for suicide may also be warranted (Table 4).

Nonpharmacologic Therapy
Psychosocial Interventions
Combined psychotherapy and pharmacotherapy is the most effective treatment for major depressive disorder. However, some data show that psychotherapy alone

Table 2: Medical Conditions Associated with Depression[8]

Endocrine	Addison's disease Cushings' disease Diabetes mellitus	Hypocalcemia Hypothyroidism Hypopituitarism	Hypercalcemia Hyperthyroidism
Infectious	AIDS General paresis (neurosyphilis) Infectious mononucleosis Influenza	Malaria Pneumonia Subacute bacterial endocarditis Toxoplasmosis	Tuberculosis Viral encephalitis Viral hepatitis
Collagen	Lupus erythematosus	Rheumatoid arthritis	
Neurologic	Alzheimer's disease Cerebral tumors Cerebrovascular disorder	Complex partial seizures Head trauma Huntington's chorea	Multiple sclerosis Parkinson's disease Sleep apnea
Miscellaneous	Abdominal cancer Alcoholism Anemia	Disseminated carcinomatosis Pancreatitis Peptic ulcer	Porphyria Postpartum state

Table 3: Medications Associated with Depression[8]

Acyclovir	Bethanidine	Fenfluramine withdrawal	Phenytoin
Acetazolamide	Chloroquine	Indomethacin	Prednisone
Adrenocorticotropic hormones	Cimetidine	Interferon	Propranolol
Alcohol	Cocaine	Interleukin-2	Reserpine
Amphetamines	Cycloserine	Isoniazid	Steroidal contraceptives
Anabolic steroids	Debrisoquine	Levodopa	Timolol
Asparaginase	Dexamethasone	Methyldopa	Valproic acid
Barbiturates	Digoxin	Ondansetron	Vinblastine
Benzodiazepines	Disulfiram	Phenothiazine antipsychotics	Vincristine

Figure 1: **Assessment of Patients with Major Depression or Dysthymic Disorder**[1]

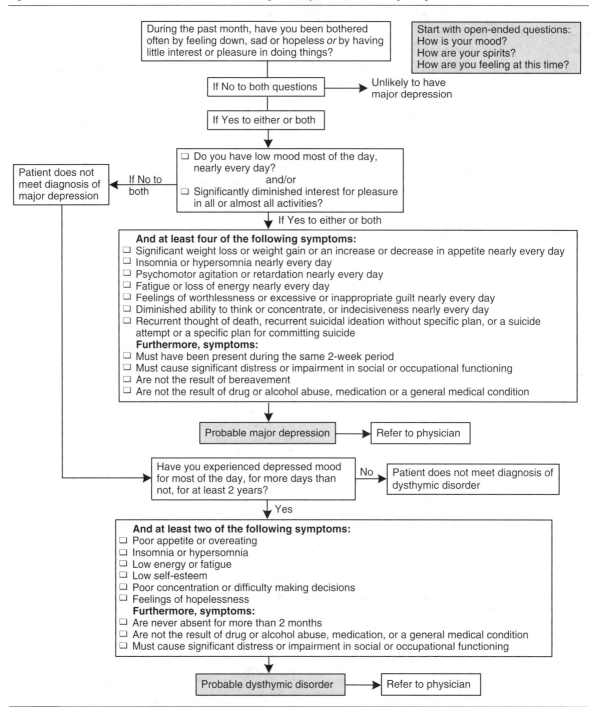

Table 4: **Risk Factors for Suicide**[13-15]

Male sex
  (particularly if unemployed, retired or single)
Drug or alcohol abuse
Impulsivity
	Feelings of helplessness and hopelessness
	Previous psychiatric treatment or
	  hospitalization for psychiatric illness
	Previous suicide attempt(s)
		Family history of suicidal behavior
		Presence of anxiety, agitation or
		  panic attacks
		Plan for suicide

is effective in patients with mild major depressive episodes. Psychotherapeutic treatments include cognitive behavioral therapy, interpersonal therapy, psychodynamic psychotherapy, marital and family therapy and group therapy.[1,16-19] Psychosocial intervention is best suited for:

• Patients with mild to moderate depressive symptoms
• Patients with significant psychosocial stressors or interpersonal difficulties
• Women who are pregnant, breastfeeding or planning to become pregnant.

Exercise and relaxation therapy complement psychosocial intervention.

Electroconvulsive Therapy (ECT)

Introduced in 1938, ECT has the highest rate of response of any form of antidepressant treatment. Appropriate candidates include:[20]

• Patients experiencing severe depressive symptoms and functional impairment
• Individuals with coexisting psychotic symptoms or catatonia
• Patients who are suicidal or who are refusing food
• Individuals with comorbid medical conditions in which the use of antidepressants is contraindicated
• Patients not responding to antidepressant treatment

Light Therapy

A 10,000-lux intensity light box slanted toward the patient's face for 30 minutes per day is the preferred short-term treatment procedure. Consider light therapy:

• For seasonal affective disorder
• As an adjunct in chronic major depressive disorder or dysthymia with seasonal exacerbations
• For patients with a history of reactivity to ambient light, hypersomnia, atypical negative symptoms and overeating of sweet food in the afternoon

Patients receiving antidepressants and light therapy should be counseled on the potential photosensitizing effect of some antidepressant medications and the need for sunscreens.[21]

Pharmacologic Therapy

The use of antidepressant medication is suggested when clinical features include a previous response to antidepressant medication, significant sleep and appetite disturbances, agitation, severe symptoms or the anticipated need for maintenance therapy. Clinical effectiveness of antidepressants is generally comparable between classes and within classes. For this reason the initial selection is usually based upon prior response, side effect profile, concomitant medical problems, potential drug interactions, cost and data from clinical trials.

• The use of a selective serotonin reuptake inhibitor (SSRI) is the drug of first choice in most patients due to ease of dosing and tolerability.
• Due to potential serious side effects and dietary restrictions, MAOIs should be restricted to patients who fail to respond to other treatments.
• MAOIs may be more effective in patients with major depressive disorder with atypical features.
• Titrating an antidepressant to full therapeutic doses is dependent on developing side effects, the patient's age and the presence of comorbid illnesses.
• Patients starting antidepressant therapy should be monitored for response to treatment, adverse effects and target symptoms (Table 5).
• In the elderly, starting and maintenance dosage of tricyclic antidepressants should generally be half that of the usual adult dosage.
• If no improvement in symptoms is observed following six to eight weeks of antidepressant therapy, consider an adjustment in the treatment regimen.

Table 5: **Monitoring Therapy for Depression**[22,23]

Monitoring parameter	Comment
Target symptoms	• Anxiety, insomnia, and decreased appetite usually begin to improve within the first week of treatment. • Increased energy and libido are often seen within 1 mo. • Depressive symptoms may take up to 8 wks to fully respond to antidepressant medication. Improvement is usually seen after 3-4 wks.
Antidepressant plasma concentration	• Allows one to assess compliance. • Allows one to determine if the patient is within therapeutic range. • Suggested plasma concentrations are available for some TCAs, bupropion and maprotiline.
Adverse effects of antidepressant therapy	• CNS (e.g., headaches, sedation, seizures, memory impairment). • Cardiovascular (e.g., hypertension, dizziness, tachycardia). For patients older than 40 an ECG is warranted prior to starting treatment with a TCA. • Gastrointestinal (e.g., nausea, vomiting, diarrhea, weight gain). • Anticholinergic effects (e.g., dry mouth, urinary retention, constipation). • Sexual dysfunction (e.g., decreased libido, impotence, ejaculatory disturbances). • Abrupt withdrawal (e.g., lethargy, nausea, headache, fever, sweating, confusion, irritability, crying, insomnia, vivid dreams, anxiety).
Emergence of suicidal ideation	• Patients are at greater risk for suicide within the first few weeks of antidepressant therapy when they begin to have more energy.
Psychometric rating scales	• Allows for rapid and reliable measurement of symptom severity.
Interviewing family member or friend	• Can provide valuable information regarding depressive symptoms as well as daily, social and occupational functioning. Permission from the patient should be obtained.

TCA = tricyclic antidepressant; CNS = central nervous system; ECG = electrocardiogram.

• Patients should be monitored weekly or twice weekly for six to eight weeks whenever a change in their treatment regimen has been made.

• The use of an SSRI or bupropion appears to be safer than tricyclic antidepressants in patients with a history of ventricular arrhythmia, subclinical sinus node dysfunction, conduction defects, prolonged QT intervals or a recent history of myocardial infarction.[24,25]

• Individuals with comorbid major depression and dementia should be prescribed an antidepressant with the lowest possible degree of anticholinergic property.

• Patients with obstructive uropathy (prostatism and other forms of bladder outlet obstruction) should be prescribed an antidepressant with a relatively low degree of antimuscarinic effects.

• Adolescents requiring antidepressant therapy should consult a pediatric psychiatrist.

Herbal Remedies (Table 6)

The last decade has seen a significant increase in the use of herbal medications for the management of chronic conditions including depression. In a recent survey the use of herbals medication in the general population increased from 3% in 1990 to about 12% in 1997.[29]

• Although considered safe and effective by most patients, the efficacy of herbal products has only recently started to be evaluated in controlled clinical trials.

• Very little information is available regarding the safety, side effects or potential drug interactions involving herbal products.

• Many patients do not recognize herbal products as drugs and may not inform their physician or pharmacist of their use.

• Use of herbal products should be queried when taking a history.

Table 6: **Herbal Remedies for Treatment of Depression**[26,27]

Common name (scientific name)	Adverse effects	Cautions/ contraindications	Drug interactions[28]	Dosage
St. John's wort (*Hypericum perforatum*)	• Photosensitivity • GI upset • Dizziness • Insomnia • Restlessness • Agitation	• Pregnancy and lactation	• Potential: ↑ MAOI effect (possible hypertensive crisis) ↑ SSRI effect (possible serotonin syndrome) ↓ cyclosporine effect (organ rejection) ↓ indinavir ↓ ethinyl estradiol and desogestrel ↓ digoxin levels	• 300-900 mg per day of standardized St. John's wort extract in divided doses

GI = gastrointestinal; MAOI = monoamine oxidase inhibitor; SSRI = selective serotonin reuptake inhibitor.

• St. John's wort, corydalis, ginkgo, lemon balm, marjoram, mug wort and scarlet pimpernel are herbals that have been used to treat depression.[26,27] Only St. John's wort has evidence supporting its effectiveness.

• St. John's wort appears to block the reuptake of serotonin, norepinephrine and dopamine.

• Studies show St. John's wort has similar efficacy and better tolerability compared to amitriptyline, imipramine and maprotiline for the treatment of mild to moderate depression.[30]

• St. John's wort is well tolerated, having no anticholinergic or sedative properties but several documented drug interactions (Table 6).

• St. John's wort may be appropriate for the individual who is unwilling to seek the attention of a physician.

• Data suggest potential efficacy of S-adenosyl-L-methionine (SAMe) for the treatment of depression.[31]

• Other natural products for which evidence of efficacy for depression is lacking are dehydroepiandrosterone (DHEA) and D-phenylalanine.

Monitoring of Therapy

Routine monitoring of patients with depression should be performed at regular intervals during antidepressant therapy. The frequency of monitoring is dependent on the severity of the target symptom(s). Initially, it may be necessary to monitor a patient's symptoms daily. Fifty to 65% of patients with depression will respond to therapy.[32] Once the acute symptoms have lessened, monitoring may be performed on a weekly or in some cases monthly basis. Table 5 lists examples of monitoring parameters to consider. Delayed onset of action of antidepressants together with symptoms of guilt, worthlessness, helplessness and hopelessness make patient education and support essential. Educate patients regarding their illness and their pharmacotherapy.

There is no clear consensus as to duration of therapy. Consider the duration and severity of the current episode as well as the number of previous episodes. Clinical guidelines recommend that patients experiencing their first episode be maintained on antidepressant therapy for at least six to nine months after remission of symptoms.[22,33] For patients with a history of multiple episodes, or inadequate treatment response, the guidelines are less clear. However, treatment with an antidepressant longer than one year after remission of symptoms is not unreasonable since these individuals are at a greater risk for a recurrence.

If the treating physician has decided to discontinue antidepressant therapy, the patient should be monitored closely and regularly for symptoms of relapse/recurrence. The patient should be assessed weekly or twice weekly for between four and six months. Patients who discontinue antidepressant therapy are at a greater risk of relapse/recurrence. Evidence suggests that, compared to patients who were maintained on antidepressants, those patients who were discontinued have a much higher relapse rate (6.24 vs. 1.85%

per month), a shorter time to 50% relapse (14.2 vs. 48.0 months), and a higher 12-month relapse risk (44.8 vs. 19.5%) (all p < 0.001).[32]

Suggested Readings

Abrams R. *Electroconvulsive Therapy*. New York: Oxford University Press; 1997.

Candro R, Edmonsdson J, Gabbard GO, Manley M, Pataki CS, Sadock VA, eds. *Kaplan and Sadock's Synopsis of Psychiatry: Behavioral Science/Clinical Psychiatry*. 8th ed. Baltimore, MD: Williams & Wilkins; 1998.

CANMAT Depression Work Group. Clinical guidelines for the treatment of depressive disorders. *Can J Psychiatry* 2001;46(suppl 1):1S-92S.

Fawcett J, Stein DJ, Jobson KO. *Textbook of Treatment Algorithms in Psychopharmacology*. West Sussex: John Wiley & Sons; 1999.

Kando JC, Wells BG, Hayes PE. Depressive disorders. In: DiPiro JT, Talbert RL, Yee GC, Matzke GR, Wells BG, Posey LM, eds. *Pharmacotherapy: A Pathophysiologic Approach*. 4th ed. Stanford, CT: Appleton & Lange;1999:1141-60.

Work Group on Major Depressive Disorder. Practice guideline for the treatment of patients with major depressive disorder (revision). *Am J Psychiatry* 2000;157(suppl 4):1-45.

References

1. *American Psychiatric Association Diagnostic and Statistical Manual of Mental Disorders*. 4th ed. Text Revision (DSM-IV-TR); Washington, DC: American Psychiatric Association; 2000.
2. Schildkraut JJ. The catecholamine hypothesis of affective disorders: a review of supporting evidence. *Am J Psychiatry* 1965;122:509-22.
3. Gastpar M, Gilsdorf U, Abou-Aleh Mt, Ngo-Khac T. Clinical correlates of response to CST: the dexamethasone suppression test in depression: a World Health Organization collaborative study. *J Affect Disord* 1992;26:17-24.
4. Shelton RC, Winn S, Ekhatore N, Loosen PT. The effects of antidepressants on the thyroid axis in depression. *Biol Psychiatry* 1993;33:120-6.
5. Kupfer DJ, Ehlers CL, Frank E, Grochocinski VJ, McEachran AB. EEG sleep profiles and recurrent depression. *Biol Psychiatry* 1991;30:641-55.
6. Krishnan KRR, McDonald WM, Escalona PR, et al. Magnetic resonance imaging of the caudate nuclei in depression. *Arch Gen Psychiatry* 1992;49:553-7.
7. Drevets WC, Videen TO, Price JL et al. A functional anatomical study of unipolar depression. *J Neurosci* 1993;12: 3628-41.
8. Candro R, Edmonsdson J, Gabbard GO, Manley M, Pataki CS, Sadock VA, eds. *Kaplan and Sadock's Synopsis of Psychiatry: Behavioral Science/Clinical Psychiatry*. 8th ed. Baltimore, MD: Williams & Wilkins; 1998.
9. Katon W, Schulberg H. Epidemiology of depression in primary care. *Gen Hosp Psychiatry* 1992;14:237-47.
10. Weissmann MM, Bland RC, Canino GJ. Cross-national epidemiology of major depression and biopolar disorder. *JAMA* 1996;276:293-9.
11. Kessler RC, McGonagle KA, Zhao S. Lifetime and 12-month prevalence of DSM-III-R psychiatric disorders in the United States: results of the national comorbidity survey. *Arch Gen Psychiatry* 1994;51:8-19.
12. Coryell W, Endicott J, Keller M. Major depression in a non-clinical sample: demographic and clinical risk factors for first onset. *Arch Gen Psychiatry* 1992;49:117-25.
13. Suokas J, Suominen K, Isometsa et al. Long-term risk factor for suicide mortality after attempted suicide—findings of a 14-year follow-up study. *Acta Psychiatr Scand* 2001;104: 117-21.
14. Qin P, Agerbo E, Westergard-Nielson N et al. Gender differences in risk factors for suicide in Denmark. *Br J Psychiatry* 2000;177:546-50.
15. Brown GK, Beck AT, Steer RA, et al. Risk factors for suicide in psychiatric outpatients: a 20-year prospective study. *Consult Clin Psychol* 2000;68:371-7.
16. Robinson LA, Berman JS, Neimeyer RA. Psychotherapy for the treatment of depression: a comprehensive review of controlled outcome research. *Psych Bull* 1990;100:30-49
17. Gloaguen V, Cottraux J, Cucherat M et al. A meta-analysis of the effects of cognitive therapy in depressed patients. *J Affect Disord* 1998;49:59-72.
18. Weissman MM, Markowitz JS. Interpersonal therapy: current status. *Arch Gen Psychiatry* 1994;51:599-606.
19. Miller IW, Norman WH, Keitner GI et al. Cognitive behavioral treatment of depressed inpatients. *Behav Ther* 1989;20: 25-47.
20. Scott AIF. Contemporary practice of electronconvulsive therapy. *Br Hosp Med* 1994;51:334-8.
21. Lam RW, Kripke DF, Gillin JC. Phototherapy for depressive disorders: a review. *Can J Psychiatry* 1989;34:140-7.
22. CANMAT Depression Work Group. Clinical guidelines for the treatment of depressive disorders. *Can J Psychiatry* 2001;46(suppl 1):1S-92S
23. Work Group on Major Depressive Disorder. Practice guideline for the treatment of patients with major depressive disorder (revision). *Am J Psychiatry* 2000;157(suppl 4):1-45.
24. Glassman AH, Rodriguez AI, Shapiro PA. The use of antidepressant drugs in patients with heart disease. *J Clin Psychiatry* 1998;29(suppl 10):16-21.
25. Roose SP, Glassman AH. Antidepressant choice in the patient with cardiac disease: lessons from the cardiac arrhythmia suppression trial (CAST) studies. *J Clin Psychiatry* 1999;55(9 suppl A): 83-87.
26. Jellin JM, Gregory P, Batz F, Hitchens, K et al. *Pharmacist's Letter/Prescriber's Letter. Natural Medicines. Comprehensive Database*. 3rd ed. Stockton, CA: Therapeutic Research Faculty; 2000.
27. Boon H, Smith M. *The Botanical Pharmacy*. Kingston, ON: Quarry Press; 1999.
28. Medical Economics Company. *PDR for Herbal Medicines*. 2nd ed. Montvale, NJ: 2000.
29. Eisenberg CM, Davis RB, Ettner SL et al. Trends in alternative medicine use in the United States, 1990-1997: results of a follow-up national survey. *JAMA* 1998;280:1569-75.

30. Whiskey E, Werneke U, Taylor D. A systematic review and meta-analysis of *Hypericum perforatum* in depression: a comprehensive clinical review. *Int Clin Psychopharmacol* 2001;16:239-52.

31. Fetrow CW, Avila JR. Efficacy of the dietary supplement of S-adenosyl-L-methionine. *Ann Pharmacother* 2001;35:1414-25.

32. Schulberg HC, Katon W, Simon GE et al. Treating major depression in primary care practice. *Arch Gen Psychiatry* 1998;55:1121-7.

33. Viguera AC, Baldessarini RJ, Friedberg J. Discontinuing antidepressant treatment in major depression. *Harv Rev Psychiatry* 1998;5(6):293-306.

Depression—Patient Information

To help you understand your depression better:

- Depression is caused by biochemical changes in the brain, often referred to as "chemical imbalance."
- Depression is not a sign of personal weakness; approximately 10% of people experience it.
- Do not blame yourself.
- Depression is highly treatable.
- Of people who seek help, three of four are treated successfully. Without treatment, you would likely get better spontaneously, but it could take months or years.
- Antidepressants must be taken for at least two to four weeks before you notice an improvement.
- For some, it can take up to six to eight weeks to feel better.
- Don't get discouraged if you don't feel better right away.
- Fifty to 65% of patients with depression respond to antidepressant therapy.
- Continue your medication even if you feel better. The depressive symptoms will likely return if the medication is discontinued too soon.
- Avoid alcohol. Many patients with major depression drink alcohol to either help themselves sleep or "calm their nerves." Although drinking a glass occasionally is not prohibited, it is important to remember that alcohol alters brain chemistry and disrupts sleep the same way a depressive episode does.
- Do not use illegal drugs, sedatives or stimulants.
- Do not make any major life changes. Any kind of problem when you are feeling bad may seem major and difficult to deal with. Problems will seem more manageable when you are feeling better.
- Get plenty of rest.

- Exercise regularly.
- Eat regularly.
- Keep socially active.
- Recovery is the rule, not the exception.
- Depression can last weeks, months or even years before getting better on its own. Antidepressants are used to shorten the length of time it takes to get over an episode.
- Whether the depression will return depends on the duration of the current episode, the number of previous episodes and whether you have a family history of depression.
- Early treatment reduces your chances of recurrent episodes.
- You will need to take your medication for four to five months after you get better if you are being treated for the first time, and up to 12 months or longer for repeat occurrences.
- Inform your physician and pharmacist about any over-the-counter medications, including herbal products, that you are taking, as they may interact.
- Do not stop taking your antidepressant without consulting your physician.
- Suddenly stopping your antidepressant will likely result in a withdrawal syndrome consisting of flu-like feelings of malaise and muscle aches, stomach or bowel upset, anxiety and irritability, mood dips, fatigue, headaches, and electric shock-like feelings throughout the body, especially in the arms and legs.
- Stopping your antidepressant should only be done under the supervision of your physician. The process requires a very gradual reduction in dosage over a period of time ranging from a few weeks to several months.

Chapter 8

Headache

Irene Worthington, BScPhm

Pathophysiology[1-6]

This chapter focuses on the most common primary headache disorders: tension-type headache, migraine and cluster headache. An extensive classification of headache disorders has been published by the International Headache Society.[1]

Tension-type Headache

Tension-type headache (TTH) is the most common type of headache. Although mental stress and tension are frequently thought to precipitate TTH, the exact pathophysiology is unknown.[2] Both peripheral (myofascial tissues) and central mechanisms contribute to pain in TTH. Some headache experts believe that TTH is a variant of migraine, since there are significant overlapping features; however, epidemiologic studies have concluded that migraine and TTH are different disorders, which coexist in many patients. The one-year prevalence of episodic TTH varies from 23 to 64%; for chronic TTH (> 15 days per month), it is 4 to 5%.

Migraine

The specific cause of migraine is unknown. Genetic factors may be involved. Migraine is a neurovascular disorder (dilation of meningeal blood vessels, CNS activation). It has been proposed that specific migraine triggers can provoke CNS dysfunction in susceptible individuals, leading to dilation of intracranial, extracerebral blood vessels and activation of the trigeminal sensory nerves (resulting in release of vasoactive peptides), with subsequent relaying of pain signals to the brain. Prevalence varies depending on age and sex: for females (peak: ages 35 to 45) about 17 to 20%; for males about 5 to 6%.

Cluster Headache

Cluster headache, a rare disorder, was previously thought to be a variant of migraine. However, it is currently classified as a distinct headache disorder. Prevalence is about 0.1%, predominantly in men. The exact pathophysiology is unknown. It has been suggested that an inflammatory process in the cavernous sinus and tributary veins results in cluster headache (nitroglycerin and other vasodilators can induce an attack of cluster headache). Activation of both the trigeminovascular and cranial parasympathetic systems appears to be involved in the pathogenesis of cluster headache.

Goals of Therapy[7,8]

- Identify potentially serious causes of headache and refer patient to physician/emergency room
- Refer patient to a physician for an accurate diagnosis of headache disorder (e.g., migraine, cluster headache, etc.)
- Relieve pain and any associated symptoms (e.g., nausea/vomiting), so that patient can return to normal functioning
- Prevent recurrence of headache
- Prevent complications of medication overuse

Patient Assessment[1,3,5-12] (Figure 1)

There are no diagnostic tests for primary headache disorders (e.g., tension-type headache, migraine, cluster headache). Diagnosis is based on symptoms, after ruling out any serious underlying disorders. The International Headache Society has established criteria for the diagnosis of various headache disorders.[1] Secondary headache disorders are those associated with organic causes (e.g., trauma, meningitis, space-

Figure 1: **Assessment and Management of Patients with Headache**[1,3,5-11]

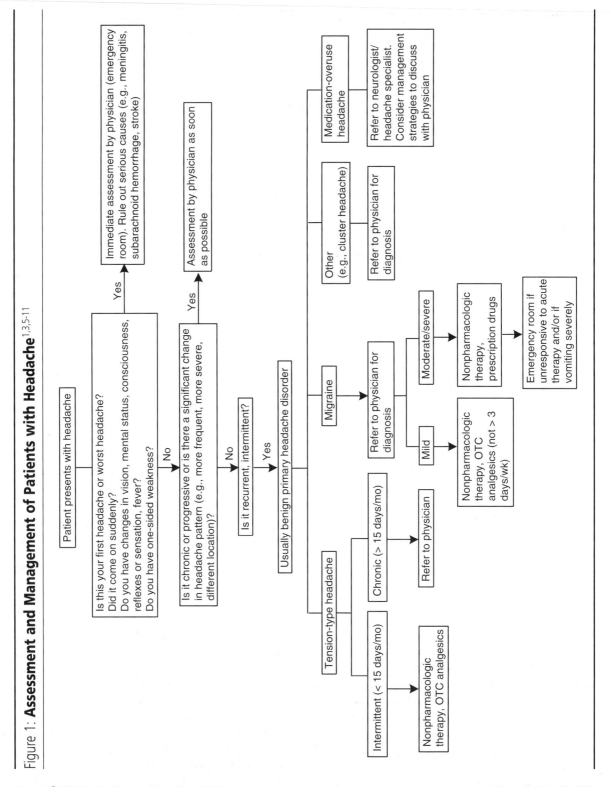

occupying lesion, etc.). Some medical procedures are associated with headache (e.g., lumbar puncture, rhinoscopy).

Patients with occasional tension-type headache do not need to see a physician unless the headaches become chronic (daily or almost daily). Patients with features of migraine should be assessed and diagnosed by a physician, to obtain appropriate treatment. Any unusual headache should be diagnosed by a physician; if the headache is very severe, with a sudden onset, immediate referral to an emergency room is necessary (see "Red Flags for Serious Headache"). A stepwise approach to headache assessment and treatment is provided in Figure 1.

Common Signs and Symptoms[4,7,13]
See Table 1 for clinical features of common headaches.

Differential Diagnosis[10-12]
- Other primary headache types: cluster headache, paroxysmal hemicrania, idiopathic stabbing headache, cold-stimulus headache, benign cough headache, benign exertional headache;
- Infectious: meningitis; encephalitis;
- Other: temporal arteritis (an important cause of headache in those over 50 years of age; associated with systemic symptoms and elevated erythrocyte sedimentation rate; if left untreated, often leads to permanent blindness); subdural hematoma; subarachnoid hemorrhage; cerebral ischemia (stroke); transient ischemic attack (TIA) after cerebral ischemia (stroke or TIA); systemic/CNS vasculitides (e.g., systemic lupus erythematosus); space-occupying lesions (e.g., brain tumor) and others
- Note: "sinus" headaches only occur in the presence of a sinus infection

Table 1: **Clinical Features of Tension-type Headache, Migraine and Cluster Headache**[3,5,9,10]

Variable	Tension-type headache	Migraine	Cluster headache[14]
Quality of headache	Pressing/tightening (nonpulsating)	Throbbing/pulsating (at least part of the time)	Penetrating
Severity	Mild to moderate	Usually moderate to severe, although can be mild	Excruciating
Location	Bilateral	Usually unilateral (can be bilateral, especially in children)	Always unilateral (supraorbital and/or temporal)
Frequency	Episodic (< 15 days/mo) or chronic (> 15 days /mo)	Episodic (variable)	Episodic headaches last 7 days to 1 yr, separated by pain-free periods lasting ≥ 14 days. Chronic: attacks occur for more than 1 yr or with headache-free intervals < 14 days.
Duration	30 min to 7 days	2-72 h	15-180 min
Aggravated by physical activity	No	Yes	No
Associated symptoms	No nausea/vomiting (anorexia may occur) *and* no photophobia and phonophobia (or one but not the other may occur)	Either nausea and/or vomiting *or* photophobia and phonophobia; may occur with or without aura (usually visual)	At least one of (on same side as headache): lacrimation, conjunctival injection, nasal congestion, rhinorrhea, miosis, ptosis, forehead/facial sweating, eyelid edema (mild or no photo/phonophobia, no vomiting)

Red Flags for Serious Headache[8,10,11]

- Severe/abrupt onset ("worst headache ever")
- Onset in middle age or older (> 40 years)
- Neurologic signs: stiff neck, focal signs, reduced consciousness
- Systemic signs: appears ill, fever, nausea/vomiting (not explained by migraine or systemic illness)
- Significant change in pattern of headaches: increased frequency and/or progressive severity
- Nocturnal occurrence or on awakening in morning; If patient consistently has headache on awakening or is awakened by a headache, there is a possibility of a brain tumor. However, migraines sometimes occur on awakening
- Onset with exercise or intercourse (may be benign or serious)

Drug-induced Headache[11,15]

Table 2 lists drugs that commonly cause headache as a side effect.

Medication-overuse Headache (Analgesic Rebound Headache/Medication Misuse Headache)[17-21]

Medication-overuse headache (MOH), formerly called "medication-induced headache," is an under-recognized condition that may occur in migraine sufferers; recognition and treatment of MOH may lead to long-term improvement in headache relief and quality of life for many patients. Frequent use (three or more days per week for several months) of analgesics can lead to MOH or chronic daily headaches in migraine sufferers. There is an association with use of acetaminophen, ASA or NSAIDs alone (much less likely to occur with NSAIDs) but MOH is more commonly associated with combination products containing barbiturates, caffeine and/or opioids. Frequent use of ergotamine (two or more days per week) or less commonly, "triptan" medications (sumatriptan, naratriptan, rizatriptan, zolmitriptan) can also result in MOH.[7,21,24] The headaches resemble tension-type headaches (migraine headaches can also be superimposed).

Treatment of MOH involves completely discontinuing the implicated drug(s), relieving withdrawal symptoms, treating recurrent headaches with migraine-specific medications (adhering to limitations in frequency of use), and possibly initiating prophylactic therapy (e.g., tricyclic antidepressants, divalproex sodium). (Note: patients taking high doses of barbiturate-containing analgesics should not abruptly discontinue them, since seizures may occur on withdrawal).

Table 2: **Drugs Associated with Headache/Migraine***[11,15-18]

Drugs causing intracranial hypertension	Drugs causing headache as a side effect
Antibiotics: Tetracycline, minocycline, trimethoprim-sulfamethoxazole, nalidixic acid	**NSAIDs:** indomethacin (also used to treat certain types of headache), diclofenac
Corticosteroids	**Nitrates:** e.g., nitroglycerin
Other: Isotretinoin Tamoxifen Cimetidine	**Beta-blockers:** e.g., atenolol, propranolol (also used for migraine prophylaxis)
	ACEIs: e.g., captopril
	Calcium channel blockers: nifedipine
	Other antihypertensives: methyldopa, reserpine, hydralazine
	H₂ antagonists: e.g., cimetidine, ranitidine
	SSRIs: e.g., fluoxetine, paroxetine, sertraline, fluvoxamine, citalopram
	Oral contraceptives and HRT (in some patients predisposed to migraine)
	Other: Caffeine (especially caffeine withdrawal) Latanoprost ophthalmic drops Cyclosporine Metronidazole Danazol

Most common drug-related causes of headache (not all inclusive).
NSAIDs = nonsteroidal antiinflammatory drugs; ACEIs = angiotensin converting enzyme inhibitors; SSRIs = selective serotonin reuptake inhibitors; HRT = hormone replacement therapy.

Ideally, patients should be referred to neurologists/ headache specialists. Community pharmacists are ideally positioned to monitor patients' use of both prescription and OTC medications, to counsel migraine patients on appropriate use of antimigraine medications and the dangers of medication overuse, to encourage patients to seek help and to provide support to patients withdrawing from medications.

Prevention[16]

Migraine attacks and other headaches are often triggered by one or more factors (Table 3).

Identification and avoidance of trigger factors in individuals are important in migraine prevention. Lifestyle changes such as maintaining regular sleeping and eating schedules, reducing stress and limiting caffeine intake (sudden decrease in consumption may lead to caffeine withdrawal headache; caffeine may help alleviate headache in some migraine sufferers) may reduce the frequency of headaches, particularly migraine. Drugs implicated in triggering headache or migraine (Table 2) should be discontinued on a trial basis if feasible.

Triggers vary among individual patients. It is not necessary for patients to avoid all potential triggers. Migraine headaches may be precipitated in some individuals by ingestion of foods containing nitrites, monosodium glutamate or aspartame, or foods con-

taining a high content of neurotransmitter precursors (e.g., tyramine, tyrosine, phenylalanine). Maintaining a diary of food ingested for 24 hours before a migraine attack may help identify food triggers.

Nonpharmacologic therapies such as relaxation therapy, biofeedback and cognitive-behavioral therapy may also be helpful in preventing migraine headaches in some individuals. (For drugs used in the prevention of migraine, see "Pharmacologic Therapy".)

Nonpharmacologic Therapy[8,16,25]

Patient education is very important in the management of headache. Provide patients with an explanation of their headache disorder. Reassure them (once the diagnosis has been confirmed by a physician in some cases) that they do not have a serious underlying cause for headaches (e.g., brain tumor). Use printed materials to reinforce verbal information. Establish realistic goals and expectations of treatment; explain benefits and limitations of various treatment options to the patient in collaboration with the patient's physician. Patients may also benefit from referral to self-help groups.

During a migraine attack, simple measures such as resting in a dark, quiet room and applying a cold cloth/ice pack to the head are helpful, although not evidence-based. Sleep often alleviates migraine

Table 3: **Migraine Triggers***[13,27]

Type of trigger	Examples
Foods and beverages that contain nitrites, MSG, aspartame or neurotransmitter precursors (e.g., tyramine, tyrosine, phenylalanine)	Aged cheeses, cured meats (e.g., hot dogs, bacon), chocolate, alcoholic beverages (especially red wine), caffeine-containing beverages, delayed meals.
Environmental	Weather changes (barometric pressure changes), bright/flickering lights, loud noise, strong odors (e.g., perfume), cigarette smoke, travel across time zones.
Chemical	Benzene, insecticides.
Hormonal	Menstruation, pregnancy (especially in first trimester), perimenopause.
Drugs	See Table 2.
Other	Sleep–wake cycle alterations, stress/anxiety (or let-down from stress), intense activity/physical exertion, sexual activity.

*Most common triggers are listed (not an exhaustive list).

headaches. There is evidence that some biobehavioral measures such as biofeedback, relaxation therapy and cognitive-behavioral therapy may help prevent migraine in some individuals. Controversial measures include chiropractic and other physical therapies, acupuncture, transcutaneous electrical stimulation, hypnosis, occipital or supraorbital nerve blockade, and homeopathic remedies.[16]

Pharmacologic Therapy

Acute/Symptomatic

Mild *tension-type* headache may not require treatment. Simple analgesics (e.g., ASA, acetaminophen) or NSAIDs (e.g., ibuprofen) will often alleviate tension-type headaches.[8]

Mild to moderate *migraine* attacks may also respond to simple analgesics or NSAIDs administered in adequate doses (Table 4). However, many migraine sufferers rely on OTC medications to the exclusion of prescription medications and do not achieve adequate pain relief.[25-29] Moderate to severe attacks of migraine often require the use of prescription medications. Overuse of analgesics by migraine sufferers (three or more days per week for several months), particularly combination products containing caffeine ± codeine ± barbiturates (e.g., butalbital), may lead to medication overuse or chronic headaches (see Medication-overuse Headache).[7]

Adjunctive drugs for the management of nausea/vomiting associated with migraine include dimenhydrinate

Table 4: **Nonprescription Analgesics for Acute Therapy of Tension-type and Migraine Headaches**[*7-9,30-33]

Drug	Adult/Pediatric dose	Selected adverse drug reactions (ADRs)/Drug interactions (DIs)	Use in pregnancy	Comments
Acetaminophen	Adult: 650-1300 mg q4h × 2 doses PRN. Pediatric: 10-20 mg/kg/dose q4h × 2 doses PRN.	ADR: potential liver (and rarely kidney) dysfunction with chronic use of high doses or with acute overdose DI: warfarin (occasional doses of acetaminophen can be used; limit intake to ≤ 2 g per day for no more than a few days)	Relatively safe—all trimesters; considered to be analgesic of first choice during pregnancy.	May be used alone or in combination with caffeine/codeine. Effective in childhood migraine. In adults, it is considered to be less effective than ASA or NSAIDs.[6] 1 g dose shown to be effective for migraine although patients with severe migraine were excluded.[31]
ASA	Adult: 650-1300 mg q4h × 2 doses PRN. Pediatric (age ≥ 12): 500-650 mg q4h × 2 doses PRN.	ADR: GI upset/ulceration/bleed DI: warfarin (↑ bleeding risk)	Relatively safe in intermittent doses during first and second trimesters; avoid use in third trimester (may be associated with prolonged gestation and labour, premature narrowing of ductus arteriosus, persistent pulmonary hypertension of the newborn).	Should not be used in children under 18 yrs of age in presence of viral illness or fever (possibility of Reye's syndrome). May be used alone or in combination with caffeine/codeine. Avoid enteric-coated preparations as this delays onset.
Ibuprofen	Adult: 400-800 mg q6h × 2 doses PRN. Pediatric: 5-10 mg/kg/dose q6h x 2 doses PRN	ADR: GI upset/ulceration/bleed DI: warfarin (↑ bleeding risk)	See ASA above	

Use of analgesics should be limited to not more than 3 days/week to avoid medication-overuse headache

and prescription drugs domperidone, metoclopramide and prochlorperazine.[5]

There are many prescription medications available for the treatment of acute migraine attacks.[7] The triptans (sumatriptan, naratriptan, zolmitriptan, rizatriptan) are considered to be the most efficacious agents for acute migraine treatment.[34] They alleviate not only headache pain but also associated migraine symptoms (nausea/vomiting, photophobia/phonophobia). The triptans are available in various delivery systems: subcutaneous injection (sumatriptan), oral tablets (all), orally disintegrating tablets (rizatriptan, zolmitriptan) and intranasal (sumatriptan). Dihydroergotamine (DHE) in nasal or injection form is also useful for migraine.[35] Evidence suggests that ergot preparations (e.g., ergotamine tartrate) have limited efficacy and excessive side effects. In contrast, DHE has proven efficacy. Various parenteral agents are used for treatment of severe migraine in the emergency room; for example, DHE with an antiemetic, chlorpromazine, prochlorperazine, ketorolac, metoclopramide,

meperidine or other opioids (not considered first-line therapy), dexamethasone.[7]

The treatment of acute attacks of *cluster headache* requires the use of oxygen or prescription medications that have a rapid onset of action (e.g., subcutaneous sumatriptan or DHE, oral zolmitriptan). OTC medications are not effective for cluster headache.[5]

Prophylactic/Preventive (Table 5)
Consider preventive therapy for migraine in the following circumstances:[7,42]
- More than two to three attacks/month, especially inadequate response to acute therapies;
- Severe attacks (any number) that significantly impair normal activity;
- Patient psychologically unable to cope with attacks;
- Optimal acute therapies have failed, are contraindicated or have produced serious side effects.

The goal of *migraine* prophylactic therapy is to reduce the frequency and severity of migraine attacks. In general, only one preventive agent is used at a time

---

Table 5: **Nonprescription Medications for Prophylaxis of Migraine Headaches**[7-9,30-32,36-42]

Drug	Adult/pediatric dose	Selected adverse drug reactions (ADRs)/drug interactions (DIs)	Use in pregnancy	Comments
Feverfew	Adults: 1-2 tablets of standardized feverfew dried leaf powder 125 mg per day, containing at least 0.2% parthenolide (e.g., Tanacet®). Pediatric: no data in children < 2 yrs	ADR: mouth ulceration, GI symptoms, contact dermatitis, "post-feverfew syndrome" following abrupt discontinuation in long-term users (e.g., headache, anxiety, insomnia, muscle and joint stiffness) DI: none documented—potential interaction with anticoagulants, antiplatelet drugs, thrombolytics (due to feverfew's inhibitory effect on prostaglandin synthesis)	No reported teratogenic effects; should be avoided—may stimulate uterine contractions and cause abortion.	Avoid use if previous contact dermatitis from plants in the Asteraceae family, including aster, chamomile, ragweed, chrysanthemum, sunflower, tansy, yarrow.
Magnesium	Adult: 600 mg/day (elemental magnesium) Pediatric: no recommendations	ADR: diarrhea, GI upset DI: None significant	Not considered to be teratogenic	Some magnesium salts are poorly absorbed; suggest citrate salt.
Riboflavin	Adult: 400 mg/day Pediatric: no recommendations	ADR: yellow discoloration of urine (benign) DI: None significant	Not considered to be teratogenic	

(in resistant cases, neurologists sometimes prescribe combinations). Medications should be started at a low dose and titrated upward to a maximally effective and tolerable dose. A trial period of two to three months is needed to assess the efficacy of most prophylactic drugs. Preventive medications may be continued for several months (sometimes years) and then withdrawn gradually to prevent rebound headaches. The choice of a prophylactic agent should take into consideration any medical conditions of the patient and contraindications (e.g., beta-blockers are contraindicated in patients with asthma). Patients should keep a diary to monitor their response to therapy.[7]

Patients should avoid overuse of acute medications as this may interfere with effectiveness of preventive migraine therapy.

Feverfew (*Tanacetum parthenium*) is a popular herbal remedy, which has been advocated for use in migraine prevention. The active constituent of feverfew is not presently known (parthenolide has been suggested as the active component). A systematic review looked at the evidence for the clinical effectiveness of feverfew using data from five randomized, double-blind, placebo-controlled trials. Several methodologic problems, such as small sample size, were identified in the trials. Although feverfew was favored over placebo in the majority of trials, it was concluded that the clinical effectiveness of feverfew in the prevention of migraine has not been established beyond a reasonable doubt.[36] Adverse effects associated with feverfew are generally mild and reversible. Mouth ulceration and GI symptoms have been reported most frequently. There are also anecdotal reports of contact dermatitis. A "post-feverfew syndrome" (rebound of migraine symptoms, anxiety, insomnia, muscle and joint stiffness) has been reported by long-time consumers following abrupt discontinuation.[36,37] Feverfew should not be taken by pregnant women as it may stimulate uterine contractions and cause abortion.[36,37]

Riboflavin (vitamin B$_2$) was investigated for migraine prophylaxis in one randomized, double-blind, placebo-controlled trial in 55 migraine patients. Riboflavin was administered in a dose of 400 mg per day for three months. The proportion of patients who had at least a 50% reduction in frequency of attacks was 50% for the riboflavin group versus 15% for the placebo group.

The exact mechanism of action is not known but may be related to its effects on mitochondrial energy metabolism (mitochondrial dysfunction, resulting in impaired oxygen metabolism, may play a role in migraine pathogenesis). Only minor adverse effects were reported in the riboflavin group (one case of diarrhea and one case of polyuria). Riboflavin can also cause a yellow discoloration of the urine (not significant).[38]

Magnesium deficiency has been suspected to play a role in the pathogenesis of migraine in up to 50% of patients. Intravenous infusion of magnesium sulfate relieves acute attacks of migraine in over 50% of patients.[39] Prophylactic oral magnesium supplementation has been shown to be effective in two double-blind studies, but ineffective in another in which lack of response may have been due to poor absorption of magnesium from the preparation used.[39-41] In one of the studies demonstrating the efficacy of magnesium, patients received 600 mg (24 mmol) of magnesium daily in the form of trimagnesium dicitrate (not available in Canada; an alternative may be magnesium citrate).[40] More definitive, large-scale studies are needed to assess the role of magnesium in migraine prophylaxis.

Various prescription medications are used for migraine prophylaxis.[7] These include beta-blockers (without intrinsic sympathomimetic activity), tricyclic antidepressants, calcium channel blockers (e.g., flunarizine, verapamil), serotonin (5-HT$_2$) receptor antagonists (e.g., pizotifen, methysergide), valproic acid/divalproex sodium, NSAIDs (used for one week per month for menstrual migraine prophylaxis), estrogen gel/transdermal patches (for menstrual migraine). Clinical trials are ongoing with several other promising agents such as topiramate, gabapentin and botulinum toxin.

For *cluster* headache, prophylactic medications (verapamil, lithium carbonate, methysergide or valproic acid) are started at the onset of the cluster period, in conjunction with corticosteroids (e.g., prednisone 60 to 80 mg per day for 2 to 3 days, followed by 10 mg decrements every 2 to 3 days) or ergotamine derivatives (daily for 2 to 3 weeks, not used within 24 hours of a triptan). Preventive medications are continued for the duration of the cluster period.

Monitoring of Therapy

Acute Therapy

Ideally medications should relieve headaches (no pain or mild pain), as well as associated nausea/vomiting and photophobia/phonophobia, within about two hours. Patients should report any adverse effects to their physician (see Table 4 for side effects and drug interactions of OTC medications).

Prophylactic Therapy

Migraine prophylactic medications should be tried for at least two months to determine efficacy. A "good" response is considered to be a 50% reduction in the frequency of migraine attacks. Patients should record attacks in a migraine diary.[4] Patients should report any adverse effects to their physician (see Table 5 for side effects associated with OTC prophylactic medications).

Resource Tips

Canadian: www.migraine.ca (under construction at print date)
www.fqmc.qc.ca/ (Quebec Migraine and Headache Foundation—French; English version under construction)

US: www.achenet.org (American Council for Headache Education)
www.ama-assn.org/special/migraine/migraine.htm (*JAMA*'s Migraine Information site)

International: www.w-h-a.org/wha/index.asp (World Headache Alliance)

Suggested Readings

Edmeads JG, Gawel MJ, Vickers J. Strategies for diagnosing and managing medication-induced headache. *Can Fam Physician* 1997;43:1249-54.

Gawel MJ, Worthington I, Maggisano A. A systematic review of the use of triptans in acute migraine. *Can J Neurol Sci* 2001;28:30-41.

Goadsby PJ, Lipton RB, Ferrari MD. Migraine – current understanding and treatment. *N Engl J Med* 2002; 346:257-70.

Pryse-Phillips WEM, Dodick DW, Edmeads JG, Gawel MJ, Nelson RF, Purdy RA, et al. Guidelines for the nonpharmacologic management of migraine in clinical practice. *CMAJ* 1998;159:47-54.

Pryse-Phillips WEM, Dodick DW, Edmeads JG, Gawel MJ, Nelson RF, Purdy RA, et al. Guidelines for the diagnosis and management of migraine in clinical practice. *CMAJ* 1997;156:1273-87.

Worthington I. Delivery systems for acute migraine medications. *Can Fam Physician* 2001;47:322-9.

Worthington I. Pediatric migraine. *Pharmacy Practice* 1999;15(3):48-57.

Zed PJ, Loewen PS, Robinson G. Medication-induced headache: overview and systematic review of therapeutic approaches. *Ann Pharmacother* 1999;33:61-72.

References

1. Headache Classification Committee, International Headache Society. Classification and diagnostic criteria for headache disorders, cranial neuralgias and facial pain. *Cephalalgia* 1998;8(suppl 7):1-96.
2. Jensen R, Olesen J. Tension-type headache: an update on mechanisms and treatment. *Curr Opin Neurol* 2000;13:285-9.
3. Saper JR. Headache disorders. *Med Clin North Am* 1999;83: 663-90.
4. Hargreaves RJ, Shepheard SL. Pathophysiology of migraine —new insights. *Can J Neurol Sci* 1999;26 Suppl 3:S12-S19.
5. Dodick DW, Campbell JK. Cluster headache: diagnosis, management, and treatment. In: Silberstein SD, Lipton, RB, Dalessio DJ, eds. *Wolff's Headache and Other Head Pain.* 7th ed. New York: Oxford University Press, 2001:283-309.
6. Lipton RB, Hamelsky SW, Stewart WF. Epidemiology and impact of headache. In: Silberstein SD, Lipton RB, Dalessio DJ, eds. *Wolff's headache and other head pain.* 7th ed. New York: Oxford University Press, 2001:85-107.
7. Pryse-Phillips WEM, Dodick DW, Edmeads JG, Gawel MJ, Nelson RF, Purdy RA, et al. Guidelines for the diagnosis and management of migraine in clinical practice. *CMAJ* 1997;156: 1273-87.
8. Purdy RA. Headache in adults. In: Gray J, ed. *Therapeutic Choices.* 3rd ed. Ottawa: Canadian Pharmacists Association; 2000:80-91.
9. Worthington I. Pediatric migraine. *Pharm Prac* 1999;15(3): 48-57.
10. Dodick D. Headache as a symptom of ominous disease. What are the warning signals? *Postgrad Med* 1997;101(5): 46-64.
11. Clinch CR. Evaluation of acute headaches in adults. *Am Fam Physician* 2001;63:685-92.
12. Campbell JK, Sakai F. Diagnosis and differential diagnosis. In: Olesen J, Tfelt-Hansen P, Welch KMA, eds. *The Headaches.* 2nd ed. Philadelphia: Lippincott, William & Wilkins; 2000:359-63.
13. Worthington I. Migraine therapy update (CE lesson). *Pharm Prac* 1995;Apr: 1-8.
14. Dodick DW, Rozen TD, Goadsby PJ, Silberstein SD. Cluster headache. *Cephalalgia* 2000;20:787-803.
15. Silberstein SD. Drug-induced headache. *Neurol Clin North Am* 1998;16:107-23.
16. Pryse-Phillips WEM, Dodick DW, Edmeads JG, Gawel MJ, Nelson RF, Purdy RA, et al. Guidelines for the nonpharma-

cologic management of migraine in clinical practice. *CMAJ* 1998;159:47-54.

17. Askmark H, Lundberg PO, Olsson S. Drug-related headache. *Headache* 1989;29:441-4.

18. Weston BC. Migraine headache asociated with latanoprost. *Arch Ophthalmol* 2001;119:300-1.

19. Edmeads JG, Gawel MJ, Vickers J. Strategies for diagnosing and managing medication-induced headache. *Can Fam Physician* 1997;43:1249-54.

20. Zed PJ, Loewen S, Robinson G. Medication-induced headache: overview and systematic review of therapeutic approaches. *Ann Pharmacother* 1999;33:61-72.

21. Turner CJ, Pryse-Phillips W. Pilot study to improve health outcomes for medication-induced headache sufferers. *Can J Clin Pharmacol* 1999;6:113-7.

22. Katsarava Z, Diener H-C, Limmroth V. Medication overuse headache. *Drug Safety* 2001;24:921-7.

23. Bahra A, Walsh M, Menon S et al. Does chronic daily headache arise de novo in association with regular analgesic use? *Cephalalgia* 2000;20:294.

24. Diener H-C, Dahlof CGH. Headache associated with chronic use of substances. In: Olesen J, Tfelt-Hansen P, Welch KMA, eds. *The Headaches*. 2nd ed. Philadelphia: Lippincott, Williams & Wilkins; 2000:871-8.

25. Rapoport AM. Emerging nonspecific migraine therapies: targets and unmet needs. *Headache* 1999;39 (suppl 2):S27-S34.

26. Sheftell FD. Role and impact of over-the-counter medications in the management of headache. *Neurol Clin* 1997; 15(1):187-98.

27. Lipton RB, Stewart WF, Goadsby PJ. Headache-related disability in the management of migraine. *Neurology* 2001;56 (suppl 1): S1-S3.

28. Edmeads J, Findlay H, Tugwell P, Pryse-Phillips W, Nelson RF, Murray TJ. Impact of migraine and tension-type headache on life-style, consulting behaviour, and medication use: a Canadian population survey. *Can J Neurol Sci* 1993; 20:131-7.

29. Lipton RB, Stewart WF. Acute migraine therapy: Do doctors understand what patients with migraine want from therapy? *Headache* 1999;39 (suppl 2):S20-S266.

30. Whiting S. Headache in children. In: Gray J, ed. *Therapeutic Choices*. 3rd ed. Ottawa: Canadian Pharmacists Association; 2000:92-100.

31. Briggs GG, Freeman RK, Yaffe SJ. *Drugs in Pregnancy and Lactation*. 5th ed. Baltimore: Williams & Wilkins; 1998.

32. Pfaffenrath V, Rehm M. Migraine in pregnancy. What are the safest treatment options? *Drug Safety* 1998;19:383-8.

33. Lipton RB, Baggish JS, Stewart WF, Codispoti JR, Fu M. Efficacy and safety of acetaminophen in the treatment of migraine. Results of a randomized, double-blind, placebo-controlled, population-based study. *Arch Intern Med* 2000; 160:3486-92.

34. Gawel MJ, Worthington I, Maggisano A. A systematic review of the use of triptans in acute migraine. *Can J Neurol Sci* 2001;28:30-41.

35. Worthington I. Delivery systems for acute migraine medications. *Can Fam Physician* 2001;47:322-9.

36. Vogler BK, Pittler MH, Ernst E. Feverfew as a preventive treatment for migraine: a systematic review. *Cephalalgia* 1998;18:704-8.

37. Chavez ML, Chavez PI. Feverfew. *Hosp Pharm* 1999;34: 436-61.

38. Schoenen J, Jacquy J, Lenaerts M. Effectiveness of high-dose riboflavin in migraine prophylaxis. A randomized controlled trial. *Neurology* 1998;50:466-70.

39. Mauskop A, Altura BM. Magnesium for migraine. Rationale for use and therapeutic potential. *CNS Drugs* 1998; 9:185-90.

40. Peikert A, Wilimzig C, Kohne-Volland R. Prophylaxis of migraine with oral magnesium: results from a prospective, multi-centre, placebo-controlled and double-blind randomized study. *Cephalalgia* 1996;16:257-63.

41. Pfaffenrath V, Wessely P, Meyer C, Isler HR, Evers S, Grotemeyer KH, et al. Magnesium in the prophylaxis of migraine—a double-blind, placebo-controlled study. *Cephalalgia* 1996;16:436-40.

42. Tflet-Hansen P, Welch KMA. General principles of pharmacological treatment of migraine. In: Olesen J, Tfelt-Hansen P, Welch KMA, eds. *The Headaches*. 2nd ed. Philadelphia: Lippincott, Williams & Wilkins; 2000:385-9.

Headache—Patient Information

Headaches are very common. They may occur during viral illness such as colds or influenza (flu).

Tension-type Headaches

- The most common type of headache is called "tension-type headache" (although it is not caused only by tension). The pain is usually mild to moderate, on both sides of the head or across the forehead, and there is a feeling of tightness or pressure in the head and sometimes, in the shoulders and back of the neck. The pain usually goes away on its own, or an over-the-counter pain reliever such as ASA, acetaminophen or ibuprofen can be taken. If these headaches occur on more than 15 days per month, see your doctor.

Migraine Headaches

- Migraine headaches are also fairly common (more common in women than in men) and tend to run in families. They usually occur on one side of the head (sometimes both, especially in children) and the pain is usually moderate to severe and throbbing. Physical activity tends to worsen the pain. Other symptoms are present — they may include nausea and/or vomiting or sensitivity to light and sound. An aura, usually visual (for example, flashes/bursts of light, zig-zag lines, dark spots surrounded by light), sometimes occurs just before the headache.
- Many things can trigger migraine attacks. These vary among individuals and may include:
—Food (such as aged cheeses, cured meats, chocolate, red wine)
—Hormones (in women — menstruation, menopause)
—Chemicals (such as MSG in foods)
—Environment (changes in weather, bright lights, loud noises, strong odors, cigarette smoke)
—Other factors (such as anxiety/stress, too much or too little sleep, not eating regularly)
—Too much caffeine (coffee, cola drinks, etc.), or especially if suddenly reducing the amount of caffeine (withdrawal); it is helpful to keep a diary to figure out possible triggers
- For treating a migraine attack, nondrug therapy such as lying down in a dark, quiet room and applying a cold cloth/ice pack to the head may be helpful. Sleep will also help. Other therapies such as biofeedback, relaxation and cognitive-behavioral therapy may help prevent migraine headaches in some people.
- For milder migraine attacks, over-the-counter pain relievers may be used (ASA, acetaminophen or ibuprofen).
- It is important not to use pain relievers on more than three days per week, to avoid rebound headaches and chronic daily headaches (also called "medication-overuse headache").
- See a physician if headaches occur daily or almost daily (these tend to be more like tension-type headaches). The pain relievers will need to be stopped, which may make the headaches worse for a while (the doctor will usually prescribe a medication to treat severe headaches).
- For more severe migraine attacks, prescription medications are usually needed. Drugs for nausea may also be used — they include dimenhydrinate (over-the-counter), metoclopramide (prescription) or domperidone (prescription). If the migraine isn't relieved by medication that can be taken at home or severe vomiting occurs, go to the emergency room.
- If migraine attacks occur frequently or are very severe or long lasting, preventive drugs, taken daily, may be prescribed by a physician.
- Some over-the-counter preventive therapies that may be helpful for some people include the herb feverfew (dose of 125 to 250 mg per day), vitamin B_2 (in a dose of 400 mg per day) and magnesium (usually in citrate form, in a dose of 600 mg per day of elemental magnesium). Talk to a physican before taking any preventive medications.

Other Headaches

There are many other less common types of headache. See a physician to diagnose these headaches. Many people who think they have "sinus" headaches are actually suffering from migraine or another type of headache. Sinus headaches only occur if a sinus infection is present.

Severe, New or Unusual Headaches

Fortunately, most headaches are not due to serious causes such as brain tumors (usually other symptoms are also present). Some types of headaches may be cause for concern. If you have a very severe headache that comes on suddenly (first or "worst" headache ever experienced), go to the emergency room right away. Also go to the emergency room if you have symptoms such as fever, stiff neck, drowsiness, confusion, seizures or general feeling of weakness, as well as headache. If you experience a new or unusual type of headache, or if there is a change in your usual headache pattern (e.g., they become more frequent or severe), see your physician as soon as possible.

An updated book on migraine, in easy-to-understand terms, can be obtained from your local bookstore: *Migraine*, by Valerie South, RN, 2001.

Chapter 9

Fever

Yvonne Shevchuk, BSP, PharmD, FCSHP

Fever, which is an elevated core body temperature, is generally considered to be caused by infection; however, noninfectious causes include inflammatory diseases, neoplasms and immunologically mediated conditions such as some drug fevers. The definition of fever varies; anything above the normal range for body temperature can be defined as fever.[1-6] In adults, an individual's body temperature varies with the time of day (normal circadian variation); it is lowest at approximately 6 am and highest between 4 and 6 pm. Fever in children is most often defined as rectal temperature > 38.0°C if the child is appropriately dressed and resting. The mean amplitude of variability is 0.5°C. Oral temperatures above 37.2°C in early morning or ≥ 37.8°C any time during the day defines fever. Outside the neonatal period, children generally have a higher temperature than adults; however, this is poorly documented.[2,7,8] Basal core temperatures decrease toward the adult range by one year of age and continue to decline until puberty. There is a direct correlation between height of fever and rate of serious bacterial infection in children. With temperatures above 40°C, there is increased likelihood of serious bacterial infection.[3]

Mild elevations in body temperature occur with exercise, ovulation, pregnancy, excessive clothing (overbundling of infants), ingestion of hot foods or liquids, and chewing gum or tobacco.

Rectal temperatures are approximately 0.6°C higher and axillary temperatures approximately 0.5 to 1.0°C lower than oral temperatures. A high fever is usually defined as a temperature greater than 40.5°C. Neurologic damage does not occur below a body temperature of 41.7°C.

Pathophysiology[1,3,4,6]

The thermoregulatory centre in the anterior hypothalamus normally controls core temperature within a narrow range by balancing heat production by muscle and liver tissues with heat dissipation from skin and lungs. With fever, the thermoregulatory set point is elevated. Endothelial cells of the organum vasculosum laminae terminalis, a network of enlarged capillaries surrounding the hypothalamus, release arachidonic acid metabolites when exposed to pyrogens in the circulation. Prostaglandin E_2, released by the hypothalamus, is thought to be the major substance producing an elevation of the thermoregulatory set point. Initially, with an elevated set point, there is vasoconstriction of peripheral blood vessels to conserve heat, shivering to increase heat production, and behavioral changes such as seeking warmer environments and clothing. When the set point is reduced, for example, by administering antipyretics or disappearance of pyrogens, there is vasodilation and sweating as well as behavioral changes such as removal of clothing.

There are both exogenous and endogenous sources of pyrogens — substances that cause fever. The most common exogenous sources are microorganisms, their products or toxins (e.g., lipopolysaccharide endotoxin of gram-negative bacteria). Exogenous pyrogens induce formation and release of endogenous pyrogens. Endogenous pyrogens or pyrogenic cytokines are polypeptides produced by host cell macrophages, monocytes and other cells. The most common are interleukin 1β, interleukin 1α and tumor necrosis factor.

Goals of Therapy[3,4]

- Provide patient comfort
- Reduce parental anxiety
- Reduce metabolic demand caused by fever in patients with cardiovascular or pulmonary disease
- Prevent or alleviate fever-associated mental dysfunction in the elderly (common practice but evidence is unclear)

Patient Assessment[1,6,7] (Figure 1)

Fever is a symptom or sign of illness, not a disease, and the reason for fever should be determined. Most commonly it is due to infection, often viral. Fever persisting longer than three days, recurrent fever or high fever (40.5°C) should be evaluated by a physician.

Once fever is established, the body initiates processes to permit homeostasis. Peripheral vasodilation causes

Figure 1: **Assessment of Patients with Fever**

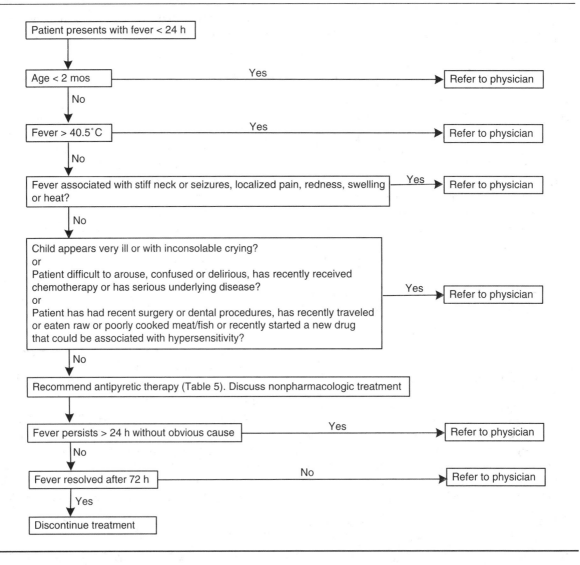

the skin to feel hot. Sweating may occur. Malaise and fatigue may be seen at higher temperatures. Headache, backache, myalgia, arthralgia, somnolence, chills and rigors may also be associated with fever.

Drug-induced fever is a symptom of hypersensitivity but can occur with other symptoms such as myalgia, chills and headache. Table 1 lists several medications associated with drug-induced fever.

Fever differs from hyperthermia, which is an increase in core temperature without an increase in hypothalamic set point. If hyperthermia is suspected, refer the patient to a physician; antipyretics are not useful (see Chapter 10).

Measurement of Body Temperature[6,7,9-20]

There are five practical ways to measure temperature in an ambulatory setting — oral, rectal, axillary, tympanic membrane and transcutaneous routes (Table 2). Oral, rectal and axillary temperatures may be taken with a standard mercury in glass thermometer or an electronic thermometer with digital display (Tables 3 and 4).

Electronic thermometers are safer and easier to use because they are faster, easier to read and avoid the environmental concerns of mercury. Generally, equilibration times require 30 to 60 seconds, while up to 10 minutes are required for standard glass thermometers. They are, however, more expensive.

Problems associated with the use of standard mercury thermometers are:

- Insufficient time is allowed for equilibration when taking the temperature (three to four minutes orally, two to three minutes rectally, and 4 to 10 minutes axillary);
- They are improperly read;
- The user fails to reset the thermometer, and
- It is incorrectly placed.

Nonpharmacologic Therapy[3,4,6,11,21-24]

Sponging increases evaporation to promote heat loss. Tepid water sponging may be useful to reduce body temperature; however, it does not reset the hypothalamic set point. Therefore, to maintain the elevated temperature the body actually works harder by shivering (results in increased oxygen consumption). As well, sponging often causes significant patient discomfort. One study showed no additional benefit from sponging after antipyretic administration.[11] If used, administer antipyretics 30 minutes before sponging to reduce hypothalamic set point.

Tepid sponging should be done with water only. Isopropyl alcohol has resulted, rarely, in hypoglycemia, intoxication and coma as a result of absorption through the skin or inhalation of fumes and is not recommended.[4,23]

Start sponging approximately 30 minutes after administration of an antipyretic in children with a temperature > 40°C. If the temperature is > 41°C, the child has a seizure, or delirium is present, sponging can be started immediately after antipyretic administration. The child should be sitting in about 5 cm of water and the skin surface continuously bathed. Total immersion in water is much less efficient as evaporation is inhibited. The water temperature should be lukewarm (29 to 32°C) but increased if shivering occurs. Generally, sponging should be carried out for at least 20 minutes.[4] Application of ice packs or cooling blankets and circulatory fans are also sometimes used in hospitalized patients.

Table 1: **Selected Drugs Associated with Fever**

Allopurinol	Digoxin	Nifedipine
Amphotericin B	Diltiazem	Oral contraceptives
Antacids	Epinephrine	Phenytoin
Antibacterials	Folic acid	Procainamide
Antibiotics	Griseofulvin	Propylthiouracil
Anticholinergics	Heparin	Quinidine
Antihistamines	Hydralazine	Quinine
Antineoplastics	Ibuprofen	Ranitidine
Antituberculars	Insulin	Salicylates
Azathioprine	Interferon	Streptokinase
Barbiturates	Iodides	Sulindac
Carbamazepine	Iron dextran	Tacrolimus
Cimetidine	Metoclopramide	Tolmetin
Clofibrate	Methyldopa	Triamterene
Corticosteroids	MAOIs	Vitamins
Cyclosporine	Neuroleptics	

Adapted with permission from Beringer PM, Middleton RK, Table 4-7 Allergic Reactions to Drugs. In: Koda-Kimble MA, Young LY, eds. *Applied Therapeutics*, 7th ed. New York: Lippincott Williams & Wilkins, 2001:4-9.

Table 2: **Methods of Measuring Body Temperature**

Rectal

This route is preferred for newborns, in children less than 5 years old when an axillary temperature is not sufficient, and when the oral route is not suitable due to mouth breathing. It is contraindicated in premature infants, the immunocompromised and in the presence of rectal anomalies, recent anorectal surgery or severe hemorrhoids. A rare complication is perforation of the rectum.

Instructions for use in children

- Shake thermometer until mercury line is below 37°C.
- Lay infant or young child face down across parent's lap.
- Lubricate anus and thermometer with petroleum jelly (pea size quantity).
- With one hand gently insert thermometer 2 to 3 cm into rectum.
- Hold buttocks closed against thermometer with other hand.
- Leave standard thermometer in place for 2 to 3 min.

Oral

This route can be used in children over 5 years old and adults; younger children may bite the thermometer or have difficulty keeping it in the closed mouth. This may also be a problem for individuals who have difficulty understanding instructions, e.g., the mentally impaired or demented elderly. Avoid the oral route when nasal breathing is difficult (e.g., due to viral upper respiratory tract infection); mouth breathing will cause spuriously low temperatures. Beverages, either hot or cold, and smoking should be avoided for at least 10 minutes prior to taking an oral temperature.

Instructions for use

- Shake thermometer until mercury line is below 37°C.
- Place thermometer on either side of mouth (between gum and cheek) or under the tongue.
- Hold in place with lips or fingers (not the teeth).
- Breathe through nose with mouth closed.
- Leave standard thermometer in place for 3 to 4 min.

Armpit

Axillary (armpit) temperatures have many disadvantages. They take a long time to measure and are affected by a number of factors including hypotension, cutaneous vasolidation and prior cooling of the patient. Axillary temperature may be a poor alternative to rectal temperatures in children aged three months to six years.[18] Although axillary temperatures are generally considered to be approximately 0.5°C lower than oral temperatures, reliable data are not available to correlate axillary with oral or rectal temperatures. The obvious advantage of axillary temperatures are that this route is very accessible, safe and less frightening to children than rectal temperatures.

Instructions for use

- Shake thermometer until mercury line is below 37°C.
- Place thermometer in apex of axilla.
- Hold elbow against chest to stabilize the thermometer.
- Leave standard thermometer in place for 4 to 10 min.

Ear[13,16,17]

Tympanic membrane thermometers (TMT) measure infrared emissions from the tympanic membrane. Because the tympanic membrane and the hypothalamus share the same blood supply, these thermometers are considered to reflect core temperature measurements. The temperature is then converted by the thermometer to reflect oral or rectal temperatures, which may lead to some inaccuracy in the temperature reading. The aiming of the ear probe and proper placement in the ear canal are important for accurate measurements. Improper placement can result in a lower temperature reading from a lower outer ear canal wall temperature. There may be a poor correlation of TMT with rectal temperatures and this route may not be sensitive enough to screen for fever in pediatric patients.[19,20] The advantages of TMT include simplicity, speed and patient acceptance. Less than two seconds is needed to obtain a reading. Other advantages include lack of external influences such as hot beverage ingestion, and no mucous membrane contact, therefore minimal risk of disease transmission. Acute otitis media and nonobstructive cerumen do not appear to affect the accuracy of TMT. A disadvantage is high cost.[19]

Transcutaneous[18-19]

The transcutaneous route uses a plastic strip that is placed on the forehead for one minute and indicates temperature by changing color. The strip contains encapsulated thermophototropic esters of cholesterol (called liquid crystals) that change color in response to temperature changes. They are easier to read and require less time than a standard thermometer, but are less reliable because skin temperature is not a reliable indicator of core temperature. The strip incorporates a correction factor for this but assumes the factor is the same in all individuals. When studied in emergency departments, they were poor predictors of fever.[14,16-18] Their accuracy is affected by ambient temperature (e.g., cold hands holding the strip and nearby heat sources such as a lamp). Because they can register afebrile temperatures in a truly febrile child, possibly delaying medical attention, their use is not recommended.

Table 3: **Normal Pediatric Temperature Ranges Associated with Measurement Technique**

Measurement technique	Normal temperature range
Rectum	36.6°C-38°C (97.9°F-100.4°F)
Mouth	35.5°C-37.5°C (95.9°F-99.5°F)
Armpit	34.7°C-37.3°C (94.5°F-99.1°F)
Ear	35.8°C-38°C (96.4°F-100.4°F)

Adapted with permission from *Pediatrics and Child Health* 2000; 5:277-278. Ref #CP00-01 http://www.cps.ca

Table 4: **Recommendations for Temperature Measuring Techniques**

Age	Recommended technique	
Birth to 2 years	First choice:	Rectum (for an exact reading)
	Second choice:	Armpit (to check for fever)
	Not recommended:	Tympanic membrane thermometers
Between 2 and 5 years	First choice:	Rectum
	Second choice:	Ear
	Third choice:	Armpit
Older than 5 years	First choice:	Mouth
	Second choice:	Ear
	Third choice:	Armpit

Adapted with permission from *Pediatrics and Child Health* 2000; 5:277-278. Ref #CP00-01 http://www.cps.ca

Other nonpharmacologic interventions include removal of excess clothing and bedding, increased fluid intake to replace increased insensible water loss in fever, maintenance of ambient temperatures around 20 to 21°C and avoidance of physical exertion.[4]

Pharmacologic Therapy[3,4,6,25-27]

There are many arguments against treating a fever.[3,4,6,9-11,28]

- Fever is an important defence mechanism; it enhances the immune response.
- Use of antipyretics may impair the use of temperature as an important clinical tool for monitoring the progress of an infection or response to antibiotics.
- Fever is usually self-limited and the most common consequences of fever are generally harmless — mild dehydration, febrile delirium, febrile seizures and discomfort.

Therefore, the decision to use antipyretics must be individualized to the patient. Reduction of fever, not

"normal" body temperature, may be the goal. Assessment of the patient should not depend solely on the elevation of temperature (Figure 1).

Acetaminophen, ASA and ibuprofen are all currently indicated to reduce fever. These drugs reduce body temperature in febrile patients by decreasing prostaglandin synthesis in the brain and reducing the hypothalamic set point. They do not lower normal body temperature. Short-term treatment with these drugs is associated with few side effects. Intermittent administration of antipyretics may exaggerate swings in temperature, which may make the individual feel worse. Use at regular intervals may improve patient discomfort and reduce the risk of increased metabolic demand with shivering.

ASA should be avoided in children less than 18 years old with a viral illness because of its association with Reye's syndrome in influenza and varicella. Reye's syndrome consists of acute encephalopathy with cerebral edema, fatty infiltration of the liver and metabolic derangements such as hypoglycemia. It occurs

Table 5: **Drug Therapy for Fever**[3,4,25,27,37-43]

	Acetaminophen	ASA	Ibuprofen
Dose			
Adults	325-650 mg q 4-6 h PRN (maximum 4 g per day)	325-650 mg q 4-6 h PRN (maximum 4 g per day)	200-400 mg q 4-6 h PRN (maximum 1.2 g per day)
Children	10-15 mg/kg q 4-6 h PRN (no greater than 5 doses per day or 65 mg/kg per day)	10-15 mg/kg q 4-6 h PRN (no greater than 5 doses per day or 65 mg/kg per day)	5 mg/kg q 6-8 h (temp < 39°C); 10 mg/kg q 6-8 h (temp > 39°C) (maximum 4 doses per day or 40 mg/kg per day)
Dosing in renal dysfunction	Clcr 10-50mL/min: extend interval from q4 to q6h Clcr < 10 mL/min: q8h	Clcr 10-50 mL/min: extend interval from q4 to q6h Clcr < 10mL/min: avoid use	No adjustment in renal dysfunction required
Onset of effect	30 min	Within 1 h	Within 1 h
Maximum temperature reduction	3 h	3 h	2-4 h
Duration	4-6 h	4-6 h	6-8 h
Side effects	• Allergic reactions (rare) • Rash • Thrombocytopenia, leukopenia, pancytopenia • Repeated dosing at or slightly above upper limit of recommended doses may result in severe hepatic toxicity • Analgesic nephropathy (individuals who use combination analgesics for prolonged periods)	• Dyspepsia, heartburn, abdominal pain, vomiting, nausea, rectal irritation (suppositories) • GI bleeding • Tinnitis or hearing loss (chronic ingestion) • Sodium and H₂O retention • Allergic reactions • Skin rash • Hepatotoxicity • Leukopenia, thrombocytopenia, agranulocytosis • Platelet dysfunction • Associated with Reye's syndrome in pediatrics • Analgesic nephropathy (individuals who use combination analgesics for prolonged periods)	• Dyspepsia, heartburn, abdominal pain, vomiting, nausea, anorexia, diarrhea • GI bleeding • Dizziness, headache, nervousness, fatigue, irritability • Aseptic meningitis • Hepatotoxicity • Skin rash • Allergic reactions • Reduced renal function, acute renal failure • Sodium and H₂O retention • Platelet dysfunction • Hemolytic anemia, thrombocytopenia, aplastic anemia, agranulocytosis

	Acetaminophen	ASA	Ibuprofen
Contraindications/Precautions	• Hypersensitivity • Chronic ethanol consumption • Malnutrition/fasting	• Children < 18 yrs with viral illness • Active GI lesions • History of recurrent GI lesions • Bleeding disorders • Thrombocytopenia • ASA hypersensitivity • Pregnancy • Concomitant ethanol use • Individuals who rely on vasodilatory renal prostaglandins, for renal function (CHF, hepatic cirrhosis with ascites, chronic renal failure, hypovolemia)	• Peptic ulcer disease, GI perforation or bleeding • Hypersensitivity • Bleeding disorders • Pregnancy • Concomitant alcohol use • Individuals who rely on vasodilatory renal prostaglandins, for renal function (CHF, hepatic cirrhosis with ascites, chronic renal failure hypovolemia)
Overdose	GI disturbance Hepatotoxicity Death	Tinnitus, hyperpyrexia, hyperventilation, acid-base disturbances, nausea, vomiting, dehydration, coma, seizures, bleeding, hepatotoxicity, renal failure, hyper- or hypoglycemia, death	GI disturbances, bleeding, CNS depression, metabolic acidosis, hypotension, bradycardia, seizures, drowsiness, diaphoresis, liver dysfunction, death. Serious toxicity from overdose is unusual
Drug interactions	Alcohol, phenytoin, barbiturates, carbamazepine, isoniazid	• Warfarin and anticoagulants • Uricosuric agents (probenecid, sulfinpyrazone) • Sulfonylureas • Corticosteroids • Methotrexate • Alcohol • Antagonism of hypotensive effects of ACEI, diuretics, beta blockers	• Warfarin and anticoagulants • Lithium • Methotrexate • Alcohol • Antagonism of hypotensive effects of ACEI, diuretics, beta-blockers
Other comments	• Rectal products slowly and incompletely absorbed • Detected in breast milk of nursing mothers but adverse events in infants not reported	• Take with food • Rectal products slowly and incompletely absorbed • Detected in breast milk	• Take with food

in otherwise previously healthy children. Since the cause of fever is unknown initially in many circumstances, avoid ASA generally in children.[29-31]

Acetaminophen is a safe and effective antipyretic with few contraindications, which can be used in any age group. Many years of clinical experience is also an advantage. Recently a loading dose of acetaminophen has been studied.[32] A 30 mg/kg loading dose in children four months to nine years of age resulted in a more rapid and sustained response and a greater reduction in temperature compared to 15 mg/kg. Although this strategy is used in some emergency departments, the safety of this practice has not been evaluated and the dose is an initial dose only; subsequent doses should be 10 to 15 mg/kg. Recommending a loading dose to parents is premature at this time. Standard dosing is provided in Table 5.

Ibuprofen, although as effective as acetaminophen, is considered a second-line agent. There is less experience with it than acetaminophen. It can cause more adverse effects than acetaminophen, is more expensive, but is less toxic in overdose. Ibuprofen may produce greater temperature reductions[33,34] and have a longer duration of action[34] than acetaminophen. Serious toxicity with short-term therapeutic doses appears to be rare.[26,35,36]

Table 5 outlines dosing, side effects, contraindications, precautions and toxicity in overdose of ASA, acetaminophen and ibuprofen.

Fever in Specific Patient Groups
Children[6,7]
Young children have an immature central nervous system thermoregulatory system, and in the first two months of life may have minimal or no fever during an infectious illness. Since neonates and infants are less able to mount a febrile response, when they do become febrile, it is more likely to indicate a major illness. After three months of age, the degree of fever more closely approximates that seen in older children.

Fever is common in children and is usually due to bacterial or viral infection. Because children have had less exposure than adults to infectious agents, they are more susceptible upon initial contact. Reactions to vaccinations may also be a cause. Compared to adults, children are more sensitive to ambient temperature

(due to a greater body surface area for heat exchange) and at higher risk for dehydration.

In children ages three months to five years, seizures occur with 2 to 5% of febrile episodes. Although simple febrile seizures are rarely associated with neurologic damage or permanent seizure disorders, they concern and frighten parents. For this reason, antipyretics are often recommended for children in this age group, particularly those with previous febrile seizures or neurologic problems. Recommending antipyretics at the first sign of fever is not effective in preventing recurrent febrile seizures even though this practice is frequently recommended.[44-46]

Patients with Cardiovascular or Pulmonary Disorders[3,39]
Increased metabolic demands which occur during the chill phase (increased metabolic rate, norepinephrine-mediated peripheral vasoconstriction, increased arterial blood pressure) may aggravate comorbid disease states in patients with congestive heart failure, coronary, pulmonary or cerebral insufficiency. Fever may result in deterioration in cognitive function and delirium.

The Elderly[47,48]
Older individuals exhibit less intense fevers in response to infection compared to younger individuals. They also become hypothermic more often when infected and have greater morbidity and mortality from infections. Fever in individuals older than 60 is less likely to be a benign febrile illness than it is in younger individuals; therefore, it is important to carefully assess fever in the elderly. The elderly are more likely to have the cardiovascular and pulmonary conditions described above. **Acetaminophen** is safer in older individuals with risk factors predisposing to GI toxicity of NSAIDs.

Pregnancy
Studies in humans suggest that exposure to fever and other heat sources during the first trimester of pregnancy is associated with increased risk of neural tube defects.[49]

Acetaminophen crosses the placenta and is relatively safe for short-term use in pregnancy when therapeutic doses are used. Use of ASA and NSAIDs can result in a number of problems. Since these drugs inhibit prostaglandin synthesis, they may interfere with labor and cause premature closure of the ductus arteriosus resulting in persistent pulmonary hypertension in the infant. Platelet aggregation is inhibited in the newborn if ASA is ingested by the mother within seven days of delivery and salicylates displace bilirubin from protein binding sites. Increased bleeding has been reported in both mothers and infants if ASA is ingested close to the time of delivery.[25]

Alternating Antipyretics

In the past, alternating acetaminophen with ASA for management of fever unresponsive to a single agent was recommended. Since ASA is no longer recommended in children and adolescents because of an association with Reye's syndrome, this practice has been abandoned. However, recommendations to alternate acetaminophen with ibuprofen have emerged.[50] This practice has not been shown to be either safe or more effective than a single antipyretic. This recommendation is often confusing to caregivers and could result in increased dosing errors.[51]

Fever Phobia

The term "fever phobia" describes unrealistic concerns and misconceptions parents have regarding fever in children.[52-54] Health care professionals should undertake educational interventions to ensure appropriate management of fever and rational use of antipyretics.

Review the following points with all parents when recommending an antipyretic preparation:

- Assist the parent in calculating the correct mg/kg dose of the drug and ensure they know the maximum number of doses which can be administered in a 24-hour period.
  In a study of 100 caregivers given a mock dosing scenario which required the caregiver to determine and measure a correct dose of acetaminophen for their child, only 40% stated an appropriate dose for their child.[55]
- Ensure the parent has and will use an appropriate measuring device.
  In the same study, only 67% of caregivers accurately measured the amount they intended to give. Forty-three percent measured out a correct amount of acetaminophen, however, 30% of these did so by accident by inaccurately measuring an improper dose.[55]

- Ask what form of product they have at home and calculate the appropriate number of mLs or tablets for the child.
  Multiple miscalculated overdoses of acetaminophen given by parents account for an important cause of acetaminophen toxicity.[56]
  Use of incorrect measuring devices, differences in medication concentrations (e.g., pediatric drops vs suspensions), use of adult formulations for pediatric patients, and unrecognized acetaminophen content in multiple ingredient cough and cold products contribute to this problem.[57]
- Ask about *other preparations*, particularly cough and cold products, they may be coadministering and ensure they are aware of the antipyretic content of these products. The coadministration of these products should be carefully monitored to ensure the *cumulative* dose is within the recommended range.

Monitoring of Therapy

Recommendations for frequent monitoring of temperature likely contribute to parental concern and fever phobia. The temperature should be taken if the patient feels warm or looks ill to determine the initial temperature. Subsequently, temperatures need not be taken more than two or three times daily unless the patient has recently received chemotherapy. If the fever persists for 24 hours without an apparent cause, or for more than three days, medical attention should be sought. The degree of illness and not the temperature should guide therapy and referral.

Monitor:

- All patients given antipyretics for development of rash or other allergic reactions.
- Patients with pre-existing comorbid illness for edema and decreased urine output.
- For other common side effects, such as GI intolerance and tinnitus (Table 5).
- To ensure appropriate doses, products and measuring devices are being used, and the patient is not receiving excessive amounts of antipyretics through use of cough and cold or analgesic products.
- To ensure the patient is not receiving interacting medications (Table 5). Recommend avoiding alcohol.

Suggested Readings

American Academy of Pediatrics, Committee on Drugs. Acetaminophen toxicity in children. *Pediatrics* 2001;108:1020-4.

American Academy of Pediatrics, Committee on Quality Improvement, Subcommittee on Febrile Seizures. Practice parameter: Long-term treatment of the child with simple febrile seizures. *Pediatrics* 1999. Available from: http://www.pediatrics.org/cgi/content/full/103/6/e86.

Crocetti M, Moghbeli N, Serwint J. Fever phobia revisited: Have parental misconceptions about fever changed in 20 years? *Pediatrics* 2001;107:1241-6.

Drwal-Klein LA, Phelps SJ. Antipyretic therapy in the febrile child. *Clin Pharm* 1992;11:1005-21.

Hersh EV, Moore PA, Ross GL. Over-the-counter analgesics and antipyretics: A critical assessment. *Clin Ther* 2000;22:500-48.

Mayoral CE, Marino RV, Rosenfeld W, Greensher J. Alternating antipyretics: Is this an alternative? *Pediatrics* 2000;105:1009-12.

Plaisance KI, Mackowiak PA. Antipyretic therapy. Physiologic rationale, diagnostic implications, and clinical consequences. *Arch Intern Med* 2000;160:449-56.

Plaisance KI. Toxicities of drugs used in the management of fever. *Clin Infect Dis* 2000;31(suppl 5):s219-23.

Simon HK, Weinkle DA. Over-the-counter medications. Do parents give what they intend to give? *Arch Pediatr Adolesc Med* 1997;151:654-6.

References

1. Gelfand JA, Dinarello CA. Fever and hyperthermia. In: Fauci AS, et al, eds. *Harrison's Principles of Internal Medicine*, 14th ed. Montreal, QC: McGraw-Hill; 1998:84-90.
2. Mackowiak PA, Bartlett JG, Borden EC, et al. Concepts of fever: recent advances and lingering dogma. *Clin Infect Dis* 1997;25:119-38.
3. Plaisance KI, Mackowiak PA. Antipyretic therapy. Physiologic rationale, diagnostic implications, and clinical consequences. *Arch Intern Med* 2000:160:449-56.
4. Drwal-Klein LA, Phelps SJ. Antipyretic therapy in the febrile child. *Clin Pharm* 1992;11:1005-21.
5. Mackowiak PA, Wasserman SS, Levine MM. A critical appraisal of 98.6°F, the upper limit of the normal body temperature, and other legacies of Carl Reinhold August Wunderlich. *JAMA* 1992;268:1578-80.
6. Alperin ER, Henretig FM. Fever. In: Fleisher GR, Ludwig S. eds. *Textbook of Pediatric Emergency Medicine*, 4th ed. Philadelphia, PA: Lippincott, Williams & Wilkens; 2000: 257-66.
7. Bonadio WA. Defining fever and other aspects of body temperature in infants and children. *Pediatr Ann* 1993;22:467-73.
8. Herzog LW, Coyne LJ. What is fever? Normal temperature in infants less than 3 months old. *Clin Pediatr* 1993;32:142-6.
9. Schmitt BD. Fever in childhood. *Pediatrics* 1984;74(suppl): 929-36.
10. Mackowiak PA. Physiological rationale for suppression of fever. *Clin Infect Dis* 2000;31(suppl 5):s185-9.
11. Newman J. Evaluation of sponging to reduce body temperature in febrile children. *CMAJ* 1985;132:641-2.
12. Mackowiak PA. Clinical thermometric measurements. In: Mackowiak PA, ed. *Fever: Basic mechanisms and management* 2nd ed. Philadelphia: Lippincott-Raven;1997:27-34.
13. Terndrup TE. An appraisal of temperature assessment by infrared emission detection tympanic thermometry. *Ann Emerg Med* 1992;21:1483-1492.
14. Lewit EM, Marshall CL, Salzer JE. An evaluation of a plastic strip thermometer. *JAMA* 1982;247:321-25.
15. Zengeya ST, Blumenthal I. Modern electronic and chemical thermometers used in the axilla are inaccurate. *Eur J Pediatr* 1996;155:1005-8.
16. Hooker EA. Use of tympanic thermometers to screen for fever in patients in a pediatric emergency department. *South Med J* 1993;86:855-58.
17. Selfridge J, Shea SS. The accuracy of the tympanic membrane thermometer in detecting fever in infants aged 3 months and younger in the emergency department setting. *J Emerg Nurs* 1993;19:127-30.
18. Scholefield JH, Gerber MA, Dwyer P. Liquid crystal forehead temperature strips. *Am J Dis Child* 1982;136:198-201.
19. Reisinger KS, Kao J, Grant DM. Inaccuracy of the Clinitemp skin thermometer. *Pediatrics* 1979;64:4-6.
20. Davis CB. Liquid crystal forehead temperature strips. *Am J Dis Child* 1983;137:87.
21. Steele RW, Tanaka PT, Lara RP, Bass JW. Evaluation of sponging and of oral antipyretic therapy to reduce fever. *J Peds* 1970;77:824-9.
22. Purssell E. Physical treatment of fever. *Arch Dis Child* 2000;82:238-9.
23. Garrison RF. Acute poisoning from use of isopropyl alcohol in tepid sponging. *JAMA* 1953;152:317-8.
24. Axelrod P. External cooling in the management of fever. *Clin Infect Dis* 2000;31(suppl 5):s224-9.
25. Hersh EV, Moore PA, Ross GL. Over-the-counter analgesics and antipyretics: A critical assessment. *Clin Ther* 2000;22: 500-48.
26. Lesko SM, Mitchell AA. An assessment of the safety of pediatric ibuprofen. A practitioner-based randomized clinical trial. *JAMA* 1995;273:929-33.
27. Clark WG. Antipyretic therapy. Clinical trials 1990 through 1995. In: Mackowiak PA, ed. *Fever: basic mechanisms and management* 2nd ed. Philadelphia, PA: Lippincott-Raven 1997:295-302.
28. Styrt B, Sugarman B. Antipyresis and fever. *Arch Intern Med* 1990;150:1589-97.
29. Fulginiti VA, Brunell PA, Cherry JD, Ector WL, Gershon AA, Gotoff SP, et al. Special report. Aspirin and Reye syndrome. *Pediatrics* 1982;69:810-12.
30. Starko KM, Ray CG, Dominguez LB, Stromberg WL, Woodall DF. Reye's syndrome and salicylate use. *Pediatrics* 1980;66: 859-64.
31. Waldman RJ, Hall WN, McGee H, Van Amburg G. Aspirin as a risk factor in Reye's syndrome. *JAMA* 1982;247:3089-94.

32. Treluyer JM, Tonnelier S, d'Athis P. Antipyretic efficacy of an initial 30mg/kg loading dose of acetaminophen versus a 15mg/kg maintenance dose. *Pediatrics* 2000;108. Available from http:// www.pediatrics.org/cgi/content/full/108/4/e73.

33. Van Esch A, Van Steensel-Moll HA, Steyerberg EW, Offringa M, Habbema JDF, Derksen-Lubsen G. Antipyretic efficacy of ibuprofen and acetaminophen in children with febrile seizures. *Arch Pediatr Adolesc Med* 1995;149:632-7.

34. Walson PD, Galletta G, Braden NJ, Alexander L. Ibuprofen, acetaminophen, and placebo treatment of febrile children. *Clin Pharmacol Ther* 1989;46:9-17.

35. Lesko SM, Mitchell AA. Renal function after short-term ibuprofen use in infants and children. *Pediatrics* 1997;100: 954-7.

36. Lesko SM, Mitchell AA. The safety of acetaminophen and ibuprofen among children younger than two years old. *Pediatrics* 1999. Available from http://www.pediatrics.org/ cgi/content/full/ 104/4/e39.

37. Whelton A. Renal effects of over-the-counter analgesics. *J Clin Pharmacol* 1995;35:454-463.

38. McIntyre J, Hull D. Comparing efficacy and tolerability of ibuprofen and paracetamol in fever. *Arch Dis Child* 1996;74: 164-7.

39. Plaisance KI. Toxicities of drugs used in the management of fever. *Clin Infect Dis* 2000;31(suppl 5):s219-23.

40. Autret E, Reboul-Marty J, Henry-Launois B, Laborde C, Courcier S, Goehrs JM et al. Evaluation of ibuprofen versus aspirin and paracetamol on efficacy and comfort in children with fever. *Eur J Clin Pharmacol* 1997;51:367-71.

41. Whitcomb DC, Block GD. Association of acetaminophen hepatotoxicity with fasting and ethanol use. *JAMA* 1994;272: 1845-50.

42. Aronoff GR, Berns JS, Brier ME et al. Drug prescribing in renal failure. *Dosing guidelines for adults*. 4th ed. Philadelphia, PA: American College of Physicians; 1999:19,79.

43. American Academy of Pediatrics Committee on Drugs. Acetaminophen toxicity in children. *Pediatrics* 2001;108: 1020-4.

44. American Academy of Pediatrics, Committee on Quality Improvement, Subcommittee on Febrile Seizures. Practice parameter: Long-term treatment of the child with simple febrile seizures. *Pediatrics* 1999. Available from http://www.pediatrics.org/cgi/content/full/103/6/e86.

45. van Stuijvenberg M, Derksen-Lubsen G, Steyerberg EW, Habbema JDF, Moll HA. Randomized controlled trial of ibuprofen syrup administered during febrile illness to prevent febrile seizure recurrences. *Pediatrics* 1998. Available from http://www.pediatrics.org/cgi/content/full/102/5/e51.

46. Camfield PR, Camfield CS, Shapiro SH, Cummings C. The first febrile seizure – antipyretic instruction plus either phenobarbital or placebo to prevent recurrence. *J Pediatr* 1980;97:16-21.

47. Bender B., Scarpace PJ. Fever in the elderly. In: Mackowiak PA, ed. *Fever: basic mechanisms and management*, 2nd ed. Philadelphia, PA: Lippincott-Raven Publishers;1997:363-73.

48. Keating HJ, Klimek JJ, Levine DS et al. Effect of aging on the clinical significance of fever in ambulatory adult patients. *J Am Ger Soc* 1984;32:282-7.

49. Milunsky A, Ulcickas M, Rothman KJ, Willett W, Jick SS, Jick H. Maternal heat exposure and neural tube defects. *JAMA* 1992;268:882-5.

50. Mayoral CE, Marino RV, Rosenfeld W, Greensher J. Alternating antipyretics: Is this an alternative? *Pediatrics* 2000;105:1009-12.

51. Mofenson HC, McFee R, Caraccio T, Greensher J. Combined antipyretic therapy: another potential source of chronic acetaminophen toxicity. *J Pediatr* 1998;133:712-13.

52. Crocetti M, Moghbeli N, Serwint J. Fever phobia revisited: Have parental misconceptions about fever changed in 20 years? *Pediatrics* 2001;107:1241-46.

53. Schmitt BD. Fever phobia: Misconceptions of parents about fevers. *Am J Dis Child* 1980;134:176-81.

54. May A, Bauchner H. Fever phobia: The pediatrician's contribution. *Pediatrics* 1992;90:851-4.

55. Simon HK, Weinkle DA. Over-the-counter medications. Do parents give what they intend to give? *Arch Pediatr Adolesc Med* 1997;151:654-6.

56. Rivera-Penera T, Gugig R, Davis J, et al. Outcome of acetaminophen overdose in pediatric patients and factors contributing to hepatotoxicity. *J Pediatr* 1997;130:300-4.

57. Heubi JE, Bien JP. Acetaminophen use in children. More is not better. *J Pediatr* 1997;130:175-7.

Fever—Patient Information

- Treat the individual, not the fever. Fever itself is rarely dangerous and fever-lowering drugs are not always required.
- Use acetaminophen or ibuprofen, not ASA, for fever in children and adolescents.
- Do not wake a sleeping child to administer drugs for fever unless the child has had previous febrile seizures.
- Do not use fever medication for more than three days without consulting a doctor.
- Encourage the person with fever to drink lots of fluids and remove excess clothing and bedding.
- Contact the doctor for:
—Fever over 40.5°C;
—Children less than two months old who have fever;
—If the child appears very ill, has a stiff neck, has a seizure, is confused or delirious, or is crying inconsolably.

- Contact the doctor if you have recently received chemotherapy.
- Read labels carefully. Use an appropriate dosage form for your child, determine the dose based on the child's weight, and use the proper measuring device.
- Use one drug; avoid alternating acetaminophen with ibuprofen.
- Check other medications, especially cough and cold, for acetaminophen or ASA content to avoid giving too much.
- Keep antipyretics and all other medications out of reach of children.

Chapter 10

Heat-related Disorders

Dorothy Tscheng, BScPhm

Heat-related illnesses are a major cause of preventable death.[1,2] The incidence of these disorders increases with higher temperature and humidity.[1] Deaths due to cardiovascular and respiratory illnesses also increase during heat waves and may not be attributed directly to the heat.[3] There is a wide spectrum of heat-related disorders, ranging from heat edema to heat stroke.

Pathophysiology

The body's thermoregulatory centre is responsible for the maintenance of core body temperature. Signals from various parts of the body keep the centre informed of the internal and external conditions. Heat illness results from an imbalance of heat generated within and absorbed by the body and its ability to dissipate excessive heat.[1,2,4]

The body eliminates heat by four different mechanisms:[1,2]

- *Evaporation* is the loss of heat through moisture from the skin or the respiratory tract system. It usually accounts for about 30% of heat loss. This mechanism becomes more important the higher the ambient temperature becomes.
- *Radiation* is the transfer of heat through electromagnetic waves. It accounts for about 65% of heat loss when ambient temperature is less than body temperature. At higher ambient temperatures, heat gain can result.
- *Conduction* is the transfer of heat through physical contact with a cooler object. It is responsible for approximately 2% of heat loss.
- *Convection* is the transfer of heat to the air and vapour. Good airflow helps promote heat loss due to convection. It accounts for about 10% of heat loss. Vasodilation contributes to heat loss by convection.

A reduction in the efficacy of any of the above mechanisms results in an increased risk of heat-related illnesses. As ambient temperature and humidity increase, heat dissipation is less efficient.

There are two types of heat stroke: classic and exertional. Exertional heat stroke, as its name depicts, usually occurs in younger, healthy individuals who have participated in strenuous physical activity. The characteristics of this type of heat stroke often differ from classical heat stroke. Sweating, acute renal failure, lactic acidosis, hypokalemia, rhabdomyolysis and disseminated intravascular coagulation are more common and hyperuricemia is more severe with the exertional type. Older patients with predisposing health risks in poor environmental conditions usually present with classical heat stroke.[2]

Risk Factors

The young and the elderly are particularly susceptible to heat-related disorders.[1,2,5] Neonates have poorly developed thermoregulatory mechanisms and produce more heat for the same level of activity compared to adults.[1,2] In addition, children do not sweat as much as adults and because of their greater surface area-to-body ratio, will gain more heat on a hot day.[6] The elderly, with their comorbid illnesses, multiple medications and poor thermoregulatory response, are predisposed to heat illnesses.[1,5] They also have decreased vasodilatory response to heat and decreased thirst response. Table 1 outlines some of the other risk factors for heat-related illnesses.

Medication-related Causes

Medications listed in Table 2 can predispose patients to heat-related disorders through various mechanisms that include:[4]

- Blockage of sweat excretion (anticholinergic effects and hypovolemic causes)

Table 1: **Risk Factors for Developing Heat-related Illnesses**[1,2]

Conditions	Behavior/Environmental Factor
Age (children, adolescents, elderly) Alcoholism Cardiac disorders Dehydration Diabetes (uncontrolled) Extensive skin disease Fever Hypertension (uncontrolled) Hyperthyroidism Obesity Parkinson's disease Peripheral vascular disease Psychiatric disorders	Activity in hot, humid conditions Lack of acclimatization Lack of air conditioning or ventilation Lack of breaks during exercise Lack of fluid intake Sleep deprivation Use of heavy clothing or equipment

- Vasoconstriction of cutaneous vessels
- Disruption of hypothalamic thermoregulation

Goals of Therapy

- Normalize body temperature
- Reduce and eliminate symptoms
- Prevent mortality

Ideally, prevention of heat-related disease is the ultimate goal.

Patient Assessment (Figure 1)

The symptoms of various heat-related problems depend on the degree or stage of the illness. Patients' complaints range from edema in the feet to more serious concerns of confusion or coma. The spectrum of disorders is described (from the mildest to the most severe) in Table 3.

If any acute neurologic symptoms of heat stroke are present, the person must be taken to the hospital immediately, preferably in an air-conditioned vehicle, to be assessed and treated. Assume the patient is suffering from heat stroke until otherwise diagnosed.[2] Differential diagnoses include but are not limited to meningitis, neuroleptic malignant syndrome, thyroid storm, drug withdrawal, serotonin syndrome, septic shock and overdose of various substances including cocaine, salicylates and antidepressants.[1]

Prevention

Prevention of heat-related illness is the primary goal. Strategies to help reduce the risk include:

- Drinking fluids (approximately 500 mL to 1.8 L) before exercise and replenishing with about 250 mL every 20 minutes during the activity. Rehydration afterward is also important. For every kilogram of weight lost (during the activity), about 4.1 L of fluids should be consumed.[1,2] Thirst should not be relied upon as a reminder to drink as some athletes will not feel thirsty until 5% of the body's fluids are lost.[2]
- Avoiding heavy outdoor activities during peak sun hours (10 am to 3 pm).
- Staying out of the sun if possible. Take as many breaks as possible in the shade or in an air-conditioned environment.[7,8]
- Wearing light-colored, lightweight clothing. Natural fibers such as cotton are good choices.[7,8]
- Acclimatizing to the environment. Gradual exposure to the ambient conditions can prevent heat-related illnesses. The average adult requires exposure to the ambient temperatures one to four hours at a time. Four to seven episodes of repeated exposure are

Table 2: **Medications that can Predispose to Heat-related Illnesses**[2,4,5]

Mechanism	Drug class
Blockage of sweat excretion	- Anticholinergics - Antipsychotics - Antihistamines - Tricyclic antidepressants - Selective serotonin reuptake inhibitors - Diuretics - Beta-blockers
Vasoconstriction of cutaneous vessels	- Alpha-agonists - Monoamine oxidase inhibitors - Sympathomimetics - Cocaine
Disruption of hypothalamic regulation	- Antipsychotics - Amphetamines (including Ecstasy)

Figure 1: **Assessment of Patients with Heat-related Disorders**[1,2,5,6]

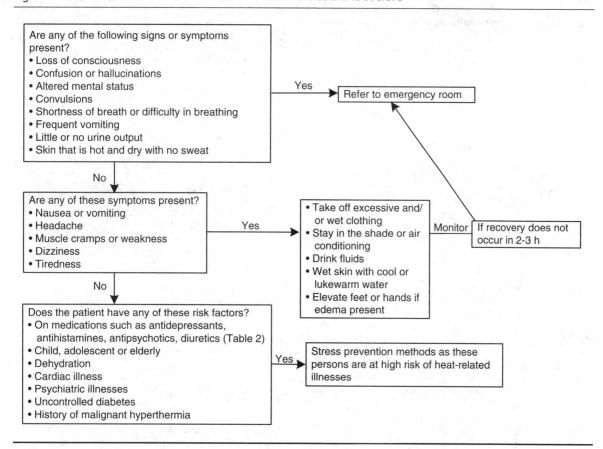

Nonpharmacologic Therapy

often required to facilitate acclimatization.[2] Children may require more exposure time/episodes.[1]

It is imperative to address heat stroke immediately. Delaying treatment results in poorer outcomes for the patient.[2] The first priority is cooling the patient using external methods. Unnecessary clothing should be removed and fanning can de done to allow for increased airflow around the patient. This will aid evaporation.[1,2] There is controversy as to whether patients should be cooled using water, wet towels or ice baths. Excessive cooling could also cause shivering, which produces more body heat. Despite the controversy, initiate some form of external cooling en route to the hospital. Internal cooling methods, such

as cold water irrigation to the stomach or rectum, are used in hospital as necessary.

Other types of heat-related illnesses are not considered emergent and can be addressed appropriately depending on the degree of the illness. Table 3 outlines various treatment options for different heat-related disorders.

Pharmacologic Therapy

Medications do not help reduce the body's internal temperature. Although not the mainstay of therapy, medications can be helpful in treating some of the complications of heat stroke. Neuroleptics (chlorpromazine) reduce the amount of shivering which in turn reduces the amount of heat produced, and

Table 3: **Heat-related Disorders—Symptoms and Therapy**[1,2,5,7]

Type of illness	Features/Symptoms	Therapy
Heat edema	• Edema in the extremities from transient vasodilation of vessels, sodium and water retention and with prolonged standing • More frequent during the summer months	• Elevate feet or hands • No specific treatment • Prevention with acclimatization
Heat cramps	• Cramps in muscles of the arms, legs and stomach are most common • Warning sign of heat exhaustion • May be due to lack of sodium in body	• Stop activity and rest in a cool, shaded area. • Oral rehydration solution containing glucose and sodium (e.g., Gatorade) or a homemade solution containing 5 mL of table salt per 0.9 L water • Lightly stretch muscles involved
Heat syncope	• Dizziness • Fainting episode	• Stop activity and rest in a cool, shaded area. • Patients often recover quickly after falling to the ground (secondary to fainting) • Slowly get up from a standing or sitting position
Heat exhaustion	• Weakness • Nausea and/or vomiting • Tachycardia, hypotension • Dizziness • Headache • Irritability • Core body temperature above 38°C but below 40.5°C	• Stop activity and rest in a cool, shaded area • Rehydrate with water or oral rehydration solution with about 1 L/h for several hours • Recovery is usually quick, within 2-3 h • Acclimatization reduces the incidence of heat exhaustion

Heat stroke	• **Medical emergency** – can result in death
	• Similar to heat exhaustion with the added feature of neurological symptoms in the majority of cases such as:
	  —Altered mental status
	  —Hallucinations
	  —Confusion
	  —Convulsions
	  —Coma
	• Core body temperature above 40.5°C
	• Medications can predispose (Table 3)
		• Stop activity immediately and rest in a cool, shaded area
		• Remove excessive clothing
		• Rehydrate
		• Ensure good air circulation around patient
		• Take to **emergency room** as soon as possible

benzodiazepines (diazepam) are used to treat seizures. Mannitol is used to promote osmotic diuresis and prevent or treat renal failure.[1] The use of these medications in this setting is beyond the scope of this reference.

Monitoring of Therapy

In preventing heat-related illnesses, athletes should ensure proper hydration (see Prevention) as thirst is an unreliable sign of body fluid loss. Voiding urine should occur at least four times daily and the urine should be light yellow.[2] Body weight can also be used

as a monitoring tool for athletes. A loss of 2 to 3% represents a mild depletion in water. Loss of more than 7% is considered severe and cessation of the activity is recommended until the athlete is rehydrated.[1]

For those not participating in activities, but who are at risk of developing heat-related disorders, monitoring of symptoms by friends and family can aid in preventing these illnesses.

Follow-up treatment for heat stroke involves monitoring of temperature, blood pressure, respiratory status, fluid status and electrolytes, and occurs in the hospital setting.[1,2] After hospital discharge, patients should avoid high ambient temperatures for up to 48 hours and be reminded to drink plenty of fluids.[1]

Suggested Readings

Barrow MW, Clarke KA. Heat-related illnesses. *Am Fam Phys* 1998;58:749-56,759.

Tscheng D. Heat-stroke and medications. *Can Pharm J* 2000;133:30-2.

References

1. Kunihiro A, Foster JDR. *Heat Exhaustion and Heat Stroke from Emergency Medicine.* Available at: www.emedicine.com. Accessed May 4, 2001.

2. Barrow MW, Clarke KA. Heat-related illnesses. *Am Fam Phys* 1998;58:749-56, 759.

3. Kilbourne EM. The spectrum of illness during heat waves. *Am J Prev Med* 1999;16:359-60.

4. Tscheng D. Heat stroke and medications. *Can Pharm J* 2000; 133:30-2.

5. Hett HA, Brechtelsbauer DA. Heat-related illness. *Postgrad Med* 1998;103:107-8,114-5,119-20.

6. Anderson SJ, Griesemer BA, Johnson MD et al. Climatic heat stress and the exercising child and adolescent. *Pediatrics* 2000;106:158-9.

7. Anonymous *Heat-Related Illness: What You Can Do To Prevent It.* Available at: www.familydoctor.org. Accessed May 4, 2001.

8. Anonymous Information from your family doctor – preventing heat illnesses. *Am Fam Phys.* Available at: www.aafp.org. Accessed May 4, 2001.

9. Kashmeery A. Exertional heat illness. *Lancet* 2000;355 (9219):1992.

Heat-related Disorders—Patient Information[5,7,9]

What is heat illness?
- Your body has ways to keep itself cool when the weather is hot or if you are exercising. When your body has difficulty doing this, a heat-related illness such as heat cramps or heat stroke can occur.

What are some of the signs that I may be suffering from a heat-related illness?
- Headache
- Nausea and/or vomiting
- Muscle weakness or cramps
- Dizziness

What can I do to prevent this from happening?
- If possible, avoid heavy outdoor activities when the sun is hottest (between 10 am and 6 pm).
- Try to stay in the shade. If you have to stay in direct sun, wear loose-fitting, light-colored clothing.
- Take several breaks from your activity.
- Drink plenty of fluids before, during and after any outdoor activity. Minimize the amount of coffee, tea, cola and alcoholic beverages.

What do I do if I do not feel well?
- Rest in the shade or in an air-conditioned environment if possible.
- Take off as much clothing as possible.
- Drink water or oral rehydration fluids.
- Wet yourself with cool or lukewarm water.
- See your doctor if you are not urinating (peeing) or sweating, if you have several episodes of vomiting, or if you start to feel confused.

What else should I do if I know I am at risk?
- Let your family and friends know that you may be at risk for heat-related illnesses. They can watch over you in case you develop symptoms.
- Wear a Medic-Alert identification bracelet or something similar.

Chapter 11

Nicotine Addiction

Melanie Rantucci, MScPhm, PhD

Pathophysiology

Tobacco dependency is the inability to discontinue tobacco use despite awareness of medical consequences.[1] Nicotine is recognized as the substance that causes the physically addictive effects of tobacco smoking. The US Surgeon General and Health Canada agree that tobacco smoking is a drug addiction and that nicotine is the drug in tobacco that causes addiction.[2,3] Nicotine addiction is so strong that opiate addicts and alcoholics claim it would be easier to do without these substances than cigarettes.[4]

Nicotine addiction involves physical factors, as well as psychologic and social components.[5] Chemical and biologic changes take place in the brain and tolerance develops with continued use. There is a craving for continued use, a tendency to increase usage, and profound physical and psychological symptoms elicited by withdrawal.[6] At the start, nicotine is poisonous and most people feel sick and dizzy, but these negative effects are quickly overcome and the body builds a tolerance to nicotine, resulting in an increase in the amount of cigarettes smoked.[2]

When smokers attempt to quit and nicotine use is discontinued, they often feel the *physical* effects of nicotine withdrawal including craving for nicotine, irritability, anxiety, difficulty concentrating, drowsiness, hunger, gastrointestinal symptoms, headaches and disturbed sleep.[7] A possible cause for the central adrenergic hyperactivity (anxiety, restlessness and craving) is excessive stimulation of neurons in the locus coeruleus region of the brain by norepinephrine.[8] Withdrawal symptoms generally peak 24 to 72 hours after the last cigarette, although rebound withdrawal can occur several weeks after complete abstinence.[9] The craving symptoms of abstinence, however, may continue for many years.[6,9]

The *psychological* habit of smoking is a result of its repetitive nature.[5] Behavioral conditioning results from the hand-to-mouth ritual with each cigarette. This behavior is repeated 250 times a day, or over 90 000 times a year for a "pack-a-day" smoker, multiplied by the number of years of smoking. The use of cigarettes in specific situations and during stress or emotional crisis also contributes to the psychological habit.

The pleasure of smoking is also a positive reinforcement.[5] Nicotine appears to produce euphoria or a "high" similar to some other addictive psychomotor stimulants. Within seven seconds of puffing on a cigarette, nicotine is delivered directly to the brain.[5] Once addicted, smokers continue to smoke to reduce unpleasant feelings arising from withdrawal, as well as to alleviate the unpleasant moods produced by stressors.[5] The weight gain associated with smoking cessation, resulting from increased hunger and eating, is also a reinforcement to continue smoking.[10]

Social situations further reinforce smoking addiction. For example, many smokers have a cigarette after a meal, while talking on the telephone or immediately on awakening. These acts are routine activities of daily living and will continue after smoking cessation. Friends and relatives may also smoke and the exsmoker may still associate with them.

As a result of the addictive nature of nicotine and the psychological and social aspects of smoking, it is understandably very difficult for smokers to quit. Only 20% of those who try to quit succeed on their first or second attempt, and up to 60% may take seven or more attempts.[6] *Relapse* is very common after periods of varying abstinence, up to 10 years, although most smokers are confirmed former smokers after two years.[2]

The health risks associated with smoking are well known and are attributable to not only the nicotine in tobacco, which causes the addiction, but also to the more than 4000 chemicals in tobacco smoke, 50 of which cause, initiate or promote cancer.[11] These include tar, ammonia, carbon monoxide, oxides of nitrogen and benzopyrene.[11]

Smoking is the single most common preventable cause of death and disability in Canada, resulting in 45 200 deaths in Canada in 1996 (29 229 male and 15 986 female), more than 20% of all deaths among Canadians.[12] Some of the important health risks associated with smoking are in Table 1.

In addition to the risk of smoking to the smoker, environmental tobacco smoke (ETS) or *second-hand smoke* puts friends and family of smokers at risk, accounting for over 300 lung cancer deaths each year.[12] The effects of ETS include eye and throat irritation, coughing, rhinitis, headaches, and various types of cancer, particularly lung cancer. It has been repeatedly linked to respiratory problems and recurrent acute otitis media in children as well as sudden infant death syndrome (SIDS).[25]

For the smoker who requires medication for various health conditions, there is added risk as a result of potential *drug interactions*. The various components of tobacco smoke may induce alterations in drug absorption, distribution, metabolism, excretion and effectiveness of many drugs. As a result, smokers may require larger doses or more frequent administration of drugs in order to maintain therapeutic blood levels. The following drugs may be affected in this way: theophylline,[26,27] tricyclic antidepressants (i.e., amitriptyline, desipramine, imipramine, nortriptyline),[26-28] selective serotonin reuptake inhibitors (SSRIs),[28] some antipsychotics (i.e., clozapine, chlorpromazine, haloperidol, fluphenazine, olanzapine, thiothixene),[28] estrogens,[26,27] warfarin,[27,29] some analgesics (i.e., pentazocine, propoxyphene),[26,27] flecainide,[26,27] benzodiazepines (i.e., chlordiazepoxide, diazepam),[26-28] propranolol[26,27] and cimetidine.[30]

Table 1: **Health Risks Associated with Smoking**

- *Cancer:* smoking accounts for about 30% of all *cancer*-related deaths. Cancer of the lung, pancreas, kidney, bladder, lip, oral cavity and pharynx, esophagus and larynx, are all increased 2-27 times for smokers compared to nonsmokers.[11]

- *Ascorbic acid:* smokers have been found to have lower serum ascorbic acid than nonsmokers (25% lower in those smoking less than 20 cigarettes daily and 40% lower in those smoking more than 20 cigarettes daily) and need twice as much vitamin C.[13]

- *Coronary artery disease and cerebral thrombosis:* smokers have two to four times higher risk of coronary artery disease, 1.5 times higher risk of cerebral thrombosis[14] and increased risk of arteriosclerotic peripheral vascular disease.[15]

- *Chronic obstructive lung disease:* oxidants in smoke particles cause reduced ciliary function and an increase in mucus production by goblet cells. Migration of inflammatory cells to the lung tissue leads to chronic obstructive lung disease including chronic bronchitis and emphysema.[16] There is also a higher incidence of lung and throat infections.[2]

- *Effects on infants:* smoking in pregnant women has been linked to *lower birth weight infants* (150 g lower on average at term) and a 25-50% increase in fetal and infant deaths, with 35% of all sudden infant death syndrome (SIDS) incidences accountable to maternal tobacco smoke.[17,18]

- *Oral diseases:* smoking increases oral diseases such as leukoplakia (white patches on oral mucosa that may become malignant) smoker's palate, impaired gingival bleeding, periodontitis and ulcerative gingivitis in addition to lip, mouth and throat cancers, resulting in death of 700 Canadians in 1996.[12,19]

- *Delayed wound healing:* possibly from cutaneous vasoconstriction, increased platelet adhesiveness and diminished proliferation of red blood cells, macrophages and fibroblasts.[20]

- *Insulin resistance:* chronic smokers have been found to have insulin resistance, with a recent study showing higher steady-state plasma glucose concentrations in smokers compared with nonsmokers in spite of similar steady-state plasma insulin concentrations.[21]

- *Impotence*, or *erectile dysfunction*: twice as likely to occur in smokers than non-smokers and exposure to second-hand smoke is a significant factor in becoming impotent.[13]

- *Ulcers:* increased incidence of bleeding and perforated ulcers.[22]

- *Musculoskeletal effects:* adversely affects bone mineral density, lumbar disk disease and the dynamics of bone and wound healing.[23]

- *Cosmetic dermatology effects:* causes premature aging of skin and wrinkling.[24]

In spite of these many risks of smoking, addiction to nicotine is common. In 1996–97, 5.8 million Canadians smoked (28.9% aged 15 or over; 31.5 % of males and 26.3% of females).[31] Although this has decreased from 1981 when 38.1% of Canadians reported smoking, more young men and women aged 15 to 19 years of age are smoking now (31% of females and 27.2% of males) than in 1989 (23.5% of females and 21.6% of males).

On the positive side, Canadian smokers are smoking fewer cigarettes per day on average (17.5 per day in 1996–97 compared to 20.6 per day in 1981) and 556 000 smokers or 10% of smokers quit smoking between 1994–5 and 1996–97, with 3% reporting that they had reduced their smoking to only occasionally.[32] *Reasons given for quitting* were overwhelmingly concerns about the effects of smoking on their physical health, although cost, pressure from family/friends and pregnancy were also reported. Unfortunately those who quit were replaced by 947 000 Canadians who became current smokers for the first time or resumed smoking between 1994–95 and 1996–97.[32]

For those who quit, there are immediate and longer term health benefits through reduced chances of developing heart disease, cancer, breathing problems and infections. Quitting before the age of 50 results in an overall reduction by half in the chances of dying in the next 15 years.[33]

Patient Assessment

Health professionals are in an ideal position to not only assist patients who want to quit smoking, but also to identify smokers and assist them in coming to a decision to quit smoking. Although most smokers (46% of those still smoking, 59% of those who have relapsed and 45% of new smokers)[32] report they would like to quit, the highly addictive nature of nicotine and smoking behavior makes quitting very difficult and relapse rates are very high. In most smoking cessation programs, a successful quit rate is considered to be between 15 and 20%, and most smokers attempt to quit several times before they finally succeed.[34] When confronted with a patient who may be eligible for a smoking cessation program, health professionals can follow the assessment plan illustrated in Figure 1.

Because the risks associated with nicotine addiction are so high, all health professionals should take the initiative to provide, at minimum, a brief intervention with patients to assess whether they are smokers. Once a patient has been identified as a smoker, it is important to proceed with an assessment that identifies which smoking cessation method would work best for the individual based on four characteristics of the smoker:[37,38]

- The extent of the person's motivation to quit
- The extent of the person's biological addiction to nicotine
- The extent of the person's psychological addiction to smoking
- Whether the smoker has tried to quit before, the method used and the outcome

Assessing the patient's motivation to quit is based on the "Stages of Change Model" of behavior change (see Chapter 3). In the *precontemplation* stage the patient is not thinking about quitting. The health professional can best help the patient by getting the patient to think and talk about smoking and to see "pros" for changing their behavior.[35] In the *contemplation* stage, the patient is thinking about quitting but not ready to quit. The health professional can help the patient to feel more committed and comfortable taking the next step, *preparation*. In the preparation stage, the patient has made the decision to quit and is getting ready. The health professional should help the patient feel confident in their decision and not to "fear failure." Once the patient is in the *action* stage where they are already involved in a quitting process, the health professional can help maintain the quitting behavior and deal with the threat of relapse as needed. Finally, when the patient is in *maintenance*, they have successfully quit but need to try to remain a non-smoker. The health professional can monitor the patient to prevent relapse or deal with it in a positive way if it does happen.[35] In dealing with a relapse, the health professional should emphasize that this attempt at quitting has been a good learning experience, and assist the patient to review the experience, identify personal strengths and weaknesses, and formulate a new quitting plan that includes strategies to deal with high-risk situations.[35]

In all stages beyond contemplation, it is useful for the health professional to proceed to assess the physical,

Figure 1: **Assessment of Patients with Nicotine Dependence**

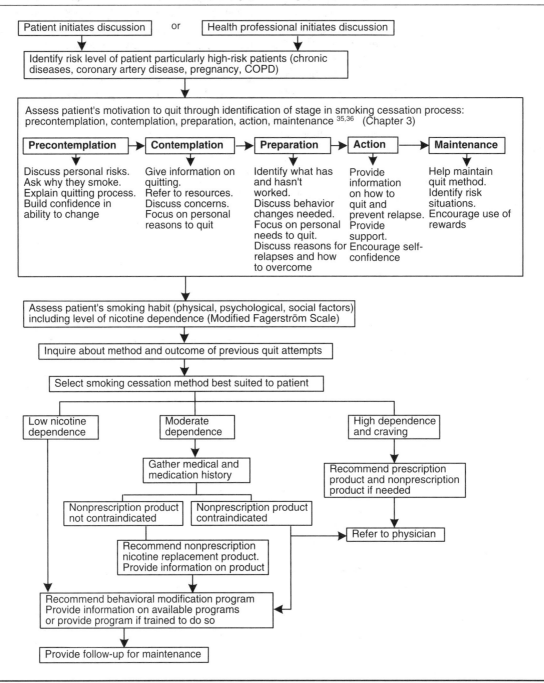

COPD = chronic obstructive pulmonary disease

psychological and social aspects of the patient's smoking habit by inquiring about:

Number of cigarettes smoked per day:
• Less than 15: light smoker
• 15-25: moderate smoker
• More than 25: heavy smoker

Times of day when smoking occurs:
• Immediately upon awakening
• During meals and coffee breaks
• With friends

Situations triggering smoking:
• Stressful situations
• Social situations
• Hunger or boredom

Social support to quit:
• Family and friends supportive

• Access to resources such as a drug benefit plan, group smoking cessation program by employer

Previous experiences quitting:
• Number of quit attempts
• Type of smoking cessation aids or programs used
• Reasons for resuming smoking
• Symptoms and intensity of nicotine withdrawal experienced

A series of questions to ask patients to assist in determining the level of nicotine dependence has been suggested by Fagerström and is adapted here in Figure 2.[39]

Having gathered this information, the health professional can determine the most appropriate smoking cessation treatment method for the patient.

Figure 2: **Modified Fagerström Nicotine Tolerance Scale**

Questions	A=0 point	B=1 point	C=2 points	Score
1. How soon after you wake up do you smoke your first cigarette?	After 30 min	Within 30 min	—	
2. Do you find it difficult to refrain from smoking in places where it is forbidden?	No	Yes	—	
3. Which of all the cigarettes you smoke in a day is the most satisfying one?	Any other than first one in the morning	First one in morning	—	
4. How many cigarettes a day do you smoke?	1-15	16-25	More than 26	
5. Do you smoke more during the morning than during the rest of the day?	No	Yes	—	
6. Do you smoke when you are so ill that you are in bed most of the day?	No	Yes	—	
7. Does the brand you smoke have a low, medium or high nicotine content?	Low	Medium	High	
8. How often do you inhale the smoke from your cigarette?	Never	Sometimes	Always	
			Total	

Score
< 5 – Low nicotine dependence
5-6 – Moderate nicotine dependence
7 – High nicotine dependence

Adapted from Fagerström KO. Measuring the degree of physical dependence to tobacco smoking with reference to individualization of treatment. *Addict Behav* 1978;3:235-41.[39]

Goals of Therapy[40]

- Assist the patient to reach the *maintenance* stage of smoking behavior change
- Assist the patient to identify their personal physical, psychological and social aspects of smoking
- Provide social support for behavior change through encouragement and assistance
- Help the patient to develop skills and assist in problem solving to achieve and maintain abstinence
- Relieve symptoms of nicotine withdrawal and craving for tobacco through pharmacologic therapy if necessary

Most commonly, smokers report quitting "on their own," through self-help either by "cold turkey" (completely stopping smoking), or through gradually cutting down on the number of cigarettes. This is relatively successful with a reported 16 to 20% quit rate (remaining abstinent at one year after quitting).[41,42] With the assistance of a cessation program of some sort, quit rates are still seldom more than 20% on average.[40] However, intensive clinical interventions (6 to 12 weeks of individual or group counseling led by a professional) are generally more successful than self-help or various kinds of public health programs (worksite, community, media) with quit rates from 20 to 40% for intensive clinical programs compared to 5 to 15% for public health programs.[43] Combining two or more methods for smoking cessation including both pharmacologic and nonpharmacologic therapies results in greater success.[41]

The US-based Agency for Health Care Policy and Research (AHCPR) conducted an extensive review of the literature on tobacco use and identified a plethora of possible components for a tobacco use program as shown in Table 2.[40] Since no single method seems to work well for everyone, the best approach is to tailor the program to the individual.

Nonpharmacologic Therapy

Nonpharmacologic therapy to treat nicotine addiction involves various behavioral interventions and alternative therapies. One or more of these methods combined may be sufficient for success in patients who are light smokers. It is also the most appropriate therapy for patients in whom pharmacologic therapy is contraindicated because of potential interaction with other medications used or because of other physical conditions such as severe heart disease or pregnancy.

Behavioral Modification Programs: Individual and Group Support Programs or Health Professional Counseling

Regardless of their level of nicotine dependence, encourage patients to participate in some sort of behavioral modification program. Light smokers may be able to quit using behavioral modification alone, but moderate to heavy smokers benefit most from the addition of pharmacologic therapy.

There are many self-help materials, group programs and counseling programs that patients can use alone and health professionals can refer patients to these. A partial list of the available programs which offer a variety of resources from booklets, to videos, to correspondence programs and materials for patients is provided in Table 3. A complete list of programs in each province is available on the Health Canada web site, "Guide to Tobacco Use Cessation Programs in Canada."[44]

Apparently only one in five smokers who are preparing to stop smoking actually seeks formal help with quitting.[45] Although smokers can become involved in self-help programs, health professionals should be providing behavioral interventions for all smokers,

---

Table 2: **Possible Components of a Tobacco Use Cessation Program**[40]

- Specialized assessment for nicotine dependence, motivation, readiness and stage of change, stress, self-efficacy, etc.
- General problem solving, coping skills, relapse prevention and stress management
- Weight, diet, nutrition counseling
- Exercise/fitness program
- Social support outside or within the program
- Aversion therapy
- Smoking reduction
- Relaxation and breathing training
- Setting a quit day
- Hypnosis
- Acupuncture
- Pharmacologic therapy
- Follow-up

---

regardless of the patient's motivation to quit. Even brief advice to quit from a primary care physician during a routine consultation has been found effective in increasing the number of smokers stopping for at least six months.[46-48] In general, greater contact between the patient and the program provider leads to greater success.[46] Programs and materials have been designed to assist health professionals in providing smoking cessation counseling to their patients, a few of which are also listed in Table 3.

Behavior programs usually involve a variety of behavior modification techniques such as relaxation training, stress management, cognitive restructuring, relapse prevention and the development of adaptive behaviors. Table 4 describes the types of behavioral support that health professionals can provide to patients who are quitting smoking.[49]

Health professionals should allow a minimum of 20 minutes, weekly for at least 4 weeks, increasing duration to more than 8 weeks where possible for improved efficacy.[49] Follow-up counseling extending to 1 or 2 years at 3, 6, 9 12, 18 and 24 months is also desirable.[45] The involvement of multiple providers is also desirable as it has been found to enhance treatment efficacy.[49]

Acupuncture

Acupuncture therapy for smoking cessation involves needles or staple-like attachments placed at strategic points under the skin on the surface of the nose or on the ear. It is based on the Chinese science of energy pathways in the body. There is no reliable scientific evidence of effectiveness in smoking cessation over the placebo effect, with most evaluations being poorly constructed, providing unreliable results.[41,50,51]

Table 3: **Smoking Cessation Programs Available in Canada for Self-Help and Health Professional Counseling**[44]

Program name	Brief description	Contact information
One Step at a Time–A Smoker's Guide to Quitting	Self-help program, by correspondence. Set of booklets for men and women	Windsor-Essex County Health Unit Tel.: (519) 258-2146 Ext 260
COMMIT Planning Guides	Brief self-help guides also available on Internet	Commit to A Healthier Brant, Brantford, ON E-mail: commit@commit.org
The Fresh Start Quit Smoking Program	16-h group program	Canadian Cancer Society Tel.: (416) 961-7223
In Control	Video and audio tape in 9 min segments over 13 days for low literacy smokers. Individual or group format	Canadian Lung Association Tel.: (613) 747-6776
New Tools for Survival, A Guide to Building Your Own Recovery	200-page manual aimed at long-term maintenance of smoking cessation	Neighbourhood Tobacco Recovery Network, Woodlawn, ON Tel.: (613) 832-1296
Guide Your Patients to a Smoke-Free Future	Materials for health professionals with various intervention options and self-help resources for distribution to patients	Canadian Council on Smoking and Health, Ottawa, ON Tel.: (613) 567-3050
BC Doctors' Stop-Smoking Project	Program to assist physicians set up a counseling program	Physicians' Stop-Smoking Project, SSP/BCMA Tel.: (604) 736-4566
How to Help Your Patients Stop Using Tobacco: A National Cancer Institute Manual for the Oral Health Team	Program to assist health professionals provide counseling programs	National Cancer Institute, US Department of Health and Human Services Tel.: (301) 496-5583

Table 4: **Behavioral Assistance That Health Professionals Should Provide**[35,45,49]

Set quit date	Ask patient to decide on a specific date to quit within the next 2 wks (if using nicotine replacement therapy) or to agree on a schedule to reduce smoking.
Suggest methods to counter the urge to smoke	Help patients to identify triggers such as coffee drinking or ash trays and suggest ways to avoid them (e.g., removing all ashtrays from house or from table in restaurant, change to drinking tea). Help patient plan distractions (e.g., exercise, relaxation techniques, low-calorie snacks).
Manage "high-risk" situations	Assist the patient to identify and develop coping skills for situations where smoking risk is highest.
Identify supports	Work with the patient to identify people or programs that can provide support for quitting.
Establish goals and rewards	Help the patient establish a goal for quitting and rewards to increase motivation.
Provide follow-up support	Monthly for 3 mos, then at 6-12 mos for successful quitters; for those who fail to quit with treatment and require additional therapy and counseling, provide closer follow-up (every 2 wks for 3 mos, then at 6, 9, 12, 18 and 24 mos).
Deal with relapse	If relapse occurs, help patient to learn from it and plan for next attempt. Assist the patient to review the experience, to identify personal strengths and weaknesses, and to formulate a new quitting plan that includes strategies to deal with high-risk situations.

Aversion Therapy

Aversion therapy is based in the concept that association of an unpleasant sensation with smoking can reduce the desire to smoke. Techniques used have included mild electric shock; breath-holding; rapid smoking; unpleasant taste, noise or smell; and imagined stimuli. There is a lack of good methodologic studies to support this type of therapy although rapid or excessive smoking has been found to be the most promising of the aversion techniques. Due to concerns about the potentially harmful effect on the heart and lungs of this method of aversion therapy, it is not recommended as a smoking cessation method.[41,51]

Hypnosis

Hypnosis is a deep, relaxed state of attention during which people are more responsive to suggestions. Hypnotherapy for nicotine addiction attempts to change a person's habits and attitudes to cigarettes. The therapist's skill and experience are very important, as are the patient's susceptibility to hypnosis and

desire to quit. Schwartz reviewed over 50 reports and critiques and concluded that there is good evidence that some success in smoking cessation can be found with hypnosis, particularly if it is combined with behavioral modification or counseling.[41] Follow-up counseling and support or combining the therapy with other smoking cessation methods may also improve the success of hypnotherapy.[41,51,52]

Laser Therapy

In laser therapy a laser beam is directed at certain key points of the body surface, as in acupuncture. This stimulation of key points apparently triggers a release of endorphins, which relieve symptoms of craving for nicotine. There have been no reliable studies to support the success of this therapy.[41,51]

Clove and Herbal Cigarettes

There are various products available in the form of cigarettes that contain ingredients other than tobacco, providing a previous smoker with the smoking behaviour without providing nicotine. However, these products, which contain cloves and various herbs, may also contain tar, carbon monoxide and various other toxins. In fact, studies have shown that clove cigarettes actually contain up to 70% of tobacco, providing nicotine and the dangers of all-tobacco cigarettes.[53,54]

Pharmacologic Therapy

Pharmacologic therapy available to assist patients in smoking cessation includes two basic types of therapy: nicotine replacement therapy and non-nicotine therapies. Products that cause an unpleasant sensation when the individual smokes and products that simulate the tracheobronchial sensations elicited by smoking are no longer available in Canada. In the United States, all smoking cessation products except those containing nicotine have been ordered off the market because of the lack of data to substantiate claims.

The purpose of pharmacologic therapy to aid smoking cessation is to reduce the physical effects of nicotine withdrawal such as irritability, anxiety, difficulty concentrating, drowsiness, hunger, GI symptoms, headaches and disturbed sleep, which peak within 72 hours and may continue intermittently for several weeks.[7] In addition, pharmacologic therapy is needed for some patients to reduce the psychological effects of withdrawal with respect to the craving for nicotine, which can last up to several years, or as some ex-smokers will attest, indefinitely.[6,9] While many patients may benefit from pharmacologic therapy, some patients may not require it to successfully quit, particularly those who are mildly addicted to nicotine. In addition, medication may be contraindicated for certain patients because of potential drug or disease interactions.

Nicotine Replacement Therapy

There are a number of different forms of nicotine medication which replace the nicotine in the cigarette, and are thus referred to as nicotine replacement therapy. Although originally supplied by prescription only, they are now available as nonprescription products in Canada. In some provinces some products are restricted to pharmacy-only sales. These products include polacrilex chewing pieces (gum) and several different brands of transdermal patches, although nasal sprays and inhalers have also been investigated.

Table 5 lists the various products and their dosages, adverse effects, drug interactions, and contraindications. In general, provided that the patient receives adequate counseling on the appropriate use of these products, the incidence of side effects or adverse effects are few. Pay particular attention to the contraindications involving heart diseases. However, given the significant risks of continued smoking, patients with heart disease and pregnant patients may be at less risk from using pharmacotherapeutic smoking cessation methods than continuing to smoke.[61,62]

The different forms of nicotine replacement therapy are generally equally effective.[46] Various studies show quit rates at 6 to 12 months of 17 to 34% for the patch versus 9 to 27% for the gum in comparison to 12% for placebo.[62] Combining behavioral programs with nicotine replacement therapy results in greater success than either treatment alone.[46] For heavy smokers who continue to suffer withdrawal symptoms while using a single nicotine patch, daily doses of nicotine may be increased up to 35 mg per day for smokers previously using 21 to 40 cigarettes a day, and up to 40 mg per day for smokers previously using more than 40 cigarettes a day, with reported safety and improved efficacy.[63-65] This may be achieved by additional chewing pieces or patches or the combination of both. It has been suggested that combining the nicotine patch and gum may provide more complete nicotine replacement since it provides a baseline steady level of nicotine with "boluses" of nicotine for flexibility and treatment of cravings. However, there have been concerns about the risk of this becoming addicting, and should therefore be used only under close supervision.[45]

Other Medications

A number of other therapeutic agents have been investigated for use in nicotine addiction. Clonidine is somewhat effective but of limited use because of significant side effects.[46,66,67] Other agents tested include tricyclic antidepressants, moclobemide, benzodiazepines, beta-blockers, lobeline, cimetidine and SSRIs, but study limitations and conflicting findings limit proper evaluation of these agents at this time.[46,55,68,69]

Bupropion, an antidepressant, has been found to be an effective smoking cessation aid.[46,47,70] It is a different approach to smoking cessation since it affects CNS

Table 5: Nonprescription Drug Therapy for Nicotine Addiction[45,55-60]

Drug	Dosage	Adverse effects[56,58,59]	Contraindications (CI)/ Drug interactions*	Comments
Nicotine Resin Complex (Nicorette® 2 mg, Nicorette Plus® 4 mg)	4 mg = 1 cigarette per hour 2 mg = ½ cigarette per hour Up to 20 pieces per day. One piece should be bitten once or twice then "parked." This is repeated for up to 30 min when desire to smoke arises. Then discard piece. Gradually reduce dose to one per day over 3 mos, continuing for maximum of 6 mos as shown in chart (a) below.	Hiccups; jaw, mouth or throat soreness; changes in taste perception; GI (indigestion, nausea, vomiting); CNS (insomnia, dizziness, irritability, headache, confusion, convulsions, depression, euphoria, numbness, paresthesia, syncope, tinnitus, weakness); CV (edema, hypertension, palpitations, tachyarrhythmias, tachycardia, chest pain); dermatologic (erythema, itching, rash, urticaria); respiratory (breathing difficulty, cough, hoarseness, sneezing, wheezing). Rare reports of miscarriage, MI, CHF, CV accident and cardiac arrest but link to Nicorette® not established. Rare severe allergic reaction.	**Contraindications:** Smoking while using this medication; immediately following postmyocardial infarction; life-threatening arrhythmia; severe angina pectoris; temporomandibular joint disease; pregnancy; breastfeeding; children under 18 years of age **Drug interactions:** Acetaminophen, caffeine, imipramine, oxazepam, pentazocine, propranolol, theophylline, insulin, adrenergic antagonists (e.g., prazosin, labetalol), propoxyphene, adrenergic agonists (e.g., isoproterenol, phenylephrine)	Should not be chewed like gum but bitten once or twice, then "parked" between cheek and gum, wait a minute, then repeat for about 30 min. Avoid use of acidic beverages while chewing as this decreases absorption (e.g., coffee, fruit juices). Excreted in breast milk.
Nicotine Transdermal Patches: 16 Hour Patches: Nicotrol® 5, 10, 15 mg; 24 Hour Patches: Habitrol® 7, 14, 21 mg; Nicoderm® 7, 14, 21 mg; Prostep® 11, 22 mg	Patch applied to non-hairy, clean, dry skin site in upper arm or hip using a different site each day. Apply upon waking and remove at bedtime, 16–24 h per day. Dosage should be started at highest strength for heavy smoker, or intermediate dose for light or moderate smoker, gradually reducing strength over a period of 6–16 wks as shown in chart (b) below. Adjustment should be made for patients under 45 kg or those with CV disease.	Skin reactions at application site (erythema, pruritus, burning, edema, blisters, rash, burning sensation); headache; weakness; flu syndrome; pain; CV (palpitations, chest pain, blood pressure changes, tachycardia); GI (abdominal pain, dyspepsia, nausea, diarrhea, constipation, dry mouth, nausea and vomiting, flatulence, stomatitis; myalgia; arthralgia; arthritis; dysmenorrhea; toothache; CNS (insomnia, dizziness, abnormal dreams, nervousness, depression, hypertonia, somnolence, paresthesia, anxiety, emotional lability); respiratory (cough, pharyngitis, rhinitis, dyspnea, sinusitis); miscellaneous (sweating, taste perversion, fatigue); allergic reaction.	**Contraindications:** Smoking while using this medication. Severe renal impairment. Immediately following post myocardial infarction; life-threatening arrhythmia; severe angina pectoris; recent cerebral vascular accident; breastfeeding; children under 18 years of age; generalized skin disorders. Relative CI: Pregnancy; atopic or eczematous dermatitis. Caution in hyperthyroidism, pheochromocytoma, insulin-dependent diabetes, active peptic ulcers, accelerated hypertension. **Drug interactions:** Acetaminophen, caffeine, imipramine, oxazepam, pentazocine, propranolol, theophylline, insulin, adrenergic antagonists (e.g., prazosin, labetalol), propoxyphene, adrenergic agonists (e.g., isoproterenol, phenylephrine).	Assess patient in first 2 wks to ensure smoking has been discontinued or medication discontinued if smoking is continuing. Benefits of smoking cessation need to be weighed against risks of nicotine replacement therapy for patients with accelerated hypertension, CV or peripheral vascular disease, pregnancy Remove patch during prolonged strenuous activity to avoid nicotine toxicity from increased absorption. Rotate patch application sites daily, preferably upper arm and upper chest.

Used patches should be folded so that medicated sides are facing and discarded safely away from reach of children or pets.

*Smoking may affect certain medications, requiring an increased dose of the medication in most cases, and nicotine replacement will continue to similarly affect medications. When smoking and nicotine replacement therapy are discontinued, medications may require adjustment to a decreased dose. [54-58]

(a) Dosage Chart for Nicotine Resin Complex[57]

Number of cigarettes smoked/day	Month 1- First 2 weeks Pieces/Day	Month 1- Second 2 weeks Pieces/Day	Month 2 Pieces/Day	Month 3 Pieces/Day	Months 4-6 Pieces/Day
20 or more	20	15	10	5	1 if the urge to smoke returns
15-19	16	12	6	3	Same as above
11-14	12	9	5	3	Same as above
10 or less	10	8	4	2	Same as above

(b) Dosage Chart for Nicotine Patches[45]

Habitrol®	Nicoderm®	Nicotrol®	Prostep®
21 mg/24 h × 3-4 wks	21 mg/24 h × 6 wks	15 mg/16 h × 8 wks	22 mg/24 h × 6-12 wks
14 mg/24 h × 3-4 wks	14 mg/24 h × 2 wks	10 mg/16 h × 2 wks	11 mg/24 h × 6-12 wks
7 mg/24 h × 3-4 wks	7 mg/24 h × 2 wks	5 mg/16 h × 2 wks	

GI = gastrointestinal; CNS = central nervous system; CV = cardiovascular; MI = myocardial infarction; CHF = congestive heart failure pathways to reduce the effects of withdrawal, particularly the craving for nicotine. The effectiveness of bupropion treatment for seven weeks versus placebo one year after quitting are reported in the range of other smoking cessation therapies (23% vs. 12%).[71] A placebo-controlled study comparing bupropion 300 mg per day alone or nicotine transdermal 21 mg per day alone versus the two combined resulted in six month and one year cessation rates of 30% and 23% respectively for bupropion alone; 18% and 12% respectively for the nicotine transdermal alone; 33% and 28% for the combined use; compared to 13% and 8% for placebo.[69] The quit rates for the combination were statistically significantly better (p < 0.05) than placebo or nicotine transdermal alone but not compared to bupropion alone. Bupropion alone was also statistically significantly better (p < 0.05) than placebo or nicotine transdermal alone.[72]

Since bupropion is an antidepressant, there are a number of contraindications including pregnancy, breastfeeding, history of seizures, anorexia or bulimia, and taking MAOIs. Patients who are alcohol-dependent, taking St. John's wort or SSRI antidepressants should exercise caution while on bupropion.[72] There are also a number of side effects ranging from the more common dry mouth and insomnia to the more rare hypertension, arthralgia, myalgia, dizziness, tremor, somnolence, bronchitis, pruritus, rash and taste perversion.[72] At this time, this drug is available only on a doctor's prescription in Canada.

As with other pharmacotherapeutic agents for smoking cessation, bupropion should be used in combination with behavioral programs to assist the quitting process.[72]

Monitoring of Therapy

Because of the large behavioral component of nicotine addiction and attempts at withdrawal, monitoring of therapy is crucial to the success of smoking cessation therapy. Ideally, through involvement in a smoking cessation program, the patient receives ongoing monitoring for a period of time by a clinician or therapist involved with the program. If a formal program that includes this service is not provided, then the pharmacist providing the medication or nurse or physician prescribing the treatment should provide this.

Smoking relapse rates are high, particularly at the beginning of smoking cessation, with 66% reportedly relapsing within 48 hours and 76% within the first week when patients attempt to self-quit.[49] As a result, follow-up should begin within the initial week following the quit date, particularly if the patient is receiving nicotine replacement therapy, in order to avoid adverse effects from excessive nicotine levels. Follow-up counseling should be provided every month for three months, then at six months, and at one year.[45] Additional monitoring should be considered for patients who are at high risk: heavily nicotine-addicted with many previous smoking cessation attempts; under severe psychosocial stress; with other addictions such as alcohol or drugs; on medication that interacts with nicotine; with history of clinical depression or schizophrenia; for whom cessation is medically urgent.[45] This more intensive monitoring should include follow-up every 2 weeks for the first 3 months, then at 6, 9, 12, 18, and 24 months.[45]

Also monitor the patient for side effects or adverse effects resulting from the pharmocotherapeutic smoking cessation therapy, and for the effectiveness of treatment in reducing or preventing nicotine withdrawal symptoms as shown in Table 6.

Advice for the Patient

Regardless of the stage that the patient is at in their decision to quit smoking, the health professional should provide advice and encouragement to the patient to quit. This should include information about the dangers of smoking, the benefits of quitting smoking, and methods and resources available to assist in quitting smoking.

Once the patient has decided to take action and a plan has been developed, the patient information provided by the manufacturers along with the medication is an excellent resource for them. Review it with patients, and encourage them in the behavioral aspects of quitting.

Resource Tips

Patients can also do a self-assessment that leads them through these questions by logging onto a web site developed by Health Canada: http:www.hc-sc.gc.ca/hecs-sesc/tobacco/index.html

Table 6: **Monitoring Therapy for Nicotine Addiction**

Parameter	Indicators/Goal/ Time frame	Monitoring	Health professional's recommended actions
Smoking	Patient reports no smoking immediately.	Daily by patient; by health professional according to schedule recommended (at 1 wk, every month for 3 mos, once at 6 mos, and 1 yr)	Inquire as to smoking level, encourage and support. If patient has a relapse, discontinue nicotine replacement therapy until patient is ready to quit again; encourage patient to reset a quit date; discuss possible reasons for relapse and help patient strategize ways to be more successful with the next quit attempt; avoid scolding the patient but rather provide empathy.
Desire to smoke	Patient reports level of desire reducing to minimal by end of therapy (3-6 mos) (craving may never completely end).	As above	Intense craving may require additional treatment (e.g., bupropion). Encourage behavioral changes to distract desire; empathize with patient's difficulty and strongly support endurance.
Nicotine withdrawal symptoms	Patient reports reduced or lack of withdrawal symptoms within 25 min to 24 h, (e.g., irritability, anxiety, difficulty concentrating, drowsiness, hunger, GI symptoms, headaches and disturbed sleep).	As above	If symptoms are bothersome, consider increasing dosage, switching or adding an alternative method of nicotine replacement therapy.
Medication adverse effects	Patient reports no adverse effects when questioned specifically throughout duration of pharmacotherapeutic treatment.	As above	If minor side effects occur, suggest ways to modify (e.g., for belching and GI upset with gum, advise slower chewing); or consider switching to an alternative method of nicotine replacement therapy. If serious adverse effect (e.g., hypertension), consider reducing dose or discontinuing medication and switching to alternative (e.g., bupropion).
Weight gain[73]	Patient reports minimal weight gain over the 6-12 mos following quitting.	Weekly by patient. By health professional according to schedule recommended as above	Reassure patient that weight gain is generally only slight (about 5 kg in first year after quitting). Encourage healthy eating habits, exercise, having healthy snacks available to deal with cigarette cravings (e.g., carrot sticks).
Stress	Patient reports minimal additional stress due to smoking cessation over 6-12 mos following quitting.	Daily by patient. By health professional according to schedule recommended as above	Assess for evidence of excessive stress by patient report or physical and behavioral evidence (weight loss, nervous habits, GI symptoms, headache). Suggest behavioral therapy (i.e., deep breathing, muscle relaxation, positive self-talk). Or refer to stress management program Encourage exercise and other distracting activities. Treat stress-related symptoms as needed (refer to physician, recommend appropriate medication to reduce stress, or treat stress-related physical symptoms).

Suggested Readings

Kuz G. Kicking butt. *Pharm Pract* 1999;15(5):50-53, 57-59, 63.

Nolan RP. Smoking cessation. In: Gray J, ed. *Therapeutic Choices*. 2nd ed. Ottawa: Canadian Pharmaceutical Association; 2000:343-49.

Roberts G, Wynn M, Smith K. Health Canada. *Guide to Tobacco Use Cessation Programs in Canada*. Health Canada Online: Available from www.hc-sc.gc.ca/hesc-sesc/tobacco/quitting/cessation/tobrpt2.html. Accessed Mar 30, 2001.

Smoking Behaviour of Canadians, Cycle 1. 1994/95 and Cycle 2, 1996/97, Who is quitting and why? *National Population Health Survey Highlights*, No. 1, Ottawa: Health Canada, January 1999. Available from www.hc-sc.gc.ca/main/lcdc/web/bc/nphs/nphs18_e.html.

Smoking Cessation. Living Smoke Free, On the Road to Quitting, Health Canada Online, Ottawa: Health Canada, updated Jan 17, 2001. Available from www.hc-sc.gc.ca/hppb/cessation/road/self_diagnosis/unit3/13.html.

Smoking in Canada during the past 16 years. *Quick Facts on Smoking in Canada*, Wired Health, Health Promotion Online. Ottawa: Health Canada, January 1999: Available from www.hc-sc.gc.ca/hppb/wired/smoking.html.

References

1. Pollin W. The role of the addictive process as a key step in causation of all tobacco related diseases (editorial). *JAMA* 1984;252:287.
2. US Department of Health and Human Services. *The Health Consequences of Smoking: Nicotine Addiction. A Report of The Surgeon General*. Rockville, Maryland: Public Health Service, Centers for Disease Control, Center for Health Promotion and Education, Office in Smoking and Health; 1988. DHHS publication no. (CDC) 88-8406.
3. Tobacco, Nicotine and Addiction: A Committee Report Prepared at the Request of The Royal Society of Canada for the Health Protection Branch, Health and Welfare Canada, 1989.
4. Hunt WA, Barnett LW, Branch LG. Relapse rates in addiction programs. *J Clin Psychol*. 1971;27:455-56.
5. Fiore M, Jorenby D, Baker T, et al. Tobacco dependence and the nicotine patch. Clinical guidelines for effective use. *JAMA* 1992;268(19)L 2687-2694.
6. Gossel TA: The Physiological and Pharmacological Effects of Nicotine. *U.S. Health Professional Supplement*, February, 1992.
7. Hughes JR, Hatsukami D. Signs and symptoms of tobacco withdrawal. *Arch Gen Psych* 1986;43:289-94.
8. William, M. Effectiveness of clonidine in smoking cesarion. *Can J Hosp Pharm* 1992;45:77-78.
9. Gourlay SG, McNeill JJ: Antismoking products. *Med J Australia*, 1990;153:699-704.
10. Coambs RB, Li S, Kozlowski L. Age interacts with heaviness of smoking in predicting success in cessation of smoking. *Am J Epidemiol*, 1992;135:240-246.
11. Monograph on the Evaluation of the Carcinogenic Risk of Chemicals to Humans. Tobacco Smoking, Vol.38. WHO. International Agency for Research on Cancer 1985, Switzerland.
12. Makomaski-Illing EM, Kaiserman MJ. Mortality Attributable to Tobacco Use in Canada and its Regions. 1994 and 1996. *Chronic Dis Can* 1999;20:111-117.3.
13. Feldman HA, Johannes CB, Derby CA, Kleinman KP, Mohr BA, Araujo AB, McKinlay JB. Erectile Dysfunction and Coronary Risk Factors: Prospective Results from the Massachusetts Male Aging Study. *Prev Med* 2000;30:328-338.
14. McGill HC. The cardiovascular pathology of smoking. *Am J Heart*. 1988;115:250-7.
15. US Department of Health and Human Services. The Health Consequences of Smoking: The Changing Cigarette. A report of the Surgeon General. Rockville, Maryland: Public Health Service, Centers for Disease Control, Center for Health Promotion and Education, 1981.
16. McCusker K. Mechanisms of respiratory tissue injury from cigarette smoking. *Am J Med* 1992;93(suppl 1A):25S-31S.
17. Southall, DP. Samuels MP. Reducing the risks in sudden infant death syndrome (editorial). *Br Med J* 1992;304: 265-266.
18. U.S. Department of Health and Human Services. Reducing the Health Consequences of Smoking: 25 years of progress. A Report of the Surgeon General, Rockville, Maryland: U.S. Department of Health and Human Services, Public Health Service, Centers for Disease Control, Center for Chronic Disease Prevention and Health Promotion, Office on Smoking and Health, 1989.
19. Christen AG. The impact of tobacco use and cessation on oral and dental diseases and conditions. *Am J Med* 1992; 93(suppl 1A):25S-31S.
20. Silverstein P. Smoking and wound healing. *Am J Med* 1992;93(suppl 1A):22S-24S.
21. Facchini FS, Hollenbeck CB, Jeppesen J. Insulin resistance and cigarette smoking. *Lancet* 1992;339:1128-30.
22. Anderson IB, Jargensen TT, Bonnevie OO, et al. Smoking and alcohol intake as risk factors for bleeding and perforated peptic ulcers. A population based cohort study. *Epidemiol* 2000;11:434-9.
23. Porter SE, Hanly EN Jr. The musculoskeletal effects of smoking. *J Am Acad Orthop Surg* 2001;9:9-17.
24. Aizen EE, Gilhar AA. Smoking effect on skin wrinkling in aged population. *Int J Dermatol* 2001 Jul;40:431-3.
25. DiFranza, JR, Lew RA. Effect of Maternal Cigarette Smoking on Pregnancy Complications and Sudden Infant Death Syndrome. *J Fam Pract* 1995;385-394
26. Schein JR. Cigarette smoking and clinically significant drug ineractions. *Ann Pharmacother* 1995;29:1139-1147.
27. Tatro DS. Effects of smoking on drug therapy. *Drug Newsletter* 1994;13:49-51.
28. Bezchlibnyk-Butleer KZ, Jeffries JJ, eds. *Clinical Handbook of Psychotropic Drugs*. 11th edition. Seattle: Hogrefe and Huber Publishers, 2001.
29. Colucci VJ, Knapp JF. Increase in international normalized ratio associated with smoking cessation. *Ann Pharmacother* 2001;35:385-386 (letter).

30. Hansten PD, Horn JR. *Drug Interactions Analysis and Management*. Missouri: Facts and Comparisons, 2001.
31. Smoking in Canada During the Past 16 Years. Quick facts on smoking in Canada, Wired Health, Health Promotion Online. Health Canada, January, 1999. Available from www.hc-sc.gc.ca/hppb/wired/smoking.html.
32. Smoking Behaviour of Canadians, Cycle 1. 1994/95 and Cycle 2, 1996/97, Who is quitting and why? National Population Health Survey Highlights, No. 1, Health Canada, January 1999: www.hc-sc.gc.ca/main/lcdc/web/bc/nphs/nphs18_e.html
33. Smoking Cessation. Living Smoke Free, On the road to quitting, Health Canada Online, Health Canada, updated Jan 17, 2001. Available from www.hc-sc.gc.ca/hppb/cessation/road/self_diagnosis/unit3/13.html.
34. Joint Statement, Tobacco: The Role of Health Professionals In Smoking Cessation, Canadian Association of Occupational Therapists, Canadian Association of Social Workers, Canadian Dental Association, Canadian Medical Association, Canadian Nurses Association, Canadian Pharmacists Association, Canadian Physiotherapy Association, Canadian Psychological Association and Canadian Society of Respiratory Therapists. *Can Pharm J* 2001;134:34-35.
35. Smoking Cessation – Living Smoke Free, Education Resources & Research, Getting Smoke-free: An information kit for community organizations working with women. understanding and using the stages of change. Health Canada Online, Health Canada, updated Jan 17, 2001. Available from www.hc-sc.ca/hppb/cessation/resou... ofessional/getting-smoke-free/change7.html.
36. DiClemente CC. Changing addictive behaviors: A process perspective. *Amer Psychol Soc* 1993;2:101-106.
37. Godenick MT. Review of available smoking cessation methods, 1989. Part I and II. *Maryland Med J* 1989;38:277-279:377-380.
38. Prochaska JO, Velicer, WF, Rossi JS, et al. Stages of change and decisional balance for 12 problem behaviors. *Health Psychol* 1994;13:39-46.
39. Fagerström KO. Measuring the degree of physical dependence to tobacco smoking with reference to individualization of treatment. *Addict Behav* 1978;3:235-41.
40. Fiore MC, Bailey WC, Cohen SJ, et al. Smoking cessation. Clinical practice guideline No.18. Rockville, MD: U.S. Department of Health and Human Services, Public Health Service, Agency for Health Care Policy and Research, April 1996, no 96-0692.
41. Shwartz, JL. Review and evaluation of smoking cessation methods: The United States and Canada, 1978-1985. National Cancer Institute: U.S. Department of Health and Human Services, Public Health Service, National Institutes of Health, 1987. Rockville, MD. NIH Publication No.87. p. 2940.
42. Fiore MC, Novotny TS, Pierce JP. Methods used to quit smoking in the United States. Do cessation programs help *JAMA* 1990;263:2760-2765.
43. Prochaska JA. A stage paradigm for integrating clinical and public health approaches to smoking cessation. *Addic Behav* 1996;21:721-732.
44. Roberts G, Wynn M, Smith K. Health Canada. Guide to tobacco use cessation pPrograms in Canada. Health Canada Online. Available from www.hc-sc.gc.ca/hppb/tobaccoreduction/bub/tobrpt l.html. Accessed March 30, 2001.
45. Bass, F. Smoking cessation. In: Gray J, ed. *Therapeutic Choices*. 1st ed. Ottawa: Canadian Pharmaceutical Association; 1995:268-75.
46. Fiore MC, Bailey WC, Cohen SJ, et al. Treating tobacco use and dependence. A clinical practice guideline. Rockville, MD: US Department of Health and Human Services, 2000
47. West R, McNeill A and Raw M. Smoking cessation guidelines for health professionals: an update. Thorax. 2000;55:987-999.
48. A clinical practice guideline for treating tobacco use and dependence: A US Public Health Service report. The tobacco use and dependence clinical practice guideline panel, staff and consortium representative. *JAMA* 2000;283:3244-3254.
49. Nolan RP. Smoking cessation. In: Gray J, ed. *Therapeutic Choices*. 2nd ed. Ottawa: Canadian Pharmaceutical Association; 2000. p. 343-49.
50. White AR, Rampes H, Ernst E. Acupuncture for smoking cessation (Cochrane Review). Cochrane Database Syst Rev 2000;3.
51. Shwartz JL. Methods for smoking cessation. *Clinics Chest Med*, 1991;12:737-753.
52. Pederson LL, Scrimgeour WG, Defcoe NM. Comparison of hypnosis plus counselling, counselling alone and hypnosis alone in a community service smoking withdrawal program. *J Consult Clinical Psychol* 1975;43:920l.
53. Illnesses possibly associated with smoking clove cigarettes, morbidity and mortality weekly report, U.S. Centers for Disease Control, 1985;34(21):297-299.
54. Information alert: Tobacco-less cigarettes, addiction research foundation, October 1993.
55. Hughes JR, Stead LF, Lancaster T. Anxiolytics for smoking cessation (Cochrane Review). Cochrane Database Syst Rev 2000;4.
56. Nicorette®, Nicorette Plus® monograph. In: Repchinsky, C, ed. *Compendium of Pharmaceuticals and Specialties*, 37th ed. Ottawa: Canadian Pharmacists Association; 2002:11 21-1123.
57. Nicorette®, Patient Information. In: Repchinsky, C, ed. *Compendium of Pharmaceuticals and Specialties*, 37th ed. Ottawa: Canadian Pharmacists Association; 2002:B169-170.
58. Nicotrol® monograph. In: Repchinsky, C, ed. *Compendium of Pharmaceuticals and Specialties*, 37th ed. Ottawa: Canadian Pharmacists Association; 2002:1123-1125.
59. Nicoderm® monograph. In: Repchinsky, C, ed. *Compendium of Pharmaceuticals and Specialties*, 37th ed. Ottawa: Canadian Pharmacists Association; 2002:1119-1121.
60. Habitrol® monograph. In: Repchinsky, C, ed. *Compendium of Pharmaceuticals and Specialties*, 37th ed. Ottawa: Canadian Pharmacists Association; 2002:711-712.
61. Benowitz N. Nicotine replacement therapy during pregnancy. *JAMA* 1991;266:3174-7.
62. Repchinsky C. Nicotine replacement therapy. *Can Pharm J* 1993;27(3):87-88.
63. Gourlay S. The pros and cons of transdermal nicotine therapy. *Med J Aust* 1994:152-9.
64. Dale LC, Hurt RD, Offord KP, et al High-dose nicotine patch therapy. *JAMA* 1995;274:135-8.
65. Dale LC, Hurt RD, Hays JT, et al. Drug therapy to aid in smoking cessation. *Postgrad Med* 1998;104.75-84.
66. Gourlay SG, Stead LF, Benowitz NL. Clonidine for smoking cessation (Cochrane Review). Cochrane Database Sys Rev 2000;3.
67. William M. Effectiveness of clonidine in smoking cessation. *Can J Hosp Pharm*. 1992;45:77-78.
68. Covey LS, Sullivan MA, Johnston JA et al. Advances in non-nicotine pharmacotherapy for smoking cessation. *Drugs* 2000;59:17-31.

69. Stead LF, Hughes JR. Lobeline for smoking cessation (Cochrane Review). Cochrane Database Syst Rev 2000;3.
70. Hughes JR, Stead LF, Lancaster T. Antidepressants for smoking cessation (Cochrane Review). Cochrane Database Syst Rev 2000;4.
71. Hurt RD, Rachs DPL, Glover ED et al. A comparison of sustained-release bupropion and placebo for smoking cessation. *N Engl J Med* 1997;337:1195-202.
72. Zyban® monograph. In: Repchinsky, C, ed. *Compendium of Pharmaceuticals and Specialties*, 37th ed. Ottawa: Canadian Pharmacists Association; 2002:1942-1945.
73. O'Hara P, Connett JE, Lee WW, et al. Early and late weight gain following smoking cessation in the Lung Health Study. *Am J Epidemiol* 1998;148:821-830.

Smoking Cessation—Patient Information

Congratulations on deciding to quit smoking! Whether this is your first time quitting, or you have tried to quit before, follow these tips to be successful.

- Set a quit date. It should be within the next two weeks. Avoid a time when you will be under stress.
- Think about why you want to quit and all the good things that you expect as a result of quitting.
- If you have tried to quit before, you have probably learned some valuable tips of what *not* to do this time. Think about what was most difficult last time, and why you gave up trying. Think about the things you need to avoid this time.
- Find a smoking cessation group or a pharmacist, nurse or doctor who you can see regularly over the next six months to a year to help you stick to your plan.
- Tell your family and friends that you are quitting. Ask them to help you to stick to your plan. If they smoke, ask them to respect your decision to quit and to not smoke in front of you. Think of things you can do to avoid smoking while with them.
- Find someone you know who does not smoke and ask them to help you to quit.
- Make a diary for a few days to keep track of when and why you smoke.
- Think of ways to avoid situations when you usually smoke.
- Think of things you can do instead of smoking; for example chewing gum, sipping water, holding a fake cigarette.
- You may put on up to five pounds of weight while quitting, so plan how you can avoid this with healthy eating and increased activity. Watch your diet, and plan to keep healthy snacks around for when you get the urge to nibble. Keep busy with healthy activities like walking or an exercise program. Starting a new activity will help to break old ways of acting when you smoked.
- If you are taking medication to help you to quit, be sure to follow the instructions carefully. If you are taking nicotine replacement therapy, *do not* continue smoking, as this is very dangerous for your health.

Respiratory Section Highlights

Chapter 12: **Allergic Rhinitis**

Prevention
    Pollen
    Outdoor and indoor molds
    House dust mites
    Animal allergens
Nonprescription agents for allergic rhinitis
    Oral antihistamines
    Mast cell stabilizers
    Decongestants
Prescription therapy
Alternative therapy
Management of allergic rhinitis in children
Management of allergic rhinitis during pregnancy and breastfeeding

Chapter 13: **Upper Respiratory Tract Infections**

The common cold
Influenza
Sinusitis
Pharyngitis
Cough
Differential diagnosis of upper respiratory tract infections
Prevention
    Influenza vaccine
    Antivirals
Pharmacologic Therapy
    Antihistamines
    Decongestants
    Antitussives
    Expectorants
    Natural products
    Antivirals
Management of the common cold and influenza in children

Chapter 12

Allergic Rhinitis

Hélène Roy, BPharm, MSc

Pathophysiology

Allergic rhinitis affects 20% of the population, and the prevalence is increasing.[1-3] There is a strong genetic predisposition; children have a 30% chance of developing allergic rhinitis if one parent is affected and 50% if both are affected.[1,4] Prevalence usually peaks in the late teens or early twenties and gradually reduces after age 45.[5] Allergic rhinitis is an unusual cause of perennial rhinitis in individuals over 65 years of age.[6]

Allergic rhinitis is characterized by inflammation of the nasal mucosa following contact with an airborne allergen. The allergic reaction is mediated by antigen-antibody responses and takes place in three phases. The first phase, sensitization, occurs on first contact with the allergen. IgE is produced and fixated to mast cells and basophils. When the subject is re-exposed to the allergen the second and third phases occur. The immediate reaction (second phase) occurs within minutes and lasts 30 to 90 minutes. Preformed and newly generated mediators (histamine; leukotrienes LTC4, LTD4, LTE4; prostaglandin D2; kinins) are released from mast cells. The late (third) phase occurs four to eight hours after exposure. It is characterized by migration of inflammatory cells (eosinophils, monocytes, macrophages and basophils) and is associated with hyperresponsiveness to inhaled irritants and allergens.[3,6]

Allergic rhinitis is either seasonal or perennial. Seasonal allergic rhinitis begins in spring and ends in fall. In general, tree pollens cause symptoms in spring, grass pollens in late spring to summer, and weed pollens in late summer to early fall.[2] Some outdoor molds may also cause seasonal allergic rhinitis. Perennial allergic rhinitis is caused by allergens present year-round, such as house dust mites, animal dander, cockroaches and indoor molds.[2] Perennial and seasonal allergic rhinitis often co-exist in the same patient.

Rhinitis may also be non-allergic. Conditions associated with non-allergic rhinitis are listed in Table 1. Drugs associated with rhinitis are listed in Table 2.

Table 1: **Possible Non-allergic Causes of Acute and Chronic Rhinitis**[6]

Acute	Chronic
Infection (viral, bacterial)	Vasomotor rhinitis
Foreign body	Nasal tumors
(more common in children)	Choanal atresia*
Drug induced (Table 2)	Nasal septal deviation
Hypothyroidism	Enlarged adenoids and tonsils
Pregnancy	CSF rhinorrhea

A congenital defect where the posterior nares do not communicate with the nasopharynx.

Table 2: **Drugs Associated with Rhinitis**[6]

ACE inhibitors	Methyldopa
ASA and other NSAIDs	Oral contraceptives
Beta-blockers	Phentolamine
Chlorpromazine	Prazosin
Cocaine (repeated use)	Reserpine
Guanethidine	Topical decongestants (overuse)

Goals of Therapy

- Prevent symptoms by avoiding exposure to allergen(s)
- Alleviate symptoms produced by the allergic response

Patient Assessment[5-9]

The sensitization phase of allergic rhinitis is asymptomatic. Symptoms of the immediate phase include paroxysms of sneezing, nasal and palatal pruritus, congestion and clear rhinorrhea. Symptoms of the delayed phase are similar but congestion predominates. Patients may also have itchy, red, watery eyes (*allergic conjunctivitis*); itchy throat; ear fullness and popping; and a feeling of pressure over the cheeks and forehead. Facial signs of allergic rhinitis are illustrated in Figure 1. The *allergic salute* is a sign more commonly seen in children, where the patient wipes the nose with the palm of the hand in a upward motion.

Presentation varies. Some patients present primarily with symptoms of sneezing and rhinorrhea, whereas others are mostly bothered by nasal blockage and have little or no itching or sneezing.[6]

The symptoms of perennial and seasonal allergic rhinitis are similar but itching of the nose, eyes and palate is more common in seasonal allergic rhinitis.[8] Symptoms of seasonal allergic rhinitis are often worst in the morning when pollen counts are highest.

Figure 1: **Facial Signs of Allergic Rhinitis**

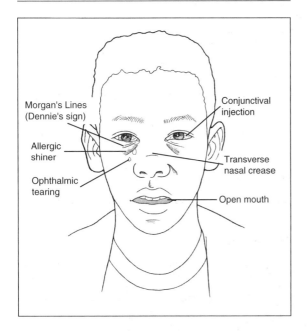

Allergic rhinitis can have a significant impact on patients' quality of life. Patients may be unable to sleep and be fatigued or have headache and difficulty concentrating.[6] Other complications of allergic rhinitis include sinusitis, otitis media and, in children, dental overbite and a high-arched palate due to chronic mouth breathing.[5,6,9]

An assessment plan for patients suffering from allergic rhinitis is illustrated in Figure 2. During the assessment, also identify precipitating factors/allergens and assess occupational exposure and response to previous therapy.

Refer patients to a physician if they have already tried appropriate nonprescription therapy for two weeks without an adequate response, or if the allergen responsible for symptoms cannot be readily identified.[5] Also refer patients to a physician if they have a fever or purulent nasal or ocular secretions, as they may have an infection.

Prevention and Nonpharmacologic Therapy[5-7]

Nonpharmacologic therapy is the first step in the management of allergic rhinitis. Environmental control can sometimes permit enough symptom control to avoid pharmacologic therapy. The benefits of environmental control may take weeks or months to fully manifest. Avoiding the responsible allergen is especially important in children because of the risk of developing new sensitivities. Avoidance measures for common allergens are presented below.

Pollen
- Keep windows and doors closed.
- If use of air conditioning is necessary, keep the unit on the indoor cycle.
- Do not use window or attic fans.
- Monitor weather reports on pollen counts, if available. Decrease outdoor exposure during periods of high pollen counts. Pollen counts tend to be highest on sunny, windy days.
- Do not dry clothing outdoors.
- Shower or bathe after outdoor activity to remove pollen from hair and skin and prevent contamination of bedding.

Figure 2: **Assessment and Initial Treatment of Patients with Allergic Rhinitis**[6,7]

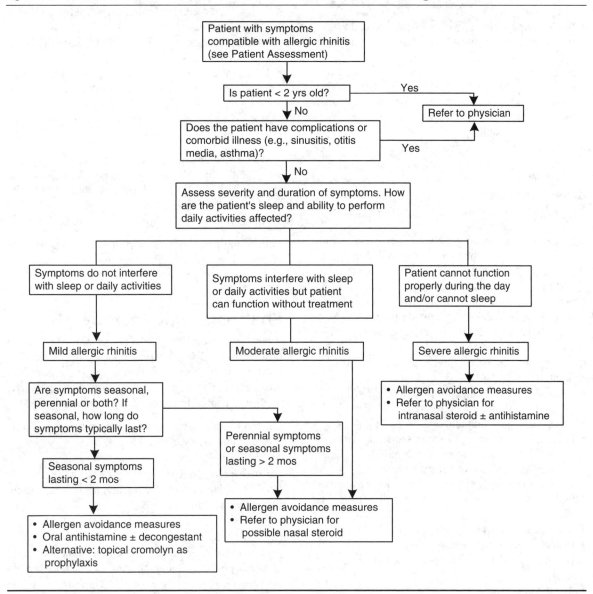

Outdoor Molds

- Remain in a closed environment as much as possible.
- If use of air conditioning is necessary, keep the unit on the indoor cycle; note however, that units can be heavily contaminated with mold.
- Use face masks for activities such as raking leaves or working with compost or dry soil; these have limited value, however, because air seeps around the edges of the mask and the mask does not protect the eyes.

Indoor Molds

- Use fungicide on sinks, shower stalls, non-refrigerated vegetable storage areas and garbage pails. A solution of equal parts household bleach and water effectively kills mold.[10]

- Avoid console humidifiers and cool mist vaporizers; if these must be used, keep them scrupulously clean.
- If the home is built over a crawl space, install a plastic vapor barrier over exposed soil and keep foundation vents open.
- If the basement is damp or tends to flood, avoid carpeting or furnishing the basement. Use a dehumidifier at all times and remove the water extracted from the air frequently; evacuate any standing water as soon as possible.
- Remove houseplants, which are a common source of mold.

House Dust Mites
- Avoid carpeting the bedroom and main living areas.
- Plastic, leather or wood furniture is best.
- Some *acaracides* (e.g., benzyl benzoate, tannic acid) appear to reduce the mite population if used regularly. However, their clinical effect is unproven and they should not be routinely recommended.[5]
- Mite-sensitive patients should avoid vacuuming or making beds. Those who must do their own cleaning should wear a facemask during cleaning and for 10 to 15 minutes afterward.
- Use a vacuum cleaner with an efficient double filtration system.
- If possible, clean while the patient is not at home.
- Keep indoor humidity between 40 and 45%.
- Minimize use of humidifiers.
- Encase all mattresses, box springs and pillows in the patient's bedroom in zippered, allergen-proof casings.
- Consider replacing old mattresses.
- Wash bedding in hot (60°C) water at least every two weeks. Cooler water temperatures will not kill dust mites.[11]
- Avoid stuffed toys that cannot be washed.
- Do not store items under the bed.
- Use window shades instead of venetian blinds.

Animal Allergens
- Strongly consider permanently removing the animal from the household. "Trial" removals are not helpful; it can take 20 weeks or longer for cat allergen levels to drop to levels comparable to homes without cats.
- If the family is unwilling to remove the animal from the home then:
  —Confining the animal to an uncarpeted room (not the patient's bedroom) with a high efficiency particulate air (HEPA) filter or electrostatic air purifier may help. If the family is unwilling to do this, then the animal must not be allowed into the patient's bedroom.
  —Washing cats weekly may help, though this is controversial;
  —Eliminate litter boxes if possible; otherwise place them in an area unconnected to the air supply for the rest of the house;
  —Keep caged pets in an uncarpeted area remote from the patient's bedroom.

Tobacco smoke can aggravate the symptoms of allergic rhinitis and should be avoided by all allergic rhinitis patients.[8] Other irritants that should be avoided include insect sprays, air pollution and fresh tar or paint.[11]

Occasionally surgery is required to manage the complications of allergic rhinitis (e.g., pronounced hypertrophy of the inferior turbinates).[7,8]

Pharmacologic Therapy[6,7,9]

When avoidance of allergens is ineffective or impractical, consider pharmacologic options. If it is possible to predict the onset of symptoms (e.g., seasonal allergic rhinitis, intermittent exposure) prophylactic medication should be started before exposure.

For more information on the management of allergic conjunctivitis, see Chapter 14.

Nonprescription Therapy
Nonprescription agents for treatment of allergic rhinitis are described in Table 3.

Oral Antihistamines
Antihistamines decrease nasal itching, sneezing, rhinorrhea, conjunctival itching and lacrimation but do not relieve nasal congestion.[12-14] They are first line treatment in mild cases of allergic rhinitis. They may be combined with a decongestant in the presence of nasal congestion. They are less effective than intranasal steroids for the symptoms of allergic rhinitis, but are generally considered better for ocular symptoms, though the evidence for this is minimal.[6,15]

Antihistamines are more effective when taken before allergen exposure. The best results are obtained with chronic dosing; therefore, patients should take the antihistamine for as long as they are in contact with the allergen.[12-14]

Antihistamines are divided into two major classes: the first and the second generation. All are equally effective. The major differences between them rest in their side effect profiles.[16-18] The first generation antihistamines cause more anticholinergic effects (dry mouth and nasal passages, difficulty voiding urine, constipation, tachycardia), drowsiness and performance impairment. Performance impairment has been documented using various measures, including reaction time, visual-motor coordination, arithmetical exercises and memory, learning and driving tests. CNS depression and impairment effects can be independent of any subjective complaints by the patient.[6,19] First generation antihistamines also impair children's learning and academic performance. Workers taking first generation antihistamines have decreased work performance and are more likely to be involved in workplace accidents. Daytime performance effects are noted even when the antihistamine is taken only at bedtime.[6]

Administration of standard doses of **loratadine** and **fexofenadine** results in an incidence of sedation equivalent to placebo. However, drowsiness has been reported to occur at higher than recommended doses or rarely in susceptible individuals at recommended doses.[6] Use of **cetirizine** in standard doses results in an incidence of sedation greater than that seen with placebo, but much less than with the first generation antihistamines.[6]

Due to their improved adverse effect profile, especially with regard to sedation and psychomotor performance, consider second generation antihistamines before first generation antihistamines for the treatment of allergic rhinitis.[6,7]

The first generation antihistamines are contraindicated in narrow-angle glaucoma, bladder neck obstruction, hyperthyroidism, cardiovascular disease and prostatic hypertrophy.

Monoamine oxidase inhibitors (MAOIs) may prolong and intensify the anticholinergic effects of the first generation antihistamines.[20] If antihistamines are combined with CNS depressants, additive CNS depressant effects may occur;[20] this may be less likely with loratidine and fexofenadine.

If tolerance develops to the therapeutic effect, changing to an agent in a different pharmacologic class may be effective.

Mast Cell Stabilizers
Sodium cromoglycate reduces itching, sneezing and rhinorrhea but is not very effective for nasal congestion.[21] It is immediately effective as prophylaxis.[6] Treatment should begin before exposure to the allergen and continue for the entire allergen season. If the treatment begins after allergen exposure, relief may be delayed up to four weeks. Sodium cromoglycate is less effective than antihistamines and corticosteroids in allergic rhinitis.

Decongestants
Decongestants are available in oral and topical formulations. Oral decongestants generally have a weaker effect on obstruction than the topical formulations.[7] When given orally decongestants are systemically absorbed. This can result in systemic side effects (Table 3). Most available agents cause blood pressure elevations in normotensive persons only at doses that significantly exceed the recommended range.[22] Elevation of blood pressure may occur at standard doses in hypertensive patients.[23]

Systemic absorption from topical formulations is very low. The side effects are mainly local (Table 3). *Rhinitis medicamentosa* can also occur if topical decongestants are used for more than three or five days.[24] Rhinitis medicamentosa is a rebound vasodilation that results in nasal congestion when the topical agent is stopped. This condition is more likely to occur with shorter-acting agents (**ephedrine** and **phenylephrine**) rather than longer-acting agents (**oxymetazoline** and **xylometazoline**). Many ways to overcome this problem have been proposed, including a slow tapering of the decongestant, a switch to intranasal corticosteroids or an abrupt discontinuation of the topical decongestant. Abrupt cessation works but is difficult because the patient is nasally congested for several days or weeks.[25]

Decongestants may be used in conjunction with antihistamines. A topical decongestant spray may be necessary for the first few days of therapy with an intranasal steroid or cromolyn if nasal congestion is present, in order to optimize medication delivery.[6]

Table 3: **Nonprescription Agents for Allergic Rhinitis**[20,21,28-32]

Medication	Dose	Pediatric dosage	Side effects			Comments
			CNS	Anticho-linergic	GI	
First-generation antihistamines						
Brompheniramine	4-8 mg q4-6h SR: 8-12mg q12-24h	0.5 mg/kg per day given in 3 or 4 divided doses	+	++	−	
Chlorpheniramine	4 mg q4-6h	0.35 mg/kg per day given in 3 or 4 divided doses	+	++	−	
Clemastine	1 mg q12h	0.05 mg/kg per day given in 2 or 3 divided doses	++	+++	+	
Cyproheptadine	4 mg q8h	0.25 mg/kg per day given in 3 or 4 divided doses	+	++	−	
Dexbrompheniramine	2 mg q4-6h SR: 4-6 mg qhs Max: 12 mg per day	2-5 yrs: 0.5 mg q4-6h 6-11 yrs: 1 mg q4-6h	+	++	−	
Dexchlorpheniramine	2 mg q4-6h	2-5 years: 0.5 mg q4-6h 6-11 years: 1 mg q4-6h	+	++	−	Interaction with monoamine oxidase inhibitors: may cause severe hypotension.
Diphenhydramine	25-50 mg q6-8h	5 mg/kg/day given in 3 or 4 divided doses	++	+++	+	
Diphenylpyraline	2 mg q4h Max: 10 mg per day	2-5 yrs: 1-2 mg q8h Max: 4 mg per day 6-11 yrs: 2 mg q6h Max: 6 mg per day	+	++	Unknown	
Doxylamine	7.5-12.5 mg q4-6h Max: 75 mg per day	2-6 yrs: 1.9-3.125 mg q4-6h Max: 18.75 mg per day 6-12 yrs: 3.75-6.25 mg q4h-6h Max: 37.5 mg per day	++	+++	Unknown	
Pheniramine	5-15 mg q4h	2-6 yrs: 3.125-3.25 mg q4-8h 6-12 yrs: 2.5-7.5 mg q4-8h	+	++	Unknown	
Pyrilamine	25-50 mg q6-8h		+	+/−	+	
Triprolidine	2.5 mg q4-6h	0.18 mg/kg per day q6-8h	+	++	−	

Second-generation antihistamines

Medication	Dose	Pediatric dosage	Side effects			Comments
Cetirizine	5-10 mg once daily	≥ 2 yrs and ≤ 40 kg: 0.25 mg/kg once daily; > 40 kg: 10 mg once daily	+/-	+/-	+	Active metabolite of hydroxyzine. If CrCl < 30 mL/min or hepatic impairment: 5 mg daily. Initial response 30 min
Fexofenadine	60 mg q12h; SR: 120 mg q24h	No data available under 12 years old	+/-	+/-	−	Active metabolite of terfenadine. Only 5% of a dose is metabolized.
Loratadine	10 mg once daily	≥ 2 yrs and ≤ 30 kg: 5 mg once daily; > 30 kg: 10 mg once daily	+/-	+/-	+	If CrCl < 30 mL/min or hepatic impairment: administer dosage every other day.

+++ High; ++ Moderate; + Low; +/- Low to none; − None

Medication	Dose	Pediatric dosage	Side effects	Comments
Mast cell stabilizer				
Sodium cromoglycate	2-4 sprays 3 to 6 times daily	5-12 yrs: 1-2 sprays 3 to 6 times daily	Local: sneezing, nasal stinging or irritation, bad taste in the mouth, epistaxis.	
Decongestants				
Oral Onset of action: 30 minutes				
Ephedrine	8 mg q6-8h	2-3 mg/kg per day given in divided doses q4-6h	Mild CNS stimulation (nervousness, excitability, restlessness, dizziness, weakness, insomnia). Peripheral vasoconstriction. Tachycardia or palpitation may occur. Blood pressure may be increased in hypertensive subjects. May adversely affect blood sugar control in diabetics.	Patients with heart disease, high blood pressure, hyperthyroidism, diabetes, angle closure glaucoma and prostatic enlargement should use oral decongestants under a physician's supervision. Concurrent use with MAOIs may cause hypertensive crisis.
Phenylephrine	10 mg q4h Max: 60 mg per day	2-5 yrs: 2.5 mg q4h Max: 15 mg per day; 6-12 yrs: 5 mg q4h Max: 30 mg per day		
Pseudoephedrine	30-60 mg q4-6h SR: 120 mg q12h Max: 240 mg per day	4 mg/kg per day given in divided doses q6h		

(cont'd)

Table 3: **Nonprescription Agents for Allergic Rhinitis**[20,21,28-32] *(cont'd)*

Medication	Dose	Pediatric dosage	Side effects	Comments
Topical	Onset of action: 5-10 minutes			
Naphazoline	0.05% solution 1-2 drops q3-6h	0.05% solution 6-12 yrs: 1 drop q6h	Burning, stinging, sneezing, dryness of the nasal mucosa. Bradycardia, tachycardia, hypotension and hypertension have been reported.	Duration of action: 4-6 h (intermediate-acting)
Oxymetazoline	0.05% solution 2-3 drops or 2-3 sprays q12h	0.025% solution 2-5 yrs: 2-3 drops q12h		Duration of action: Up to 12 h (long-acting)
Phenylephrine	0.25% or 0.5% solution 2-3 drops or 2-3 sprays q3-4h	0.125% solution 1-6 yrs: 2-3 drops q4h 0.25% solution 6-12 yrs: 2-3 drops q4h		Duration of action: Up to 4 h (short-acting)
Xylometazoline	0.1% solution 2-3 drops or 2-3 sprays q8-10h	0.05% solution 2-12 yrs: 2-3 drops or sprays q8-10h		Duration of action: Up to 12 h (long-acting)

MAOI = monoamine oxidase inhibitor; SR = sustained release

Prescription Therapy
Corticosteroids

Intranasal steroids are more effective against the nasal symptoms of allergic rhinitis than either oral antihistamines or nasal cromoglycate. Unlike oral antihistamines, they are not effective against allergic conjunctivitis. Intranasal steroids are the drug of choice for moderate to severe or persistent allergic rhinitis, and for mild allergic rhinitis that does not respond to antihistamines.[6,7] Nasal steroids are often combined with antihistamines to treat severe or resistant cases of allergic rhinitis.[6,7] However, there is little to no clinical evidence to support this practice.[15]

Short courses of oral corticosteroids may be required for severe cases of allergic rhinitis unresponsive to other treatment.[6,7]

Immunotherapy

Immunotherapy may be indicated when the exposure to allergens is significant and unavoidable, and when the symptom complex is severe enough to warrant the time, expense and slight risk of anaphylaxis.[6,26]

Other Prescription Therapies

Intranasal **ipratropium** bromide is effective for rhinorrhea secondary to allergic rhinitis but not other symptoms.[7] **Oral antileukotrienes** may be effective in the management of allergic rhinitis but this requires further study.[6] The intranasal antihistamine **levocabastine** is effective for sneezing, nasal pruritus and rhinorrhea. It has a rapid onset of action (< 15 minutes), but must be used two to four times daily.[7]

Alternative Therapies

There are insufficient data to recommend any herbal treatment for allergic rhinitis.[27]

Homeopathic preparations of *Galphimia glauca* may be effective in the treatment of allergic rhinitis and allergic conjunctivitis. Because adverse effects are rare with homeopathic remedies, this may be considered as an alternative to conventional treatment.[27]

Children

The principles of management of allergic rhinitis in children are similar to those for adults. In children less than two years of age, nasal saline drops or spray may be used to clear nasal passages before eating or sleeping.[7] Most oral antihistamines and nasal cromolyn are considered safe and effective in children over two years of age,[7] though there is limited information on the use of fexofenadine in children under 12 years of age. Table 3 provides dosage guidelines and lower

Table 4: **Monitoring Therapy for Allergic Rhinitis**

Symptoms	Monitoring	Endpoint of therapy	Actions
Allergic symptoms (sneezing, runny nose, itchy and watery eyes, congestion, rhinorrhea)	**Patients:** daily **Pharmacist/Physician:** Next pharmacy visit or by telephone 1 wk later	Patient able to perform daily activities. Patient able to sleep.	If nonprescription therapy ineffective after 1 wk, optimize allergen avoidance and medication dose (if applicable). If symptoms not controlled after a further week of therapy, refer to a physician.[9]
Drowsiness (antihistamine)	**Patient:** daily. **Pharmacist/Physician:** Next pharmacy visit or by telephone when checking for efficacy		Switch to a less sedating antihistamine. If using cetirizine, could give dose at bedtime.
Insomnia (oral decongestant)	**Patient:** daily **Pharmacist/Physician:** 1 wk	No insomnia.	Change medication schedule so last dose taken 4-6 h before bedtime or discontinue medication.
High blood pressure (oral decongestant)	**Physician or Nurse:** Monitor blood pressure of hypertensive patients twice in the first week[29]	No elevation in blood pressure above baseline.	Stop decongestant if blood pressure elevated above baseline.

age limits for nonprescription agents. Nasal steroids are also effective and generally considered safe in children over four years of age.[7] However, some nasal steroids may have a temporary negative effect on the growth of children. It is uncertain if there is any long-term effect on height. If nasal steroids are used, use the lowest possible dose, monitor growth and use other therapies (e.g., antihistamines) to minimize the dose of steroid required for symptom control.[6,7] Decongestants are not recommended for use in children.[6,7]

Pregnancy[6,33,34]

Nasal cromoglycate and nasal beclomethasone are both considered safe for use during pregnancy.[6,33] Information on nasal steroids other than beclomethasone is lacking. With the exception of brompheniramine, neither the first- nor the second-generation antihistamines have been associated with teratogenic effects in pregnancy; however, the first-generation antihistamines are favored because of substantially greater experience with these agents. Both oral and topical decongestants are considered second-line agents during pregnancy, though more information is needed to clarify their safety. Immunotherapy generally should not be started during pregnancy. Courses of immunotherapy that have started prior to conception may be continued if they are providing benefit and not causing systemic reactions; doses should not be increased during pregnancy.

Breastfeeding[34,35]

The American Academy of Pediatrics (AAP) considers fexofenadine, loratadine and triprolidine to be usually compatible with breastfeeding. Adverse effects have been reported in a breastfeeding infant whose mother was taking clemastine. Based on this information the AAP recommends that clemastine be used with caution during lactation. Information on the use of other antihistamines during breastfeeding is not available.

Due to its low molecular weight, phenylephrine would be expected to pass into breast milk; the effects of this exposure on a nursing infant are unknown. Information on the use of other topical decongestants during breastfeeding is not available.

The AAP considers pseudoephedrine to be usually compatible with breastfeeding. There is no available information on the use of other oral decongestants during breastfeeding.

Information on the use of topical sodium cromoglycate during breastfeeding is not available, though the manufacturer recommends it be used with caution.[36]

Monitoring of Therapy

Table 4 provides a monitoring plan framework that should be individualized.

Advice for the Patient

Counsel all patients on allergen avoidance. In addition, patients who require drug therapy should receive counseling regarding proper use of the medication, expected results and management of side effects (Table 4).

Suggested Readings

Dykewicz MS, Fineman S, eds. Diagnosis and management of rhinitis: complete guidelines of the Joint Task Force on Practice Parameters in Allergy, Asthma and Immunology. *Ann Allergy Asthma Immunol* 1998;81:478-518.

May JR. Allergic rhinitis. In: Dipiro JT, Talbert RL, Yee GC, Matzke GR, Wells BG, Posey LM, eds. *Pharmacotherapy: A Pathophysiologic Approach.* 4th ed. Connecticut: Appleton and Lange; 1999: 1479-88.

Simon PA. Acute and chronic rhinitis. In: Young LY, Koda-Kimble MA, eds. *Applied Therapeutics: The Clinical Use of Drugs.* 6th ed. Vancouver, WA: Applied Therapeutics; 1995:21.2-22.2.

Slater JW, Zechnich AD, Haxby DG. Second-generation antihistamines: a comparative review. *Drugs* 1999;57:31-47.

van Cauwenberge P, Bachert C, Passalacqua G et al. Consensus statement on the treatment of allergic rhinitis. *Allergy* 2000; 55: 116-34.

References

1. Nash DR. Allergic rhinitis. *Pediatric Ann* 1998;27:799-808.
2. Naclerio RM. Allergic rhinitis. *N Engl J Med* 1991;325:860-9.
3. Howard PH. ABC of allergies: pathogenic mechanisms:a rational basis for treatment. *BMJ* 1998;316:758-61.
4. Meltzer EO. Treatment options for the child with allergic rhinitis. *Clin Pediatr* 1998;37:1-10.
5. Larsen JS. Antihistamines and quality of life in allergic rhinitispatients. *US Pharm* 2001 May: 87-96.

6. Dykewicz MS, Fineman S, eds. Diagnosis and management of rhinitis: complete guidelines of the Joint Task Force on Practice Parameters in Allergy, Asthma and Immunology. *Ann Allergy Asthma Immunol* 1998;81:478-518.

7. van Cauwenberge P, Bachert C, Passalacqua G et al. Consensus statement on the treatment of allergic rhinitis. *Allergy* 2000;55:116-34.

8. Payton KB, Hebert J, Clarke KD, eds. Canadian Rhinitis Symposium: a multidisciplinary approach to the management of rhinitis. *CMAJ* 1994;151 (4 Suppl): 1-25.

9. Tkachyk SJ. New treatments for allergic rhinitis. *Can Fam Physician* 1999;45:1255-60.

10. John Hopkins University. The John Hopkins Allergy and Asthma web page. *Mold control in the house*. Available at http://www.hopkins-allergy.org/rhinitis/therapeutics-house.html. Accessed December 20, 2001.

11. National Institute of Allergy and Infectious Disease (US). *Treating people with allergic diseases*. Available at http://www.niaid.nih.gov/publications/allergens/treating.htm. Accessed December 20, 2001.

12. Haaksma EEJ, Leur R, Timmerman H. Histamine receptors: subclass and specific ligands. *Pharmacotherapy* 1990;47:73-104.

13. Slater JW, Zechnich AD, Haxby DG. Second-generation antihistamines: a comparative review. *Drugs* 1999;57:31-47.

14. Simons FE, Simons KJ. The pharmacology and use of H1-receptor antagonist drugs. *Drug Therapy* 1994;330:1663-70.

15. Nielsen LP, Mygind N, Dahl R. Intranasal corticosteroids for allergic rhinitis. *Drugs* 2001;61(11):1563-79.

16. Horak F, Stubner UP. Comparative tolerability of second generation antihistamines. *Drug Saf* 1999;20:385-401

17. Simon FER. H1-receptor antagonists: comparative tolerability and safety. *Drug Saf* 1994;10:350-80.

18. Walsh GM, Annunziato L, Frossard N et al. New insights into the second generation antihistamines. *Drugs* 2001;61:207-36.

19. Weiler JM, Bloomfield JR, Woodworth GG et al. Effects of fexofenadine, diphenhydramine and alcohol on driving performance. A randomized, placebo-controlled trial in the Iowa driving simulator. *Ann Intern Med* 2000;132:354-63.

20. Novak KK, ed. *Drug Facts and Comparisons*. St. Louis, MO: Facts and Comparisons, 2002:700.

21. Simon PA. Acute and chronic rhinitis. In: Young LY, Koda-Kimble MA, eds. *Applied Therapeutics: The Clinical Use of Drugs*. 6th ed. Vancouver: Applied Therapeutics; 1995:21.2-21.22.

22. Johnson DA, Hricik JG. The pharmacology of alpha-adrenergic decongestants. *Pharmacother* 1993;13:110S-15S.

23. Chua SS, Benrimoj SI, Gordon RD et al. A controlled clinical trial on the cardiovascular effects of pseudoephedrine in hypertensive patients. *Br J Clin Pharmacol* 1989;28:369-72.

24. Kanfer I, Dowse R, Vuma V. Pharmacokinetics of oral decongestants. *Pharmacotherapy* 1993;13:116S-28S.

25. Graf P. Rhinitis medicamentosa: aspects of pathophysiology and treatment. *Allergy* 1997;52:28-34.

26. The College of Physicians and Surgeons of Manitoba. Guideline number 304. *Allergy: testing and therapy*. Available at http://www.umanitoba.ca/colleges/cps/_Guide/304.html. Accessed December 20, 2001.

27. Ernst E, ed. *The Desktop Guide to Complementary and Alternative Medicine: an Evidence Based Approach*. Mosby: Toronto, 2001.

28. May JR. Allergic rhinitis. In: Dipiro JT, Talbert RL, Yee GC, Matzke GR, Wells BG, Posey M, eds. *Pharmacotherapy: A Pathophysiologic Approach*. 4th ed. Conneticut: Appleton and Lange; 1999:1479-88.

29. Ashton, LW Antihistamines. In: Anderson PO, Knoben JE, Troutman WG, eds. *Handbook of Clinical Drug Data*. 9th ed. Conneticut: Appleton and Lange; 1999:735-48.

30. Pachorek RE. Cough and cold. In: Anderson PO, Knoben JE, Troutman WG, eds. *Handbook of Clinical Drug Data*. 9th ed. Conneticut: Appleton and Lange; 1999:754-9.

31. Taketomo CK, Hodding JH, Kraus DM, eds. *Pediatric Dosage Handbook*. 8th ed. Cleveland, OH: Lexi-Comp; 2001-2002.

32. McEvoy GK, ed. *AHFS Drug Information 2001*. Bethesda, MD: American Society of Health-System Pharmacists; 2001.

33. Mazzotta P. Loebstein R. Koren G. Treating allergic rhinitis in pregnancy. Safety considerations. *Drug Saf* 1999;20:361-75.

34. Briggs GG, Freeman RK, Yaffe SJ. *Drugs in Pregnancy and Lactation*. 5th ed. Baltimore, MD: Williams and Wilkins, 1998.

35. American Academy of Pediatrics. Policy statement: The transfer of drugs and other chemicals into human milk. *Pediatrics* 2001;108(3):776-89.

36. Product Information. Cromolyn Nasal Solution. Pharmascience, 2001.

Allergic Rhinitis—Patient Information

The most important thing you can do to feel better is to avoid the cause of your allergies. Some helpful tips are given below. If you do not know what causes your allergies, see your doctor.

If you are allergic to *pollen*:
- Keep the windows and doors of your house closed.
- If you need to use air conditioning, keep the unit on the indoor cycle.
- Do not use window or attic fans.
- Check weather reports on pollen counts, if they are available. Avoid spending time outdoors when pollen counts are high. Pollen counts tend to be highest on sunny, windy days and in the morning.
- Do not dry your clothing outdoors.
- Shower or take a bath after outdoor activity to remove pollen from your hair and skin and to keep it from getting into your bedding.

If you are allergic to *outdoor molds*:
- Stay indoors as much as possible.
- If you need to use air conditioning, keep the unit on the indoor cycle; note that air conditioning units can be heavily contaminated with mold.
- Use facemasks while raking leaves or working with compost or dry soil.

If you are allergic to *indoor molds*:
- Use a solution of equal parts household bleach and water on sinks, shower stalls, non-refrigerated vegetable storage areas and garbage pails to kill mold.
- Avoid using humidifiers and cool mist vaporizers; if these must be used, clean them often.
- If your home is built over a crawl space, install a plastic vapor barrier over exposed soil and keep the foundation vents open.
- If your basement is damp or tends to flood, do not put carpet or furniture there; use a dehumidifier at all times and empty it of water often; drain any standing water as soon as possible.
- Do not keep houseplants.

If you are allergic to *dust mites*:
- Do not put carpet in your bedroom or main living areas.
- Plastic, leather or wood furniture is best.
- Avoid vacuuming or making beds. If you must do your own cleaning wear a facemask during cleaning and for 10 to 15 minutes afterward.
- If possible, have someone else clean the house while you are not at home.
- Use a vacuum cleaner with an efficient double filtration system.
- Keep indoor humidity between 40 and 45%. A little machine called a hygrometer can measure the humidity in your house. These can be found at hardware stores and home centres.
- Avoid using humidifiers and cool mist vaporizers.
- Encase all mattresses, box springs and pillows in your bedroom in zippered, allergen-proof casings.
- Consider replacing old mattresses.
- Wash your bedding in hot (60°C) water at least every two weeks. Cooler water will not kill dust mites.
- Do not keep stuffed toys that cannot be washed.
- Do not store items under your bed.
- Use window shades instead of venetian blinds.

If you are allergic to a *pet*:
- Strongly consider permanently removing the animal from your house.
- If this is not acceptable then:
  —Keeping the animal in a room where there is no carpet (not your bedroom) and where you have installed a HEPA or electrostatic air purifier may help. If this is not possible then the animal must be kept out of your bedroom at all times;
  —Washing cats weekly may help, though this has not been proven;
  —Get rid of litter boxes if possible; if not, put them in an area not connected to the air supply for the rest of the house;
  —If the animal lives in a cage, keep it in a room without carpet far away from your bedroom.

If avoiding the cause of your allergies does not make you feel better or if your allergies are interfering with your sleep or your daily activities, you may need medication. Your pharmacist can help you pick the best medication for you.

Instructions for Using Nasal Sprays or Drops

Nasal sprays

1. Gently blow your nose.
2. With your head upright, close one nostril by pressing a finger on the side of your nose. Spray the medication into the open nostril, breathing in through your nose while quickly squeezing the bottle.
3. Do the same thing on the other side.
4. Blow your nose in three to five minutes. For severe congestion, a second application of decongestant may now be applied if needed.
5. Rinse the tip of the spray bottle with hot water, but try not to get any water in the bottle.
6. Do not use this product more than is recommended.

Nose drops

1. Have the child gently blow their nose.
2. Lie the child on their back, on a bed with the child's head hanging slightly over the side.
3. Insert the dropper about 0.8 cm (1/3 inch) into a nostril and instill the recommended number of drops. The child should remain in this position for approximately five minutes. Tilt head from side-to-side.
4. Apply the solution to the other nostril in the same way.
5. Blow the nose three to five minutes later.
6. Alternatively, drops can be administered with the head tilted backward, followed by moving the head toward the knees, holding for a few seconds, and then returning to the upright position
7. Rinse the dropper with hot water and return it to the bottle. Although hard to do, avoid touching the dropper to the nostril.
8. Do not use this product more than is recommended.

Adapted from Taylor JG. The common cold. In: Carruthers-Czyzewski P, ed. *Self-Medication: Reference for Health Professionals*. Ottawa, ON: Canadian Pharmaceutical Association, 1992:191-212.

Chapter 13

Upper Respiratory Tract Infections

Hélène Roy, BPharm, MSc

Pathophysiology

The Common Cold

The common cold is a viral infection. Six different types of viruses, including 200 serotypes, can be responsible. Rhinoviruses (30 to 50%) and coronaviruses (10 to 20%) are the most frequently involved. Less common are respiratory syncytial virus (RSV), adenovirus, parainfluenza and enterovirus.[1-3]

The common cold occurs frequently. Preschool children average five to seven episodes annually and an adult two to three. It is estimated that 40% of time lost from work and 30% of absences from school are due to the common cold.[1,4,5] It can occur at any time of year but is less common during the summer months. Rhinoviruses are more prevalent during fall and spring, and coronaviruses during mid-winter and early spring.[1]

Infection is transmitted by hand-to-hand contact and via aerosol particles. Contact between the virus and nasal mucosa appears to be important for initiation of the infection. The increase in vascular permeability (with leakage of serum into the nasal mucosa and nasal secretion) and glandular secretion that follows is responsible for symptoms.[1] The mechanisms by which these changes occur are not clear. The host defense response seems to play a primary role. There is both a humoral and cellular immune response. No increase in histamine concentration is noted.[1] Viral replication peaks in 48 hours but viral shedding can continue for up to three weeks.[1]

Complications of the common cold include otitis media and sinusitis.[6]

Influenza

Influenza is a viral infection normally seen between November and April.[7] The infection is primarily transmitted via aerosol particles.[8] Viral replication occurs in the superficial epithelium of the airway tract. Symptoms are related to the presence of the virus in the airway (cough, sore throat, nasal discharge) or to the host immune response (chills, fever). Two types of viruses cause serious infection in humans, influenza A and B.[9] Though influenza A is more common and tends to cause more severe illness, it is impossible to differentiate between influenza A and B clinically.[9,10] Many subtypes of both influenza A and B exist, and these are classified according to their surface antigens. Immunity to one subtype does not confer protection against another subtype and mutations occur often.[7] Complications of influenza include pneumonia and death. Each year influenza and pneumonia are responsible for 70,000 to 75,000 hospitalizations and 6700 deaths in Canada.[11] Persons at high risk of experiencing complications due to influenza are described in Table 1.

Table 1: **Persons at High Risk of Complications Due to Influenza**[12]

Adults and children with chronic cardiac or pulmonary disorders severe enough to require regular medical follow-up or hospital care.

Any resident of a nursing home or other chronic care facility, regardless of age.

Persons over 65 years of age

Adults and children with chronic conditions, such as diabetes mellitus or other metabolic disease, cancer, immunodeficiency or immunosuppression, renal disease, anemia or hemoglobinopathy.

Sinusitis

Acute sinusitis is characterized by inflammation of the sinuses in response to infection or allergy and may be influenced by anatomical abnormality.[13,14] One to five per cent of common colds are complicated by acute sinusitis. This increases to 5 to 10% in children.[15] Events that introduce microorganisms into the sinuses, such as dental extraction, may be precipitants. Viral or bacterial infections, as well as allergic rhinitis, disrupt mucociliary transport and may also cause sinusitis. 70% of sinusitis is caused by *S. pneumoniae* or *H. influenzae*.[14] *M. catarrhalis* is also a common pathogen in children.[16,17]

The condition is considered chronic if symptoms persist more than three months. Risk factors for developing chronic sinusitis are: anatomical abnormalities (e.g., deviation of the nasal septum, septal spurs, hypertrophic turbinates, nasal polyps); conditions that affect the normal function of the mucociliary sinus epithelium (e.g., cystic fibrosis); and conditions that affect the normal immune defenses of the upper respiratory tract. Sixty per cent of chronic sinusitis is caused by *H. influenzae*. Other responsible organisms are *S. aureus*, alpha-hemolytic streptococcus, *Bacteroides* species, *Veillonella* species, *Corynebacterium* species, *P. aeruginosa* (patients with nasal polyps or cystic fibrosis) and fungi (diabetic or immunocompromised patients).[13,14]

Complications of acute sinusitis include periorbital and orbital cellulitis, orbital abcess, blindness and cavernous sinus thrombosis.[18] Complications of chronic sinusitis can include mucoceles (airless, expanded sinuses) and nasal polyps.[18]

Pharyngitis

Acute pharyngitis is an inflammatory syndrome of the pharynx. Many bacterial and viral organisms are capable of inducing pharyngitis, either as a single manifestation or as part of a more generalized illness.[19] Pharyngitis may be present in Epstein-Barr infection, influenza, the common cold, measles, varicella, allergic rhinitis and sinusitis, or may be due to exposure to irritating substances or environmental pollutants, ingestion of caustic substances or direct trauma to the pharynx. Among bacterial causes, group A beta-hemolytic streptococcus (GABHS) is by far the most commonly implicated (15 to 30% of cases in children and 5 to 10% in adults). Pharyngitis due to GABHS is usually seen during the winter and early spring. Suppurative complications (peritonsillar or retropharyngeal abscess, cervical lymphadenitis, otitis media, mastoiditis and sinusitis), rheumatic fever and

post-streptoccocal glomerulonephritis may occur secondary to bacterial pharyngitis.[20] Rheumatic fever is prevented by treatment of GABHS within 10 days of onset of the infection.[15]

Cough

Cough is present in many respiratory diseases. It can result from a wide range of chemical and mechanical stimuli. The cough is produced by a reflex arc. First, receptors in the head, neck and chest are stimulated. The information is transmitted to the cough centre in the medulla via the afferent limb of the vagus nerve. This results in increased neural activity in the efferent pathway to both the expiratory musculature and airway.[21] Common causes of cough are listed in Table 2.

Table 2: **Common Causes of Cough**[22]

Asthma
Chronic bronchitis
Congestive heart failure
Drugs (e.g., ACE inhibitors)
Emphysema
Foreign body
Gastroesophageal reflux
Inhaled chemical irritants
Post nasal drip (sinusitis, allergic rhinitis)
Upper/lower respiratory tract infection

Goals of Therapy

- Alleviate symptoms
- Eradicate infection or shorten the duration of infection
- Prevent complications of the infection

Patient Assessment (Figure 1)

Common conditions that present with upper respiratory tract symptoms are described in Tables 3 and 4.

Some important points to note are described below:
- In pharyngitis, compared to the common cold, the onset of throat pain is more rapid and the pain is more severe.
- Prolonged nasal congestion and purulent drainage are consistent with possible sinusitis; especially if accompanied by fever, headache and facial pain.

Table 3: **Differential Diagnosis of Upper Respiratory Tract Infections**[6,7,10,13,19,21]

Symptom	Common cold	Allergic rhinitis	Influenza	Sinusitis	Pharyngitis
Nasal discharge and congestion	Clear at the beginning, then can become mucopurulent. Nasal congestion is common.	Abundant; aqueous and clear. Nasal congestion may be present.	Clear at the beginning, than mucopurulent. Nasal congestion is rare.	Persistent, purulent rhinorrhoea. Colored (yellow, green)	Rare
Fever	Rare	No	Yes (38-40°C) Sudden onset	Possible	Yes
Sore throat	Common. Mild (dry, scratchy, sore)	No	Sometimes	No	Severe, sudden onset
Cough	Mild to moderate. Dry at the beginning; often changes to productive as the cold progresses	No	Common. Unproductive	No	Rare
Headache	Rare	Via sinus congestion	Yes	Via sinus congestion	
General aches and pain	Mild	Earaches, especially in children	Common (myalgia)	Rare	Possible
Other		Pruritus (palate, nose, eyes). Sneezing, lacrimation, allergic shiners,* allergic salute†	Fatigue, weakness, chills.	Facial tenderness; jaw and tooth pain	
Duration	Usually 5-7 days but 25% last 14 days	As long as exposed to the allergen	10 days	Days to weeks	3 days

*Allergic shiners: dark circles under the eyes.
†Allergic salute: upward rubbing of the nose.

Figure 1: **Assessment of Patients with Upper Respiratory Tract Symptoms**[2,15,23-26]

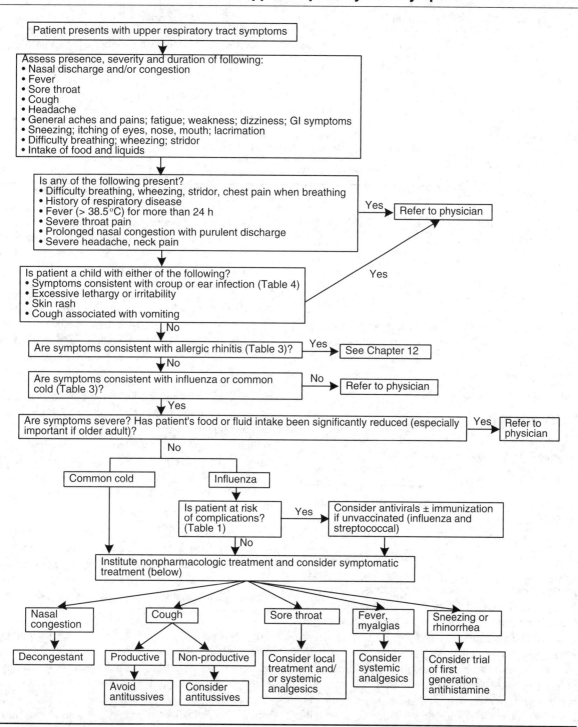

Table 4: **Croup and Otitis Media in Children**[25,27-29]

Condition	Croup	Otitis media
Possible signs and symptoms	Barking, seal-like cough, usually unproductive Gradually worsening inspiratory stridor Dyspnea Fever Hoarseness	Fever, especially one beginning several days after the start of a cold Earache or child tugging at or fingering ear Irritability and/or lethargy Vomiting Purulent drainage from ear
Other characteristics	Fluctuating course with rapid improvements and declines; symptoms often worse at night. Prodrome (2-5 days) consisting of mild fever, rhinorrhea, malaise, sore throat and cough	

- Cough persisting longer than three weeks should be assessed by a physician.[30]

Patients suffering from the common cold usually first complain of discomfort of the throat (dryness, scratchiness), followed by nasal congestion and rhinorrhea. Nasal discharge is clear and watery at the beginning and becomes mucopurulent as the infection progresses. Cough may be present and may persist for one to two weeks. Usually dry at the beginning, it often becomes productive.

Prevention

Direct contact (hand-to-hand) is the major mode of transmission of rhinovirus and coronavirus. *Routine handwashing* decreases the incidence of the common cold.[1] Handwashing has less impact on influenza transmission because the virus is mostly transmitted by small aerosol particles. Proper handwashing technique is described in the Patient Information sheet.

Annual vaccination is the most effective way to prevent influenza and it complications. The vaccine is modified each year according to the viruses expected to circulate in the population that year. The efficacy of the vaccine depends on the degree of antigenic match between the vaccine virus and the circulating virus. Healthy school-age children and adults respond well to vaccination, whereas preschool children, the elderly and the immunocompromised respond less well.[12] In general, with a good antigenic match, influenza vaccination prevents influenza illness in 70 to 90% of healthy children and adults and is

approximately 70% effective in preventing hospitalization for pneumonia and influenza in the community-dwelling elderly.[12] Vaccination also reduces rates of illness and numbers of physician visits and sick days in healthy, working adults.[31]

Protection is generally achieved approximately two weeks after vaccine administration. Immunity usually lasts less than one year. In the elderly, antibody levels may fall below protective levels in less than four months.[12]

Vaccination is recommended for individuals at high risk of complications due to influenza (Table 1). It is also recommended for people capable of transmitting influenza to those at high risk, such as health care workers and household contacts (including children) of people at high risk who either cannot receive the vaccination or may respond inadequately to it (e.g., elderly, immunocompromised).[12]

The optimal time for vaccination is mid-October to November. However, if this time frame is missed, vaccination should be performed at any opportunity that becomes available prior to the end of the flu season.[12] The vaccine is safe in all stages of pregnancy and during lactation.[12]

Amantadine is 70 to 90% effective in preventing illness due to influenza A, but is not effective against influenza B.[12] Situations where amantadine prophylaxis is recommended are described in Table 5. Amantadine prophylaxis should not replace annual influenza vaccination in groups for whom vaccine is recommended.

Table 5: **Indications for Amantadine Prophylaxis of Influenza A**[12]

Control of institutional outbreaks of influenza A.

In people at high risk during an outbreak when vaccine is unavailable, contraindicated, or unlikely to be effective due to poor antigenic match between the vaccine virus and the outbreak virus.

To provide protection while waiting for an antibody response in people at high risk who are vaccinated late.

In combination with vaccination in people at high risk who are not expected to have sufficient immune response to the vaccine.

For people who provide care to high risk people during an outbreak, but who have not been vaccinated.

The neuraminidase inhibitors **zanamivir** and **oseltamivir** are approximately 75% effective in preventing clinically defined influenza, and 60% effective in preventing laboratory confirmed influenza.[32] Their optimal use remains undefined.

Another method traditionally advised for the prevention of cold and flu transmission is coughing or sneezing into a tissue, then promptly throwing it away.[33] The effectiveness of this maneuver has not been studied.

Nonpharmacologic Therapy[5]

For the common cold, influenza, pharyngitis and sinusitis, nonpharmacologic treatment consists of bed rest, good hydration and increased humidity (> 50%). Irritated nasal tissue may be soothed with commercial **nasal saline solutions** or a home-made solution (5 mL of salt in 250 mL of warm water).[34] **Petrolatum** may be applied to a raw nose to increase patient comfort.

Pharmacologic Therapy

Nonprescription agents used in the management of upper respiratory tract infections are described in Table 6.

Antihistamines

The use of antihistamines in the management of the common cold is controversial. The efficacy of antihistamines for this indication is limited because histamine is not involved in the pathology of this infection. Due to their anticholinergic properties, first generation antihistamines may be marginally helpful in managing rhinorrhea associated with the common cold.[23,41] However, concern exists that making mucus thicker may make secretions more difficult to expel, leading to increased congestion of the nose and/or chest. The adverse effect profile of the first generation antihistamines must also be considered when evaluating the risk-benefit ratio of these drugs for this indication.

Second generation antihistamines have no effect on symptoms of the common cold.

Decongestants

The decongestants are sympathomimetic agents. They can relieve nasal congestion associated with the common cold, influenza and sinusitis.

Single doses of nasal decongestants are moderately effective in relieving nasal congestion due to the common cold in adults. There is no evidence that regular use is helpful so recommend single or as-needed use only. There is no published evidence that decongestants are effective in children under 12 years of age.[42]

Decongestants are available in oral and topical formulations. Side effects differ between oral and topical formulations (Table 6). Oral decongestants are generally not recommended in patients with hypertension. While most available agents cause blood pressure elevations in normotensive persons only at doses that significantly exceed the recommended range, elevation of blood pressure may occur at standard doses in hypertensive patients.[43,44]

Rhinitis medicamentosa is a rebound vasodilation that occurs after prolonged regular use (three to five days) of topical decongestants and results in nasal congestion when the topical agent is discontinued. This condition is more likely to arise with shorter-acting agents (ephedrine and phenylephrine) rather than longer-acting agents (oxymetazoline, xylometazoline). Many treatments for this problem have been proposed including a slow reduction in use of the decongestant, a switch to inhaled corticosteroid or an abrupt discontinuation of the topical decongestant. Abrupt cessation works but is difficult because the patient will be congested for several days or weeks.[45]

Topical decongestants should not be used in children under six months of age because they are obligate

Table 6: **Nonprescription Medications for Upper Respiratory Tract Infections**[35-40]

Drugs	Adult dose	Pediatric dose	Adverse effects	Interactions	Comments
Oral	Onset of action: 30 minutes				
Pseudoephedrine	30-60 mg q4-6h SR: 120 mg q12h Max: 240 mg per day	2-5 yr: 15 mg q6h Max: 60 mg per day 6-12 yr: 30 mg q6h Max: 120 mg per day	Mild CNS stimulation (nervousness, excitability, restlessness, dizziness, weakness, insomnia). Peripheral vasoconstriction. Tachycardia or palpitation may occur. Blood pressure may be increased in hypertensive patients. May adversely affect blood sugar control in diabetics	Concurrent therapy with MAOIs may cause hypertensive crisis.	Patients with heart disease, high blood pressure, hyperthyroidism, diabetes, angle-closure glaucoma or prostatic enlargement should be directed to a physician before using an oral decongestant.
Ephedrine	12.5-25 mg q3-4h Max: 150 mg day	2-6 yrs: 2-3 mg/kg per day in 4-6 divided doses 7-11 yrs: 6.25-12.5 mg q4h Max: 75 mg per day > 12 yrs: 12.5-50 mg q3-4h Max: 150 mg per day			Low therapeutic index. Patients with heart disease, high blood pressure, hyperthyroidism, diabetes, angle-closure glaucoma or prostatic enlargement should be directed to a physician before using an oral and decongestant.
Phenylephrine	10 mg po q4h				Patients with heart disease, high blood pressure, hyperthyroidism, diabetes, angle-closure glaucoma or prostatic enlargement should be directed to a physician before using an oral decongestant.
Topical	Onset of action: 5-10 min				
Phenylephrine	0.25% or 0.5% solution 2-3 drops or 2-3 sprays q3-4h	1-6 yrs: 0.125% solution, 2-3 drops q4h 6-12 yrs: 0.25% solution, 2-3 drops q4h	Local burning and stinging, sneezing, dryness of the nasal mucosa. Rhinitis medicamentosa when used for more than three to five days. Bradycardia, tachycardia, hypertension and hypotension have been reported.		Duration of action: up to 4 h (short acting)
Naphazoline	0.05% solution 1-2 drops q3-6h	6-12 yrs: 0.05% solution, 1 drop q6h			Duration of action: 4-6 h (intermediate acting)
Oxymetazoline	0.05% solution 2-3 drops or 2-3 sprays q12h	2-5 yrs: 0.025% solution, 2-3 drops q12h			Duration of action: up to 12 h (long acting)
Xylometazoline	0.1% solution 2-3 drops or 2-3 sprays q8-10h	2-12 yrs: 0.05% solution, 2-3 drops or sprays q8-10h			Duration of action: up to 12 h (long acting)

Antitussives

Drug	Dose (adult)	Dose (pediatric)	Onset	Adverse effects	Drug interactions	Comments
Dextromethorphan	60-120 mg per day given in divided doses q6-8h	1-2 mg/kg per day given in divided doses q6-8 h	15-30 min	Generally well tolerated. Occasional drowsiness and nausea	– MAOI (including moclobemide): serotonin syndrome – Inhibitors of CYP 2D6 (e.g., fluoxetine, quinidine): increase dextromethorphan levels	Causes less sedation than codeine and other opioids. Dextromethorphan 15-30 mg = codeine 8-15 mg as antitussive
Codeine	10-20 mg/dose q4-6h Max: 120 mg per day	1-1.5 mg/kg per day given in divided doses q4-6h	1-2 h	Drowsiness, sedation, nausea, vomiting, constipation	CNS depressants	Causes less sedation than hydrocodone. Metabolized to morphine

Expectorants

Drug	Dose (adult)	Dose (pediatric)	Onset	Adverse effects	Drug interactions	Comments
Guaifenesin	200-400 mg q4h Max: 2.4 g per day	12 mg/kg per day given in divided doses q4h		Side effects are rare. Drowsiness, nausea and vomiting have been reported at high doses		

MAOI = monoamine oxidase inhibitor; CYP 2D6 = cytochrome P450 2D6

nose breathers and if rebound congestion occurs it could cause obstructive apnea.

Antitussives

Antitussives are commonly used to treat cough although there is little evidence to demonstrate their efficacy.[22,46] Some studies have shown that they are no more effective than placebo in the treatment of cough associated with the common cold or other acute upper respiratory tract infections.[47-49]

Antitussives are not recommended when a cough performs a useful function. If they are given to a patient with a productive cough, more mucus is retained.[22]

Expectorants

Expectorants are reported to reduce sputum viscosity and allow a more effective removal of secretions from the respiratory tract.[22] Again, there is a lack of evidence to support their efficacy. They do not thin sputum or increase sputum volume, even at doses higher than recommended.[22] Good hydration with oral liquids and humidified air is, perhaps, the best expectorant that can be recommended.

NSAIDs

NSAIDs are used in respiratory conditions to reduce associated headaches, sore throat and fever. Usual analgesic/antipyretic doses are used. These agents do not alter viral shedding or antibody response.[50]

Natural Products
Echinacea [51-55]

Echinacea is hypothesized to stimulate the immune system and is widely used to prevent and treat the common cold and other respiratory infections.[51] Three species of echinacea are available: *Echinacea angustifolia*, *Echinacea purpurea* and *Echinacea pallida*. *E. purpurea* is the most frequently studied, but *E. angustifolia* is most commonly used in North America. Numerous studies have been performed to evaluate the efficacy and safety of echinacea for this indication. Though it appears to be safe, current evidence regarding its efficacy is inconclusive.[53-55]

The suggested dose is 1 g three times daily. Treatment should begin at the first sign of symptoms and continue at least 10 to 14 days.[51] Echinacea is generally well-tolerated. Adverse effects are rare but have included allergy, nausea and dizziness, tingling of the tongue and excessive salivation. Concurrent treatment with hepatotoxic medication should be avoided since cases of hepatotoxicity have been related to echinacea use. Echinacea is contraindicated in patients with immunosuppression, including AIDS, or autoimmune diseases or taking immunosuppressant medication. Safety in pregnancy or during lactation has not been established.

Zinc [56-61]

Zinc gluconate or acetate lozenges have been postulated to decrease the duration and severity of the common cold. In vitro, zinc has the capacity to inhibit viral replication. However, evidence for its efficacy in vivo is inconsistent.[56-60]

If zinc is used, the lozenge should contain at least 13.3 mg of elemental zinc and be free of agents that chelate zinc and inhibit its absorption, such as citric acid and tartaric acid. Treatment should begin within 48 hours of symptom onset. The dose is one lozenge every two hours while awake for the duration of the cold. Common side effects are bad taste, mouth irritation, nausea and diarrhea. Side effects and the frequency of dosing frequently lead to discontinuation of therapy. Zinc has been reported to cause mouth irritation and gastric erosions. It should be avoided in cases of aphthous or peptic ulcers. Zinc may decrease absorption of tetracyclines or quinolones; avoid concomitant therapy.

Vitamin C (Ascorbic Acid) [2]

It is a popular belief that large doses of vitamin C can prevent the common cold; there is no reliable evidence that this is the case. However, a recent systematic review concluded that high dose vitamin C (> 1 g daily) may shorten the duration of the common cold by approximately half-a-day.[62] The clinical significance of this is debatable.

Prolonged intake of more than 1 g per day of vitamin C may cause oxaluria, uricosuria, renal stones, diarrhea, or, if abruptly discontinued, rebound scurvy.

Antivirals
Neuraminidase Inhibitors [32,63-66]

Oseltamivir and zanamivir inhibit neuraminidase, an enzyme essential for the replication of influenza A and B. Neuraminidase inhibitors reduce symptom severity and decrease the duration of the flu symptoms by 1 to 1.5 days if started within 48 hours of symptom onset. They are also effective in prevention.[63-65]

Amantadine[66]

Amantadine is effective for the prophylaxis of illness due to influenza A, but not influenza B (see Prevention). It also decreases the severity of symptoms and shortens the duration of illness due to influenza A by about one day if started within 48 hours of symptom onset. Its use is limited by its prominent CNS side effects.

Other Agents

Anesthetics such as benzocaine, phenol or menthol may reduce the sensitivity of peripheral nocireceptors. They have been used as decongestants and antitussives, but evidence for their efficacy is poor.

Lozenges, by their demulcent effect on the throat and their ability to increase salivation, may reduce the discomfort of a sore throat.

Children[23,25,67]

Acetaminophen is the preferred agent for relief of aches and pains or fever greater than 38.5°C. **Ibuprofen** may also be used. **ASA** should be avoided due to its association with Reye's syndrome. See Chapter 9 for more information on the management of fever.

Other cough and cold remedies should be avoided in children under two years of age. Therapeutic strategies of use in these individuals are:
- Prop the child upright to sleep in the daytime (e.g., in a car seat) to help prevent nasal congestion.
- Use **saline drops** and a nasal aspirator to suction mucus from the nasal passages.
- Use a humidifier to keep the oropharynx moist (avoid steam vaporizors, which can cause burns if the child tips it over).

In older children, **dextromethorphan** can be used to treat nonproductive coughs, though evidence of efficacy in children is absent. There is no published evidence that decongestants are effective in children under 12 years of age;[42] topical formulations are preferred over oral formulations by some clinicians because of their relative lack of systemic effects.[25]

Pregnancy and Lactation

See Chapter 53.

Use of Combination Products

In some situations, combination products may be practical and enhance patient compliance by reducing the number of medications the patient must take. However, it is almost always preferable to choose single-ingredient products. Combination products do not allow flexibility. During the course of an illness, some ingredients will become not-indicated as some symptoms resolve but with a combination product, the patient will continue to take the useless medication. Sometimes formulations do not contain appropriate ratios of one product compared to another; to reach a therapeutic dosage of one ingredient it is necessary to take too high a dose of another ingredient.

Monitoring of Therapy

Table 7 contains information on monitoring therapy.

Advice for the Patient

Counsel patients regarding:
- Nonpharmacologic therapy
- Proper use of medication
- Expected results and management of side effects
- When to contact a physician

Suggested Readings

Bisno AL. Acute pharyngitis. *N Engl J Med* 2001;344: 205-11.

Evans KL. Recognition and management of sinusitis. *Drugs* 1998;56:59-71.

National Advisory Committee on Immunization. Statement on influenza vaccination for the 2001-2002 season. *Can Comm Dis Rep* 2001 Aug 1;27 (ACS-4):1-24.

Smith MB, Feldman W. Over-the-counter cold medications: a critical review of clinical trials between 1950 and 1991. *JAMA* 1993;269:2258-63.

Turner RB. The common cold. *Pediatric Ann* 1998; 27:790-5.

References

1. Turner RB. The common cold. *Pediatric Ann* 1998;27:790-5.
2. Mossad SB. The common cold. *BMJ* 1998;317:33-36.
3. Saroea HG. Common colds. Causes, potential cures, and treatment. *Can Fam Physician* 1993;39:2215-20.

Table 7: **Monitoring Therapy for the Common Cold and Influenza**

Symptoms	Monitoring	Endpoint of therapy	Actions
Common cold symptoms (congestion, rhinorrhea, cough, sore throat)	**Patients:** daily **Pharmacist:** Next pharmacy visit or by telephone 2-3 days later	Patient able to perform daily activities. Patient able to sleep	Optimize nonpharmacologic measures. Change treatment.
Insomnia (oral decongestant)	**Patients:** daily **Pharmacist:** 1 wk	No insomnia	Change medication schedule or discontinue medication.
High blood pressure (oral decongestant; hypertensive patients only)	**Physician or Nurse:** Monitor blood pressure 2 times in the first week.	No elevation in blood pressure above baseline	Stop decongestant if blood pressure elevated above baseline.
Drowsiness (antihistamine)	**Patients:** daily **Pharmacist:** Next pharmacy visit or by telephone when checking for efficacy	No drowsiness	Discontinue treatment.
Drowsiness (antitussive)	**Patients:** daily **Pharmacist:** Next pharmacy visit or by telephone when checking for efficacy.	No drowsiness	Change medication schedule or treatment.

4. Keast DH, Marshall JN, Stewart MA, Orr V. Why do patients seek family physicians' services for cold symptoms? *Can Fam Physician* 1999;45:335-40.

5. Lowenstein SR, Parrino TA. Management of the common cold. *Adv Intern Med* 1987;32:207-34.

6. Pray WS. Allergic rhinitis vs. the common cold. *US Pharm* 1999;24(1). Available at: http://www.uspharmacist.com/NewLook/DisplayArticle.cfm?item_num=152. Accessed March 6, 2002.

7. Cate TR. Clinical manifestation and consequences of influenza. *Am J Med* 1987;82:15-9.

8. Anonymous. Prevention and control of influenza: recomendations of the Advisory Committee on Immunization Practices (ACIP) *MMWR* 1998;47 (RR-6):1-26.

9. Anonymous. Prevention and treatment of influenza A & B. Therapeutics Letter 2000 Nov/Dec. Therapeutics Initiative, Vancouver, BC.

10. Nahata MC, O'Mara NB. Viral infections. In: Koda-Kimble MA, Young LL, eds. *Applied Therapeutics: The Clinical Use of Drugs.* 7th ed. New York, NY: Lippincott, Williams and Wilkins, 2001:70-1 to 70-18.

11. Canadian Consensus Conference on Influenza. *Can Comm Dis Rep* 1993;19-17:136-142.

12. National Advisory Committee on Immunization. Statement on influenza vaccination for the 2001-2002 season. *Can Comm Dis Rep* 2001 Aug 1; 27: ACS-4.

13. Low DE, Desrosiers M, McSherry J et al. A practical guide for the diagnosis and treatment of acute sinusitis. *CMAJ* 1997;156:1S-14S.

14. Evans KL. Recognition and management of sinusitis. *Drugs* 1998;56:59-71.

15. Reed BD. Sinusitis and pharyngitis. In: Taylor RB, ed. *Family Medicine: Principles and Practice.* 4th ed. New York, NY: Springer-Verlag, 1994:294-303.

16. Wald ER. Sinusitis. *Pediatric Ann* 1998;27:881-8.

17. Temple ME, Nahata MC. Pharmacotherapy of acute sinusitis in children. *Am J Health-Syst Pharm* 2000;57:663-8.

18. Hayes RO. Pediatric sinusitis: when it's not just a cold. *Clinician Reviews* 2001;11(10):52-9. Available at: http://www.medscape.com/CPG/ClinReviews/2001/v11.n10/c1110.01.haye-01.html. Accessed December 4, 2001.

19. Bisno AL. Acute pharyngitis. *N Engl J Med* 2001;344:205-11.

20. Dajani A, Taubert K, Ferrieri P, Peter G, Shulman S. Treatment of acute streptococcal pharyngitis and prevention of rheumatic fever: a statement for health professionals. *Pediatrics* 1995;96:758-64.

21. Richer M, Deschênes M. Upper respiratory tract infections. In: Dipiro JT, Talbert RL, Yee GC, Matzke GR, Wells BG, Posey LM, eds. *Pharmacotherapy: A Pathophysiologic Approach.* 4th ed. Connecticut: Appleton and Lange, 1999: 1479-88.

22. Irwin RS, Curley FJ, Bennet FM. Appropriate use of antitussives and protussives. *Drugs* 1993;46:80-91.

23. Hook R. Treating the common cold. *Pharm Post* 1999 Oct; CE Lesson.

24. Blanchard N. Pediatric infectious diseases. In: Koda-Kimble MA, Young LL, eds. *Applied Therapeutics: The Clinical Use of Drugs.* 7th ed. New York, NY: Lippincott Williams and Wilkins, 2001:94-1 to 94-24.

25. Canadian Paediatric Society. *A parent's guide to colds and flu in children.* Available at: http://www.cps.ca/english/statements/ID/id91-03.htm. Accessed October 25, 2001.

26. Canadian Paediatric Society. Caring for Kids page. *The common cold.* Available at: http://www.cps.ca/english/carekids/childhoodillnessess/CommonCold.htm. Accessed May 9, 2001.

27. Baumgardner DJ. Communicable diseases of children. In: Taylor RB, ed. *Family Medicine: Principles and Practice.* 4th ed. New York, NY: Springer-Verlag, 1994:134-144.

28. Hall CB, McBride JT. Acute laryngotracheobronchitis (croup). In: Mandell GL, Bennett JE, Dolin R, eds. *Mandell, Douglas & Bennett's Principles and Practice of Infectious Diseases.* 5th ed. Toronto: Churchill Livingstone, 2000:663-9.

29. Klein JO. Otitis externa, otitis media and mastoiditis. In: Mandell GL, Bennett JE, Dolin R, eds. *Mandell, Douglas & Bennett's Principles and Practice of Infectious Diseases.* 5th ed. Toronto: Churchill Livingstone, 2000:669-75.

30. Irwin RS, Madison JM. The diagnosis and treatment of cough. *N Engl J Med* 2000;343(23):1715-21.

31. Ahmed F, Singleton JS, Franks AL. Influenza vaccination for healthy young adults. *N Engl J Med* 2001;345(21):1543-7.

32. Jefferson T, Demicheli V, Deeks J, Rivetti D. Neuraminidase inhibitors for preventing and treating influenza in healthy adults (Cochrane Review). In: *The Cochrane Library*, Issue 2, 2001. Oxford: Update Software.

33. Bélanger D. The common cold. *Can Pharm J* 2000 Oct; 133 (8):19.

34. Simon PA. Acute and chronic rhinitis. In: Young LY, Koda-Kimble MA, eds. *Applied Therapeutics: The Clinical Use of Drugs.* 6th ed. Vancouver, WA: Applied Therapeutics, 1995; 21-2 to 21-22.

35. Hansten PD, Horn JT. *Drug Interactions Analysis and Management.* St. Louis, MO: Facts and Comparisons, Inc., 2001.

36. Taketomo CK, Hodding JH, Kraus DM, eds. *Pediatrics Dosage Handbook.* 8th ed. Cleveland, OH: Lexi-Comp, 2001.

37. Pachorek RE. Cough and cold. In: Anderson PO, Knoben JE, Troutman WG, eds. *Handbook of Clinical Drug Data.* 9th ed. Conneticut: Appleton and Lange, 1999:754-9.

38. May JR. Allergic rhinitis. In: Dipiro JT, Talbert RL, Yee GC, Matzke GR, Wells BG, Posey M, eds. *Pharmacotherapy: A Pathophysiologic Approach.* 4th ed. Conneticut: Appleton and Lange, 1999:1479-88.

39. Pentel P. Toxicity of over-the-counter stimulants. *JAMA* 1984;252:1898-1903.

40. Pray WS. BP effects of nasal decongestants. *US Pharm* 2000; 25(2):18-26. Available at: http://uspharmacist.com/New Look/DisplayArticle.cfm?item_num=475. Accessed March 12, 2002.

41. Hendeles L. Efficacy and safety of antihistamines and expectorants in nonprescription cough and cold preparations. *Pharmacotherapy* 1993;13:154-8.

42. Taverner D, Bickford L, Draper M. Nasal decongestants for the common cold (Cochrane Review). In: *The Cochrane Library*, Issue 1, 2001. Oxford: Update Software.

43. Chua SS, Benrimoj SI, Gordon RD, et al. A controlled clinical trial on the cardiovascular effects of single doses of pseudoephedrine in hypertensive patients. *Br J Clin Pharmacol* 1989;28:369-72.

44. Johnson DA, Hricik JG. The pharmacology of alpha-adrenergic decongestants. *Pharmacotherapy* 1993;13:110S-5S.

45. Graf P. Rhinitis medicamentosa: aspects of pathophysiology and treatment. *Allergy* 1997;52:28-34.

46. Schroeder K, Fahey T. Over-the-counter medications for acute cough in children and adults in ambulatory settings (Cochrane Review). In: *The Cochrane Library,* Issue 3, 2001. Oxford: Update Software.

47. Freestone C, Eccles R. Assessment of the antitussive efficacy of codeine in cough associated with common cold. *J Pharm Pharmacol* 1997;49:1045-9.

48. Sause RB. OTC products to relieve coughs. *US Pharmacist* 1994;19:33-7.

49. Taylor JA, Norvack AH, Almquist JR, Roger JE. Efficacy of cough suppressants in children. *J Pediatr* 1993;122:799-802.

50. Sperber SJ, Hendley O, Hayden FG, Riker DK, Sorrentino JV, Gwaltney Jr JM. Effects of naproxen on experimental rhinovirus colds; a randomized, double-blind, controlled trial. *Ann Intern Med* 1992;117:37-41.

51. Giles JT, Palat CT, Chien SH, Chang ZG, Kennedy DT. Evaluation of echinacea for treatment of the common cold. *Pharmacotherapy* 2000;20:690-7.

52. Grimm W, Müller HH. A randomized controlled trial of the effects of fluid extract of Echinacea purpurea on the incidence and severity of colds and respiratory infections. *Am J Med* 1999;106:138-42.

53. Jurgens TM. Echinacea. In: Chandler F, ed. *Herbs; Everyday Reference for the Health Professional.* Ottawa: Canadian Pharmacists Association, 2000:102-5.

54. Ernst E, ed. *The Desktop Guide to Complementary and Alternative Medicine; an Evidence-based Approach.* London, UK: Harcourt Publishers Inc, 2001:102-3.

55. Melchart D, Linde K, Fischer P, Kaesmayr J. Echinacea for preventing and treating the common cold (Cochrane Review). In: *The Cochrane Library*, Issue 4, 2001. Oxford: Update Software.

56. Potter YJ, Hart LL. Zinc lozenges for the treatment of common colds. *Ann Pharmacother* 1993;27589-92.

57. Marshall S. Zinc gluconate and the common cold. *Can Fam Physician* 1998;44:1037-42.

58. Mossad SB, Macknin ML, Medendorp SV, Mason P. Zinc gluconate lozenges for treating the common cold. *Ann Inter Med* 1996;125:81-8.

59. Garland ML, Hagmeyer KO. The role of zinc lozenges in the treatment of the common cold. *Ann Pharmacother* 1998;32: 63-9.

60. Jackson JL, Peterson C, Lesho E. A meta-analysis of zinc salts lozenges and the common cold. *Arch Intern Med* 1997;157: 2373-6.

61. Hulisz DT. Zinc and the common cold: What pharmacists need to know. *US Pharm* 1999;24(3). Available at: http://www.uspharmacist.com/NewLook/DisplayArticle.cfm?item_num=161. Accessed March 6, 2002.

62. Douglas RM, Chalker EB, Treacy B. Vitamin C for preventing and treating the common cold (Cochrane Review). In: *The Cochrane Library*, Issue 1, 2001. Oxford: Update Software.

63. Hayden FG, Osterhaus A, Treanor JJ et al. Efficacy and safety of the neuraminidase inhibitor zanamivir in the treatment of influenzavirus infections. *N Engl J Med* 1997;337:874-80.

64. Bardsley-Elliot A, Noble S. Oseltamivir. *Drugs* 1999;58: 851-60.

65. Calfee DP, Hayden FG. New approach to influenza chemotherapy: neuraminidase inhibitors. *Drugs* 1998;56: 537-53.

66. Couch RB. Prevention and treatment of influenza. *New Engl J Med* 2000;343(24):1778-87.

67. American Academy of Pediatrics. Policy statement: use of codeine- and dextromethorphan-containing cough remedies in children. *Pediatrics* 1997;99(6):918-20.

Common Cold and Influenza—Patient Information

To help you to feel better:
- Drink lots of fluids
- Use a vaporizer or humidifier
- Soothe your irritated nose with a saline solution

Handwashing

Washing your hands often will help keep you from getting the cold or flu, or spreading it to other people. Wash your hands before cooking or eating, feeding a baby or child, giving someone medication, and after wiping your nose (when possible).

What is a good handwashing routine?
1. Wet your hands under running water.
2. Using soap, scrub your hands for 20 seconds (the time it takes to sing *Twinkle, Twinkle Little Star*).
3. Rinse your hands under running water for 10 seconds.
4. Dry your hands with a clean towel.

Medications for Colds and Flu

Many medications for colds and flu are available without a prescription. Ask your pharmacist if medication can help you or not.

The common cold and the flu are viral infections. Antibiotics will not help you get better.

See a doctor if:
- You have trouble breathing, *or*
- You make strange sounds when you breathe, *or*
- You have a severely sore throat, *or*
- You have a lung disease such as asthma, emphysema or chronic bronchitis, *or*
- You have a fever for more than 24 hours, *or*
- Your cold or flu lasts for more than 7 to 10 days

Take a child to the doctor if:
- They seem to have an earache, *or*
- They have a high fever (temperature above 39°C or 102°F), *or*
- They seem overly sleepy, *or*
- They seem overly cranky or fussy, *or*
- They have rapid breathing or trouble breathing, *or*
- They have a cough that lasts more than 10 days, *or*
- They have a skin rash

Eye Care Section Highlights

Chapter 14: **Eye Conditions**

Eyelid conditions
- Anatomy and physiology of the eyelid
- Hordoleum
- Chalazion
- Blepharitis
- Eyelid hygiene

Conjunctivitis
- Acute bacterial conjunctivitis
- Hyperacute bacterial conjunctivitis
- Chronic bacterial conjunctivitis
- Viral conjunctivitis
- Seasonal allergic conjunctivitis (SAC)
- Causes of conjunctivitis

Dry eye

Chapter 15: **Contact Lens Care**

- Common visual problems
- Types of contact lenses
- Contact lens solutions
- Contact lenses-related problems
- Proper care of lenses
- Prevention of complications
- Comparative features of rigid gas permeable (RGP) and soft lenses
- Systemic drug interactions with contact lenses
- Local drug interactions with contact lenses

Chapter 14

Eye Conditions

Anne M. Friesen, BSc(Pharm), MSc

Eyelid Conditions

Pathophysiology

Eyelids and lashes protect the globe (eyeball) from foreign bodies and injuries and help maintain a wet corneal surface. The eyelid is a complex structure of skin, muscle and fibrous tissue. The skin of the eyelid is among the thinnest anywhere on the body, which allows for the mobility of the eyelids. Underneath the skin lies loose, areolar tissue that is capable of significant edema and swelling. The next layer is the orbicularis muscle, responsible for closing the eyelids and innervated by the seventh cranial nerve.[1,2]

Posteriorly in the eyelid is the tarsus, a dense fibrous connective tissue plate that supports the lid margins and forms the skeleton of the eyelid (Figure 1).[1,2] Modified sebaceous glands, known as meibomian glands, are contained within the tarsal plates and secrete the lipid layer of the tear film. There are 30 to 40 glands in the upper lid and 20 to 30 in the lower lid.[3]

The glands of Zeis and Moll lie in the anterior section of the eyelid. Zeis's glands are modified sebaceous glands that are associated with the lash follicles. Moll's glands are modified sweat glands whose ducts open either into a lash follicle or directly onto the anterior lid margin between the lashes (Figure 2).[3]

Figure 1: **Anatomy of the Eyelids and Anterior Eye**

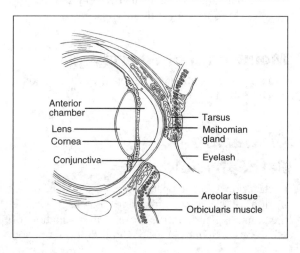

Figure 2: **Cross-Section of Upper Eyelid**

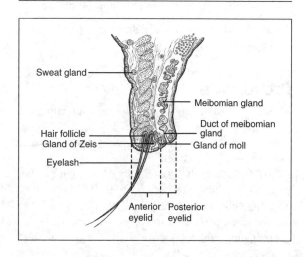

Hordeolum

Pathophysiology

A hordeolum (sty, stye) is an infection of the eyelid glands. Even though it is the most common eyelid infection in ophthalmology, its exact prevalence is unknown. When the glands of Zeis or Moll are involved, the infection is smaller and more superficial. In this type of infection, referred to as an external hordeolum, the lesion always points toward the skin. A larger swelling usually involves the meibomian glands, and is called an internal hordeolum. This lesion can point either to the skin or to the conjunctival surface. It generally has a more prolonged course than an external hordeolum because it rarely drains spontaneously. Microbiologic cultures are seldom required for either type of hordeolum since the most common infecting organism is *S. aureus*.[1,2,4-6]

Goals of Therapy

- Resolve infection
- Prevent recurrence
- Prevent transmission to other eye or to household contacts

Patient Assessment

Patients with hordeolum present with unilateral, localized lid swelling, tenderness and erythema. The amount of discomfort increases with the degree of lid swelling. Hordeola are often associated with blepharitis and have a tendency to recur in these patients.[2,4]

An algorithm for the assessment of eye conditions is presented in Figure 3.

Prevention

A common sense approach to avoid infecting the fellow eye or transmitting the infection to other persons in the household includes the following instructions for the patient:

- Avoid touching the eyes and wash the hands after any contact with the infected eye.
- Change compresses and towels after each use.
- Take care not to allow the tip of eye drop bottles or ophthalmic ointments to touch the eye or eyelashes.

Conscientious attention to treating symptoms of blepharitis may help to decrease the incidence of recurrent hordeola.

Nonpharmacologic Therapy[1,2,3,6]

External hordeola drain spontaneously, but **warm compresses** applied for 10 to 15 minutes three or four times a day will hasten resolution, which usually occurs within 48 hours.[2]

A single study showed that a hard-boiled egg retained heat longer than a warm compress.[7] The authors suggest that a hard-boiled egg wrapped in a handkerchief or compress is a convenient and cost-effective way to apply heat to the eyelid. The same egg can be reboiled prior to each application.[7]

Referral to a physician is required for hordeola that do not spontaneously drain within 48 hours. In these situations incision and drainage may be required.

Pharmacologic Therapy[1,2,3,6]

Nonprescription Therapy

Self-medication with nonprescription ophthalmic antibacterials is not necessary and is not recommended.

Prescription Therapy

After incision and drainage, a physician may prescribe an ophthalmic antibacterial ointment such as **bacitracin** or **erythromycin**, applied to the conjunctival sac several times a day, to help prevent further infection. If cellulitis develops or if the infection is severe, oral antibacterials such as **erythromycin**, **cloxacillin**, or **tetracycline** may be prescribed.

Monitoring of Therapy

Table 1 provides a monitoring plan, which should be individualized.

Chalazion

Pathophysiology

A chalazion is an idiopathic, sterile, chronic inflammation of a meibomian gland. Blockage of the meibomian gland orifices results in stagnation of sebaceous secretions. A lesion develops over a period

Figure 3: **Assessment of Patients with Eye Conditions**

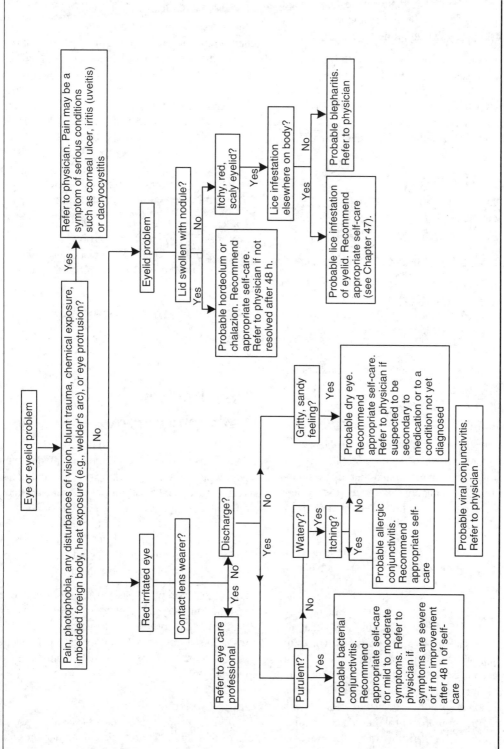

of weeks and is characterized by painless, localized swelling. Most chalazia point toward the conjunctival surface, causing conjunctival redness and swelling.

Chalazia are more common in people with blepharitis, acne rosacea or seborrheic dermatitis. These patients are also at greater risk for the development of multiple or recurrent chalazia. Patients with recurrent or persistent chalazion should be evaluated for more serious conditions such as meibomian gland carcinoma.[1-3]

Goals of Therapy

- Resolve lesion
- Prevent recurrence

Patient Assessment

The initial symptoms of chalazion (mild inflammation and tenderness) may resemble hordeolum, but without the acute inflammatory signs. Large chalazia may press on the eyeball and cause astigmatism or visual distortion.[1,2]

An algorithm for the assessment of eye conditions is presented in Figure 3.

Prevention

Encourage patients who have recurrent chalazia associated with blepharitis to maintain good lid hygiene (see Blepharitis, nonpharmacologic therapy). Patients with dermatologic conditions like acne rosacea and seborrheic dermatitis should be encouraged to maintain treatments for these conditions.

Nonpharmacologic Therapy[1,2,3,8,9]

Approximately 25% of chalazia resolve spontaneously. Initial treatment for chalazion is similar to that for hordeolum, especially for small lesions. **Warm compresses**, applied several times a day, are used to soften sebaceous secretions that may be blocking meibomian gland orifices. Refer patients to a physician if resolution does not occur within a few days of initiating warm compress treatment. Immediate referral is required for patients with a painful chalazion or impaired vision.

Pharmacologic Therapy[1-3,8,9]

Nonprescription Therapy

Self-medication with nonprescription ophthalmic antibacterials is not necessary and is not recommended.

Prescription Therapy

Larger chalazia may require surgical excision, intralesional steroid injections, or both. These procedures should be performed by an ophthalmologist. When excision is required, the ophthalmologist makes a vertical incision on the conjunctival surface, followed by careful curettement of the gelatinous material.

Topical antibacterials or corticosteroid drops may be prescribed after surgery to prevent infection and decrease inflammation. The presence of cellulitis is an indication for the use of systemic antibacterials.

Monitoring of Therapy

Table 1 provides a monitoring plan, which should be individualized.

Blepharitis
Pathophysiology

Blepharitis is a chronic condition that usually affects the eyelids bilaterally. Although the different types can be defined as anterior and posterior, blepharitis often occurs as a mixed condition in patients, making it difficult to accurately diagnose and treat. It can also be associated with chronic dermatologic conditions such as acne rosacea and seborrheic dermatitis. These conditions must also be addressed for optimal control over the ocular effects of blepharitis.[1-6]

Long-term complications of this chronic disorder include physical damage to the eyelids as well as damage to the cornea. Inflammation of the cornea can result in scarring, loss of surface smoothness and loss of visual acuity. If the inflammation is severe, corneal perforation may occur.[1-6]

Anterior Blepharitis[1-6]

Staphylococcal blepharitis is usually caused by *S. aureus* or *S. epidermidis*. Patients present with inflammation and erythema along the anterior margin of the eyelid. The lid margins are scaly, with crusts and tiny ulcerations around the lashes. In chronic inflammatory staphylococcal blepharitis, loss of eyelashes (madarosis) may occur. Complications of staphylococcal blepharitis include recurrent hordeola or chalazia, epithelial keratitis of the lower third of the cornea, and marginal corneal infiltrates.

Seborrheic blepharitis (nonulcerative) presents with less inflammation and redness along the anterior border of the eyelid and the scales are more oily or greasy than in staphylococcal blepharitis. Seborrheic blepharitis is often associated with seborrheic dermatitis affecting other parts of the body.

Although two types of anterior blepharitis have been identified, it is more common for patients to present with a mix of staphylococcal and seborrheic types. Patients with either form of anterior blepharitis also show a predisposition to developing conjunctivitis.

Posterior Blepharitis[1-6]
Meibomian gland dysfunction can lead to inflammation of the posterior aspect of the eyelid (closer to the eyeball). This is a bilateral, chronic condition that sometimes coexists with anterior blepharitis.

Meibomian seborrhea is characterized by excessive glandular secretions. Symptoms can include photophobia, burning sensation, an excessively oily or foamy tear film and froth on the lid margin. Although they may be difficult to detect, small oil globules may be sitting at the meibomian gland orifices on the lid margin. There are usually few signs of inflammation.

Meibomianitis is characterized by inflammation and obstruction of the meibomian glands. Signs include diffuse or localized inflammation of the posterior lid margin. In chronic cases the meibomian gland orifices become obstructed and the posterior lid margin may become thick, rounded and notched. When pressure is applied over the glands, a soft cheesy substance is expressed. In very severe cases the glands are so blocked that no secretions can be expressed.

Goals of Therapy
- Reduce inflammation and discomfort associated with blepharitis
- Reduce the risk of recurrence of severe symptoms

- Reduce the risk of complications such as conjunctivitis and keratitis

Patient Assessment
Generally, symptoms of blepharitis include irritation, burning and itching of the lid margins. There may also be a foreign-body sensation in the eye. Patients may complain of a sandy or gritty sensation in the eyes that is worse upon awakening. This is because during sleep the inflamed eyelids lie against the cornea, tear secretion decreases, and inflammatory mediators have several hours to act on the surface of the eye.[1-6] See also Pathophysiology, anterior and posterior blepharitis.

An algorithm for the assessment of eye conditions is presented in Figure 3.

Prevention
Blepharitis is almost always a chronic condition that frustrates patients and physicians. Inadequate instruction and noncompliance with lid hygiene are the most common reasons for treatment failure.[10] Patients need to be encouraged to maintain a long-term lid hygiene program as this helps prevent exacerbations and long-term complications. Treatment of dermatologic disorders elsewhere in the body, such as seborrheic dermatitis, is important in achieving long-term control of blepharitis.[4,10]

Nonpharmacologic Therapy[2,3,5,11]
Treatment for all types of blepharitis consists of regular and long-term **eyelid margin hygiene**:
1. Warm compresses, applied to closed eyelids for 5 to 10 minutes, help to melt solidified material in the glands.
2. Gentle scrubbing of the lid margin follows. The patient should be instructed not to scrub the conjunctiva or the outer lid area, only the lid margin. The patient can use either warm water with a facecloth, a commercial eyelid scrub (e.g., Eyescrub®, Lid-Care®, or Blepharoshampoo®), or a few drops of baby shampoo in a small amount of warm water.
3. Mechanical expression, performed by an ophthalmologist, may be necessary to decrease the amount of irritating lipids within the glands.

Lid hygiene may be required on a daily basis immediately after initial diagnosis or during periods of exacerbation, but may be reduced to twice a week once control has been achieved. This decision should be made by the treating physician. Very few patients will be able to completely discontinue a lid hygiene regimen.

Pharmacologic Therapy[2,3,5,10]

Nonprescription Therapy

Topical nonprescription antibacterials should be used only on the advice of a physician.

Prescription Therapy

Pharmacologic treatment of anterior blepharitis may include topical antistaphylococcal antibiotics, used after eyelid cleansing. Antibacterial ointments, applied on the lid margins, are preferred to drops because of increased contact time between the drug and tissues. Ointments that cover gram-positive organisms, such as **bacitracin** and **erythromycin**, are applied one to four times a day for one to two weeks. If effective,

treatment can be reduced to once a day at bedtime for a further four to eight weeks. Treatment should be continued for a month after all signs of inflammation have subsided.

Short-term treatment with weak corticosteroids (e.g. **prednisolone** 0.125% twice daily) or **corticosteroid/antibacterial** combinations may be necessary during exacerbations.

In posterior blepharitis, patients may require systemic antibacterial therapy for several weeks or even months, in addition to lid hygiene. **Tetracycline**, **doxycycline**, or **minocycline** is usually the drug of choice. **Erythromycin** is an alternative when tetracyclines are contraindicated. However, its efficacy has not been as well established as that of the tetracyclines.

Monitoring of Therapy

Table 1 provides a monitoring plan, which should be individualized.

Conjunctivitis

Pathophysiology

The conjunctiva is a thin, translucent tissue layer that lines the inside of the eyelids (palpebral portion) and the outer aspect of the globe (bulbar portion) (Figure 1). It is a relatively elastic tissue that covers the episclera, the sclera and the uveal tissue layers. The conjunctiva is exposed to many microorganisms and other environmental factors because of its location. The combined action of the tears and eyelids protect the conjunctiva by trapping and diluting debris and organisms, then flushing the tears into the nasolacrimal duct.[10,12]

Conjunctivitis is a general term that refers to any inflammatory condition of the membrane that lines the inside of the eyelids and covers the exposed surface of the sclera. The inflammation can be hyperacute, acute or chronic in presentation and can be caused by infections or noninfectious material. Conjunctivitis is the most common cause of red eye worldwide.[11,12]

Infections, both bacterial and viral, are responsible for the majority of cases of conjunctivitis. Other causes of conjunctivitis are listed in Table 2.[11,12]

Patient Assessment

An algorithm for the assessment of eye conditions is presented in Figure 3.

Typically, patients present with a foreign body sensation in the eye. Other descriptions of symptoms include a scratching or burning sensation, a feeling of fullness around the eyes, itching and mild photophobia. There is some degree of redness in the conjunctiva, as well as some type of discharge. Often the eyes are crusty or sticky after sleeping.[3,11-13]

Signs and symptoms of the most common types of conjunctivitis are listed in Table 3.

Acute Bacterial Conjunctivitis

Although acute bacterial conjunctivitis is usually self-limiting and resolves within two weeks, appropriate treatment shortens the course of the disease to one to three days, decreases person-to-person spread and decreases the risk of more serious corneal complications.[11,12] The most common causative organism is *S. aureus*, but *S. pneumoniae* and *H. influenzae* are also common, especially in children.[10,13,14] Most patients can be treated empirically with good results. However, cultures may be required in certain patient groups, especially young children and debilitated patients, since these patients may demonstrate non-specific or indeterminate clinical signs.[11]

Goals of Therapy

- Cure infection
- Prevent transmission to other persons
- Prevent complications

Nonpharmacologic Therapy[6,10-14]

The conjunctival sac can be irrigated with sterile saline or a commercial eye wash product as necessary to remove conjunctival secretions. Eyelids that are stuck together in the morning should be soaked with a warm compress and opened carefully. The patient and family need to pay attention to personal hygiene to avoid transmitting the infection (see Infections of the Eyelids or Conjunctiva—Patient Information). Contact lens wear should be stopped and contact lens wearers should be referred to a physician because of their increased risk of developing serious infections.

Pharmacologic Therapy[6,10-14]

Nonprescription Therapy

For typical adult cases of bacterial conjunctivitis, **polymyxin B/gramicidin** eyedrops (e.g., Polysporin®, Optimyxin®) can be instilled in the affected eye(s) two to four times a day for seven to ten days. A ribbon of **polymyxin B/bacitracin** ophthalmic ointment can be applied to the inside of the lower lid

one to three times a day for seven to ten days. Generally, treatment should continue for two days after symptoms have resolved.

If there is no improvement within 48 hours of starting treatment, refer the patient to a physician. All children with conjunctivitis should be referred to a physician.

Prescription Therapy

The empiric treatment of choice includes broad spectrum antibacterial drops such as **trimethoprim/ polymyxin B**, or ophthalmic ointments containing **erythromycin** or **bacitracin**. Adults and adolescents generally prefer ophthalmic drops, but ointments may be better tolerated by young children, who may not be bothered by ointment-induced blurred vision and who may find drop administration irritating.

Sulfacetamide sodium 10% solution is still commonly prescribed for conjunctivitis because it is inexpensive and well-tolerated. However, reports of bacterial resistance may make this bacteriostatic agent less useful.

Aminoglycosides (**neomycin**, **gentamicin**, **tobramycin**) provide good gram-negative coverage, but relatively poor gram-positive coverage. Toxicity to the corneal epithelium can occur, especially with prolonged use, and **neomycin**, in particular, has been associated with local allergic reactions.

Chloramphenicol, available in solution and ointment form, was a popular antibacterial in the past. It has largely been replaced by other agents because of its association with aplastic anemia when given systemically.

Fluoroquinolone antibiotics (**ciprofloxacin**, **ofloxacin**, **norfloxacin**) should be reserved for serious infections such as bacterial keratitis. Also, their poor coverage of *Streptococcus* species makes them unsuitable for the treatment of simple acute bacterial conjunctivitis.

Monitoring of Therapy

Table 1 provides a monitoring plan, which should be individualized.

Table 1: **Monitoring Therapy for Selected Eye Conditions**[1-6,10-12,15,16]

Eye Condition	Monitoring	Goals/Endpoint of Therapy	Actions
Hordeolum	**Patient:** daily **Pharmacist:** after 48 h	Spontaneous drainage within 48 h.	If drainage does not occur within 48 h, refer patient to a physician. Refer patient to a physician if any increase in pain or signs of infection.
Chalazion	**Patient:** daily **Pharmacist:** after 2-3 days	Resolution of chalazion within a few days	If spontaneous drainage does not occur, refer to a physician. For patients with blepharitis, encourage regular lid hygiene* to prevent chalazion recurrence.
Blepharitis	**Patient:** daily during exacerbation. Less often when controlled **Pharmacist:** each pharmacy visit in chronic disease. Within 1 wk if patient requires anti-infective therapy	Control inflammation and discomfort. Reduce the risk of severe, long-term complications.	Encourage compliance with lid hygiene regimen.* Ensure that patients scrub only the margin of the eyelid and do not scratch the eyeball or conjunctiva. Refer to a physician if new onset of blepharitis is suspected. Refer exacerbations to a physician to assess need for anti-infective or other therapy.
Bacterial conjunctivitis	**Patient:** daily **Pharmacist:** within 2 days of initiating drug therapy	Resolution of infection. A decrease in signs and symptoms should occur within 48 h.	*Adults:* Refer to a physician if no improvement within 48 h. *Children:* Refer to a physician. Do not recommend self-treatment.
Chronic bacterial conjunctivitis	**Patient:** daily **Pharmacist:** each pharmacy visit	Control of infection. Reduce the risk of long-term complications.	As for blepharitis
Viral conjunctivitis (adenovirus)	**Patient/family:** daily **Pharmacist:** within 1 wk of initiating treatment	Ease symptoms while infection resolves. Prevent transmission to others.	Refer to a physician for initial assessment to rule out other viral causes. If decongestant or lubricant drops cause irritation, discontinue use or suggest a preservative-free product.
Seasonal allergic conjunctivitis	**Patient:** daily **Pharmacist:** within 3 days of initiating drug therapy	Ease patient discomfort. Stop inflammatory process. Prevent allergy in future seasons.	If decongestant or lubricant drops cause irritation, discontinue use or suggest a preservative-free product. Refer to a physician if no improvement within 3 days, or if symptoms persist despite treatment. Refer to a physician if symptoms are severe.

See Blepharitis, Nonpharmacologic Therapy.

Hyperacute Bacterial Conjunctivitis

This infection is most commonly seen in neonates or sexually active young people (15 to 24 years old). It is a severe, sight-threatening ocular infection caused by *N. gonorrhoea, N. meningitidis,* or *N. gonorrhoea,* subsp. *N. kochii.* It is characterized by a copious, yellow-green, purulent discharge, redness, irritation and tenderness to palpation. Symptoms are rapidly progressive, leading to severe corneal damage, perforation and loss of vision if there is any delay in treatment. When infants are affected, they typically develop bilateral discharge three to five days after birth. Transmission of the organism occurs during vaginal delivery. However, infant infection rates are generally low because of the routine use of ophthalmic antibiotic ointments immediately after delivery. In adults the organism is usually transmitted from the genitalia to the hands and then to the eyes.[6,11-13]

Goals of Therapy

- Cure infection
- Prevent transmission to other persons
- Prevent complications (preserve eyesight)

Nonpharmacologic Therapy[6,11-13]

Immediate referral to a physician or emergency department is required. After treatment has been initiated, nonpharmacologic therapy as in acute bacterial conjunctivitis can be used.

Pharmacologic Therapy[6,11-13]

Nonprescription Therapy

Physician referral is imperative. Nonprescription medication use is inappropriate.

Prescription Therapy

Treatment consists of immediate Gram staining of specimens, followed by systemic and ophthalmic antibacterials and saline irrigation. In adults, **ceftriaxone** 1 to 2 g intramuscularly is the therapy of choice. **Spectinomycin** or oral **ciprofloxacin** can be used in patients allergic to penicillin.

Chronic Bacterial Conjunctivitis

This is defined as a condition that lasts four weeks or longer. It is often associated with blepharitis, and is sometimes found in conjunction with facial seborrhea, acne rosacea, nasolacrimal duct obstruction or chronic dacryocystitis. *S. aureus* and *M. lacunata* are most commonly involved, the latter occurring in clusters in women who share contaminated makeup.[3,6]

Goals of Therapy

- Control infection
- Treat underlying cause
- Prevent complications

Nonpharmacologic Therapy[6,11,12]

Treatment is similar to the treatment of blepharitis. Eyelid hygiene and warm compresses are important as a daily routine. Contaminated facial care products and makeup should be discarded.

Pharmacologic Therapy[6,11,12]

Nonprescription Therapy

Because chronic bacterial conjunctivitis has a protracted course with periods of exacerbation, treatment with nonprescription products without a physician's recommendation is inappropriate.

Prescription Therapy

Topical antibacterials are used during periods of exacerbation. Oral **tetracycline** may benefit patients with meibomian gland dysfunction or acne rosacea, except in pregnant or nursing women and children. Treating acne rosacea with topical **metronidazole** may ameliorate the associated conjunctivitis.

Monitoring of Therapy

Table 1 provides a monitoring plan, which should be individualized.

Viral Conjunctivitis

Patients with viral conjunctivitis usually present with an acutely red eye, watery discharge, conjunctival swelling, soreness or pain, foreign body sensation and mild photophobia. There may be tenderness around the preauricular node. Occasionally, patients may have subconjunctival hemorrhage.[11]

Both eyes may be affected at the same time, or the second eye may become infected a few days after the first. If this happens, the infection is usually more severe in the first eye. The most common causative

---

Table 2: Causes of Conjunctivitis[3,11,12]

Bacterial
Hyperacute
  N. gonorrhoea
  N. meningitidis
  N. gonorrhoea subsp. N. kochii
Acute
  S. aureus
  S. pneumoniae
  H. influenzae
Chronic
  S. aureus
  M. lacunata

Chlamydial
Trachoma (C. trachomatis)

Viral
Adenovirus
Herpes simplex virus

Rickettsial (rare)

Fungal (rare)

Parasitic (rare)

Immunologic
Immediate Hypersensitivity Reactions
  Hay fever
  Vernal keratoconjunctivitis
  Atopic keratoconjunctivitis
  Giant papillary conjunctivitis
Delayed hypersensitivity reactions
Autoimmune Disease
  Keratoconjunctivitis sicca with Sjögren's Syndrome
  Ocular cicatricial pemphigoid

Chemical or Irritative
Iatrogenic
  Miotics
  Idoxuridine
  Preservatives
  Contact lens solutions
Occupational
  Acids
  Alkalies
  Smoke
  Wind
  UV light

Unknown Etiology
Ocular rosacea
Psoriasis
Stevens-Johnson syndrome (erythema multiforme major)
Kawasaki disease
Superior limbic keratoconjunctivitis

Associated with Systemic Disease
Thyroid disease
Gouty conjunctivitis
Carcinoid conjunctivitis
Sarcoidosis
Tuberculosis
Syphilis

Secondary to Dacryocystitis or Canaliculitis

Table 3: Signs and Symptoms of Conjunctivitis[3,11-13]

Clinical findings	Viral	Bacterial	Allergic
Itching	Minimal	Minimal	Severe
Redness	Generalized	Generalized	Generalized
Discharge	Profuse, serous	Moderate, mucopurulent or purulent	Moderate, serous or mucoid

---

organism is *adenovirus*. Viral infections are highly contagious and can be spread through respiratory tract-to-eye, finger-to-eye, or instrument-to-eye (physician's office) contact, and via contaminated swimming pools. Some patients have an associated respiratory tract infection.[6,11-13]

The incubation period ranges from 2 to 14 days and the infection can last from two to four weeks.[13]

Herpes simplex (HSV) and *herpes zoster* can also cause viral conjunctivitis. The risk of progressive keratitis is higher with these types of infection.

Goals of Therapy

Adenovirus:
- Relieve symptoms
- Prevent transmission to others

HSV or herpes zoster:
- Cure infection
- Prevent complications
- Prevent transmission

Nonpharmacologic Therapy[3,6,11]

All patients with suspected viral conjunctivitis should be referred to a physician to determine the cause.

Treatment of adenovirus conjunctivitis is supportive. Warm or cold compresses may increase patient comfort. Instruct patients to avoid direct contact with other persons for at least seven days after the onset of symptoms.[11] Children should be kept out of school until there is no ocular discharge (a minimum of one week).

Pharmacologic Therapy[3,6,11]

Nonprescription Therapy
Ocular decongestants and/or lubricants may be useful in improving patient comfort.

Prescription Therapy
Antiviral agents are not indicated in adenovirus infection. Corticosteroid eye drops may prolong the course of the disease by allowing viral proliferation and should not be used unless under the direction of an ophthalmologist.

Treatment of HSV or herpes zoster infection usually consists of topical (**trifluridine**) and oral (**acyclovir, famciclovir, valacyclovir**) antiviral agents.[6,11,12]

Monitoring of Therapy

Table 1 provides a monitoring plan, which should be individualized.

Seasonal Allergic Conjunctivitis (SAC)
Pathophysiology

The most common type of allergic conjunctivitis is seasonal allergic rhinoconjunctivitis, also known as hay fever. Patients experience ocular itching, tearing, redness and mild eyelid swelling.[3,11,12] Although ragweed is the most common airborne cause of allergic rhinitis, grass pollen is considered the most common cause of ocular symptoms.[15]

Nonpharmacologic Therapy[3,11,12,15,16]

Allergen avoidance is an important first step in the treatment of SAC. Grassy fields, trees and flowers should be avoided and windows should be kept closed to prevent pollens from entering the home. Cold compresses over the eyes offer considerable relief of symptoms, especially ocular pruritus.

Pharmacologic Therapy[3,11,12,15,16]

Nonprescription Therapy
Oral antihistamines have been used successfully in the treatment of SAC. Topical therapy is presented in Table 4.

Refer patients with moderate to severe SAC, or those who do not respond to nonprescription treatment within 72 hours, to a physician.

Prescription Therapy
Levocabastine and **emedastine** are histamine H_1 antagonists with a rapid onset of action. They are more effective than antihistamine/vasoconstrictor combinations or oral antihistamines in relieving itchy, watery eyes. **Olopatadine** possesses both antihistaminic and mast cell stabilizing activity. **Nedocromil**

Table 4: **Topical Nonprescription Drug Therapy of Seasonal Allergic Conjunctivitis (SAC)**[3,11,12,15,16]

Drug	Dose	Expected Clinical Benefit	Comments
Balanced salt solution	Irrigate eyes several times a day.	Allergen dilution and decrease in allergen-conjunctiva contact time.	First-line treatment of SAC. Refer to physician if no improvement within 72 h.
Ocular lubricants e.g., methylcellulose polyvinyl alcohol	1 drop 2-4 times daily	Allergen dilution and decrease in allergen-conjunctiva contact time.	First-line treatment of SAC. Benzalkonium chloride as preservative may irritate eyes, especially if used ≥ 4 times per day. Refrigeration of dropper bottle may improve soothing effect. Refer to physician if no improvement within 72 h.
Decongestants e.g., naphazoline phenylephrine oxymetazoline tetrahydrozoline	1-2 drops every 3-4 h when necessary, up to 4 times a day	Decrease in eye redness and eyelid edema through vasoconstriction. No improvement in underlying allergic response.	Second-line treatment of mild to moderate SAC. Contraindicated in angle-closure glaucoma. May cause burning/stinging upon instillation. Rebound redness may occur with prolonged used.
Antihistamine/decongestant combinations e.g, decongestants listed above, plus: antazoline pheniramine pyrilamine	1-2 drops every 3-4 h when necessary, up to 4 times a day	Decrease in eye redness, itching, eyelid edema and tearing. Generally more effective than decongestant alone, especially in reducing itching.	Second-line treatment of mild to moderate SAC. See decongestants, above.
Mast cell stabilizer e.g., sodium cromoglycate	1-2 drops 4 times daily	Prevents histamine release from mast cells. Regular use during allergy season will prevent redness, itching and eyelid edema.	Second-line treatment of mild to moderate SAC. May take up to 10 days for maximum effect. Must be started before the allergy season to prevent symptoms.

and **lodoxamide** are mast cell stabilizing agents that have demonstrated effectiveness in alleviating the signs and symptoms of SAC.

Nonsteroidal antiinflammatory eyedrops such as **ketorolac** can decrease the amount of ocular itching and conjunctival redness in SAC.

Severe cases of SAC may require the use of topical **corticosteroids** or other immunomodulatory agents.

Ideally these patients would be under the care of an ophthalmologist.

Monitoring of Therapy

Table 1 provides a monitoring plan, which should be individualized.

Dry Eye

Pathophysiology

The tear film is a three-layered structure less than 10 mm thick with a volume of 7 ± 2 μl. The outermost layer is composed of lipids secreted by the meibomian glands. It covers the entire free surface of the tear fluid and is important in stabilizing the tear film and slowing the evaporation of the aqueous layer. The middle layer is aqueous and is the thickest part of the tear film. It contains inorganic salts, glucose, urea, trace elements, and the antibacterial proteins, lactoferrin and lysozyme. The mucin layer is formed by goblet cells in the conjunctiva. It lies adjacent to the cornea and stabilizes the tear film by interacting with epithelial layers in the cornea and conjunctiva and the aqueous layer. It also removes waste materials such as mucus threads and fibrils.[2,17,19]

Dry eye can generally be classified into five etiological categories (Table 5):
- *Aqueous deficiency* – decreased lacrimal gland secretion. This can be caused by disorders such as Sjögren's syndrome[19-21]; anticholinergic agents can also inhibit lacrimal gland secretion.[22]
- *Mucin deficiency* – damage or inflammation of goblet cells can be caused by conditions such as erythema multiforme.[18] Long-term use of topical antiglaucoma medications (Table 5) has been rarely associated with the development of ocular cicatricial pemphigoid, a disease characterized by chronic, treatment-resistant conjunctivitis that results in progressive scarring and shrinking of the eyelids (cicatrization), severe dry eye, and eventual blindness.[23,24]
- *Lipid deficiency* – a decreased lipid layer is common in patients with blepharitis.[19] Recent evidence also suggests that meibomian gland dysfunction may

be partly responsible for dry eye in Sjögren's syndrome.[25]
- *Impaired lid function* – contact lens wear can impair proper tear film distribution across the eye by interfering with the blinking process.[17,18]
- *Epitheliopathies* – defects in the corneal epithelium that can impair tear film stability. There is some indication that epithelial turnover is controlled by the autonomic nervous system. Anticholinergic medications may interfere with this control mechanism.[17,18]

Severe or chronic dry eye, also known as keratoconjunctivitis sicca (KCS), can lead to serious ocular surface disease if left untreated. Persistent dry spots on the cornea can predispose the eye to bacterial infection. Corneal ulceration, thinning, or perforation are possible. Subsequent scarring of the cornea may markedly reduce vision.[2,26]

Goals of Therapy

- Ease patient discomfort and minimize symptoms
- Prevent or delay complications
- Educate patients about their condition and encourage compliance, especially those with long-term disease

Patient Assessment

An algorithm for the assessment of eye conditions is presented in Figure 3.

Patients with dry eye may complain of a foreign body sensation in the eye. Words like "sandy" or "scratchy" are used to convey this feeling. Eyes often feel like they are burning, itchy or tired. Other symptoms include photophobia, blurred vision, redness, discomfort and difficulty in moving the lids. Although most patients state that their eyes feel dry, some will report increased tearing. This is a reflex tearing that does little to increase comfort. Unlike blepharitis and conjunctivitis, dry eye symptoms tend to worsen over the course of the day.

Prevention

Warn patients receiving medications that may cause dry eye about this potential and how to treat it if it occurs. Contact lens wearers need to pay careful attention to proper cleaning and wear of their lenses (see Chapter 15). People involved in concentration activities (e.g., computer work, video games) often forget to blink, and may need to be reminded to do so. Those suffering from chronic blepharitis should be encouraged to maintain lid hygiene to decrease the occurrence of dry eye. Patients with autoimmune or dermatologic diseases (e.g., Sjögren's syndrome, rheumatoid arthritis, acne rosacea) could be asked about any symptoms of dry eye. Because of the severity of dry eye that can be associated with these diseases, referral by their treating physician to an ophthalmologist may be suggested to optimize therapy and prevent complications.

Nonpharmacologic Therapy

Nonpharmacologic therapy of dry eye may involve environmental changes. As tobacco smoke is a common cause of eye irritation, encourage patients to avoid smoking and smoky rooms. Humidifiers can improve conditions for dry eye sufferers, especially in winter. Moisture chamber spectacles, or ski or swim goggles can also be worn to increase humidity in the eye area as well as decrease the evaporation of tears. A moistened gauze placed inside the goggles helps maintain a moist environment. A cool, moist washcloth placed over closed eyelids may provide short-term relief.[2,17,20,22]

Tear duct (punctal) occlusion may be used in severe or chronic dry eye to prevent drainage of existing tears via the nasolacrimal ducts. Punctal plugs, inserted by an ophthalmologist trained in this technique, are used to assess whether a patient will

benefit from this treatment. It is possible to dislodge the plugs, especially if patients rub their eyelids. Therefore, nasolacrimal occlusion for eye drop instillation is not recommended or required in patients with punctal plugs. Permanent occlusion is achieved through heat or electrocautery.[17,27]

Pharmacologic Therapy

Nonprescription Therapy

Pharmacologic therapy generally begins with administration of nonprescription **artificial tear solutions**. The choice of agent depends on the severity of disease and the underlying cause. In general terms, treatment begins with either a volume-enhancing agent to supplement suboptimal tear production or a contact-enhancing agent to help retain existing tears.

Although numerous products are available, the best therapy is still achieved through a trial and error approach. This can be frustrating, both for the patient and for the physician. A one to two week trial of eye drops is needed to determine the subjective efficacy of the product (i.e., patient comfort, improvement in symptoms).[4,28]

An ideal tear replacement product would possess the following properties:[17]

- Electrolytes (sodium, potassium, calcium, bicarbonate) in concentrations similar to that of normal tears.
- An osmolarity of 200 to 280 mOsm to dilute the abnormally high osmolarity of tears in dry eye patients, often > 312 mOsm (normal tear osmolarity is 300 mOsm).
- pH of 7.4 to 7.7.
- Viscosity of < 20 centipoise (cps). (Water is 0.7 cps.)
- No cytotoxicity. Ethylenediaminetetraacetic acid (EDTA), an additive in some eye drops, can damage corneal epithelial cells.
- Preservative-free. Benzalkonium chloride, the most common preservative in eye preparations, can be toxic to the corneal epithelium.[17,29] Other preservatives, such as polyquaternium-1 (Polyquad[R]) or sodium perborate, may be safer alternatives.[30,31]

Substituted Cellulose Ethers
Carboxymethylcellulose 1% provides a higher viscosity solution than **methylcellulose, hydroxyethylcellulose, hydroxypropylcellulose**, or **hydro-**

xypropylmethylcellulose and is effective in improving severe ocular symptoms.[18,32] The higher viscosity produces more blurring of the vision, however, and may be more appropriate for night time use.

Polyvinyl Polymers

Polyvinyl alcohol 1.4% solution is much less viscous than methylcellulose 0.5% solution and may be preferred by some patients. Polyvinylpyrrolidone appears to form an artificial layer that mimics mucin, making it useful for eyes deficient in mucin and water.[18]

Sodium Hyaluronate

Sodium hyaluronate is a polysaccharide polymer that acts as a viscoelastic solution at physiologic pH, with a viscosity 500,000 times that of saline. An injectable form is often used in intraocular surgical procedures. Ophthalmic solutions in concentrations of 0.1 to 0.5% have been successful in treating symptoms of dry eye.[18,19]

Ointments

Petrolatum-containing ophthalmic ointments have a longer retention time in the eye than drops but can

---

Table 5: **Causes of Dry Eye**[2,17,18,33-35]

Aqueous Deficiency

Congenital
  Riley-Day Syndrome
  Congenital alacrima
  Trigeminal nerve aplasia

Acquired
  Sjögren's Syndrome
  Sarcoidosis
  Leukemia, lymphoma
  Hemochromatosis
  Progressive systemic sclerosis
  Graft vs host disease
  Menopause
  Androgen or prolactin deficiency

Infection
  Mumps
  HIV-AIDS complex
  Epstein-Barr virus

Injury
  Surgical removal of lacrimal gland
  Noxious agents (e.g., tobacco smoke, exhaust fumes)
  Irradiation
  Chemical burns

Medications
  Anticholinergic/antimuscarinic agents (e.g., scopolamine, atropine)
  First generation antihistamines (e.g., chlorpheniramine)
  ß-blockers (e.g., propranolol, timolol)
  Diuretics (e.g., hydrochlorothiazide, indapamide)
  Isotretinoin
  Niacin (in doses used to treat hyperlipidemia)
  Oral contraceptives
  Phenothiazine antipsychotics (e.g., chlorpromazine)
  Tricyclic antidepressants (e.g., amitriptyline)

Mucin Layer Deficiency

Vitamin A deficiency

Conjunctival shrinkage
  Erythema multiforme

  Stevens-Johnson syndrome
  Ocular cicatricial pemphigoid

Chronic conjunctivitis
  Trachoma

Allergic conjunctivitis

Medications
  topical epinephrine
  topical echothiophate iodide
  topical timolol

Topical pilocarpine

Chemical burns

Irradiation

Lipid Layer Deficiency

Blepharitis

Advanced age

Meibomian gland dysfunction
  Acne rosacea

Medications
  Isotretinoin

Impaired Lid Function

Eyelid abnormalities
Ectropion or entropion
Keratinization of lid margin
Lagophthalmos

Decreased or absent blinking
  Neurologic disorders
  Hyperthyroidism
  Contact lenses
  Herpes simplex keratitis

Proptosis

Conjunctival abnormalities
  Pterygium

Epitheliopathies

Anticholinergic medication

cause unacceptable blurred vision. This limits their application to bedtime use for most patients. Only severe dry eyes require daytime administration.[17,18]

Carbomer resins are synthetic high molecular weight polymers of acrylic acid crosslinked to a polyalkyl polyether. Carbomer 940 aqueous gel is significantly more effective than both placebo and polyvinyl alcohol 1.4% solution.[36,37] Although carbomer 940 acts like an ointment, it causes less blurred vision than petrolatum-based ophthalmic ointments.

Artificial Tear Inserts

Water-soluble **hydroxypropylcellulose** is available as an insert to be placed in the conjunctival sac. It dissolves over several hours, allowing long-term ocular lubrication. Blurred vision is common for the first few hours, but it is preservative free. Manual dexterity and education are required for proper instillation.[17,18]

Prescription Therapy

Oral **pilocarpine** is indicated for the treatment of dry eye associated with Sjögren's syndrome.[38] Other treatments that have been investigated for severe dry eye include topical **acetylcysteine**[2,17,18] (removes excessive mucus), topical **methylprednisolone**[39], topical cyclosporine[40], topical estradiol[41], and periorbital intramuscular injections of botulinum toxin.[42]

Monitoring of Therapy[2,4,17,18,28]

Patients with intermittent symptoms of dry eye can be treated effectively with one or more of the numerous ocular lubricants available. Refer to a physician if symptoms do not resolve or if they worsen within a few days.

Signs of preservative toxicity include stinging upon instillation and conjunctival inflammation. If these symptoms are present, the patient may need to be directed to another product, or to their physician for assessment. Patients who require more than four applications per day for long periods of time should use a preservative free product to prevent toxicity.

Periodic assessment of eye drop and ointment instillation technique (see Proper Use of Eye Drops, Proper Use of Eye Ointments—Patient Information) will help patients make best use of the agents. Devices such as the Auto-Drop® and Auto-Squeeze® (Owen Mumford,

www.owenmumford.com) are usually available through local wholesalers and can be offered to patients to aid in ocular medication administration.

Resource Tips

Mayo Clinic.com, Diseases and Conditions A to Z, www.mayoclinic.com/findinformation/diseases and conditions/index.cfm

Eye Care Links
www.seeintl.org/eyecare.html

St. Luke's Cataract and Laser Institute
www.stlukeseye. com

Suggested Readings

Fechner PU, Teichmann KD. *Ocular therapeutics – pharmacology and clinical application*. Thorofare: SLACK Inc., 1998.

Morrow GL, Abbott RL. Conjunctivitis. *Am Fam Physician* 1998;57:735-46.

Rhee DJ, Pyfer MF, eds. *The Wills Eye Manual. Office and emergency room. Diagnosis and treatment of eye disease*. 3rd ed. New York, NY: Lippincott Williams & Wilkins; 1999.

Thielen TL, Castle SS, Terry JE. Anterior ocular infections: an overview of pathophysiology and treatment. *Ann Pharmacother* 2000;34:325-46.

Vaugh D, Asbury T, Riordan-Eva P, eds. *General Ophthalmology*. 15th ed. Stamford, CT: Appleton & Lange; 1999.

References

1. Rubin S, Hallagan L. Lids, lacrimals, and lashes. *Emerg Med Clin North Am* 1995;13:631-48.
2. Sullivan JH, Crawford JB, Witcher JP. Lids, lacrimal apparatus, and tears. In: Vaugh D, Asbury T, Riordan-Eva P, eds. *General Ophthalmology*. 15th ed. Stamford, CT: Appleton & Lange; 1999:74-91.
3. Kanski JJ. *Clinical Ophthalmology*. 4th ed. Boston: Butterworth-Heinemann; 1999.
4. Shields SR. Managing eye disease in primary care. Part 2. How to recognize and treat common eye problems. *Postgrad Med* 2000;108(5):83-6, 91-6.
5. Raskin EM, Speaker MG, Laibson PR. Blepharitis. *Infect Dis Clin North Am* 1992;6:777-87.
6. Thielen TL, Castle SS, Terry JE. Anterior ocular infections: an overview of pathophysiology and treatment. *Ann Pharmacother* 2000;34:325-46.
7. Freedman HL, Preston KL. Heat retention in varieties of warm compresses: a comparison between warm soaks,

hard-boiled eggs and the Re-Heater. *Ophthalmic Surg* 1989;20:846-8.

8. Cottrell DG, Bosanquet RC, Fawcett IM. Chalazions: the frequency of spontaneous resolution. *BMJ* 1983;287:1595.

9. Smythe D, Hurwitz JJ, Tayfour F. The management of chalazion: a survey of Ontario ophthalmologists. *Can J Ophthalmol* 1990;25:252-5.

10. Baum J. Infections of the eye. *Clin Infect Dis* 1995;21:479-86.

11. Morrow GL, Abbott RL. Conjunctivitis. *Am Fam Physician* 1998;57:735-46.

12. Schwab IR, Crawford JB. Conjunctiva. In: Vaugh D, Asbury T, Riordan-Eva P, eds. *General Ophthalmology*. 15th ed. Stamford, CT: Appleton & Lange; 1999:92-118.

13. Jackson WB. Differentiating conjunctivitis of diverse origins. *Surv Ophthalmol* 1993;38 (suppl):91-104.

14. Weiss A, Brinser JH, Nazar-Stewart V. Acute conjunctivitis in childhood. *J Pediatr* 1993;122:10-4.

15. Bielory L. Allergic and immunologic disorders of the eye. Part II: ocular allergy. *J Allergy Clin Immunol* 2000;106:1019-32.

16. Hingorani M, Lightman S. Therapeutic options in ocular allergic disease. *Drugs* 1995;50:208-21.

17. Fechner PU, Teichmann KD. *Ocular therapeutics – pharmacology and clinical application.* Thorofare: SLACK Inc., 1998.

18. Jaanus SD. Lubricants and other preparations for ocular surface disease. In: Bartlett JD, Jaanus SD, eds. *Clinical Ocular Pharmacology*. 3rd ed. Boston, Mass.: Butterworth-Heinemann, 1995:355-67.

19. Semes L. Diagnosis and primary care management of tear film deficiencies. *Optom Clin* 1995;4:87-104.

20. Friedlaender MH. Ocular manifestations of Sjögren's Syndrome: keratoconjunctivitis sicca. *Rheum Dis Clin NA* 1992;18:591-608.

21. Oxholm P, Prause JU, Schiodt M. Rational drug therapy recommendations for the treatment of patients with Sjögren's Syndrome. *Drugs* 1998;56:345-53.

22. Asbell PA, Torres MA. Therapeutic dilemmas in external ocular diseases. *Drugs* 1991;42:606-15.

23. Fiore PM, Jacobs IH, Goldberg DB. Drug-induced pemphigoid. *Arch Ophthalmol* 1987;105:1660-3.

24. Baudouin C, Pisella PJ, Fillacier K, et al. Ocular suface inflammatory changes induced by topical antiglaucoma drugs. *Ophthalmol* 1999;106:556-63.

25. Shimazaki J, Goto E, Ono M, et al. Meibomian gland dysfuntion in patients with Sjögren Syndrome. *Ophthalmol* 1998;105:1485-8.

26. Pflugfelder SC. Advances in the diagnosis and management of keratoconjunctivitis sicca. *Curr Opin Ophthalmol* 1998;9:50-3.

27. Cohen EJ. Punctal occlusion. *Arch Ophthalmol* 1999;117:389-90.

28. Gilbard JP. Dry eye, blepharitis and chronic eye irritation: divide and conquer. *J Ophthalmic Nurs Technol* 1999;18:109-15.

29. Gobbels M, Spitznas M. Corneal epithelial permeability of dry eyes before and after treatment with artificial tears. *Ophthalmol* 1992;99:873-8.

30. Lopez BD, Ubels JL. Quantitative evaluation of the corneal epithelial barrier: effect of artificial tears and preservatives. *Curr Eye Res* 1991;10:645-56.

31. Lopez BD, Ubels JL. Artificial tear composition and promotion of recovery of the damaged corneal epithelium. *Cornea* 1993;12:115-20.

32. Allergan. Celluvisc (carboxymethylcellulose 1%) product information. Irvine; 1991.

33. Jaanus SD, Bartlett JD, Hiett JA. Ocular effects of systemic drugs. In: Bartlett JD, Jaanus SD, eds. *Clinical Ocular Pharmacology*. 3rd ed. Boston, Mass.: Butterworth-Heinemann; 1995:957-1006.

34. Semes LP, Clompus RJ. Diseases of the lacrimal system. In: Bartlett JD, Jaanus SD, eds. *Clinical Ocular Pharmacology*. 3rd ed. Boston: Butterworth-Heinemann; 1995:601-30.

35. Fraunfelder FT. *Drug-induced Ocular Side Effects*. 4th ed. Baltimore: Williams & Wilkins; 1996.

36. Sullivan LJ, McCurrach F, Lee S, et al. Efficacy and safety of 0.3% carbomer gel compared to placebo in patients with moderate-to-severe dry eye syndrome. *Ophthalmol* 1997;104:1402-8.

37. Marner K, Mooller PM, Dillon M, et al. Viscous carbomer eye drops in patients with dry eyes. Efficacy and safety. A randomized, open, cross-over, multicentre study. *Acta Ophthalmol Scand* 1996;74:249-52.

38. Vivino FB, Al-Hashimi I, Khan Z. Pilocarpine tablets for the treatment of dry mouth and dry eye symptoms in patients with Sjögren Syndrome. *Arch Intern Med* 1999;159:174-81.

39. Marsh P, Pflugfelder SC. Topical nonpreserved methylprednisolone therapy for keratoconjunctivitis sicca in Sjögren Syndrome. *Ophthalmol* 1999;106:811-6.

40. Liegner JT, Yee RW, Wild JH. Topical cyclosporine therapy for ulcerative keratitis associated with rheumatoid arthritis. *Am J Ophthalmol* 1990;109:610-2.

41. Sator MO, Joura EA, Golaszewski T, et al. Treatment of menopausal keratoconjunctivitis sicca with topical oestradiol. *Br J Obstet Gynaecol* 1998;105:100-2.

42. Spiera H, Asbell PA, Simpson DM. Botulinum toxin increases tearing in patients with Sjögren's Syndrome: a preliminary report. *J Rheumatol* 1997;24:1842-3.

Using Eye Products—Patient Information

- For external use only.
- Never share your eye products with another person.
- Close containers tightly after use.
- Store in a cool, dark place. Some products have to be stored in the refrigerator. Check with your pharmacist.
- Discard the product:
  —If it changes color or appearance
  —If it was opened more than one month ago, or
  —Immediately after use if it is a single (or unit) dose package (without preservatives); it is intended for a single use only—do not reuse leftover product.
- Keep out of reach of children.
- If you are having difficulties administering your eye product, have a family member or friend assist you, or ask your pharmacist about devices that might help.
- Thoroughly wash hands before and after using the product.

- Never contaminate the container tip by allowing it to touch the eyes, eyelids, eyelashes, fingers or counter surface. This applies to the cap of the container as well. Replace the cap as soon as possible.
- Use only as directed.
- Some products may temporarily blur vision; be careful while driving or performing other hazardous tasks.
- Discontinue the medication and see your eye care professional if:
  —You experience eye pain;
  —Your eyes are sensitive to light;
  —You experience visual changes;
  —The eye irritation and redness continues;
  —Self-medicating for more than 48 hours (with anti-infectives) or 72 hours (with other agents) does not clear up the condition or the condition worsens, or
  —Without treatment the condition has lasted longer than 48 hours.

Proper Use of Eye Drops—Patient Information

- Wash hands thoroughly.
- Carefully remove the bottle cap, trying not to contaminate the rim or the inside of the cap (lay it on its side on a clean, dry tissue).
- Tilt head back or lie down.
- If the medication is a suspension, shake the bottle before using it. Ask your pharmacist if you're not sure.
- While your eyes are open, gently pull down on the lower eyelid to form a pouch.
- Holding the bottle almost horizontally, approach your eye from the side. This reduces the risk of accidentally hitting the eye with the tip of the bottle.
- Hold the tip near the eyelid but at least 2.5 cm (1 inch) away. Do not touch the lids or lashes with the tip of the bottle.
- Look upwards by moving your eyes only. (Looking up moves the centre of the eyeball away from where the drop is going and will keep your eye from blinking hard when the drop goes in.)
- Instil one drop into the pouch of the lower eyelid. Hold this position to let the drop fall as deeply as possible into the pouch.
- Look down for several seconds and then slowly release the lower lid. Looking down brings the centre of the eye into maximum contact with the medication. (This is especially important for infections of the cornea.)
- Gently close (do not squeeze) the eyes for at least 30 seconds (up to five minutes). A tissue may be used to blot around the eye, but do not rub. Closing the eye keeps the medication in contact with the eye for as long as possible. If the eye is closed too tightly, the medication may be squeezed out.
- Applying gentle pressure across the bridge of the nose with your thumb and index finger may also help keep medication from going down the tear duct. If you have recently undergone eye surgery, ask your eye doctor whether pressure should be applied to the bridge of your nose.
- Before opening the eye, blot away excess medication. Do not rub the eye. Try not to blink.
- Do not rinse the tip of the eye drop bottle. Replace the bottle cap.
- Wash hands thoroughly.
- If more than one drop is prescribed, wait three to five minutes between drops. This ensures the first drop is not flushed away and the second drop is not diluted by the first.

Figure 4: **Eye Drop Instillation**

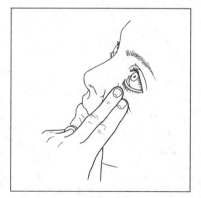

Step 1: *Gently pull down on the lower eyelid to form a pouch.*

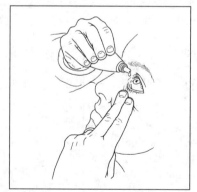

Step 2: *Hold bottle horizontally, approach the eye from the side. Hold tip at least 2.5 cm away from the eyelid.*

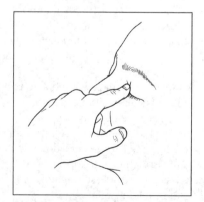

Step 3: *Keep eye closed for at least 30 seconds (up to 5 minutes). Apply gentle pressure to the bridge of the nose. If you had eye surgery recently, ask the doctor before applying pressure.*

Patient Self-Care (PSC), 2002

- If more than one medication is used, wait 5 to 10 minutes between different medications.
- If you have problems with balance or dizziness, lie down or sit down in a very stable position to use your drops. This will reduce the risk of falling.
- If you have tremors or arthritis, devices are available that can help you administer eye drops. Discuss this with your pharmacist or eye care professional.

- Eye drop bottles usually contain a preservative to prevent contamination of the medication. However, the bottles can become contaminated over time, especially if the bottle tip has come into contact with the eye or the eyelashes. A good rule of thumb is to throw out any bottles that have been open for a month or more.

Proper Use of Eye Ointments—Patient Information

- Wash hands thoroughly.
- Hold the tube in your hand for a few minutes to warm the ointment and help it flow better. Remove the container cap (lay it on its side on a clean, dry tissue).
- When opening the tube for the first time, squeeze out and discard the first 0.25 cm (0.1 inches) of ointment as it may be too dry.
- Tilt head back or lie down.
- While your eyes are open, gently pull down on the lower eyelid to form a pouch.
- Holding the tube almost horizontally, approach your eye from the side. This reduces the risk of accidentally hitting the eye with the tip of the tube.
- Hold the tip near the eyelid but at least 2.5 cm (1 inch) away. Do not touch the lids or lashes with the tip of the tube.
- Look upwards by moving your eyes only. (Looking up moves the centre of the eyeball away from where the ointment is going and will keep your eye from blinking hard when the ointment goes in.)
- Place 0.6 to 1.25 cm (0.25 to 0.5 inches) of ointment into the pouch of the lower eyelid. It is not necessary to place the ointment along the entire length of the pouch.
- Gently close the eye for one to two minutes and roll the eyeball in all directions.
- Replace the container cap.
- After the ointment is used, vision may be blurred for a few minutes; do not drive or operate machinery until blurriness disappears.
- Using a clean tissue, remove excess ointment from the eyelid margins.
- Wash hands thoroughly.
- If both an ointment and eye drop are used, use the eye drop first. Wait at least five minutes before using the ointment.

- If different types of ointments are to be used, wait at least 10 minutes before using the second one.
- If ointments are to be applied to the outer eyelids, place the ointment on a sterile cotton-tipped applicator and apply to the lid.
- Eye ointments usually contain a preservative to prevent contamination of the medication. However, the tubes can become contaminated over time, especially if the tip has come into contact with the eye or the eyelashes. A good rule of thumb is to throw out any tubes that have been open for a month or more.

Figure 5: **Eye Ointment Instillation**

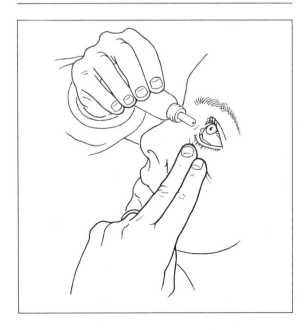

Infections of the Eyelids or Conjunctiva— Patient Information

- See your eye care professional if:
  —You have pain, altered vision or severe redness;
  —This is a recurrent condition;
  —You have an underlying disease (e.g., diabetes);
  —Self-treatment longer than 48 hours with anti-infectives does not clear up the condition;
  — The condition worsens with treatment;
  —Without treatment the condition has lasted longer than 48 hours.
- Use separate facecloths, towels, pillows and sheets from other family members since the infection may spread. Use a fresh facecloth and towel for each cleaning.

- Do not use an eye patch unless recommended by your eye care professional.
- If you need to use a device to help instil your eye drops, wash it with soap and warm water after each use.
- Cosmetics (e.g., mascara) can be a source of reinfection.
- Wash your hands before and after touching your eyes.
- For eye infections, it is important that the eye area is cleaned, especially before applying any medication. This is particularly true when there is a sticky discharge or an eyelid infection (clean the lids thoroughly).

Special Advice for Instilling Eye Drops in Children— Patient Information

Positioning
Have the child lie down and close the eyes.

Alternate Positioning Method:
For infants and small children who may not cooperate, an alternative method can be tried. Sit on the floor and have the child sit on your lap—legs astride yours—facing you. While supporting the back and head, gently lower the child backward until they are lying along your legs. You have the option of having your own legs at an angle toward your body. Several options are then available, according to the control desired. With the child lying down, hold the head with one hand and instil drops with the other on the side you are holding. In very resistant cases, the child's head may be gently clamped between your legs, and the feet wedged against your body under your arms. Either procedure can be done with the assistance of a third person.

Instillation
Wash your hands thoroughly. Approach the eye holding the container horizontally, resting the hand on the

child's cheek to prevent injury to the eye if the child moves suddenly.

Instil the drop(s) properly (see Proper Use of Eye Drops—Patient Information).

Alternate Instillation Methods:
1. Use the *closed eye method:* Place the drop on the eyelid in the inner corner of the eye, then have the child open the eye so the drop falls in by gravity. (This method is also useful for adults with a strong blink reflex.)
2. Pull the lower lid down and instil the drop through the lashes, avoiding touching the bottle to the lashes.
3. If the instillation of drops or ointment application is important (e.g., to treat an infected eye), it is better, although not ideal, to get some drops or ointment on the lids and lashes (keeping the lids closed momentarily) and allow the preparation to seep onto the surface of the eye, than for no drops or ointment to be used at all.

Chapter 15

Contact Lens Care

David Wing, BSP, MS and Ken Gellatly, OD

Pathophysiology

Hyperopia and myopia are errors in refraction where parallel rays of light do not focus properly on the retina. In *hyperopia* (farsightedness), light focuses behind the retina, causing near objects to be blurry while distant objects are focused. In *myopia* (near-sightedness), light focuses before reaching the retina, causing near objects to be focused and distant objects to be blurry. In *astigmatism*, the shape of the eye or cornea is oval or elliptical, causing parallel rays of light to intersect at two different points. *Presbyopia* is part of natural aging where control of the state of contraction of the ciliary muscle for accommodation is decreased, resulting in progressive decline in clear vision for near objects. In *aphakia*, the lens is absent, either congenitally, or more likely, due to surgery for removal of a cataract (loss of transparency of lens). Aphakic individuals have reduced near and far vision.

Contact Lenses

Contact lenses can correct hyperopia, myopia, astigmatism, presbyopia and aphakia. Contact lenses are foreign bodies that sit on a tear cushion and do not actually contact the eye as implied by their name. As tears constantly bathe the cornea, supplying oxygen, contact lenses act as physical barriers producing progressive hypoxia and edema. Whether clinical symptoms result depends on duration of wear, compliance with the care regimen, lens materials, lens design and fit.

Contact lenses offer many advantages over eyeglasses:[1,2]
- An entire field of view in focus;
- Natural appearance;
- No fogging from temperature changes, perspiration or weather;
- No annoying reflections and peripheral obstructions.

The two major types of contact lenses are rigid gas permeable (RGP) and soft. The longevity of a single set of lenses is classified according to replacement schedule:
- Conventional (more than one year);
- Planned replacement (lenses replaced at a fixed interval; e.g., every two weeks, every month or every three months);
- Daily disposable (brand new lenses inserted every day).

Types of Contact Lenses

Table 1 compares some of the important features of RGP and soft lenses.

Rigid Gas Permeable Lenses

The RGP lens combines the optical qualities and durability of PMMA (polymethyl methacrylate, the original hard lens, which is now obsolete) with the oxygen permeability and comfort of soft lenses.[3] RGP lenses have a sufficiently high oxygen permeability to prevent clinically observable corneal edema with normal wear. Hence, better long-term visual acuity and in general, fewer complications are achieved than with either PMMA or soft lenses. RGP lenses have replaced the original PMMA lenses as the standard of care for hard lenses.

Soft Lenses

Soft lenses are made of a flexible polymeric material, usually hydroxyethyl methacrylate (HEMA) with a high capacity for water absorption.[4,5] Their main advantage over RGP lenses is increased comfort. This is due to their flexibility (which increases with increasing water content), soft thin edges and hydrophilic nature, all of which allow normal tear exchange with each blink reflex.

Unfortunately, these lenses have an open matrix which concentrates tear film lipoproteins, ophthalmic preparations, environmental pollutants, chemical vapors, oil and dust from fingers, cosmetics and some contact lens solution preservatives, all of which can lead to ocular irritation. Soft lens materials also tend to develop lens deposits (i.e., accumulation of proteins and lipids) more rapidly than RGP lens materials.

Wear Schedules[6,7]

In the *conventional* wearing schedule, lenses are replaced at an interval of greater than one year. Due to compliance problems (e.g., inadequate cleaning, disinfection and rinsing; reuse of old solutions; poor hygiene; using lenses for a longer time than recommended), *planned replacement programs* (PRPs) were developed.

In a PRP, lenses are worn on a daily basis (although PRPs can also include extended-wear lenses) and disposed of at a fixed interval (e.g., every two weeks, monthly or quarterly) as determined by the eye care professional.

Advantages of PRPs include:
- More frequent insertion of a new, sterile lens;
- Lower cost because of reduced need for solutions (multipurpose solutions can replace single purpose solutions);
- Improved vision (from more frequent replacement);
- Improved comfort (deposits are reduced, which increases lens wettability and reduces dryness);
- Improved compliance (from increased monitoring);
- More convenience (multipurpose solutions can be used, in association with increased monitoring);
- Fewer complaint-related office visits (reduction in giant papillary conjunctivitis, acute red eye and infective or inflammatory keratitis);
- Fewer problems associated with lost lenses (wearer has immediate access to a new set of lenses) or damaged lenses (wearer has no need to keep an old spare pair of lenses on hand).

In addition to supplied lenses, a disposable system that includes solutions and storage cases that are replaced at regular intervals may decrease the risk of ocular infections.

Daily disposables are sterile soft lenses that are opened fresh each day, worn and then disposed of in the evening. These lenses, which require no regular solutions for daily care, offer advantages for wearers who may have compliance problems with one of the other wear schedules.[8]

Extended-wear is defined as continuous use of a contact lens for 24 hours or more. The lenses are usually soft; however, RGP lenses are increasing in use for extended-wear schedules. Early uncontrolled trials suggested that the rate of serious complications was not excessive and many wearers adopted extended-wear schedules. However, extended-wear of contact lenses was eventually implicated in promoting microbial keratitis.[9] The most likely causes are increased protein accumulation, decreased flushing of bacteria during sleep and decreased immunologic activity during sleep. To decrease the frequency of infection, the FDA recommends that extended-wear soft lenses be worn for a maximum of seven days before removal for cleaning or disposal.[10]

Goals of Contact Lens Care
- Optimize vision
- Promote lens longevity and comfort
- Minimize complications such as eye irritation and infection

Patient Assessment

Use the following questions and answers to identify potential problems and aid in appropriate and timely referral to eye care professionals.

What type of contact lenses are you wearing?
The lens type (RGP or soft) determines the care regimen. Solutions for either lens type from the same manufacturer can likely be interchanged. However, patients should consult their eye care professional for confirmation.

Do you have any of the following symptoms:
- Pain when inserting or wearing the lenses or after wearing them?
- Burning that causes excessive tearing?

Table 1: **Comparative Features of Rigid Gas Permeable (RGP) and Soft Contact Lenses**

Characteristics	Soft lenses	RGP lenses
Composition	Hydroxyethyl-methacrylate (HEMA) is the most common polymer	PMMA/silicone, fluoro-silicone acrylate
Water content (%)	29 to 85 (hydrophilic)	Up to 2 (hydrophobic)
Life expectancy of lens (years)	2	5
Solution requirements	Only soft lens solutions	Only RGP solutions
Visual acuity	Good	Excellent
Cost		
initial	Similar	Similar
maintenance	More	Less
Gas permeability	Less	More
Adaptability (days)	< 1	5 to 10
Daily wear time (hours)	12	> 12
Extended wear (days)	Up to 7	Up to 7
Initial comfort	Most	Intermediate
Long-term comfort	Intermediate	Most
Strength	Fragile	Strong
Accumulation of deposits from tear film	Most susceptible	Least susceptible
Effect of humidity	Easily affected	Minimally affected
Risk of microbial contamination	Greatest	Slight

- Inability to keep your eyes open?
- Severe or persistent haze, fog or halos while wearing the lenses?
- Redness, irritation or itching?

These symptoms may be due to poor lens fit, damaged lenses, improper handling, microbial conjunctivitis, solution or lens intolerance, ocular or systemic disease, or improper lens care. Painful lid swelling and photophobia may be due to overwear. If any of these symptoms occur, patients should discontinue lens wear and consult their eye care professional.

How long have you worn lenses?
Every contact lens wearer experiences discomfort during the first few weeks while the eyes adapt. Since it may not be obvious at first which problems are significant, wearers should contact their eye care professional.

What medications are you taking? (Tables 2 and 3)
Any ophthalmic preparation should be used only on the advice of an eye care professional, who will specify whether the medication should be used while the lens is in place. Almost any ophthalmic product that is not specifically designed for use with contact lenses will cause temporary discomfort.

Numerous systemic medications can alter eye dynamics sufficiently to warrant therapeutic intervention. Sedatives (including alcohol), hypnotics, antihistamines and muscle relaxants can affect the eyelid, producing incomplete blinking or a decreased rate of blinking. Antihistamines, anticholinergics, tricyclic antidepressants and diuretics can decrease tear volume, leading to significant discomfort.

If you wear soft lenses, what method of disinfection did your eye care professional recommend?
Knowledge of the disinfection method makes it possible to reinforce the instructions of the eye care professional and prevent wearers from using solutions not designed for their method of disinfection. There are two forms of chemical disinfection: oxidizing agents (i.e., hydrogen peroxide) and disinfecting agents (e.g., polyquaternium-1, polyaminopropyl-

biguanide, polyhexanide, alkytriethanolammonium chloride and sorbic acid).

What products do you use for the care of your lenses?

Eye care professionals recommend specific products for lenses. Pharmacists can identify and correct inappropriate substitution of products. Refer the wearer to an eye care professional if there is any confusion or uncertainty regarding which solutions to use.

Describe how you use your lens care products.

Noncompliance is the greatest threat to eye comfort and lens life. Inadequate cleaning and disinfection cause about 50% of all problems associated with contact lenses. To ensure wearers are compliant, ask them to describe their care regimen (Figure 1).

What measures do you take before reinsertion after the lens has been dropped?

Unfortunately, wearers often pick up the lens and promptly reinsert it along with whatever the lens has collected. RGP lenses should be rinsed with an aerosol saline solution and soft lenses with an appropriate rinsing solution before being reinserted.

Prevention of Complications

Taking proper care of contact lenses is crucial in maintaining optimal eye health. The ideal contact lens care system would be economical, easy to use and free of side effects and would maintain all types of contact lenses in a clean and sterile state.[11] While such a system does not exist, newer systems combined with improved contact lens technology (e.g., daily disposables) and compliance-enhancing programs (e.g., PRPs) have brought the standard of practice closer to the ideal. Figure 1 outlines the steps required to maintain contact lenses.

Noncompliance is the greatest threat to eye health and lens life. Unfortunately, noncompliance rates of 40 to 90% have been reported.[12] Common forms of noncompliance include inadequate cleaning or rinsing before disinfection, and economizing by using old solutions. Solution contamination, inadequate lens disinfection, manipulation of the lens in the eye and poor hygiene increase the exposure of the eye to pathogens, which can lead to microbial keratitis and corneal ulcers.

Contact Lens Solutions

General Principles

When contact lenses are purchased, the eye care professional usually gives the wearer a starter kit containing a complete lens care system.[13] Once the sample kit is finished, wearers tend to replace their solutions with the same brand if the solutions have been compatible with the eye. Otherwise, a different set of solutions is recommended by the eye care professional on a trial basis. This trial and error scenario is repeated until the effect of the solutions on the corneal epithelium, as viewed by a biomicroscope, is considered acceptable by the eye care professional. Advise wearers to always use solutions from a single manufacturer unless otherwise instructed by their eye care professional. Manufacturers formulate each component of a care regimen to be compatible with each of the other components. The effect of substituting even one solution from a different manufacturer is not predictable, even if it has the same active ingredients in the same concentration. In addition, all solutions that are recommended by an eye care professional will have been found to be compatible with the wearer. Unpreserved aerosol saline is the only product that can be substituted by the wearer.[14]

Cleaning Solutions

The most important step in the proper care of all contact lenses is cleaning, which optimizes visual acuity, comfort, eye health and lens life.[15] Debris from numerous sources collects on the lens from the moment of insertion. The longer the interval between cleanings, the greater the risk of complications (e.g., blurred vision, ocular discomfort, local allergic reactions, ocular infection or blindness). The two main types of cleaning solutions are surfactants (which remove loose debris) and protein cleaners (which remove imbedded protein). Protein cleaners are primarily used for soft lenses.

Surfactants

Since many contact lens contaminants are not water-soluble, rinsing is inadequate.[16] Surfactants emulsify and suspend organisms and other debris, reducing contamination and facilitating disinfection (the presence of debris can inactivate disinfectants). Proper cleaning and rinsing can remove more than 99.9% of the contaminants prior to disinfection.[15]

Figure 1: **Steps for Proper Care of Contact Lenses**[*†]

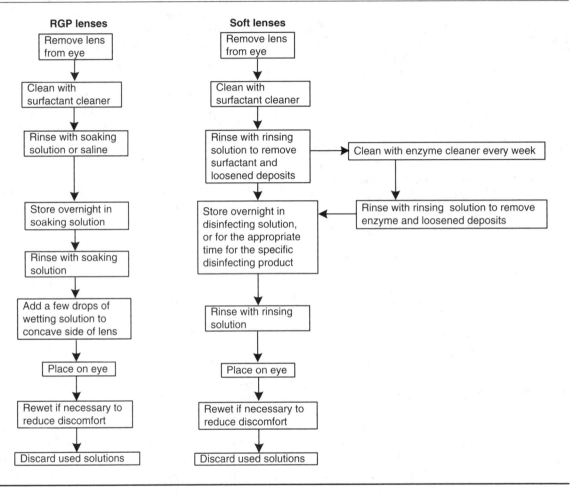

*There may be variations to these generic regimens (e.g., an enzyme cleaner may not be required in a PRP).
†With multipurpose solutions, two (usually cleaning and disinfecting) or more functions are combined in one formulation.

Daily surfactant cleaning is similar for soft and RGP lenses. For soft lenses, preservatives that do not concentrate in the lens (e.g., polyquaternium-1) are used. Immediately after lens removal, a few drops of solution are applied to each lens surface. The lenses are cleaned in the palm of the hand using the index finger in a circular motion for 30 to 60 seconds. Vigorous friction rubbing between the thumb and forefinger for 30 to 60 seconds is an alternative method. The surfactant is then thoroughly rinsed off with a rinsing solution before disinfection. If an enzyme cleaner is used, the surfactant cleaner is used first since it acts on the lipids that may hide protein deposits, making the enzyme cleaner more effective. Surfactants must be thoroughly rinsed off the lens and hands to minimize the risk of chemical keratoconjunctivitis, stinging, allergic reactions, conjunctival hyperemia and eyelid edema.[16]

Unorthodox cleaners include toothpaste, baking soda, laundry detergent, hair shampoo and skin cleaners.[17] These nonsterile products can leave long, deep, jagged scratches on lenses and are not recommended.

Protein Cleaners

With soft lens use, protein accumulates from the first day of wear and may produce decreased visual acuity, ulcerative keratitis and giant papillary conjunctivitis (GPC), an inflammation of the lining of the upper eyelid thought to be an allergic reaction to protein deposits.[18] Symptoms of GPC include redness of the upper eyelid along with multiple white bumps, mucous discharge and blurred vision. In addition, *P. aeruginosa* adheres more readily if a soft lens has a mucin or a protein and mucin coating.[19] This bacterium has been implicated in causing microbial keratitis or corneal ulcers, with possible visual impairment. The incidence of corneal ulcers can be reduced significantly with weekly enzyme cleaning. For RGP lenses, enzyme cleaning is optional and is generally redundant when surfactants are properly used.

Most enzyme cleaners contain papain, pancreatin or subtilisin. Enzymes remove protein deposits by catalyzing the natural breakdown of debris into simple compounds, which become softer and easier to remove by cleaning or rinsing. The lens must be rubbed to effectively remove the broken-down protein molecules. Enzymes generally require 6 to 12 hours to work. Enzyme tablets should be dissolved only in sterile saline, although subtilisin can be dropped into hydrogen peroxide during disinfection.[20]

The use of enzymes does not obviate the need for daily surfactant cleaning since enzymes cannot remove nonprotein deposits. A surfactant removes the nonprotein debris and enables the enzyme to exert its effect. Optimal lens cleaning involves the daily use of a surfactant followed by weekly enzyme cleaner.[18]

Disinfecting Solutions

A disinfectant actively kills microorganisms on lenses while a preservative maintains the sterility of a solution against outside insult.[21] Most disinfecting solutions for soft lenses contain disinfectants and preservatives. Some also contain surfactants but in a lower concentration than in cleaning solutions, so disinfecting still requires a separate cleaning step.

Chemical Disinfection

There are two basic forms of chemical disinfection solutions for soft lenses: oxidizing agents (i.e., hydrogen peroxide) and disinfecting agents (e.g., polyquaternium-1, polyaminopropylbiguanide, alkyl-

triethanolammonium chloride and sorbic acid). Sorbic acid (or potassium sorbate), combined with an EDTA (ethylenediaminetetraacetic acid) salt, is not a chemical disinfection system, but rather a soaking and rinsing system for both RGP and soft lenses. Benzalkonium chloride (BAC) and chlorobutanol are used in solutions for RGP lenses only because they are adsorbed by the HEMA polymer in soft lenses, with subsequent rapid release causing ocular tissue damage.[21]

Chemical disinfection of soft lenses is similar to the soaking process for RGP lenses, as the lenses are soaked (or stored) overnight, in a chemical disinfecting solution.[22] All soft lenses can be chemically disinfected with the appropriate solution. After disinfection, soft lenses must be thoroughly rinsed with at least 25 mL of rinsing solution (usually normal saline or a multipurpose solution) before lenses are inserted into the eye. With RGP lenses, saline or the disinfecting solution itself is used for rinsing. Any kind of water (e.g., tap, bottled, distilled) is not recommended for any lens because of potential accumulation of minerals in the lens and possible microbial contamination.[22,23]

Hydrogen peroxide was once one of the more popular chemical disinfectants for soft lenses[24] but now represents less than 10% of chemical disinfection systems.[25] Its use has declined with the advent of the more convenient multipurpose solutions. However, when used properly, hydrogen peroxide is the most effective chemical disinfectant and produces the mildest ocular response when properly neutralized. Oxidizing agents are inherently unstable and, in the presence of organic debris, form free radicals that attach to debris and disperse it.[26] The effervescence is a secondary means of removing debris from the lens matrix. Following disinfection, hydrogen peroxide is neutralized by a platinum catalyst, sodium pyruvate, catalase, thiosulfite, or by rinsing and dilution. These systems are either "one-step" (where neutralization occurs automatically) or "two-step" (where the wearer initiates neutralization). Despite its strong cleaning action, all hydrogen peroxide manufacturers recommend the adjunctive use of daily cleaners and weekly enzyme cleaners. Hydrogen peroxide does not affect the tints of contact lenses, although hydrogen peroxide first aid products may cause tints to fade. Hydrogen peroxide first aid products are not designed for ophthalmic use and may contain impurities, stabilizers and other additives that irritate ocular tissue.[27,28]

Wetting and Rewetting Solutions[29]

Accessory solutions provide wetting/rewetting, lubrication and cushioning functions in various combinations. Wetting/rewetting agents are artificial tears preserved with chemicals that are compatible with soft lenses. Lubrication and cushioning actions are imparted by viscosity agents, large colloidal molecules that increase resistance to flow, holding the tears in the eyes and reducing the drying-out effect of solutions. They produce a cushioning and lubricant effect between the lens and eyelid and between the lens and cornea. Unlike wetting solutions, they do not enhance the flow of tears over the cornea.

Solutions in this class have all three properties to varying degrees. Since the clinical significance of these differences is unknown, their uses are interchangeable.

Soft Lenses

Soft lenses tend to dry out through the day, especially in a dry or polluted environment. Up to 75% of soft lens wearers experience this symptom.[30] Additional risk factors for dry eye include: use of diuretics or hormones (e.g., oral contraceptives), lack of adequate tearing (due to age), certain conditions (e.g., rheumatoid arthritis and to a lesser extent hypertension), air conditioning and low humidity. Rewetting solutions can be used to relieve dryness, but should be limited to one drop every four to five hours. More frequent use can result in red, irritated eyes and a foreign body sensation. No one product is consistently superior to any other, although unpreserved solutions are generally recommended because they minimize the potential for allergic reactions. Lubricants have not been found to be significantly superior to saline.[30] Artificial tears that are not specifically formulated for contact lenses should not be used for rewetting soft lenses because most contain preservatives (e.g., BAC) that can accumulate in the lens matrix.

RGP Lenses

RGP lenses require wetting to reduce the foreign body sensation upon insertion.[31] The mucin layer of the tear film contains highly hydrated polysaccharides that wet the lens. However, this deposition can take up to 15 minutes to develop, during which time the wearer experiences discomfort. A wetting and cushioning solution minimizes the transitional discomfort until the eyes adjust. The solution is applied to the concave side of the lens immediately before insertion. Wetting agents reduce surface tension between tears and the contact lens or between tears and the cornea, allowing tears to spread evenly. Although natural saliva has excellent wetting properties, it contains many potential pathogens and should *never* be used as a wetting agent.

Saline

Saline is available in preserved or unpreserved formulations (unit-dose or multi-dose).[32] Preserved saline minimizes the risk of contamination during repeated use. Unpreserved unit-dose saline eliminates potential sensitivity reactions to preservatives. However, microbial contamination can occur if the solution stands for longer than one hour or if it is used improperly. Multi-dose aerosol nonpreserved saline is equally effective in preventing sensitivity reactions and remains sterile for the life of the product. Before each use of aerosol saline, a small amount of saline should be dispensed and discarded, since the saline inside the mechanism is open to the outside environment and may be contaminated.[33]

Multipurpose Solutions[34,35]

The eye care professional may recommend as many as five single purpose products or as few as one all-purpose product. To increase convenience, many products combine two or more functions in a single solution. Although some researchers suggest that cleaning is compromised with the use of multipurpose solutions, clinical evaluations of multipurpose products for both soft and RGP lenses have shown they improve compliance and exhibit acceptable cleaning efficacy, leading to their wide acceptance. There appear to be no specific problems associated with multipurpose solutions although the incidence of sensitivity would be expected to be greater (due to the presence of more chemicals) than that of single purpose solutions.

Lens Cases

Contact lenses should be stored in their cases, completely covered by disinfecting solution.[36] If they dry out, the lens shape can temporarily change, rendering the lens useless until it can regain its original shape.

Storage cases must be maintained with the same vigilance as lenses, since a dirty case will nullify the previous steps taken in the care of contact lenses. Storage cases should be kept clean by routine (at least monthly) boiling in water for 10 minutes. The lens case must be allowed to cool for 30 to 45 minutes before replacing the lenses. If the case is not cleaned by boiling at least once a month, it should be replaced monthly. Even if it is cleaned properly on a regular basis, it should be replaced every three months. Fortunately, lens case replacement is being incorporated into PRPs. The soaking solution should be replaced daily and the case flushed of old solution and air-dried before adding new solution.[37] About

Table 2: **Systemic Drug Interactions with Contact Lenses**

Drug	Effect on Lenses
Oral contraceptives	Lens intolerance (increased sensitivity and awareness of lenses because of corneal and lid swelling from estrogen, and altered tear composition resulting in decreased lubricating ability of tears)
Antihistamines Hypnotics Sedatives	Decrease in blink rate (blinking is required to maintain hydration in soft lens wearers and helps supply oxygen to the cornea in RGP lens wearers)
Muscle relaxants	Incomplete blinking
Anticholinergics Antihistamines Maprotiline Tricyclic antidepressants	Decreased tear volume (leading to irritation and deposits in soft lens wearers, and corneal drying in RGP lens wearers).
Propoxyphene napsylate plus acetaminophen	Soft lens adherence from decreased tear volume
Isotretinoin	Itching and decreased wear time in soft lens wearers
ASA	Ocular irritation and redness in soft lens wearers
Dopamine Nitrofurantoin Phenazopyridine Phenolphthalein Rifampin Sulfasalazine Tetracycline	Discoloration of soft lenses

Table 3: **Local Drug Interactions with Contact Lenses**

Drug	Effect on soft lenses
Phenylephrine Tetrahydrozoline	Dark discoloration of lens with repeated use
Fluorescein Rose bengal	Concentration of diagnostic agent in lenses
Benzoyl peroxide	Fading of tinted lenses

40% of bacterial eye infections among contact lens wearers can be attributed to carrying cases.

Monitoring of Therapy

Pharmacists can help contact lens wearers optimize lens care by providing information on the many systemic and ophthalmic medications that can affect contact lenses by altering eye shape, affecting the blink reflex, altering tear volume and composition, concentrating in the lens or by discoloring the lens (Tables 2, 3).[38-65] Inform the wearer that drug-lens interactions are possible and can negatively affect the success of contact lens wear. All wearers should maintain a current list of their medications, and show it to their eye care professional.

Suggested Readings

Dart J. Extended-wear contact lenses, microbial keratitis, and public health (editorial). *Lancet* 1999;354: 174-5.

Levey SB, Cohen EJ. Methods of disinfecting contact lenses to avoid corneal disorders. *Surv Ophthalmol* 1996;41:245-51.

Sankaridurg PR, Sweeney DF, Sharma S et al. Adverse events with extended wear of disposable hydrogels: results for the first 13 months of lens wear. *Ophthalmology* 1999;106:1671-80.

Silbert JA. A review of therapeutic agents and contact lens wear. *J Am Optom Assoc* 1996;67:165-72.

Smith SK. Patient noncompliance with wearing and replacement schedules of disposable contact lenses. *J Am Optom Assoc* 1996;67:160-4.

References

1. Alberta Association of Optometrists. Contact lenses. Available from http://www.optometrists.ab.ca/guide/contacts.htm.
2. Contact Lens Manufacturers Association. Wouldn't you rather wear contacts than glasses? Available from http://www.contactlenses.org/clsglasses/htm. Accessed Aug 24, 2000.
3. Anonymous. Contact lenses now. *Drug Ther Bull* 1988;26: 39-40.
4. Lum VJ, Lyle WM. Chemical components of contact lens solutions. *Can J Optom* 1981;43:136-51.
5. Mandell RB. *Contact Lens Practice.* Springfield: CC Thomas, 1981:495-518.
6. Lane I. Daily disposable: putting them into practice. *Rev Optom* 1995;132(4):66-68.
7. Gellatly KW. Disposable contact lenses: a clinical performance review. *Can J Optom* 1993;55:166-73.
8. Nason RJ, Boshnik EL, Cannon WM et al. Multisite comparison of contact lens modalities. Daily disposable wear in successful contact lens wearers. *J Am Optom Assoc* 1994;65: 774-80.
9. Schein OD, Glynn RJ, Poggio EC et al. Microbial Keratitis Study Group. The relative risk of ulcerative keratitis among users of daily-wear and extended-wear soft contact lenses. A case-control study. *N Engl J Med* 1989;321:773-8,824-6.
10. Vilforth JC. The Food and Drug Administration is requesting manufacturers of cosmetic extended-wear soft contact lenses to indicate a recommended wearing time in the product labeling (News). *Arch Ophthalmol* 1989;107:969.
11. Jantzi JD, Jantzi JA. Contact lens care systems and eyecare. Available from http://www.pharmacyconnects.com/content/phpost/1998/09-98/ce-09-98.htm.
12. Claydon BE, Efron N. Non-compliance in contact lens wear. *Ophthalmol Physiol Optics* 1994;14:356-364.
13. Smith RE, MacRae SM. Contact lenses—convenience and complications (editorial). *N Engl J Med* 1989;321:824-6.
14. Shovlin J. Don't let patients "mix and match" solutions. *Optom Manage* 1994;May:61.
15. Sibley MJ, Shih KL, Hu JC. The microbiological benefit of cleaning and rinsing contact lenses. *Int Contact Lens Clin* 1985;12:235-42.
16. Sibley MJ. Cleaning solutions for contact lenses. *Int Contact Lens Clin* 1982;9:291-4.
17. Diefenbach CB, Seibert CK, Davis LJ. Analysis of two "home remedy" contact lens cleaners. *J Am Optom Assoc* 1988;59: 518-21.
18. Morgan JF. Maintenance and care of soft lenses. In: Ruben M, ed. *Soft contact lenses: clinical and applied technology.* Toronto, ON: J Wiley & Sons, 1978:285-90.
19. Aswad MI, John T, Barza M et al. Bacterial adherence to extended wear soft contact lenses. *Ophthalmol* 1990;97: 296-302.
20. Breen W, Fontana F, Hansen D et al. Clinical comparison of pancreatin-based and subtilisin-based enzymatic cleaners. *Contact Lens Forum* 1990;15:32-8.
21. Ernst RR. Sterilization by heat. In: Block SS, ed. *Disinfection, sterilization and preservation.* Philadelphia, PA: Lea & Febiger, 1977:481-521.
22. Sibley MJ. Disinfection solutions. *Int Ophthalmol Clin* 1981; 21:237-47.
23. Penland RL, Wilhelmus KR. Microbiologic analysis of bottled water: is it safe with contact lenses? *Ophthalmology* 1999; 106:1500-3.
24. Holden B. A report card on hydrogen peroxide for contact lens disinfection. *CLAO J* 1990;16(1 suppl):s61-4.
25. Johnson & Johnson Vision Care. 2000 survey data. Markham, ON.
26. Gasset AR, Ramer RM, Katzin D. Hydrogen peroxide sterilization of hydrophilic contact lenses. *Arch Ophthalmol* 1975;93:412-5.
27. Gordon KD. The effect of oxidative disinfecting systems on tinted hydrogel lenses. *Can J Optom* 1989;51:175-6.
28. Anonymous. Contact lens questions and answers. Generic peroxide. *Rev Optom* 1986;123:77.
29. Weissman BA, Tari LA. A solution for the dry eye. *Contact Lens Forum* 1982;Feb:5-7.
30. Efron N, Golding TR, Brennan NA. The effect of soft lens lubricants on symptoms and lens dehydration. *CLAO J* 1991;17:114-9.

31. Mauger TF, Hill RM. Solutions that soothe. *Contact Lens Forum* 1982; Feb:75-7.
32. Harris MG, Higa CK, Lacey LL et al. The pH of aerosol saline solution. *Optom Vis Sci* 1990;67:84-8.
33. Donzis PB. Corneal ulcer associated with contamination of aerosol saline spray tip. *Am J Ophthalmol* 1997;124:394-5.
34. Mulford MB, Houlsby RD, Langston JB et al. Rigid lens care revisited. *Contact Lens Forum* 1980;Sept:33-43.
35. Roth HW, Roth-Wittig M. Multipurpose solutions for soft lens maintenance. *Int Contact Lens Clin* 1980;7:92-5.
36. Simmons PA, Edrington TB, Hsieh L et al. Bacterial contamination rate of soft contact lens cases. *Int Contact Lens Clin* 1991;18:188-91.
37. Larragoiti ND, Diamos ME, Simmons PA et al. A comparative study of techniques for decreasing contact lens storage contamination. *J Am Optom Assoc* 1994;65:161-3.
38. Anonymous. Contact lens questions and answers. Fading away. *Rev Optom* 1985;122:89.
39. Fraunfelder FT. *Drug-induced ocular side effects and drug interactions.* Philadelphia, PA: Lea & Febiger; 1982:251.
40. Garber JM. "Film" solution (letter). *Contact Lens Forum* 1980;Sept:15.
41. Krezanoski JZ. Topical medications. *Int Ophthalmol Clin* 1981;21:173-6.
42. Lea SJH, Loades J, Rubinstein MP. The interaction between hydrogel lenses and sodium fluorescein. Theoretical and practical considerations. *Acta Ophthalmol* (Copenh) 1989;67:441-6.
43. Miller D, Brooks SM, Mobilia E. Adenochrome staining of soft contact lenses. *Ann Ophthalmol* 1976;8:65-7.
44. Miranda MN, Garcia-Castineiras S. Effects of pH and some common topical ophthalmic medications on the contact lens Permalens. *CLAO J* 1983;9:43-8.
45. Sugar J. Adenochrome pigmentation of hydrophilic lenses. *Arch Ophthalmol* 1974;91:11-2.
46. Kaufman A. The effects of contraceptives on contact lens performance. *Contact Lens J* 1980;6:15-8.
47. Petursson GJ, Fraunfelder FT, Meyer SM. Pharmacology of ocular drugs. 6. Oral contraceptives. *Ophthalmol* 1981;88:368-71.
48. Aucamp A. Drug excretion in human tears and its meaning for contact lens wearers. *South Afr Optom* 1980;39:128-36.
49. Barber JC. Management of the patient with dry eyes. *Contact Intraocul Lens Med J* 1977;3:10-5.
50. Bergmanson JPG, Rios R. Adverse reaction to painkiller in hydrogel lens wear. *J Am Optom Assoc* 1981;52:257-8.
51. Chang FW. The possible adverse effects of over-the-counter medications on the contact lens wearer. *J Am Optom Assoc* 1977;48:319-23.
52. Farber AS. Ocular side effects of antihistamine-decongestant combinations. *Am J Ophthalmol* 1982;94:565.
53. Fraunfelder FT. *Drug-induced ocular side effects and drug interactions.* Philadelphia, PA: Lea & Febiger, 1982:88-97,112-31,165-70,186-7, 190-4, 206-7,297-305,306-8,311-5.
54. Garston M. When meds disrupt contact lens wear. *Rev Optom* 1993;Apr:49-50.
55. Harris J, Jenkins P. Discoloration of soft contact lenses by rifampicin (letter). *Lancet* 1985;2:1133.
56. Koffler BH, Lemp MA. The effect of an antihistamine (chlorpheniramine maleate) on tear production in humans. *Ann Ophthalmol* 1980;12:217-9.
57. Lemp MA, Hamill JR Jr. Factors affecting tear film breakup in normal eyes. *Arch Ophthalmol* 1973;89:103-5.
58. Litovitz GL. Amitriptyline and contact lenses (letter). *J Clin Psychiatry* 1984;45:188.
59. Lyons RW. Orange contact lenses from rifampin (letter). *N Engl J Med* 1979;300:372-3.
60. Miller D. Systemic medications. *Int Ophthalmol Clin* 1981;21:177-83.
61. Onofrey B. The odd case of the blurry-eyed cruise passenger. *Rev Optom* 1991;Oct:93.
62. Riley SA, Flegg PJ, Mandal BK. Contact lens staining due to sulphasalazine (letter). *Lancet* 1986;1:972.
63. Simmerman JS. Contact lens fitting after Accutane treatment. *Rev Optom* 1985;122:102.
64. Troiano G. Amitriptyline and contact lenses (letter). *J Clin Psychiatry* 1985;46:199.
65. Valentic JP, Leopold IH, Dea FJ. Excretion of salicylic acid into tears following oral administration of aspirin. *Ophthalmol* 1980;87:815-20.

Contact Lens Care—Patient Information

Care of Rigid Gas Permeable (RGP) and Soft Lenses

- Carefully follow the care regimen prescribed for you.
- If you suspect problems or have any questions, contact your eye care professional.
- Use oil-free soap to wash your hands well and then dry them before handling your lenses. Dirt and germs on your hands can be transferred to your lenses.
- Keep your fingernails short to prevent tearing and scratching your lenses.
- If you remove lenses over a sink, close or cover the drain to avoid losing your lenses.
- Each solution is made for a special purpose. Use RGP lens solutions for RGP lenses only and soft lens solutions for soft lenses only.
- Do not use any household products, such as detergents, soaps, shampoos, skin cleansers or toothpaste to clean your lenses.
- Never use saliva to wet your lenses; it contains bacteria that can cause infection.
- Never rinse with any kind of water (e.g., tap, bottled, distilled) after your lenses have been cleaned or disinfected.
- Do not use solutions from different manufacturers, unless your eye care professional recommends otherwise, because the solutions may not be safe to use together.
- Do not use contact lens products after their expiry date.
- Keep all contact lens products out of the reach of children.
- Thoroughly clean and rinse lenses after you remove them and before you disinfect them. Most bacteria are removed with this important first step.
- Thoroughly rinse off cleaners or disinfectants before inserting the lens into the eye. Residues can have harmful effects on the eye and lens.
- Use fresh disinfecting (soaking) solutions every day.
- Avoid contaminating bottle tips by practising good hygiene and not touching the tip to anything.
- Thoroughly clean, rinse and air-dry the contact lens case each morning after inserting your lenses. Clean the case by boiling it at least once a month and replace it at least every three months.

- Do not wear contact lenses to the hairdresser. If worn under a hair dryer, the hot air will cause mucus and tears to dry and harden on the lenses.
- Do not wear lenses while swimming because they may wash out. Soft lenses can stick to the eye when exposed to swimming pool water.
- Wear protective eye gear if you participate in contact sports.
- Do not wear daily-wear lenses longer than the recommended time and remove them daily.
- If there is unexpected redness, swelling, pain or irritation, stop wearing your lenses and contact your eye care professional.
- If you use daily-wear lenses, visit your eye care professional at least once every six months.
- If you use extended-wear lenses, visit your eye care professional at least once every two to three months.

Special Instructions for Soft Lenses

- Rinse your hands thoroughly after washing. Soap residues can stick to soft lenses.
- Do not use discolored enzyme products.
- If you want to change solutions, contact your eye care professional.
- Remove your lenses before applying medicinal eye drops. Afterward, do not reinsert your lenses for at least one hour unless otherwise instructed by your eye care professional.
- When storing your lenses, carefully centre the lenses in the case and close the lid tightly.
- If your lenses become stuck together, moisten them with saline or daily cleaner before sliding them apart.
- If a lens tears, save the pieces because your eye care professional will want to be sure that none of the pieces have become lodged in your eye. Some companies replace torn lenses.
- If you fall asleep with your lenses on, moisten them with lubricating drops before removing them from your eyes.
- Wait one hour before reinserting your lenses if you have been swimming.

Special Instructions for RGP Lenses

- Never rub your eyes while wearing your contact lenses.
- Do not rinse your lenses under hot water; they could change shape.

Contact Lenses and Cosmetics—Patient Information

- Do not apply cosmetics if eyes are swollen, red or infected.
- Use a good quality "water-resistant" mascara that does not flake off (instead of "waterproof" mascara, which likely contains oils). Problems occur if mascara gets on or underneath lenses.
- Use oil-free and fragrance-free eye makeup.
- Apply eye makeup sparingly and remove it daily. Cream eye shadows are preferred over powdered shadows.
- Make sure anyone giving you advice on cosmetics knows that you wear contact lenses.
- Never share eye cosmetics; another person's bacteria may be dangerous to your eyes.
- When using hair dyes, bleaches, perm lotions or medicated shampoos, remove your lenses.
- Spray deodorants and hairsprays can irritate your eyes. Particles accumulating on your lenses can cause discomfort, and your lenses might have to be replaced. Protect your lenses by closing your eyes when you spray, then walk away from the area. Use pump sprays if possible.
- If you have to remove your lenses temporarily while wearing make-up, you can avoid smearing your make-up if you tilt your head to one side after putting your lenses back in. This makes the tears run to the side.
- Before handling your lenses, scrub your hands and fingers thoroughly to remove all cosmetics, including nail polish, nail polish remover, perfumes, colognes, lotions and suntan oil.
- Apply cosmetics, nail polish, hand creams and perfumes *after* inserting lenses.
- Remove lenses *before* removing makeup.

Ear Section Highlights

Chapter 16: **General Ear Conditions**

Signs and symptoms associated with various ear conditions
Hearing loss
Ear pain
Ear drainage
Drugs associated with ototoxicity
Complications of ear piercing
Foreign bodies
Otitis media
Barotrauma
Impacted cerumen
Agents to remove excessive or impacted cerumen

Chapter 17: **Otitis Externa**

Types of otitis externa
Drugs for otitis externa

Chapter 18: **Vertigo and Dizziness**

Conditions causing vertigo
Medications that often cause dizziness
Nonprescription drugs for vertigo

Chapter 19: **Tinnitus**

Assessment of patients with tinnitus

General Ear Conditions

Yvonne Shevchuk, BSP, PharmD, FCSHP

Signs and Symptoms

There are many conditions that result in ear symptoms. Figure 1 provides an algorithm for patient assessment and Table 1 describes signs and symptoms associated with various otic conditions. Signs and symptoms commonly associated with, but not limited to, ear disease include:

Hearing Loss[1-3]

Hearing loss is classified as *conductive* hearing loss or *sensorineural* hearing loss. Conductive hearing loss occurs when sound is prevented from gaining access to the inner ear. It may result from diseases of the external or middle ear. Examples include otitis externa, impacted cerumen, upper respiratory tract infections, otitis media, foreign objects or water trapped in the ear, and tumors. Rupture of the tympanic membrane due to acute otitis media or trauma also produces hearing loss. Sensorineural hearing loss involves the inner ear or cochlea, the auditory nerve or a central nerve lesion. These conditions are not managed by self-care. Drugs associated with ototoxicity can also produce hearing loss (Table 2).

Upper respiratory tract infections (e.g., common cold) commonly cause reduced hearing. Unless hearing loss is identified as due to impacted cerumen or an upper respiratory tract infection, all patients with hearing loss should be referred to their physician for assessment.

Ear Pain (otalgia)[1,2,7,9]

Otalgia is usually associated with inflammation of the external or middle ear, but pain may be referred to the ear from other sites such as the teeth, temporomandibular joint, pharynx or sinuses. If pain is persistent or lasts more than a few days, refer the patient for medical evaluation.

Ear Drainage (otorrhea)[1]

Otorrhea may be caused by something as simple as a scratch in the ear to serious medical conditions. Otorrhea is often a sign of otitis externa, otitis media with perforation of the tympanic membrane, or drainage from the middle ear from tympanostomy tubes. Bloody drainage can occur with several conditions, including trauma, neoplasm and foreign bodies. Clear drainage may be from the middle ear or a cerebrospinal fluid leak. Drainage resulting from mild otitis externa (e.g., eczematous) may be self-treated; however, unless this is specifically identified as the cause, the patient should be referred to a physician.

Tinnitus, Vertigo and Dizziness

These symptoms are discussed in detail in Chapter 18, Vertigo and Dizziness, and in Chapter 19, Tinnitus.

Miscellaneous Conditions Affecting the Ear

Conditions affecting the auricle such as lacerations, burns, frostbite, dermatitis, and infections are amenable to self-treatment if not severe (see Chapters 41, 47 and 48). Refer the patient to a physician if these are not easily distinguishable by history and appearance.

Complications of Ear Piercing[19]

Ear piercing complications are common. Mild bacterial infections secondary to piercing can be managed with local therapy: cleansing, warm compresses, topical antibiotics, and removal of the earring. Allergic dermatitis is managed by avoidance of the inciting compound (nickel or gold) and may include short-term use of a mild topical corticosteroid. See Ear Piercing—Patient Information for guidelines to reduce

Figure 1: **Assessment of Patients with Ear Complaints**[1-18]

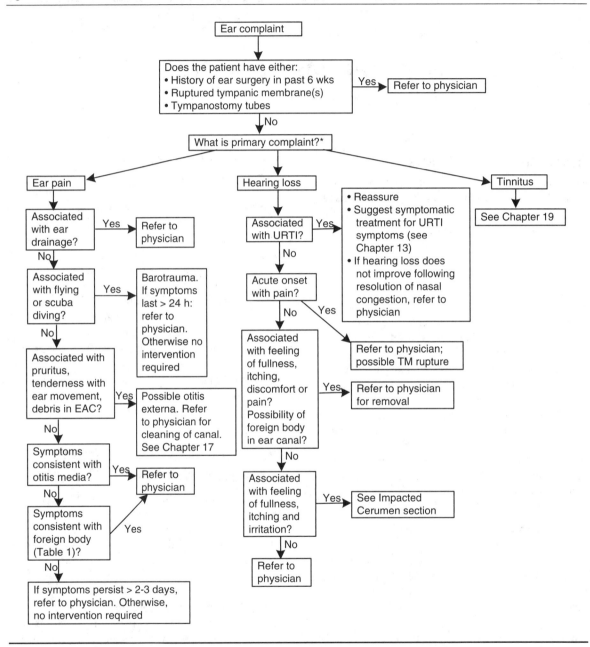

EAC = external auditory canal; TM= tympanic membrane; URTI= upper respiratory tract infection
Ear conditions often present as a constellation of symptoms (Table 1). The predominant symptom often varies between individuals. For this reason, more than one path of this algorithm may apply to a particular case.

Table 1: **Signs and Symptoms Associated with Various Ear Conditions**

Condition	Pain	Pruritus	Discharge	Hearing loss	Comments
Ruptured tympanic membrane	Yes (sudden, sharp)	No	Yes	Yes (abrupt)	May be associated with acute otitis media, barotrauma and other conditions
Impacted cerumen	Rarely unless infected	Frequent	Rarely unless infected	Yes (gradual)	May be described as fullness or pressure
Acute bacterial otitis externa	Yes (acute onset)	Sometimes	Frequent	Sometimes	Associated with excessive moisture, trauma to EAC , attempts to scratch or remove wax from EAC. Pain with chewing, movement of auricle
Eczematous otitis externa	Sometimes	Yes	Sometimes (crusting, oozing)	Sometimes	Characteristic features of underlying dermatologic condition may be present (e.g., psoriatic plaques; erythema and scaling with atopic dermatitis). May become secondarily infected
Otitis media	Yes (abrupt onset)	No	Yes if TM ruptures	Sometimes	Primarily in children. Pain relieved with rupture of TM. Commonly preceded by viral URTI
Foreign body	Yes	Sometimes	If becomes infected	Yes	Fullness and pressure in the ear
Barotrauma	Yes	No	Yes if TM ruptures	Yes	Associated with air travel (descent) and diving. Tinnitus and vertigo also may be present

EAC = external auditory canal; TM = tympanic membrane; URTI = upper respiratory tract infection
Adapted from Torsher L. Ear care products. In: Carruthers-Czyzewski P, ed. *Nonprescription Drug Reference for Health Professionals.* Ottawa, ON: Canadian Pharmaceutical Association, 1996:155.

the risk of ear piercing complications and information on caring for the ears after piercing.

Foreign Bodies[2,7,8]
Foreign bodies in the ear canal are more frequent in children than adults. Often the patient will give a history of a foreign object entering the ear. Patients experience pain, which may be dull or severe, a feeling of fullness or pressure in the ear and loss of hearing. Insects are particularly annoying because of their movement. They may be drowned with mineral oil or alcohol before removal. Foreign objects should be removed by a physician. Caution patients not to try removing objects by syringing especially if they are organic (e.g., beans, peas, insects) because they may swell, or if the objects are sharp because

scratching of the canal or perforation of the tympanic membrane may result.

Otitis Media[7,9-11]
Acute otitis media (AOM) is an infection of the middle ear cavity and is one of the most frequent bacterial infections in childhood. It is most commonly due to *S. pneumoniae*, *H. influenzae* or *M. catarrhalis.* Most children experience at least one episode by the age of two. Symptoms include acute ear pain (often unilateral and developing over a few hours), fever and reduced hearing. Tugging or pulling on the ears is often described, but this is a very nonspecific sign. Children too young to complain of pain or pressure in the ears may display irritability, excessive fussiness, poor feeding and disrupted sleep patterns. Acute otitis

Table 2: **Some Drugs Associated with Ototoxicity**[4,5]

More commonly reported

Aminoglycosides
– Neomycin, kanamycin, amikacin, netilmicin, gentamicin,
  tobramycin, streptomycin
Antineoplastics
– Cisplatin, nitrogen mustard, methotrexate, vincristine, bleomycin,
  dactinomycin
Antiparasitics
– Quinine, chloroquine
	ASA/Nonsteroidal anti inflammatory drugs
	Loop diuretics
	– Ethacrynic acid, furosemide, bumetanide
	Macrolides
	– Erythromycin, clarithromycin
	– Azithromycin
	Tetracyclines
	– Doxycycline, minocycline
	Vancomycin

Less commonly reported

Carbamazepine Cimetidine Cyclosporine Deferoxamine Diazoxide Enalapril Famotidine	Lidocaine Omeprazole Propylthiouracil Pyrimethamine Quinidine Valproic acid

media is more common in the winter months. A recent history of viral upper respiratory tract infection is often present.

Eighty per cent of children experience spontaneous symptomatic relief with placebo or no drug therapy.[9] In several European countries, AOM is managed with aggressive analgesic therapy and not routinely treated with antibiotics unless the child fails to respond in 72 hours. In North America, antibiotic therapy is the standard; however, in an era of increasing antimicrobial resistance, there is some movement towards "watchful waiting." Watchful waiting is 48 to 72 hours of analgesic therapy in children with low risk of serious sequelae (older than two years of age, mild or unilateral AOM, without severe pain or systemic toxicity, normal host, no otorrhea, no history of chronic or recurrent AOM, and availability of good follow-up).[10,12]

Therapy

- If antibiotics are used, systemic therapy is required; topical agents are not used in AOM.
- Adequate analgesia with usual doses of acetaminophen or ibuprofen is important (see Chapter 9).
- Local heat application (heating pad or hot water bottle) may be beneficial, but should be used cautiously and with close supervision in children to avoid burns. A young child should never sleep with a hot water bottle or heating pad. Instillation of warmed oils may also provide short-term symptomatic relief, but should not be used if the tympanic membrane is ruptured. Warming should be done by rolling the bottle between the palms; other methods such as placing the bottle in a glass of warm water or using the microwave oven should be avoided — serious burns have been reported.
- Topical anesthetic agents do not reach adequate concentrations in the middle ear, so the effects are similar to those of warmed oil. Because they may cause local hypersensitivity reactions, their use is not recommended.
- Decongestants and antihistamines do not speed the resolution of effusion and can have significant adverse effects in children.[13,14] Although they may be used to treat the signs and symptoms of accompanying viral respiratory tract infections (see Chapter 13), make it clear to parents that they are not of benefit for the ear infection.

For a more complete discussion of acute otitis media, see the Suggested Readings.

Barotrauma[2,7,8,15]

Otic barotrauma , also referred to as *aerotitis media*, occurs when an individual cannot equalize the pressure gradient between the middle ear and the atmosphere. This occurs with air travel (descent) and underwater diving. The eustachian tube closes, causing a painful pressure change in the middle ear and extravasation of fluid and blood into the middle ear space. Tympanic membrane perforation may result. The symptoms are a sensation of ear blockage followed by ear pain, tinnitus, vertigo, and conductive hearing loss. The condition may last two or three days and usually resolves spontaneously. Treatment includes analgesics for pain, decongestants to encourage opening of the eustachian tube and attempts at auto-inflation using the *Valsalva maneuver* (forced expiration keeping the mouth tightly closed and the nostrils pinched) or the *Toynbee maneuver* (holding the nose and swallowing hard with the mouth closed). The Valsalva maneuver may cause syncope or cardiac arrhythmia and should not be recommended to patients with cardiac disease.

More severe injury can occur with deep sea dives. Occasionally surgery may be required.

If symptoms of barotrauma do not subside in 24 hours, or if bloody fluid drains from the ear, indicating a ruptured tympanic membrane, refer the patient to their physician.

Poor functioning of the eustachian tube can result in failure of pressure equilibration during descent while flying. This may be due to congenital and anatomic conditions, but upper respiratory tract infections, eustachian tube edema resulting from allergies, chronic middle ear disease and nasal chamber edema during pregnancy also produce eustachian tube dysfunction. Flying should be postponed in these individuals if at all possible. The eustachian tube also does not function normally while an individual is asleep.

Beginning early in the descent, individuals should swallow, yawn and auto-inflate frequently. They should ensure they are awakened prior to descent. Children can be given gum to chew or candy to suck; small children can be given a bottle or breastfed during descent to reduce discomfort.

Nasal sprays and oral decongestants are often recommended to prevent barotrauma. In adults **pseudoephedrine** 120 mg sustained release formulation taken 30 minutes before flying has been shown to reduce pain, blockage, and hearing loss in individuals with a history of ear discomfort,[16,17] but oxymetazoline nasal spray is not better than placebo.[16] One mg/kg of pseudoephedrine administered 30 to 60 minutes prior to departure is no better than placebo in children aged six months to six years.[18] Other decongestants have not been studied. The most appropriate recommendation by the pharmacist is 60 mg (regular release) or 120 mg (sustained release) of oral pseudoephedrine in adults. Administration 30 minutes prior to takeoff is appropriate for short flights. Because it is the descent which causes problems, on long international flights, pseudoephedrine should be taken 30 to 60 minutes prior to anticipated arrival time. Drowsiness in some individuals was the only adverse effect reported in clinical trials specific to barotrauma. The contraindications and precautions are the same as for individuals using decongestants for other purposes (see Chapter 13).

Impacted Cerumen
Pathophysiology[2,7,20-22]

The skin lining the lateral two-thirds of the external auditory canal (EAC) contains hair follicles, ceruminous and sebaceous glands. Ear wax (cerumen) is composed of secretions from these glands mixed with exfoliated squamous epithelium. Cerumen functions to lubricate and protect the ear; it is water repellent, preventing maceration of the EAC, and is bacteriostatic. It is normally secreted in small amounts and moves out of the ear by the action of cilia, talking and chewing. The ear is usually self-cleaning. The external opening can be cleaned using a washcloth over the index finger. Discourage attempts at removing ear wax with cotton-tipped applicators, hair pins, matches, fingernails and other objects. This may push wax further into the canal causing impaction.[20,23]

Accumulation of ear wax may:[20,21]
- Result in inability to see the tympanic membrane (required when attempting to diagnose middle ear conditions);
- Cause impaction of wax;
- Produce hearing loss;

- Produce discomfort, pain or vertigo;
- Contribute to infection.

Factors that disrupt the normal migration of cerumen to the outer EAC increase the risk for impaction and include:[23]
- Older age: ceruminous glands atrophy, creating drier cerumen that is more difficult to expel from the ear;
- Abnormally narrow or mishaped EAC;
- Numerous ear canal hairs;
- Hearing aids;
- Bony growths in the canal (osteophyte or osteoma).

A history of previous impaction is also a risk factor.

Goals of Therapy
- Remove impacted cerumen to relieve symptoms
- Avoid damage to the EAC
- Prevent future impaction

Patient Assessment
Figure 2 illustrates the assessment of a patient who likely has impacted cerumen.

Figure 2: **Assessment of Patients with Impacted Cerumen Symptoms**[23,24]

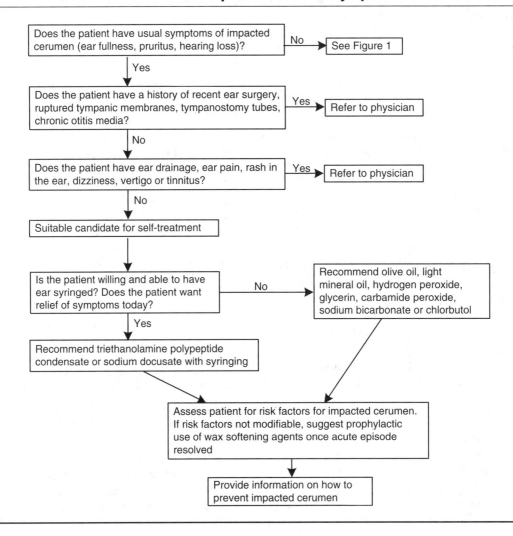

Question the patient regarding the common symptoms of cerumen impaction (sensation of fullness in the ear, hearing loss and discomfort) and risk factors for impaction. There is often a history of attempted removal of wax with cotton-tipped swabs or other foreign objects, which have actually pushed the wax further into the ear and exacerbated symptoms. If there is discharge from the ear, co-existing otitis externa may be present (see Chapter 17). Refer the patient to a physician if the ear has been injured, the tympanic membrane is perforated, there is a history of recent ear surgery, the patient has tympanostomy tubes, there is drainage from the ear, hearing loss, tinnitus or dizziness or if the patient is a child.

Nonpharmacologic Therapy

Since the ear is generally self-cleaning, products or techniques to aid in cerumen removal should be recommended only when the physician has requested their use (for example, when there is a need to see the tympanic membrane) or for symptomatic relief. Discourage use by the patient to simply "keep the ears clean."

A common method used to remove ear wax is syringing the ear with water at body temperature, with or without prior instillation of ear drops to soften the wax. Syringing can be done in the physician's office, emergency department or at home by a caregiver. It is difficult to perform the procedure on oneself and this should not be recommended.

Complications of syringing include failure to remove wax, pain or discomfort, vertigo, otitis media or otitis externa, and perforation of the tympanic membrane.[20,23,24]

Syringing is contraindicated if the tympanic membrane is perforated. Steps outlining proper syringing technique are found in Impacted Cerumen (Ear Wax)—Patient Information.

Pharmacologic Therapy

A number of agents enhance removal of wax from the ear (Table 3). These products are instilled for the required period of time, after which the wax is allowed to be expelled naturally or the ear syringed to remove the softened wax. Few studies exist to provide evidence of their effectiveness. Studies comparing

Table 3: **Agents to Remove Excessive or Impacted Cerumen**[8,21-25]

Agent	Dose	Comments
Softening agents • Olive oil • Light mineral oil • 3% hydrogen peroxide (diluted up to ½ with water) • Glycerin • Carbamide peroxide 6.5% • 15% sodium bicarbonate • Chlorbutol 5%	4-6 drops in the ear canal twice daily for 3-7 days	Generally not irritating Effects are delayed Hearing loss and fullness may initially be exacerbated due to swelling of wax Wax may be allowed to be expelled naturally or ear may be syringed after 3-7 days These agents may be instilled periodically (daily or 2-3 times weekly) for prevention of impaction
Triethanolamine polypeptide condensate	4-6 drops in the affected ear canal for 10-15 min **followed by syringing**	Less effective than docusate sodium; equivalent to olive oil. A poor wax disintegrator in vitro If successful, effects are immediate If left in canal for longer periods, irritation and hypersensitivity can occur
Docusate sodium 10 mg/mL	1 mL in the affected ear for 10-15 min	Effective wax disintegrator in vitro and in a clinical trial No commercial preparation available Allowed to drain out of ear by gravity; if wax still present then syringe ear

the effectiveness of various agents to each other or to syringing are poorly done and not easily compared, making it difficult to recommend one agent over another.

One trial compared sodium bicarbonate in glycerol, sterile water and a combination product containing chlorbutol 5%, paradichlorobenzene 2% and arachis oil 57.3%. All three preparations were instilled twice daily for five days. They significantly increased clearance of wax from the ears by natural expulsion and reduced the need for syringing.[20] The chlorbutol product that is commercially available contains oil of terbinth (turpentine oil), paradichlorobenzene and peanut oil. Turpentine is a rubefacient and counterirritant used topically to provide analgesia. It can cause skin irritation. Paradichlorobenzene gives the characteristic smell to moth balls and is used to repel insects. Their inclusion in a product used to remove ear wax is questionable. Arachis oil may induce allergic reactions and patients allergic to peanuts should not use this product.

Commercially prepared otic products are available in a dropper bottle. If preparations such as olive oil are chosen, the patient should purchase a dropper and instil the substance in a manner similar to normal drops. "Home remedies" such as dilutions of hydrogen peroxide or solutions of sodium bicarbonate should be freshly prepared and used immediately.

Olive oil, light mineral oil, hydrogen peroxide, glycerin or sodium bicarbonate are sometimes recommended in individuals prone to cerumen impaction as preventive therapy.

For instructions on proper instillation of ear drops, see Chapter 17, Ear Drops—Patient Information.

Monitoring of Therapy

Relief of symptoms (ear fullness, hearing loss, discomfort) should occur as soon as the wax is expelled with products like triethanolamine polypeptide condensate or docusate sodium. Relief may occur gradually after five to seven days with wax-softening products. The pharmacist can follow-up with the patient at this time. If relief does not occur, refer the patient to a physician. If irritation of the canal occurs, use of the product should be discontinued. This is generally sufficient; however, if the irritation is severe

or otitis externa develops appropriate treatment may be required. Initially, hearing loss or fullness may be exacerbated due to swelling of wax within the canal.

Suggested Readings

Otitis Media

Del Mar C, Glasziou P, Haymen M. Are antibiotics indicated as initial treatment for children with acute otitis media? A meta-analysis. *BMJ* 1997;314:1526-9.

Dowell SF, Butler JC, Giebink GS et al. Acute otitis media: management and surveillance in an era of pneumococcal resistance – a report from the drug-resistant *Streptococcus pneumoniae* therapeutic working group. *Pediatr Infect Dis J* 1999;18:1-9.

Erramouspe J, Heyneman CA. Treatment and prevention of otitis media. *Ann Pharmacother* 2000;34:1452-68.

Barotrauma

Csortan E, Jones J, Haan M et al. Efficacy of pseudoephedrine for the prevention of barotrauma during air travel. *Ann Emerg Med* 1994;23:1324-7.

Newbegin C, Ell S. Ear barotrauma after flying and diving. *Practitioner* 2000;244:96-105.

Impacted Cerumen

Meador JA. Cerumen impaction in the elderly. *J Gerontol Nurs* 1995;21(12):43-5.

Sharp JF, Wilson JA, Ross L, Barr-Hamilton RM. Ear wax removal: a survey of current practice. *BMJ* 1990;301:1251-3.

References

1. Kenna M. The ear. In: Behrman RE, Kliegman RM, Jenson HB, ed. *Nelson Textbook of Pediatrics.* 16th ed. Philadelphia: WB Saunders Company; 2000:1938-59.
2. Jackler RK, Kaplan MJ. Ear, nose and throat. In: Tierney LM, McPhee SJ, Papadakis MA, eds. *Current Medical Diagnosis and Treatment 2001.* 40th ed. New York: Lange Medical Books/McGraw Hill; 2001:217-31.
3. Weber PC, Klein AJ. Hearing loss. *Med Clin North Am* 1999;83:125-37.
4. Fortune DS, Haynes DS, Hall JW. Tinnitus. Current evaluation and management. *Med Clin North Am* 1999;83:153-62.
5. Seligmann H, Podoshin L, Ben-David J, Fradis M, Goldsher M. Drug-induced tinnitus and other hearing disorders. *Drug Safety* 1996;14:198-212.
6. Baloh RW. The dizzy patient. *Postgrad Med* 1999;105:161-172.

7. Arnett A. Pain-earache. In: Fleisher GR, Ludwig S, eds. *Textbook of Pediatric Emergency Medicine*. 4th ed. Philadelphia: Lipincott Williams and Wilkins; 2000:453-8.

8. Gossel TA, O'Hara JD. Counseling patients to treat ear afflictions. *US Pharm.*; 1993:18(12):26-35.

9. Rosenfeld RM, Vertrees JE, Carr J et al. Clinical efficacy of antimicrobial drugs for acute otitis media: Metaanalysis of 5400 children from thirty-three randomized trials. *J Pediatr* 1994;124:355-67.

10. Del Mar C, Glasziou P, Haymen M. Are antibiotics indicated as initial treatment for children with acute otitis media? A meta-analysis. *BMJ* 1997;314:1526-9.

11. Nix De. Upper respiratory infections. In: Herfindal ET, Gourley DR, ed. *Textbook of Therapeutics Drug and Disease Management*. 7th ed. Philadelphia: Lippincott Williams and Wilkins; 2000:1392-94.

12. Van Buchem FL, Peeters MF, van't Hof MA. Acute otitis media: a new treatment strategy. *BMJ* 1985;290:1033-7.

13. Mandel EM, Rockette HE, Bluestone CD, Paradise JL, Nozza RJ. Efficacy of amoxicillin with and without decongestant-antihistamine for otitis media with effusion in children. *N Engl J Med* 1987;316:432-7.

14. Cantekin EI, Mandel EM, Bluestone CD et al. Lack of efficacy of a decongestant-antihistamine combination for otitis media with effusion ("secretory" otitis media) in children. *N Engl J Med* 1983;308: 297-301.

15. Newbegin C, Ell S. Ear barotrauma after flying and diving. *Practitioner* 2000;244:96-105.

16. Jones JJ, Sheffield W, White LJ, Bloom MA. A double-blind comparison between oral pseudoephedrine and topical oxymetazoline in the prevention of barotrauma during air travel. *Am J Emerg Med* 1998;16:262-4.

17. Csortan E, Jones J, Haan M et al. Efficacy of pseudoephedrine for the prevention of barotrauma during air travel. *Ann Emerg Med* 1994;23:1324-7.

18. Buchanan BJ, Hoagland J, Fischer PR. Pseudoephedrine and air travel-associated ear pain in children. *Arch Pediatr Adolesc Med* 1999;153:466-8.

19. Torsher L. Ear care products. In: Carruthers-Czyzewski P, ed. *Nonprescription Drug Reference for Health Professionals*. Ottawa, ON: Canadian Pharmaceutical Association, 1996: 149-61.

20. Keane EM, Wilson H, McGrane D, Coakley D, Walsh JB. Use of solvents to disperse ear wax. *Br J Clin Pract* 1995;49:71-2.

21. Singer AJ, Sauris E, Viccellio AW. Ceruminolytic effects of docusate sodium: a randomized, controlled trial. *Ann Emerg Med* 2000;36:228-32.

22. Meheta AK. An in-vitro comparison of the disintegration of human ear wax by five cerumenolytics commonly used in general practice. *Br J Clin Prac* 1985;39:200-3.

23. Meador JA. Cerumen impaction in the elderly. *J Gerontol Nurs* 1995;21(12):43-5.

24. Sharp JF, Wilson JA, Ross L, Barr-Hamilton RM. Ear wax removal: a survey of current practice. *BMJ* 1990;301:1251-3.

25. Chaput de Saintonge DM, Johnstone CI. A clinical comparison of triethanolamine polypeptide oleate-condensate ear drops with olive oil for the removal of impacted wax. *Br J Clin Prac* 1973;27:454-5.

Ear Candling—Patient Information

Ear candling or coning involves placing a cone-shaped device into the ear and lighting the end. The person lies on their side, a collecting plate is placed above the ear, and the candle is inserted through a hole in the plate and into the ear canal. The candle is lit, allowed to burn down for several minutes and after the candle is blown out a cotton swab is used to remove ear wax.

The candles are made of linen or cotton and soaked in wax or paraffin and allowed to harden. Some waxes contain herbs or other substances. Home-made candles may be made of wax-soaked newspaper and cones of pottery into which herbal smoke is blown. The procedure is said to remove earwax and other impurities by creating a vacuum that draws wax and debris out of the canal, inner ear, sinuses and brain.

Candling is purported to be useful for a long list of purposes including cleaning the ear canal, relieving sinus pressure, purifying the mind, relieving earaches, curing swimmers ear, curing Meniere's disease, relieving vertigo, and stabilizing emotions, to name a few.

In reality, candling does not produce a vacuum so substances are not drawn out of the canal. Because of the nature of ear wax, the negative pressure required to pull wax from the canal would pierce the eardrum. Also, there is no connection between the outer ear and other areas such as the sinuses or brain that would allow impurities to be drawn out.

Candling is not only ineffective, it is also dangerous. There is risk of fire, injury to the ear, and facial and ear burns. The sale of ear candles in Canada is illegal.

Ear Piercing—Patient Information*

Guidelines to Reduce the Risk of Ear Piercing Complications

- Piercing should be done only by individuals with proper training and sterile equipment. Home-pierced ears have a higher rate of infection and complication.
- Do not pierce the ears of children under five years of age. Earrings tend to get caught during play and proper hygiene is difficult.
- Individuals with valvular heart disease, diabetes, glomerulonephritis or a history of rheumatic fever should not have their ears pierced, as the risk of systemic infection is increased.
- Individuals with a history of keloid formation should not have their ears pierced.
- Avoid the use of earrings containing nickel or gold in newly pierced ears to reduce risk of allergic dermatitis.
- Studs should be made in a single piece from surgical grade stainless steel.
- Before the procedure, earlobes should be cleaned with alcohol and allowed to dry, or cleansed with chlorhexidine soap.

Care of the Ears Following Piercing

- Wipe twice daily with rubbing alcohol for the first six weeks. Be sure to get between stud and skin on the front, and between earring back and skin on the back of the lobe.
- Examine ears carefully after they are pierced, watching for redness, swelling or rash, and feel the lobes for cysts or nodules. Consult a physician promptly if any of the above develop.
- Chlorhexidine soap may be used in place of alcohol to prevent drying and cracking of earlobes.
- Do not turn or twist earrings; this increases the risk of infection. Leave studs in place for six weeks.
- Ensure all shampoo is rinsed well from ear areas, and avoid use of hair sprays and perfumes until lobes are well healed.
- At end of healing period, the earlobe may be lubricated with soap and water to allow easy removal of the stud.
- Once earlobes are healed, wash daily with soap and water, just as one would wash the face.
- Wash earrings with soap and water prior to each use.

*Adapted from Torsher L. Ear care products. In: Carruthers-Czyzewski P, ed. *Nonprescription Drug Reference for Health Professionals.* Ottawa, ON: Canadian Pharmaceutical Association, 1996:149-61.

Impacted Cerumen (Ear Wax)—Patient Information

- Ears are generally self-cleaning; wax removal is not usually necessary.
- Objects placed in the ear canal can push wax further in and cause hearing loss, discomfort, and impaction of wax.
- Olive oil, vegetable oil, light mineral oil, or a commercial ear drop preparation is sometimes needed to help soften ear wax and aid in removal.
- Some products require instillation of drops twice daily for several days before the wax softens enough to come out on its own (olive oil, vegetable oil, light mineral oil, carbamide peroxide).
- Some products (triethanolamine polypeptide condensate) should remain in the ear for only 15 minutes before they are syringed out.
- Make sure you know how to use the product safely before you leave the pharmacy.
- Do not syringe ears yourself; this may damage the ear. Have someone help you.
- Stop using the product if irritation occurs.

- If you have repeated problems with ear wax, using olive oil, vegetable oil, light mineral oil, or sodium bicarbonate solution two to three times a week may prevent the problem.

How to Syringe the Ears
- **Never attempt to flush out the ear canal if there is any possibility the ear drum has burst.**
- It is difficult to perform this procedure on yourself; get help from a friend.
- Fill ear syringe with water at body temperature.
- Hold a basin just below the ear to catch the outflow. Lay a towel over the shoulder.
- Straighten the ear canal by gently pulling upwards and backwards on the ear (in a child pull downwards and backwards).
- Insert the ear syringe just into the opening of the ear canal.
- Direct stream of water along the upper surface of the ear canal so that the returning flow pushes the ear wax out from behind. Use gentle force only.

Chapter 17

Otitis Externa

Yvonne Shevchuk, BSP, PharmD, FCSHP

Pathophysiology[1-8]

Otitis externa (OE) is defined as inflammation of the external auditory canal (EAC) and is often due to infection. The EAC is warm, dark and prone to becoming moist. This provides an excellent environment for bacteria or fungi to proliferate, particularly if the EAC is traumatized. Otitis externa can be categorized as acute diffuse, acute localized, chronic, eczematous or necrotizing.

Acute Diffuse OE

Predisposing factors for acute diffuse OE include:[5,7]

- Too little cerumen – cerumen provides antibacterial action by physically protecting the canal and maintaining a low pH;
- Too much cerumen – can lead to occlusion and maceration;
- Moisture (swimming, bathing, water sports, perspiration, increased humidity) – macerates underlying skin and raises pH;
- Trauma to EAC (fingernails, cotton-tipped swabs, other foreign objects, overzealous wax removal) – abrasion and laceration allowing inoculation of organisms;
- Chronic dermatologic disorders;
- Hearing aids;
- Narrow, hairy ear canal.

The most common etiology of acute otitis externa is bacterial infection. Fungal overgrowth occurs in approximately 10% of cases. The two most common microorganisms causing acute otitis externa are *Pseudomonas aeruginosa* and *Staphylococcus aureus*.

Bacterial OE produces otalgia, pruritus and tenderness, especially on movement of the ear. These symptoms may be more intense than those seen with fungal OE. Fever and regional lymphadenopathy may be present. Fungal OE may be asymptomatic or may produce pruritus and fullness in the ear. It classically occurs after prolonged treatment of bacterial OE with antibiotics which alter the bacterial flora of the EAC. The EAC may contain black, grey, bluish green, yellow or white fungal elements and debris.

Acute Localized OE (furunculosis)

This is an acute localized "boil" in the ear canal usually due to *S. aureus*. It produces localized pain, itching, edema, erythema and possibly a fluctuance or abscess. The pain subsides when the boil comes to a head and bursts.

Chronic OE

Chronic OE is characterized as a thickening of the external auditory canal skin secondary to low grade infection and inflammation. There is usually unrelenting pruritus, mild discomfort and dry flaky skin in the EAC with lack of cerumen.

Eczematous OE

Eczematous OE may be due to a variety of skin conditions, including atopic, seborrheic or contact dermatitis, psoriasis, lupus erythematosus, neurodermatitis, and infantile eczema. Lesions typically occur elsewhere on the body, especially the head and neck, as well as the auricle and EAC. Appearance may range from mild erythema and scaling with atopic dermatitis to the typical adherent scales of psoriasis (see the Dermatology section for a more complete description of the lesions). The most common symptom is pruritus, although erythema, edema, crusting and oozing may be present. The lesions may become secondarily infected with bacteria or fungi.

Necrotizing (malignant) OE

This is an infection which extends to the mastoid or temporal bone and is usually seen in diabetic or immunocompromised patients.

This chapter focuses on the management of acute diffuse otitis externa.

Goals of Therapy

- Eliminate pathogenic microorganisms
- Control pain
- Restore the canal to normal health so it resists infection – return to normal acidic pH and adequate cerumen

Patient Assessment[5,8]

Acute otitis externa is characterized by ear discomfort or pain (otalgia) and discharge in or coming from the ear (otorrhea). The discomfort can range from pruritus to severe pain. The pain is often worse with motion of the ear, including movement caused by chewing. If the canal becomes occluded by edema and debris, a feeling of ear fullness and hearing loss can occur. Determining the type of OE (infectious versus noninfectious) can be assisted by the description of the signs and symptoms above and the presence of contributing factors (e.g., history of swimming or trauma to the EAC), or the presence of dermatologic conditions on the body other than the EAC.

One of the most important principles of management is proper cleansing of the canal, in order for topical treatment to be effective. Cleansing must be done by a physician. Therefore, if there is significant edema or debris in the EAC, refer the patient to a physician.

Nonpharmacologic Therapy[5,7]

Adequate cleansing of the canal with removal of debris is required so that topical therapy can be effective. This is done by the physician and may have to be done frequently. If the canal is not patent, ear wicks may be inserted to reduce edema and swelling and provide a mechanism for drug delivery to the canal. These may remain in place for two to five days. Pain management is an important consideration and nonpharmacologic measures may include use of heating pads, hot water bottles or hot packs.

Pharmacologic Therapy[5,7]

Topical therapy is the mainstay of therapy, although in more severe cases, when infection has spread beyond the EAC or when otitis media co-exists, systemic antibiotics may be required. Topical therapy options include acidifying agents, antibiotics alone or antibiotics combined with corticosteroids (Table 1). There are no comparative trials suggesting one approach is better than another, therefore the choice appears to be determined by physician and patient preference, the side effect profile of the agents and cost. Some sources recommend "drying" the ear with an acidifying agent prior to a course of antibiotic therapy; however, the acidifying agents used in OE do have antibacterial properties. Acidification of the ear canal with **2% acetic acid** or Burow's solution (**0.5% aluminum acetate**) is often effective. Household **vinegar** can be diluted 1:1 with propylene glycol or isopropyl alcohol for use as an acidifier.

Antibiotic drops are available as both otic and ophthalmic preparations. Both nonprescription and prescription products are available. Otic products are more acidic than ophthalmic preparations and may cause burning on instillation. If a patient cannot tolerate otic preparations, ophthalmic preparations may be more comfortable. Preparations for treatment of otitis externa may contain steroids which act to reduce inflammation and edema and may resolve symptoms more quickly. However, this has not been shown in all studies and steroids may occasionally be topical sensitizers.

One particular concern with topical therapy of acute otitis externa is the potential ototoxicity of aminoglycosides. This is a documented adverse effect of systemically administered aminoglycosides. With topical administration, if the tympanic membrane is intact, the risk is extremely small. Risk factors for ototoxicity include using the product for more than one week and continued use after otorrhea has subsided.[9-11] Topical fluoroquinolones have not been associated with ototoxicity.

Enough drops to fill the canal (three to four drops) should be instilled four times daily (most products except fluoroquinolones). Therapy should continue for three to four days after symptoms resolve; usually five to seven days, but up to 14 days may be needed. For information on correct instillation of ear drops see Ear Drops—Patient Information.

Otitis externa can be very painful. Usual doses of acetaminophen or ibuprofen can be used for

Table 1: **Drugs for Otitis Externa**[5,7,9-11,13-16]

Acidifying agents

Preparation	Rx or OTC	Comments/Advantages/Disadvantages
Aluminum acetate 0.5%/ benzethonium chloride 0.03%	OTC	Broad spectrum antibacterial Antiinflammatory and astringent Restores acidity to canal Non-irritating May produce burning on instillation Lower cost than antibiotics Used for prevention and treatment Benzethonium Cl has antiseptic properties; added as a preservative
Acetic acid 2%/ benzethonium chloride 0.02%	OTC	Broad spectrum antibacterial Restores acidity to canal Can be irritating to inflamed canal Possibly ototoxic Lower cost than antibiotics Used for prevention and treatment Benzethonium Cl has antiseptic properties; added as a preservative

Antibiotics

Preparation	Rx or OTC	Comments/Advantages/Disadvantages
Gentamicin otic soln	Rx	Aminoglycosides active against gram-negative organisms (e.g., *Pseudomonas*) and *S. aureus*
Tobramycin ophth soln	Rx	Neomycin not active against *Pseudomonas* Potentially ototoxic, particularly with perforated TM or use >1 week
Neomycin/polymyxin B, gramicidin	Rx	Neomycin – contact dermatitis in 15% of patients Gramicidin and polymixin B – see below
Gramicidin/polymyxin B	OTC	Gramicidin – active against gram-positive organisms Polymixin B – active against gram-negative organisms Potentially ototoxic
Ciprofloxacin ophth soln	Rx	Active against many gram-negative organisms including *P. aeruginosa* and some gram-positive (*S. aureus*)
Ofloxacin ophth soln	Rx	Not associated with ototoxicity Well tolerated Twice daily dosing Expensive

Antiinflammatory agents

Preparation	Rx or OTC	Comments/Advantages/Disadvantages
Betamethasone disodium phosphate	Rx	Antiinflammatory properties reduce swelling and edema Steroid alone for dermatologic causes of AOE; if bacterial combine with acidifier or antibiotic
Dexamethasone	Rx	May cause hypersensitivity reactions

Combined antibiotic/antiinflammatory

Preparation	Rx or OTC	Comments/Advantages/Disadvantages
Framycetin/Gramicidin/ Dexamethasone	Rx	Framycetin – Aminoglycoside See comments above
Gentamicin/Betamethasone	Rx	
Neomycin/Hydrocortisone	Rx	

(cont'd)

Table 1: **Drugs for Otitis Externa**[5,7,9-11,13-16] (cont'd)

Preparation	Rx or OTC	Comments/Advantages/Disadvantages
Combined antibiotic/antiinflammatory (cont'd)		
Polymixin B/Neomycin/ Hydrocortisone	Rx	
Ciprofloxacin/Hydrocortisone	Rx	
Other		
Polymyxin B/Lidocaine	OTC	Lidocaine may cause topical hypersensitivity reactions; do not use with ruptured TM Oral analgesics preferred
Antipyrine/Benzocaine	OTC	Benzocaine – may produce topical hypersensitivity reactions; – do not use with ruptured TM Antipyrine – mild anaesthetic; can cause burning and itching Oral analgesics preferred
Isopropyl alcohol 95%/ Glycerin 5%	OTC	Useful drying agent, but painful when used in acute otitis externa Use for prevention

OTC = over-the-counter; Rx = prescription, TM = tympanic membrane, AOE = acute otitis externa

analgesia. Although some otic preparations contain topical anesthetics, the efficacy of these agents has not been determined and topical hypersensitivity reactions can occur. If topical anesthetic agents are used in addition to other topical therapy, this will dilute the acidifier or antibiotic present in the canal. Avoid their use in otitis externa. Systemic analgesics and local application of heat are preferred recommendations.

Fungal otitis externa often responds to cleansing and acidification alone, although specific antifungal agents (amphotericin B, clotrimazole) may also be used.

Eczematous otitis externa is managed by treating the underlying dermatologic disease (e.g., seborrhea, psoriasis, acne).[12] Contact dermatitis commonly occurs on or in the ears and grooming products (e.g., shampoos, hair sprays, and hair dyes) are common allergens. Hearing aids and earplugs may also cause dermatitis of the EAC. Neomycin is one of the most common topical medications that can produce allergic contact dermatitis.[13] It is a common ingredient in otic preparations. Patients sensitive to neomycin may also react to gentamicin and tobramycin. Cosensitization (not true antigenic cross-sensitivity) to bacitracin in

these products may also occur. Other agents commonly placed in the ear that are reported to cause contact dermatitis include benzocaine, propylene glycol, and triethanolamine polypeptide condensate. Management includes avoiding the offending agent, aluminum acetate solution to dry oozing lesions, and reacidification of the canal or symptomatic therapy with topical corticosteroid.

Prevention of Recurrence

Give individuals who develop acute otitis externa information on how to prevent a recurrence:

- After swimming or bathing, dry the external canal with a blow dryer on low setting or by instillation of acidifying or alcohol drops.
- Avoid overzealous cleansing and scratching of the ear canal.
- Use a bathing cap while swimming.
- Ear plugs may be used to keep the ears dry, but they may also act as a local irritant.
- Avoid water sports for at least 7 to 10 days after acute otitis externa.

Monitoring of Therapy

Symptoms should be significantly reduced by day three of therapy and should be completely resolved in a week. Occasionally up to 14 days of treatment is needed. Follow-up with the patient in three to five days to ensure symptoms are improving and at the end of treatment to ensure resolution. If symptoms worsen or do not resolve, the patient may be reacting to the medication (contact dermatitis), a superinfection may have developed or the diagnosis may be incorrect. Refer the patient to their physician.

Advice for the Patient

Counsel patients on:

- Prevention of recurrences;
- Methods of pain control;
- Correct use of ear drops;
- Possible side effects of treatment and their management (Table 1);
- When to see the doctor.

Suggested Readings

Bojrab DI, Bruderly T, Abdulrazzak Y. Otitis externa. *Otolaryngol Clin North Am* 1996;29:761-82.

Sander R. Otitis externa: a practical guide to treatment and prevention. *Am Fam Physician* 2001;63:927-36, 941-2.

Shea CR. Dermatologic diseases of the external auditory canal. *Otolaryngol Clin North Am* 1996;29: 783-93.

References

1. Gossel TA, O'Hara JD. Counseling patients to treat ear afflictions. *US Pharm* 1993;18(12):26-35.
2. Kenna M. The ear. In: Behrman RE, Kliegman RM, Jenson HB, eds. *Nelson Textbook of Pediatrics*. 16th ed. Philadelphia: WB Saunders Company; 2000:1938-59.
3. Jackler RK, Kaplan MJ. Ear, nose and throat. In: Tierney LM, McPhee SJ, Papadakis MA, eds. *Current Medical Diagnosis and Treatment 2001*. 40th ed. New York: Lange Medical Books/McGraw Hill; 2001:217-231.
4. Arnett A. Pain-earache. In: Fleisher GR, Ludwig S, eds. *Textbook of Pediatric Emergency Medicine*. 4th ed. Philadelphia: Lippincott Williams and Wilkins; 2000:453-8.
5. Sander R. Otitis externa: A practical guide to treatment and prevention. *Am Fam Physician* 2001;63:927-36, 941-2.
6. Mirza N. Otitis externa. Management in the primary care office. *Postgrad Med* 1996;99:153-8.
7. Bojrab DI, Bruderly T, Abdulrazzak Y. Otitis externa. *Otolaryngol Clin North Am* 1996;29:761-82.
8. Boustred N. Practical guide to otitis externa. *Aust Fam Physician* 1999;28:217-21.
9. Guthrie RM, ed. Diagnosis and treatment of acute otitis externa: an interdisciplinary update. *Ann Otol Rhinol Laryngol* 1999;108 (Suppl 176):1-18.
10. Thorp MA, Kruger J, Oliver S, Nilssen ELK, Prescott CAJ. The antibacterial activity of acetic acid and Burow's solution as topical otological preparations. *J Laryngol Otol* 1998;112:925-8.
11. Marais J, Rutka JA. Ototoxicity and topical eardrops. *Clin Otolaryngol* 1998;23:360-7.
12. Shea CR. Dermatologic diseases of the external auditory canal. *Otolaryngol Clin North Am* 1996;29:783-93.
13. Fraki JE, Kalimo K, Tuohimaa P, Aantaa E. Contact allergy to various components of topical preparations for treatment of external otitis. *Acta Otolaryngol* 1985;100:414-8.
14. Hannley MT, Denneny JC, Holzer SS. Use of ototopical antibiotics in treating 3 common ear diseases. *Otolaryngol Head Neck Surg* 2000;122(6):934-40.
15. Bath AP, Walsh RM, Bance ML, Rutka JA. Ototoxicity of topical gentamicin preparations. *Laryngoscope* 1999;109(7 Pt 1):1088-93.
16. Simpson KL, Markham A. Ofloxacin otic solution. A review of its use in the management of ear infections. *Drugs* 1999;58:509-31.

Otitis Externa—Patient Information

- Otitis externa, or "swimmer's ear," is an infection of the ear canal. Symptoms are itching or pain in the ear and drainage. Plugging and hearing loss can occur.
- Too much water (from bathing, swimming, water sports) or removal of protective ear wax makes the skin in your ears more easily infected.
- Skin conditions can also occur in the ear canal and cause otitis externa.
- Placing objects like cotton-tipped applicators or fingernails in the ear canal can scratch the skin and cause an infection.
- Treatment is usually with ear drops, but the doctor may have to clean the canal for the drops to work.
- Most drops need to be used four times a day.
- Use drops until all symptoms are gone for three days.
- Symptoms are usually much better in three days and should be gone in 10 days.

- Keep your ears as dry as possible – take a bath instead of a shower, avoid swimming and water sports until the treatment is done. Don't poke fingers or other objects into your ears.

To prevent otitis externa from happening again:
- Keep the ear canal as dry as possible:
  —Use bathing caps when swimming;
  —Dry ears with a towel after swimming or bathing and then use a blow dryer on low setting or vinegar or alcohol drops in the ear.
- Do not clean ear wax out of your ears:
  —Ears are usually self-cleaning and the wax protects against infection. If ear wax is causing pain, see your doctor or pharmacist.
- Do not put anything in the ear canal except ear drops. Fingernails, cotton-tipped swabs, and other objects irritate and damage skin, making infection more likely.

Ear Drops—Patient Information*

- Warm the ear drops to body temperature by holding the bottle in your hands for a few minutes. Do *not* heat the drops in hot water because this could cause pain and dizziness.
- The person administering the ear drops should wash their hands with soap and water.
- The ear drops must be kept clean. Do not touch the dropper against the ear or anything else that could contaminate it.
- Shake the bottle before use if necessary.
- Tilt your head or lie on your side so that the ear you are treating is facing up.

In *adults and children over 3 years*:
- Gently pull the top of the ear *up and back*.

In *children under 3 years*:
- Gently pull the top of the ear *down and back*.

NOTE: Pulling the top of the ear will help to straighten the ear canal so that the ear drops can reach the eardrum.

- Place the prescribed number of drops into the ear. Do not insert the dropper into the ear canal as it may cause injury.
- Remain in the same position for a short time (5 to 10 minutes) after you have administered the drops. This will allow the ear drops to run down into the ear canal.
- Dry the ear lobe if there are any ear drops on it.

General Instructions
If you must administer drops in both ears, wait about 5 to 10 minutes before placing the drops in the second ear. This will help keep the medicine in the ear canal of the first ear for at least 5 to 10 minutes before you have to tilt your head to put drops in the other ear. It is generally not recommended that cotton be placed in the ear after the ear drops have been instilled because the cotton can soak up the drug.

---

*Reprinted with permission of Key Porter Books from *Understanding Canadian Prescription Drugs* by Dorothy L. Smith © 1992.

Chapter 18

Vertigo and Dizziness

Yvonne Shevchuk, BSP, PharmD, FCSHP

Pathophysiology[1-8]

Dizziness refers to a variety of sensations such as lightheadedness, fainting, spinning and giddiness. Vertigo is defined as a sensation of motion where there is none or an exaggerated sense of motion in response to a given bodily movement. It is the cardinal symptom of vestibular disease as a result of lesions or disturbances in the inner ear, eighth cranial nerve or vestibular nuclei and their pathways in the brain stem and cerebellum. Vertigo is usually accompanied by varying degrees of nausea and vomiting as well as pallor and perspiration. It may be acute, chronic or recurrent.

Dizziness has a number of causes unrelated to ear conditions including cardiovascular conditions (e.g., arrhythmias, hypertension), metabolic or endocrine conditions (e.g., anemia, diabetes), psychiatric conditions and neurological conditions (e.g., migraine, head injury).[9]

Specific conditions that produce vertigo include:
- *Viral neurolabyrinthitis:*[7,8] a self-limiting condition that manifests as vertigo of sudden onset, nausea, ataxia and nystagmus. The condition is preceded by a nonspecific viral illness. The vertigo reaches a peak within a few days and then gradually subsides over a few days to weeks. Hearing loss can vary from none (referred to as *vestibular neuritis*) to profound. The patient should keep still for the first few days to avoid exacerbating symptoms and use vestibular suppressants and antiemetics. After a few days, medications should be withdrawn and walking encouraged to stimulate vestibular compensation.
- *Benign paroxysmal postural vertigo:*[7,8] the most common type of vertigo. Symptoms of vertigo and nystagmus are precipitated by movement or position change of the head. The condition is thought to be caused by the presence of debris or small crystals of calcium carbonate within the semicircular canals. The vertigo is brief, lasting less than one minute, and hearing loss and tinnitus are not usually present. Symptoms disappear in a few weeks but may recur. Specific physical treatment is much more beneficial than drug therapy.[10]
- *Meniere's disease:*[7,8,11,12] characterized by intermittent vertigo, sensorineural hearing loss, tinnitus and/or a feeling of fullness in the ear. The vertigo has an acute onset, and persists from 30 minutes to several hours. The exact cause is unknown, but the condition is associated with distension of the endolymphatic compartment of the inner ear secondary to accumulation of endolymph. The frequency of attacks is variable, but they tend to occur in clusters with a mean of 6 to 11 clusters per year. When symptoms occur, they can be managed with vestibular suppressants and antiemetics. Salt restriction and diuretics (e.g., hydrochlorothiazide-triamterene; loop diuretics are avoided) may reduce the frequency of attacks. The benefits of betahistine, a histamine agonist are not well-established although the drug is commonly used for Meniere's disease.[11] Flunarizine, a calcium channel blocker, is used in Europe.[13]

Drug-induced causes of dizziness are listed in Table 1. Ototoxic drugs may also produce vertigo (see Table 2, Chapter 16).

Goals of Therapy[7]
- Reduce or eliminate symptoms of vertigo
- Reduce or eliminate nausea and anxiety
- Avoid compromising the process of vestibular compensation (i.e., allowing the brain to find a new sensory equilibrium despite the vestibular lesion)

Table 1: **Medications That Often Cause Dizziness**

Class of Medication	Probable Mechanism	Example
α_1-Adrenergic antagonists	Orthostatic hypotension	Prazosin
Alcohol	Hypotension, osmotic effects	Wine, cough syrups
Aminoglycosides	Ototoxicity	Gentamicin
Anticonvulsants	Orthostatic hypotension	Carbamazepine
Antidepressants	Orthostatic hypotension	Desipramine
Anti-Parkinsonian medication	Orthostatic hypotension	Levodopa
Antipsychotics	Orthostatic hypotension	Olanzapine
β-Blockers	Hypotension or bradycardia	Atenolol
Calcium-channel blockers	Hypotension, vasodilation	Verapamil
Class la antiarrhythmics	Torsades de pointes	Procainamide
Digitalis glycosides	Hypotension	Digoxin
Diuretics	Volume contraction, vasodilation	Hydrochlorothiazide
Narcotics	Central nervous system depression	Morphine, propoxyphene
Oral sulfonylureas	Hypoglycemia	Tolazamide
Vasodilators	Hypotension, vasodilation	Hydralazine

Reproduced with permission from Sloane PD et al. Dizziness: state of the science. *Ann Intern Med* 2001;134:823-32.

Patient Assessment

Drug-induced causes for vertigo and dizziness should always be sought. All patients with vertigo should be assessed by a physician. If the vertigo is accompanied by numbness, tingling or weakness in any part of the body, visual disturbances, confusion or difficulty speaking, this is an emergency and the patient should call 911 or an ambulance. The patient may be experiencing a transient ischemic attack or stroke.

Nonpharmacologic Therapy

Nonpharmacologic therapy depends on the cause of the vertigo;
- *Epley maneuver* for benign paroxysmal postural vertigo.[10] The Epley maneuver is a specific sequence of head position changes performed by a physician that moves particles into the posterior semicircular canal toward the utricle;
- Vestibular rehabilitation is a physical therapy program to improve balance, eye-hand coordination, and habituate the patient to feelings of dizziness;
- Salt restriction for Meniere's disease;
- Bedrest for acute viral neurolabyrinthitis;
- Surgery is indicated in selected cases, often as third-line therapy after drugs and physical therapy have failed.

Pharmacologic Therapy

Drug therapy for vertigo is symptomatic; in the majority of cases the mechanism of the vertigo is unknown and specific therapy can therefore not be determined. Unless a specific cause of vertigo is known (e.g., Meniere's disease), the choice of pharmacologic agent for treatment depends on the adverse effect profile of the drug, presence of contraindications and cost. Most drugs used in vertigo down-regulate vestibular excitability (i.e., they are vestibular suppressants).[2-4,6,7,9] Table 2 describes nonprescription agents used to treat vertigo. Prescription drugs used to treat vertigo include benzodiazepines, betahistine and flunarizine.[11,13,14] Evidence of efficacy through well-controlled trials is lacking.

Although these drugs may reduce vertigo, they also reduce vestibular function in the normal ear, which is a disadvantage. Vestibular suppressants reduce or slow down vestibular compensation and prevent the CNS from receiving the necessary feedback to facilitate compensation.[7,9] For this reason, anticholinergics, antihistamines and benzodiazepines are not intended for long-term use. In most cases the duration of treatment would be a week or less.

Table 2: **Nonprescription Drugs for Vertigo**[3,6,7,9]

Drug	Dose	Common side effects	Comments
Dimenhydrinate	25-50 mg PO q6h or 100 mg PR q8h	Drowsiness, confusion, anticholinergic effects (dry mouth, mydriasis, blurred vision, constipation, urinary retention, confusion)	Also have antiemetic effects. Avoid combining with CNS depressants. Contraindicated in angle closure glaucoma, prostatic hypertrophy, and urinary retention.
Meclizine	25-50 mg PO q4-6h	Drowsiness, confusion, anticholinergic effects (see Dimenhydrinate), extrapyramidal reactions. Anticholinergic effects less than scopolamine.	
Promethazine	25-50 mg PO, or PR q4-6h (nausea) (BID for vertigo)	Drowsiness, confusion, anticholinergic effects (see Dimenhydrinate), extrapyramidal reactions	
Scopolamine	0.6 mg PO q4-6h or transdermal patch 1 q72h	Drowsiness, anticholinergic effects (see Dimenhydrinate)	

Monitoring of Therapy

Vertigo is often self-limiting. Evaluate the need for continued use of medication frequently. Determine the severity, duration and frequency of the vertigo. Monitor the patient for relief of vertigo and associated symptoms such as nausea, vomiting and anxiety. If no improvement of vertigo is noted, drug therapy should be discontinued. Patients should also be monitored for adverse effects such as drowsiness and anticholinergic effects.

Advice for the Patient

Counsel patients who receive drug therapy regarding:
- Expected duration of treatment;
- Management of side effects (Table 2);
- Instructions not to combine drug therapy with alcohol.

Suggested Readings

Derebery MJ. The diagnosis and treatment of dizziness. *Med Clin North Am* 1999;83:163-77.

Rascol O, Hain TC, Brefel M et al. Antivertigo medications and drug-induced vertigo. A pharmacologic review. *Drugs* 1995;50:777-91.

Sloane PD, Coeytaux RR, Beck RS, Dallara J. Dizziness: state of the science. *Ann Intern Med* 2001; 134:823-32.

References

1. Kenna M. The ear. In: Behrman RE, Kliegman RM, Jenson HB, eds. *Nelson Textbook of Pediatrics*. 16th ed. Philadelphia: WB Sauders Company; 2000:1938-59.
2. Jackler RK, Kaplan MJ. Ear, nose and throat. In: Tierney LM, McPhee SJ, Papadakis MA, eds. *Current Medical Diagnosis and Treatment 2001*. 40th ed. New York: Lange Medical Books/McGraw Hill; 2001:217-231.
3. Derebery MJ. The diagnosis and treatment of dizziness. *Med Clin North Am* 1999;83:163-77.
4. Daroff RB, Martin JB. Faintness, syncope, dizziness, and vertigo. In: Fauci AS et al, eds. *Harrison's Principles of Internal Medicine*. 14th ed. Montreal: McGraw-Hill Health Professionals Division; 1998:100-7.
5. Seidman MD, Jacobson GP. Update on tinnitus. *Otolaryngol Clin North Am* 1996;29:455-65.
6. Baloh RW. The dizzy patient. *Postgrad Med* 1999;105:161-72.
7. Rascol O, Hain TC, Brefel M et al. Antivertigo medications and drug-induced vertigo. A pharmacologic review. *Drugs* 1995;50:777-91.
8. Austin DF. Noninflammatory diseases of the labyrinth. In: Ballenger JJ, ed. *Diseases of the Nose, Throat, Ear, Head and Neck*. 14th ed. Philadelphia: Lea and Febiger; 1991:1193-212.
9. Brandt T. Management of vestibular disorders. *J Neurol* 2000; 247:491-99.
10. Froehling DA et al. The canalith repositioning procedure for the treatment of benign paroxysmal positional vertigo: a randomized controlled trial. *Mayo Clin Proc* 2001;75:695-700.
11. James AL, Burton MJ. Betahistine for Meniere's disease or syndrome (Cochrane Review). In: *The Cochrane Library*, Issue 4, 2001. Oxford: Update software.
12. Foster CA. Vestibular disorders. In: Jafek BW, Murrow BW, eds. *ENT Secrets*. 2nd ed. Philadelphia: Hanley and Belfus, Inc; 2001: 81-6.
13. Haid T. Evaluation of flunarizine in patients with Meniere's disease. *Acta Otolaryngol* 1988;460:149-53.
14. Parfitt K, ed. *Martindale. The Complete Drug Reference*. 32nd ed. London: Pharmaceutical Press; 1999: 411.

Vertigo—Patient Information

Vertigo is a kind of dizziness where you feel like you are moving but you really are not. It often makes people feel sick to their stomach.

Vertigo can be caused by many things, including viral infections and inner ear problems. Sometimes it goes away on its own. Other times the body learns to ignore the feeling. **Anyone with vertigo should see a doctor to find out what is causing it.**

Medications can be used to treat vertigo and any upset stomach it causes. These do not fix the underlying problem. They may even keep your body from learning to ignore the vertigo.

If you suffer from attacks of vertigo, avoid potentially hazardous activities such as climbing ladders, driving and operating machinery.

Here are some important points about the medications used to treat vertigo:

- They may cause drowsiness or blurred vision; use caution driving and operating dangerous machinery.
- Dry mouth may occur; chewing on sugarless candy or gum may help relieve this dryness.
- They may cause constipation; drink plenty of water and eat high-fibre foods.
- Don't combine them with alcohol or other drugs that might make you drowsy or less alert.
- If you notice anything unusual or if side effects really bother you, talk to your pharmacist or doctor.

Chapter 19

Tinnitus

Yvonne Shevchuk, BSP, PharmD, FCSHP

Pathophysiology[1-5]

Objective tinnitus is caused by a sound produced within the head due to either vascular (e.g., arteriovenous malformations, arterial bruits) or mechanical (e.g., palatal myoclonus, patulous eustachian tube) causes. *Subjective* tinnitus, which is more common, is the perception of sound or noise without any external stimulation. It may be described as buzzing, ringing, roaring, whistling or hissing. Continuous bilateral high-pitched tinnitus is most commonly associated with chronic noise exposure, presbycusis (age-associated hearing loss) and ototoxic drugs. Hearing loss is commonly present. The most important treatment is avoidance of excessive noise, ototoxic agents (see Table 2, Chapter 16), and other factors that may cause cochlear damage. Other than otological and drug-induced causes, neurologic (e.g., closed head injury, post-meningitis), metabolic (e.g., hyperthyroidism, hypothyroidism, hyperlipidemia), psychiatric and dental disease may also cause tinnitus.

Goals of Therapy

- Treat the underlying medical condition if possible
- Correct hearing loss if correctable
- Reduce or eliminate tinnitus
- Improve the patient's quality of life

Patient Assessment

Drug-induced causes of tinnitus should always be sought and the patient's physician made aware of any possible drug causes identified. Review the patient's drug history, both current and past, for potentially ototoxic drugs. All patients with tinnitus lasting greater than 24 hours should be assessed by a physician. The severity of tinnitus and the impact on the patient's quality of life should be assessed.

Nonpharmacologic Therapy

- Avoid loud noises. Use noise protectors if loud noise cannot be avoided
- Avoid caffeinated beverages and stimulants
- Stop smoking (significant reduction in tinnitus may be noted with caffeine and nicotine avoidance)
- Use masking techniques or devices (an external noise is used to cover the tinnitus)
- Use hearing aids in patients with hearing loss (the increased sound from the hearing aid may mask the offending tinnitus)
- Try stress management and biofeedback

Pharmacotherapy

Many drugs have been studied in the management of tinnitus but drug therapy has only a minor role to play in its management. Tocainide, carbamazepine, baclofen, lamotrigine, misoprostol, nicotinamide, betahistine and iontophoresis of lidocaine were all found in randomized controlled trials to show no benefit over placebo.[6] Alprazolam- and nortriptyline-treated patients improved compared to placebo.

Ginkgo biloba has been studied in the management of tinnitus. In at least two trials, one trial that was for tinnitus alone, it was no more effective than placebo.[7,8] However, it may be useful in tinnitus associated with vascular insufficiency.[9,10] The recommended dose is 120 to 160 mg per day of ginkgo leaf extract divided into two or three doses. Adverse effects of ginkgo biloba include mild GI complaints, headache, dizziness, palpitations and allergic skin reactions. The drug is also associated with bleeding and seizures. Ginkgo biloba may increase the risk of bleeding when combined with warfarin or antiplatelet drugs; advise patients to avoid this combination.

A number of other herbal products (examples include bupleurum, feverfew, cordyceps, glossy privet, goldenseal, ground ivy, lycium, melatonin, poria mushroom, vitamin A, and zinc) are also claimed to be useful for tinnitus, but no evidence to confirm or refute this use exists.[9]

Monitoring of Therapy

If drug therapy is attempted, monitor carefully to determine any therapeutic benefit. The subjective nature of tinnitus makes this particularly difficult. Drugs providing little benefit should be discontinued.

Advice for the Patient

Counsel patients on:
- Nonpharmacologic therapy
- Expected results of drug therapy
- Possible side effects and their management

Suggested Readings

Dobie RA. A review of randomized clinical trials in tinnitus. *Laryngocope* 1999;109:1202-11.

Fortune DS, Haynes DS, Hall JW. Tinnitus. Current evaluation and management. *Med Clin North Am* 1999;83:153-62.

Schleuning AJ. Management of the patient with tinnitus. *Med Clin North Am* 1991;75:1225-37.

Seligmann H, Podoshin L, Ben-David J, Fradis M, Goldsher M. Drug-induced tinnitus and other hearing disorders. *Drug Safety* 1996;14:198-212.

References

1. Kenna M. The ear. In: Behrman RE, Kliegman RM, Jenson HB, eds. *Nelson Textbook of Pediatrics*. 16th ed. Philadelphia: WB Sauders Company; 2000:1938-59.
2. Jackler RK, Kaplan MJ. Ear, nose and throat. In: Tierney LM, McPhee SJ, Papadakis MA, eds. *Current Medical Diagnosis and Treatment 2001*. 40th ed. New York: Lange Medical Books/McGraw Hill; 2001:217-231.
3. Fortune DS, Haynes DS, Hall JW. Tinnitus. Current evaluation and management. *Med Clin North Am* 1999;83:153-62.
4. Seidman MD, Jacobson GP. Update on tinnitus. *Otolaryngol Clin North Am* 1996;29:455-65.
5. Schleuning AJ. Management of the patient with tinnitus. *Med Clin North Am* 1991;75:1225-37.
6. Arnett A. Pain-earache. In: Fleisher GR, Ludwig S, eds. *Textbook of Pediatric Emergency Medicine*. 4th ed. Philadelphia: Lipincott Williams and Wilkins; 2000:453-8.
7. Holgers KM, Axelsson A, Pringle I. Ginkgo biloba extract for the treatment of tinnitus. *Audiology* 1994;33:85-92.
8. Drew S, Davies E. Effectiveness of ginkgo biloba in treating tinnitus: double blind, placebo controlled trial. *BMJ* 2000;322:73-5.
9. Jellin JM, ed. *Natural Medicines Comprehensive Database*. 3rd ed. Stockton, CA: Therapeutic Research Faculty; 2000.
10. Ernst E, Stevinson C. Ginkgo biloba for tinnitus: a review. *Clin Otolaryngol* 1999;24:164-7.

Tinnitus—Patient Information

Tinnitus is the sensation of hearing an abnormal sound in the ears. It may be a ringing, clicking, buzzing, hissing or whistling. Tinnitus may be caused by a number of things, including medications. If you take medications, check with your pharmacist to see if they may be connected to the problem. See a doctor if your tinnitus lasts longer than 24 hours.

There are a number of non-drug measures that may help to manage tinnitus. These include avoiding smoking, caffeine and stimulants, using noise to mask tinnitus, using hearing aids and stress management or biofeedback.

One important thing you can do is to avoid loud noises. Use ear protection if you must be exposed to loud noises.

In some people drug therapy may be tried. If you do try a medication, make sure you have information about its possible side effects.

Do not take ginkgo biloba for tinnitus if you are on warfarin or drugs that hamper platelet function, like ASA, ticlopidine or clopidogrel.

Gastrointestinal Conditions
Section Highlights

Chapter 20: **Nausea and Vomiting**

> Motion sickness
> Pregnancy-associated nausea and vomiting
> > Hyperemesis gravidarum
> Chemotherapy-associated nausea and vomiting
> Medication-induced nausea and vomiting
> > Opioid-induced nausea and vomiting
> Nonprescription antiemetic agents

Chapter 21: **Constipation**

> Acute and chronic constipation
> Constipation in infants and children
> Constipation during pregnancy
> Instructions for administering an enema
> Long-term use of laxatives
> Dietary fibre in selected foods
> Agents for treatment and prevention of constipation

Chapter 22: **Diarrhea**

> Diarrhea not related to travel
> > Oral rehydration therapy
> > Diarrhea in children
> > Diarrhea during pregnancy
> > Nonprescription agents for diarrhea
> Travelers' diarrhea
> > Preventive measures
> > Nonprescription agents for the prevention and management
> > of travelers' diarrhea

Abdominal Pain Assessment

Chapter 23: **Dyspepsia and GERD**

> Preventive and nonpharmacologic treatments for dyspepsia and GERD
> Antacids
> Alginic Acid
> Nonprescription H_2-receptor antagonists

Chapter 24: **Gas and Cramps**

Nonprescription drugs used to treat gas and cramps

Chapter 25: **Irritable Bowel Syndrome**

Treatment approach to specific subtypes of IBS
Constipation predominant
Diarrhea predominant
Bloating and gas predominant

Chapter 26: **Infant Colic**

Behavioral management strategies for parents of crying babies
Baby massage for infant colic
Behavioral management
Environmental manipulation
Dietary manipulation
Pharmacologic therapy for infant colic
Monitoring therapy for infant colic
Sample colic diary

Perianal Symptom Assessment

Chapter 27: **Hemorrhoids**

Drug therapy of hemorrhoids

Chapter 28: **Pinworms**

Diagnosis of pinworm
Nonprescription drug therapy of pinworm infection
Monitoring therapy for pinworms

Chapter 29: **Ostomy Care**

Types of ostomy
Appliances and accessories
Common problems
Foods with implications for ostomy patients
Medication use
Lifestyle considerations

Chapter 20

Nausea and Vomiting

Peter Loewen, BSc(Pharm), PharmD

Pathophysiology[1,2]

Nausea is the unpleasant sensation of the imminent need to vomit and may or may not lead to vomiting. Vomiting is the forceful expulsion of gastric contents with contraction of the abdominal and chest wall musculature.[1] Retching or "dry heaves" is the same physiologic process as vomiting, but without expulsion of gastric contents due to lack thereof, or less coordinated or less marked reverse peristalsis against a closed glottis.

The American Gastroenterological Association recognizes nausea and vomiting (N&V) as a symptom of over 75 different conditions;[1] some of these are listed in Table 1. This chapter addresses the most commonly encountered causes of N&V in general practice. Syndromes that have a high incidence of N&V, such as migraine, are addressed in other chapters.

The pathophysiology of N&V is complicated by the involvement of numerous neurotransmitters and nerve systems arising from different organs and activated by a variety of stimuli (Figure 1). Because of this, it is often difficult to determine which stimulus is most responsible for a patient's symptoms and to design a therapeutic plan.

Complications of prolonged or severe N&V include esophageal rupture, Mallory-Weiss tears, dehydration, hypokalemia, hypomagnesemia, hypo- or hypernatremia, metabolic alkalosis, malnutrition and dental caries.

Motion Sickness

Motion sickness, also known as airsickness, seasickness or carsickness, is extraordinarily common: 58% of children experience car-sickness; 29% of airline pilots have incapacitating airsickness,[2] 50% of space shuttle astronauts get spacesickness, and up to 100% of

Table 1: Selected Causes of Nausea and Vomiting[1,3-5]

Appendicitis	Irritable bowel syndrome
Cholangitis	Nonulcer dyspepsia
Cholecystitis	Noxious odors
Chronic renal dysfunction/uremia	Pancreatitis
Diabetic ketoacidosis	Peptic ulcer disease
Drugs	Postoperative nausea and
Gastric outlet obstruction	vomiting
Gastroenteritis	Pregnancy
Gastroparesis	Pyelonephritis
Head trauma	Vestibular disorders
Increased intracranial pressure	(including motion sickness)
Intestinal obstruction	Viral hepatitis (acute)

travelers on ships experience seasickness.[6] It is rare in children under two years of age.[6]

Motion sickness begins with a feeling of "stomach awareness," followed by increased salivation, belching, and, if the stimulus persists, nausea, pallor, sweating, and vomiting or retching.[1,6]

Theories of the cause of motion sickness centre around a mismatch between the motion one expects to occur (either through visual cues or previous experiences) and the actual motion sensed by the vestibular apparatus in the ear. The vertical component to the motion is believed to be most important in causing motion sickness, and also that the frequency of the movement must be relatively slow and prolonged to cause it.[7] This may explain why ship travel, characterized by low-frequency continuous heaving, is such a potent cause of motion sickness while traveling in a speedboat is not.

Neurotransmitters thought to be most responsible for motion sickness include histamine, acetylcholine and

Figure 1: **Pathways Involved in Nausea and Vomiting**

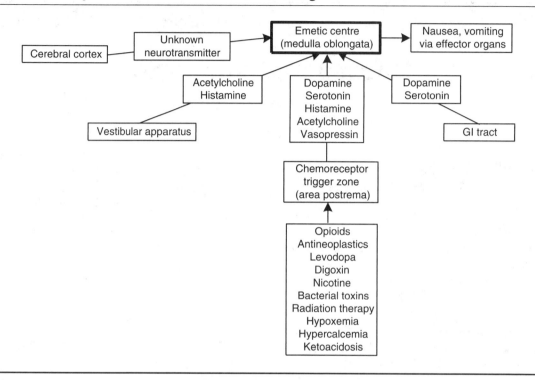

dopamine, and drugs used for treatment are aimed at modulating receptors for these chemicals.

Postchemotherapy Nausea and Vomiting (PCNV)
N&V associated with chemotherapy is divided into three types: acute, delayed and anticipatory. Whether acute or delayed N&V is experienced depends most strongly on the actual chemotherapy drug(s) administered and their dosage and infusion rate.

Some acute postchemotherapy N&V facts:
- Occurs during the first 24 hours after administration of cancer chemotherapy.
- Occurs in > 90% of patients receiving highly-emetogenic chemotherapy regimens (e.g., cisplatin, cyclophosphamide).
- May begin within 30 minutes of administration of therapy (e.g., mechlorethamine) and usually does not persist beyond 24 hours.
- The neurotransmitter most responsible is serotonin (5-HT$_3$ receptors) while type 2 dopamine receptors are of lesser importance.[8]

- Chemotherapy and radiation therapy cause entero-chromaffin cells lining the GI tract to release serotonin in large amounts, activating 5-HT$_3$ receptors in the GI tract which stimulate the vomiting centre in the medulla oblongata (Figure 1).

Delayed postchemotherapy N&V facts:
- Begins at least 24 hours after administration of chemotherapy and may last longer than 120 hours.[8]
- Cisplatin and cyclophosphamide are the most commonly used drugs that cause acute as well as delayed N&V, often with a N&V-free period in between. With cisplatin the incidence of delayed nausea and/or vomiting may be as high as 80%.[9]
- Serotonin is less important in delayed N&V and other causes, including conversion of the drug to emetogenic metabolites, are possible but poorly understood.

Anticipatory vomiting facts:
- A conditioned or learned response to previously poorly managed nausea and vomiting in chemotherapy patients.[8]

- Occurs in 25 to 50% of patients by the fourth course of chemotherapy.
- Occurs before, during or immediately after chemotherapy administration but before acute N&V would be expected to occur.

Pregnancy-associated Nausea and Vomiting (PANV)

Also known as "morning sickness," nausea and vomiting are both common in pregnancy, affecting 70% and 60% of women respectively.[10] These symptoms are normal in pregnancy. Several theories on the role of N&V in pregnancy have been put forward, but the best supported is that it serves to protect mother and fetus from foods that might be potentially dangerous. Meat, fish, poultry, and eggs — all of which carry the risk of infectious diseases — produce the most aversion in North America. Morning sickness is less common in societies that do not eat such foods.[11] Another theory is that N&V stimulates production of neurohormones that preferentially partition nutrients to the fetus, ensuring normal fetal growth.[12] Progesterone and estrogen are also believed to play a role in PANV.[13] Women who have morning sickness are significantly less likely to have miscarriages, and those who vomit are even less likely to have miscarriages than those who only have nausea.[11,12]

Symptoms typically begin 39 days after the last menses and persist for 45 days, although 9% of women have N&V that persists beyond 20 weeks gestation.[14] N&V may occur at any time of day and be constant throughout the day.

Hyperemesis gravidarum is a serious condition affecting 1 to 5% of pregnancies. It is characterized by intractable vomiting beginning in the first trimester and possibly continuing throughout the pregnancy. Vomiting may lead to dehydration, electrolyte disturbances, and eventually weight loss and muscle wasting. This condition can threaten the survival of the fetus and the mother, and requires early identification and treatment. Such symptoms must also prompt investigation for specific diseases such as urinary tract infections, thyrotoxicosis and hepatitis.[10] Hyperemesis gravidarum is diagnosed only when other possible causes of nausea and vomiting have been ruled out.

Postoperative Nausea and Vomiting (PONV)

Postoperative nausea and vomiting affects up to 80% of patients undergoing procedures such as hysterectomy, laparoscopy, orthopedic surgery, ophthalmologic, ear/nose/throat and breast surgery.[13] Other types of surgery are associated with lower, but often significant, incidences of PONV. It is defined as nausea and/or vomiting or retching occurring within 24 or 48 hours of the end of the procedure. Numerous risk factors have been identified including female sex, obesity, previous PONV, preoperative anxiety, age 6 to 16 years, longer duration of the procedure, quantity of opioid administered during the procedure, use of barbiturates for induction of anesthesia, use of nitrous oxide for anesthesia, and uncontrolled postoperative pain.[13]

Nausea and/or vomiting may be present in the recovery room immediately following surgery or may begin several hours later. Besides the obvious unpleasantness for the patient, PONV can sometimes result in overnight hospital stays when day-case surgery was planned, interfere with pain management efforts, lead to wound dehiscence if vomiting or retching occurs following abdominal procedures or result in fluid and electrolyte imbalances.

Because opioid analgesics are commonly administered postoperatively and cause significant nausea themselves, it is often difficult to determine the cause of N&V.

Almost all of the known mechanisms for N&V (dopaminergic, serotonergic, cholinergic, histaminergic, cortical) may be active to varying degrees in patients who experience PONV.[8,15]

Medication-induced Nausea and Vomiting

Almost all medications are capable of producing nausea and, to a lesser degree, vomiting. Some of the most commonly used and/or emetogenic nonchemotherapy drugs are listed in Table 2.

The mechanisms by which most drugs cause N&V are unknown and probably range from extensions of their pharmacologic action (e.g., anticholinergic drugs which slow down gastrointestinal persistalsis such as amitriptyline) to direct irritation of the gastrointestinal tract (e.g., NSAIDs) to toxic stimulation of the vomiting centre (e.g., L-dopa, nicotine, opioids).

Table 2: **Commonly Used Drugs That Frequently Cause Nausea and/or Vomiting**[1,16]

Antiinflammatory:	Anticonvulsants:
ASA	Phenytoin
NSAIDs	Carbamazepine
Auranofin	Valproic acid
Colchicine	Phenobarbital
Cardiovascular:	**Others:**
Digoxin	Acyclovir
Amiodarone	Levodopa
Procainamide	Narcotic analgesics
Beta-blockers	Oral contraceptives
Calcium channel blockers	Sulfonylureas
	Theophylline
Antibiotics:	
Antituberculars	
Erythromycin	
Tetracycline	
Sulfonamides	

This chapter addresses only opioid analgesics specifically.

Narcotic-induced N&V facts:[1,17]
- Forty to 70% of patients receiving narcotics experience nausea.
- N&V are most common during the first few days of therapy and tolerance develops rapidly thereafter.
- N&V may be more associated with lower doses of morphine than higher doses, although evidence to support this observation is scarce.
- There is little evidence of differences between narcotics in their propensity to cause N&V, although individuals may respond differently to different agents.
- Opioids may case N&V by stimulating afferent input into the vomiting centre, via the vestibular apparatus, the cerebral cortex, or the chemoreceptor trigger zone.

Goals of Therapy

- Reduce or eliminate symptoms of nausea
- Prevent complications of nausea
- Prevent or reduce frequency of vomiting
- Prevent complications of vomiting

Patient Assessment

Figure 2 depicts an approach to patient assessment for N&V.

Nonpharmacologic Therapy

General nonpharmacologic measures for managing N&V include eating small meals, avoiding spicy foods and noxious odors and reducing physical activity. If pain and nausea coexist, successful treatment of the pain often reduces the nausea.

Maintaining fluid intake helps prevent dehydration and electrolyte disturbances. The amount of fluid required depends on the amount lost through vomiting and/or diarrhea. Water and potassium are the most important components to replace. Generally 3 to 5 L per day of water should be taken orally in a patient who vomits several times daily. Some of this may be taken in the form of citrus juices since they contain significant amounts of potassium. Generally 30 to 40 mEq (2 to 2.5 g) of potassium are required per day.[20] If the patient is already hypokalemic, 50 to 100 mEq (3.2 to 6.4 g) may be required initially for repletion. Orange or grapefruit juice usually contains 6 to 8 mEq of potassium per 250 mL glass.[21] Apple juice contains about 4 mEq per glass. When renal function is not severely impaired, there is little danger of inducing hyperkalemia.

Commercial fluid and electrolyte replacement solutions may be used as an alternative in an attempt to achieve the same objectives, especially when drinking juices is not palatable.

Motion Sickness[6,22]
- Avoid eating a large meal within three hours of travel.
- Avoid dairy products and foods high in protein, calories, or sodium before travel.
- Avoid alcohol, smoking and disagreeable odors.
- Avoid visual stimuli that commonly precipitate motion sickness, such as reading and watching videos during travel.
- While traveling, focus on a stable external object or the horizon.
- While on a boat, stay in a central location least susceptible to motion.
- While in a vehicle, sit in a front seat with a clear forward view.

Figure 2: **Assessment of Patients with Nausea and Vomiting**

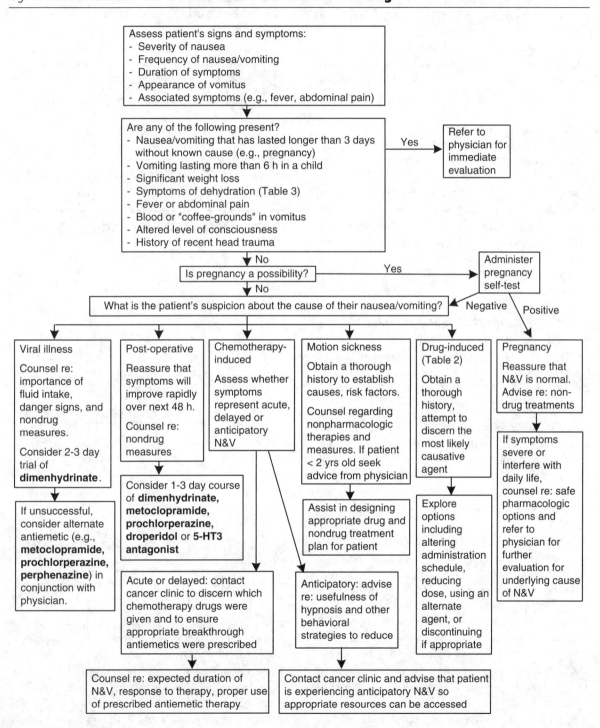

Assess patient's signs and symptoms:
- Severity of nausea
- Frequency of nausea/vomiting
- Duration of symptoms
- Appearance of vomitus
- Associated symptoms (e.g., fever, abdominal pain)

Are any of the following present?
- Nausea/vomiting that has lasted longer than 3 days without known cause (e.g., pregnancy)
- Vomiting lasting more than 6 h in a child
- Significant weight loss
- Symptoms of dehydration (Table 3)
- Fever or abdominal pain
- Blood or "coffee-grounds" in vomitus
- Altered level of consciousness
- History of recent head trauma

Yes → Refer to physician for immediate evaluation

No

Is pregnancy a possibility? → Yes → Administer pregnancy self-test

No

What is the patient's suspicion about the cause of their nausea/vomiting?

Negative | Positive

Viral illness

Counsel re: importance of fluid intake, danger signs, and nondrug measures.

Consider 2-3 day trial of **dimenhydrinate**.

If unsuccessful, consider alternate antiemetic (e.g., **metoclopramide, prochlorperazine, perphenazine**) in conjunction with physician.

Post-operative

Reassure that symptoms will improve rapidly over next 48 h.

Counsel re: nondrug measures

Consider 1-3 day course of **dimenhydrinate, metoclopramide, prochlorperazine, droperidol** or **5-HT3 antagonist**

Chemotherapy-induced

Assess whether symptoms represent acute, delayed or anticipatory N&V

Acute or delayed: contact cancer clinic to discern which chemotherapy drugs were given and to ensure appropriate breakthrough antiemetics were prescribed

Motion sickness

Obtain a thorough history to establish causes, risk factors.

Counsel regarding nonpharmacologic therapies and measures. If patient < 2 yrs old seek advice from physician

Assist in designing appropriate drug and nondrug treatment plan for patient

Anticipatory: advise re: usefulness of hypnosis and other behavioral strategies to reduce

Drug-induced (Table 2)

Obtain a thorough history, attempt to discern the most likely causative agent

Explore options including altering administration schedule, reducing dose, using an alternate agent, or discontinuing if appropriate

Pregnancy

Reassure that N&V is normal. Advise re: non-drug treatments

If symptoms severe or interfere with daily life, counsel re: safe pharmacologic options and refer to physician for further evaluation for underlying cause of N&V

Counsel re: expected duration of N&V, response to therapy, proper use of prescribed antiemetic therapy

Contact cancer clinic and advise that patient is experiencing anticipatory N&V so appropriate resources can be accessed

- If in a car, drive rather than be a passenger.
- Increase ventilation and exposure to cool fresh air.
- Minimize head movement by pressing head into headrest.
- Foods promoted as having antimotion sickness activity include: apricot juice, carrot juice, unroasted pumpkin or squash seeds, parsley, and peppermint tea.[23] No controlled trials of any of these remedies have been published.
- Although widely promoted for its antinausea effects, ginger root (candied, powder, capsules, tea infusion) is devoid of antimotion sickness effects.[24]
- SeaBands® acupressure wristbands are inferior to scopolamine and similar to placebo for preventing motion sickness.[25] Intense acupressure at the P6 acupressure point is effective for preventing motion sickness, but the technique is not practical for everyday use.[26] More information on P6 can be found in Nonpharmacologic Therapy of Pregnancy-associated Nausea and Vomiting.

Postchemotherapy Nausea and Vomiting (PCNV)
Although potent antiemetic medications are usually required in patients receiving highly emetogenic chemotherapy, hypnosis reduces anticipatory nausea and reduces the amount of antiemetic medication required in both children and adults.[27]

Particularly for anticipatory N&V, other behavioral maneuvers aimed at producing relaxation, diverting attention and enhancing feelings of control may be effective.[8]

Pregnancy-associated Nausea and Vomiting[10] (PANV)
Although not well-studied, the following measures may be recommended to reduce N&V associated with pregnancy:
- Alter diet to emphasize small, bland, frequent meals avoiding fatty, fried or spicy foods.
- Eat at times of the day when nausea is less severe.
- Eat before getting out of bed in the morning.
- Avoid the smell of food and spend less time in the kitchen.[28]
- Drink small amounts of fluid regularly between meals.
- Discontinue iron supplements temporarily as they may contribute to N&V.

Table 3: **Symptoms of Dehydration in Children and Adults**[18,19]

Children	Adults
- Dry mouth, tongue and skin - Few or no tears when crying - Decreased urination (less than 4 wet diapers in 24 h) - Sunken eyes - Grayish skin - Sunken soft spot (fontanel) in infants - Decreased skin turgor (Figure 3)	- Increased thirst - Decreased urination - Feeling weak or light-headed - Dry mouth/tongue

Figure 3: **Decreased Skin Turgor**

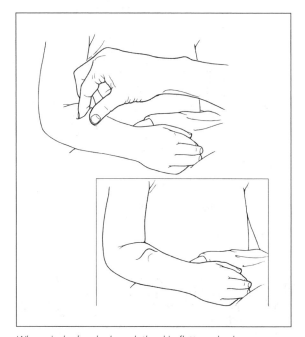

When pinched and released, the skin flattens slowly.

- In patients with frequent vomiting, maintenance of fluid and electrolyte status orally or intravenously is essential.
- Several studies have demonstrated efficacy of P6 acupressure or acupuncture, particularly for reducing nausea.[29,30] This point is also known as Nei Guan ("inner guard") and is the sixth point along the pericardial meridian, hence abbreviated as P6.

P6 is anatomically located about 5 cm proximal to the distal crease of the wrist, between the tendons of palmaris longus and flexor carpi radialis of either forearm (Figure 4). The point can be stimulated with the tip of a finger with or without moderate pressure massaging. There is no consensus regarding how long or how often to apply the pressure, but some practitioners recommend 5 to 10 minutes of pressure at least four times daily.[30] Patients may be taught to do this themselves. (Note that this technique is different from the one shown to be effective for motion sickness.) Wearing SeaBands® continuously is an alternative, but some studies (in motion sickness) have shown less efficacy than manual pressure, they tend to slip out of position, and some patients find them too conspicuous.

- Reassurance that nausea and vomiting are normal, not harmful to the fetus (perhaps even beneficial), and usually subsides as the pregnancy progresses, may be helpful to patients.

Figure 4: **P6 Acupressure Point**

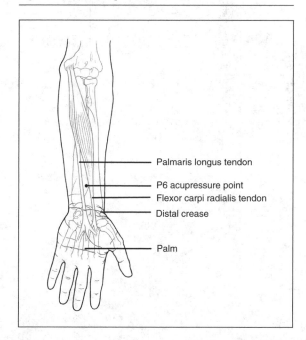

Palmaris longus tendon

P6 acupressure point
Flexor carpi radialis tendon
Distal crease

Palm

Postoperative Nausea and Vomiting (PONV)

General measures that may be useful in preventing PONV include avoiding significant intake of food for 48 hours postoperatively, slow and gradual increase in physical activity postoperatively, avoiding noxious odors and stimuli, and maintaining adequate hydration. Smoothly transporting the patient from the post-anesthetic recovery room to the ward is also important.

Nonpharmacologic treatments that have been studied and found effective include smelling peppermint oil,[31] P6 acupressure (described above),[32] and applying an isopropyl alcohol swab under the nose for several seconds.[33] Comfort measures such as cool cloths and sucking on ice chips may also be beneficial.

Pharmacologic Therapy

For treatment of N&V not associated with any of the conditions specifically discussed in this chapter, such as viral gastroenteritis, there is no evidence that one antiemetic is superior to another. The initial choice should be made on the basis of availability (i.e., nonprescription versus prescription status), previous response, available routes of administration, cost, adverse effects, and patient preference. These criteria often result in dimenhydrinate being tried first.

If symptoms are worsened by movement, it may be surmised that acetylcholine is a significant contributor and anticholinergic agents such as **dimenhydrinate** may be tried first. If symptoms are associated with a feeling of fullness in the stomach, a prescription prokinetic such as **metoclopramide** or **domperidone** may be a logical starting point. If patients fail to respond to these initial measures, selection of other antiemetics is based on adverse effects, available routes of administration, patient preference and cost. Give consideration to trying agents with different mechanisms of action if combinations of antiemetics are to be used.

Nonprescription agents used in the management of nausea and vomiting are described in Table 4.

Motion Sickness

Since acetylcholine and dopamine are thought to be the most important neurotransmitters causing motion sickness, it follows that anticholinergic and anti-dopaminergic drugs are fairly effective in controlling it. Like all causes of nausea and vomiting, prevention is more effective than treatment of established N&V.

Table 4: **Nonprescription Antiemetic Agents**[6,8,14,16,34]

Agent	Main uses	Onset	Dose	Drug Interactions	Adverse effects
Dimenhydrinate	All types (except PCNV)	30 min	Adult: 50-100mg PO q4-6h PRN Child 6-12y: 25-50 mg PO q6-8h PRN Child 2-6y: 12.5-25 mg PO q6-8h PRN	Alcohol and any other medication that causes drowsiness may enhance sedative effects of the antihistamine, increase confusion, ataxia, and paradoxical excitation (if this would otherwise have occurred).	Sedation, constipation, blurred vision, paradoxical excitation in children
Diphenhydramine	MS, PANV, General		Adult: 25-100 mg q4-6h PO PRN Child 6-12yrs: 25 mg PO q4-6h PRN (max 300 mg per day)		
Meclizine	MS, General		Adult: 25-50 mg PO q24h		
Promethazine	All types		Adult: MS: 12.5-25 mg PO/PR q24h PRN PONV: 12.5-25 mg PO/PR q4h PRN Child: MS: 6.25-12.5 mg PO/PR q24h PRN	Alcohol and other CNS depressants (additive effects)	Sedation, somnolence, akathisia, acute dystonic reactions, tremor/pseudo-parkinsonism, rash, agitation, blurred vision, hypotension, dizziness
Pyridoxine (Vitamin B₆)	PANV	1-2 h	10-25 mg three times daily	None known	None
Scopolamine	MS	4 h	Adult: 1 patch every 72 h. Should not be used in children	Sedatives, anticholinergics (additive effects)	Sedation, constipation, dry mouth, blurred vision, rash, allergic contact dermatitis, eye irritation if hands touch eyes after handling patch. Marked CNS disturbances (e.g., disorientation, delirium) can occur in susceptible patients. The elderly are at increased risk of CNS effects.

General = potentially useful for most causes of N&V besides the ones specifically mentioned; PCNV = postchemotherapy N&V; MS = motion sickness; PANV = pregnancy-associated N&V.

- For short duration of exposure, **dimenhydrinate** taken 30 minutes beforehand is effective for most patients. **Diphenhydramine** is an alternative.
- Longer-acting preparations such as **meclizine** or a **scopolamine** transdermal patch applied at least four hours before exposure may be effective.
- For more severe or refractory nausea, **promethazine** or the prescription drugs perphenazine, chlorpromazine and metoclopramide may be helpful.
- If alertness is required, transdermal scopolamine or oral promethazine have been combined with the prescription products dextroamphetamine (a controlled substance) or ephedrine. These combinations have been used in extreme situations (e.g., by airline pilots) after the patient has become thoroughly accustomed to their CNS effects, as these may be unpredictable.[35]
- The most appropriate agent for *children* older than two years is dimenhydrinate given one hour before exposure, then every six hours as needed. Diphenhydramine may also be used as an alternative and may help children sleep better while traveling.[6] Some children experience paradoxical excitability with these agents, so a test dose should be administered well before traveling.[6]
- Since dimenhydrinate is recommended by Canada's *Motherisk* program for augmenting Diclectin® therapy in pregnancy[36] and it is considered generally safe in pregnancy, it can be considered for intermittent therapy of motion sickness in pregnant patients. Phenothiazines are also commonly used in pregnancy in many countries, although less safety data are available.

Postchemotherapy Nausea and Vomiting (PCNV)

Nonprescription antiemetics are not useful in either the treatment or prevention of PCNV. Effective prescription agents are available and include the 5-HT$_3$ antagonists, corticosteroids, benzodiazepines, prochlorperazine, metoclopramide, haloperidol and dronabinol.

Pregnancy-associated Nausea and Vomiting (PANV)

Since the thalidomide tragedy of the 1960s, women and their caregivers have considered pharmacologic treatment of N&V a last resort. The voluntary withdrawal of the combination product Debendox® (or Bendectin®) in 1983 over unsubstantiated concerns of teratogenicity fuelled this trepidation.[37] Interestingly, following withdrawal of Bendectin®, hospitalizations for hyperemesis gravidarum rose by 50% in the US and Canada.[10]

When nonpharmacologic methods fail to control N&V, there is a role for medications to help relieve symptoms and prevent weight loss, dehydration and hospitalization. In patients with hyperemesis gravidarum, the combination of intravenous fluids and antiemetic drugs is often necessary.

- The prescription combination product Diclectin®, containing 10 mg each of pyridoxine (vitamin B$_6$) and doxylamine is the drug of choice for PANV in Canada. Consistent evidence in over 200,000 pregnancies demonstrates its safety and efficacy.[14,38,39]
- Pyridoxine alone may safely reduce PANV[38] and may be used in place of Diclectin® in those women who prefer a "natural" remedy or for whom doxylamine is contraindicated.
- Although studied in fewer pregnancies than Diclectin®, dimenhydrinate, hydroxyzine, prochlorperazine, chlorpromazine, and promethazine have not demonstrated teratogenicity and can be given orally, rectally or parenterally.[14] Promethazine is the most commonly used antiemetic for PANV in Australia.[40]
- Other prescription agents that may be effective include corticosteroids, metoclopramide and ondansetron. Data on these agents are limited but reassuring.[39]
- If vomiting continues despite these therapies and/or where hospitalization for rehydration is required or being considered, administer **thiamine** orally (25 to 50 mg three times daily) or intravenously (100 mg once weekly) to prevent Wernicke's encephalopathy.[10]
- Powdered **ginger root** 250 mg four times daily is superior to placebo for treating hyperemesis gravidarum[41] and regular morning sickness.[42] High quality human safety data are not available for ginger. Studies of extremely high concentrations of ginger in pregnant rats have either shown no negative effects on fetuses[43] or increased rates of fetal loss.[44] The relevance of this conflicting data to humans is unknown. The dose used (1000 mg per day) is similar to the daily dietary intake of ginger in many cultures.[41]

Postoperative Nausea and Vomiting (PONV)

- The most effective strategy to manage PONV is to prevent it by identifying high-risk patients and giving antiemetic prophylaxis at the time of induction or discontinuation of anesthesia.[45]
- Appropriate prophylaxis therapies include 5-HT$_3$ antagonists, droperidol, and to a lesser extent, prochlorperazine. Use of these agents in combination with dexamethasone 8 to 10 mg IV intraoperatively enhances their efficacy.[46]
- Treatment of established PONV has not been thoroughly studied, but available evidence and experience supports the use of the following agents as needed postoperatively: 5-HT$_3$ antagonists, metoclopramide, perphenazine, prochlorperazine, droperidol, and to a lesser extent, dimenhydrinate.

Opioid-induced Nausea and Vomiting

Therapeutic options include:

- Altering the administration schedule so nausea does not interfere with meals;
- Reducing the dose of narcotic as low as possible;
- If pain is not controlled, attempting an increase in dosage since nausea is sometimes caused by pain;
- Consider switching to another narcotic at 75% of the equivalent daily dose. No solid evidence for differences between narcotics exist in terms of emetogenicity, but patient responses are highly variable;
- Addition of an antiemetic drug is often helpful, although the possibility of additive CNS side effects must be carefully weighed;
- Appropriate antiemetic agents include: metoclopramide, diphenhydramine, dimenhydrinate, perphenazine, prochlorperazine, promethazine, domperidone, haloperidol, chlorpromazine, atropine, scopolamine, and possibly the 5-HT$_3$ antagonists;
- No specific antiemetic has been demonstrated to be more useful than any other for narcotic-induced N&V so selection must be made on the basis of safety, cost, available routes of administration, and patient preference;
- In patients receiving opioids for chronic pain states, changes to the drug therapy regimen should be made as part of a team approach, closely involving the other providers caring for the patient.

Monitoring of Therapy (Table 5)

Efficacy

For all of the conditions discussed, monitoring therapy involves close attention to the patient's description of the nausea response, changes in frequency of vomiting, and vigilant monitoring for emergence of serious complications such as weight loss, dehydration, changes in mental status (which may signal electrolyte disturbances), and blood loss from any source. Assess adherence to nonpharmacologic measures when response to therapy is suboptimal.

Safety

Table 4 shows the most common adverse effects of the nonprescription antiemetic agents. If a patient experiences an intolerable adverse effect, consider dosage reduction, switching to another agent or relying on nondrug measures alone.

- Regardless of the drug, if it is effective but sedation is bothersome, try reducing the dose to find the minimum effective dose.
- If the drug is effective but causes paradoxical excitability, try reducing the dose to find the minimum effective dose.
- If PONV persists beyond 48 hours postoperatively, patients should consult their surgeon or other physician for guidance. The most common cause of nausea and vomiting > 48 h postoperatively is opioid analgesics.

Advice For the Patient

Counsel all patients with nausea and vomiting regarding:

- Warning signs of when medical attention should be sought;
- Reassurance that the nausea and/or vomiting will improve with time;
- Nonpharmacologic measures to improve N&V, tailored to the specific cause in their case;
- Possible adverse effects of drug therapy, especially sedation, which may preclude performing activities requiring mental alertness such as driving or operating dangerous machinery;
- Instructions not to combine antiemetic medications with alcohol, and

Table 5: **Monitoring Therapy for Nausea and Vomiting**

Symptoms	Monitoring	Endpoint of therapy	Actions
Pregnancy-associated nausea	**Patient:** continuously **Pharmacist:** day 3	Minimal/no nausea	If taking dimenhydrinate or pyridoxine and inadequate response after 3 days, refer for prescription for Diclectin.®
Pregnancy-associated vomiting	**Patient:** continuously **Pharmacist:** day 3	Vomiting does not interfere with daily activities and does not result in other morbidity (dehydration, weight loss, electrolyte disturbances)	If taking dimenhydrinate or pyridoxine and inadequate response after 3 days, refer for prescription for Diclectin.®
Motion sickness	**Patient:** whenever exposed to stimulus **Pharmacist:** after next visit	Minimal/no nausea. No vomiting	Depending on the drug being used, increase dosage, ensure dose given 30-60 min before stimulus. If nonprescription drugs ineffective, refer for prescription.
Postoperative N&V	**Patient:** continuously for 72 h after surgery **Pharmacist:** for 72 h after surgery	Minimal or no nausea, no vomiting during 48-h postoperative period	If dimenhydrinate ineffective after two doses, refer for prescription.
Opioid-induced N&V	**Patient:** continuously **Pharmacist:** daily	Minimal or no nausea. No vomiting	If dimenhydrinate ineffective, refer for prescription for effective antiemetic or narcotic dosage adjustment.
Symptoms of dehydration (Table 3)	**Patient:** continuously **Pharmacist:** daily	No symptoms of dehydration	If symptoms of dehydration occur, refer to physician immediately.

• Instructions to wash their hands after handling the scopolamine patch as severe eye irritation or mydriasis can occur if the eyes are touched.

Resource Tips

Motherisk web site: www.motherisk.org
Nausea and Vomiting in Pregnancy Helpline: 1-800-436-8477

Suggested Readings

American Gastroenterological Association. AGA Technical Review on nausea and vomiting. *Gastroenterology* 2001;120:263-86.

ASHP Commission on Therapeutics. ASHP therapeutic guidelines on the pharmacologic management of nausea and vomiting in adult and pediatric patients receiving chemotherapy or radiation therapy or undergoing surgery. *Am J Health-Syst Pharm* 1999; 56:729-64.

Gahlinger PM. Motion sickness. *Postgrad Med* 1999; 106(4):177-84.

Nelson-Piercy C. Treatment of nausea and vomiting in pregnancy. *Drugs* 1998;19:155-64.

O'Mahony S, Coyle N, Payne R. Current management of opioid-related side effects. *Oncology* 2001;15: 61-82.

References

1. American Gastroenterological Association. AGA Technical Review on nausea and vomiting. *Gastroenterology* 2001;120: 263-86.
2. James M, Green R. Airline incapacitation survey. *Aviat Space Environ Med.* 1991;62:1068-72.
3. Friedman LS, Isselbacher KJ. Nausea, vomiting and indigestion. In: Fauci AS, Braunwald E, Isselbacher JK, et al., eds. *Harrison's Principles of Internal Medicine.* 14th ed. New York, NY: McGraw-Hill; 1998:230-6.
4. Taylor AT. Nausea and vomiting. In: DiPiro JT, Talbert RL, Yee GC, et al., eds. *Pharmacotherapy: A Pathophysiologic Approach.* 4th ed. Stamford TC: Appleton and Lange 1999: 586-98.
5. Lyndley C. Nausa and vomiting. In: Koda-Kimble MA, Young LY, eds. *Applied Therapeutics: The Clinical Use of Drugs.* 7th ed. New York, NY: Lippincott, Williams and Wilkins, 2001:6-1 to 6-17.
6. Gahlinger PM. Motion sickness. *Postgrad Med* 1999;106: 177-84.
7. Bles W, Bos JE, Kruit H. Motion sickness. *Curr Opin Neurol* 2000;13:19-25.
8. ASHP Commission on Therapeutics. ASHP therapeutic guidelines on the pharmacologic management of nausea and vomiting in adult and pediatric patients receiving chemotherapy or radiation therapy or undergoing surgery. *Am J Health-Syst Pharm* 1999;56:729-64.
9. Kris MG, Gralla RJ, Clark RA, et al. Incidence, course, and severity of delayed nausea and vomiting following the administration of high-dose cisplatin. *J Clin Oncol* 1985;3: 1379-84.
10. Nelson-Piercy C. Treatment of nausea and vomiting in pregnancy. *Drugs* 1998;19:155-64.
11. Flaxman SM, Sherman PW. Morning sickness: a mechanism for protecting mother and embryo. *Q Rev Biol* 2000;75: 113-48.
12. Huxley RR. Nausea and vomiting in early pregnancy: its role in placental development. *Obstet Gynecol* 2000;95:779-82.
13. Kenny GNC. Risk factors for postoperative nausea and vomiting. *Anaesthesia* 1994;49(suppl):6-10.
14. Mazzotta P, Gupta A, Maltepe C, Koren G, Magee L. Pharmacologic treatment of nausea and vomiting during pregnancy. *Can Fam Physician* 1998;44:1455-7.
15. Andrews PL. Physiology of nausea and vomiting. *Br J Anaesth* 1992;69(Suppl1):S2-S19.
16. McEvoy GK. *American Hospital Formulary Service Drug Information 2001.* Bethesda, MD: American Society of Health-System Pharmacists, 2001.
17. O'Mahony S, Coyle N, Payne R. Current management of opioid-related side effects. *Oncology* 2001;15:61-82.
18. Canadian Paediatric Society. *Dehydration and diarrhea.* Available at: http://www.caringforkids.cps.ca/babies/Dehydration.htm. Accessed December 12, 2001.
19. Pace B. JAMA patient page — preventing dehydration from diarrhea. *JAMA* 2001;285(3):362.
20. Health World Online. *Potassium.* http://www.healthy.net/asp/templates/article.asp? PageType=article&ID=2063. Accessed March 18, 2002.
21. Joshipura KJ, Ascherio A, Manson JE, et al. Fruit and vegetable intake in relation to risk of ischemic stroke. *JAMA* 1999;282:1233-9.
22. Lindseth G, Lindseth PD. The relationship of diet to airsickness. *Aviat Space Environ Med* 1995;66:537-41.
23. Zoltan R. *Encyclopedia of Natural Healing.* Blaine, WA: Natural Life Publishing, 1998:969-71.
24. Stewart JJ, Wood MJ, Wood CD, et al. Effects of ginger on motion sickness susceptibility and gastric function. *Pharmacology* 1991;42:111-20.
25. Bruce DG, Golding JF, Hockenhull N, Pethybridge RJ. Acupressure and motion sickness. *Aviat Space Environ Med* 1990;61:361-5.
26. Hu S, Stritzel R, Chandler A, Stern RM. P6 acupressure reduces symptoms of vection-induced motion sickness. *Aviat Space Environ Med* 1995;66:631-4.
27. Handel DL. Complementary therapies for cancer patients: what works, what doesn't, and how to know the difference. *Texas Medicine* 2001;97:68-73.
28. Abraham S. Nausea and vomiting in pregnancy. *Curr Ther* 1006;37:41-8.
29. Vickers AJ. Can acupuncture have specific benefits on health? A systematic review of acupuncture antiemesis trials. *J R Soc Med* 1996;89:303-11.
30. Belluomini L, Litt RC, Lee KA, et al. Acupressure for nausea and vomiting in pregnancy: a randomized, blinded study. *Obstet Gynecol* 1994;84:245-8.

31. Tate S. Peppermint oil: a treatment for postoperative nausea. *J Adv Nurs* 1997;26(3):543-9.

32. Lee A, Done ML. The use of nonpharmacologic techniques to prevent postoperative nausea and vomiting: a meta-analysis. *Anesth Analg* 1999;88:1362-9.

33. Smiler BG. Isopropyl alcohol for transport-related nausea. *Anesth Analg* 1998;87:1211-7.

34. Clinical Pharmacology 2000. Gold Standard Multimedia. 2001.

35. Gillingham KK, Previc FH. Spatial orientation in flight. In: DeHart RL, ed. *Fundamentals of Aerospace Medicine.* 2nd ed. Baltimore: Lippincott Williams & Wilkins, 1996:309-97.

36. Magee LA. The safety and effectiveness of antiemetic therapy for NVP. In: Koren G, Bishai R, eds. *Nausea & Vomiting of Pregnancy: State of the art 2000.* Motherisk, 2000. Available at http://www.nvp-volumes.org.

37. Pastuszak A. Doxylamine/pyridoxine for nausea and vomiting of pregnancy. *Can Pharm J* 1995;128:39-42.

38. Jewell D, Young G. Interventions for nausea and vomiting in early pregnancy (Cochrane Review). In: The Cochrane Library, Issue 2, 2001. Oxford: Update Software.

39. Bishai R, Mazzotta P, Atanackovic G, et al. Critical appraisal of drug therapy for nausea and vomiting of pregnancy: II. Efficacy and safety of diclectin. *Can J Clin Pharmacol* 2000;7:138-43.

40. Abraham S. Nausea and vomiting in pregnancy. *Curr Ther* 1996;37:41-8.

41. Fischer-Rasmussen W, Kjaer SK, Dahl C, et al. Ginger treatment of hyperemesis gravidarum. *Eur J Obstet Gynecol Reprod Biol* 1991;38:19-24.

42. Vutyavanich T, Kraisarin T, Ruangsri R. Ginger for nausea and vomiting in pregnancy: randomized, double-masked, placebo-controlled trial. *Obstet Gynecol* 2001;97(4):577-82.

43. Weidner MS, Sigwart K. Investigation of the teratogenic potential of a zingiber officinale extract in the rat. *Reprod Toxicol* 2001;15(1):75-80.

44. Wilkinson JM. Effect of ginger tea on the fetal development of Sprague-Dawley rats. *Reprod Toxicol* 2000;14(6):507-12.

45. Frighetto L, Loewen PS, Dolman J, Marra CA. Cost-effectiveness of prophylactic dolasetron or droperidol vs rescue therapy in the prevention of PONV in ambulatory gynecologic surgery. *Can J Anaesth* 1999;46:536-43.

46. Henzi I, Walder B, Tramer M. Dexamethasone for the prevention of postoperative nausea and vomiting: a quantitative systematic review. *Anesth Analg* 2000;90:186-94.

Motion Sickness—Patient Information

Some suggestions that may help with motion sickness:

- Avoid eating a large meal within three hours of travel.
- Avoid dairy products and foods high in protein (e.g., meat or nuts), calories or salt before travel.
- Increase ventilation and get more cool fresh air.
- Avoid alcohol, smoking and disagreeable odors.
- Avoid reading and watching videos while traveling.
- While traveling, focus on the horizon or an object that is outside the car, plane or boat that does not move.
- Try pressing your head into the headrest.
- While on a boat, try to stay in the middle of the boat.
- While in a vehicle, sit in a front seat with a clear forward view.
- If in a car, drive rather than be a passenger.

Some people feel these ideas may be helpful, but since there is no proof that they work, try them after the suggestions above:

- Eat/drink apricot juice, carrot juice, unroasted pumpkin or squash seeds, parsley, and/or peppermint tea.

- Try ginger root. This comes as candied ginger, powder, capsules and tea infusion.
- Try SeaBands® acupressure wristbands.

If your pharmacist or doctor has provided medication for you to use for motion sickness, here are some facts:

- Do not take your anti-nausea medication with alcohol.
- All anti-nausea medications can cause drowsiness. Do not drive a car or operate dangerous machinery while under the influence of these medications. They are as dangerous as alcohol when driving.
- If you need to be alert and take anti-nausea medication, talk to your pharmacist or doctor about other medications that may be helpful for you.
- Other side effects commonly caused by antinausea medications include dizziness, shakiness, anxiety, blurred vision and constipation. Your pharmacist can tell you more about the specific side effects of the medication you are taking.
- When children take anti-nausea medications, they sometimes get very excitable instead of drowsy. Be sure to test the medication on the child prior to traveling to see what effects it has on them.

Morning Sickness—Patient Information

It is important for you to understand that nausea and vomiting are *completely normal* during the first 12 weeks after your last period (the first part of your pregnancy). In fact, women who have nausea and vomiting are less likely to have a miscarriage.

Some suggestions to help you cope with nausea or vomiting:

- Alter your diet so that you eat small, bland, frequent meals. Avoid fatty, fried, or spicy foods.
- Try eating at times of the day when nausea is less severe.
- Try eating before getting out of bed in the morning.
- Avoid the smell of food and try to spend less time in the kitchen.
- Drink small amounts of fluid regularly between meals.
- Discontinue iron supplements temporarily as they often contribute to N&V.
- Try taking powdered ginger root 250 mg four times daily. Your pharmacist can help you select a high quality ginger product.
- Talk to your doctor about trying acupressure.

Remember: Morning sickness usually gets better as your pregnancy progresses!

There are several medications to treat nausea which have proven to be safe in millions of pregnancies without increasing the risk of birth defects. If your nausea or vomiting is not tolerable after trying the above, talk to your pharmacist or doctor about safe and effective medications you can use for nausea during your pregnancy.

When should you worry about nausea and vomiting?
- When vomiting does not respond to any of the treatments provided.
- If you are losing weight, or not gaining weight as you should be.
- When you vomit any amount of blood.
- If you cannot keep fluids down and you feel very thirsty or feel faint when you get up from lying down. This may mean you are dehydrated.

If you experience any of these, you should visit your doctor immediately. One to five percent of pregnant women have severe vomiting and require special treatment to prevent dehydration.

The University of Toronto's Motherisk program has a toll-free helpline if you have questions or concerns about nausea and vomiting in pregnancy. **Call 1-800-436-8477**. They also have an excellent web site with information about morning sickness and many other issues: www.motherisk.org

You can learn more about eating healthy during pregnancy from your local public health department, or at:
http://www.health.gov.ab.ca/public/nutrit/preg.html.

Chapter 21

Constipation

Janie Bowles-Jordan, BScPhm

Pathophysiology

Constipation is generally defined as infrequent and/or unsatisfactory defecation twice weekly or less; this number is subjective, varying among age groups and nationalities.[1] Though this definition focuses on the frequency of defecation, patients may describe constipation as straining to defecate, passing hard stools or incomplete defecation. Some patients incorrectly believe that a daily bowel movement is normal and that anything less means they are constipated. In fact, the average number of bowel movements for adults in the Western world varies from three daily to one every three days.[2] The average frequency of bowel movements for children varies according to age and is summarized in Table 1. Functional constipation refers to constipation with no identifiable cause (e.g., metabolic, organic, pharmacologic). Diagnostic criteria for chronic functional constipation are described in Table 2.

Table 1: **Average Frequency of Bowel Movements for Children**[3]

Age	Bowel movements per week	Bowel movements per day
0-3 mos		
Breastfed	5-40	2.9
Formula-fed	5-28	2.0
6-12 mos	5-28	1.8
1-3 yrs	4-21	1.4
> 3 yrs	3-14	1.0

Reproduced with permission from Fontana M, et al. Bowel frequency in healthy children. *Acta Paediatrica Scandinavica* 1989;78:682-4.

Table 2: **ROME II Diagnostic Criteria for Functional Constipation**[4]

At least 12 wks, which need not be consecutive, in the preceding 12 mos of 2 or more of:
• Straining in > 25% of defecations;
• Lumpy or hard stools in > 25% of defecations;
• Sensation of incomplete evacuation in > 25% of defecations;
• Sensation of anorectal obstruction/blockade in > 25% of defecations;
• Manual maneuvers to facilitate > 25% of defecations (e.g., digital evacuation, support of the pelvic floor); and/or
• < 3 defecations per week.

Loose stools are not present, and there are insufficient criteria for IBS.

Reproduced with permission from Thompson WG, et al. Functional bowel disorders and functional abdominal pain. *Gut* 1999;45 (Suppl2):II43-II47.

Normal colonic motility combines segmenting contractions that promote mixing of luminal contents, propagating contractions that propel them short distances and high amplitude contractions that transport them long distances. Constipation results from disordered movement through the colon and/or anorectum. It may be due to GI motor problems (Table 3), or may be secondary to structural, neurologic or metabolic abnormalities or drug therapy (Table 4).

Constipation (both chronic and acute) affects 2 to 28% of the population, with a higher reported incidence in women.[9] The prevalence increases dramatically in both genders over age 65. A minority of patients seek medical care, accounting for 2.5 million annual visits in the United States.[2] Eighty-five per cent of these physician visits result in a prescription for a laxative or cathartic.[2]

Table 3: **GI Motor Problems Associated with Primary Constipation**[1,5]

Slow transit constipation (colonic inertia)	Decrease in high amplitude propagating contractions leading to prolonged fecal residues in the ascending colon +/- increased uncoordinated motor activity in the distal colon.
Pelvic floor dysfunction	Normal colonic movement but retention of feces for prolonged periods in the rectum.
Megarectum and megacolon	Dilation of the rectum or colon leading to atonic bowel, blunted rectal sensation and decreased defecation forces.
Rectoceles	Misdirection of stool into pouches in the rectovaginal septum where part of the rectum protrudes into the vagina.
Hirschsprung's disease	Congenital aganglionosis of the distal intestine; often limited to the rectosigmoid area.

Table 4: **Secondary Causes of Constipation**[1,6-8]

Diseases associated with chronic constipation	Drugs associated with constipation
Neurogenic disorders	Amantadine
Autonomic neuropathy	Anticonvulsants
Diabetes mellitus	Anticholinergics
Intestinal pseudo-obstruction	Antidiarrheal agents
Multiple sclerosis	Antihistamines
Parkinson's disease	(first generation)
Spinal cord injury	Antipsychotics
Stroke	Phenothiazines
Nonneurogenic disorders	Barbiturates
Hypothyroidism	Benzodiazepines
Hypercalcemia	Beta-blockers
Systemic sclerosis	Calcium channel blockers,
Pregnancy	especially verapamil
Panhypopituitarism	Cation-containing agents
Irritable bowel syndrome	Aluminum
Chronic renal failure/uremia	Barium
Cystic fibrosis	Bismuth
Anatomic obstructions	Calcium
Diverticulosis	Iron
Malignant tumor	Cholestyramine
Stricture	Clonidine
Psychiatric	Diuretics
Depression	5-HT$_3$ antagonists
Eating disorder	(e.g., ondansetron)
Pain secondary to anal fissures,	Lithium
hemorrhoids and other	NSAIDs
anorectal conditions	Opioids
	Polystyrene sodium sulfonate
	Pseudoephedrine
	Tricyclic antidepressants
	(Amitriptyline>Nortriptyline)
	Vinca alkaloids

Constipation has been associated with fewer years of education, low caloric intake, greater number of medications used, lower socioeconomic status, physical and sexual abuse, and a sedentary lifestyle.[2,9-11] Low dietary fibre or fluid intake is not associated with an increased risk of constipation.[2,12]

Constipation affects up to 31% of women in late pregnancy.[13] Causes include the use of calcium and iron supplements, high levels of circulating progesterone, and the effect of the gravid uterus pushing on the colon.[14]

In cancer patients, the prevalence of constipation is 50% and this rises to 78% in palliative patients. Tumor compression of the large intestine or interference with colonic neural innervation are the usual mechanisms involved.[15] These problems are seen in primary and metastatic bowel tumors, peritoneal mesothelioma, pelvic cancer, and malignant ascites. Table 5 summarizes causes of constipation in cancer patients.

Table 5: **Causes of Constipation in Cancer Patients**[15]

Tumor compression of large intestine
Tumor interference with colonic neural innervation
Hypercalcemia secondary to bone metastases
Hormonal changes
Chemotherapy, either directly or indirectly due to poor hydration and nutritional status resulting from nausea and vomiting
Direct intestinal radiation
Opioid use

Some factors leading to acute constipation may include traveling, attempting toilet training (in children), and ignoring the urge to defecate. Withholding feces can lead to prolonged fecal stasis in the colon, with absorption of fluid and an increase in the size and consistency of stools. The passage of large hard stools can stretch the anus and habituate the rectum to the stimulus of the fecal mass, and the urge to defecate subsides.[16]

Complications resulting from untreated or chronic constipation include fecal impaction, anal fissures, hemorrhoids and megacolon. Rare complications include intestinal perforation, volvulus and, in the bedbound elderly, stercoral ulceration (pressure necrosis of the rectal or sigmoid mucosa due to a fecal mass; rectal bleeding and perforation occur rarely).

Goals of Therapy[17]

- Establish regular bowel movements
- Eliminate straining
- Avoid complications of constipation
- Use laxatives appropriately

Patient Assessment

Symptoms of constipation include infrequent defecation; abdominal distension; nausea; vomiting; anorexia; early satiety; stools that are small, hard, and/or difficult to evacuate; and incomplete rectal emptying. Patients suffering from chronic constipation may also lose weight.

Fecal impaction is the inability to pass a hard collection of stool. Symptoms of impaction include rectal discomfort, anorexia, nausea, vomiting, abdominal pain, urinary frequency, and both fecal and urinary overflow incontinence. Physically or mentally incapacitated persons and the elderly are at particular risk of impaction, as are those who require long-term use of medications associated with constipation (Table 4).

Large or frequent purchases of laxatives, a history of frequent cycles of constipation and diarrhea, or complaints of constipation despite use of laxatives may indicate laxative abuse. Refer patients exhibiting these characteristics to a physician. Other exclusions to self-care include recent abdominal surgery and a suspected eating disorder (e.g., bulimia nervosa).[18]

A general assessment plan for patients with constipation is illustrated in Figure 1.

Prevention[1,7,19,20]

The following strategies may be used to prevent constipation:
- High-fibre diet. The American Dietetic Association recommends a daily fibre intake of 25 to 30 g for adults. Few adults consume this level; 10 g per day of total dietary fibre is often sufficient as a daily minimum goal.[7,19] Table 6 lists the fibre content of some common foods.
- Minimum fluid consumption of 1500 mL of water or juice daily.
- Regular, private toilet routine.
- Heed the urge to defecate.
- Use of a prophylactic laxative if using constipating medication.
- Moderate physical activity may be helpful, though this has not been proven.[1]

Nonpharmacologic Therapy[2,6,20,21]

The following nonpharmacologic strategies may be helpful in managing constipation:
- Increase caloric intake in patients with low-calorie diets. This improves colonic transit time but does not help pelvic floor dysfunction.[22]
- Patients should establish a regular bowel regimen by attempting to have a bowel movement at the same time each day. Colonic activity is highest in the morning and after meals, making after breakfast the best time for a bowel movement.
- Patients should consume a high fibre diet. The target is 25 to 30 g of fibre daily. Table 6 lists the fibre content of some common foods. Patients with poor dentition can eat foods that are easy to chew such as bran muffins, bran cereal, fibre biscuits, applesauce and baked beans. Fibre-enriched formulations of nutritional supplement drinks are available for those patients unable to prepare meals, or as snacks between meals.
- If adult patients are unable to attain the recommended goal for dietary fibre, two to six tablespoonfuls (30 to 90 mL) of **wheat bran** daily taken

Figure 1: **Assessment of Patients with Constipation**

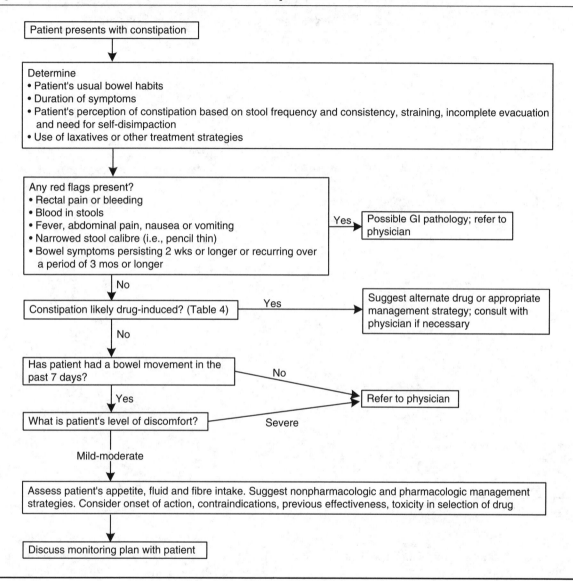

Patient presents with constipation

Determine
- Patient's usual bowel habits
- Duration of symptoms
- Patient's perception of constipation based on stool frequency and consistency, straining, incomplete evacuation and need for self-disimpaction
- Use of laxatives or other treatment strategies

Any red flags present?
- Rectal pain or bleeding
- Blood in stools
- Fever, abdominal pain, nausea or vomiting
- Narrowed stool calibre (i.e., pencil thin)
- Bowel symptoms persisting 2 wks or longer or recurring over a period of 3 mos or longer

Yes → Possible GI pathology; refer to physician

No

Constipation likely drug-induced? (Table 4)

Yes → Suggest alternate drug or appropriate management strategy; consult with physician if necessary

No

Has patient had a bowel movement in the past 7 days?

No → Refer to physician

Yes

What is patient's level of discomfort?

Severe → Refer to physician

Mild-moderate

Assess patient's appetite, fluid and fibre intake. Suggest nonpharmacologic and pharmacologic management strategies. Consider onset of action, contraindications, previous effectiveness, toxicity in selection of drug

Discuss monitoring plan with patient

with a 250 mL glass of water or juice can be used to supplement dietary fibre.
- Prune and other juices containing sorbitol (e.g., apple, pear) may also be helpful.
- Because inactivity is associated with constipation, exercise has been advocated as a treatment option. Though not clearly shown to be effective, it is still worth recommending for many preventive health reasons.[1]
- Weight loss is suggested for the treatment of chronic constipation in overweight patients. Like exercise, this has not been proven but is still worth recommending.[1] The goal is to reach a weight compatible with a body mass index (BMI) of 18.5 to 24.9 (see

Table 6: **Dietary Fibre in Selected Foods**

Food	Serving size	Fibre content	
		g/serving	g/100 g
Whole bran cereal	30 g	9–10	30–33
Fruit & Fibre	40 g	5.5–6.2	13.8–15.5
Weetabix	35 g	4.6	13.1
Bran Flakes	30 g	4.4–5.3	14.7–17.7
Grapenuts	30 g	3.6	12
Shredded Wheat Spoon Size	30 g	4	13.3
Shredded Wheat Biscuits	25 g	3.2	12.8
Frosted Mini Wheats	30 g	2.9	9.7
Shreddies	30 g	2.7	9.0
Cheerios	30 g	1.5–2.5	5.0–8.3
Captain Crunch	30 g	0.8	2.7
Rice Crispies	30 g	0.3	1
Corn Flakes	30 g	0.8	2.7
Whole wheat bread	2 slices	2.5	4.8
Enriched white bread	2 slices	0.9	1.7
Spinach, cooked, drained	125 mL	10	6
Beans, white, cooked	100 mL	6	7
Beans, green or yellow, cooked	125 mL	2	3
Potatoes, cooked in skin	1 long	5	2
Potatoes, peeled, boiled	1 long	2	1
Broccoli, cooked	250 mL	4	4
Peas, cooked	125 mL	3	5
Brussels sprouts, cooked	4	2	3
Carrots, raw	1	2	3
Carrots, sliced, cooked	100 mL	2	3
Parsnips, cooked, mashed	100 mL	3	3
Tomato, raw, unpeeled	1	2	2
Cabbage, red or green, raw, chopped	100 mL	1	3
Cauliflower, raw, chopped	100 mL	1	2
Celery, inner sticks, raw	3	1	2
Banana	1	3.9	
Orange	1	2.6	
Grapefruit	0.5	0.7	

Adapted from Farmer PS. Gastrointestinal products. In: Carruthers-Czyzewski P, ed. *Nonprescription Drug Reference for Health Professionals.* Ottawa, ON: Canadian Pharmaceutical Association, 1996:293.

Chapter 33 for more information on weight loss and the BMI).

Patients with chronic constipation often benefit from a program of bowel retraining. This involves developing a regular schedule for defecation and modifying behavior with respect to diet and exercise as described above. Patients should not repress the urge to defecate or spend prolonged periods of time at the toilet. Patients may need to place a footstool in front of the toilet to elevate their thighs, thus placing the pelvis in the optimum position for defecation.[6,21,23]

Biofeedback and relaxation training can be useful in the treatment of constipation due to pelvic floor dysfunction. This trains patients to relax their pelvic floor muscles and to coordinate relaxation and pushing during defecation.[6,9]

Nonpharmacologic Management (Children)

- Children over the age of two should try to obtain a dietary level of fibre equal to or greater than their age plus 5 g per day.[20]
- In infants, juices that contain sorbitol (e.g., prune, apple, pear) can increase the frequency of bowel

movements and water content of stools. Barley malt extract (2 to 10 mL in 250 mL milk or juice) or corn syrup can be used as stool softeners.[16]

- Children with functional constipation should be encouraged to attempt defecation 5 to 15 minutes after each meal until they have their bowel movement for that day.[16,24]
- Biofeedback may be beneficial for the treatment of a small subgroup of children with intractable constipation.[16]

Pharmacologic Treatment[1,2,7,9,25,26]

There are five basic groups of laxatives: bulk, emollient, saline, osmotic and stimulant. The individual agents within each class are described in Table 7.

- Few trials have compared the effectiveness of different types of laxatives and the data that are available show no statistically significant difference between treatments. The majority of the data available is from nursing homes and hospitals instead of community-based centres, limiting its applicability to the general population.
- Bulk laxatives are considered the safest agents and are suitable for long-term use.
- Each dose of a bulk-forming laxative should be administered with at least 250 mL of water or juice to prevent fecal impaction and/or esophageal obstruction.
- Avoid long-term use of other agents, if possible (see Long-term Use of Laxatives).
- Saline laxatives should be administered with sufficient water to prevent dehydration.[26]
- Stimulant laxatives are usually administered at bedtime.
- Suppositories should be moistened with lukewarm water before insertion and retained as long as possible.[28]

Acute and chronic constipation require different management. *Chronic constipation* is treated in a step-wise approach (Table 8). The optimal management of *acute constipation* has not been well studied; a reasonable approach is to base therapy on the patient's level of discomfort. If a patient is very uncomfortable, then an agent with a relatively quick onset of action is preferred. Otherwise, the preferred approach is a trial of a bulk laxative plus nonpharma-

cologic measures. If constipation is not relieved within 48 hours, add an agent with a quicker onset of action.

If fecal impaction is present, it must be relieved before maintenance treatment can begin. This may be done manually using a local anesthetic lubricant and/or by inserting a tap water, phosphate, saline or mineral oil enema daily for up to three days.[1] Soapsuds enemas should be avoided because of an irritant effect on the colonic mucosa that may result in proctitis or colitis.[8] If the stool is higher than can be reached with enemas and the patient has no sign of bowel obstruction, use polyethylene glycol orally to disimpact the patient.[19] Patients should not self-disimpact unless trained to do so.

Instructions for Administering an Enema
The patient should:
- Lubricate the enema nozzle if it is not pre-lubricated.
- Lie on their left side with knees bent.
- Insert the enema nozzle into the rectum, with the nozzle pointing towards the navel.
- Gently squeeze the container until the dose is expelled; if discomfort is felt at this point, the flow is probably too fast.
- Retain the solution until definite abdominal cramping is felt.

Herbal Therapy

There is little evidence to support the efficacy and/or safety of the following herbals: aloes, buckthorn, dandelion, flaxseed, licorice and rhubarb. Yellow dock is an effective laxative but its safety has not been definitively established.[29,30]

Homeopathic Therapy

No clinical trials could be found investigating the use of homeopathy in constipation. Some commonly used remedies include alumina, byronia, calcarea carbonica, conium, lycopodium, natrum muriaticum, nux vomica, sepia and silicea.[31]

Children

The overwhelming majority of children with chronic constipation suffer from functional constipation – a cycle of pain on defecation, fecal retention and

Table 7: **Agents for Treatment and Prevention of Constipation**[1,2,6,7,16,21,25-28]

Agent	Dose	Onset of action	Drug interactions	Adverse effects	Comments
Bulk forming					
Psyllium	Adults: 7 g (15-30 mL) 1-3 times daily with 250 mL of water or juice. Children > 6 yrs: 7.5-15 mL 1-3 times daily with 250 mL of water or juice	12-72 h	Do not take within 2 h of other medication or the effect of the other medication may be reduced.	Generally well tolerated; some flatulence, bloating common at start of therapy. This can be minimized by starting with a low dose and gradually increasing. Anaphylaxis, asthma and other allergic reactions have been reported. Allergic reactions may occur in up to 18% of health care workers with occupational exposure to psyllium.[26] Other adverse reactions reported include esophageal obstruction and fecal impaction.	Contraindicated if partial mechanical obstruction of GI tract. Inappropriate for fluid restricted patients or patients with dysphagia, esophageal strictures or partial obstructions of GI tract. Adequate administration of fluid with each dose important to prevent esophageal obstruction and/or fecal impaction. When used to treat chronic functional constipation may take 2-3 mos for maximum effect.
Sterculia gum	Adults: 7-28 g divided into 1-3 doses. Consult physician for children under 12 yrs of age	12-72h	Do not take within 2 h of other medication or the effect of the other medication may be reduced.	Rare allergic reactions. Bloating, flatulence	
Polycarbophil	Adults: 4-6 g daily divided into 1-4 doses	12-72 h	Do not take within 2 h of other medication or the effect of the other medication may be reduced.	Generally well-tolerated, some flatulence, bloating. Other adverse reactions reported include esophageal obstruction and fecal impaction.	
Methylcellulose	Adults: 2 g (15 mL) 1-3 times daily	12-72 h			
Bran	Adults: Initially 30-90 mL per day, followed by 250 mL of fluid. Some patients require up to 250 mL bran daily	3-5 days	May interfere with absorption of iron, calcium and fat-soluble vitamins	Diarrhea, bloating, flatulence	Reduces total cholesterol and risk of colon cancer. Can be added to yogurt, cereals, soups or applesauce. If patient has celiac disease use rice bran.

Hyperosmotic

Glycerin suppository Adult: 2.6 g/ suppository Children: 1.44 g/ suppository	1 suppository PR daily to BID or prn. Insert high into rectum and retain for 15 min if possible.	0.25-1 h		Rectal irritation	
Lactulose	Pediatric: 1-3 mL/kg daily in divided doses.* Adult 15-30 mL daily- BID.	24-48 h	Slower absorption of medication from the intes- tine due to acidification. Ideally, do not take within 2 h of other medication.	Flatulence and abdominal cramps are common, especially at the beginning of therapy. Nausea is more common with higher doses. Diarrhea is a sign of overdosage.	Many patients find sweet taste intolera- ble. Avoid in patients who require a galactose-free diet. 667 mg lactulose = 147 mg galactose, < 80 mg lactose. Not absorbed systemically; has less than 80 mg/dose of other sugars. Can be used by diabetics.
Sorbitol 70% solution	Pediatric: 1-3 mL/kg in divided doses.* Adult: 15-30 mL daily- BID.	24-48 h	Slower absorption of med- ication from the intestine due to acidification. Ideally, do not take within 2 h of other medication.	Flatulence, abdominal cramps, nausea, diarrhea.	Cost-effective alternative to lactulose

Saline

Magnesium hydroxide 400 mg/5 mL, 800 mg/5 mL	Pediatric: 80-240 mg/kg per day.* Adult: 15-30 mL once or twice daily	0.5-3 h	May reduce bioavailability of digoxin and the tetracy- clines	Risk of hypermagnesemia increased with overdose and in infants and those with renal impairment. Hypokalemia may also occur with prolonged use or overdose.	Caution with dehydration. Not recom- mended with cardiac or renal disease
Magnesium citrate	Pediatric maintenance: < 6 yrs: 1-3 mL/kg once daily (on physician advice only). 6-12 yrs: 100-150 mL per day.* >12 yrs: 150-300 mL per day.* Adult: 75-150 mL daily as laxative. 300 mL once as cathartic. Drink 250 mL water before and after each dose.	0.5-3 h	May reduce bioavailability of digoxin and the tetracy- clines	Risk of hypermagnesemia increased with overdose, in infants and those with renal impairment. Hyperkalemia has occurred.	Caution with dehydration. Not recom- mended with cardiac or renal disease. Chill solution before administration for greater palatability.

(cont'd)

Should not exceed recommended adult dose.

Table 7: **Agents for Treatment and Prevention of Constipation**[1,2,6,7,16,21,25-28] (cont'd)

Agent	Dose	Onset of action	Drug interactions	Adverse effects	Comments
Sodium phosphate oral	< 5 yrs age on physician's advice only. Adults (laxative): 20-30 mL once or twice daily diluted in 125 mL water and followed by another 250 mL water for the relief of occasional constipation Adults (cathartic): 45 mL once	0.5-3 h		Hyperphosphatemia has occurred; risk increased in the elderly and those with impaired renal function. Hypocalcemia, hypokalemia and hypernatremia have also been reported.	Best taken on an empty stomach upon rising, 30 min before a meal, or at bedtime. Not recommended for pregnant or nursing women. Not recommended for sodium restricted patients. Caution with renal or cardiac disease. Often used as a cathartic prior to surgery or GI procedures.
Enemas					
Tap water enema	Not recommended < 2 yrs age. Adult: 500 mL PR	5-15 min		Water intoxication and dilutional hyponatremia have occurred in children, the elderly and patients with megacolon. Risk of mechanical trauma to rectal wall.	Use warm, but not hot, tap water.
Phosphate enema	< 2 yrs: avoid. 2-12 yrs: 60 mL as a single dose. Under a physician's supervision doses of 6 mL/kg (up to 135 mL) have been used. Adult: 120 mL as a single dose	2-15 min		Abdominal distention, vomiting. Risk of mechanical trauma to rectal wall. Hypophosphatemia and hypocalcemia have occurred; most common in patients with renal dysfunction or when enema is retained too long.	Avoid in patients with potential for prolonged retention (e.g., paralytic ileus, congenital megacolon) and those with cardiac disease, renal dysfunction or pre-existing electrolyte abnormalities.
Mineral oil enema	Not recommended < 2 yrs age. Pediatric: disimpaction 15-30 mL/yr up to 240 mL. Adult: 100-250 mL PR daily	4-8 min		Incontinence. Risk of mechanical trauma to rectal wall	

Lavage

Polyethylene glycol	Maintenance in older children: 5-10 mL/kg per day Adult disimpaction: 2 L daily for 2 days Adult maintenance for chronic constipation: 200 mL 1-3 times daily	0.5-1h	Nausea, retching, bloating, abdominal cramps, vomiting and anal irritation. Rarely aspiration pneumonia, pulmonary edema and Mallory-Weiss tears have occurred	Commonly used prior to colonoscopy.

Lubricant/emollient

Mineral oil	< 1 yr old: not recommended (see comments). > 1 yr old: disimpaction: 15-30 mL/yr of age up to 240 mL daily.† Maintenance: 1-3 mL/kg per day.* Adult: 15-45 mL QHS while sitting up	6-8 h	Reduced absorption of vitamins A,D,E and K. Increased anticoagulant effect due to decreased absorption of vitamin K. Do not use with docusate, which increases absorption of mineral oil	Can be mixed with fruit juice or carbonated beverage. Not recommended for periods > 1 wk. Light mineral oil should not be used internally. Young children may be at higher risk of aspiration. Due to aspiration risk, not recommended for those who are bedridden or have swallowing difficulties, gastric retention or GERD. Crosses placenta. Has caused hemorrhagic disease of the newborn; not recommended for prolonged periods in pregnancy. Minimally absorbed but not metabolized; accumulates in tissues with repeated use

Stimulants

Senna 8.8 mg sennosides/5 mL; 8.6 mg, 12 mg sennosides/tab; 30 mg supp	2-6 yrs: 2.5-7.5 mL per day. 6-12 yrs: 5-15 mL per day. Adult: 2-4 tablets (17-34 mg) daily in 1-4 divided doses (max dose 8 tabs per day). Pregnancy: 1-2 tabs hs (max dose 4 tabs per day). Children > 25 kg: ½ supp QHS Adult: 1 supp qhs	PO: 6-12 h PR: 5 min	Abdominal pain, diarrhea, hypokalemia, allergic reactions and, rarely, proctitis and idiosyncratic hepatitis	Anthraquinone. Excreted into breast milk. May discolor urine red to pink or brown to black

(cont'd)

Should not exceed recommended adult dose.
†Under physician's supervision.

Table 7: **Agents for Treatment and Prevention of Constipation**[1,2,6,7,16,21,25-28] (cont'd)

Agent	Dose	Onset of action	Drug interactions	Adverse effects	Comments
Cascara sagrada 325 mg/5 mL; 320-487.5 mg tabs, capsules	Not for use in children. Adult: 2-5 mL or 0.3-1 g (tabs) at bedtime	6-12h		Abdominal discomfort, diarrhea, hypokalemia, allergic reactions.	Avoid in pregnancy. Aromatic formulation contains 0.2% alcohol. Anthraquinone. Excreted into breast milk. May discolor urine red to pink or brown to black.
Bisacodyl 5 mg tablets	≥ 2 yrs: 5 mg PO at hs. Doses of up to 15 mg at hs have been used under a physician's supervision. Adult:10 mg PO at bedtime	6-12 h	Should not be used by patients taking proton pump inhibitors or H₂-receptor antagonists; do not take within one hour of antacids.	Abdominal pain, cramps, diarrhea, hypokalemia. Rectal administration may cause rectal irritation or burning.	Preferred stimulant for long-term use in opioid users. Appears in breast milk. Tablets should not be crushed, broken or chewed.
10 mg suppository 10 mg microenema	< 2 yrs: ½ supp PR. 2 yrs or older: ½-1 supp PR. 6-12 yrs: ½ enema daily PRN. Adult: 1 enema or supp daily PRN	30 min			
Castor oil	< 2 yrs: Not recommended. 2-6 yrs: Use only on advice of physician. 2-12yrs: 5-15 mL at bedtime. Adult:15-60 mL at bedtime	2-6 h		Cramping and abdominal pain common. May stimulate uterine contractions during pregnancy. Hypokalemia and hypernatremia have occurred.	Contraindicated in pregnancy. Due to purgative action, normally reserved for emergency use or pre-procedure.
Stool softening					
Docusate sodium Docusate calcium	100 mg once or twice daily. 240 mg once or twice daily	12-72 h	Absorption of mineral oil may be increased.	Usually well tolerated. Mild, transient nausea or GI cramps may occur. Occasional rash.	Use with bulk laxatives. Evidence poor regarding efficacy of stool softeners; primary role is in prevention. Most useful to soften hard stools; no documented laxative action.

Table 8: **Management of Chronic Constipation**[1,7,9]

Step I	Unless a modifiable cause is identified, chronic constipation is initially managed by patient education, lifestyle modification, and dietary changes, including fibre supplementation (i.e., bran) and/or bulk-forming laxatives. Fibre intake should be increased gradually every 7-10 days. Saline laxatives and/or enemas may be used as rescue treatment if no bowel movement has occurred for two consecutive days.
Step II	After a 4-6 wk trial, if the problem persists second line agents such as an osmotic or saline laxative may be added.
Step III	Third-line agents such as emollients and stimulants should be limited to short-term use after other agents have failed. This is due to the high incidence of side effects from these classes.

chronic rectal distension.[32] Management of constipation specific to the treatment of infants and children is presented below.

Infants[16]
- The use of enemas is not recommended in infants.
- Rectal disimpaction of infants can be achieved with glycerin suppositories.
- Lactulose or sorbitol can be used as stool softeners.
- Mineral oil and stimulant laxatives are not recommended for infants.

Children One Year of Age or Older[16]
Magnesium hydroxide, mineral oil, lactulose and sorbitol are considered safe and effective in this population by the North American Society for Pediatric Gastroenterology and Nutrition. It should be noted, however, that young children are at increased risk of lipoid pneumonia due to aspiration of mineral oil.[33] Senna and bisacodyl may be used as rescue medication when other agents are ineffective. Disimpaction can be achieved with either oral or rectal medication, including enemas.

Pregnancy
The use of fibre supplements during pregnancy increases the frequency of defecation and leads to softer stools.[34] Stimulant laxatives are more effective than bulk-forming laxatives but may cause more side effects. Other laxatives have not been studied in this population.

Dietary supplements (e.g., bran) and bulk laxatives are the agents of choice. Osmotic laxatives and magnesium hydroxide are considered safe for intermittent use as second-line agents.[14,35] Stimulant laxatives are reserved for when other agents have failed.[35]

Docusate has traditionally been added if fibre supplementation has failed during pregnancy but there is little evidence to support this practice.

Breastfeeding[36,37]
Cascara, magnesium sulfate and senna are the only laxatives that have been identified by the American Association of Pediatrics as "usually compatible" with breastfeeding. Information assessing the transfer of other laxatives into breast milk is not available.

Laxatives that are not absorbed are considered first-line therapy. These include the bulk-forming and osmotic agents. Due to their favorable adverse effect profile and lower cost, bulk-forming laxatives are preferred, followed by magnesium salts such as magnesium hydroxide. Cascara sagrada and senna are acceptable second-line agents. If stimulant laxatives are used, monitor the infant for loose stools.

Cancer Patients
Stimulant laxatives are the mainstay of therapy, with enemas used intermittently. Do not use bulk forming laxatives or patients will impact.[38] Hyperosmotic agents often incite nausea. If the patient has not passed a stool in more than three days, refer the patient to a physician to rule out impaction.

In neutropenic or thrombocytopenic patients, avoid rectal manipulation to prevent infection or bleeding; give oral laxatives and cathartics only.

Long-term Use of Laxatives
Most patients suffering from constipation will self-medicate. They often overuse laxatives resulting in a pendulum effect between constipation and diarrhea. This type of abuse is present in about four per cent of

laxative users.[2] Long-term use of stimulant laxatives has traditionally been discouraged based on tests linking long-term use to damage of the enteric nervous system in the myenteric plexus and smooth muscles of the colon. However, these tests are technically difficult to perform and the results have not been confirmed by newer technologic methods. Even if neurologic damage does exist, there is no evidence that it is due to laxative use; it might be the cause of the constipation rather than a side effect of long-term laxative use. Many experts now believe that the risks of long-term stimulant laxative use have been overemphasized, and that if used no more than two or three times weekly they are safe and effective.[1,39] However, due to the side effects of cramping and increased cost of stimulant laxatives compared to other classes, it is still best to reserve stimulants for third-line therapy when previous treatment has failed.

Melanosis coli is a melanotic hyperpigmentation of the colonic mucosa that occurs after long-term use of the anthraquinones. It is benign and reverses 3 to 12 months after discontinuation of the laxative.[1,6,8,26]

Other side effects of laxative overuse include various electrolyte abnormalities. Hypermagnesemia, hypernatremia and hyperphosphatemia can occur due to accumulation of absorbed ions. Hypernatremia can also arise when large volumes of osmotic laxatives cause substantial water loss from the gastrointestinal tract. Hypokalemia may result as the body tries to regain fluid losses by activating the renin and aldosterone system thereby retaining sodium and excreting potassium in the feces and urine.[39]

Chronic constipation may cause long-term impairment of bowel motility and dependency on laxatives to stimulate motility. Slowly weaning the patient from a stimulant laxative to bulk-forming and/or osmotic laxatives may improve long-term control. Once chronic constipation is relieved the bowel may recover some contractile function, and the stimulant can be tapered and finally discontinued after a regular pattern has been developed. However, patients experiencing long-standing constipation with years of bowel stretching may have permanently lost muscle contractility and may require both a stimulant laxative and a bulk-forming laxative to maintain regularity. The level of medication used in severe constipation is greater than usual maintenance doses. Once a good bowel regimen is reestablished, recommend the lowest effective dose to minimize side effects.

Monitoring of Therapy

Table 9 provides a monitoring plan framework that should be individualized.

Table 9: **Monitoring Therapy for Constipation**

Symptoms	Monitoring	Endpoint of therapy	Actions
Inability to have bowel movement	Acute constipation: **Patient:** daily. **Pharmacist:** After 1-3 days of therapy, depending upon the agent chosen	Full bowel movement.	If fibre and nonpharmacologic measures are unsuccessful in 3 days, add agent with quicker onset of action. If other laxative not effective, or if patient has not had a bowel movement in 7 days, refer to physician.
	Chronic constipation: As above plus— **Patient:** keep daily bowel log (see sample). **Pharmacist:** Check with patient weekly for 4 wks.	Chronic constipation: As above, plus patient should have established regular bowel patterns after one month.	Chronic constipation: If patient has not established regular patterns after one month, treatment plan should be reassessed.
Bloating, cramping	Acute constipation **Patient:** daily. **Pharmacist:** day 3.	Bloating and cramping should be relieved shortly after full bowel movement occurs.	If full bowel movement has occurred but bloating and cramping are not relieved, refer to physician.

The use of a daily bowel log may be helpful in patients with chronic constipation, including children. A sample log is included at the end of this chapter.

Advice for the Patient

All patients should receive counseling regarding:
- Normal variation in frequency of bowel movements;
- Nonpharmacologic methods of treating and preventing constipation, and
- When they should contact a physician.

In addition, all patients who require drug therapy should receive counseling regarding:
- The expected onset of action of the laxative and what to do if constipation is not relieved, and
- Usual side effects of the medication.

Suggested Readings

American Dietetic Association. Position of the American Dietetic Association: health implications of dietary fiber. *J Am Dietetic Assoc* 1997;97(10):1157-9.

Baker SS, Liptak GS, Colletti RB, et al. Constipation in infants and children: evaluation and treatment. A medical position statement of the North American Society for Pediatric Gastroenterology and Nutrition. *J Ped Gastroenterol Nutr* 1999;29:612-26.

Locke III GR, Pemberton JH, Phillips SF. American Gastroenterological Association technical review on constipation. *Gastroenterology* 2000; 199(6):1766-78.

References

1. Wald A. Constipation. *Adv Gastroenterol* 2000;84(5):1231-46.
2. Locke III GR, Pemberton JH, Phillips SF. AGA technical review on constipation. *Gastroenterology* 2000;119:1766-78.
3. Fontana M, Bianch C, et al. Bowel frequency in healthy children. *Acta Paediatric Scand* 1987;78:682-4.
4. Thompson WG, Longstreth GF, Drossman DA, et al. Functional bowel disorders and functional abdominal pain. *Gut* 1999;45(Suppl II): 1143-47.
5. Youssef NN, DiLorenzo C. Childhood constipation: evaluation and treatment. *J Clin Gastroenterol* 2001;33(3):199-205.
6. Wong PWK, Kadakia S. How to deal with chronic constipation; A stepwise method of establishing and treating the source of the problem. *Postgrad Med* 1999;106(6):199-210.
7. Abyad A, Mourad F. Constipation: Common sense care of the older patient. *Geriatics* 1996;51(12):30.
8. Longe RL, DiPiro JT. Diarrhea and constipation. In: DiPiro JT, Talbert RL, Yee GC, Matzke GR, Wells BG, Posey LM, eds. *Pharmacotherapy: A Pathophysiologic Approach*. 4th ed. Stamford, CT: Appleton and Lange, 1999:599-613.
9. Locke III GR, Pemberton JH, Phillips SF. American Gastroenterological Association medical position statement: guidelines on constipation. *Gastroenterology* 2000;119:1761-6.
10. Everhart JE, Go VLW, Johannes RS, et al. A longitudinal survey of self-reported bowel habits in the United States. *Dig Dis Sci* 1989;34:1153-62.
11. Johanson JF, Sonnenberg A, Koch TR. Clinical epidemiology of chronic constipation. *J Clin Gastroenterol* 1989;11:525-36.
12. Towers AL, Burgio KL, Locher J, et al. Constipation in the elderly: influence of dietary, psychological and physiological factors. *J Am Geriatr Soc* 1994;42:701-6.
13. Greenhalf JO. Laxatives in the treatment of constipation in pregnant and breastfeeding mothers. *Practitioner* 1973;210: 259-65.
14. Bonapace ES, Fisher RS. Constipation and diarrhea in pregnancy. *Gastroenterol Clin North Am* 1998;27(1):197-211.
15. Bisanz A. Managing bowel elimination problems in patients with cancer. *ONF* 1997;24(4):679-86.
16. Baker S, Liptak GS, Colletti RB. Constipation in infants and children: evaluation and treatment. A medical position statement of the North American Society for Pediatric Gastroenterology and Nutrition. *J Ped Gastroenterol Nutr* 1999;29: 612-26.
17. Chaun H. Constipation. In: Jean Gray, ed. *Therapeutic Choices*. 1st ed. Ottawa, Canada: Canadian Pharmacists Association, 1995:702-7.
18. Waller D. Binge eating. *BMJ* 2001;322:343.
19. Prather C, Ortiz-Camacho P. Evaluation and treatment of constipation and fecal impaction in adults. *Mayo Clin Proc* 1998;73:881-7.
20. American Dietetic Association. Position of the American Dietetic Association: health implications of dietary fiber. *J Am Dietetic Assoc* 1997;97(10):1157-9.
21. Thompson WG. Constipation: A physiological approach. *Can J Gastroenterol* 2000; 14 (Suppl D):155D-162D.
22. Chiarioni G, Bassotti G, Monsignori A, et al. Anorectal dysfunction in constipated women with anorexia nervosa. *Mayo Clin Proc* 2000;75(10):1015-9.
23. Chiotakakou-Faliakou E, Kamm MA, Taminiau JA, Buller HA. Biofeedback provides long term benefit for patients with intractable, slow and normal transit constipation. *Gut* 1998; 42:517-21.
24. van der Plas RN, Benninga MA, Taminiau JA, Buller HA. Treatment of defaecation problems in children: the role of education, demystification and toilet training. *Eur J Pediatr* 1997;156:689-92.
25. Petticrew M. Effectiveness of laxatives in adults. *Effective Health Care* 2001;7(1):1-12. Available at www.york.ac.uk/inst/crd/ehc71.pdf. Accessed April 11, 2002.
26. Brunton LL. Agents affecting gastrointestinal water flux and motility; emesis and antiemetics; bile acids and pancreatic enzymes. In: Hardman JG, Limbird LE, eds. *Goodman and Gilman's The Pharmacologic Basis of Therapeutics*. 9th ed. New York, NY: McGraw-Hill, 1996:917-36.
27. Minaker K, Harai D. Constipation in the elderly. *Hospital Practice* 1995:67-76.
28. McEvoy GK, ed. *American Hospital Formulary Service Drug Information 2001*. Bethesda, MD: American Society of Health-System Pharmacists, 2001.
29. Ernst E, ed. *The Desktop Guide to Complementary and Alternative Medicine*. New York, NY: Mosby, 2001.
30. Jellin JM, ed. *Natural Medicines Comprehensive Database*. Stockton, CA: Therapeutic Research Faculty, 1999.

31. Boon H, Smith M. *Health Care Professional Training Program in Complementary Medicine*, Botanica Consulting Inc. 1998,126-133.
32. Anonymous. Paediatric constipation: Guidelines for referral to a paediatric surgeon. *Paediatric Child Health* 2001;6(1): 21-2.
33. Novak KK, ed. *Drug Facts and Comparisons*. St. Louis, MO: Facts and Comparisons, 2002.
34. Jewell DJ, Young G. Interventions for treating constipation in pregnancy (Cochrane Review). *Cochrane Library*, Issue 2, 2001.
35. Smith J, Taddio A, Koren G. Drugs of choice for pregnant women. In: Koren G, ed. *Maternal-Fetal Toxicology: A Clinician's Guide*. 2nd ed. New York, NY: Marcel-Dekker, Inc., 1994.
36. Hagemann,TM. Gastrointestinal medications and breastfeeding. *J Hum Lact* 1998;14(3):259-62.
37. American Academy of Pediatrics. The transfer of drugs and other chemicals into human milk. *Pediatrics* 2001;108(3): 776-89.
38. Hveld JL. Cancer care: preventing and treating constipation. *Nursing* 1995;25(3):26-7.
39. Xing JH. Adverse effects of laxatives. *Dis Colon Rectum* 2001;44:1201-9.

Constipation—Patient Information

What is a normal bowel movement?
A normal bowel movement can occur up to three times a day or only three times a week. This is different from person to person. A normal bowel movement should be soft, hold its shape and be easy to pass.

Causes of Constipation
Constipation can be caused by many things, including prescription and nonprescription medications. If you take medication, check with your pharmacist to see if it could be making you constipated. Other things that can cause constipation are diseases and emotional factors such as depression. Often though, constipation is due to simple factors such as not going to the bathroom when you have the urge.

To Prevent Constipation:
- Drink at least six to eight 250 mL glasses of water daily.
- Eat a balanced diet that is high in fibre and includes fruit, vegetables and bran. Foods high in fibre include 100% bran cereal, beans, peas, raspberries and broccoli.
- Exercise regularly.
- Try to have a bowel movement at the same time each day. For many people the best time is shortly after breakfast.

- Go to the bathroom when you have the urge; waiting will cause problems. Do not rush; take time to pass the entire stool.

Using Laxatives
The most natural way to regulate your bowels is by eating a healthy diet and following the tips described above. Sometimes however, a laxative is needed. The safest laxatives for most people are bulk forming laxatives like psyllium. These should work within three days. If this is too long to wait, other laxatives are available that work more quickly. Do not use these other laxatives for more than a week unless your doctor tells you to. Talk to your pharmacist about which laxative is best for you.

When to See Your Doctor
You should see your doctor right away if you are constipated *and*:
- You have not had a bowel movement for seven days, *or*
- You are extremely uncomfortable because you are constipated, *or*
- You have pain in your rectum (back passage) or rectal bleeding, *or*
- You have a fever, your belly hurts or you feel like throwing up, *or*
- Your bowel movements are thin as a pencil, *or*
- You have a problem with your bowels that lasts longer than two weeks or keeps coming back.

Daily Bowel Log

Date	Number of bowel movements and consistency of each (for example hard, soft, loose)	Straining (yes/no)	Complete movement (yes/no)	Fibre and fluid intake (number of glasses juice/ water and servings of fibre)	Methods used to treat constipation

Chapter 22

Diarrhea

Antonietta Forrester, BScPhm

Diarrhea Not Related to Travel

Pathophysiology

Diarrhea is the unusually frequent excretion of watery stools. It is associated with loss of electrolytes and loss of fecal matter at a rate of approximately > 200 gm/24 hours.[1] Losses of greater than 500 mL/24 hours are indicative of *secretory* diarrhea. Decreased fluid absorption or increased fluid secretion can lead to dehydration, which can ultimately lead to death particularly in children and the elderly. Diarrhea can be either acute or chronic. *Acute* diarrhea lasts less than 14 days and is often caused by infectious agents, drugs or food toxins. Diarrhea is considered *chronic* if it lasts longer than 14 days or if there are repeated episodes of diarrhea lasting less than 14 days each. Chronic diarrhea is often indicative of an inflammatory process (e.g., ulcerative colitis). Other causes of chronic diarrhea include ischemia, infections, radiation or chemotherapy, and maldigestion or malabsorption of fat or carbohydrates.

Although there are no specific statistics on the prevalence of diarrhea in adults,[2] the illness is thought to be underreported. Diarrhea is common in the pediatric population. American statistics indicate that children under five years of age experience 1.3 to 2.7 episodes of diarrhea yearly.[3] This data can be extrapolated to the Canadian population.

Aside from dehydration, complications of diarrhea include electrolyte imbalances, hemorrhoids and rectal prolapse. Diarrhea often results in a decreased ability to perform daily activities.

The most common causes of acute diarrhea are bacterial and viral infections. A list of major bacterial agents can be found in the Travelers' Diarrhea section later in this chapter. Infectious viral agents include:[4]

- Rotavirus—responsible for causing severe diarrhea in infants and children, and the most common cause of gastroenteritis among children worldwide.[5]
- Norwalk-like virus—responsible for milder form of diarrhea affecting older children and adults
- Adenovirus
- Astrovirus
- Calcivirus

Acute childhood diarrheal pathogens are transmitted by close contact and in particular the oral-fecal route. Childcare settings are a common place for diarrheal episodes.

Drugs are also a common cause of diarrhea (Table 1). In particular, broad-spectrum antibiotics such as penicillins, cephalosporins and erythromycins are implicated in altering the bacterial flora of the gut resulting in diarrhea. This usually occurs two to three days after starting the antibiotic and resolves when the antibiotic is discontinued. An uncommon but potentially serious adverse reaction to an antibiotic altering gut flora is antibiotic-induced *psuedomembranous colitis*, associated with the anaerobic organism *C. difficile*. The agents most commonly implicated as causes of pseudomembranous colitis are clindamycin, ampicillin and the cephalosporins,[8] although any antimicrobial agent can cause it, including those used to treat it. The condition usually develops 4 to 10 days after initiation of the antibiotic and is characterized by

Table 1: **Drugs Associated with Diarrhea**[6,7]

Acarbose
Alcohol
Antacids—magnesium salts
Antibiotics (most common)
Anticoagulants
Antihypertensives—especially propranolol
Antimetabolites—especially colchicine
Cardiovascular drugs—especially digoxin
Cholestyramine
Cholinergics
Cimetidine
Cytotoxic agents—especially 5-FU plus interferon or
    leucovorin
Domperidone
HIV medications—especially nelfinavir
Lactose-containing pharmaceuticals
Lactulose
Metoclopramide
Misoprostol
NSAIDs—especially naproxen
Orlistat
Potassium supplements
Prostaglandins
SSRIs—especially paroxetine
Sulfasalazine
Ticlopidine

significant loss of fluid, fever and abdominal pain. It is most commonly treated with **metronidazole** or oral **vancomycin**.[9]

Diarrhea may be associated with intolerance to food components, such as lactose or gluten, or with food allergies. Foods that contain large amounts of sorbitol or mannitol can cause an osmotic diarrhea.[4]

Other causes of diarrhea include: nervousness or anxiety, tumors, opiate withdrawal, rapid increase of fibre in the diet, enteral nutritional supplements, deficiencies of specific nutrients such as vitamin A and zinc,[10] excesses of specific nutrients such as vitamin C, inflammatory bowel disease, irritable bowel syndrome, diabetes.[4,6]

Goals of Therapy

- Determine the specific etiology and treat appropriately
- Decrease the symptoms and re-establish normal stools
- Avoid complications such as dehydration

Patient Assessment

Aside from frequent loose stools, symptoms of infectious diarrhea may include nausea, vomiting, abdominal pain, headache, fever, chills and malaise.

Question patients with repeated episodes of diarrhea about any relationship between symptoms and consumption of dairy or grain products. If such a relationship exists, refer the patient to a physician or dietician to rule out lactose or gluten intolerance (see Nutrition Appendix 1).

An assessment plan for patients suffering from diarrhea not related to travel is illustrated in Figure 1.

Prevention

- Eliminate/discontinue drugs causing diarrhea.
- Avoid lactose-containing products if lactose intolerance is suspected or diagnosed.
- Avoid gluten-containing products if celiac disease is diagnosed.
- Encourage handwashing after going to the toilet or changing a diaper and before preparing and eating food. Transmission of GI infections in the childcare setting is reduced significantly if infection control procedures are followed. High compliance with handwashing decreases episodes of diarrhea by 66%.[13]
- Prevent food poisoning:[14]
  — Avoid milk and fruit juices that are unpasteurized.
  — Cook foods thoroughly, especially red meat, poultry and eggs.
  — Eat foods soon after they have been cooked so that pathogens do not have time to grow.
  — Rinse foods that are not cooked before they are eaten (i.e., fresh fruits and vegetables) under running water.
  — Keep hot foods hot (60°C) and cold foods cold (4°C).
  — When preparing raw meats and poultry, keep them separated from cooked food, fresh fruits and vegetables.
  — Use separate cutting boards for raw meats and vegetables.
  — Reheat foods completely when serving leftovers.
  — Wash hands with hot, soapy water before and after preparing food.

Figure 1: **Assessment of Patients with Diarrhea Not Related to Travel**[4,11]

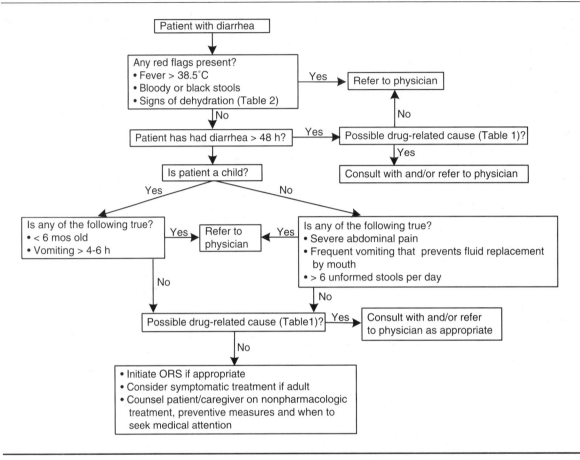

ORS = oral rehydration solution

— Use mild solution of water and soap to clean counters, cutting boards and utensils.
— Protect food from insects and animals.

Nonpharmacologic Therapy

Rehydration and maintaining electrolyte balance are the cornerstones of therapy for diarrhea.[15] Oral rehydration therapy (ORT) can treat the majority of patients with diarrhea as well as prevent most diarrhea-related complications.[3] Oral rehydration solution (ORS) takes advantage of the sodium/glucose-coupled active absorption mechanism. It is composed of sodium and glucose in the concentration

and osmolality of the luminal fluid. It is recommended by the World Health Organization (WHO) and should be used early, particularly when treating children and the elderly. The WHO formula for ORS is included in Table 3 as are those of the commercially available Gastrolyte® and Pedialyte®. The use of fruit juices, pop or tea with sugar is unsuitable due to the high carbohydrate concentration of these drinks. Homemade oral rehydration solutions can also be used although this is discouraged because mixing errors often occur. Examples of homemade ORS recipes are described in Table 4.

ORT is contraindicated in the following instances:[17]
• Protracted vomiting despite small frequent feedings

Table 2: **Symptoms of Dehydration in Children and Adults**[11,12]

Children	Adults
• Dry mouth, tongue and skin	• Increased thirst
• Few or no tears when crying	• Decreased urination
• Decreased urination (less than 4 wet diapers in 24 h)	• Feeling weak or light-headed
• Sunken eyes, cheeks or abdomen	• Dry mouth/tongue
• Grayish skin	
• Sunken soft spot (fontanel) in infants	
• Decreased skin turgor (Figure 2)	
• Irritability or listlessness	

Figure 2: **Decreased Skin Turgor**

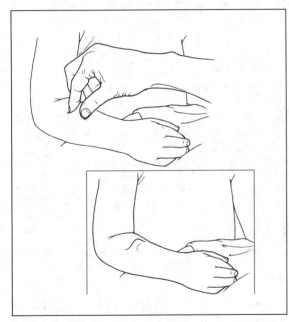

When pinched and released, the skin flattens slowly.

• Worsening diarrhea and an inability to keep up with losses
• Stupor or coma
• Intestinal ileus

Rapid refeeding with age-appropriate foods should immediately follow rehydration.[15] Withholding food for bowel rest, formula dilution and systematic elimination of lactose are no longer standard recommendations.

Pharmacologic Therapy

Antidiarrheal medications are indicated for relief of debilitating symptoms that accompany diarrheal illness. Nonprescription agents useful in the management of diarrhea are described in Table 5.

Prescription therapies for diarrhea include:
• Cholestyramine: useful in treatment of bile acid-induced diarrhea[1]
• Codeine: doses necessary for antidiarrheal effect not attainable with nonprescription products (result in acetaminophen overdose)
• Clonidine: effective against diarrhea associated with opioid withdrawal and diabetic autonomic neuropathy[1]
• Diphenoxylate with atropine: less effective than loperamide[21]
• Octreotide: useful in diarrhea due to chemotherapy, short bowel syndrome, neuroendocrine tumors, AIDS–associated diarrhea and other chronic diarrhea not responding to standard treatment[22-24]

Probiotics

Probiotics are live microorganisms (bacteria and yeast) that exert a beneficial effect by improving the balance of the host's flora.[25,26]

There are few well-designed clinical trials of the use of probiotics to treat or prevent diarrhea. However, *L. rhamnosus* strain GG has been shown to reduce the duration of diarrhea due to rotavirus in children[26] and decrease the incidence of antibiotic-associated diarrhea in children.[27,28]

The standardized brewer's yeast Hansen CBS 5926 may be useful for diarrhea. It can have some activity against *C. difficile* and enterotoxigenic *E. coli*. It

Table 3: **Composition of ORS Preparations**

Component	WHO	Gastrolyte®	Pedialyte®
Sodium (mmol/L)	90	60	45
Potassium (mmol/L)	20	20	20
Chloride (mmol/L)	80	60	35
Bicarbonate (mmol/L)	30	0	0
Citrate (mmol/L)	0	30	30
Glucose (g/L)	20	20	25

Table 4: **Recipes for Homemade Oral Rehydration Solution**[16]

	Ingredients	Amount
Recipe #1	Fruit juice	240 mL (1 cup)
	Honey (pasteurized)	2.5 mL (1/2 tsp)
	Salt	0.5 mL (1/8 tsp)
	Baking soda	1 mL (1/4 tsp)
Recipe #2	Purified water	1 L (4 cups)
	Salt	5 mL (1 tsp)
	Sugar	40 mL (8 tsp)

reduces water and electrolyte influx into the intestines stimulated by *V. cholerae* toxin and can increase the activity of intestinal disaccharides, saccharides, maltase and lactase to alleviate symptoms of diarrhea. These results may not be applicable to brewer's yeast in general.[29]

Most probiotics appear relatively safe. There have been isolated reports of serious adverse effects, including one case report of liver abscess due to *L. rhamnosus* in a 74 year old diabetic. Probiotics should be used cautiously in patients who are immunosuppressed or have a badly damaged GI tract.[25]

It is interesting to note that dairy products and many commercially available probiotics may contain organisms that, unlike *L. rhamnosus* strain GG, have not been shown to survive in the human GI tract.[25] Product standardization can also be a problem.

Products may contain microorganisms not listed on the label or contain quantities of microorganisms other than that listed.[30]

Herbal Remedies

Popular herbal choices for the treatment of diarrhea include german chamomile, carob, marshmallow, slippery elm and bayberry. None are particularly effective even though there are anecdotal reports, especially in folk medicine.

Herbs useful in the management of travelers' diarrhea are discussed in Travelers' Diarrhea, Pharmacologic Therapy.

Children

In most cases diarrhea in children is self-limiting and non-life-threatening. However, death can result from dehydration brought about by diarrhea.

The treatment of childhood diarrhea focuses on correcting dehydration. ORT is the most effective treatment for children with acute diarrhea. Oral rehydration salts are readily available, effective, safe and economical but are underutilized.[31] Underutilization may be due to the inconvenience of ORT administration in the practice setting and a preference for intravenous versus oral rehydration.

Breastfeeding should be continued during episodes of diarrhea[15] and ORS should be offered. If a child is not being breastfed, all food and drink should be withheld and ORS given as described in Table 6. ORT should start as soon as diarrhea begins and continue until diarrhea is less frequent.

Table 5: **Nonprescription Agents for Diarrhea**[1,18-20]

Drug	Dosage	Adverse effects	Drug interactions	Comments
Attapulgite	3-6 yrs: 300 mg initially, then 300 mg after each BM. Max: 2100 mg per day. 6-12 yrs: 600-750 mg initially, then 600-75 mg after each BM. Max: 4200 mg per day > 12 yrs and adults: 1200-1500 mg initially, then 1200-1500 mg after each BM. Max: 8400 mg per day	Well-tolerated		May be useful for treatment of mild to moderate acute diarrhea. Not to be used for more than 2 days unless directed by a physician.
Bismuth subsalicylate (BSS)	30 mL q 30 min Max: 8 doses per day	Black tongue/stools, tinnitus	Avoid in patients taking anticoagulants or salicylates, probenecid, methotrexate.	Used to treat chronic idiopathic diarrhea with a reduction in stool weight and frequency.
Loperamide	Adult: 4 mg stat then 2 mg after each loose BM Max: 16 mg per day	Abdominal cramps or discomfort, drowsiness, dizziness, dry mouth, skin rash.		Contraindicated in children under age 2. Not recommended for children under 12 yrs except on the advise of a physician. Avoid in acute dysentery (i.e., fever and bloody stools). Discontinue if symptoms persist longer than 48 hours. Opiate-like CNS effects have been observed in children under 3 yrs of age. Monitor patients with hepatic dysfunction for signs of CNS toxicity.
Psyllium	5 mL (5-6 g) q12h	Cramping, flatulence		Separate administration of other medications by 2 h. Contraindicated in patients with dysphagia. Allergic reactions have occurred. Esophageal obstruction has occurred when insufficient liquid was administered with the dose.

BM=bowel movement.

Even if a child refuses ORS by the cup or bottle, the solution is to be given by a medicine dropper or small teaspoon. If vomiting occurs, ORS should be continued with a spoon giving 15 mL every 10 to 15 minutes until vomiting stops, then resuming with the regular amount (Table 6). If vomiting does not stop after four to six hours, the child should receive medical attention.

Early refeeding should begin within six hours of beginning ORS. For infants who are formula-fed, start with small, frequent feedings of the child's usual formula. Should the diarrhea persist for five days, switch to a soy-based formula as lactose intolerance may be suspected.[17]

For older children, early refeeding with age-appropriate, previously tolerated foods is recommended.[15,17] After 24 to 48 hours, the child's normal diet can resume. It may take 7 to 10 days for stools to become completely formed. Restricting a child to a complex carbohydrate diet (e.g., BRATT diet: bananas, rice, applesauce, tea and toast) is inappropriate.[32]

For dehydrating, persistent diarrhea the use of hypo-osmolar oral rehydration solutions (e.g., Gastrolyte®, Pedialyte®) is beneficial and superior to iso-osmolar ORS.[33] Hypo-osmolar ORS results in a shorter period of diarrhea, less stool output and less need for maintenance therapy.

Pregnancy

Diarrhea in pregnancy is mainly due to viral or bacterial causes and is usually self-limiting. Maintenance of fluid intake is important. The use of loperamide to treat diarrhea during pregnancy is not associated with an increased risk of major malformations.[34]

The Elderly

The elderly are particularly susceptible to dehydration due to diarrhea. Nursing homes are similar to childcare settings where pathogens are spread by the oral-fecal route. Prompt rehydration is essential in limiting damage to vital organs.

Monitoring of Therapy

Table 7 provides a monitoring plan framework that should be individualized.

Table 6: **Administration of ORS to Non-breastfed Infants**[11]

Age of child	Amount of ORS to give
0-6 mos	30-90 mL every hour
6-24 mos	90-125 mL every hour
> 2 yrs	125-250 mL every hour

Table 7: **Monitoring Therapy for Diarrhea**

Symptoms	Monitoring	Endpoints	Actions
Loose, watery stools	**Patient:** regularly as long as symptoms persist. **Pharmacist:** ask for symptom report; call patient within 48 h to see if symptoms have resolved	Resolution of symptoms. Return to usual bowel evacuation pattern	Antidiarrheal medications may be necessary within first 2 days to alleviate symptoms. If symptoms persist beyond 48 h, seek medical attention.
Signs of dehydration (Table 2)	**Patient:** continually	No signs of dehydration	If signs of dehydration (Table 2) occur despite ORS, refer to physician.
Fever or blood in stools	**Patient:** regularly as long as symptoms persist	No fever; no blood in stools	Refer to physician if this occurs.

Travelers' Diarrhea

Pathophysiology

Travelers' diarrhea is an illness that affects 20 to 50% of two-week travelers from industrialized countries to developing countries like Latin America, Asia and Africa.[35] It is generally self-limiting and even without treatment usually resolves within three to four days. For the most part it is non-life-threatening; however, infants, the elderly, patients with severe chronic diseases (e.g., chronic renal failure, congestive heart failure, insulin dependent diabetes mellitus, inflammatory bowel disease) and immunocompromised hosts may suffer dire consequences. It is known by many names including Montezuma's revenge, GI trots, Turkey trots, turista and Delhi belly. It is defined by three or more loose, unformed stools per day along with at least one symptom of enteric infection such as fever, abdominal cramps, nausea, fecal urgency or dysentery.[36] Caused by bacteria, viruses and parasites, it is primarily spread by the fecal-oral route. Infectious agents responsible for travelers' diarrhea (Table 8) vary depending on the geographical area visited as well as the time of year. Factors associated with an increased likelihood of acquiring travelers' diarrhea include adventurous eating habits, gastric hypo-chlorhydria, immunodeficiency and a relative lack of gut immunity seen in younger individuals.[16]

Goals of Therapy

- Educate travelers before they reach their destination in developing countries so as to avoid diarrheal illness
- Educate travelers on effective treatment regimens in case they experience symptoms
- Shorten the period of suffering and minimize interruption of vacation and/or business plans
- Prevent complications such as dehydration

Patient Assessment

The assessment and management of travelers' diarrhea is illustrated in Figure 3.

Prevention

The incidence of travelers' diarrhea can be minimized by choosing appropriate foods and avoiding those associated with the illness (Table 9).

Table 8: **Common Causes of Travelers' Diarrhea**[16]

Bacterial
Aeromonas spp.—common in Thailand
Campylobacter jejuni—common in Mexico, Thailand, Morocco (dry winter)
Enterotoxigenic *Escherichia coli* (ETEC)—common in Latin America, Africa
Plesiomonas spp.
Salmonella spp.
Shigella spp.
Vibrio cholerae—common in India, Ecuador, Bali and Indonesia
Yersinia spp.

Viral
Norwalk virus
Rotavirus

Parasitic
Cryptosporidium parvum—common in Russia
Cyclospora cayetanensis—common in Nepal
Entamoeba histolytica
Giardia lamblia—common in Russia and Nepal

Table 9: **Food and Travelers' Diarrhea**[16,21]

Safe foods/ beverages	Unsafe food/ beverages
Piping hot food	Buffet food at room temperature
Peeled fruit (preferably done by self)	Fresh soft cheese
	Food from street vendors
Cooked vegetables	Cold salads
Carbonated beverages (with no ice cubes)	Leafy and/or raw vegetables
	Uncooked, cold sauces
Boiled or bottled water	Unpeeled fruit
Pasteurized milk (if properly stored)	Raspberries/strawberries/ watermelon
	Ice cubes/chips
	Undercooked hamburger/meat/fish
	Shellfish
	Large reef fish from the Caribbean and South Pacific (e.g., snapper, barracuda, grouper, jack, moray eel)
	Custards, mousses, mayonnaise, hollandaise sauce

Figure 3: **Self-management of Travelers' Diarrhea**[16,37]

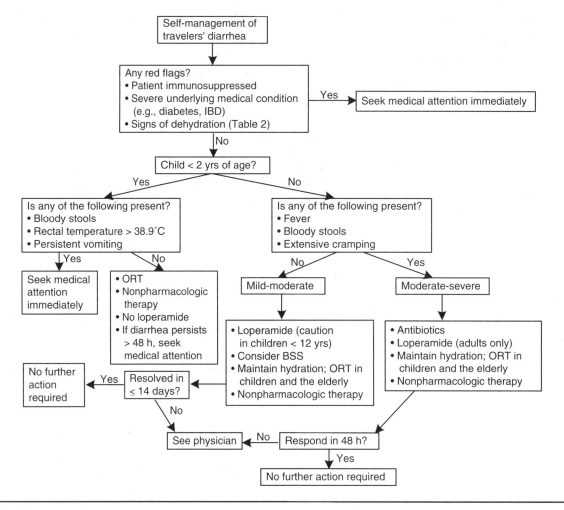

BSS = bismuth subsalicylate

Other measures that travelers should follow include:
- Follow the adage "Boil it, cook it, peel it or forget it."
- Use purified water or water from the hot tap to brush teeth.
- Wash hands frequently while traveling, particularly before handling or consuming food (if soap and water are unavailable, consider using commercially available waterless hand sanitizing agents).[16]
- Avoid drinking the water while swimming.
- Avoid drinking local water (although some resort areas have their own filtration system to purify water).

- Drink bottled beverages in their original containers and ensure the cap is sealed.
- Bismuth subsalicylate is 60 to 65% effective as a prophylactic agent[16] (Table 10) and may be used to prevent travelers' diarrhea.

Consider antibiotic prophylaxis in selected cases:
—People who cannot tolerate even a brief illness (e.g., elite athletes, business or political travelers);
—People at high risk of travelers' diarrhea due to achlorhydria, gastrectomy or history of repeated episodes of severe travelers' diarrhea;

Table 10: **Nonprescription Agents for Prevention and Treatment of Travelers' Diarrhea**[16,20,21,38]

Drug	Dosage	Adverse effects	Drug interactions	Comments
Bismuth subsalicylate (BSS)	Prevention: 2 × 262 mg tabs or equivalent suspension QID Treatment: 2 × 262 mg tabs or equivalent suspension every 30 min × 8 doses	Black tongue/stools, tinnitus	Avoid in patients taking anticoagulants or salicylates, probenecid, methotrexate. Can interfere with absorption of doxycycline (which may be used for malaria prevention)	Avoid in patients with history of ASA allergy. Limit prophylaxis to 3 wks. Not for children < 2 yrs.
Loperamide	Prevention: Not recommended. Treatment: 4 mg stat then 2 mg after q loose BM Max: 16 mg per day	Abdominal pain or discomfort, drowsiness or dizziness, dry mouth, skin rash		Contraindicated in children < 2 yrs. Caution in children < 12 yrs. Drug of choice as antimotility agent for treatment of travelers' diarrhea.

—Those who are immunosuppressed;

—Those with chronic illness at increased risk of experiencing complications due to travelers' diarrhea (see Pathophysiology).

Typhoid vaccine is recommended for travelers who will have significant exposure to contaminated food and water in smaller cities and villages or rural areas off the usual tourist routes. **Cholera vaccine** may be of benefit to health care workers in endemic areas or aid workers in refugee camps, but it is not recommended for most travelers.[16]

Methods for purifying untreated water are discussed in Appendix D: Information for the Traveler.

Nonpharmacologic Therapy

Travelers are advised to maintain and possibly increase their fluid intake during bouts of diarrhea, though dehydration is not a major concern. Health Canada suggests that children and the elderly use ORS, while healthy adults maintain hydration with canned juices, purified water, carbonated soft drinks or clear salty soups to maintain light-colored urine and relieve thirst.[16]

Pharmacologic Therapy

Nonprescription agents for the prevention and treatment of travelers' diarrhea are described in Table 10. **Golden seal** (*Hydrastis canadensis*) has been used to treat travelers' diarrhea. The primary active constituent is thought to be **berberine**. There are limited human data to support the efficacy of golden seal or berberine in the treatment of infectious diarrhea. The dose of berberine sulfate used in clinical studies was 400 mg per day given in one to four doses. The adult dose of dried herb is 0.5 to 1 g, three times daily. Safety in children or during breastfeeding has not been established. Golden seal is contraindicated during pregnancy. The use of golden seal extracts appears safe. However, administration of high doses of berberine may result in serious adverse effects (e.g., hypertension, seizures, respiratory failure).[39,40]

Antibiotics useful in treating travelers' diarrhea include the quinolones, azithromycin and cefixime. Trimethoprim/sulfamethoxazole is of limited use due to widespread resistance.[16] Prior to departure, travelers should see a physician for appropriate antibiotics for use in case of diarrhea while traveling.

Monitoring of Therapy[16,37]

Patients can monitor their condition based on the frequency and severity of symptoms. They can expect a fairly brief illness if they take medication and in some cases even without medication. Monitoring includes reduction of loose, watery stools to ≤ 1 per day within two to three days. Medical attention should be sought if the patient develops signs of dehydration, or if a child less than two years of age develops bloody stools, a rectal temperature > 38.9°C or persistent vomiting. Should symptoms persist longer than 14 days once back from vacation, a physician should be consulted.

Suggested Readings

Diarrhea

The American Academy of Pediatrics. The management of acute gastroenteritis in young children. *Pediatrics* 1996;97(3):424-35.

Brandt LJ, Greenwald D, eds. Acute and chronic diarrhea: a primer on diagnosis and treatment. Available at: http://www.acg.gi.org/acg-dev/physicianforum/gifocus/diarrhea.html.

Guerrant RL, Van Gilder T, Steiner TS, et al. Practice guidelines for the management of infectious diarrhea. *Clin Inf Dis* 2001;32:331-51.

Yassin SF, Young-Fadok TM, Zein NN, Pardi DS. *Clostridium difficile*-associated diarrhea and colitis. *Mayo Clin Proc* 2001;76:725-30.

Travelers' Diarrhea

Andsell VE, Ericsson CD. Prevention and empiric treatment of travelers' diarrhea. *Med Clin North Am* 1999;83(4):945-73, vi.

Committee to Advise on Tropical Medicine and Travel. Statement on travelers' diarrhea. *Can Comm Dis Rep* 2001, Mar 15;27(ACS-3):1-12.

References:

1. Fedorak RN. Diarrhea. In: Gray J, ed. *Therapeutic Choices.* 3rd ed. Ottawa, ON: Canadian Pharmacists Association; 2000:874-81.
2. Sandler RS, Stewart WF, Liberman JN, Ricci JA, Zorich NL. Abdominal pain, bloating & diarrhea in the United States: prevalence & impact. *Dig Dis Sci* 2000;45(6):1166-71.
3. Ladinsky M, Duggan A, Santosham M, Wilson M. The World Health Organization oral rehydration solution in US pediatric practice: a randomized trial to evaluate parent satisfaction. *Arch Pediatr Adolesc Med* 2000;154(7):700-5.
4. Brandt LJ, Greenwald D, eds. *Acute and chronic diarrhea: a primer on diagnosis and treatment.* Available at: http://www.acg.gi.org/acg-dev/physicianforum/gifocus/diarrhea.html. Accessed April 26, 2001.
5. Nappert G, Barios JM, Zello GA, Naylor JM. Oral rehydration solution therapy in the management of children with rotavirus diarrhea. *Nutr Rev* 2000;58(3 pt1):80-7.
6. Bisanz A. Managing bowel elimination problems in patients with cancer. *ONF* 1997;24(4):679-86.
7. Thomas RE, Wyer M. Nausea, vomiting, diarrhea and constipation. In: Herfindal ET, Gourley DR, Lloyd Hart L, eds. *Clinical Pharmacy and Therapeutics.* 4th ed. Philadelphia, PA: Williams and Wilkins, 1998:306-7.
8. Yassin SF, Young-Fadok TM, Zein NN, Pardi DS. *Clostridium difficile*-associated diarrhea and colitis. *Mayo Clin Proc* 2001;76:725-30.
9. Gerding DN. Treatment of *Clostridium difficile*-associated diarrhea and colitis. *Curr Top Microbiol Immunol* 2000;250:127-39.
10. Mehta DI, Blecker U. Chronic diarrhea in infancy and childhood. *J LA State Med Soc* 1998;150(a):419-29.
11. Canadian Paediatric Society. Caring for kids page. *Dehydration and diarrhea.* Available at: http://www.caringforkids.cps.ca/babies/Dehydration.htm. Accessed October 25, 2001.
12. Pace B. Preventing dehydration from diarrhea. *JAMA* 2001; 285(3):362.
13. Roberts L, Jorm L, Patel M, Smith W, Douglas RM, McGilchrist C. Effect of infection control measures on the frequency of diarrheal episodes in childcare: a randomized, controlled trial. *Pediatrics* 2000;105(4 Pt 1):743-6.
14. Canadian Paediatric Society. Caring for kids page. *How to avoid food poisoning.* Available at: http://www.caringforkids.cps.ca/eating/FoodPoisoning.htm. Accessed October 25, 2001.
15. Kaila M, Onnela T, Isoauri E. Treatment of acute diarrhea in practice. *Acta Paediatr* 1997;86(12):1340-4.
16. Committee to Advise on Tropical Medicine and Travel. Satement on travellers' diarrhea. *Can Comm Dis Rep* 2001, Mar 15;27(ACS-3).
17. Canadian Paediatric Society. Oral rehydration therapy and early refeeding in the management of childhood gastroenteritis. *Can J Paediatrics* 1994; 1(5):160-4.
18. Zaid MR, Hasan M, Khan AA. Attapulgite in the treatment of acute diarrhea: a double-blind placebo–controlled study. *J Diarrhoeal Dis Res* 1995;13(1):44-6.
19. Repchinsky C, ed. *Compendium of Pharmaceuticals and Specialties 2002.* Ottawa, ON: Canadian Pharmacists Association; 2002.
20. Repchinsky C, ed. *Compendium of Nonprescription Products 2001.* Ottawa, ON: Canadian Pharmacists Association; 2001.
21. Andsell VE, Ericsson CD. Prevention and empiric treatment of traveler's diarrhea. *Med Clin North Am* 1999;83(4):945-73, vi.
22. Fried M. Octreotide in the treatment of refractory diarrhea. *Digestion* 1999;60(Suppl 2):42-6.
23. Baille-Johnson HR. Octreotide in the management of treatment-related diarrhea. *Anticancer Drugs* 1996;7(Suppl 1):11-5.
24. Cascinu S. Management of diarrhea induced by tumors or cancer therapy. *Curr Opin Oncol* 1995;7(4):325-9.
25. Elmer GW. Probiotics: "Living drugs". *Am J Health-Syst Pharm* 2001; 58:1101-9.

26. Alvarez-Olmos MI, Oberhelman RA. Probiotic agents and infectious diseases: a modern perspective on a traditional therapy. *Clin Inf Dis* 2001;32:1567-76.

27. Arvola T, Laiho K, Torkkeli S, et al. Prophylactic *Lactobacillus* GG reduces antibiotic associated diarrhea in children with respiratory infections: a randomized study. *Pediatrics* 1999; 104(5):e64. Available at: http://www.pediatrics.org/cgi/content/full/104/5/e64. Accessed March 13, 2002.

28. Vanderhoof JA, Whitney DB, Antonson DL, Hanner TL, Lupo JV, Young RJ. *Lactobacillus* GG in the prevention of antibiotic-associated diarrhea in children. *J. Pediatr* 1999;135(5): 535-7.

29. Jellin JM, ed. *Natural Medicines Comprehensive Database.* 2nd ed. Stockton, CA: Therapeutic Research Faculty, 1999.

30. Hamilton-Miller JMT, Shah S, Smith CT. "Probiotic" remedies are not what they seem. *BMJ* 1996;312:55-6.

31. Guandalini S. Treatment of acute diarrhea in the new millennium. *J Pediatr Gastroenterol Nutr* 2000;30(5):486-9.

32. American Academy of Pediatrics. The management of acute gastroenteritis in young children. *Pediatrics* 1996;97(3): 424-35.

33. Dutta P, Mitra U, Dutta S, et al. Hypo-osmolar oral rehydration salts solution in dehydrating perisistent diarrhea in children: double-blind, randomized, controlled clinical trial. *Acta Paediatr* 2000;89(4):411-6.

34. Einarson A, Mastroiacovo P, Arnon J, et al. Prospective, contolled, multicentre study of loperamide in pregnancy. *Can J Gastroenterol* 2000;14(3):185-7.

35. Castelli F, Beltrame A, Carosi G. [Principles and management of the ambulatory treatment of traveller's diarrhea]. *Bull Soc Pathol Exot* 1998;91(5 pt 1-2):452-5.

36. Danzinger LH, Itokasu GS. Gastrointestinal infections. In: Young LL, Koda-Kimble MA, eds. *Applied Therapeutics: The Clinical Use of Drugs.* 6th ed. Vancouver, WA: Applied Therapeutics Inc., 1995.

37. Committee to Advise on Tropical Medicine and Travel. Persistent diarrhea in the returned traveller. *Can Comm Dis Rep* 1998 Jan1;24(ACS-1).

38. Caeiro JP, DuPont HL, Albrecht H, Ericsson CD. Oral rehydration therapy plus loperamide versus loperamide alone in the treatment of traveler's diarrhea. *Clin Infect Dis* 1999; 28(6):1286-9.

39. Ernst E, ed. *The Desktop Guide to Complementary and Alternative Medicine.* New York, NY: Mosby, 2001.

40. Smith M. Golden seal. In: Chandler F, ed. *Herbs: Everyday Reference for Health Professionals.* Ottawa, ON: Canadian Pharmacists Association/Canadian Medical Association, 2000:139-41.

Diarrhea—Patient Information

Almost everyone has diarrhea at some time in their life. It is especially common in children, who may have diarrhea two or three times a year. Diarrhea is usually caused by an infection or food poisoning but may also be due to drugs, food intolerance, disease, stress or anxiety.

Here are some things you can do to help protect yourself against diarrhea due to infections or food poisoning:

- Wash your hands after going to the toilet or changing a diaper, and before eating or preparing food.
- Do not drink milk or fruit juices that have not been pasteurized (check the label).
- Cook foods thoroughly, especially red meat, poultry (chicken and turkey) and eggs.
- Eat food soon after it is cooked so that germs do not have time to grow on it.
- Rinse fresh fruits and vegetables under running water before you eat them.
- Keep hot foods hot (60°C) and cold foods cold (4°C).
- Keep raw meat and poultry away from cooked food and fresh fruit and vegetables, especially while preparing food.
- Use separate cutting boards for raw meats and other foods.
- If serving leftovers, make sure they are reheated all the way through.
- Use soap and water to clean counters, cutting boards and utensils.

If you do get diarrhea, make sure you get enough fluids. This is especially important in children and older people, and in people with chronic medical conditions. These people should use special mixtures of water and salts (called oral rehydration solutions) to make sure they do not get dehydrated. Talk to your pharmacist to see if you should use these, or if medication would help with your diarrhea.

See a doctor if *any* of the following is true:
- You have a high fever (over 38.5°C or 101°F);
- Your bowel movement has blood in it or looks black;
- Your diarrhea lasts longer than two days;
- You have severe pain in your belly;
- You cannot keep fluids down;
- You have more than six bowel movements in one day;
- You feel dehydrated (very thirsty, weak or lightheaded, dry mouth or tongue, not urinating as often as usual).

Children with diarrhea should *also* see a doctor if:
- They are less than six months old, *or*
- They have vomiting that lasts longer than four to six hours, *or*
- They seem dehydrated. Children may be dehydrated if they have a dry mouth or tongue, they have no tears when they cry, they have less than four wet diapers in 24 hours, their eyes or soft spot are sunken, they are irritable or have low energy.

Travelers' Diarrhea—Patient Information

Travelers to developing countries in areas such as Latin America, Asia and Africa may develop diarrhea during the course of their trip. This is almost always due to contaminated food or water and usually gets better on its own in a few days without causing serious problems.

If you travel to one of these areas you should bring an antidiarrheal and a thermometer. Your pharmacist can help you choose the right antidiarrheal for you. Before you travel talk to your doctor about antibiotics. Many people bring antibiotics with them to take in case they do get diarrhea. A few people need to take medication to prevent diarrhea from happening at all.

Here are some things you can do to prevent diarrhea while traveling:

- Only eat foods and drink fluids that are unlikely to make you sick. These are:
  —piping hot foods
  —fruit you peel yourself
  —cooked vegetables
  —carbonated beverages (with no ice cubes)
  —boiled or bottled water
  —pasteurized milk (properly stored).

- Avoid foods likely to make you sick. These include:
  —buffet foods at room temperature
  —fresh soft cheese
  —food from street vendors
  —cold salads
  —raw vegetables
  —uncooked/cold sauces
  —unpeeled fruit
  —raspberries, strawberries, watermelon
  —ice cubes
  —undercooked meat or fish
  —shellfish
  —large reef fish such as snapper, barracuda, grouper, jack and Moray eel
  —custards, mousses, mayonnaise and hollandaise sauce.
- Remember the saying "Boil it, cook it, peel it or forget it."
- Wash your hands, especially before you eat.
- Avoid drinking water while swimming
- Do not drink local water.
- Drink bottled beverages from their original containers and make sure the cap is properly sealed.

Talk to your pharmacist about what to do if you have diarrhea while you are away.

Abdominal Pain Assessment

Peter Thomson, BSc(Pharm), PharmD

Abdominal pain can be a non-specific symptom arising from a variety of sites. The abdomen itself contains a diverse group of organs and tissues. The GI tract starts at the mouth and extends to the anus. Sites that contribute to the majority of GI tract complaints include the esophagus, stomach, liver, gall bladder, pancreas and intestines. Common causes of abdominal pain are listed in Table 1.

Abdominal pain may involve a variety of symptoms including dyspepsia, nausea and heartburn. Virtually everyone experiences abdominal symptoms on an intermittent basis. Fortunately, the vast majority of symptoms are benign in nature.

Abdominal pain is one of the most common reasons for a physician visit. However, most sufferers do not seek physician help and self-medicate with OTC products. It is estimated that recurrent upper abdominal pain or discomfort occurs in approximately 25% of the public in western countries. Heartburn adds approximately another 15% to that total.[1]

Irritable bowel syndrome (IBS) and nonulcer dyspepsia (NUD) are the most common functional disorders of the GI tract. The major difference between IBS and dyspepsia is the lack of colonic involvement in dyspepsia. IBS pain may be referred below the umbilicus whereas dyspepsia pain is usually referred to the epigastrium. Together they account for roughly half of all referrals to outpatient gastroenterology clinics.[2]

Figure 1 provides an overview of an approach to abdominal pain.

Patient Assessment

Signs of Serious GI Pathology

Pharmacists must recognize common symptoms associated with serious GI pathology and refer these patients for medical attention. In a study of over 150 patients who developed gastric or esophageal cancer under the age of 55 years, over 97% had at least one the following symptoms of serious GI pathology: dysphagia, weight loss (> 3 kg over six months), persistent vomiting, bleeding, anemia, hematemesis or melena.[4] Additional factors for serious GI pathology include: age $\geq$ 50 years (especially if new onset dyspepsia or change in symptoms), jaundice, cancer history (strong family history), anemia, multiple treatment failures and recent dramatic changes in symptoms. Fever and chills can represent an infectious source of abdominal pain requiring medical assessment.

Assessment of Patient Acuity

If no signs of serious GI pathology are apparent, undertake a systematic assessment of abdominal pain.

Table 1: Common Conditions Associated with Abdominal Pain*

Cancer	Irritable bowel syndrome (IBS)
Cholelithiasis	Myofascial pain
Chronic pancreatitis	Nonulcer (functional) dyspepsia (NUD)
Crohn's disease	Peptic ulcer disease (PUD)
Gastroesophageal reflux disease (GERD)	Ulcerative colitis

Excluding the acute abdomen.

Figure 1: **Assessment of Patients with Abdominal Pain**

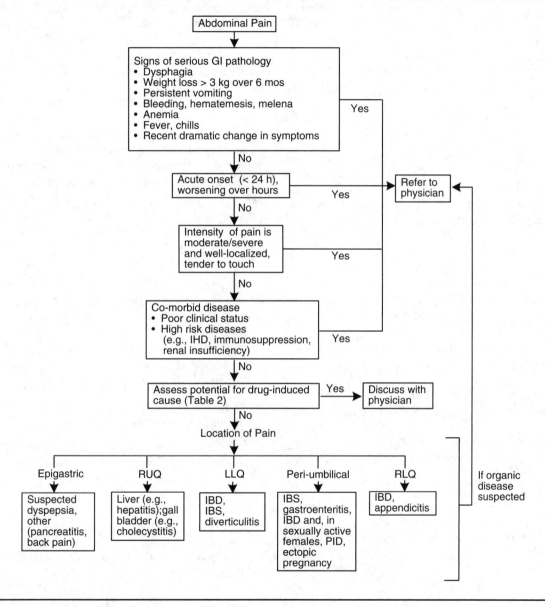

IBD = inflammatory bowel disease
IBS = irritable bowel syndrome
PID = pelvic inflammatory disease

IHD = ischemic heart disease
RUQ = right upper quadrant

LLQ = left lower quadrant
RLQ = right lower quadrant

Key assessment issues include location, triggers, intensity of pain and comorbid diseases. Acute (< 24 hours), well-localized, moderate or severe pain, worsening over hours and tender to touch usually indicates a need for medical attention. Triggers of pain such as medications and foods may suggest specific disorders such as peptic ulcer disease (PUD), gastroesophageal reflux disease (GERD), lactase deficiency or celiac disease. Intolerance to foods can give rise to abdominal pain. Spicy foods, citrus fruits and foods with a high fat content are examples. Postprandial pain is often associated with overindulgence. High fat intake and certain foods can produce indigestion and trigger symptoms of IBS. Review timing of pain with meals, and current medications (including herbals and vitamins). Evaluate alcohol and recreational drug use (if appropriate). Certain disease states such as renal failure and congestive heart failure cause abdominal pain.

Medications are commonly associated with abdominal pain (Table 2). Comorbid diseases can produce or mimic abdominal pain. Some medical conditions that may warrant physician assessment include ischemic heart disease, immunosuppression (e.g., cancer, HIV, drug-induced), psychiatric disorders (e.g., depression) and renal insufficiency. Patients on immunosuppressants are particularly noteworthy as infectious causes of abdominal pain may arise that initially have fewer or less severe manifestations of the pathology compared to non-compromised individuals (e.g., fever, pain). Extremes in age (very elderly, infants < 1 month old) are often less tolerant of stress and require closer evaluation and monitoring.[5]

Location of Abdominal Pain

Pain may be localized to different areas of the abdomen. This may help determine the likely cause of pain. More importantly, it may assist in assessing when to refer a patient for medical care. Sources of epigastric pain include GERD, PUD, NUD and pancreatitis (which also causes back pain). Right upper quadrant pain often involves the liver or gall bladder. Hepatitis and biliary colic require medical assessment. Left upper quadrant pain may involve the spleen or splenic flexure. Periumbilical pain may be due to conditions involving the pelvic organs (e.g., pelvic

inflammatory disease or ectopic pregnancy), gastroenteritis or inflammatory bowel disease (IBD). Causes of right lower quadrant pain include appendicitis. Small bowel obstructions (usually nausea and vomiting also present), inflammatory bowel disease (IBD), IBS and diverticulitis can appear as both right or left lower quadrant pain.[5]

Caveats to Abdominal Pain Assessment

In many cases, the cause of acute abdominal pain varies with patient age as well as comorbid medical conditions. There is a considerable overlap in symptoms among many of the common disorders that cause abdominal pain. For example, over 80% of IBS patients will also exhibit symptoms of dyspepsia.[6] Moderate to intense pain is not a characteristic feature of dyspepsia. Likewise in biliary tract disease and pancreatitis, the pain is usually acute and more intense in nature.[6]

Recurrent abdominal pain occurs in approximately 10% of school-aged children. Pain is usually periumbilical and varies in intensity. Nausea and vomiting may occur but weight loss is uncommon. In over 90% of cases there is no organic cause. Stress (e.g., school) may be a component. Drug therapy is generally not recommended.[7]

Suggested Readings

Silen W. Abdominal pain. In: Fauci AS, Braunwald E, Isselbacher KJ, et al., eds. *Harrison's Principles of Internal Medicine*. 14th ed. New York, NY: McGraw-Hill, 1998:65-68.

References

1. AGA Technical Review: Evaluation of Dyspepsia. *Gastroenterol* 1998;114:582-95.

Table 2: **Some Medications Commonly Associated with Abdominal Pain**

Amiodarone (especially loading dose)	Metformin
Antibiotics	NSAIDs (including COX-2 Inhibitors)
Anticonvulsants	Neuroleptics
Antineoplastics	Opioids
Antiretrovirals	SSRIs
Iron supplements	Sulfasalazine

2. Jones J, Boorman J, Cann P et. al. British Society of Gastro-enterology guidelines for the management of the irritable bowel syndrome. *Gut* 2000;(suppl II):ii 1-19.

3. Silen W. Abdominal pain. In: Fauci AS, Braunwald E, Isselbacher KJ, et al., eds. *Harrison's Principles of Internal Medicine*. 14th ed. New York, NY: McGraw-Hill, 1998:65-68.

4. Gillen D, McColl KE. Does concern about missing malignancy justify endoscopy in uncomplicated dyspepsia in patients aged less than 55? *Am J Gastroenterol* 1999;94:75-9.

5. Glasgow RE, Mulvihill SJ. Abdominal pain, including the acute abdomen. In: Feldman M, Scherschmidt BF, Sleisenger MH, eds. *Gastrointestinal and Liver Disease*. 6th ed. Philadelphia, PA: WB Saunders, 1998:80-89.

6. McQuaid K. Dyspepsia. In: Feldman M, Scherschmidt BF, Sleisenger MH, eds. *Gastrointestinal and Liver Disease*. 6th ed. Philadelphia: WB Saunders, 1998:105-16

7. Hay WW. Recurrent abdominal pain. In: Hay WW, Hayward AR, Levin MJ, Sondheimer JM, eds. *Current Pediatric Diagnosis and Treatment*. 14th ed. Old Tappan, NJ: Appleton and Lange, 1998:550-552.

Chapter 23

Dyspepsia and GERD

Peter Thomson, BSc(Pharm), PharmD

Dyspepsia is the most common gastrointestinal complaint seen by family practitioners. Additionally, likely less than 25% of individuals with dyspepsia seek physician assessment.[1] Dyspepsia itself is a symptom complex rather than a specific disease entity and commonly refers to pain or discomfort centred in the upper abdomen. Patients often use terms such as heartburn, indigestion, gas, bloating and nausea to describe dyspepsia. It arises from both organic and functional sources (Table 1). Organic refers to an actual pathologic source. Functional dyspepsia, also known as nonulcer dyspepsia (NUD), refers to dyspepsia of at least three months' duration with no definitive structural or biochemical explanation.[2] It is estimated that 29% of Canadians have dyspepsia.[3] The most feared pathology in this regard is cancer. However, both esophageal and gastric cancer are uncommon in the North American population, especially in those younger than 55 years of age.

Pathophysiology

Dyspepsia can be caused by numerous factors (Table 1). Some medications associated with dyspepsia are listed in Table 1. Dyspepsia can be triggered by large meals, irritant foods or alcohol consumption. For most patients symptoms are minor and infrequent. Two subsets of patients with dyspepsia are those with functional dyspepsia and gastroesophageal reflux disease (GERD).

Functional Dyspepsia

Nervous system pathways are involved in functional dyspepsia, which is associated with an increased sensitivity to organ distension. Although motility disorders arise frequently in functional dyspeptics,[4] there is poor correlation between the delayed gastric emptying and both symptoms of delayed emptying and response to prokinetic agents.[1] This should not be confused with organic causes of dyspepsia where

Table 1: **Causes of Dyspepsia**[1]

Organic (40%):
    Peptic ulcer disease (15-25%)
    Reflux esophagitis (5-15%)
    Gastric or esophageal cancer < 2%, (estimated that in all dyspeptics presence of a curable GI cancer is 0.001%)
    Other diseases: e.g., cholecystitis, pancreatitis, celiac disease, Crohn's disease, sarcoidosis, hypothyroidism, hypercalcemia, hepatoma, intestinal angina, renal failure, diabetic gastroparesis
    Food intolerance: e.g., lactase deficiency, allergies (rare), spicy/irritant foods – coffee, acidic juices, peppermint
    Medications: e.g., alendronate, amiodarone, antibiotics, NSAIDs (including COX-2 inhibitors), iron
    Herbals: e.g., garlic, feverfew, chaste tree berry, white willow
    Infections: e.g., CMV, *G. lamblia, S. stercoralis*
Functional (nonulcer) dyspepsia (60%)

pathologic changes in GI motility are known (e.g., diabetic gastroparesis). Both motor and sensitivity changes in the GI tract are postulated pathophysiologic mechanisms of NUD. It does not appear that acid production in the stomach is a major contributor to dyspepsia,[4] although some dyspepsia is secondary to acid reflux.

Psychosocial factors involved in NUD are not easily quantified. There appears to be a subgroup of patients who have an actual psychiatric diagnosis such as depression or an anxiety disorder. As well, NUD patients often have impairment in quality of life. The contribution of psychosocial issues to the prevalence and severity of NUD is of considerable debate.

Gastroesophageal Reflux Disease (GERD)

GERD is defined as the retrograde spilling of the gastric contents (including acid and pepsin) into the esophagus. Everyone has some degree of reflux, especially after meals. It becomes pathologic only when associated with symptoms or complications.

Two issues are paramount in regards to GERD. Firstly, patients may experience discomforting symptoms which include acid regurgitation, pain and heartburn. Secondly, structural damage may arise. Esophagitis can potentially lead to complications such as strictures, *Barrett's esophagus* and esophageal cancer. Common complications are bleeding (anemia) and weight loss. Some patients may develop aspiration. Barrett's esophagus involves the replacement of squamous epithelium with columnar epithelium. It occurs in 5 to 12% of GERD patients and is related more to duration of GERD than severity. Barrett's is an identifiable risk for adenocarcinoma (5 to 10%). Adenocarcinoma is a feared complication of GERD as its five year survival rate is less than 10%.

The incidence of GERD is rising in North America. It is difficult to define the exact incidence as many individuals with GERD do not seek medical attention. As well, there is no single gold standard for the diagnosis of GERD. In some surveys, over 40% of the population experience monthly symptoms of the disorder with roughly half that amount experiencing symptoms on a weekly basis.[2] Table 2 lists some of the potential risk factors for the development of GERD.

Table 2: **Risk Factors for GERD**

Nutrition	Decrease LES pressure (e.g., high fat meal) Increase TLESRs (e.g., gastric distension from carbonated drinks)
Pregnancy	
Obesity	
Increasing age	
Disease states: Sjögren's syndrome, possibly asthma	
Drugs that decrease LES pressure (e.g., alpha- and beta-blockers, alcohol, anticholinergics, benzodiazepines, calcium channel blockers, narcotics, nitrates, nicotine, theophylline)	

LES: lower esophageal sphincter
TLESR: transient lower esophageal sphincter relaxation

Classic features of injury to the esophagus are pain and difficulty in swallowing (*odynophagia* and *dysphagia*), and heartburn. Esophagitis is reported in approximately 30% of newly diagnosed cases of patients with classic symptoms of GERD. In the majority of cases the inflammation is mild.[5]

Heartburn (*pyrosis*) and acid regurgitation are the key symptoms in GERD. Unfortunately heartburn may not correlate well with esophagitis. Chest pain may be a symptom of GERD as well as myocardial ischemia. Like angina, in GERD the pain may radiate to the neck. Heartburn is often worse with bending over, lying down and eating fatty meals. Atypical signs of GERD include morning hoarseness, cough, hiccups and wheezing that are associated with upper airway manifestations of GERD. This may affect the pharynx, larynx and other parts of the respiratory tract.

The pathophysiology of GERD involves a complex set of factors that have interrelated effects. The esophagus is cleared by peristalsis which is stimulated by esophageal dilatation. Decreased peristalsis can arise in certain situations such as during sleep.

Lower esophageal sphincter (LES) pressures may be normal or lower in individuals with GERD. GERD can be a self-perpetuating disease as it reduces esophageal peristalsis and LES pressure. Delayed gastric emptying can increase the frequency of reflux and the volume of gastric contents that is refluxed. Delayed emptying can arise in infants.

It is now known that other factors are involved besides LES pressure and gastric emptying. Two major ones are transient lower esophageal sphincter relaxations (TLESRs) and hiatus hernia (HH). TLESRs are independent of swallowing and are much more prolonged events than LES relaxation with swallowing. Mediated by the vagus nerve, they are increased by stomach distension, fatty food ingestion and smoking. Subjects with GERD have more frequent periods of reflux with their TLESRs. An HH occurs with the herniation of the stomach above the diaphragm. HH is not a major factor in initiating heartburn but is a key factor related to TLESRs. The larger the HH, the greater the frequency of the TLESR period. Roughly 30% of adults have HH with increased age and 30% have heartburn but the combination of both features is much less common.

Damage to the esophagus is related not only to composition of reflux (e.g., acid, pepsin) but also the duration of time the reflux is in contact with esophageal mucosa. With acid and other refluxate exposure the esophagus becomes damaged. Approximately one-third of untreated GERD patients have endoscopic evidence of inflammation (esophagitis). A refluxate with a pH less than 4 is associated with a higher incidence of severe disease. Over 80% of all reflux events with acid present in the esophagus are not sensed by the patient.[5]

Goals of Therapy

- Prevent recurrence of symptoms
- Alleviate symptoms

Patient Assessment

Figure 1 depicts an assessment plan for patients with dyspepsia. For uninvestigated dyspepsia, patient assessment should start with a review of alarm features (see Assessment of Abdominal Pain) and symptoms. If alarm features are not present take a history to rule out obvious sources of dyspepsia. Refer patients to a physician when serious pathology (e.g., peptic ulcer disease) is suspected. Refer patients with previous significant GI pathology for physician assessment in most cases, as well as patients with suspected upper airway manifestations of GERD. Symptoms of the latter include chronic cough (at least three weeks), globus sensation, wheezing, morning hoarseness, laryngitis and hiccuping. These symptoms usually necessitate intensive acid suppressive therapy.

Figure 1: **Assessment of Patients with Dyspepsia**[6,7]

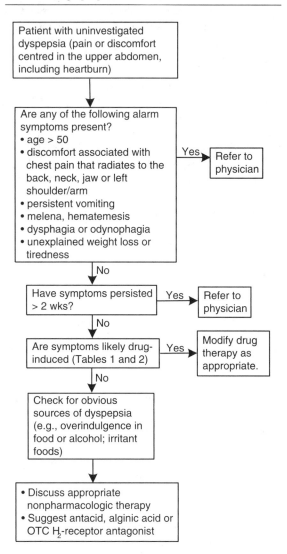

Nonpharmacologic Therapy

Overall, lifestyle modifications have not been well studied in a manner to assert their efficacy. Still many patients derive symptomatic benefit from inexpensive and usually simple measures. Some recommendations are provided in Tables 3 and 4. These likely have their greatest impact in patients with mild symptoms.[6]

Pharmacologic Therapy

Patients with moderate to severe or frequent symptoms of GERD should be treated with proton pump inhibitors, prokinetic agents or prescription doses of H_2-receptor antagonists. Antacids or sodium alginate can be used for breakthrough symptom control in these patients.

Few trials indicate that any therapy is of proven benefit for functional dyspepsia. Despite this, up to 98% of patients who seek medical help will be prescribed a drug. The natural history of functional dyspepsia is such that the majority of patients relapse without therapy.[2] However, only a minority of patients require continuous chronic therapy with prescription agents (i.e., proton pump inhibitors, prokinetic agents, H_2RAs). Of those requiring long-term therapy, a significant portion will have difficulty achieving complete symptom relief.[1]

Patients with minor or intermittent symptoms may use either an antacid, sodium alginate or nonprescription H_2-receptor antagonist (H_2RA) as symptomatic therapy.

Nonprescription agents used in the management of dyspepsia and GERD are described in Tables 5 and 6.

Antacids

There is little evidence to support the use of antacids in functional dyspepsia despite their widespread use.[11] In GERD, relief of heartburn occurs in approximately 20% of patients and the esophagus is protected from gastric contents for roughly 1.5 hours.[13] Antacids do provide therapeutic benefits in peptic ulcer disease (PUD) but their inconvenience (frequent dosing, volume and taste of suspensions) makes other acid suppression therapy more attractive. There are four basic types of antacids available: sodium bicarbonate and salts of aluminum, calcium and magnesium. In the most commonly available salt forms, the order of potency (based on weight) is aluminum hydroxide (least potent), followed by magnesium hydroxide, sodium bicarbonate and calcium carbonate (most potent). Some products contain a combination of salts, especially aluminum and magnesium. The rationale for the **aluminum–magnesium combination** is to offset the tendency of the respective agents to cause constipation and diarrhea. Table 5 provides an

---

Table 3: **Preventive and Nonpharmacologic Treatments for Dyspepsia**[1,8]

Lifestyle modifications:

Smaller, more frequent meals	Avoid foods that precipitate events
Quit smoking	Reduce alcohol intake
Reduce caffeine intake	Obtain ideal body weight
Stress reduction	Avoid lying down right after meals

Psychological:
Stress reduction management and other behavioral therapies
Patient reassurance in regards to the benign nature of the disorder

---

Table 4: **Lifestyle Modifications in the Treatment of GERD**[8]

Avoid foods which delay gastric emptying or increase acid exposure:

    chocolate, onions, carminatives (spearmint, peppermint), high fat meals. Limit excessive alcohol and nicotine consumption.

    Avoid lying down following meals, or eating before bedtime

Avoid large meals

Elevate head of bed roughly 10 cm

Avoid exercising or bending on a full stomach

Avoid tight-fitting clothes around the waist

Obtain ideal body weight (somewhat controversial)

Table 5: **Antacids**[9-12]

Antacid	Adverse effects	Drug interactions	Comments
Aluminum hydroxide	Constipation common. Hypophosphatemia has occurred with prolonged use or high doses. With long-term use in endstage renal disease can cause dementia and osteomalacia.	↓ absorption of quinolones, tetracyclines, digoxin, iron, isoniazid. May also decrease serum concentrations of ASA but only when large doses of ASA are used.	Avoid use in patients prone to constipation or bowel obstruction. Avoid long-term use in those with renal disease.
Calcium carbonate	Constipation, belching, flatulence. In high doses can cause milk-alkali syndrome or hypercalcemia.		Stimulates gastrin release, thereby increasing acid production. Up to 10% systemically absorbed. Calcium carbonate 500 mg = elemental calcium 200 mg.
Magnesium salts	Diarrhea common. May cause hypermagnesemia in those with renal dysfunction. Renal stones have been reported with the trisilicate salt.		Available as hydroxide, carbonate and trisilicate salts. Avoid use in those with renal failure.
Aluminum/magnesium combinations	Diarrhea. Long-term use in end-stage renal disease may cause osteomalacia and dementia. May cause hypermagnesemia in those with renal dysfunction		Avoid high doses or prolonged use in those with renal dysfunction. Constipating effect of aluminum is meant to offset the diarrhea-producing action of magnesium, but in most patients diarrhea predominates.
Alginic acid/antacid combinations	Adverse effects are those of the antacid		Available in combination with aluminum, magnesium and calcium antacids

overview of the different products and precautions with each agent. **Sodium bicarbonate** is only suitable for occasional use because of its high sodium content. It should be avoided in hypertension, CHF, renal dysfunction, edema, cirrhosis, pregnancy and other situations where excess sodium intake may be harmful. Adverse effects include flatulence, belching and abdominal distension. Sodium bicarbonate can also cause metabolic alkalosis, which may become significant in patients with renal dysfunction or with high doses or prolonged use.

Dosing equivalency amongst antacids is based upon their ability to neutralize a molar amount of acid, which is called the *acid neutralizing capacity (ANC)*. Doses of 10-40 mEq ANC are commonly recommended for functional dyspepsia in adults. GERD usually requires doses ranging from 80-160 mEq ANC. ANCs are dependent on the formulation and quantity of each antacid. Doses are therefore individual to each preparation. Because ANCs are not provided in

Canadian labeling information or product monographs, antacid doses are often based on manufacturers' recommendations. The most common dose is 10 to 20 mL or 2 to 4 tabs after meals and at bedtime, as needed. Doses used in GERD are higher (e.g., 30 mL one hour after meals and at bedtime).

Antacids are available in a variety of formulations. Suspensions have a greater acid neutralizing ability than solids because of their smaller particle size so are the preferred formulation if the patient can tolerate the taste.[10] Some tablet formulations overcome this difference by incorporating more active ingredient per dose. Other factors to consider in product selection include concomitant clinical conditions and cost. Sodium content is important in salt-sensitive patients Fortunately most products have a low sodium content.

Calcium carbonate is generally the preferred agent in patients with compromised renal function as these patients often have hypocalcemia and hyper-

Table 6: **Nonprescription H$_2$ Receptor Antagonists**[12]

Drug	OTC Dose	Drug Interactions	Adverse Effects	Comments
Famotidine	Adults and children ≥ 12 yrs: 10 mg prn. For prevention of acid-related symptoms associated with the consumption of food and/or beverage: 10 mg, 10-15 min before eating. Repeat prn. Max: 20 mg per day	No significant drug interactions	Headache and dizziness	Therapy should not exceed 2 wks of continuous treatment without medical consultation. Antacids may be given concomitantly if needed.
Ranitidine hydrochloride	Adults and children ≥ 16 yrs: 75 mg prn. For prevention of symptoms brought on by consuming food or beverages: 75 mg 30-60 min before eating a meal expected to cause symptoms. Max: 150 mg per day	Antacids – concurrent administration of antacid of medium to high potency (75 mEq) is not recommended. Do not take antacids within 0.5-1 h of ranitidine ingestion. Ketoconazole – Do not take ranitidine for at least 2 h after ketoconazole. Sucralfate – Take high doses of sucralfate 2 h after ranitidine administration.	Headache, nausea, vomiting and diarrhea	Patients are advised to consult their physician if symptoms get worse or continue after 2 wks of treatment. Use by children under 16 yrs of age should be supervised by a physician.

phospatemia. Patients with compromised renal function are predisposed to developing the *milk alkali syndrome*, a rare event associated with calcium carbonate use. This syndrome refers to the development of hypercalcemia, metabolic acidosis and renal insufficiency. Symptoms include nausea, vomiting, weakness and decreased mental status. Chronic ingestion of calcium carbonate may cause hypophosphatemia in predisposed patients. These are generally patients with poor dietary intake of phosphates such as malnourished alcoholics. Characteristic features of hypophosphatemia include muscle weakness, tiredness and, in its most severe form, breathing difficulties and heart failure.

Magnesium based antacids should be avoided in renal failure and limited in the elderly due to the risk of hypermagnesemia. Signs of magnesium toxicity include nausea and vomiting, flushing, drowsiness and muscle weakness.

Although antacids appear to be of limited to no benefit in NUD,[14,15] adequate doses (based on acid neutralizing capacity of agent) can raise the gastric pH sufficiently to prevent pepsin activation.[8] Antacids maintain an increased stomach pH only while they are in the stomach so the duration of effect is dependent on the gastric emptying time. After a large meal, the duration of effect may be one to three hours. On an empty stomach it may be less than one hour.[8] If the dose of antacid neutralizes 90% of stomach acid the pH only rises one full point (e.g., pH 1.3 to 2.3).[10] Despite the lack of evidence, many clinicians feel that antacids may resolve some dyspeptic symptoms (e.g., heartburn) related to the presence of acid in the stomach.[10] The lower esophageal sphincter pressure may also increase with the use of antacids, likely due to increased gastric pH.[8] Antacids have limited data to support their role in placebo-controlled trials.[8]

Alginic Acid
Alginic acid acts by physical means and tends to form a layer on top of the gastric contents. The rationale for its action is to be preferentially refluxed into the esophagus over other gastric contents, thereby

decreasing esophageal exposure to acid and bile. Evidence of this agent's ability to prevent or reverse esophageal injury is lacking. In short-term trials, the combination of alginic acid with an antacid has not produced a therapeutic advantage over antacid alone.[16]

H$_2$ Receptor Antagonists

OTC doses of H$_2$RAs decrease the frequency of night-time awakenings for GERD. Overall, symptom relief appears similar to antacids but the duration of effect is longer.[14] All H$_2$RAs appear to have similar efficacy.

Pregnancy and Lactation

See Chapter 53.

Monitoring of Therapy

Patients with symptoms that persist for more than two weeks should be referred to a physician. As well, patients with symptoms incompletely relieved by antacids and H$_2$RAs and recurring over a number of times per year should be referred.

Advice for the Patient

Counsel patients on:
- Nonpharmacologic interventions.
- Expected side effects and their management.
- Seeing a doctor if the condition lasts more than two weeks or if alarm features appear.

Suggested Readings

Bytzer P, Talley NJ. Dyspepsia. *Ann Intern Med* 2001; 134:815-22.

Dent J, Brun J, Fendrick AM, et al. An evidence-based appraisal of reflux disease management—the Genval Workshop Report. *Gut* 1999;44 (Suppl 2): S1-S16.

DeVault KR, Castell DO, et al. Updated guidelines for the diagnosis and treatment of gastroesophageal reflux disease. *Am J Gastroenterol* 1999;94(6): 1434-42.

van Zanten SJOV, Flook N, Chiba N, et al. An evidence-based approach to the management of uninvestigated dyspepsia in the era of *Helicobacter pylori. CMAJ* 2000;162 (12 Suppl): S3-S23.

References

1. McQuaid K. Dyspepsia. In: Feldman M, Scherschmidt BF, Sleisenger MH, eds. *Gastrointestinal and Liver Disease*. 6th ed. Philadelphia: WB Saunders, 1998:105-16.
2. AGA technical review: evaluation of dyspepsia. *Gastroenterol* 1998;114:582-95.
3. Tougas G, Chen Y, Hwang P, Liu MM, Eggleston A. Prevalence and impact of upper gastrointestinal symptoms in the Canadian population. *Am J Gastroenterol* 1999;94: 2845-54.
4. Bytzer P, Talley NJ. Dyspepsia. *Ann Intern Med* 2001;134: 815-822.
5. Fass R. Nonerosive reflux disease. Medscape Gastroenterology 2001;3(1). Available at: http://www.medscape.com/viewarticle/412762_6. Accessed Feb. 15, 2002.
6. van Zanten SJOV, Flook N, Chiba N, et al. An evidence-based approach to the management of uninvestigated dyspepsia in the era of *Helicobacter pylori. CMAJ* 2000;162 (12 Suppl): S3-S23.
7. Balestrini S. Help for heartburn. *Pharm Practice* 1996;12(2): 42-50.
8. Kitchen LI, Castell DO. Rationale and efficacy of conservative therapy for gastroesophageal reflux disease. *Arch Intern Med* 1991;151:448-53.
9. Hansten PD, Horn JT. *Drug Interactions: Analysis and Management*. St. Louis, MO: Facts and Comparisons, 2002.
10. McEvoy GK, ed. *AHFS Drug Information 2001*. Bethesda, MD: American Society of Health-System Pharmacists, 2000.
11. Maton PN, Burton ME. Antacids revisited. A review of their clinical pharmacology and recommended therapeutic use. *Drugs* 1999;57:855-70.
12. Repchinsky C, ed. *Compendium of Nonprescription Products 2001*. Ottawa, ON: Canadian Pharmacists Association, 2001.
13. DeVault KR. Overview of medical therapy for gastroesophageal reflux disease. *Gastro Clin N Am* 1999;28: 831-845.
14. Fisher RS, Parkman HP. Management of nonulcer dyspepsia. *N Engl J Med*; 1998;339:1376-81.
15. Holtmann G, Talley NJ. Functional dyspepsia. Current treatment recommendations. *Drugs* 1993;45:918-30.
16. Lanza FL, Sibley CM. Role of antacids in the management of disorders of the upper gastrointestinal tract. Review of clinical experience 1975-1985. *Am J Gastroenterol* 1987;82: 1223-1241.

Dyspepsia—Patient Information

Symptoms such as heartburn occur in virtually everyone. They tend to recur, are episodic and are not associated with an increased risk of serious diseases such as cancer.

See a physician if you experience any of the following:
- Severe abdominal pain
- Pain on the side of your abdomen that persists in the same spot
- Unexplained weight loss of more than 3 kg in the past six months
- New feelings of shortness of breath or chronic tiredness
- Difficult or painful swallowing
- Persistent vomiting
- Coughing up blood
- Blood in the stool or black, tarry stools

Your symptoms should not require more than two weeks of continuous medication every six months. If your symptoms are more frequent, last longer than two weeks or if there is incomplete response to therapy, see your doctor.

Liquid antacids should be shaken well and can be taken before or after meals.

Chapter 24

Gas and Cramps

Peter Thomson, BSc(Pharm), PharmD

Pathophysiology

Belching arises from air swallowed into the gastrointestinal (GI) tract. Gas may result from impaired absorption in the small intestine. Some substances metabolized in the large intestine cause bloating.[1] Bacteria in the colon can also produce gas from the conversion of sugars and proteins. Some foods may be prone to producing gas, such as beans and broccoli. Another source of gas in the intestines is swallowed air. This can occur more frequently following lying down after meals, causing air to become trapped below the lower esophageal sphincter with resulting bloating and pain.

Most gas that is belched comes from the esophagus rather than the stomach.[2] The ability to belch may be impaired by previous GI surgery (e.g., hernia repair) and body position (e.g., lying down).

Gas in the intestines (usually around 200 mL) comes from swallowed air, intestinal production and transfer from the circulation.[2] The passage of gas is an important physiologic function. In fact, the inability to pass gas may be a hallmark of serious GI pathology (e.g., small bowel obstruction). A normal number and volume of flatulence is not well defined. Generally, 10 to 15 episodes of flatulence per day is considered normal in a young adult. In the elderly, passage of flatulence may occur more frequently but this is not well defined.[3]

There is a poor correlation between the volume of gas in the intestines and patient symptoms. Patients complaining of excess gas often have only small volumes of gas present. There appears to be an increased nervous system sensitivity to intestinal volume (or distension) in these patients.[2] Pain from gas can arise anywhere in the abdomen. Irritable bowel syndrome (IBS) is a common functional disorder in those patients who have abdominal pain due to the presence of gas (see Chapter 25).[3]

Two common dietary sources of intestinal gas are lactose and nonabsorbable carbohydrates. A deficiency of lactase in the GI tract permits lactose to reach the colon where it is metabolized into fatty acids and two gases: hydrogen and carbon dioxide.[3] *Lactase deficiency* is primarily an acquired disorder, more commonly seen in older children and adults. Common causes include infectious gastroenteritis, giardiasis and celiac disease. Approximately 15% of Caucasians and 40% of Asians in the US are lactase deficient.[4] Common symptoms associated with lactose intolerance are bloating, flatulence and diarrhea. Patients may undergo testing to confirm the diagnosis (lactose tolerance test, hydrogen breath test).

Foul-smelling flatulence does not arise from common gases in the GI tract. Rather, trace amounts of other gases such as methyl sulfides and indole are responsible.[3] Sulfur is a component of many foul-smelling gases.

Infant colic refers to severe, paroxysmal crying in otherwise healthy, well-fed infants (see Chapter 26).

Goals of Therapy

- Relieve symptoms (pain, bloating, abnormal flatulence and belching)
- Educate patient regarding preventive measures

Patient Assessment (Figure 1)

A patient complaint of excess gas, either belching or flatulence, is very subjective. Usually the complaint results when there is an increase from what they perceive as their normal amount. Excess gas may arise

Figure 1: **Assessment of Patients with Gas and Cramps**

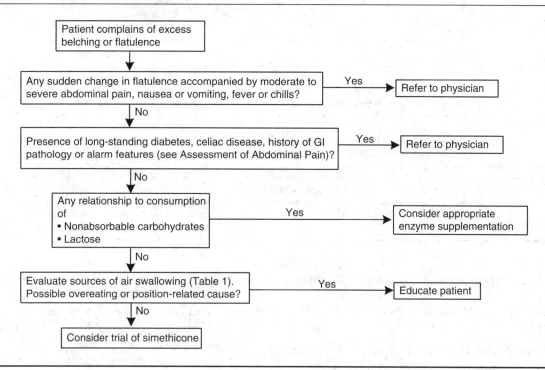

Patient complains of excess belching or flatulence

↓

Any sudden change in flatulence accompanied by moderate to severe abdominal pain, nausea or vomiting, fever or chills? — Yes → Refer to physician

↓ No

Presence of long-standing diabetes, celiac disease, history of GI pathology or alarm features (see Assessment of Abdominal Pain)? — Yes → Refer to physician

↓ No

Any relationship to consumption of
• Nonabsorbable carbohydrates
• Lactose — Yes → Consider appropriate enzyme supplementation

↓ No

Evaluate sources of air swallowing (Table 1). Possible overeating or position-related cause? — Yes → Educate patient

↓ No

Consider trial of simethicone

from dietary sources. Evaluate dietary sources such as nonabsorbed carbohydrates found in some vegetables and beans. Baked beans do increase the volume of flatulence. As well, consider any history of milk intolerance (i.e., lactose intolerance).

Actual pathology may arise from motility disorders and from disorders that affect the GI tract. Refer patients with a history of pathology that may affect the GI tract or any alarm features of abdominal pain (see Abdominal Pain Assessment) to a physician. Long-standing diabetes may lead to the development of gastroparesis, usually associated with nausea and vomiting. Suspect celiac disease in patients with diarrhea, weight loss and tiredness (anemia).

Abdominal fullness and pain arising when standing and relieved on lying down may be due to decreased tone of the rectus muscle. Previous childbirth and abdominal surgeries are risk factors for this condition.[3]

When evaluating flatulence, it is important to elucidate a history from the patient. New, sudden changes in flatulence, associated with moderate to severe abdominal pain, nausea or vomiting, fever or chills warrant physician referral. New symptoms of flatulence lasting more than a few days, especially if fever or chills are present, should raise the concern of intestinal parasites such as *G. lamblia* ("beaver fever"). Question patients about sources of drinking water in these circumstances. Prokinetic drugs may increase the number of episodes of flatulence per day.[2]

Nonpharmacologic Therapy

With belching, seek sources of swallowed air. Table 1 provides a list of some common causes. Some patients gulp air with each belch. This is often associated with multiple small belches over seconds. Educating the patient to stop gulping air with each belch should relieve this. Even telling the patient to stop belching should help.[3] Other sources of air swallowing are postnasal drip, poorly fitting dentures and excess salivation (e.g., chewing gum, chomping on cigars) and ingestion of gas-producing or releasing substances

Table 1: **Causes of Gas Disorders**[3]

Primary disorder	Potential causes	Treatment
Belching	Postnasal drip	Decongestant
	Poorly fitting dentures	Properly fitting dentures
	Increased salivation from cigar smoking, chewing gum and hard candies	Reduce intake
	Carbonated beverages	Reduce intake
Flatulence	Poorly absorbed carbohydrates (e.g., broccoli, cabbage, beans, cauliflower)	Reduce intake Alpha-D-galactosidase
	Sorbitol and fructose (e.g., sugarless gum, artificial sweeteners)	Reduce intake
	Lactase deficiency (milk products)	Reduce intake Lactase replacement

(e.g., carbonated beverages, sodium bicarbonate). Encourage patients to eat their meals slowly to decrease the likelihood of gulping air when they swallow.

The feeling of bloating with the desire to belch can simply be due to overeating. Very large meals ingested in the late evening may make patients more symptomatic. Eating less and earlier in the day may reduce this. Abdominal cramping may arise from a number of dietary and pharmaceutical sources, such as osmotic laxatives.

Alpha-D-galactosidase supplements (e.g., Beano®) may be used prior to the ingestion of nonabsorbable carbohydrates such as those found in brown beans. Beano® has established efficacy in reducing symptoms of flatulence associated with bean ingestion but evidence for other unabsorbed carbohydrates (e.g., broccoli, cauliflower and cabbage) is lacking.[3] The manufacturer suggests a role for a wider variety of alpha-linked sugar-containing products including cereals, nuts, grains, most legumes and cruciferous vegetables. Enzyme products should not be put on hot foods (i.e., too hot to eat or during cooking) as heat renders the enzyme inactive. Instruct patients to place the liquid enzyme on the first spoonful of food.

Lactase supplementation taken with or prior to ingestion of lactose (e.g., dairy products) can prevent flatulence in patients with lactase deficiency. The amount of supplementation required is dependent on the amount of lactose ingested. Milk products still must be taken in moderation as large doses of lactose will not be completely broken down by the lactase supplement. Liquid drops of the enzyme can be added to a carton of milk and left stored for 24 hours in the fridge to break down the lactose. Lactaid® milk is readily available. Some dairy products may not produce symptoms (e.g., yogurt may contain lactase-producing bacteria). Dieticians can supply charts with the lactose content of dairy products to assist patients with their food selections. Following infectious gastroenteritis, it may be a number of months before lactase activity returns to normal.

Pharmacologic Therapy (Table 2)

Simethicone acts by preventing bubbling of liquids in the stomach. It does not appear to be absorbed from the GI tract and does not appear to have any significant adverse effects. Data are lacking for a clear benefit with this agent for belching.[3]

In patients with abdominal pain associated with intestinal gas, prokinetic agents such as metoclopramide or domperidone may provide symptomatic relief.[2] In most cases, prescription drug therapy is not employed unless there is underlying pathology affecting GI motility.

Table 2: **Nonprescription Drugs Used to Treat Gas and Cramps**[5,6]

Generic names	Usual adult dose/meal	Adverse effects
Alpha-D-galactosidase	150-450 GalU with the first bite of food	Rare allergic reactions (rash, pruritus)
Lactase	3000-9000 FCC lactase units	No apparent adverse effects from product itself; large doses of lactose incompletely hydrolyzed
Simethicone	80-160 mg	None reported

GalU = galactose units; FCC = Food Chemical Codex

Alternative Therapy

Peppermint probably acts by reducing lower esophageal sphincter pressure, theoretically making it easier to pass gas from the stomach into the esophagus. This pressure reduction potentially could increase the likelihood of GERD.

Garlic and ginger are other alternative products promoted for treatment of intestinal gas. However, there is insufficient evidence to recommend their use.

Monitoring of Therapy

Refer patients with symptoms persisting for more than one to two weeks despite therapy to a physician.

Exclusion diets (e.g., of lactose or nonabsorbed carbohydrates) should be monitored for effective resolution of symptoms. Monitor quantity of supplements used to assess if there is symptomatic relief with the agents. If symptoms persist, both diet and other sources of the triggers should be more rigourously evaluated (e.g., lactose in medications and herbals).

Suggested Readings

Clearfield HR. Clinical intestinal gas syndromes. *Prim Care* 1996;23:621-628.

Strocchi A, Levitt MD. Intestinal gas. In: Feldman M, Scherschmidt BF, Sleisenger MH, eds. *Gastrointestinal and Liver Disease*. 6th ed. Philadelphia, PA: WB Saunders, 1998:153-160.

References

1. Camilleri M. Management of the irritable bowel syndrome. *Gastroenterology* 2001;120:652-68.
2. Strocchi A, Levitt MD. Intestinal gas. In: Feldman M, Scherschmidt BF, Sleisenger MH, eds. *Gastrointestinal and Liver Disease*. 6th ed. Philadelphia, PA: WB Saunders, 1998:153-160.
3. Clearfield HR. Clinical intestinal gas syndromes. *Prim Care* 1996;23:621-628.
4. Ulshen M. Malabsorptive disorders. In: Behrman RE, Kliegman RM, Jensen HB, eds. *Nelsons's Textbook of Pediatrics*. 16th ed. Toronto, ON: WB Saunders, 2000:1159-71.
5. Repchinksy C, ed. *Compendium of Nonprescription Products*. Ottawa, ON: Canadian Pharmacists Association, 2001.
6. McEvoy GK, ed. *American Hospital Formulary Service Drug Information 2001*. Bethesda, MD: American Society of Health-System Pharmacists, 2001.

Gas and Cramps—Patient Information

Excess belching (burping) is often caused by swallowed air or things you eat that release gas. Some things you can do to help are:

- Do not chew gum or cigars.
- Do not drink carbonated beverages such as colas.
- Eat your meals slowly.

If you feel bloated, avoid eating large meals, especially late in the day.

If your gas and cramps seem to be related to food, talk to your pharmacist. There may be a medication that may help you.

See your doctor if:

- Your symptoms persist for more than one to two weeks.
- You experience unintended weight loss.
- Your stools dramatically change in color (e.g., pale white stools, black tar-like) or contain blood.

Changing what you eat may help. Check with a health professional before making changes to your diet.

Chapter 25

Irritable Bowel Syndrome

Peter Thomson, BSc(Pharm), PharmD

Generalizations about irritable bowel syndrome (IBS) are difficult as patient presentation varies. The key features of IBS are abdominal pain associated with an altered bowel pattern. Symptoms of IBS include bloating, cramping and diarrhea that often follow eating. IBS is commonly defined as abdominal pain or discomfort for at least 12 weeks, that need not be consecutive, in the past 12 months that has two of the following three features: relieved by defecation, onset associated with a change in stool frequency or onset associated with a change in stool form.[1] Other symptoms that help to substantiate the diagnosis of IBS are alterations in stool frequency, form or passage; abdominal bloating or distension or passage of mucus in the stool.[1] Symptoms of IBS not related to the GI tract include tiredness, insomnia, dysuria and back pain.[2]

IBS can be divided into diarrhea or constipation predominant subtypes. Unfortunately, subtype differentiation does not correlate with pathophysiologic features on a consistent basis[2] and some symptoms are found in both subtypes of IBS.

Likely three-quarters of all IBS sufferers do not seek medical care. Patients more likely to seek a physician are those with more pain and those with more psychological symptoms.[2,3] The frequency at which IBS is found in a population depends on whether it is defined as meeting the diagnostic criteria of IBS (approximately 3%) or just presence of its symptoms (up to 20%).[4] Females are more likely to seek medical help for IBS but there does not appear to be recognizable risk factors based on sex or race. IBS accounts for about 25% of all gastroenterology specialist appointments.[4]

Pathophysiology

There are a variety of pathophysiologic changes in subgroups of patients with IBS. These include altered neurologic function and sensitivity to stimuli, altered GI motility (including both large and small bowel) and abnormal psychosocial features.

Nociceptive inputs for the GI tract provide input to pain centres that are augmented by psychosocial factors leading to the patient's sensation and interpretation of pain.[5] Patients are often found to have increased sensitivity to distension. This has been seen in the rectum, ileum and esophagus.[2,3] Pain may be associated with altered motility in the small intestine. An altered balance of neurotransmitters in the GI tract may also be involved. Stress is known to cause changes in GI motility in both the small and large intestine.[3]

Within referral clinics, reports of psychological features can be high, with over half of patients meeting the clinical criteria for depression.[6] In addition, anxiety and somatization disorders also appear more frequently in patients with IBS. Abuse (physical, sexual) may be reported in one-third of subjects. In IBS patients who do not seek physician assessment, it is not certain that these psychological features are present.

Patients frequently report food intolerance in IBS yet the incidence of food allergies is uncommon. Approximately 10% of IBS patients may be lactose intolerant. Eliminating lactose from the diet usually does not resolve the symptoms of IBS.[2] Bile acids are proposed precipitants in IBS.

After an acute illness with a GI pathogen (e.g., *Campylobacter, Shigella, Salmonella*), some individuals may develop persistent IBS symptoms. Likely less than one-third of IBS can be related to an infectious precipitant.[4]

Goals of Therapy

- Improve quality of life by minimizing (not eliminating) symptoms
- Reassure patient regarding benign nature of IBS

Patient Assessment (Figure 1)

Refer patients with alarm features (see Abdominal Pain Assessment) or blood in the stool to a physician for assessment. Also consider the duration and course of symptoms. If symptoms are recurrent over months to years they are suggestive of a functional GI disorder

Figure 1: **Assessment of Patients with Irritable Bowel Syndrome**

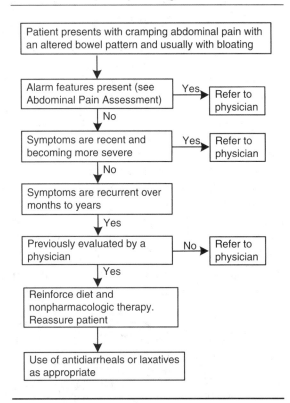

such as IBS. Symptoms of recent onset or becoming steadily more severe, especially over a short time period, are suggestive of an organic GI disorder (e.g., inflammatory bowel disease) that requires physician assessment. Most patients with symptoms of IBS should initially undergo a basic diagnostic work-up by a physician to rule out organic GI disorders such as infections.

Acute flares of IBS may be altered by removing triggers and dealing with psychological issues that affect the patient. A careful medication history should be performed on all patients. Prescription medications, OTCs and herbals all can be potential sources of GI adverse effects.

The most common foods associated with triggering IBS are wheat and dairy products. Other reported triggers include other grains (corn and oats), caffeine, alcohol and fat.[7] Contributing factors can include simple sugar alternatives such as lactose, fructose (e.g., fruit juices), sorbitol (e.g., sugar free gum) and excess or insufficient intake of dietary fibre.

The most important complications of IBS are the loss of productivity and consumption of health care resources related to the disorder. Many patients see a number of different physicians and other health care providers. Unrealistic expectations can arise, especially with regard to drug therapy. The patient's goals may be unrealistic and goal planning with the patient and other health providers is an important part of the treatment plan. Prevention is difficult to achieve on a consistent basis.

Nonpharmacologic Therapy

Patient symptoms are a guide to most therapeutic plans (e.g., pain, bloating, gas, diarrhea, constipation). A key component of the therapeutic plan is patient reassurance. The likelihood of a serious organic GI disease such as cancer is likely no different in IBS than the general population. In general, therapies are likely to offer only limited relief over the long term. Counseling patients on the high likelihood for recurrence is important.

Nondrug therapies for IBS include regulating dietary fibre and lactose intake, stress management and counseling for psychological issues. Fibre may provide beneficial effects through a number of mechanisms such as reducing pressure within the intestines, leading to less pain, and reducing gas and bloating by binding bile salts. Lactose intolerance should be considered and consumption of dairy products may be decreased, at least on a trial basis.

Avoidance of lifestyle triggers such as excess caffeine or fruit intake is a usual component of the treatment plan. Exclusion diets are of limited benefit and probably are most helpful in reducing gas.[4] If patients insist on dietary restrictions they should be monitored to avoid nutritional deficiencies. This may be accomplished with guidance from a dietician. There appears to be a high placebo response to exclusion diets.

Pharmacologic Therapy

There are virtually no well-designed, placebo-controlled trials evaluating drug therapies in IBS.[8] In general, drug therapies are only marginally more effective than placebo over the long term. Short-term results over a few weeks may be dramatic as there is a high placebo response (roughly 50%) to therapy in IBS.[7] To date, only psychological and dietary treatments have been found to provide benefits over the long term.[2] With any therapy that is initiated, four

weeks is generally considered the minimum length needed to determine efficacy.

Coexisting features of a psychiatric illness do not appear to affect the response to antidepressants. **Antidepressants** appear most effective in patients with more pain-related symptoms than abnormal bowel habit symptoms.[6] There are no clear data establishing therapeutic superiority amongst the antidepressants. Patient response to antidepressants may vary so trying a different antidepressant may be worthwhile.

Antispasmodics may provide some relief in IBS patients with abdominal pain, distension or bloating. They include dicyclomine, clidinium, pinaverium, trimebutine and hyoscine. Their mechanism of action is thought to be through relaxation of smooth muscle. Generally, they are not recommended for regular use as tolerance appears to develop, but may be used up to twice daily as needed for acute flares.[4] Other treatments of abdominal pain include serotonin (5-HT) receptor agonists (e.g., 5-HT$_4$) and antagonists (e.g., 5-HT$_3$). The use of alternative therapies including herbals appears to be higher in IBS than in some organic GI disorders.[4]

Nonprescription agents used in the management of IBS are described in Table 1.

Table 1: **Nonprescription Therapy for IBS**[3,9,10,13]

Drug	Dose	Adverse effects	Comments
Dicyclomine	10-20 mg TID-QID PRN abdominal pain	Dry mouth, drowsiness, constipation, confusion, blurred vision	Avoid in patients with tachyarrhythmias, angle-closure glaucoma, urinary retention, hyperthyroidism. The elderly are more susceptible to adverse effects. Has been used in doses of up to 40 mg QID
Loperamide	2-4 mg up to four times daily	Abdominal cramps, drowsiness, dry mouth, nausea and vomiting, skin rash	Individual dose varies; can cause constipation. No significant drug interactions
Magnesium hydroxide	30-60 mL per day	Diarrhea. Risk of hypermagnesemia increased in patients with renal dysfunction.	Avoid in patients with renal dysfunction
Lactulose	15-60 mL per day in one or two divided doses	Flatulence, abdominal cramps, diarrhea. Nausea more common with higher doses	May cause bloating. No significant drug interactions

General Treatment Approach for Specific Subtypes of IBS[4]

Constipation Predominant
The available evidence does not clearly establish the benefit of bulking agents in constipation predominant IBS.[11] However, fibre supplementation is commonly used as first line treatment. Initiate therapy with dietary measures that increase fibre intake such as bran or psyllium. Assess the patient's current diet to see if optimal fibre intake is already present (i.e., 20 to 30 g per day). Patients who fail fibre ($\geq$ 30 g per day) should be considered for use of an osmotic laxative such as magnesium hydroxide or lactulose.

Diarrhea Predominant IBS
Antidiarrheals are usually tried, **loperamide** being the most common. **Codeine** is an alternative. In patients with diarrhea symptoms the target intake of fibre is usually 30 g per day. Patients should generally start at a lower intake and gradually increase their fibre to reach this goal. Lactose intolerance should be excluded in all patients with diarrhea predominant IBS. The bile salt binding agent **cholestyramine** is used mostly in patients with bile salt malabsorption but may be tried in these patients as well.

Bloating and Gas Predominant IBS
This form is usually managed using dietary changes (i.e., limitation of fibre intake and avoidance of gas-producing vegetables). **Antispasmodics** are most commonly used in this form of IBS. **Antidepressants** may also have a role. Evidence for use of promotility agents is uncertain. Peppermint oil has been used but evidence of benefit is inconclusive.[11] Agents under investigation include neurokinin, alpha$_2$-antagonists, κ-opioid agonists, M3-receptor antagonists and alpha$_2$-agonists.[12]

Monitoring of Therapy

Monitor diets as they often become more restrictive over time. Many patients associate symptom changes with their diet. Advise patients of the alarm features of serious GI pathology (see Abdominal Pain Assessment).

Symptoms often recur or present differently over the course of time. In more difficult cases, patient dissatisfaction with care increases. A long-term care plan for the patient is important as they frequently seek new alternative sources of heath care to deal with persisting or recurrent symptoms. Good communication with other health care providers is especially important in this difficult-to-manage group of functional GI disorder patients.

Most therapeutic trials should be at least one month in length. Antidepressants often require six weeks or more to assess their effectiveness. More than one antidepressant is often tried as interpatient variability in response may occur.

Resource Tips

American Gastroenterology Association. Digestive Health Resource Center: http://www.gastro.org/public/digestinfo.html.

Suggested Readings

Miller SJ, Heck AM. Irritable bowel syndrome. *US Pharm* 2000;25(11 Suppl): 3-13. Also available at: http://www.uspharmacist.com/newlook/ce/ibs/lesson.CFM.

Talley NJ, Stanghellini B, Heading R, et al. Functional gastroduodenal disorders (ROME II). *Gut* 1999;45 (suppl 2): II37-42.

References

1. Thompson WG, Longstreth GF, Drossman DA, Heaton KW, Irvine EJ, Muller-Lissner SA. Functional bowel disorders and functional abdominal pain. *Gut* 1999;45 (suppl II): II43-47.
2. Jones J, Boorman J, Cann P, et al. British Society of Gastroenterology guidelines for the management of the irritable bowel syndrome. *Gut* 2000;47 (suppl II): II 1-19.
3. Horwitz BJ, Fisher RS. The irritable bowel syndrome. *N Engl J Med* 2001;344:1846-50.
4. Camilleri M. Management of the irritable bowel syndrome. *Gastroenterology* 2001;120(3):652-68.
5. Drossman DA. Diagnosing and treating patients with refractory functional gastrointestinal disorders. *Ann Intern Med* 1995;123:688-97.
6. Clouse RE. Antidepressants for functional gastrointestinal syndromes. *Dig Dis Sci* 1994;39:2352-63.
7. American Dietetic Association/Dieticians of Canada. *Manual of Clinical Dietetics.* 6th ed. Chicago, IL: American Dietetic Association, 2000.
8. Akehurst R, Keltenthaler E. Treatment of irritable bowel syndrome: a review of randomised controlled trials. *Gut* 2001; 48(2):272-82.

9. Paterson WG, Thompson WG, Vanner SJ, et al. Recommendations for the management of irritable bowel syndrome in family practice. *CMAJ* 1999;161(2):154-60.

10. Miller SJ, Heck AM. Irritable bowel syndrome. *US Pharm* 2000; 25(11 Suppl): 3-13. Also available at: http://www.uspharmacist.com/newlook/ce/ibs/lesson.CFM. Accessed Feb. 14, 2002.

11. Jailwala J, Imperiale TF, Kroenke K. Pharmacologic treatment of the irritable bowel syndrome: a systematic review of randomized, controlled trials. *Ann Intern Med* 2000;133: 136-147.

12. De Schryver AMP, Samsom M. New developments in the treatment of irritable bowel syndrome. *Scand J Gastroenterol Suppl* 2000;232:38-42.

13. McEvoy GK, ed. *American Hospital Formulary Service Drug Information 2001.* Bethesda, MD: American Society of Health-System Pharmacists, 2001.

Irritable Bowel Syndrome—Patient Information

- IBS is usually a chronic disorder that tends to recur unpredictably. It is unlikely that any therapy will completely resolve all symptoms for the rest of your life.
- It is not associated with a higher risk of serious gastrointestinal diseases, like stomach cancer.
- Keep track of the frequency of stools if they are irregular. See your doctor if the stools dramatically change in color (e.g., pale white or black tar-like stools) or contain blood.
- See your doctor if you unintentionally lose weight greater than 3 kg (about six or seven pounds) over six months.

- Stress may aggravate the condition. Try to develop techniques to help reduce stress.
- See your doctor if symptoms are very severe or persist for more than three days in a row.
- Avoid caffeine; sugarless gums or candies and eating too much fruit.
- Changing your lifestyle may help to decrease the frequency of symptoms. Try diet restrictions only after talking with a health care professional.

Chapter 26

Infant Colic

Shelita Dattani, BSc(Pharm), PharmD

Pathophysiology

Colic is reported in approximately 10 to 20% of healthy infants.[1,2] The most accepted definition of colic is the Wessel "rule of three" which defines colic as unexplained paroxysmal bouts of fussing and crying that last more than three hours a day, for more than three days a week, and for greater than three weeks.[1,3]

The term colic is imprecise and frequently overused. Although crying is an integral component of colic, a behavioral definition includes increased motor activity and altered patterns of sleeping and eating.[1,4] It is often associated with clenched fists, reddening of the face, drawing up of the legs, abdominal distension and flatus.[1] Occasionally, excessive regurgitation and vomiting can occur.[1,5,6]

The diagnosis of colic is considered when an otherwise thriving infant presents with crying. It usually starts around the second week of life and is most common in infants aged four to six weeks. It gradually improves and becomes uncommon at three to four months of age and beyond. A normal diurnal variation has been noted, with crying more often in the late afternoon or evening. Males and females are affected with equal frequency and infants from families with higher socioeconomic status seem to be more affected.[1,3,7] Limited data suggest that colic may be more likely in babies whose mothers smoke.[7] Colic occurs in both breastfed and formula-fed babies.[1,7]

The proposed causes of colic include organic, behavioral and psychological components (Table 1).[4] A combination of these factors may be implicated in any given infant. Some experts feel that colic may be best viewed as a clinical manifestation of normal emotional development, in which an infant has diminished capacity to regulate crying duration.[4,8] Parents will become frustrated if they try to pinpoint the exact cause of the baby's colic.

Goals of Therapy[4,7]

- Provide parental reassurance as necessary
- Minimize parental stress and frustration and help strengthen coping skills
- Control symptoms associated with colic
- Emphasize the importance of consoling the infant, even if efforts seem fruitless. Do not advocate a "wait it out" approach—this may interfere with parent-child bonding
- Provide information on community support to give parents the opportunity to share and consult with other parents

Table 1: **Proposed Causes of Infant Colic**[1,7,9]

Proposed cause	Possible rationale
Organic	Carbohydrate intolerance, intestinal gas, motility disorder, gastroesophageal reflux, immature central and autonomic nervous system, milk or food allergy.
Behavioral	Improper feeding or feeding technique, smoking in the home.
Psychological	Inadequate social network, parental anxiety and stress, maternal postpartum depression.

Patient Assessment

Table 2 lists some common causes of crying and their symptoms, and provides some basic management strategies to deal with the problem once obvious sources of crying have been eliminated (e.g., dirty diaper, hunger). Crying is one of the few ways a baby can communicate, and the parental response reassures the infant that someone is listening. The strategies below can be attempted in any order. If the baby continues to cry, parents should move on to another strategy and not persist in any one measure.[4]

An assessment plan for infants with colic is illustrated in Figure 1. If crying persists after the parents undergo a trial of simple management strategies, refer them to their physician who will want to perform a complete history and physical examination to rule out any organic causes of crying or underlying medical conditions.

Nonpharmacologic Therapy

Nonpharmacologic therapy is the mainstay of treatment of colic. Since the cause of colic is unknown, there are as many nonpharmacologic treatments as there are proposed etiologies. Furthermore, there is a lack of evidence to support the efficacy of these interventions.[5] Pharmacists and other health care professionals should take a holistic approach when advising parents of treatment strategies. Remind parents that any given strategy may or may not work and that flexibility is essential to success.

Table 2: **Behavioral Management Strategies for Parents of Crying Babies**[1,4,10]

Problem	Symptoms	Potential strategies
Hunger	Crying between feedings. Inadequate weight gain	Hunger periods often do not follow a regular pattern. Increase feeding frequency as needed and do not be concerned about overfeeding.
Need to suck	Refusing bottle or breast. Baby may want to suck	Use a pacifier or allow baby to suck on fist or fingers if that is comforting.
Overheating	Crying when tightly swaddled or layered	Loosen covers, reduce clothing, reduce room temperature.
Need for attention or physical contact	Crying or fussiness when left alone	Hold, rock or cuddle baby. Do not worry about spoiling the infant or contributing to a bad habit.
Insomnia	Crying, inability to sleep at bedtime	Avoid excessive stimulation or arousal before bedtime.
Tired	Crying or fussiness when handled	Put the baby down in a dark, quiet room. Unless crying excessively, babies can be left alone for short intervals to see if they will fall asleep on their own. Babies who are crying loudly should be picked up and held or rocked quietly until they fall asleep.
Lack of stimulation	Crying or fussiness when left alone	Play with the baby, provide a visual or auditory distraction, or place baby in an infant seat or swing where there is a lot of activity (e.g., kitchen).
Ear infection	Crying or irritability; infant may be fingering or pulling on ear. Infant may not be sleeping or eating well. May be accompanied by or preceded by a cold. Occasionally, fluid may be draining out of the ear canal. Fever may be present (if temperature > 39°C, refer to physician immediately even if other symptoms of ear infection are absent).	Refer to physician.
Teething	Crying, excessive salivation, inflamed gums. Typically begins after 5 mos of age.	Provide teething rings or biscuits.

Figure 1: **Assessment of Infants with Suspected Colic**

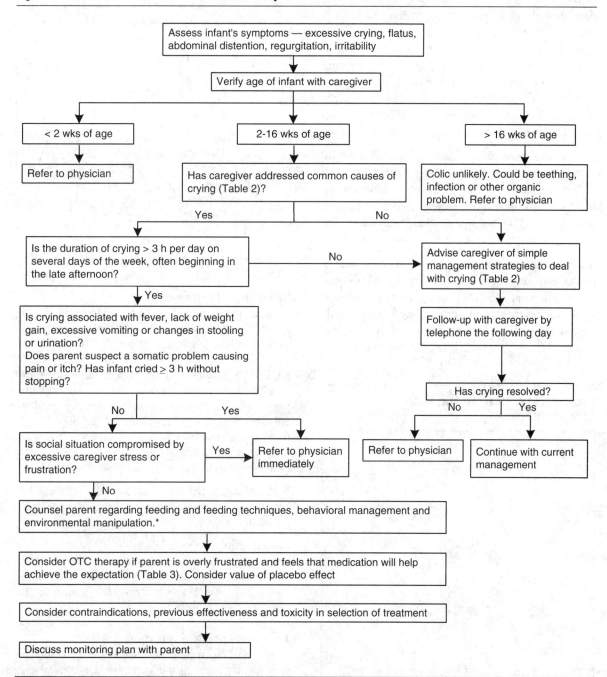

Recommend that caregiver maintain a colic diary for 48 to 72 hours that documents crying and fussing spells and associated symptoms. Parents should also log sleeping, feeding, playtime and bowel movements in this diary. (See Patient Information.)

Physical Methods

Methods that have been attempted include gentle pressure to the abdomen, carrying, rocking, swaddling, skin-to-skin contact, use of infant carriers and massage. There are several forms of massage, including whole-body massage and belly massage (infant facing downward in one hand with bottom in highest position. Parent starts from the navel and massages abdomen in clockwise motion).[6,11,12] Figures 2 and 3 illustrate the correct method of belly massage.

Babies who demonstrate possible gastric distress by pulling their legs up and arching their backs may derive some relief if their legs are gently pushed back and forth, in an altering or "bicycle" motion. Repetitive motion relaxes infants and physical contact from the parent or caregiver may have a calming effect.[1,4]

Warm baths and hot water bottles covered with a cloth may relieve rectal spasm. Parents should test hot water with a finger before pouring it into a hot water bottle, to prevent burning and scalding.[4] Heating pads should not be used due to the risk of burning the infant.

Figure 2: **How to Hold the Baby**

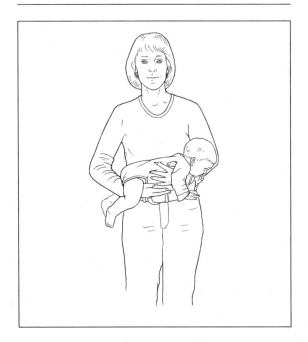

Figure 3: **How to Massage the Baby**

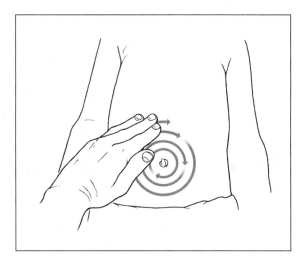

Behavioral Management

A **colic diary** that documents crying and fussing spells can help parents and the health care professional create a management strategy by helping to establish some patterns in the infant's day. Parents can log their behaviors, look for patterns and then try to modify these behaviors to see if the situation improves. A routine schedule for feeding, holding, playtime and general care can be developed once patterns are established. At the very least, keeping a diary gives a parent a better sense of control and a clearer perspective of a frustrating situation.[1,13]

It is imperative that the caregiver has sufficient rest breaks when symptoms can no longer be tolerated. Parental tension will make everyone's distress worse.

Even though colic itself is usually self-limiting for the infant, it can take some time to repair the parent-infant attachment relationship. The physician may refer the family to mental health professionals, such as counselors or psychologists.[1,4]

Environmental Manipulation

"White noise" may be comforting to some infants. This may involve running the vacuum cleaner or placing the infant securely in a car seat on the top of the washer or the dryer. Many colicky infants will stop crying and fall asleep when riding in a car. Car-ride simulation devices are also available.[1]

The smooth, repetitive motion of baby swings may pacify anxious infants.

If parents try a series of calming techniques without using any one consistently for at least a day, the infant may get overstimulated, which can make the colicky situation worse. Other parents give up trying and withdraw from their infants, which can lead to a spiraling of parent and infant stress.[1,4]

Dietary Manipulation

The majority of the dietary manipulations recommended below require specialized follow-up, and although pharmacists may suggest attempting these strategies, most are not likely to be involved in implementing them.

Breastfeeding

Breastfeeding should be continued as weaning a colicky infant to formula can result in symptoms worsening.[1]

Some infants with colic may have symptoms caused at least in part by allergy.[14] Some data demonstrate that symptoms of colic may improve when cow's milk is removed from the mother's diet.[1,14] Therefore, health care professionals may advise mothers to avoid all cow's milk protein and dairy products for one to two weeks. If a mother decides to do this, recommend calcium supplements.

Foods noted to aggravate colic in breastfed infants include cabbage, broccoli, caffeine, citrus fruit and chocolate. There are limited data suggesting that eliminating these foods from the mother's diet for a period of time may help with colicky symptoms.[1,14,15]

Formula Feeding

Substituting traditional formulas with soy or hypoallergenic formula may reduce duration of crying by approximately 20%. The majority of infants who do not respond to soy formulas later respond to hypoallergenic formula.[14,15] Lactose-reduced formula has not been shown to reduce crying in colicky newborns.[4,7,14,15] The addition of fibre to formula is not effective.[7,14]

If formula changes are made, they should not be pursued if symptoms do not improve after one week.[4] Frequent formula changes are not recommended.[9]

Feeding Techniques

There are many simple techniques that can be helpful in feeding a colicky bottle-fed infant.

- To prevent regurgitation and promote the exit of swallowed air, infants should be held in a vertical position during feeding with the head higher than the feet.[1,15,16]
- It is also important to use the correct bottle and nipple size for the infant's age. Curved bottles allow the infant to be fed while sitting up, and bottles with a collapsible bag may decrease air swallowing. Pharmacists can recommend changing the nipple of the bottle to one with a smaller hole or anticolic design to prevent frequent colic attacks. The effects of these measures have not been formally studied.[1]
- Infants should be burped in an upright position, with the baby held over the shoulder or in a gentle chin grasp. Burping should be encouraged after every 30 to 60 mL of formula or after every 5 to 10 minutes of breastfeeding.[1,4]

Pharmacologic Therapy

Over the years, different medications have been recommended for the management of colic. The efficacy of pharmacologic agents in the treatment of colic is difficult to assess due to the highly subjective nature of the problem, conflicting results and high placebo effect noted in clinical trials.[5,14] Furthermore, the age of the patient group and fear of possible harm to the infant limit research into medications that are safe and effective.[11]

Table 3 describes various pharmacologic therapies for colic. A herbal tea containing a mixture of chamomile, balmmint, fennel, licorice and vervain has also been used with some success. However, the commercial preparation studied is not available in Canada and the amount of each herb that was contained in the tea is unknown.

If pharmacologic therapy is tried:

- Ensure that nonpharmacologic measures have been used to their fullest potential
- Use the lowest effective dose
- Use intermittent dosing only when necessary based on symptoms
- Be aware that the agents available provide questionable benefit and are not routinely recommended in the treatment of colic

Table 3: **Pharmacologic Therapy for Infant Colic**[1,4,7,14]

Agent	Effective dose	Mechanism of effect	Onset	Side effects	Comments
Gripe water	2.5-5 mL as necessary with or after each feeding Maximum: 40 mL per 24 h	Contains carminatives such as anise oil, dill oil and fennel oil, which are proposed to help in elimination of gas. Also contains sodium bicarbonate which reacts with gastric acid to form carbon dioxide and water. The gas formed actually increases infant's flatulence.	Within minutes (exact onset unknown)	Flatulence	Not recommended — no proven clinical benefit. Some products contain small percentage of alcohol. Alcohol-free products are available.
Dicyclomine 2 mg/mL syrup	Infants over 6 mos of age: 5-10 mg 3-4 times per day given 15 min before feeding. Maximum: 40 mg per day. Dilute syrup with equal volume of water.	Anticholinergic — alters gastrointestinal motility and relieves smooth muscle spasm. Has been shown to decrease duration of crying up to 45% in colicky infants.	60-90 min	Drowsiness, blurred vision, constipation, dry mouth, difficult urination	Contraindicated in infants **less than 6 mos** of age because of association with apnea and seizures in small infants. Since colic is unlikely in infants > 16 wks of age, infants should be assessed by a physician prior to treatment with dicyclomine. Concomitant use of other agents with anticholinergic activity (i.e., antihistamines) may increase potential of adverse effects. May antagonize effects of metoclopramide if used concurrently.
Simethicone 40 mg/mL liquid	0.25-0.5 mL with or after each feeding as necessary. May be added to formula or given directly from dropper. Maximum: 6 mL per 24 h	Based on the possible etiology of gas in colic. Antiflatulent — alters surface tension of mucus and allows entrapped gas bubbles to coalesce and be more easily released by the mouth or anus.	Within minutes (exact onset unknown)	None, due to lack of systemic absorption	Minimal proven clinical benefit. May be useful because of potential placebo effect.
Sucrose	Mix 5 mL in 30 mL of water (12%) and give 2 mL to infant via dropper. Increase concentration to 25-50% if necessary.	Proposed analgesic effect in infants. Short acting — response lasts less than 30 minutes.	Within minutes (exact onset unknown)	None reported	Limited data shows 63% of infants respond with decrease in symptoms. More research is needed before it can be recommended. If solution is not administered right away, store in refrigerator and inspect for changes in appearance before administration. Do not substitute with honey because of risk of botulism in infants.

Inappropriate Pharmacologic Therapy

Table 4 lists agents previously used in the treatment of infant colic, but now considered inappropriate due to questionable efficacy and/or unacceptable adverse effects.

Monitoring of Therapy

Table 5 provides a framework for a monitoring plan that should be individualized for each patient.

Table 4: **Inappropriate Pharmacologic Therapy of Infant Colic**[1,4,11,17]

Drug	Selected adverse effects	Comments
Alcohol	Alcoholic gastritis, intoxication, hypoglycemia	Efficacy unknown
Diphenhydramine	Sedation, constipation, urinary retention	Efficacy unknown
Sedative (e.g., barbiturates, chloral hydrate)	Excessive sedation, respiratory depression	Limited efficacy
Combinations of sedatives and anticholinergics (e.g., hyoscyamine/atropine/scopolamine/ phenobarbital)	Sedation, respiratory depression, constipation, urinary retention	Questionable efficacy

Table 5: **Monitoring Therapy for Infant Colic**[1,4,13]

Symptoms	Monitoring	Endpoint of therapy	Actions
Excessive crying	**Parent:** daily — log behavior in a colic diary to assess patterns. Document associated symptoms. **Pharmacist or health care provider:** after 3 days or at next pharmacy visit. Review diary with parent.	Decrease in frequency or duration of crying episodes to less than 3 h per day, less than 3 days per week	If current treatment strategy is not effective, try another strategy based on patterns noted in diary. If still ineffective after 3 days, refer to a physician to rule out organic etiology for crying. If crying is associated with fever, vomiting or significant change in stool or urination pattern, or if infant cries for ≥ 3 h without stopping, refer to physician immediately.
Parental anxiety	**Parent:** daily **Pharmacist or health care provider:** after 3 days or at next pharmacy visit	Decrease in parental anxiety and frustration. Improved parental coping skills	Reassure parents and reemphasize coping strategies. Remind them to take "time out" rest periods away from the infant. If they continue to seem frustrated or overwhelmed, refer to a physician for counseling.
Infant agitated or not able to fall asleep	**Parent:** daily — log behavior in diary and document associated symptoms. **Pharmacist or health care provider:** after 3 days or at next pharmacy visit. Review diary with parent.	Infant able to fall asleep. Infant calm before bedtime or naptime	If environmental manipulation or other soothing techniques are ineffective after 3 days, refer to a physician for thorough history and physical. If associated with fever, excessive vomiting, or significant change in stool or urination pattern, refer to physician immediately.
Refusal to eat or fussiness after eating	**Parent:** daily — log behavior in diary and indicate whether related to other symptoms such as gas, fever, constipation. Monitor weight daily. **Pharmacist or health care provider:** after 3 days or at next pharmacy visit. Review weight with parent and check for signs of dehydration (e.g., decrease in urination, sunken eyes or fontanel, poor skin turgor).	Less or minimal fussiness after eating. No weight loss or signs of dehydration	If ineffective after 3 days of intervention, refer to a physician for thorough physical assessment. Suggest that caregiver discuss alterations in maternal diet or formula to rule out allergenic component to colic. If weight loss or signs of dehydration are evident in the infant, refer to physician immediately.

Advice for the Patient

Counsel caregivers of colicky babies regarding:
- When to seek medical advice
- Nonpharmacologic management strategies
- Proper use of any drug therapy chosen
- Expected results of any drug therapy and management of side effects

Resource Tips

Parents can call their regional health department's parent-child information line or their local children's hospital hotline for more information on community support for parents of colicky babies.

Internet-based information on colicky infants:
- Canadian Paediatric Society: www.cps.ca
  Searchword: colic
- My Web MD: www.mywebmd.com
  Searchword: colic

Suggested Readings

Balon AJ. Management of infantile colic. *Am Fam Physician* 1997;55(1):235-42.

Berkowitz CD. Management of the colicky infant. *Compr Ther* 1997;23(4):277-280.

Garrison MM, Christakis DA. Early childhood: colic, child development, and poisoning prevention: A systematic review of treatments for infant colic. *Pediatrics* 2000;106:184-90.

Gervais A. Colic. *Can Pharm J* 1996;129(7): 27-28.

Larsen JH. Infants' colic and belly massage. *Practitioner* 1990;234:396-7.

Pray WS. Infant colic: the therapeutic puzzle. *US Pharm* 1997;22(3):20-24.

References

1. Berkowitz CD. Management of the colicky infant. *Compr Ther* 1997;23(4):277-80.
2. Sferra TJ, Heitlinger LA. Gastrointestinal gas formation and infantile colic. *Pediatr Clin North Am* 1996;43(2):489-510.
3. Reust CE, Blake RI Jr. Diagnostic workup before diagnosing colic. *Arch Fam Med* 2000;9(3):282-3.
4. Balon AJ. Management of infantile colic. *Am Fam Physician* 1997;55(1):235-42.
5. Gervais A. Colic. *Can Pharm J* 1996;129(7):27-28.
6. Gervais A. Colic. *Can Pharm J* 1998;131(2):23.
7. Clemons RM. Issues in newborn care. *Prim Care* 2000;27 (1):251-67.
8. Barr RG. Colic and crying syndromes in infants. *Pediatrics* 1998;102(5 Suppl E):1282-6.
9. Gurry D. Infantile colic. *Aust Fam Physician.* 1994;23(3): 337-46.
10. Farmer PS. Gastrointestinal products. In: Carruthers-Czyzewski P, ed. *Nonprescription Drug Reference for Health Professionals.* Ottawa: Canadian Pharmaceutical Association, 1996:289-90.
11. Pray WS. Infant colic: the therapeutic puzzle. *US Pharm* 1997;22(3):20-24.
12. Larsen JH. Infants' colic and belly massage. *Practitioner* 1990;234:396-7.
13. Personal Communication. Barry Lester, PhD, Director of Infant Development Center, Professor in Departments of Psychiatry and Pediatrics, Brown University.
14. Garrison MM, Christakis DA. Early childhood: child development and poisoning prevention. A systematic review of treatments for infant colic. *Pediatrics* 2000;106:184-90.
15. Lucassen PL, Assendelft WJ, Gubbels JW, et al. Effectiveness of treatments for infantile colic: systematic review. *BMJ* 1998; 316:1563-9.
16. Hopkins RG. Infantile colic. *J Fam Pract* 1985;21(3):175.
17. Management of infantile colic. *Drug Ther Bull* 1992;30 (4):15-6.

Infant Colic—Caregiver Information

- Colic is common. The cause is not known. In most babies, it goes away by the time they are three-to-four-months old.
- Colic does not mean that your baby is ill or has a disease.
- Don't take your baby's colic personally. Your baby is not mad at you or rejecting you.
- Maintain a colic diary for about two or three days to help establish patterns to your infant's fussy periods. It may help you and your doctor create a management plan and also give you a sense of control over the situation.
- You may have to try several different approaches such as holding your baby, warm baths, rocking, music, or car rides, before you find the one that consoles your baby. Remember that what works on one day may not work on the next day. Try to be flexible in your approach.
- Having a colicky baby can be very stressful and overwhelming. Take time for yourself and don't feel guilty. Ask your spouse, a grandparent or a babysitter to watch the baby for a period of time every few days while you enjoy a rest break.

If you are thinking of using nonprescription medication to treat your infant's colic:
- —Be aware that there is little proof that the available medications work.
- —Do not use the medication for more than a few days and only use it when your baby has symptoms. If it is not providing relief, stop using it.

- —Use a calibrated dropper or an oral syringe instead of a teaspoon or tablespoon to administer liquid medication to your infant. This will ensure that your baby is getting the most accurate dose of medication. Read the label carefully to make sure that you are giving the right dose. Clean droppers and syringes with soap and water and store the parts in a clean, dry place. Tightly close medication bottles and keep out of the reach of children.
- —If using a dropper: Be sure to measure the liquid at eye level and give it to your baby quickly, because droppers tend to drip.
- —If using an oral syringe: Measure the liquid, then hold the syringe with the tip pointing up and tap air bubbles toward the end. Push the plunger gently to force air out and check that you have the correct amount of medication in the syringe. Squirt the medication in the back of your baby's mouth, where it is less likely to spill out.

You should see a doctor if:
- —Your baby develops a fever, is vomiting or regurgitating excessively, is having difficulty breathing, or if there is any change in the stool or urination pattern, *or*
- —Your baby cries for 3 hours without stopping, *or*
- —You have tried all of the other strategies for more than three days, *or*
- —You feel so overwhelmed that you are worried that you are going to harm your baby.

Sample Colic Diary for Parents

Hour	Crying ("C" for crying or "F" for fussy) — note length and intensity of crying spell	Other symptoms (for example, gas or arching back)	Comments (for example, hungry, tired) — indicate or note sleeping, feeding, crying, stooling and playtime patterns in this column	Measures you use to console your baby (for example, holding, car-ride, change in feeding technique)
0600				
0700				
0800				
0900				
1000				
1100				
1200				
1300				
1400				
1500				
1600				
1700				
1800				
1900				
2000				
2100				
2200				
2300				
2400				
0100				
0200				
0300				
0400				
0500				

Gastrointestinal Conditions

Perianal Symptom Assessment

Patricia Carruthers-Czyzewski, BScPhm, MSc (Pharmacology)

Patients may erroneously attribute any perianal symptom to hemorrhoids. In fact these symptoms may be due to a number of conditions, ranging in severity from poor hygiene to colorectal cancer. An assessment plan for patients reporting perianal symptoms is illustrated in Figure 1. All too often, patients seeking relief with nonprescription agents have delayed consulting a pharmacist or physician until the symptoms have become unbearable and the condition has advanced to the point where medical referral is necessary.

Table 1: Patients at High Risk of Colorectal Cancer[5]

- Those over 50 yrs of age
- Those with a history of colorectal cancer or adenomatous polyposis
- Those with a family history of familial adenomatous polyposis or hereditary nonpolyposis colon cancer
- Those with IBD
- Those with a strong family history (either cancer or polyps in a first-degree relative < 60 yrs old or two first-degree relatives of any age)

References:

1. Turnbull GK, Vanner SJ, Burnstein M. The colon. In: Thomson ABR, Shaffer EA, eds. *First Principles of Gastroenterology: The Basis of Disease and an Approach to Management.* Available at: http://www.gastroresource.com/GITextbook/en/chapter11/11-4.htm. Accessed November 15, 2001.
2. Henley CE. Diseases of the rectum and anus. In: Taylor RB, ed. *Family Medicine Principles and Practice.* 4th ed. New York, NY: Springer-Verlag, 1994:717-24.
3. Pfenniger JL, Zainea GG. Common anorectal conditions: Part I. Symptoms and complaints. *Am Fam Physician* 2001;63(12):2391-8.

Figure 1: Assessment of Patients with Perianal Symptoms[1-4]

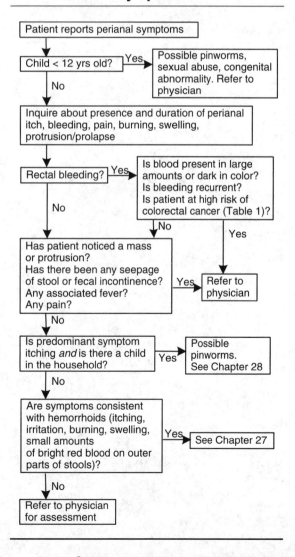

4. Pfenniger JL, Zainea GG. Common anorectal conditions: Part II. Lesions. *Am Fam Physician* 2001;64(1):77-88.

5. American Cancer Society. *Can colon and rectum cancer be found early?* Available at: http://www.cancer.org/eprise/ main/docroot/ped/ped_2?sitearea=PED&level=1. Accessed November 16, 2001.

Chapter 27

Hemorrhoids

Patricia Carruthers-Czyzewski, BScPhm, MSc (Pharmacology)

Pathophysiology

Hemorrhoids are often described as varicose veins in the anal canal. However, hemorrhoids are not veins at all, they are displaced anal cushions. The cushions are normal structures that have a rich arterial supply leading directly into distensible venous spaces. They help seal the upper anal canal and contribute to continence.

Hemorrhoids can be classified as internal, external or mixed hemorrhoids (Figure 1). Internal hemorrhoids originate above the dentate/pectinate/anorectal line and may be further classified into four stages (see below). Internal hemorrhoids should not cause pain unless complications develop, since this area has no nerve fibres. External hemorrhoids originate below

the dentate line and can cause pain, since this area is well innervated by pain fibres. The term "mixed hemorrhoids" is used when internal and external hemorrhoids coexist.[1]

Internal hemorrhoids can be classified symptomatically according to their degree of formation. First-degree hemorrhoids swell in the anal cushion due to straining and are usually painless. During the second stage, a small part of the anal mucosa or cushion may protrude at the anus during defecation. After the bowel movement, the hemorrhoid spontaneously returns to its normal position. Third-degree hemorrhoids remain in the prolapsed position after defecation, but may be replaced manually within the anus. Fourth-degree hemorrhoids cannot be replaced after a bowel movement, and thus create a permanent bulge at the anus. This condition is quite painful, and it is usually at this stage that individuals should consult their physician. Fourth-degree hemorrhoids are at risk of thrombosis and gangrene.[2]

Hemorrhoids are common. Fifty-eight to 86% of individuals will have hemorrhoids at some point in their lives.[3,4] A US survey showed a prevalence of 4.4% in the general population. The incidence of hemorrhoids may be overestimated. Some studies have indicated that when patients complain of hemorrhoids, only 50% actually have simple hemorrhoids; other problems include thrombosed hemorrhoids in approximately 18.5% of patients with anal complaints, fissures in 8% and miscellaneous problems in 23%.[5]

Many factors may be associated with the development of hemorrhoids: constipation, diarrhea, pregnancy, and possibly type of work and physical exertion.[5,6] Straining, usually as a result of constipation, is the main contributing factor. When the individual tries to pass small, firm stools, the intrarectal pressure rises,

Figure 1: **Hemorrhoids**

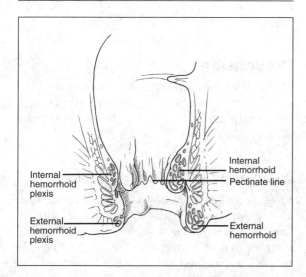

blocking the venous return from the anal canal and leading to more straining. The shearing action of the fecal mass passing over the area causes a loosening of the underlying connective tissue. Diarrhea, either acute or chronic, can also cause hemorrhoids due to futile and protracted straining.

Heredity is not an important factor. The only connection between heredity and hemorrhoids is the similarity of diet and personal habits in members of the same family.[6]

Pregnancy is believed to precipitate the onset of hemorrhoids in susceptible women. The woman who experiences hemorrhoids in the last few months of pregnancy may have become symptomatic due to increased abdominal pressure, allowing already existing hemorrhoids to present themselves. Other possibilities are that during pregnancy there may be a softening of the elastic tissue that supports anal cushions or that the woman may be more constipated. In any case, these hemorrhoids usually resolve after parturition.

Other possible causes of hemorrhoids include increased abdominal pressure due to heavy lifting and prolonged standing or sitting. Prolonged periods of time on the toilet can increase the risk of hemorrhoids; in this position, the perineum is relaxed and the anal cushions are unsupported.[6] The prevalence of hemorrhoids gradually increases with age. This continues until the seventh decade of life, when the prevalence begins a slow decline.[6] Evidence of any of these risk factors as primary causes of hemorrhoids is nonexistent. Rather, it is probable that each can worsen asymptomatic hemorrhoids that are already present.[6]

Hemorrhoids are found primarily in populations consuming the western world's diet, one high in white flour, sugar and fibre-depleted carbohydrate foods. However, fibre intake and the prevalence of hemorrhoids are not associated.

Goals of Therapy

- Relieve symptoms
- Prevent complications
- Promote good bowel habits and hygiene

Patient Assessment

For some patients, the first symptom is a painful mass at the anus lasting several days to weeks (thrombosed hemorrhoid), sometimes accompanied by the sudden relief of pain following rupture of the skin overlying the thrombus and bleeding. Other symptoms include itching, swelling and burning. Swelling is probably the main cause of pruritus. Individuals often have fecal soiling of underwear. Prolapse often coincides with the beginning of a troublesome amount of discharge as a result of increased mucus production. The degree of discomfort experienced by the patient is dependent on the type of hemorrhoids and their severity. Internal hemorrhoids lack nerves and are painless. When hemorrhoids bleed, the blood is usually bright red and seen on the outer part of stools after defecation. The patient does not usually bleed at other times.

Refer patients to their physician:
- If the patient mentions prolapse that must be manually replaced;
- If there is rectal bleeding and
  —Blood is present in large amounts *or*
  —The blood is dark in color *or*
  —Bleeding is recurrent *or*
  —The patient is at high risk of colorectal cancer (see Table 1, Perianal Symptom Assessment);
- If patients are under the age of 12 (may be a sign of birth abnormality, pinworms, sexual abuse);
- If the problem persists for more than seven days.

Since many patients delay seeking help for hemorrhoids until symptoms have become unbearable, referral to a physician is often required.

Prevention

The most important preventive measure is to avoid constipation (see Chapter 21). One should not remain on the toilet more than one to two minutes. Straining should be avoided.

Nonpharmacologic Therapy

Fibre supplementation may help relieve constipation and relieve pruritus related to fecal soilage. Adding fibre to the diet (total of 20 to 30 g per day) is usually adequate to relieve symptoms of hemorrhoids in individuals with first- and second-degree hemorrhoids.

If these general measures do not relieve hemorrhoidal symptoms, advise the individual to use a Sitz bath three to four times daily. Sitz baths help relieve irritation and pruritus. Their effectiveness may in part be related to relaxation of the internal anal sphincter. A Sitz bath consists of a tub of warm water (about 46°C) in which the individual sits for 15 minutes at a time. Plastic Sitz baths may be fitted over the toilet seat rim for greater convenience.

Any prolapsed hemorrhoids must be replaced with a moistened tissue. After each bowel movement, the anorectal area should be cleaned with soap and water and wiped with a wet toilet tissue.

Surgical hemorrhoidectomy may be required for treatment failures and is primary therapy for third- and fourth-degree hemorrhoids and for acute thrombosed hemorrhoids.[3]

Surgical hemorrhoidectomy is the most definitive treatment; less than 3% of individuals undergoing this procedure experience recurrence. More than 80% of people respond to medical treatment, rubber-banding or infrared coagulation; these methods cause much less discomfort and entail much less time off work than does hemorrhoidectomy.[1]

Pharmacologic Therapy[7-9]

Pharmacologic treatment is directed towards relief of symptoms. A variety of hemorrhoidal products is available. These provide only relief; none are curative. Hemorrhoidal products can provide short-term relief of pain, burning, itching, discomfort and irritation while swelling subsides and healing occurs. Many of the commercially available hemorrhoidal products are formulated in a lubricating or emollient base with combinations of two or more active ingredients, including local anesthetics, antiinflammatory agents, protectants, counterirritants, astringents, vasoconstrictors, wound-healing agents, and antiseptics. Table 1 describes nonprescription agents used in the management of symptoms due to hemorrhoids.

The safest ingredients are the protectants, vasoconstrictors and zinc sulfate.

Local anesthetics are included in some topical hemorrhoidal preparations to relieve pain. If used for less than seven days, local anesthetics are relatively safe and may relieve pain. Longer duration of use increases the risk of contact dermatitis. Good evidence of their efficacy is lacking.[7] Penetration of intact skin by local anesthetics is generally poor, but with excessive application to the rectal mucosa, absorption can occur.[7] Adverse effects associated with systemic use of local anesthetics include CNS (restlessness, excitement, nervousness, paresthesias, dizziness, tinnitus, blurred vision, nausea and vomiting, muscle twitching and tremors, convulsions) and cardiovascular (hypotension, bradycardia) effects.[7] Products containing local anesthetics should be used only in the perianal region or the lower anal canal to reduce systemic absorption. To prevent a suppository from slipping into the rectum, advise the patient to not insert it too far up and to lie down on their side after insertion to prevent it from slipping out.

Hydrocortisone is used for temporary relief of itchy anal areas and as an antiinflammatory agent in the treatment of hemorrhoids.[8] Hydrocortisone should not be used for longer than one week, to reduce the likelihood of side effects such as mucosal atrophy.

Antiseptics are used as an adjunct to good personal hygiene and are generally used in cases where mild discomfort is the main symptom. If symptoms include itchiness, pain and/or burning, the choice of a product depends on the severity of the symptoms. For mild symptoms, ointments or suppositories without hydrocortisone, such as **zinc sulfate**, are generally recommended. If there is lots of itching and discharge, a preparation with **hydrocortisone** can be recommended.

Other agents frequently included for their soothing properties include various **bismuth salts**, **zinc oxide** and **hamamelis**.

Hemorrhoidal preparations are available in a variety of dosage forms: creams, ointments, suppositories, aerosols, cleaning pads and sticks. Ultimately, the choice of delivery form lies with the consumer or physician. Many people prefer suppositories, but these products are often not effective because they tend to slip into the rectum and melt, thus bypassing the anal canal where the medication is needed. In general, creams and ointments are preferable to suppositories. They are easy to apply and usually contain the same or similar ingredients as suppositories.

Table 1: **Drug Therapy of Hemorrhoids: Components of Hemorrhoidal Products**[7-9]

Active ingredient	Concentration found in OTC products (ointments, creams, suppositories)	Dose	Adverse effects	Comments
Antiinflammatory agents				
Hydrocortisone	0.5% ointment	May be applied every morning and evening and after each bowel movement	Mucosal atrophy (more common with prolonged use)	Should not be used for longer than 7 days
Astringents: *used to relieve irritation and burning sensation*				
Bismuth	Subgallate: 1% ointment Subcarbonate: 5% ointment; 50 mg/suppository	May be applied up to 6 times daily after each bowel movement		Added to preparations for its soothing effect
Hamamelis water (Witch hazel)	10-50% ointment/cream; available as pads or wipes	May be applied up to 6 times daily after each bowel movement		
Zinc oxide	5-10% ointment/cream; 225-250 mg suppository	May be applied up to 4-6 times daily after each bowel movement		
Zinc sulfate	0.5% oint/cream; 10 mg suppository	May be applied up to 6 times daily after each bowel movement		
Local anesthetics: *temporarily relieve itching, irritation and discomfort*				
Benzocaine	1-4.5% ointment/cream; 50 mg suppository; also in aerosols and sticks	May be applied up to 6 times daily	Allergic reactions, locally and systemically; local reactions (burning and itching). Contact dermatitis	Ester type
Dibucaine	0.5-1% ointment/cream; 2.5 mg suppository	Administered each morning and evening and after each bowel movement. Max: 30 g ointment/24 h	Allergic reactions, locally and systemically; local reactions (burning and itching)	Amide type
Pramoxine	1% ointment/cream; 20 mg suppository	Administered each morning and evening and after each bowel movement	Allergic reactions, locally and systemically; local reactions (burning and itching)	Exhibits less cross-sensitivity because it does not have the usual amide or ester structure

Antiseptics: inhibits microbial growth; considered adjunctive therapy to good personal hygiene

Agent	Strength/form	Dosing	Comments	
Domiphen	0.05% ointment/cream			

Protectants: provide a physical barrier to irritation and prevent excessive water loss from tissues

Agent	Strength/form	Dosing	Comments	
Glycerin	10% ointment	Applied up to 4 times per day		
Shark liver oil	3% ointment/cream; 66 mg suppository	May be applied every morning and evening and after each bowel movement		Value as protectant is accepted
White petrolatum		Applied up to 4 times per day		
Zinc oxide	5-10% ointment/cream; 225-250 mg suppository	Applied up to 4-6 times per day		

Vasoconstrictors: constrict blood vessels; used temporarily to reduce swelling of hemorrhoidal tissue

Agent	Strength/form	Dosing	Comments	
Ephedrine	0.1-0.31% ointment/cream; 20 mg suppository	Applied up to 4 times per day	Possible systemic absorption if applied to abraded skin (see naphazoline). May cause nervousness, tremor, sleeplessness, nausea and loss of appetite	Onset of action ranges from a few seconds to 1 min and duration of action is 2-3 h. Theoretically may interact with MAOIs, including RIMAs (increased systemic adverse effects of vasoconstrictor). No published reports. Caution if heart disease, hypertension, thyroid disease, diabetes, prostatic hypertrophy
Naphazoline	0.04% ointment	May be applied every morning and evening and after each bowel movement	Possible systemic absorption if applied to abraded skin (increased blood pressure, CNS disturbances, cardiac arrhythmia, aggravation of symptoms of hyperthyroidism)	
Phenylephrine	0.25% gel	May be applied every morning and evening and after each bowel movement	Possible systemic absorption if applied to abraded skin (increased blood pressure, CNS disturbances, cardiac arrhythmia, aggravation of symptoms of hyperthyroidism)	

Wound-healing agents: may accelerate tissue healing and provide relief of symptoms

Agent	Strength/form	Dosing	Comments	
Shark liver oil	3% ointment/cream; 66 mg suppository	May be applied every morning and evening and after each bowel movement		Contains a form of vitamin A. Value as wound healer is equivocal
Yeast	1% ointment/cream; 22 mg suppository	May be applied every morning and evening and after each bowel movement		Insufficient evidence to confirm efficacy

MAOI = monoamine oxidase inhibitor; RIMA = reversible inhibitor of monoamine oxidase inhibitor type A

Nonprescription hemorrhoidal products for external use should be applied sparingly. They should not be inserted into the rectum. Before any hemorrhoidal product is applied, the anorectal area should be washed with mild soap and warm water, rinsed thoroughly and gently dried by patting or blotting with toilet tissue or a soft cloth.

Nonprescription hemorrhoid products should never be used on anyone under the age of 12, unless recommended by a doctor.

Oral analgesics, such as **acetaminophen**, may provide relief of mild discomfort or pain. Management of constipation also decreases discomfort during defecation.

Alternative Therapies

Bioflavonoids, particularly **diosmin** and **hesperidin**, have demonstrated efficacy in the treatment of hemorrhoids, presumably for their supposed action on venous capillary walls.[4] These preparations are considered safe.[4]

There is little evidence to support the topical use of **horse chestnut** for hemorrhoids, but it may be effective when used orally in doses of 100-150 mg **aescin** daily in divided doses. Adverse effects have included pruritus, nausea, stomach complaints, bleeding, nephropathy and allergic reactions. Horse chestnut and aescin are contraindicated during pregnancy and in patients who are breastfeeding or have bleeding disorders. In addition, it may interact with ASA and other antithrombotics.[10,11]

Pregnancy

Correcting constipation and taking Sitz baths are usually helpful in reducing the discomfort from hemorrhoids. External medications are preferred over those inserted into the rectum because the drugs can be well absorbed from the rectal mucosa. Products containing local anesthetics and corticosteroids should be avoided during pregnancy, except under the supervision of a physician, as their systemic absorption could have consequent effects on the fetus.[12]

Monitoring of Therapy

Assess relief of symptoms such as itching, pain or burning. Check with the patient in one week. If there is no relief within seven days, if symptoms worsen, or if bleeding, protrusion or seepage occur, refer the patient to a physician.

Advice for the Patient

Counsel patients regarding:
- Nonpharmacologic therapy
- Management of constipation, if applicable (see Chapter 21)
- Proper use of any medication chosen
- Possible side effects and their management
- When to see a physician

Suggested Readings

Cocchiara JL. Hemorrhoids: A practical approach to an aggravating problem. *Postgrad Med* 1991; 89(1): 149-52.

Hulme-Moir M, Bartolo DC. Hemorrhoids. *Gastroenterol Clin North Am* 2001; 30(1):183-97.

References

1. Pfenninger JL, Zainea GG. Common Anorectal Conditions: Part I. Symptoms and complaints. *Am Fam Physician* 2001; 63:2391-98; and Part II: Lesions. *Am Fam Physician* 2001;64: 77-88.
2. Brisinda G. How to treat haemorrhoids. Prevention is best; haemorrhoidectomy needs skilled operators. *BMJ* 2000;321: 582-3.
3. Hulme-Moir M, Bartolo DC. Hemorrhoids. *Gastroenterol Clin North Am* 2001;30(1):183-97.
4. MacKay D. Hemorrhoids and varicose veins: a review of treatment options. *Altern Med Rev* 2001;6(2):126-40.
5. Mazier WP. Hemorrhoids, fissures and pruritus ani. *Surg Clin N Amer* 1994;74:1277-92.
6. Pray WS. Hemorrhoids: self-care vs. physician care. *US Pharmacist* 2001;26(5):22-30.
7. Parfitt K, ed. *Martindale: The Complete Drug Reference*. 32nd ed. London, UK: Pharmaceutical Press, 1999.
8. McEvoy GK, ed. *AHFS Drug Information*. Bethesda, MD: American Society of Health-System Pharmacists, 2001.
9. Repchinsky C, ed. *Compendium of Nonprescription Products*. Ottawa, ON: Canadian Pharmacists Association, 2001.
10. Ernst E, ed. *The Desktop Guide to Complementary and Alternative Medicine*. London, UK: Harcourt Publishers Ltd., 2001.
11. Jellin JM, ed. *Natural Medicines Comprehensive Database*. 2nd ed. Stockton, CA: Therapeutic Research Faculty, 1999.
12. McCombs J, Cramer MK. Pregnancy and lactation: therapeutic considerations. In: DiPiro JT, Talbert RL, Yee GC, et al., eds. *Pharmacotherapy: A Pathophysiologic Approach*. 4th ed. Stamford, CN: Appleton & Lange, 1999:1303.

Hemorrhoids—Patient Information

Hemorrhoids are a common problem. They may be brought on by many things, including constipation, diarrhea, pregnancy, heavy lifting, and standing or sitting for long periods of time. Hemorrhoids can cause itching, burning and irritation around the anus. They can also bleed when you have a bowel movement.

Here are some things you can do to help:
- Avoid constipation by drinking lots of fluid and eating a healthy diet that is high in fibre.
- Don't sit on the toilet for long periods of time.
- Do not strain to have a bowel movement.

See your doctor if any of the following happen:
- The hemorrhoid does not go back in place after a bowel movement;
- You have bleeding from your rectum (back passage);
- The problem lasts longer than seven days;
- Stool or mucus leaks from your rectum between bowel movements.

Medications may help to control the symptoms of hemorrhoids, but do not fix the problem. Talk to your pharmacist for advice on which product may be best for you.

Pinworms

Patricia Carruthers-Czyzewski, BScPhm, MSc (Pharmacology)

Pathophysiology[1,2]

Enterobiasis, commonly called pinworm or seat-worm,[3] is an intestinal infection with *Enterobius vermicularis* (formerly *Oxyuris vermicularis*). Although the adult worms resemble white cotton threads about 1 cm in length, the name threadworm is best reserved for *Strongyloides stercoralis*.

Humans are the only natural host of *E. vermicularis*. Cats and dogs have been shown to hold eggs on their fur, probably as a result of dust contamination (e.g., shaking bedclothes in their presence) but there is no evidence they can act as carriers of the infection.[2,4]

E. vermicularis is an infection of the large intestine and transmission follows ingestion of mature eggs. The larvae mature in the gut in approximately one to two months. The eggs are not released into the gut contents but the mature female migrates to the anus at night and lays its eggs on the perianal or perineal skin. The eggs become infective within six hours and are transferred from the perianal region to night clothes, bedding, dust and air. The most common mode of transmission is on hands and under fingernails, either through scratching or handling infected clothes and linen.[1] Eggs can remain infective for up to 20 days.[5] The adult worm has a life span of about six weeks and, if reinfection can be prevented, the infection is self-limiting.

Pinworm is one of the few intestinal nematodes common in temperate climates and is particularly common in young children. Pinworms are a common infection in children 5 to 10 years of age and uncommon in children less than two years old. An estimated one-third of Canadian children will be infested during their childhood. It is the most common intestinal parasite seen in the primary care setting, regardless of race, socioeconomic or cultural circumstances.[1,6]

Enterobiasis is more prevalent in temperate and cold climates because of less frequent bathing and infrequent changing of underclothing.[4] It is facilitated by factors such as overcrowding in schools and family groupings as well as inadequate personal and community hygiene. The infestation is more common in homosexual men.[2] Other high risk populations include institutionalized patients, residents of native reserves, and travelers to areas of high incidence, such as India and Iran.

Despite the high prevalence of pinworms, it is a rather innocuous parasite. Consequences of infection include loss of sleep, discomfort due to symptoms, and embarassment due to the social connotations of having "worms." Only rarely have infections been associated with significant pathology, including appendicitis, chronic salpingitis and ulcerative lesions of the small and large intestine.[1]

Goals of Therapy

- Relieve itching
- Eliminate the infection
- Promote good hygiene

Patient Assessment

Though many infections are asymptomatic, enterobiasis is often associated with perianal or perineal itching.[1] The itching is worse at night, when the females lay eggs that are attached to the perianal area by a sticky substance that causes pruritus. The itching may contribute to insomnia. Often, an entire family is affected. Other symptoms, particularly in heavy infestation, include anorexia, irritability, and abdominal pain. Scratching may cause skin irritation, and in more serious cases, eczematous dermatitis, bleeding or secondary bacterial infection of excoriated skin. If the worm migrates to the genital area in females, vulvovaginitis, vaginal discharge and irritation may be seen.[7] Enuresis has also been attributed to pinworms.[4] Although symptoms may alert the parent or patient to a potential problem, studies have shown no difference in the incidence of "classic" symptoms in infected and noninfected children.[1] This reinforces the need for actual viewing of the pinworm or its ova for definite diagnosis (see Diagnosis of Pinworm).

Refer all those with suspected pinworm infestation to a physician so the diagnosis can be confirmed. This is especially important in pregnant women, children under 12, and those with renal or hepatic impairment.

Diagnosis of Pinworm[1,3,6]

Pinworm diagnosis is contingent on visual identification of either the ova or the worm itself. The two most common methods are described below.

Inspection of the perianal area: Parents may observe the worms during ovipositing by putting the child to bed without underpants and using a flashlight to examine the anus after the child has been sleeping for one hour. Worms obtained by the parents should be placed in alcohol or vinegar and brought to the clinic or doctor for confirmation of the diagnosis.

Scotch-tape test (cellulose-tape slide test): This test is performed at home in the morning before defecation or washing. A piece of transparent adhesive tape is pressed on the perianal skin, then stuck to a slide to be examined under a microscope. Diagnosis is confirmed by identification of pinworm ova. The test may have to be repeated several times. A single examination will confirm the diagnosis in 50%, three exams in 90%, and five exams in 99% of cases.

Prevention[2]

Prevention is difficult. However, proper hygiene, including handwashing after going to the toilet, after scratching the perianal area and before eating, is helpful.

Nonpharmacologic Therapy[7]

As with prevention, proper hygiene is an important component of nonpharmacologic management of pinworm infestations. If ingestion of eggs can be avoided, the infection is self-limiting. In practice, however, this is difficult to achieve and pharmacologic therapy is usually necessary for eradication.

Nonpharmacologic measures should always be used as adjunctive therapy in combination with any drug treatment. These include:
- Bathing each morning;
- Regular cleaning of bedding, night clothes, underwear and hand towels;
- Changing night clothes and sheets at the start of each treatment course;
- Handwashing and fingernail cleaning, especially prior to meals and after using the bathroom or scratching the perianal area;
- During the week following treatment, all family members should wear cotton underpants that have been washed in hot soapy water. These should be worn day and night and changed twice daily;
- Cleansing of the floors of sleeping quarters as thoroughly as possible with household cleaner and water or by airing and vacuuming around beds, curtains, and other articles in the bedroom where the highest concentrations of eggs are likely to occur;
- Frequent washing of the toilet seat;
- Avoiding shaking linens or clothing prior to washing, and
- Discouraging thumb sucking.

Cleaning or vacuuming the entire house or washing the sheets every day is probably not effective in preventing reinfection.[8]

Pharmacologic Therapy (Table 1)

A confirmed diagnosis is recommended before pharmacologic treatment is initiated, to minimize unnecessary exposure to potential adverse effects of the anthelminthics. Pinworm infections respond readily to drug therapy, but reinfection is common.[6] Two factors that contribute to the high treatment failure rate are that medication kills only the adult worms and has no effect on developing eggs and larvae, and that any eggs swallowed after the drug is given will develop and cause infection.

Table 1: **Nonprescription Drug Therapy of Pinworm Infection**[3,9]

Drug	Dosage	Adverse effects	Drug interactions	Comments
Piperazine adipate	**Adults and children > 1 yr old:** 65 mg/kg (hydrate) daily for 7 days; repeat in 2 wk. **Maximum:** 2.5 g per day (hydrate). Note: repeat treatment consists of a second 7-day course beginning 7 days after the first course ends (i.e., 2 wks from initial dose).	Nausea, vomiting, abdominal cramps and diarrhea. CNS effects such as transient dizziness, paresthesia, some incoordination and difficulty in focusing may be experienced. May exacerbate seizure disorders. Hypersensitivity reactions such as rash, fever and joint pain have occurred.	Phenothiazines (produce increased extrapyramidal effects), chlorpromazine (potential risk of seizures) and pyrantel pamoate (antagonistic effect)	Cure rate 85-90%. Should not be used in epileptics. Can be used in pregnancy. Do not use in patient with impaired renal or hepatic function. 65 mg/kg hydrate equals 78 mg/kg adipate. Maximum 3 g per day adipate.
Pyrantel pamoate	**Adults and children > 1 yr of age:** 11 mg/kg (base) single dose; repeat in 2 wk. **Maximum:** 1 g (base)	Anorexia, nausea, vomiting, abdominal cramps, diarrhea, headache, dizziness, drowsiness; transient elevation of aspartate aminotransferase (AST) has been reported.	Piperazine adipate: antagonistic effect	11 mg/kg base equals 31.9 mg/kg pyrantel pamoate. Maximum 2.9 g per day pamoate. Cure rate 90-100%. Liquid form should be shaken well before use. Avoid with liver disease or pregnancy.
Pyrvinium pamoate	**Adults and children > 1 year old:** 5 mg/kg (base) single dose; repeat in 2 wk. **Maximum:** 350 mg per day (base)	Diarrhea, nausea, vomiting, abdominal cramps, dizziness, photosensitivity		5 mg/kg base equals 7.5 mg/kg pyrvinium pamoate. Maximum 525 mg per day pamoate. Well-tolerated. Tablets should be swallowed whole to avoid staining the teeth. Will color stools red for 24-48 h after dose. Will also stain any vomitus and possibly clothes.

In general, the drug of choice is **pyrantel pamoate**.[7] It results in higher cure rates than **piperazine** with minimal side effects, and unlike **pyrvinium** it does not stain feces red. Regardless of the agent chosen, all household members should be treated since the probability of their being infested is high.[2] Treatment of symptomatic household members should be repeated to decrease the likelihood of reinfection (Table 1). The use of laxatives to facilitate removal of pinworms after anthelminthic therapy is not necessary .

The prescription drug of choice is **mebendazole**, as a single 100 mg dose (repeated after one to two weeks) for adults and children over two years old. Mebendazole has minimal side effects and, in this regard, compares favorably to the nonprescription anthelminthics. Some reports suggest it is more effective than other anthelminthics (e.g., piperazine).[5,6] It cannot be used in pregnancy.

Asymptomatic pregnant women should be treated after delivery since there are no harmful effects to mother or fetus from the infection. When a pregnant woman is symptomatic and natural cure by scrupulous attention to personal hygiene is unlikely, **piperazine** is a reasonable choice; this is based on limited evidence of its safe use in some pregnant women.[9] However, whenever possible, treatment should be delayed until at least the second trimester.[2,10]

Monitoring of Therapy

Table 2 provides a monitoring plan framework, which should be individualized.

Advice for the Patient

Counsel patients regarding:
- Proper use of the drug and need for any repeat doses;
- The need to treat all household members;
- Adjunctive nonpharmacologic measures, and
- Expected results of drug therapy and management of side effects (Table 2).

Suggested Readings

Cook G. *Enterobius vermicularis* infection. *Gut* 1994; 35:1159-62.

Table 2: **Monitoring Therapy for Pinworms**

Symptoms	Monitoring	Endpoint of Therapy	Actions
Perianal itching	**Patient:** daily **Pharmacist:** day 7	Resolution of itching	If itching has not resolved within 7 days of starting medication, repeat treatment. If itching has not resolved within 7 days of beginning second course, refer to physician.
Rash, fever, joint pain (piperazine)	**Patient:** daily **Pharmacist:** day 7	No rash, fever or joint pain	If rash, fever or joint pain occur, discontinue therapy and contact physician.
Nausea, vomiting, diarrhea, abdominal cramps.	**Patient:** daily **Pharmacist:** day 1 after treatment	Minimal GI effects	If adverse GI effects interfere with functioning or persist more than 7 days after treatment ends, contact physician.
Dizziness, drowsiness	**Patient:** daily **Pharmacist or health care provider:** day 1 after treatment	Minimal drowsiness or dizziness	Caution patient not to drive or use hazardous machinery until effect of drug is known. If symptoms interfere with function or persist more than 24 h after treatment, contact physician.

References

1. Mahmoud AA. Intestinal nematodes (roundworms). In: Mandell GL, Bennett JE, Dolin R, eds. *Mandell, Douglas and Bennett's Principles and Practice of Infectious Diseases.* 5th ed. Philadelphia, PA: Churchill Livingstone, 2000:2938-43.
2. Cook, GC. *Enterobius vermicularis* infection. *Gut* 1994;35: 1159-62.
3. Health Canada. *Labelling standard: anthelminthics.* Available at: http://www.hc-sc.gc.ca/hpb-dgps/therapeut/zfiles/english/guides/label/drug/anthelmi_e.html. Accessed November 20, 2001.
4. Russell LJ. The pinworm. *Enterobius vermicularis. Prim Care* 1991;18(1):13-24.
5. Grencis RK, Cooper ES. Enterobius, Trichuris, Capillaria, and hookworm including *Ancylostoma caninum. Gastroenterol Clin North Am* 1996;25(3):579-97.
6. Juckett G. Common intestinal helminths. *Am Fam Physician* 1995;52(7):2039-48.
7. Center for Disease Control, Division of Parasitic Diseases. *Parasites and health: enterobiasis.* Available at: http://www.dpd.cdc.gov/dpdx/HTML/Frames/A-F/Enterobiasis/body_Enterobiasis_page 2.htm. Accessed November 20, 2001.
8. Center for Disease Control, Division of Parasitic Diseases. *Fact sheet: pinworm infection.* Available at: http://www.cdc.gov/ncidod/dpd/parasites/pinworm/factsht_pinworm.htm. Accessed November 20, 2001.
9. McEvoy GK, ed. *American Hospital Formulary Service Drug Information 2001.* Bethesda, MD: American Society of Health-System Pharmacists, 2001.
10. Leach FN. Treatment of threadworm infestation during pregnancy. *Arch Dis Child* 1990;65:399-400.

Pinworms—Patient Information

Pinworms are a bothersome infection, not a disease. They are very common during childhood and are easily spread from one person to another. The eggs from the worms can live on objects such as sheets and clothing and are too small to be seen with the naked eye. A person catches the infection from the hands of an infected person or from touching objects infected with the eggs. People with pinworms may notice that their anus is very itchy, or that they have belly pain, do not sleep well or are irritable. Many people with pinworms have no signs of the infection. If one person in a household has pinworms, everyone may have them, even if they have no signs of infection.

Do not use medication to treat pinworms unless you know for sure that you or someone you live with has them. If you do need medication, it is important to take it in the correct dose and exactly as directed. Check with the pharmacist to make sure the directions are clear. Medication usually needs to be repeated about two weeks after the first dose to be sure the infection is gone.

Besides taking medication, here are some things you should do to help keep pinworms from coming back:
- Everyone in the house should keep their nails short.
- Everyone should wash their hands and scrub their nails after using the toilet and before meals.
- Wash underwear and sleepwear daily to destroy the eggs.
- Wear pyjamas or pants at night to make it harder to scratch the itchy area while you are asleep.
- Fold bedclothes or clothes before washing them. Do not shake them. This will help stop the spread of eggs.
- Do not use disinfectants to kill the eggs. They do not work.

Chapter 29

Ostomy Care

Marie Berry, BScPharm, BA, LLB

Types of Ostomy

An ostomy is an artificial opening made surgically in the body. The opening itself is called a stoma, derived from the Greek word *stoma*, meaning mouth. A colostomy involves the colon, an ileostomy the ileum or small intestine, and a urostomy the urinary tract. Ostomies may be permanent or temporary. The type of ostomy depends upon the condition being treated. A person who has had an ostomy surgery is known as an *ostomate*.

Half a million North Americans have ostomies and over 90,000 ostomy operations are performed each year in the United States and Canada. No particular age or ethnic group has more ostomies, but in general more women than men have ostomies.

The older the adult the more likely the ostomy surgery will be a colostomy because of cancer or obstruction related to disease. Ileostomies are more common in young women, especially those resulting from inflammatory bowel disease.

To construct an ileostomy, the entire colon and possibly part of the ileum is removed. Usually the ileum end is brought to the skin surface. There are two variations of ileostomy where this is not the case:

- *ileoanal reservoir* ("S" or "J" pouch): The rectum is left intact; the ileum is refashioned into an internal pouch and the end of the ileum may be pulled through the rectum;
- *continent ileostomy:* An internal pouch is created from the ileum that is emptied by the patient, thus the patient is continent.

Crohn's disease and ulcerative colitis are the most common reasons for an ileostomy. An ileostomy may also be required because of trauma, cancer, familial polyp disease, or necrotizing enterocolitis.

To construct a colostomy, part of the colon is removed and the GI tract ends with a portion of the colon. The different types of colostomy are illustrated in Figure 1. A colostomy may be required due to obstruction of the colon or rectum, genetic malformation, trauma, radiation colitis, loss of anal muscle control, diverticulitis, or cancer of the colon or rectum. Colorectal cancer is the most common indication for this procedure. Temporary colostomies are sometimes performed to allow a diseased or surgically repaired bowel to heal, and once the bowel has healed it is reversed.

Colostomies and ileostomies show a characteristic discharge, as described in Table 1.

Urostomies (urinary diversions) are most common in infants and the elderly. They are performed to correct bladder loss or dysfunction resulting from genetic malformation, cancer or neurogenic bladder. These provide for elimination of urine through an opening in the abdominal wall. Because urine always remains liquid and is discharged continuously, urostomy surgery usually requires an appliance. There are many types of urostomies:

- Ileal and colonic conduits (more common): The ileum or colon is used to fashion the conduit into which the ureters are implanted (Figure 2). Mucus shreds may be seen in urine because the bowel has been used.
- Ureterostomy (uncommon) (Figure 2): The ureters are brought to the skin surface; with time the ureters tend to narrow.
- Nephrostomy: Urine is diverted directly from the kidneys; may be temporary in the case of ureter obstruction.
- Cystotomy: Urine is diverted from the bladder.
- Continent urostomy: A pouch is formed using the cecum which is emptied by the insertion of a catheter.

Table 1: **Description of Discharge from Different Colostomies and Ileostomies**

Ileostomy	Initially the discharge is liquid. With time, as the ileum becomes more absorptive, the discharge becomes semi-soft. The discharge is continuous, odorous, and contains enzymes that may cause skin irritation. An appliance must be worn at all times.
Ascending colostomy (uncommon)	The discharge is semi-soft; an appliance must be worn at all times.
Transverse colostomy (commonly used for temporary colostomies)	The discharge is soft to semi-liquid, malodorous, and irritating; an appliance must be worn at all times.
Descending and sigmoid colostomies (more common)	Discharge is pasty. Irrigation may be an option and an appliance may not be needed.

Patient Assessment

A healthy stoma is shiny, wet, and either dark pink or red (see photo on page PS-1). It has no pain sensation because it does not contain nerve fibres. The size in adults ranges from 2 to 5 cm depending upon the portion of the bowel or urinary tract used. After surgery, it shrinks gradually over several months to its permanent size.

A careful history and inspection of the ostomy site can help to determine if the patient is experiencing a problem. See Common Problems for more information.

Goals of Ostomy Care

- Prevent common problems such as skin irritation
- Identify and resolve common problems with ostomies and stoma care
- Minimize the impact of the ostomy on the patient's daily life

Appliances and Accessories

Appliances

An appliance is used to collect waste at the stoma. Not all stomas require appliances. The ideal ostomy appliance permits effective drainage with no leakage, does not damage skin, and is odor-free.

An ostomy appliance includes the pouch, which collects waste, and the faceplate and flange, which together attach the pouch to the stoma (Figure 3). Appliances are available in both pediatric and adult sizes.

Pouch

Pouches are available in different lengths and capacities to contain the varying amounts of waste material. Pouches may be open-ended (drainable) or close-ended (not drainable) (Figure 4). Whether a drainable or non-drainable pouch is selected depends upon the site of the stoma, the consistency of the discharge, and whether the task of draining and cleaning the pouch is acceptable to the individual. Open-ended appliances afford frequent emptying and are more often used for ileostomies and when a colostomy is not regulated.

Most pouches have an odor filter; built-in adhesives and skin barriers are also common features. Some pouches have a fabric backing for comfort. Clear, opaque, or decorated pouches are available and the choice depends upon the individual's eyesight and preference.[1]

Flange

A flange is the rim or edge that surrounds the opening in the pouch. Flanges are sized depending upon the size of the stoma. Flanges are also available in different sizes, shapes (e.g., round, oval) and convexities, and in rigid or flexible formats to accommodate different body contours and stoma sizes, shapes and locations.

Faceplate

The faceplate surrounds the stoma and attaches the appliance to the stoma. As with flanges, the correct size and shape of faceplate is important and there is a wide variety to choose from.

Figure 1: **Colostomies**

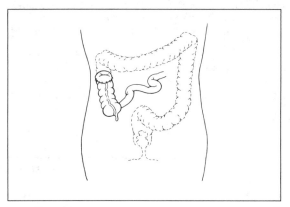

Ascending colostomy

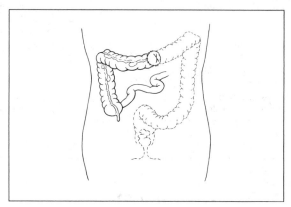

Transverse colostomy

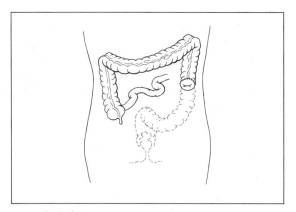

Descending colostomy

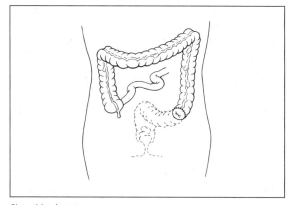

Sigmoid colostomy

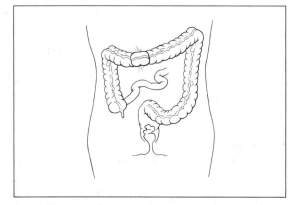

Loop colostomy

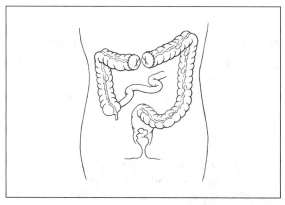

Double-barrel colostomy

Figure 2: **Urostomies**

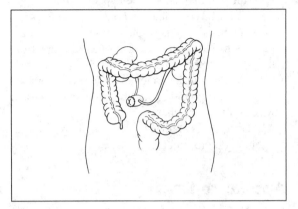

Ileal conduit

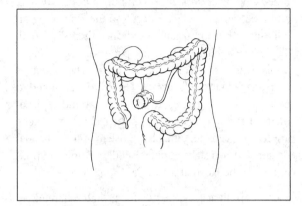

Colonic conduit

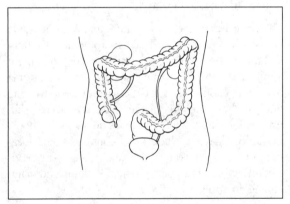

Unilateral ureterostomy

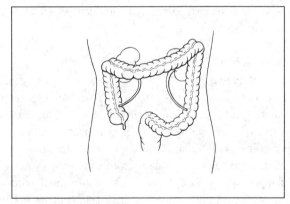

Bilateral ureterostomy

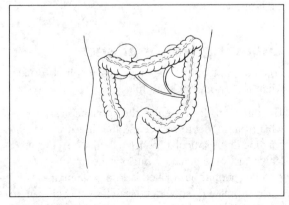

Transureteroureterostomy

One-piece vs. Two-piece (Figure 4)

Appliances are available as both one- and two-piece units. One-piece appliances combine a pouch, flange, and faceplate and attach directly to the skin using an adhesive. They are usually used once then discarded. Two-piece appliances have a separate faceplate that is applied to the ostomy with adhesive. The pouch is then attached to the faceplate. These are well-suited to individuals in whom excessive removal and replacement of the appliance irritates their skin. Two-piece appliances can be difficult to use if either manual dexterity or eyesight is diminished. Two-piece appliances can be cleaned for reuse.

Some appliance systems have interchangeable pouches, and some disposable pouches can be attached to some types of face plates. While this ability to interchange appliance components exists within a manufacturer's line of products, it does not usually extend among various manufacturers.

Accessories

Skin Barriers

Skin barriers help keep the skin surrounding a stoma intact, protecting it and keeping it dry. They are usually combinations of pectin, gelatin and cellulose and are available as wafers, powders and pastes. Wafer skin barriers are often incorporated directly into flanges and/or faceplates. They are essential with urostomies because urine can cause skin damage. It is a good idea to test a skin barrier before using it. Applying the product to an inconspicuous area of skin for 48 hours is usually sufficient to determine if there is any sensitivity.

Adhesives

Adhesives are applied either as cement, which must be allowed to dry before the appliance is attached, or as a pad. Some adhesives include skin barriers in their formulations. Some ostomy pouches have adhesive integrated into the flange and/or faceplate, making application simple.

Adhesives are the most common cause of allergies. A patch test should be performed prior to use as described in Skin Barriers.

Other Accessories

- Sometimes adhesive tape is used to position an appliance. If so, it should be hypoallergenic.
- Belts are used sometimes to hold a pouch in place. Ostomy belts are most often used by urostomy patients to reduce the strain on the adhesive from the weight of the urine in the pouch.
- Solvents are available to remove adhesives, however they are drying and should be used sparingly and washed off thoroughly.
- Appliance covers prevent rustling and prevent skin irritation due to rubbing.

Appliance Fit

Note: Measurement of the stoma and fitting an appliance are beyond the scope of this chapter and should only be performed by individuals with specialized training in this area.

The correct appliance fit is paramount. A fitting guide is usually included with each appliance to help determine the correct size based on the stoma. An appliance with an opening smaller than the stoma may cause abrasion of the stoma and poor wearing time. If the opening is larger than the stoma, skin excoriation can result. Other considerations in choosing an appliance include body contour, stoma location, presence of skin creases and scars, and type of ostomy.[2] Obesity can be a problem in fitting and maintaining an appliance.

The type of appliance may change post-surgically as the stoma heals, and as body contour changes due to weight changes, aging, pregnancy or concurrent medical conditions.

Changing the Appliance

Routine emptying of the pouch is required, usually when it is about one-third full.

The directions for changing the appliance vary somewhat from model to model and the directions accompanying the particular pouch should be consulted. However, some general principles do apply:

- Hands should be washed before beginning.
- The appliance should be carefully peeled off to avoid damaging the skin.

Figures 3a and 3b: **Placement of a Two-piece Ostomy Appliance**

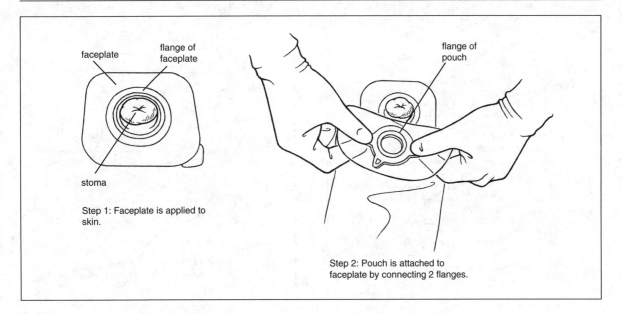

faceplate

flange of
faceplate

flange of
pouch

stoma

Step 1: Faceplate is applied to
skin.

Step 2: Pouch is attached to
faceplate by connecting 2 flanges.

- The stoma and peristomal skin should be gently washed with warm water and soap, then thoroughly dried.
- Soap must be completely washed off.
- Alcohol should not be used to clean the peristomal skin.
- All adhesive areas should be in contact with skin.
- All skin folds should be smoothed out.
- Once applied, the appliance should be pressed gently into place.

Irrigation

Irrigation is sometimes an alternative to wearing an appliance. It is less expensive and affords some control of fecal outflow. In irrigation, squirting water through the stoma into the intestine stimulates peristalsis which forces waste out. It is usually performed in the bathroom with an irrigation bag, which is much like an enema bag.

In addition to an irrigation bag, irrigation systems include an irrigation sleeve, faceplate, and stoma cone. The stoma cone is used with its pointed end inserted into the stoma to act like tubing, but to prevent bowel perforation, which could accompany the

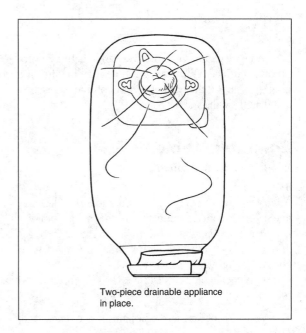

Two-piece drainable appliance
in place.

use of tubing alone. The irrigation sleeve, attached to the faceplate, carries the waste material to the toilet.

When not being irrigated, a stoma cap or even a pad is all that is required to cover the stoma. Irrigation is

Figure 4: **Ostomy Applicances**

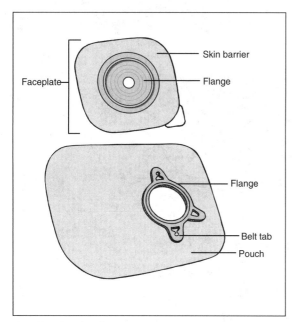

Two-piece closed appliance.

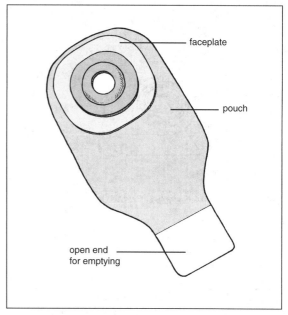

One-piece drainable appliance.

performed regularly, the interval ranging from every one to four days. A convenient time may be after the largest meal of the day, because of the peristalsis stimulated by the meal.

Common Problems

Peristomal Skin Problems

Allergies

Adhesives are the most common cause of allergies, and allergic contact dermatitis is the most common manifestation (itching, burning or stinging, redness and areas of moist, denuded skin).[3] A switch to another adhesive or appliance may be necessary. A skin barrier may help, but it needs to extend beyond the damaged area.

The majority of modern appliances are latex-free, reducing the risk of a latex allergy.

Infections

Infections can occur under the faceplate. These may be bacterial or fungal in nature; culture and sensitivity testing may be needed to identify the pathogen responsible and ensure appropriate treatment. Proper maintenance is important in preventing infections.

Ostomy sites are susceptible to fungal infections with *Candida* species because they provide a warm, moist environment conducive to fungal growth. The primary symptom of *Candida* infection is itching, accompanied by a red rash with satellite lesions.[4] With an unchecked infection, skin excoriation and additional skin irritation can occur. Use of broad spectrum antibiotics can contribute to *Candida* infections by changing the normal flora; thus knowing a patient's history of medication use is important.

Nystatin powder may be used to treat *Candida* infections. The appliance is applied directly over the powder, with any excess powder brushed off. Usually antifungal powder is continued for one week after the *Candida* infection clears. Treatment may be extended further if the individual is being treated with antibiotics.

Refer any ostomate with symptoms of infection, either those of *Candida* infection or fever, chills, foul odor from the stoma or purulent drainage, to a wound ostomy and continence nurse (WOCN) or physician for assessment.

Skin Damage
The most common peristomal skin problem is sore skin, usually the result of too frequent removal of the appliance. The skin around the stoma becomes damaged – red, swollen, burning, itchy. Skin damage may be also related to mechanical irritation caused by a poor fitting appliance, a stoma that is difficult to access, or clothing that is too tight.

Skin Excoriation
Skin excoriation is abrasion of the skin by digestive enzymes which may result in bleeding, painful skin. (See photo on page PS-1.) The most common cause is an appliance that is too big for the stoma and allows leakage. Lax replacement or maintenance may also result in waste material containing digestive enzymes coming into contact with skin. Choosing the proper size of appliance, routine maintenance of the appliance, and use of a skin barrier will avoid the problem.

Folliculitis
Folliculitis is an inflammation of hair follicles around the stoma and is characterised by redness at the base of hair follicles. Too aggressive removal of an appliance may also pull hair from follicles resulting in inflammation and infection. Shaving the area surrounding the stoma will prevent folliculitis. An electric razor is preferred because it will leave the skin intact. Clipping the hair is an alternative if shaving with an electric razor does cause skin damage.

Leakage
Ill-fitting or badly applied appliances result in leakage around the seal. Proper fit and maintenance of the appliance are therefore the solution.

Bleeding
Bleeding of the stoma is usually due to aggressive cleaning. Proper cleaning technique is required – gentle yet thorough. If bleeding persists, it may be an indication that the original disease has recurred, or that a new condition is developing. Referral is necessary.

Odor
Diet is the most common source of odor. Identifying what food is causing the odor and changing the diet usually solves the problem (Table 2). Pouches usually have an odor barrier and thus are considered odor-free, provided they are changed regularly, emptied as needed, cleaned properly, are without flaws or pinholes, and are reliably sealed. Emptying a pouch is often accompanied by odor.

Deodorants are available to help control odor. These are placed into the pouch after each emptying. Oral deodorants, such as activated charcoal, chlorophyllin copper complex and bismuth subgallate, act on the digestive system to eliminate odors from digested foods.

Gas
Some appliances have safety valves with charcoal filters – the gas is released and the charcoal absorbs odors. Strategies for decreasing gas include:
• Using an antacid;
• Eating yogurt;[5]
• Eating slowly and chewing food well;
• Avoiding drinking from a straw;
• Avoiding chewing gum;
• Limiting intake of gas-producing foods, especially prior to social occasions (Table 2).

Crystalline Phosphate Deposits
Crystalline phosphate deposits may build up on urostomies, making the stoma fragile, and cutting into the mucosa. These deposits are the major cause of blood in a urostomy pouch. Vinegar mixed with one-third to two-thirds water can be dabbed on the stoma when the appliance is cleaned to dissolve the crystals. Acidifying the urine by consuming foods such as cranberry juice or even ascorbic acid will reduce the formation of these deposits.

Fluid and Electrolyte Depletion
Ileostomates lack a normal reserve capacity for absorption of water, sodium and potassium, and should be advised to take extra fluid and electrolytes after exercise and in hot weather. Specialized fluid and electrolyte replacement drinks used by athletes are ideal. Some individuals need routine potassium supplementation and particular attention should be paid to plasma potassium levels if a diuretic is used.

Table 2: **Foods with Implications for Ostomy Patients**[5]

Bulk-forming foods: celery, coconut, coleslaw, foods with seeds or kernels (e.g., corn), dried fruits, nuts, meats in casings, popcorn, whole grains, whole vegetables, wild rice.

Gas-forming foods: beer, broccoli, brussel sprouts, cabbage, carbonated drinks, cauliflower, corn, cucumbers, dairy products, dried beans, mushrooms, onions, peas, radishes, spinach, string beans, yeast.

Diarrhea-causing foods: broccoli, beer (other alcoholic beverages are not common offenders), green beans, highly seasoned food, raw fruit, spinach.

Odor-forming foods: asparagus, beans, broccoli, cabbage, eggs, fish, garlic, onions, peas, some spices, turnips.

To avoid dehydration, fluid intake must be sufficient. This is especially important during illness and for infants. Signs and symptoms of dehydration and common electrolyte abnormalities are summarized in Tables 3 and 4.

Constipation

Individuals with colostomies are prone to constipation; fluid, fibre and exercise are recommended to avoid this problem. The causes of constipation are diverse, but it is often related to medications or diet (see Chapter 21). Laxatives should be used only under the supervision of a WOCN or physician.

Diarrhea

Ostomates with diarrhea may be at increased risk of fluid and or electrolyte imbalances (Tables 3 and 4). Fluid intake should be increased; oral rehydration solutions may be used to replenish electrolytes. Refer an ostomate with diarrhea to a WOCN or physician.

Structural Problems

Fistula Formation, Prolapse and Retraction

Fistula formation appears as leakage around the base of the stoma, causing skin erosion. All fistula formation should be investigated as it may be an indication of an underlying disease or condition (e.g., inflammatory bowel disease, cancer, abscess formation, trauma, foreign body retention). The underlying problem should be addressed. Sometimes surgical refashioning of the stoma is required.

Inward retraction of the stoma or prolapse of the stoma and/or bowel outwards may occur. Either may be due to the way the stoma was originally fashioned or to major changes in the individual's weight. Anything that increases abdominal pressure (e.g., coughing, pregnancy) increases the risk of prolapse. If the bowel is prolapsed, strangulation can occur. A prolapse should be reduced, and sometimes surgery is required.

Retraction may be controlled by the use of a convex appliance, but as with a prolapse, surgery may be needed.[10]

Table 3: **Symptoms of Dehydration in Children and Adults**[6,7]

Children	Adults
• Dry mouth, tongue and skin • Few or no tears when crying • Decreased urination (less than 4 wet diapers in 24 h) • Sunken eyes • Grayish skin • Sunken soft spot (fontanel) in infants • Decreased skin turgor (see Figure 3, Chapter 20)	• Increased thirst • Decreased urination • Feeling weak or light-headed • Dry mouth/tongue

Table 4: **Symptoms of Hyponatremia and Hypokalemia**[8,9]

Hyponatremia	Hypokalemia
Nausea, malaise, headache, lethargy, confusion, obtundation	Muscle weakness, fatigue, shortness of breath, decreased sensation in arms and legs, abdominal bloating (secondary to paralytic ileus)

Stenosis

Stenosis is a narrowing of the stoma, usually caused by formation of scar tissue due to the surgical construction, ischemia, active bowel disease, or dermatitis. Dilation and/or surgery may be required for correction.

Diet (Table 2)

Unless there are medical contraindications, individuals can eat a normal, varied diet, making their own adjustments to omit foods that change the consistency of the feces or cause odor or gas.[11] The foods most often cited as causing odor, gas, or frequent watery discharge are brans, fish, onions, carbonated beverages and beer.

People with an ileostomy will notice that high fibre foods remain undigested. Sometimes this undigested food can cause a blockage or obstruction of the stoma. These foods should be introduced into the diet one at a time. Eating them in small quantities, chewing well and drinking fluids with them will help avoid problems. Symptoms of obstruction include cramping, abdominal pain, vomiting, stoma swelling, and watery foul-smelling waste material. If an obstruction is suspected, refer to a physician.

Medication Use

With an ostomy, GI transit times for medication are altered, which may in turn affect the medication's pharmacokinetics. Extended release formulations may be unsuitable, and some medications are implicated in specific complications seen with ostomies (e.g., broad spectrum antibiotics increase the risk for fungal infections). Table 5 summarizes some medication concerns.

Lifestyle Considerations

Assure ostomates that they can wear their ordinary clothing and that if the pouch is changed and emptied as necessary it will not be visible. Women can continue to wear control top panty hose, but an elastic girdle may need adapting with an opening to prevent pressure on the stoma and pouch.

An ostomy does not interfere with exercise, sport, occupational work or sexual activity. There are specialized stomal caps and pouches that are intended for wear when swimming. A smaller sized pouch or even emptying the regular sized pouch, along with bathing suits of patterned fabric or boxer trunks for men, may help an ostomy patient feel more comfortable on the beach.[12]

Bathing and showering is possible with or without the appliance in place. Soap and water will not injure a stoma, but bath oils and soaps may leave a greasy film that can prevent the appliance from adhering. If a long soak in the bathtub is contemplated and the stoma will be below the water line, a cap can be used to prevent water from seeping into the stoma and the bowel. A wearer who wishes to attach a night drainage system to their appliance will require a freestanding holder or one that slides between the box spring and mattress.

Traveling with an Ostomy

When traveling, individuals with ostomies should always carry their ostomy supplies in their hand luggage and ensure they have sufficient supplies. Manufacturers of ostomy supplies will provide travelers with addresses for supplies at the travelers' destinations.

Resource Tips

WOCNs, formerly enterostomal therapy nurses, work with physicians in hospital and/or community settings, and are invaluable resources. Usually, an ostomy patient will have consulted with a WOCN pre- and post-surgery.

Some of the many organizations that provide patient support and/or educational material are listed below.

United Ostomy Association of Canada Inc.
Telephone: 1-888-969-9698
Web site: www.ostomycanada.ca

United Ostomy Association
Web site: www.uoa.org

International Ostomy Association
Web site: www.ostomyinternational.org

Wound, Ostomy, and Continence Nurses Society
Web site: www.wocn.org (more suitable for health care professionals)

Table 5: **Medication Concerns in Ostomy Patients**

Drugs that may have increased adverse effects

Antibiotics	Broad spectrum antibiotics may alter the normal flora of the intestinal tract resulting in diarrhea or fungal infections of the skin surrounding the stoma
Antimotility drugs	May cause constipation in colostomies and some ileostomies
Antidiarrheals	May cause constipation in colostomies
Antacids	Aluminum-containing antacids can cause constipation in colostomies; calcium-containing antacids can cause calcium stone formation in urostomies and ileostomies; magnesium-containing antacids can cause diarrhea in ileostomies
Corticosteroids	As an immunosuppressant can delay healing
Diuretics	May cause excess fluid loss and dehydration; with ileostomies fluid balance and electrolyte levels should be monitored
Laxatives	May result in perforations of colostomies, stool softeners are preferred; enemas should not be used with colostomies or ileostomies; avoid laxatives
Opioids	May cause constipation
Salt substitutes	May cause hyponatremia with ileostomies
Stool softeners	May cause diarrhea with ileostomies
Sulfa drugs	Crystallization in the kidney may be more prominent if the individual is having difficulty with fluid and electrolyte balance; more common with urostomies. Good fluid intake is required

Drugs that may be ineffective because they are poorly absorbed

Vitamins A, D, E, K, B_{12}	Can occur with extensive resection of the ileum[5]

Drug formulations that may be problematic

Enteric-coated or timed-release formulations	May pass through the intestinal tract intact; checking in the pouch for undissolved tablets will identify the problem; alternatives include chewable tablets and liquids. Avoid time-release preparations, especially with an ileostomy
Drugs that discolor the feces	For example, iron (black), bismuth (greenish black), salicylates (pink to red or black), senna (yellow), aluminum-containing antacids (whitish or speckled)

Crohn's and Colitis Foundation of Canada
Telephone: 1-800-387-1479
E-mail: ccfc@netcom.ca
Web site: www.ccfc.ca

Canadian Cancer Society
E-mail: ccs@cancer.ca
Web site: www.cancer.ca

Suggested Readings

A Professional's Guide for Counselling Ostomy Patients. Princeton, NJ: ConvaTec; 1998.

Hampton BG, Bryant RA. Ostomies and continent diversions. *Nursing Management*, 1992.

Patient Education Series: Managing your Colostomy. Libertyville, IL: Hollister Inc.; 1997.

References:

1. Mitchel JV. A clinical pathway for ostomy care in the home: process and development. *J Wound Ostomy Continence Nurs* 1998;25(4):200.

2. Rozen BL. The value of a well-placed stoma. *Cancer Pract* 1997;5(6):347.

3. ConvaTec Connection. *Preventing and managing peristomal skin problems.* Available at: http://www.convatec.com/ en_CA/education/preventative/index.html. Accessed August 29, 2001.

4. Bradley M, Pupiales M. Essential of ostomy care. *Am J Nurs* 1997;97(7):38.

5. American Dietetic Association/Dietitians of Canada. *Manual of Clinical Dietetics.* 6th ed. Chicago: 2000.

6. Canadian Paediatric Society. Caring for Kids page. *Dehydration and diarrhea.* Available at: http://www.caringforkids. cps.ca/babies/Dehydration.htm. Accessed October 25, 2001.

7. Pace B. Preventing dehydration from diarrhea. *JAMA* 2001; 285(3):362.

8. Singer GG, Brenner BM. Fluid and electrolyte disturbances. In: Fauci AS, Braunwald E, Isselbacher KJ, et al., eds. *Harrison's Principles of Internal Medicine.* 14th ed. New York, NY: McGraw-Hill, 1998:265-77.

9. Schultz NJ, Slaker RA. Electrolyte homeostasis. In: DiPiro JT, Talbert RL, Yee GC, Matzke GR, Wells BG, Posey LM, eds. *Pharmacotherapy: A Pathophysiologic Approach.* 4th ed. Stanford, CT: Appleton & Lange, 1999:890-917.

10. Metcalf C. Stoma care: empowering patients through teaching skills. *Br J Nurs* 1999;8(9):593.

11. Wood S. Nutrition and stoma patients. *Nurs Times* 1998;94 (48):65.

12. Aron S, et al. Self perceptions about having an ostomy: a postoperative analysis. *Ostomy Wound Manage* 1999;45 (4):46.

Diabetes Section Highlights

Chapter 30: **Diabetes Care**

Prevention of diabetes
Diagnosis
Key self-care goals for patients with diabetes
Eye care
Care of the kidneys
Dental care
Pneumonia and influenza vaccinations
Diabetic neuropathy
Cardiovascular health and hypertension in the diabetic patient
Skin care
Foot care
Managing hypoglycemia
Insulin absorption and care

Diabetes Appendix: **Diabetes Care Devices**

Diabetes management
Blood glucose levels
Blood glucose monitoring
  Testing/frequency of testing
  Blood lancing devices
  Characteristics of blood glucose monitors
  Testing with a blood glucose monitor
  Troubleshooting blood glucose monitors
Urine glucose monitoring
Ketone monitoring
Insulin administration devices and diabetes supplies
Teaching checklist

Diabetes Care

Maryann Hopkins, BSP, CDE

The Canadian Diabetes Association (CDA) estimates there are over two million Canadians with diabetes mellitus (about 6% of the population). CDA also suggests that many Canadians have diabetes but have not been diagnosed and that over the next few years the prevalence of diabetes will increase. In order to establish the true scope of diabetes in Canada, the National Diabetes Surveillance System has been in development since 1996. It will enable the ongoing surveillance of diabetes in Canada, including the health outcomes (morbidity, mortality) of those with this condition as well as the incidence, prevalence, and use of health care resources by those with diabetes. Diabetes is a serious health problem and a leading cause of death, new blindness and kidney disease in Canada. In 1999, the federal government allocated $115 million to establish a Canadian Diabetes Strategy to deal with this major health issue.

Pathophysiology[1]

The Clinical Practice Guidelines for the Management of Diabetes in Canada define diabetes as a "metabolic disorder characterized by the presence of hyperglycemia due to defective insulin secretion, insulin action or both."[1]

The cause of *type 1 diabetes* is multifactorial; both genetics and environment contribute. Development follows several stages. An environmental trigger occurs, often in the presence of certain Human Leukocyte Antigen (HLA) genes, which initiates an autoimmune process; i.e., an insulinitis develops and humoral and cellular immune responses are observed against islet antigens. Beta cells in the pancreas are progressively unable to produce insulin, and overt diabetes mellitus develops.

Type 2 diabetes is distinctly different from type 1.[1-3] Heredity plays a major role in its development. A noninflammatory beta cell abnormality occurs which diminishes the insulin secretory ability of the pancreas; therefore, the beta cells do not respond appropriately to hyperglycemia. A decreased sensitivity to insulin is paramount to the disease, exhibiting itself as insulin resistance in the liver and peripheral tissues. For instance, insulin circulating in the blood normally suppresses the production of glucose by the liver; however, in type 2 diabetes, the liver is less sensitive to insulin so it persistently produces glucose, raising fasting blood glucose levels. The specific mechanism by which insulin resistance occurs in the tissues is not fully known.

Gestational diabetes is first recognized or has its onset during pregnancy. Those with gestational diabetes are at high risk of developing type 1 or type 2 diabetes in subsequent years.

Although not an official classification, recent literature has coined the term "type 1 1/2 diabetes" which describes a group of patients with diabetes that clinically fits the pattern of type 2 diabetes but frequently exhibits diabetes-associated antibodies, indicating an autoimmune disease.[4,5] For example, patients with latent autoimmune disease in adults (LADA) exhibit insulin resistance, elevated glucagon levels and a slowly progressing autoimmune effect on the beta cells which results in an increased likelihood of need for insulin injections.[6]

Diabetes mellitus may also be caused by other endocrine diseases (e.g., Cushing's disease, acromegaly), drugs (Table 1) or toxins, other genetic defects, or infections.

There do not seem to be strong known risk factors for the development of type 1 diabetes. A slightly increased risk seems to exist if a close family member (mother, father, sibling) has diabetes and a significantly increased risk is present if an identical twin has the condition. Table 2 describes possible risk factors for type 1 diabetes. Table 3 lists known risk factors for type 2 diabetes.

Table 1: **Examples of Drugs Known to Induce Hyperglycemia**[7]

Alpha interferon	Pentamidine
Beta-blockers	Phenytoin
Cyclosporine	Tacrolimus
Diazoxide	Thiazide diuretics
Glucocorticoids	Thyroid hormones
Nicotinic acid	

Table 2: **Risk Factors for Type 1 Diabetes Mellitus**[1]

- Ethnicity/race (more common in the Caucasian population)
- Genetic susceptibility
- Unknown environmental factors (perhaps a virus, some foods)

Table 3: **Risk Factors for Type 2 Diabetes Mellitus**[8]

- Aboriginal, African, Asian or Hispanic descent
- Age > 45 yrs
- Close family member with diabetes
- Gestational diabetes
- Giving birth to a baby larger than 4000 g
- High blood pressure or cardiac disease
- High cholesterol or high triglycerides
- Impaired glucose tolerance (blood glucose is between 7.8 and 11 mmol/L) 2 h after a 75 g glucose load/fasting blood glucose < 7 mmol/L
- Obesity
- Physical inactivity

Prevention

First-degree relatives of someone with type 1 diabetes may have detectable immune abnormalities or reduced first phase insulin secretion during an intravenous glucose tolerance test. This indicates that they are in the asymptomatic phase of type 1 diabetes.

Potential strategies to prevent further development of type 1 diabetes in these patients have been attempted.

Several trials have been undertaken; however, there are no known successful strategies to prevent type 1 diabetes mellitus.[1]

Prevention of Type 2 Diabetes Mellitus

Two of the modifiable risk factors for developing type 2 diabetes are obesity and lack of physical activity. No studies have demonstrated prevention of type 2 diabetes in the long term; however, weight loss accomplished by healthy eating and increased physical activity have been shown to at least delay the onset of type 2 diabetes in the short term. Pharmacologic interventions have also been attempted. For instance, the Diabetes Prevention Program (a randomized, controlled trial with over 3000 American patients) has provided data to determine the success of lifestyle interventions or use of metformin in the short term (three years) in patients considered high risk for the development of type 2 diabetes.[9] Participants had impaired glucose tolerance, and at least one of the following criteria: age over 60, history of gestational diabetes, a first degree relative with diabetes, member of a minority group at high risk. The baseline risk of diabetes in patients with impaired glucose tolerance is 1 to 10% per year.[10] Corresponding to this, 10% of patients in the placebo or standard group developed diabetes per year.[10] Participants who lost 5 to 7% of their body weight and maintained physical activity on average 30 minutes per day reduced their risk of developing diabetes by 58%. Those who took metformin 850 mg twice daily reduced their risk by 31%. The study was stopped a year early as it was clear that both arms of the study (lifestyle changes and metformin) were successful interventions when compared to placebo.

A smaller randomized controlled study in Finland (the Finnish Diabetes Prevention Study, with over 500 patients) also studied patients with impaired glucose tolerance associated with an annual rate of progression to diabetes of 1 to 10%.[11] The study design assumed a 35% cumulative incidence of diabetes over the six-year period.[12] Researchers had five goals in the intervention arm: weight reduction (5% or more); reduction of fat intake to less than 30% of energy intake; reduction of saturated fat intake to less than 10% of energy intake; an increase in fibre intake to 15 g per 1000 calories, and an increase in exercise to 30 minutes per day. The incidence of diabetes was 58% less in the intervention group and those who achieved more of the goals had a lower incidence of diabetes whether they were in the control or intervention group.[12] Previous studies in China[13] and Sweden[14] showed similar results with lifestyle interventions, but these studies had methodological weaknesses.[11]

Diagnosis

The diagnosis of diabetes mellitus is based on laboratory blood tests and symptoms of high blood glucose; however, not all patients experience the classic symptoms of diabetes (Table 4). For example, the elderly are often asymptomatic or attribute symptoms of diabetes to aging or other illnesses.

Table 4: **Classic Symptoms of Diabetes Mellitus**

• Blurred vision	• Nocturia
• Fatigue	• Polydipsia
• Frequent infections	• Polyuria
• Hunger	• Weight loss

Diagnostic Criteria for Diabetes Mellitus[1]

The diagnosis of diabetes mellitus is dependent upon blood glucose levels obtained in the laboratory. Capillary blood glucose readings that fall within the criteria for diagnosis of diabetes should be confirmed with plasma glucose levels.

- Random plasma glucose $\geq$ 11.1 mmol/L *and* classic symptoms

or

- Fasting plasma glucose (no caloric intake for at least eight hours) $\geq$ 7 mmol/L

or

- A plasma glucose level two hours after a 75 g glucose load $\geq$ 11.1 mmol/L

Target levels for blood glucose have been established (Table 5).[1] Evidence that optimal blood glucose control can decrease the severity and frequency of diabetes-related complications comes from the Diabetes Control and Complications Trial (DCCT) for those with type 1 diabetes and the United Kingdom Prospective Diabetes Study (UKPDS) for those with type 2 diabetes.[15,16]

Goals of Therapy

- Develop a healthy lifestyle
- Prevent long-term microvascular and macrovascular complications
- Establish a regular medical follow-up schedule based on established recommendations
- Avoid symptoms of high or low blood sugars according to established targets
- Recognize, prevent and treat hypoglycemia

To achieve these broad goals, targets for metabolic control and hypertension have been devised by various expert groups.[17,18]

A systematic review of controlled trials revealed that several professional and organizational interventions improved the process of patient care and patient outcomes.[19] Many of the interventions were complex and multifaceted. The authors concluded that systems aimed at structured and regular review of diabetic patients improved patient care and that diabetes education led to improvements in patient outcomes.

Eye Care

The development of diabetic retinopathy is related to the duration of diabetes. Nearly all those with type 1 and more than 60% of those with type 2 diabetes will have some degree of diabetic retinopathy after having diabetes for 20 years.[20] Both macular edema and cataracts are more frequent in the diabetic population.[1]

Blindness is one of the most feared long-term complications of diabetes. Several factors predict progression of retinopathy including pregnancy (in type 1 diabetes), high blood pressure, high lipid levels, long duration of diabetes and high glycated hemoglobin levels.[1] In the DCCT, intensive insulin therapy in type 1 diabetic patients reduced or prevented the development of diabetic retinopathy.[20] Of the 726 patients included in the primary prevention cohort, 24% treated with conventional therapy suffered retinopathy versus 7% with intensive therapy (NNT=6). In the secondary prevention group with 715 patients, 41% of

Table 5: **Targets for Metabolic Control for Adults**

	Ideal (Nondiabetic)	Optimal	Suboptimal	Inadequate
Fasting or premeal (mmol/L)	3.8-6.1	4.0-7.0	7.1-10.0	Higher than 10.0
1 or 2 h after meals (mmol/L)	4.4-7.0	5.0-11.0	11.1-14.0	Higher than 14.0
Glycated hemoglobin	≤ 100%	≤ 115%	116-140%	> 140%

patients using conventional therapy had progression of retinopathy compared to 21% in the intensive therapy group (NNT=5).[21]

The UKPDS in type 2 diabetic patients revealed that every percentage point decrease in glycated hemoglobin resulted in a 35% reduction in the risk of microvascular complications including retinopathy and nephropathy.[20] Recommendations to prevent or delay the onset of diabetic retinopathy, or to prevent vision loss in the diabetic population are listed below.

Eye Care Recommendations for the Diabetic Patient[1,20]

- Screening/evaluation for retinopathy should be done annually five years after the onset of diabetes in post-pubertal patients with type 1 diabetes (after age 15).
- Screening for retinopathy should be performed for all patients at the time of diagnosis of type 2 diabetes. Follow-up should be at least every two years unless severity dictates more frequent evaluation.
- Women with type 1 diabetes should have an ophthalmic evaluation prior to becoming pregnant when possible, in the first trimester and throughout the pregnancy as needed based on perceived changes.
- Those with hypertension should comply with lifestyle and drug therapy for high blood pressure. Recommended lifestyle modification including dynamic exercise for 50 to 60 minutes three to four times per week; moderate alcohol intake (defined as no more than two drinks per day, or 14 drinks per week for males, nine drinks per week for females); stress reduction, weight loss (BMI ≤ 20-25) and moderate restriction of salt equivalent to an intake of 90 to 130 mmol per day.[18]

- Those with abnormal cholesterol levels (Table 7) should comply with cholesterol-lowering drug therapy as well as lifestyle changes. (Self-Care Strategies for Cardiovascular Health for Diabetic Patients.)
- People with diabetes should try to achieve optimal blood sugar levels (Table 5).
- Changes in vision should be reported to the physician or ophthalmologist.
- Encourage diabetic patients to stop smoking as tobacco use accelerates the development of microvascular complications of diabetes.[22]

Care of the Kidneys

The number one cause of end-stage renal disease in Canada is diabetic nephropathy.[1] Approximately 20 to 30% of those with type 1 or 2 diabetes develop some degree of nephropathy; however, fewer with type 2 progress to end-stage renal disease.[23] Early detection of microalbuminuria, early intervention strategies (e.g., use of ACE inhibitors and blood glucose normalization), and cardiovascular risk elimination help to arrest progression of the nephropathy.[1,24] A reduction in mortality from 94 to 45% has been seen with appropriate treatment of hypertension in type 1 diabetic patients.[23]

Self-Care Strategies to Prevent Diabetic Nephropathy[1,18]

- Screen for microalbuminuria in those with type 1 diabetes five years after diagnosis (after the age of 15) and annually thereafter.
- Screen for microalbuminuria in those with type 2 diabetes at the time of diagnosis and annually thereafter.
- Screening: If trace proteins or a negative dip-stick protein result is found in the urine, a micro-

albuminuria test is recommended. Screening for microalbuminuria should be performed with an albumin:creatinine ratio in a random daytime urine sample. If > 2.8 (females) or > 2 (males) the test should be repeated and confirmed in two of three measurements over three months. If there is still uncertainty, confirm with a timed urine collection that measures the rate of microalbuminuria.[1]

- Maintain optimal blood sugar (Table 5).
- Comply with hypertension treatment and have regular blood pressure checks.
- Reduce or eliminate all modifiable risks for heart disease e.g., smoking, excessive alcohol intake, stress, obesity, high cholesterol and blood pressure, physical inactivity.
- Obtain advice from a dietitian to determine appropriate protein intake. A reduced protein intake is thought to delay worsening of kidney failure.
- Seek prompt treatment for symptoms of bladder infections.

Dental Care

Those with poor blood glucose control and individuals who have had diabetes for many years are at higher risk for infections of periodontal tissue and increased calculus formation.[3] To prevent dental complications, diabetic patients should have dental visits annually or as often as their dentist recommends, brush and floss at least twice daily and use other dental cleaning aids as recommended by their dentist. Good glycemic control helps to minimize dental problems.

Pneumonia and Influenza Vaccinations

Diabetic patients are at increased risk for mortality and morbidity associated with *S. pneumoniae* and should receive the pneumococcal vaccine once. There is insufficient evidence to support revaccinating the diabetic patient unless there is the additional risk of:

- Having sickle-cell disease or debilitating cardiovascular or pulmonary disease;
- Having chronic renal disease, hepatic cirrhosis, HIV infection;
- Being immunocompromised (e.g., post-organ transplant) or asplenic.

In these patients, a one-time revaccination is recommended five years after initial vaccination in those over the age of 10.[25]

Like other patients with chronic diseases, diabetic patients should receive the influenza vaccine yearly.

Diabetic Neuropathy

Diabetic neuropathy can affect many areas of the body and will develop within 10 years in 40 to 50% of those with type 1 or 2 diabetes.[1] The most common type affects the feet, legs or hands producing symptoms such as tingling, numbness, aching, sharp, stabbing pain and other abnormal sensations. The neuropathy can lead to serious consequences such as foot or leg ulcerations or amputations. Other types of diabetic neuropathy include autonomic neuropathies such as gastroparesis and those causing bladder dysfunction, erectile dysfunction, sweating abnormalities and postural hypotension.

Self-Care Strategies to Prevent or Delay Progression of Diabetic Neuropathy[15,22,26,27]

- Encourage patients to maintain optimal blood glucose control (Table 5).
- Offer help with smoking cessation.
- Patients should avoid alcohol intake.
- Suggest annual screening for peripheral neuropathy by physicians, diabetes nurse educators or foot specialists. (See Diabetes Appendix for a simple test patients can use at home.)
- Educate patients to avoid injury by testing water temperature with the elbow rather than hands or feet.

Cardiovascular Health and Hypertension in the Diabetic Patient

Morbidity and mortality are two to four times higher in age and sex matched groups in the diabetic population than the nondiabetic population.[1] The risks of the vascular complications related to diabetes are increased in the hypertensive patient.[18] Table 6 summarizes cardiovascular disease risk in diabetic individuals.

Table 6: **Cardiovascular Disease Risk in the Diabetic Population**[1]

Condition/Description	Comments
Coronary artery disease	Twofold increase in men; 3- to 4-fold increase in women with diabetes
Stroke	Twofold increase in men; 3- to 4-fold increase in women with diabetes
Silent ischemia	More common in diabetic individuals
Infarction outcome	Worse in those with diabetes
Congestive heart failure	Greater risk in both males and females post myocardial infarction
Recurrent infarction	Fourfold increased risk in diabetic population
Risk of arrhythmias	Twofold greater risk

Those over the age of 30 with diabetes have a very high risk of developing coronary artery disease.[1] The lipid targets in Table 7 are considered optimal for the diabetic patient. If measured values are above the target levels, antilipemic medications and lifestyle changes should be implemented.[17]

Table 7: **Lipid Targets for the Diabetic Patient > 30 Years of Age**[17]

LDL-C level	< 2.5 mmol/L
Total cholesterol:HDL ratio	< 4
Triglyceride level	< 2 mmol/L

Self-Care Strategies for Cardiovascular Health for Diabetic Patients[2,17,18,22,28,29]

- Individuals with diabetes and abnormal cholesterol levels (Table 7) or high blood pressure (Table 8) should adopt a "heart healthy" lifestyle by getting regular physical activity, achieving and maintaining a healthy body weight, consuming alcohol only in moderation, eating a low fat/low salt/high fibre diet, not smoking, and reducing stress.

Table 8: **Blood Pressure in the Diabetic Population**[18]

- Those with blood pressure readings (BP) greater than 140/90 mm Hg should be treated to attain a target blood pressure of less than 130/80 mm Hg

- Those with BP readings of 130/80–139/89 and target-organ damage should receive treatment to a target of less than 130/80 mm Hg

- Diabetic patients should maintain optimal blood glucose control (Table 5).
- People with diabetes should have regular blood pressure check-ups and may benefit from home blood pressure monitoring.
- Those with diabetes should comply with antihypertensive and antilipemic medications.
- Diabetic individuals should have fasting cholesterol levels measured every one to three years as needed.
- Consider low dose acetylsalicylic acid (ASA) (81 to 325 mg) once a day in high-risk individuals over the age of 30 years and in those with heart disease. Even patients with severe stages of diabetic retinopathy who are at risk for vitreous hemorrhage are candidates for ASA treatment. Trials investigating ASA use specifically in the diabetic population are lacking. However, subset analyses of 145 secondary prevention trials suggest a reduction in stroke, myocardial infarction and vascular deaths and support the use of ASA in those with diabetes at high risk for cardiovascular events.[28]

Skin Care

Hyperglycemia, poor circulation due to vascular abnormalities and peripheral neuropathy contribute to impairing host defenses against infection.[3] Diabetic patients are predisposed to an increased risk of skin infections and a slower rate of healing.[3] Therefore, careful skin care is important in order to prevent serious skin problems. Table 9 suggests strategies for skin care in the diabetic population.

Foot Care

Individuals with diabetes are more prone to develop serious foot problems than the general population.

Table 9: **Skin Care Strategies for the Diabetic Patient**

Activity/Condition	Comment
Bathing	Patients should bathe daily with a mild soap. Avoid harsh chemicals including iodine-containing products, astringents or any agent which may worsen peripheral neuropathy or circulation e.g., alcohol, tobacco. Check water temperature with elbows not hands or feet to avoid burns
Cuts and abrasions	Keep clean; use paper tape to hold a sterile dressing or wrap gauze around wound as required
Dry skin	Use a moisturizing lotion or cream*
Existing skin problems	Ensure these are cared for and are healing
Inspect the skin daily (total body)	Check for dry, cracked skin, irritation, injury, and infection
New skin problems	Refer to physician
Sun exposure	Encourage sun safety by suggesting sunscreen and limiting exposure to sun

Moisturizing products often contain urea or alpha hydroxy-related compounds (e.g., lactic acid). See Table 6 in Chapter 41.

Foot ulcers and amputations are a major cause of disability and morbidity in those with diabetes.[1,30] It is estimated that 15% of those with diabetes will develop a lower limb ulcer during their lifetime and 14 to 20% of these will require an amputation.[31,32] Complications of diabetes such as vascular abnormalities, peripheral neuropathy and structural deformities of the feet contribute to the development of these complications.

- Peripheral neuropathy, characterized by numbness, tingling, weakness and reduced sweating decreases the sensation to pain that would normally be protective. This lack of sensation makes an individual with diabetes vulnerable to undetected injury from trauma, heat or irritation.
- Poor circulation prevents adequate nourishment or oxygenation to the tissues. This leads to dry cracked skin, changes in nail growth, and prevents or delays healing of wounds or ulcers. Encourage smoking cessation.[26]
- Improperly fitted shoes can put pressure or repetitive stress on foot deformities (e.g., hammer toes, calluses, boney prominences) found in the diabetic population. This can lead to foot ulcers.

Clinical practice guidelines[31] for diabetic foot disorders and a consensus statement on diabetic foot wound care[32] guide management of diabetic foot problems. Treatment involves assessment and evaluation, appropriate debridement, pressure relief (off-loading), wound management with dressings appropriate to the type of wound, management of infection and ischemia, medical management of comorbidities and surgical interventions if needed.[31] Prevention of an initial lesion and prevention of recurrent wounds is of utmost importance. The individual with diabetes must practise careful foot care on a daily basis. There are many strategies that reduce the risk of severe foot problems and amputations. (See Self-Care of the Feet for Diabetic Patients—Patient Information.)

Managing Hypoglycemia

One of the most serious adverse events associated with diabetes treatment regimens is hypoglycemia. Those with diabetes who are taking oral antidiabetic agents or insulin are at risk for a hypoglycemic reaction and should learn how to recognize and treat it. Teach patients to recognize the early signs and symptoms of hypoglycemia and to treat immediately with a fast-acting sugar source. Develop strategies to prevent hypoglycemic reactions. For example, some patients may need to take immediate-acting insulin after eating if insulin dose adjustments do not prevent reactions; meals and snacks should be on time; physical activity should be planned in advance.

Early signs and symptoms of hypoglycemia include:
- Sweating
- Hunger
- Shakiness
- Palpitations
- Anxiety, irritability, mood or behavior changes
- Numb lips or tongue
- Headache

If untreated, hypoglycemic symptoms may progress to:
- Blurred vision
- Confusion
- Slurred speech
- Convulsions
- Coma
- Death

Some medications which may contribute to hypoglycemia are listed in Table 10.

It is estimated that up to 25% of type 1 diabetic patients may experience hypoglycemia unawareness, in which the patient loses the autonomic warning signs of low blood sugar.[33] Avoiding hypoglycemic episodes increases beta-adrenergic sensitivity, thus restoring hypoglycemia awareness.[33]

Diabetic patients on acarbose experiencing a hypoglycemic reaction must use commercially available glucose tablets or gel, or a lactose source of sugar (e.g., milk). Acarbose delays the absorption of other types of sugars. Some examples of commercially available products include:
- Insta-glucose® gel (one 30 mL tube provides 10 g dextrose)
- BD Glucose® tablets (one tablet contains 5 g glucose)
- Dextrosol® tabs (one tablet contains 2.75 g glucose and a total of 3 g carbohydrates)

Table 10: **Examples of Drugs Known to Induce Hypoglycemia**

Alcohol
Beta-blockers
Pentamidine
Quinine/Quinidine (High doses e.g., 600-800 mg q8h)
Salicylates (high doses e.g., 4-6 g per day in adults)

See also Treatment of Hypoglycemic (Low Blood Sugar) Reactions—Patient Information.

Pharmacologic Therapy

Insulin

In order to achieve normal blood glucose levels, those with type 1 diabetes mellitus require exogenous insulin. Those with type 2 diabetes also require insulin therapy if an adequate trial of meal planning and exercise is not successful, oral antidiabetic agents are not effective or when there is a physical stress such as surgery or pregnancy.

The insulin dose, type of insulin required and the time of day the insulin needs to be administered depends on individual circumstances.

Table 11 describes some of the common insulin regimens used in the management of diabetes.

Various insulin products are available in Canada. Their characteristics are listed in Table 12.

Insulin Absorption

Several factors play a role in how the insulin will act. For example, factors affecting insulin absorption are:
- Site used to inject (fast to slower: abdomen, arms, thigh, buttock);
- Massage of the site;
- Exercise of the site of injection;
- Temperature of insulin (cold insulin absorbs more slowly);
- Lipohypertrophy (accumulation of fat at injection sites) or lipoatrophy (loss of subcutaneous tissue at the injection site). These conditions can be avoided by rotating injection sites.

Care of Insulin
- Unopened insulin may be kept refrigerated until its expiry date.
- Opened insulin that has been stored in the refrigerator should be discarded after one month (a slight potency loss occurs after 30 days if the vial has been in use).[36]
- Opened insulin in vials may be kept at room temperature, out of direct sunlight, away from fluctuating temperature changes for one month.[34] Insulin in cartridges may be stored according to manufacturer's recommendations (e.g., up to one month at ambient temperatures; for Novolin brand

Table 11: **Some Common Insulin Regimens**[1]

Regimen	Advantages	Disadvantages
Single daily injections (usually bedtime NPH, Lente or Ultralente combined with oral agents during the day)	• Reduces the nightly output of glucose by the liver • Induces less weight gain than insulin-only regimen • Patient starts the day with lower blood glucose, enhancing overall diabetes management • Easy method to start patients on insulin	• Only appropriate for those with an endogenous supply of insulin • Daytime blood glucose may not be optimal
Split mixed regimens (usually short- or rapid-acting insulins with NPH before breakfast and supper)	• Good control obtained • Convenient—only 2 injections per day	• Less flexibility (must adhere to schedule) • More difficult to schedule exercise without eating more (increased risk of weight gain) • May need snacks (increased risk of weight gain) • Risk of fasting hyperglycemia (NPH effects do not last until morning) • Risk of hypoglycemia in the late afternoon
Intensive insulin regimen (usually basal insulin is NPH or Ultralente given once or twice daily and either immediate-acting or short-acting insulin is given at mealtimes)	• Optimal control possible • Flexibility for mealtimes • Useful for those with shift work or unpredictable lifestyle	• Requires frequent blood sugar monitoring • Requires extensive training • Inconvenience of multiple injections • Increased risk of weight gain

Table 12: **Characteristics of Insulin and Analogues**[34,35]

Class	Type	Onset (h)	Peak (h)	Duration (h)
Rapid-acting	Lispro/Aspart	0.5-0.75	0.75-2.5	3.5-4.75
Short-acting	• Human insulin regular, Toronto	0.5-1	0.75-4.5	5-7.5
	• Pork insulin	0.5	2-4	5-7
Intermediate-acting	• Human insulin —NPH —Lente	 1-2 2-4	 4-12 7-15	 12-24 12-24
	• Pork insulin —NPH —Lente	1-3	6-12	24-28
Long-acting	Human insulin • Ultralente	3-4	8-16	24-28

Note: For details of the various insulins see specific products in the Compendium of Pharmaceuticals and Specialties, *published annually by the Canadian Pharmacists Association.*
For a listing of available insulins see the Compendium of Self-Care Products, *published annually by the Canadian Pharmacists Association. Onset, peak and duration may vary depending on product and patient characteristics.*

up to 37°C) or in the refrigerator.[34] All insulin should be protected from heat and freezing and excessive shaking or vibration (e.g., avoid the glove compartment of a car).

- Insulin that has clumps, is difficult to mix, has a frosted appearance or clear insulin that has a color change or cloudy look should be discarded.
- Insulin should not be stored in the luggage hold of an airplane and should be kept in an insulated container if traveling in winter or summer temperatures.

Nonprescription Therapy in the Diabetic Patient

Individuals with diabetes often select OTC remedies for minor ailments or diabetic complications. It is important for them to seek medical attention for more severe health problems before they become catastrophic; however, many minor conditions may be safely treated with the same OTC choices used by the general public.

Instruct diabetic patients to use low sugar/sugar-free products as many liquid pharmaceuticals may contain significant amounts of sugar. Low calorie options (i.e., 14 calories or less per dose) should be selected whenever possible. Also, frequency of glucose monitoring may have to be increased during illness to avoid loss of glucose control.

Occasional use of OTC *analgesics* has little or no effect on blood sugar levels, however analgesic doses of ASA and ibuprofen can adversely affect blood pressure. Regular use of acetaminophen and ASA can exacerbate chronic renal failure in a dose-dependent manner.[37] As a result, patients with diabetes requiring regular analgesia should be referred to their physicians. Topical capsaicin has successfully reduced the pain associated with peripheral neuropathy, although sometimes the effect is not seen for three to four weeks. Its use may be associated with burning and itching.[38]

Oral *decongestants* should be avoided in diabetic patients with hypertension, but data linking them to a rise in blood sugars is weak.[39,40] Another reason for cautious use in diabetic patients is the vasoconstriction caused by these agents, which can be more significant in those with vascular complications related to the disease such as poor circulation. Topical decongestants are less likely to raise blood pressure than oral decongestants but should be used with caution, if at all, in diabetic patients.[39]

Diabetic patients experiencing heartburn, indigestion or reflux can be treated with OTC *H₂-receptor antagonists* or with low sugar/sugar-free *antacids*. However, diabetes management may be complicated if significant gastroparesis is present. Encourage patients to discuss use of these nonprescription medications with their physician.

Constipation or diarrhea can be treated with the usual OTC remedies (e.g., bulk-forming sugar-free fibres, loperamide.) However, repeated constipation or diarrhea may signal gastroparesis that requires referral to a physician.

Sweeteners

Many products sold in the pharmacy contain either nutritive or non-nutritive sweeteners. Nutritive sweeteners such as sucrose, fructose, and sugar alcohols (e.g., xylitol, mannitol, sorbitol) and non-nutritive sweeteners such as aspartame, acesulfame K (potassium), sucralose, cyclamate and saccharin, can be incorporated into a well-balanced meal plan provided they are used in moderation. **Saccharin** and **cyclamate** should be avoided in pregnant and lactating women.

Sugar substitutes are regulated as food additives in Canada. Although some of these sweeteners have energy value, because they are extremely sweet only a very small amount is required in medicinal products. The effect on blood glucose is minimal if the dose contains less than 60 kJ/14 cal and less than 2.5 g of carbohydrate (see Table 7 in Chapter 33).

Alcohol

Alcohol may be incorporated into a diabetes meal plan provided blood glucose and lipids are appropriately controlled and there are no other contraindications to alcohol ingestion. Acceptable limits are defined as up to two drinks per day in men and non-pregnant, non-lactating females with diabetes.

- Increased physical activity and reduced food intake with alcohol ingestion can increase the risk of hypoglycemia.
- Those who use insulin or insulin secretagogues (e.g., sulfonylureas, repaglinide, nateglinide) should eat a carbohydrate-containing food when drinking alcohol to avoid delayed hypoglycemia.[41]
- Inform patients on metformin that acute and chronic ingestion of large quantities of alcohol can

contribute to the development of lactic acidosis, but that an occasional drink of alcohol is unlikely to be problematic.

- Alcohol contributes 29 kJ or 7 cal/g, and can therefore contribute to weight gain. Alcohol-containing medications are unlikely to contribute to poor blood glucose management or weight gain when used in moderation.

Alternative Therapy

Numerous plant remedies and dietary supplements are promoted to lower blood glucose levels.[42] Current evidence does not support the use of herbal remedies in diabetes.[43,44]

Several case reports and small studies of *chromium* in doses of 200 to 1000 µg per day have shown some lowering of blood glucose. Chromium has been associated with sleep disturbance if taken at bedtime, and possible renal insufficiency with high doses.[43] *Gymnema sylvestre* (400 mg per day) has also been shown to lower blood glucose.[44] *American ginseng* has demonstrated significant postprandial blood glucose lowering using 3 g prior to a 25 g glucose challenge.[45] *Konjac Mannan* has demonstrated improved metabolic control by improving blood glucose levels in insulin resistant patients.[46] In all of these cases, long-term results are lacking.

Resource Tips

Patients can find useful information from the Canadian Diabetes Association: www.diabetes.ca.

Suggested Readings

American Diabetes Association: Clinical practice recommendations 2001. *Diabetes Care* 2001. Available at: http://journal.diabetes.org/CareSup1Jan01.htm.

American Diabetes Association web site: www.diabetes.org.

Canadian Diabetes Association web site: www.diabetes.ca.

Gerstein HC, Haynes RB, eds. *Evidence-based Diabetes Care.* Hamilton-London (ON): BC Decker Inc.; 2001

Kahn CR, Weir GC, eds. *Joslin's Diabetes Mellitus.* 13th ed. Malvern (PA): Lea & Febiger;1994.

1998 clinical practice guidelines for the management of diabetes in Canada. *CMAJ* 1998;159 (suppl 8).

References

1. 1998 clinical practice guidelines for the management of diabetes in Canada. *CMAJ* 1998;159 (suppl 8).
2. Haire-Joshu D. *Management of Diabetes Mellitus: Perspectives of Care Across the Life Span.* 2nd ed. St. Louis, Missouri: Mosby-Year Book; 1996.
3. Davidson JK. *Clinical Diabetes Mellitus: A Problem Oriented Approach.* 3rd ed. 1999.
4. Juneja R, Palmer JP. Type 1½ diabetes: Myth or reality? *Autoimmunity* 1999;29:65-83.
5. Brooks-Worrell BM, Juneja R, Minokadeh A, Greenbaum CJ, Palmer JP. Cellular immune responses to human islet proteins in antibody-positive type 2 diabetic patients. *Diabetes* 1999;48:983-88.
6. Carlsson A, Sundkvist G, Groop L, Tuomi T. Insulin and glucagon secretion in patients with slowly progressing autoimmune diabetes (LADA). *J Clin Endocrinol Metab* 2000;85:76-80.
7. Young LY, Koda-Kimble, eds. *Applied Therapeutics The Clinical Use of Drugs.* 7th ed. Vancouver, Washington: Applied Therapeutics; 2000:48-87.
8. Canadian Diabetes Association. *Aged 45 and Older?* (pamphlet) March 3, 2000.
9. National Institute of Diabetes and Digestive and Kidney Disease. *Diet and Exercise Dramatically Delay Type 2 Diabetes; Diabetes Medication Metformin also Effective.* NIDDK clinical alert: 2001 (August 8).
10. National Institute of Diabetes and Digestive and Kidney Diseases. *Diabetes Prevention Program. Questions and Answers.* Available at: www.niddk.nih.gov/patient/dpp/dpp-qta.htm. Accessed March 2002.
11. Tataranni PA, Bogardus C. Changing Habits to Delay Diabetes. *N Engl J Med* 2001;344(18):1390-1.
12. Tuomilehto J, Lindstrom J, Eriksson JG et al. Prevention of type 2 diabetes mellitus by changes in lifestyle among subjects with impaired glucose tolerance. *N Engl J Med* 2001; 344(18):1343-50.
13. Pan XR, Li GW, Hu YH et al. Effects of diet and exercise in preventing NIDDM in people with impaired glucose tolerance. The Da Qing IGT and Diabetes study. *Diabetes Care* 1997;20(4):537-44.
14. Eriksson KF, Lindgarde F. Prevention of type 2 (non-insulin-dependent) diabetes mellitus by diet and physical exercise. The 6-year Malmo feasibility study. *Diabetologia* 1991; 34(12):891-8.
15. The Diabetes Control and Complications Trial Research Group. The effect of intensive treatment of diabetes on the development and progression of long-term complications in insulin-dependent diabetes mellitus. *N Engl J Med* 1993;329: 977-86.
16. UK Prospective Diabetes Study (UKPDS) Group. Intensive blood-glucose control with sulphonylureas or insulin compared with conventional treatment and risk of complications in patients with type 2 diabetes (UKPDS 33). *Lancet* 1998; 352:837-53.
17. Fodor G, Frohlick JJ, Genest JJG, McPherson PR. Recommendations for the management and treatment of dyslipidemia. *CMAJ* 2000;162(10):1441-7.

18. The Canadian Hypertension Recommendations Working Group. *The 1999, 2000, 2001 Canadian Hypertension Recommendations.* Available at: www.chs.md.

19. Renders CM, Valk GD, Griffin SJ et al. Interventions to improve the management of diabetes in primary care, outpatient, and community settings. *Diabetes Care* 2001 Oct; 24.

20. American Diabetes Association. Diabetic retinopathy. *Diabetes Care* 1999 Jan;22(suppl 1).

21. *Intensive Insulin Therapy Reduced Microvascular and Neurologic Outcomes in Type 1 Diabetes Mellitus.* ACP Journal Club. 1994 Mar-Apr;120:30. Revised Oct. 1999.

22. Haire-Joshu D, Glasgow RE, Tibbs TL. Smoking and diabetes. *Diabetes Care* 1999;22(11).

23. American Diabetes Association. Diabetic nephropathy. *Diabetes Care* 1999;22(suppl 1).

24. Effects of ramipril on cardiovascular and microvascular outcomes in people with diabetes mellitus: results of the HOPE study and MICRO-HOPE substudy. *Lancet* 2000;355(9200): 253-9.

25. Canadian Immunization Guide. 5th ed. Ottawa: Canadian Medical Association. Minister of Public Works and Government of Canada; 1998.

26. American Diabetes Association. Preventive foot care in people with diabetes. *Diabetes Care* 1999;22(suppl 1).

27. American Diabetes Association. Nutrition recommendations and principles for people with diabetes mellitus. *Diabetes Care* 1999;22(suppl 1).

28. American Diabetes Association. Aspirin therapy in diabetes. Position statement. *Diabetes Care* 2001;24(suppl 1).

29. Gerstein HC, Haynes RB eds. Evidence-based diabetes care. Hamilton-London (Ontario): BC Decker; 2001.

30. American Diabetes Association. Preventive foot care in people with diabetes. Position statement. *Diabetes Care* 2001; 24(suppl 1).

31. Frykberg RG, Armstrong DG, Giurini J et al. Diabetic foot disorders. *Foot Ankle Surg* 2000;39 (5):(suppl).

32. American Diabetes Association. Consensus development conference on diabetic foot wound care. *Diabetes Care* 1999;22(8).

33. Fritsche A, Stefan N. Häring H et al. Avoidance of hypoglycemia restores hypoglycemia awareness by increasing beta-adrenergic sensitivity in type 1 diabetes. *Ann Intern Med* 2001;134:729-36.

34. Repchinsky C, ed. *Compendium of Pharmaceuticals and Specialties*, 36th ed. Ottawa, ON: Canadian Pharmacists Association; 2002:805.

35. Boctor MA. Diabetes mellitus. In: Gray J, ed. *Therapeutic Choices.* 3rd ed. Ottawa: Canadian Pharmacists Association; 200:617.

36. American Diabetes Association: Clinical practice recommendations 1998. *Diabetes Care* 1999;21(suppl 1).

37. Fored CM, Ejerblad E, Lindblad P et al. Acetaminophen, aspirin, and chronic renal failure. *N Engl J Med* 2001;345(25): 1801-8.

38. Chrubasik S, Roufogalis B. Efficacy and safety of topical capsaicin preparations. *Austr J Pharmacy* 2002;83:42-4.

39. Young LY, Koda-Kimble. eds. *The Clinical Use of Drugs.* 7th ed. Vancouver, Washington: Applied Therapeutics; 2001:48-86-87.

40. Pray WS. BP effects of nasal decongestants. *US Pharm* 2000;25(2):18-24.

41. Wolever T, Barbeau MC, Charron S et al. Guidelines for the nutritional management of diabetes mellitus in the new millennium: a position statement by the Canadian Diabetes Association. *Can J Diabetes Care* 23(3):56-69.

42. Gori M, Campbell RK. Natural products and diabetes treatment. *Diabetes Educ* 1998;24(2):201-8.

43. Diabetes mellitus. Micromedex Health Care Series 2001; June:108.

44. Boon G. Botanical medicine and diabetes. *Can Diabetes* 2000;13(3):3-6.

45. Vuksan V, Sievenpiper JL, Koo VY et al. American ginseng (panax quinquefolius l) reduces postprandial glycemia in nondiabetic subjects and subjects with type 2 diabetes mellitus. *Arch Intern Med* 2000;160(7):1009-13.

46. Vuksan V, Sievenpiper J, Owen R et al. Beneficial effects of viscous dietary fibre from konjac-mannan in subjects with the insulin resistance syndrome. *Diabetes Care* 2000;23(1): 9-13.

47. Canadian Diabetes Association. *Kids with Diabetes in Your Care: A Practical Guide.* Available at: www.diabetes.ca.

Self-Care Recommendations
for Diabetic Patients—Patient Information

- Wear diabetes identification at all times.
- Aim to achieve and maintain a healthy weight.
- Keep blood pressure and cholesterol levels at the target you and your physician have established.
- Keep blood sugar levels at your target range.
- Do not smoke. Smoking increases rates of illness and death in diabetic patients.
- Follow a healthy, well-balanced meal plan. Ask to see a dietitian to establish a plan.
- Establish a regular exercise regimen with your doctor's recommendations. Wear proper footwear and inspect feet after exercising. Do not exercise if you are having unusual problems controlling your blood sugar levels, or in extreme heat or cold.
- Get advice on how to take care of your feet. (See Self-Care of the Feet for Diabetic Patients—Patient Information).

- See your doctor if you have difficulty sensing heat or cold or if you feel tingling in your hands or feet.
- Have an influenza vaccine each fall and have the "pneumonia" vaccine once.
- Have regular check-ups with your doctor, dentist and eye specialist.
- Learn about diabetes through a diabetes education program.
- Ask your doctor about medications used to prevent damage to your heart and kidneys.
- Become a knowledgeable health care consumer (e.g., ask questions, get a second opinion if you have any concerns).

Experiencing a Hypoglycemic (Low Blood Sugar)
Reaction[41,47]—Patient Information

- Be aware of early signs and symptoms of hypoglycemia including sweating, hunger, shakiness, palpitations, anxiety, irritability, mood or behavior changes, numb lips or tongue and headache.
- Always carry a source of fast sugar (e.g., glucose tablets or gel, juice box or a regular soft drink) and a snack (e.g., six crackers and cheese or peanut butter)
- At the first signs of low blood sugar, promptly treat with one of the following:
  —1/2 to 3/4 cup of orange juice
  —4 to 5 LifeSaver® candies (chewed)
  —3 to 5 sugar cubes, or 3 teaspoonsful of honey, table sugar or syrup
  —1/2 to 3/4 cup regular soft drink
- If you don't feel better or your blood glucose level is less than 4 mmol/L 10 to 15 minutes after you have treated your reaction, treat with one of the above options again. After this, if your blood sugar level is still low call a physician or go to the nearest emergency department.

- If your blood sugar is over 4 mmol/L and the next meal or scheduled snack is 30 minutes or more away, eat a snack of six crackers and one ounce of cheese or one slice of bread and a tablespoonful of peanut butter.
- If you are unable to swallow, someone else should administer a thick sugar source (e.g., honey, syrup, cake frosting) in the area between the cheek and the gums (carefully to prevent aspiration). Get medical treatment as soon as possible.
- If you are taking acarbose (Prandase) you must use glucose in the form of commercially available tablets or gel such as Insta-glucose, Dextrosol tabs, BD Glucose Tablets or a lactose source (e.g., milk) for hypoglycemia as other sugars are not absorbed quickly enough because of the medication.
- Teach family members and friends to administer glucagon in situations when hypoglycemia does not respond to the above treatment. The package insert for glucagon gives specific directions on this.

Patient Self-Care (PSC), 2002

Self-Care of the Feet
for Diabetic Patients[3]—Patient Information

1. Inspect
- Inspect feet daily, checking for scratches, cracks between toes, blisters, corns, sores, temperature changes, color changes and swelling. If you cannot see all parts of your feet, use a mirror or have another person assist with the inspection.
- Your doctor should perform a foot inspection at each appointment. Other health care professionals may include foot checks during your appointments.

2. Bathe
- Wash feet daily with warm, not hot, soapy water. Check water temperature with your elbow as you may not be able to detect an accurate temperature with hands or feet.
- Do not soak feet longer than 10 minutes. The feet must then be thoroughly dried, especially between the toes.

3. Moisturize
- Apply moisturizer to the tops and bottoms of the feet. Do not apply lotions, creams or oils between toes; instead apply a foot powder sparingly to this area to absorb excess sweat.

4. Trim
- Trim toenails straight across or have a professional cut nails. File the sharp edges with an emery board. Do not cut calluses or corns with razor blades, scissors or any other sharp object. Avoid chemical corn and callus removers which may damage the area. Only professionals specially trained in foot care should treat these problems.

5. Shoes and Socks
- Always wear shoes and clean, soft, socks or nylons. Do not wear socks that have been mended or that have holes or seams that may irritate the foot. Check the insides of shoes for sharp objects or rough spots before wearing them. Select shoes that fit well. Avoid sandals, plastic shoes, pointed toes and high heels. Break in new shoes slowly (e.g., 30 minutes the first day, 60 minutes the next day and so on).

6. Keep Feet Warm
- Wear socks to bed if feet are cold. Avoid frostbite. Do not use heating pads or hot water bottles and do not warm feet by the fireplace.

7. Circulation
- Avoid tight socks and other garments or devices that may impair circulation to the legs or feet. Avoid smoking and drinking alcohol. Maintain a healthy body weight and do not cross legs when sitting.

8. Injuries/Infections
- Report any injury or change in feet or legs to a physician so that treatment can be started as soon as possible. Start treatment for athlete's foot at the first sign of infection.

9. Exercise
- A routine of safe exercises (recommended by your physician) helps to improve circulation.

10. Control
- Good blood glucose control, cholesterol management and blood pressure regulation helps to maintain healthy feet and legs.

Diabetes Care Devices

Roger Larouche, BScPharm

Diabetes Management

The primary goals of therapy are to maintain health and avoid acute and long-term complications. Diabetes is a chronic disease; the diabetic patient requires regular medical assessment and laboratory testing to ensure optimal health. There is evidence that decreasing blood glucose levels to near normal range reduces the frequency of microvascular complications.[1,2]

Blood Glucose Levels

Optimal levels approach normal values and are associated with low risks of developing complications (Table 1). However, in some cases, these levels may be impossible to attain because of the possibility of severe side effects,[2] (e.g., hypoglycemia, diminished quality of life, cost).

Suboptimal levels can be attained by the vast majority of patients; for some, these levels will represent the best control attainable.

Inadequate glucose levels require reassessment and readjustment of therapy since these levels are associated with a markedly increased risk of chronic complications.

According to the most recent clinical practice guidelines for the management of diabetes in Canada, fasting plasma glucose levels used as diagnostic criteria of diabetes have been lowered from 7.8 mmol/L to 7.0 mmol/L. This lower figure more accurately represents the risk of a 2-hour plasma glucose of ≥ 11.1 mmol/L. These values are predictors of the development of microvascular complications.[3-5] As well, patients with fasting plasma glucose levels between 6.1 and 7.0 mmol/L show a greater risk of developing diabetes mellitus and cardiovascular disease than the general population. This evidence supports the use of self-monitoring of blood glucose.

Blood Glucose Monitoring

Daily monitoring by a diabetic patient improves the ability to control glucose levels,[6,7] and allows assessment of the effect of diet, exercise and changes in treatment regimen.

All available devices test a capillary blood sample which is whole blood. Meanwhile, laboratories use venous plasma glucose as the benchmark (plasma is whole blood without the red blood cells). Blood glucose monitors are adjusted to give results which

Table 1: **Levels of Glucose Control for Adults**

	Ideal (Nondiabetic)	Optimal	Suboptimal	Inadequate
Fasting or premeal	3.8-6.1	4.0-7.0	7.1-10.0	Higher than 10.0
1 or 2 h after meals	4.4-7.0	5.0-11.0	11.1-14.0	Higher than 14.0

All values expressed in mmol/L.

correlate with lab test results. Blood glucose self-monitoring devices should be verified annually and should not differ by more than 15% from a simultaneous laboratory measurement of a fasting venous blood sample.[8]

Canadian consensus guidelines state that blood glucose monitoring is an essential component of the therapeutic plan for all type 1 diabetic patients, all type 2 diabetic patients treated with insulin, and all previously diabetic pregnant women or those with gestational diabetes mellitus. It is an integral component of therapy for the majority of type 2 diabetic patients. Blood glucose monitoring can even be a useful component of therapy for type 2 diabetic patients treated by diet and exercise therapy.

Frequency of Testing

Health care professionals can assist in determining the frequency and timing of blood glucose measurements. Factors to consider are the potential benefits of monitoring versus cost and pain associated with the procedure.[9]

Patients with type 1 and type 2 diabetes receiving intensive insulin therapy should monitor blood glucose in order to adjust insulin doses. With intensive therapy, testing is performed before each meal, two hours postmeal and before bedtime.

Under more stable conditions, testing twice a day may be suitable. To have regular information on the whole day using twice-daily testing, patients should test with the following frequency: day 1 – before breakfast and supper; day 2 – before lunch and bedtime.

Encourage patients with type 2 diabetes using diet and exercise or taking oral agents to test periodically. Testing should also reflect premeal, postmeal and bedtime results.

Patients should test more often (e.g., up to six times per day) if:
- At any time the patient or contacts are in doubt of blood glucose control;
- Results are over 15 mmol/L;
- In case of illness;
- Any medication changes;
- Traveling (in same or different time zones), or
- Before and after vigorous exercise.

Testing

Major advancements in technology in the past 30 years have rendered blood glucose monitoring simple, easy and affordable. The price of glucose monitors has fallen drastically in recent years due to competition amongst manufacturers. As a result, better testing has led to improved outcomes for diabetic patients.[1,2] Of course, for accurate results, it is imperative that patients master the proper techniques of blood glucose monitoring.

Patients should track their results in a journal or log and share this information with their physician and other health care providers. In optimal self-monitoring of blood glucose, the patient is educated on the use of a monitor, interprets the results and modifies treatment based on current blood glucose levels according to individual guidelines provided by health care professionals.[10]

Blood Lancing Devices

The first step in blood glucose monitoring is obtaining a blood sample. A capillary blood sample is collected by puncturing the skin with a lancet which is a small needle of varying gauge or size. Lancets can be hand-held or patients can choose a spring-loaded device. When the lancing device is triggered, the needle is projected into the skin and retracts.

Since diabetic patients are more susceptible to infection, the area must be well-cleansed. Washing hands with soap and water is acceptable. When traveling, patients can use alcohol swabs instead. Lancets should not be used more than once, as a used lancet is more likely to cause infection and pain.

Most lancing devices have a depth adjustment. The majority of models are pen-shaped and accept a variety of lancets. However, some lancets can only be used by a precise lancing device. For example, Softclix® pens use Softclix® lancets.

When lancing, apply the pen on the skin exerting gentle pressure and press the trigger. Some triggers are stiffer and noisier than others. First-time users should trigger and load the device in the air a few times before lancing the skin, in order to "tame" the mechanism. Site rotation is also important. Frequent users will rotate between fingers; occasional, right-handed users might prefer lancing the left hand and vice versa. Holding the hands together, the target area is the skin visible between the fingernail and the area touching the other finger. Lancing can be painful but some devices may cause less discomfort. It is helpful if people recommending the devices take the opportunity to test them if possible. For information on available lancing devices see the *Compendium of Self-Care Products*, published annually by the Canadian Pharmacists Association.

Characteristics of Blood Glucose Monitors

Because of the many options available, health care professionals can assist diabetic patients in choosing an appropriate device based on consideration of the following factors.

Blood glucose monitors are available using two different technologies:

- *Sensor* or *electrochemical technology*: Blood is drawn through capillary action into the reaction zone where it encounters a small current; the resulting electrical output is measured. These meters do not require cleaning after use.
- *Reflectance technology*: Blood contacts a chemical, causing a change of color. The resulting color is analyzed. Most monitors using this technique require cleaning of the optic window, making the devices less user-friendly. Patients or health care professionals should consult the owner's manual for proper cleaning techniques.

Blood is usually obtained by a finger puncture with capillary blood being applied onto a test strip. Some models suggest alternate sites for blood glucose readings, such as the forearm. Special considerations and techniques apply for alternate sites.

Calibration, or coding the blood glucose monitor, is the process of programming the monitor to a new box of test strips. In some cases, calibration is as simple as inserting the test strip. Some monitors require pushing a button or inserting a code key for calibration.

Screen size is important for the many visually impaired diabetic patients. While some screens may be too small, others are large enough to display graphs.

Opening the packaging on individually foil-wrapped strips or devices with very small strips may present a problem for patients with arthritis.

Some strips cannot be touched on the areas where the blood sample is deposited or on the electrodes. More user-friendly monitors have *touchable strips*, which will not be affected by contact with these areas.

Battery life varies according to the frequency of use of the monitor and its other options. Most monitors inform users of a low battery situation. Even if batteries indicate a low charge, readings are precise. Changing batteries does not automatically cause a loss of accumulated data.

When using a monitor, operating and storing temperature range must be respected. Humidity and altitude are also important. If improperly stored, strips can give erroneous results because of exposure to humidity or temperatures outside the specified range.

All monitors are covered by a warranty and provide a 30- to 60-day satisfaction or money back guarantee. For information on available blood glucose monitors see the *Compendium of Self-Care Products*, published annually by the Canadian Pharmacists Association.

Testing with a Blood Glucose Monitor

Health care professionals assisting patients with blood glucose monitors must have a thorough knowledge of the available products. Demonstrations and detailed owner's manuals are available. As well, a quick reference guide is available with each monitor for rapid consultation.

Troubleshooting Blood Glucose Monitors

Although the newer monitors are easier to use, patients may still experience difficulties. Many monitors provide directions or error codes that patients or health care professionals can verify in the owner's manual or discuss with the manufacturer's technical support team.

Most problems are due to:

- Errors in user technique;
- Improper meter calibration. Check calibration number on strip container;
- Outdated or poorly stored strips. Check manufacturer's specifications regarding temperature, light and humidity;
- Inadequacy of blood samples, e.g., size, traces of alcohol used to clean puncture site;
- Dirty monitor window (reflectance models);

- Not respecting temperature and humidity requirements;
- Change in patient's situation, e.g., illness, stress, pregnancy, which can produce unexpected but accurate results;
- Changes in medications (including OTC).

Diabetes Management Software

With the appropriate interface, data can be downloaded from a blood glucose monitor to a computer. The software will enable the patient to see the information in different presentations, such as patient profiles, log books, means, variations, deviations from pre-set goals, charts, standard day, and insulin doses. This information can be printed. The software is available through the manufacturer; some health professionals may also offer this service. The software can be downloaded from manufacturers through the Internet, but a connection is still required between the glucose monitor and the computer (Table 2).

Urine Glucose Monitoring

Because blood glucose monitoring can be costly, painful and time-consuming, some situations may require urine glucose monitoring. Presence of glucose in the urine is the spill-over of blood glucose the kidneys could not adequately filter. Urine testing is not ideal as it does not reflect present blood glucose levels and will not indicate the presence of hypoglycemia.

Different reacting tablets and strips are available to test urine glucose. These are mostly visual identification methods, so patients must watch precise elapsed time when testing.

Ketone Monitoring

When insulin levels fall too low, the body shifts from carbohydrate to fat metabolism. Ketones are a by-product of this process. Normally ketones are excreted by the kidneys, but in this circumstance, elimination is not rapid enough and ketones accumulate in the bloodstream causing the blood to become acidic. The levels of blood glucose continue to rise, causing *diabetic ketoacidosis (DKA)* which is accompanied by the following symptoms: thirst, dry mouth and frequent urination; nausea and vomiting; blurred vision; pain in the abdomen; and fruity-smelling breath.

DKA occurs more often in type 1 diabetics but can also occur in type 2 diabetic patients. If blood glucose $\geq$ 15 mmol/L, check ketone levels. Ketones should also be tested during illness or pregnancy.[9]

Urine ketones are tested with strips. Again, the results are visual and precise elapsed time when testing is important. Blood ketones can also be monitored. Patients should check with health professionals for interpretation of results and an appropriate therapeutic plan. For information on available urine glucose and ketone tests see the *Compendium of Self-Care Products*, published annually by the Canadian Pharmacists Association.

Insulin Administration Devices

Syringes are required to measure the number of units of insulin to be administered. Various sizes and measurement increments are available. The 100-unit size has 2-unit increments for measuring larger doses, while the 50- and 30-unit syringes have 1-unit increments. The choice of syringes should be based on the total amount of insulin to be administered, remembering the smaller syringes will offer a more accurate

---

Table 2: **Examples of Available Software**

Manufacturer	Glucose monitor	Software
Abbott	Precision® QID, Precision® Xtra	PrecisionLink
Bayer	Dex®, Elite® XL	WinGlucofact Data Management
LifeScan	FastTake®, One Touch® Profile, One Touch® Ultra, SureStep®	In Touch Diabetes Management
Roche Diagnostics	AccuSoft Advantage®, AccuSoft Manager®	AccuChek Compass

measurement. The patient must also be comfortable while holding the syringe.

Needles vary in length and diameter. The shortest available needles are 5 mm; the longest, 12.7 mm. The diameter will vary from 27 to 31 gauge with higher numbers indicating a smaller diameter. The gauge (G) is related to length: shorter needles will tolerate a higher gauge, therefore causing less resistance in skin penetration and discomfort for the patient. While this is a physical and a psychological advantage, especially with children, short needles are not suitable for all patients. Obese patients using shorter needles must monitor blood glucose closely. Waiting three to five seconds before taking any needle out of the skin after injection will prevent insulin leakage from the injection site. If five seconds is not sufficient, this interval should be prolonged.

Reusing needles diminishes the point sharpness and removes the silicon coating. It may also lead to micro-traumas which are linked to nodule formation.

Insulin pens look like large fountain pens. Instead of retrieving the insulin from vials, the pen uses insulin cartridges available in two sizes that contain 150 and 300 units of human insulin.
Insulin pens are ideal for:
• Travelers;
• Patients on a frequent insulin administration program;
• Patients on a very low number of units per day;
• Those concerned with environmental waste, and
• Visually impaired patients, since they can count the clicks made when selecting the number of units to administer.

Insulin pens have limitations:
• Patients using more than 70 units per dose may need to measure and inject twice since pens only measure up to 70 units.
• Patients who require a mix of insulins (different from those commercially available) need separate pens and must inject the insulins separately.

Insulin pens should be kept at room temperature (between 0 and 30ºC), but unused cartridges can be refrigerated. Patients should understand the particular technique associated with the use of the pen. It is also advisable to keep a few syringes at home in case of a pen malfunction.

Note: Presently, there are two major companies in the pen/cartridge market and patients must be aware the *cartridges are not interchangeable.* Also, patients must know if their pens require 150 or 300 unit cartridges (1.5 mL and 3 mL) as only the appropriate cartridge size will fit the pen.

To prevent contamination, spillage or formation of air bubbles, needles should only be used once and not left in the insulin cartridge between injections.

More recent technology offers pens with electronic memory which displays dose and time of last injection. Newer pens also prevent measuring a larger dose than is actually left in the cartridge. For a listing of insulin delivery systems see the *Compendium of Self-Care Products,* published annually by the Canadian Pharmacists Association.

Insulin pumps allow the patient to receive insulin on a 24-hour basis, mimicking the body's normal insulin production. The pumps are programmable, allowing manual override for special needs. Patients selected to use insulin pumps should be fully capable of understanding the illness as well as the technical aspects involved. The pump delivers insulin through a thin plastic tubing called an infusion set. At the end of the tube is a needle which is inserted in the skin, usually the abdomen, and changed every two or three days. To confirm availability, check with local diabetic specialists, diabetic associations or a supplier (e.g., Auto Control Medical).

Auto-injecting devices are available for those who have difficulty inserting a needle; a spring-loaded mechanism automatically inserts the needle in the skin. The patient simply pushes the plunger to deliver the insulin. Some devices will insert the needle and deliver the insulin automatically. *Jet injectors* "blow" insulin through the skin without a needle. They are more precise in delivering the desired dose of insulin but are costly, not always covered by insurance programs and need proper adjustment to reduce risks of pain and bruising.

Magnifying devices enlarge the entire length of the scale on the syringe for those who are visually impaired. They also guide the needle into the insulin vial and help detect air bubbles.

Insulin measuring devices are helpful for the visually impaired or for those who need help measuring the amount of insulin required in a syringe. This device guides the needle in the vial and permits the user to feel or hear by a "click" the number of units entering the syringe; it also aids the mixing of two insulins.

Plastic syringe cases allow transport of pre-filled syringes without accidentally applying pressure to the plunger. They are available for one or seven syringes. This tool is excellent for health care professionals who pre-fill and deliver insulin to patients with special needs.

Travel kits organize all diabetic needs in one place. For patients traveling in areas of extreme temperature, most travel kits contain ice packs.

Disposing of needles/syringes in an environmentally-friendly manner is an important issue. Another key point is safe disposal to avoid injury or re-use of diabetic supplies. From manual needle disposal to electronic systems (NeedleSAFE™), these devices cut the needle from the syringe enabling the user to dispose of the used syringes in household waste.

Other disposals include biomedical waste containers, which are tamper-proof and should be disposed of through normal biomedical waste retrieval channels.

Miscellaneous Supplies

Patients should write their results in a logbook. Health professionals can use the information to guide treatment. A logbook also offers the advantage of adding such pertinent comments as illnesses, alcohol consumption and nonprescription medication use.

Sensory foot exams help detect peripheral neuropathy. Patients, caregivers or health care professionals can perform a simple test by pressing a 10 g Semmes-Weinstein monofilament lightly against the foot to determine any loss of sensation.[11,12] Studies support the stratification of patients into a high or low risk of ulceration or amputation based on this simple test.

Four to ten per cent of people with diabetes will develop a foot ulcer. Special shoes or socks may lower risks of foot complications. Socks should provide extra cushion and warmth while wicking perspiration away from the feet. Acrylic socks are recommended as cotton socks hold moisture on the skin.[13] They must also be well-adjusted in order not to cut circulation and have no rough seams. Some of

these special socks are, in fact, a "sock in a sock." They provide a reduced risk of blisters, callous or corn formation, because friction will occur between layers of the sock instead of between layers of skin. Fibers will absorb humidity and cushion the feet.

In case of hypoglycemia, patients can treat the condition by consuming a food or beverage with high sugar content. Dextrose gels or tablets (*sugar supplements*) provide an exact amount of sugar, offering a convenient and rapid solution. Encourage patients to carry these supplements at all times. Close contacts should also be familiar with the use of these supplements in case the patient is unable to self-administer.

Glucagon is a hormone that counteracts the action of insulin. A glucagon injection releases a burst of glucose into the blood, thereby easing the symptoms of low blood sugar. Glucagon kits, containing a preloaded syringe, are mainly for use by family or friends in treating a severe insulin reaction in patients unable to take sugar by mouth. Medical attention should follow for patients not recovering after a few minutes.

Hypoglycemia alarms are available for type 1 diabetic patients who experience hypoglycemic episodes characterized by headache, irritability, trembling, sweating and rapid heart beat. The alarm, which is especially useful during sleep when symptoms may not be identified, is triggered by electrodes detecting perspiration; it emits a beep to wake or alert the patient.

Resource Tips[14]

Canadian Diabetes Association: www.diabetes.ca

American Diabetes Association: www.diabetes.org

Blood Glucose Meters: www.mendosa.com/meters.htm

National Institute of Diabetes and Kidney Disease: www.niddk.nih.gov

Diabetes in control: www.diabetesincontrol.com

For information on insulin pumps: www.insulin-pumpers.org

For software inquiries: Contact the manufacturer or check www.mendosa.com/software.htm

Teaching Checklist:

Patient's name	Monitor brand
Patient's address	Monitor model

Health Care Professional	First time user:
User's profile: *(type 1 or type 2 diabetic)*	Monitor exchange:

A. Objectives of blood glucose monitor (E)*	• Why are we testing	☐
	• What are we testing	☐
	• How are we testing	☐
	• When should we test	☐
B. Preparations (P)*	• Get supplies ready	☐
	• Check calibration (adjust calibration) and expiry date	☐
	• Press the On button and/or insert a strip	☐
C. Getting a sample (P)	• Always clean the puncture site	☐
	• Lancing device, depth adjustment	☐
	• Puncture area and site rotation	☐
	• Blood sample size	☐
D. Getting the result (P)	• Drawing the sample on/in the strip	☐
	• Read and write the results in logbook	☐
	• Add pertinent comments to the logbook	☐
E. Maintenance (E)	• Disposing of lancets and strips	☐
	• Control solutions and annual test with lab test	☐
	• Check strips	☐
	• Cleaning if necessary	☐
	• Batteries	☐
	• Warranty	☐
Comments:		

E: explanation only   P: explanation and practice

References

1. Ohkubo Y, Kishikawa H, Araki E et al. Intensive insulin therapy prevents the progression of diabetic microvascular complications in Japanese patients with non-insulin-dependent diabetes mellitus: a randomized prospective 6-year study. *Diabetes Res Clin Pract* 1995;28:103-17.
2. Diabetes Control and Complications Trial Research Group (DCCT). The effect of intensive treatment of diabetes on the development and progression of long-term complications in insulin-dependent diabetes mellitus. *N Engl J Med* 1993;329: 977-86.
3. Report of the Expert Committee on the Diagnosis and Classification of Diabetes Mellitus. *Diabetes Care* 1997;20:1-15.
4. McCance DR, Hanson RL, Charles MA et al. Comparison of tests for glycated haemoglobin and fasting and two-hour plasma glucose concentrations as diagnostic methods for diabetes. *BMJ* 1994;308:1323-8.
5. Engelgau MM, Thompson TJ, Herman WH et al. Comparison of fasting and 2-hour glucose and HbA1c levels for diagnosing diabetes: diagnostic criteria and performance revisited. *Diabetes Care* 1997;20:785-91.
6. Cox DJ, Kovatchev BP, Julian DM et al. Frequency of severe hypoglycemia in insulin-dependent diabetes mellitus can be predicted from self-monitoring blood glucose data. *J Clin Endocrinol Metab* 1994;79:1659-62.
7. Schiffrin A, Suissa S. Predicting nocturnal hypoglycemia in patients with type 1 diabetes treated with continuous subcutaneous insulin infusion. *Am J Med* 1987;82:1127-32.
8. Bertrand S, Aris-Jilwan N, Reddy S et al. Recommendations for the use of self-monitoring of blood glucose in diabetes mellitus. *Can J Diabetes Care* 1996;20:14-6.
9. Goldstein DE, Little RR. Monitoring glycemia in diabetes: short-term assessment. *Endocrinol Metab Clin North Am* 1997;26:475-86.
10. 1998 clinical practice guidelines for the management of diabetes in Canada. *CMAJ* 1998;159:S1-S29
11. Vinik AI, Suwanwalaikorn S, Stansberry KB et al. Quantitative measurement of cutaneous perception in diabetic neuropathy. *Muscle Nerve* 1995;18:574-84.
12. Diabetic foot screening instructions. *Pharm Lett* Mar 2000; (16).
13. Scheffler NM. *Foot Know-How.* Available at: www.diabetes. org/Diabetes/breast/98July/pg64.htm. Accessed Dec 2001.
14. Fournier Y. Les meilleurs sites sur le diabète. *Qué Pharm* 48(5)2001:364-6.

Photo Section Highlights

1. Healthy Stoma; Chapter 29, Ostomy Care.

2. Peristomal Skin Excoriation; Chapter 29, Ostomy Care.

3. Athlete's Foot; Chapter 38, Athlete's Foot.

4. Corns; Chapter 39, Corns, Calluses, Bunions and Ingrown Toenails.

5. Plantar Warts; Chapter 40, Plantar Warts.

6. Atopic Dermatitis; Chapter 41, Dermatitis.

7. Actinic Keratoses; Chapter 44, Cosmetic Dermatology.

8. Erythema Infectiosum (Fifth Disease); Chapter 45, Viral Skin Infections.

9. Gianotti-Crosti Syndrome; Chapter 45, Viral Skin Infections.

10. Chickenpox (Varicella); Chapter 45, Viral Skin Infections.

11. Gianotti-Crosti Syndrome; Chapter 45, Viral Skin Infections.

12. Hand-Foot-Mouth Disease; Chapter 45, Viral Skin Infections.

13. Herpes Zoster; Chapter 45, Viral Skin Infections.

14. Acute Generalized Exanthematous Pustulosis (AGEP); Chapter 46, Drug-induced Skin Reactions.

15. Hypersensitivity Syndrome Reaction; Chapter 46, Drug-induced Skin Reactions.

16. Serum Sickness-like Reaction; Chapter 46, Drug-induced Skin Reactions.

17. Folliculitis; Chapter 47, Skin Infections and Infestations.

18. Candidiasis (Intertrigo); Chapter 47, Skin Infections and Infestations.

19. Scabies; Chapter 47, Skin Infections and Infestations.

20. Tinea Corporis; Chapter 47, Skin Infections and Infestations.

21. Warts; Chapter 47, Skin Infections and Infestations.

22. Lyme Disease Lesion; Chapter 48, First Aid Treatment of Skin Conditions.

23. Leukoplakia; Chapter 61, Aphthous Ulcers.

24. Aphthous Ulcer; Chapter 61, Aphthous Ulcers.

25. Establishing Successful Latch; Chapter 32, Infant Nutrition.

26. Seborrheic Dermatitis; Chapter 42, Dandruff, Seborrhea and Psoriasis.

27. Acneiform Eruption; Chapter 46, Drug-induced Skin Reactions.

28. Toxic Epidermal Necrolysis; Chapter 46, Drug-induced Skin Reactions.

29. Impetigo; Chapter 47, Skin Infections and Infestations.

30. Pityriasis Versicolour; Chapter 47, Skin Infections and Infestations.

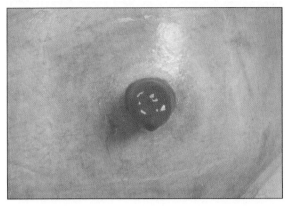

1. **Healthy Stoma**; Chapter 29, Ostomy Care. Courtesy of Convatec.

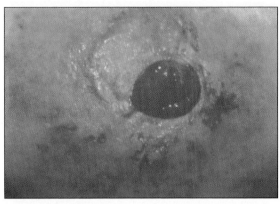

2. **Peristomal Skin Excoriation**; Chapter 29, Ostomy Care. Courtesy of Convatec.

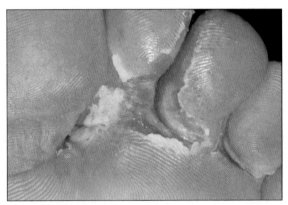

3. **Athlete's Foot**; Chapter 38, Athlete's Foot. Courtesy of SPL/Publiphoto.

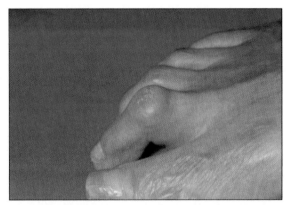

4. **Corns**; Chapter 39, Corns, Calluses, Bunions and Ingrown Toenails. Courtesy of Dr. P. Marazzi/SPL/Publiphoto.

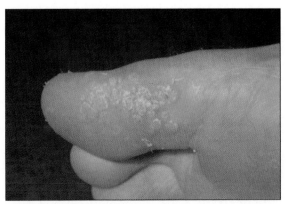

5. **Plantar Warts**; Chapter 40, Plantar Warts. Courtesy of Dr. P. Marazzi/SPL/Publiphoto.

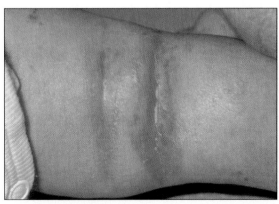

6. **Atopic Dermatitis**; Chapter 41, Dermatitis. Courtesy of Dr. P. Marazzi/SPL/Publiphoto.

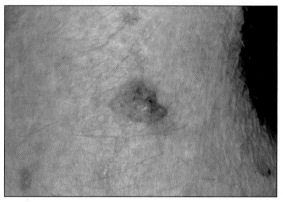

7. **Actinic Keratosis**; Chapter 44, Cosmetic Dermatology. Courtesy of Dr. P. Marazzi/SPL/Publiphoto.

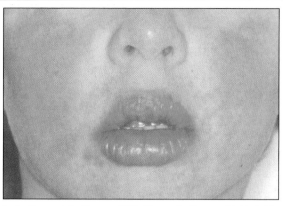

8. **Erythema Infectiosum (Fifth Disease)**; Chapter 45, Viral Skin Infections. Courtesy of Bernice Krafchik.

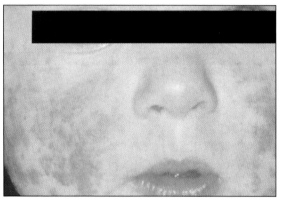

9. **Gianotti-Crosti Syndrome**; Chapter 45, Viral Skin Infections. Courtesy of Bernice Krafchik

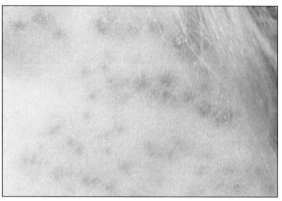

10. **Chickenpox (Varicella)**; Chapter 45, Viral Skin Infections. Courtesy of Bernice Krafchik.

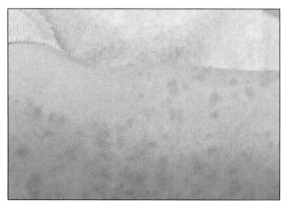

11. **Gianotti-Crosti Syndrome**; Chapter 45, Viral Skin Infections. Courtesy of Bernice Krafchik..

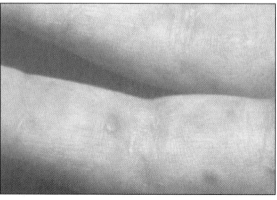

12. **Hand-Foot-Mouth Disease**; Chapter 45, Viral Skin Infections. Courtesy of Bernice Krafchik.

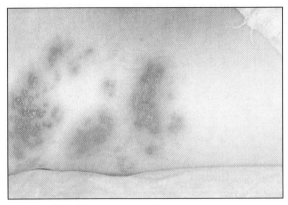

13. **Herpes Zoster**; Chapter 45, Viral Skin Infections. Courtesy of Bernice Krafchik.

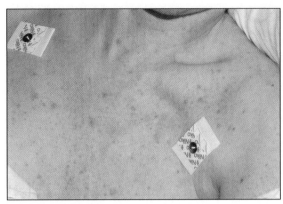

14. **Acute Generalized Exanthematous Pustulosis (AGEP)**; Chapter 46, Drug-induced Skin Reactions. Courtesy of Dr. John R. Sullivan.

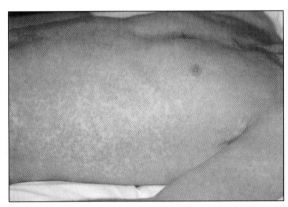

15. **Hypersensitivity Syndrome Reaction**; Chapter 46, Drug-induced Skin Reactions. Courtesy of Dr. John R. Sullivan.

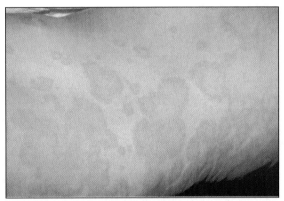

16. **Serum Sickness-like Reaction**; Chapter 46, Drug-induced Skin Reactions. Courtesy of Dr. John R. Sullivan.

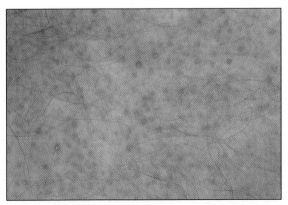

17. **Folliculitis**; Chapter 47, Skin Infections and Infestations. Courtesy of Dr. Chris Hale/SPL/Publiphoto.

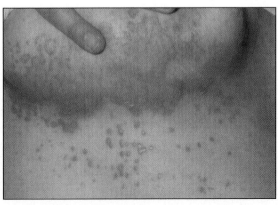

18. **Candidiasis (Intertrigo)**; Chapter 47, Skin Infections and Infestations. Courtesy of Dr. P. Marazzi/SPL/Publiphoto.

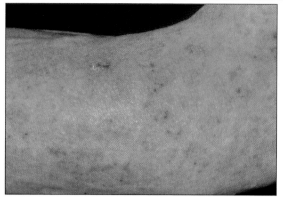

19. **Scabies**; Chapter 47, Skin Infections and Infestations. Courtesy of Dr. P. Marazzi/SPL/Publiphoto.

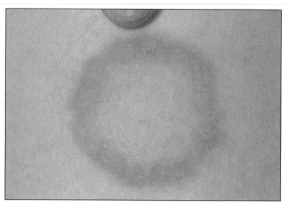

20. **Tinea Corporis**; Chapter 47, Skin Infections and Infestations. Courtesy of SPL/Publiphoto.

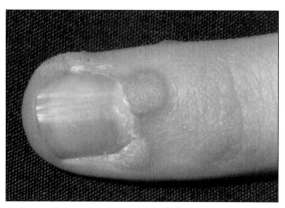

21. **Warts**; Chapter 47, Skin Infections and Infestations. Courtesy of Dr. P. Marazzi/SPL/Publiphoto.

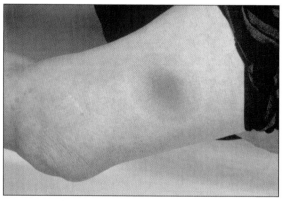

22. **Lyme Disease Lesion**; Chapter 48, First Aid Treatment of Skin Conditions. Courtesy of SPL/Publiphoto.

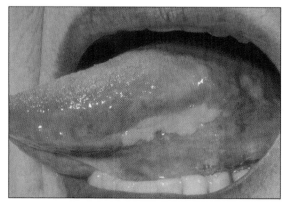

23. **Leukoplakia**; Chapter 61, Aphthous Ulcers. Courtesy of Dr. P. Marazzi/SPL/Publiphoto.

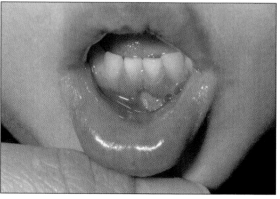

24. **Aphthous Ulcer**; Chapter 61, Aphthous Ulcers. Courtesy of Dr. P. Marazzi/SPL/Publiphoto.

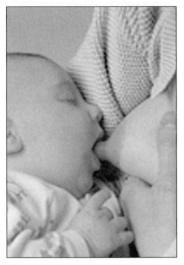

25. **Establishing Successful Latch**; Chapter 32, Infant Nutrition. Courtesy of Medela, Inc.

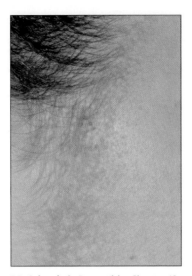

26. **Seborrheic Dermatitis**; Chapter 42, Dandruff, Seborrhea and Psoriasis. Courtesy of Dr. P. Marazzi/SPL/Publiphoto.

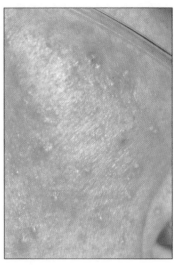

27. **Acneiform Eruption**; Chapter 46, Drug-induced Skin Reactions. Courtesy of Dr. John R. Sullivan.

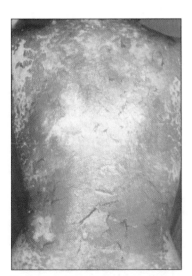

28. **Toxic Epidermal Necrolysis**; Chapter 46, Drug-induced Skin Reactions. Courtesy of Dr. John R. Sullivan.

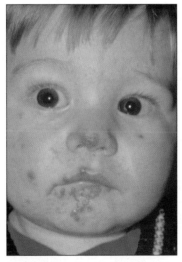

29. **Impetigo**; Chapter 47, Skin Infections and Infestations. Courtesy of Dr. P. Marazzi/SPL/Publiphoto.

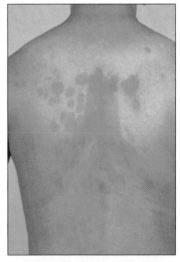

30. **Pityriasis Versicolor**; Chapter 47, Skin Infections and Infestations. Courtesy of St. Bartholomew's Hospital/SPL/Publiphoto.

Nutrition Section Highlights

Chapter 31: **Basic Nutrition**

Essential dietary components
Fat soluble vitamins
Water-soluble vitamins
Major and trace minerals
Nonessential dietary components
Preventive supplementation
Therapeutic supplementation
Calcium/fibre/iron/chelates
Food labels
Common nutrient content terms
Canada's Food Guide to Healthy Eating

Chapter 32: **Infant Nutrition**

Breastfeeding
  Physiology of breastfeeding
  Contraindications/challenges
  Benefits of breastfeeding
  Establishment of breastfeeding
  Common problems
  Drugs and breastfeeding
  Ancillary breastfeeding products
Infant Formula
  Choosing infant formula
Bottle-feeding formula or breastmilk
Vitamin and mineral supplementation of infants
Weaning and transition to solid food

Chapter 33: **Weight Management**

Classification of overweight and obesity
Medications associated with weight gain
Assessment of obesity and underweight
Warning signs of anorexia and bulimia
Diet therapy—nutrient content comparison
Artificial sweeteners
Inappropriate medications for weight loss

Nutrition Appendix 1: **Special Diets**

Sodium-restricted diet
Potassium-modified diet
Fat-restricted diet
Lactose-restricted diet
Gluten-restricted diet
Fibre-modified diet
High-calorie, high-protein diet
Purine-restricted diet
Tyramine-controlled diet

Nutrition Appendix 2: **Sports Nutrition**

Nutrition for the competitive athlete
Fluid needs during exercise
Nutritional supplements and ergogenic aids

Chapter 31

Basic Nutrition

Carole Beveridge, BScPhm, RNCP

Definitions

Nutrition is the study of foods and their constituents — their ingestion, digestion, absorption, transport and utilization — and includes the action, interaction and balance of food constituents as they pertain to human health and disease.[1] Its role is to sustain life, provide energy, promote growth and replace loss.

Energy is needed by the body for maintenance of body composition and function, for physiological processes involved in food absorption, for performing work and for adapting to various environmental stresses.

Carbohydrates, lipids and **proteins** are *macronutrients*. In addition to providing *micronutrients* (i.e., vitamins and minerals) they are the main sources of energy. Carbohydrates and proteins each supply approximately 4 kcal of energy/g, and lipids 9 kcal/g.[2]

Current guidelines suggest a daily energy intake in the range of 1800 kcal per day to 3200 kcal per day to ensure sufficient intake of nutrients.[3] Table 1 outlines current guidelines for estimating energy requirements based on age and gender; note that energy needs increase during growth and pregnancy to allow for synthesis of new tissue.

Excess or deficient energy intake can lead to underweight or overweight and increased health risks. The *Body Mass Index (BMI)* calculated as weight (kg)/ height (m)[2], is used to describe the relationship of body mass to height (see Chapter 33).

The terms "essential" and "nonessential" are used to describe whether nutrients are available endogenously or exogenously.[1] Essential nutrients are considered necessary to human life and cannot be manufactured by the body itself. They are described below.

Water comprises approximately 60% of adult body weight and provides the medium for all body fluids, including blood, lymph, digestive juices, urine and perspiration. Functions of water are numerous including regulation of body temperature, transport of electrolytes and nutrients, safe elimination of toxins and waste products.[3] Fluids in dietary food and drink provide the primary source.

Table 1: **Estimated Basal Energy Requirements in Adults**

Gender	Age	Calculation*
Male	18-30 yrs	kcal/day = (15.3 × weight) + 679
	30-60 yrs	kcal/day = (11.6 × weight) + 879
	> 60 yrs	kcal/day = (8.8 × weight) + (1128 × height) - 1071
Female	18-30 yrs	kcal/day = (14.7 × weight) + 496
	30-60 yrs	kcal/day = (8.7 × weight) + 829
	> 60 yrs	kcal/day = (9.2 × weight) + (637 × height) - 302

Weight in kg; height in m.
Reprinted with permission from the World Health Organization. American Dietetic Association/Dietitians of Canada. *Manual of Clinical Dietetics.* 6th ed. Chicago: 2000 (Table 1.17). WHO Technical Report Series No. 724.

Requirements: Water requirements average approximately 2.5 L daily, but can easily increase fivefold in extreme conditions of hot weather or heavy exercise.[4]

Typically, daily turnover of water is approximately 4% of total body weight, even without perspiration. Daily fluid requirements based on body weight can be estimated as follows:[5]

100 mL per kg body weight for first 10 kg

plus 50 mL per kg body weight for next 10 kg

plus 20 mL per kg body weight for each kg above 20 kg

Thirst is the body's primary mechanism for ensuring adequate hydration; however, up to 2% of body weight can be lost before this mechanism becomes activated. *Dehydration* is defined as the loss of at least 1% of body weight as a result of fluid loss. Its progression can be marked by a number of signs and symptoms such as dry mouth, dizziness and delirium.

A 10% loss of body water through excessive vomiting, diarrhea or sweating can pose a significant health risk and lead to electrolyte depletion, while a 20% loss can be fatal.[1] Drugs such as alcohol and diuretics can aggravate fluid imbalance.

Dehydration in children through prolonged vomiting and/or diarrhea is a significant health concern. Isonatremic dehydration, with loss of both potassium and sodium occurs in approximately 80% of cases and is typically managed using oral rehydration solutions. Hypernatremic dehydration (15%) and hyponatremic dehydration (5%) can usually be similarly managed, provided fluid is replaced over six to eight hours and a balanced electrolyte solution is used.[6] (See Chapter 20, Nausea and Vomiting, and Chapter 26, Infant Colic, for a discussion of dehydration.)

Carbohydrates serve as the body's major energy source and the sole energy source for the central nervous system. Carbohydrates provide structure to cell components in addition to assisting in regulation of protein and lipid metabolism.[7,8] As the body's preferred energy source, carbohydrates are efficiently absorbed for immediate use or easily converted to storage forms, such as glycogen in the muscle and liver or fatty acids in adipose tissue.[3,9] Consumption of *complex carbohydrates*, a primary source of dietary fibre and beta-carotene, is encouraged due to its association with a lower incidence of heart disease and cancer.[3] In addition, complex carbohydrates such as whole grains typically have a lower *glycemic index* than processed forms, resulting in better satiety and more stable blood sugar levels.

Typically 40 to 50% of the North American diet is provided by carbohydrates in the form of fruits, grains, vegetables and refined sugar; ready availability, low cost and ease of storage influence their widespread consumption.

Requirements: Current guidelines recommend that 55% of energy be provided in the form of carbohydrates.[3]

Protein is the most plentiful substance in the body after water. Protein consists of large molecules that are broken down into *amino acids* during digestion. The main role of protein is the construction of body protein including the growth and repair of muscles, blood, internal organs, skin, hair and nails. Eggs, milk, meat, fish and poultry are sources of protein.[7] Foods considered to be *complete proteins* contain all of the nine *essential amino acids* in the correct ratio to maintain *nitrogen balance* — the difference between nitrogen ingestion and excretion and a measure for tissue growth, degradation or maintenance.[3] A *vegetarian diet* can supply all of the essential amino acids, provided a variety of complementary grains and legumes are included.[1] The body synthesizes protein based on the availability of essential amino acids, leaving any unused molecules to be burned as energy or converted to fat.[10]

Requirements: Current guidelines suggest the average adult protein requirement is approximately 0.6 g/kg body weight or 20% of daily caloric intake.[3]

Lipids are the most concentrated energy source in our diets. Fatty acids, which are simple lipids, are designated as *saturated, unsaturated* or *polyunsaturated* on the basis of their physical and functional properties. The *essential fatty acids*, linoleic acid and linolenic acid, belong to the *omega-6* and *omega-3* family of unsaturated fatty acids, respectively. Although they are required for normal physiologic function, they cannot be synthesized endogenously.[10] **Triglycerides** comprise 95% of the fats found in foods; they are the storage form of fat and the primary fat in the blood. Excess intake is stored in the form of adipose tissue.

Fats act as carriers for the fat-soluble vitamins (A, D, E and K), as a cushion of protection to internal organs, and as a thermal blanket against the environment. They also have a role in satiety, by helping to control the rate of digestion in the stomach.[7] Growing evidence links intake of essential fatty acids to health benefits, notably cardiovascular: polyunsaturated fats, particularly omega-6 fats, assist in reducing total cholesterol levels while omega-3 fats may facilitate improved blood pressure and triglyceride levels.[5,11]

Derived from both animal and plant sources, linoleic acid is commonly found in vegetable oils, nuts and seeds. In North America, intake predominates over the omega-3 fatty acids due to limited intake of primary food sources that include flax, pumpkin seeds, walnuts, and cold water fish.[10]

Requirements: Dietary lipids, primarily saturated fatty acids, are linked to elevated blood cholesterol and the development of atherosclerosis, a risk factor in coronary heart disease.[3] In addition, dietary fat is associated with cancer incidence and mortality, particularly cancer of the breast, colon and prostate.[12]

Current guidelines recommend that energy from fat should be limited to 30% of total daily caloric intake and saturated fatty acids specifically, no more than 10%.[13] Unsaturated fatty acids actually lower serum cholesterol; increasing consumption relative to saturated fat intake in conjunction with lowering LDL cholesterol provides additional protection against heart disease.[5]

Fibre is a component of complex carbohydrate that is largely indigestible; it consists of both soluble and insoluble factions. Although technically not a nutrient, there is growing evidence that associates a high fibre diet with lower incidence of heart disease and certain cancers.[3]

In addition to facilitating bowel function, several other benefits are attributed to a high fibre diet. *Insoluble fibre* acts as a bulking agent to shorten intestinal transit time, a potential benefit in reducing both constipation and colorectal cancer risk.[14] *Soluble fibre*, such as mucilages and pectins, can slow gastric emptying, assisting in satiety and blood sugar control; additionally it improves serum cholesterol levels.[15] Good sources of insoluble fibre include cereal grains and apples while soluble fibre is found in foods such as bananas, oatmeal and seeds.

Intake should be increased gradually along with increased fluid intake to maximize benefit and avoid

GI complaints. Excessive intake (greater than 35 g per day) should be avoided due to GI intolerance and risk of interference with absorption of minerals such as calcium, iron, magnesium and phosphorus.[7]

Requirements: The North American diet is typically low in fibre due to high intake of processed carbohydrates and foods from animal sources. Current guidelines recommend intake of 20 to 35 g daily, preferably through a variety of food sources rather than supplements.[3]

Vitamins are organic molecules important for biochemical transformations. There are 13 known vitamins, organized into two groups: the fat-soluble vitamins A, D, E and K, and those that are water-soluble, the B-complex vitamins and vitamin C.

Minerals are naturally occurring inorganic elements which typically perform structural and catalytic roles.[1] Unlike vitamins, minerals often become incorporated within structures and existing chemicals of the body. Although lacking in caloric or energy value, micronutrients are critical for health, playing specific roles in energy transfer and tissue synthesis.[4] Vitamins typically perform a regulatory rather than a structural function, with the ability to exert hormone-like functions and assist in the protection of cell membranes.

Minerals have three main roles in the body:[4] structural, in the formation of bones and teeth; functional, in maintaining normal heart rhythm, muscular contractility, neural conductivity and acid-base balance; and regulatory, in cellular metabolism, including the activation of enzymes and hormones.

With few exceptions, essential micronutrients cannot be synthesized within the human body and must be obtained from food or supplements.[1] Some vitamins such as beta-carotene are ingested in their provitamin or precursor form and are converted to the active substance within the body.

Requirements: A daily dietary source of water-soluble vitamins is recommended because of humans' limited ability for storage. Fat-soluble vitamins require protein carriers in the blood and are not readily excreted but stored in the liver and fatty tissue, thus having the potential for toxicity. The water-soluble vitamins, on the other hand, travel unattached in the blood and lymph, and are excreted in the urine. Except at high doses, toxic symptoms are unlikely. Health Canada provides guidelines to ensure adequate vitamin and mineral intake for the population. *Recommended Nutrient Intake (RNI)* is defined as the level of dietary intake thought to be sufficiently adequate to meet the requirements of almost all individuals in a group with specified characteristics, taking into account individual variability. Of necessity the RNI exceeds the requirement of almost all individuals.[13]

Currently, *Dietary Reference Intake (DRI)* standards are being developed cooperatively by American and Canadian representatives and are expected to replace the RNI. Unlike older standards, the DRI is based on scientific data and provides a range of values from optimal to maximum. For definitions of various dietary intakes as well as further details on recommended levels of individual intakes see the *Compendium of Pharmaceuticals and Specialties*, published annually by the Canadian Pharmacists Association.

Tables 2, 3 and 4 outline relevant information for the key micronutrients.

Nonessential Dietary Components

Alcohol

Alcohol (ethanol) intake at moderate levels elevates the level of high-density lipoprotein (HDL) in serum and lowers the amount of serum lipoprotein (a). Both effects favor a decrease in cardiovascular disease risk.[24] Present recommendations suggest that moderate alcohol intake, defined as less than or equal to 14 drinks per week for men and nine drinks per week for women, lowers cardiovascular risk.[25] However, excess intake can negatively influence both nutritional status and physiological parameters such as blood glucose, blood pressure and triglycerides.[3] Alcohol provides 7 kcal of energy per g; guidelines recommend a maximum intake of 5% of total energy or two drinks per day, whichever is less.[15]

Aluminum

Found in soil, water and air, aluminum is unavoidable. Aluminum compounds are commonly used as food additives as well as in water treatment. Concern for aluminum toxicity is mounting as evidence of its potential for neurotoxicity and involvement in various neurologic diseases, including Alzheimer's, increases.[26]

Because of reduced renal function, elderly patients using maximum doses of aluminum-containing antacids are at risk of high intake levels. Presently, it is not known how significantly aluminum consumption can affect the nervous system except in dialysis encephalopathy where high levels of aluminum in dialysis fluids and antacids contribute to dementia.[26] Guidelines encourage improved awareness and reduced exposure where possible.[3]

Aspartame

As a well-known artificial sweetener, aspartame is used in a variety of foods. Evidence continues to associate increased availability and intake of simple sugars in the diet with increased tooth decay, in addition to possible links with diabetes, obesity and coronary heart disease. As a result, artificial sweeteners have become an increasingly popular alternative to sugar. Whether or not usage has reduced caloric or simple sugar intake is controversial; recent claims suggest that high-intensity sweeteners do not facilitate weight reduction and may actually stimulate appetite.[3] Evidence suggests that current consumption levels are within acceptable levels of less than 40 mg/kg of body weight per day.[3]

Caffeine

Caffeine occurs in chocolate, drugs and various beverages with an average concentration of 80 mg per cup. As a stimulant, intake of greater than 500 mg is associated with adverse effects including irritability, nervousness, nausea and insomnia.[27] Current recommendations suggest caffeine intake from all sources be limited to no more than the equivalent of four cups of coffee (approximately 400 to 450 mg) per day.[3] Table 5 lists the caffeine content of common foods and beverages.

Cholesterol

As a basic structural component of the cellular membrane, a number of critical substances originate from cholesterol, including bile acids for the absorption of fat, antiinflammatory hormones such as cortisone, sex hormones such as progesterone, estrogen, and testosterone, and vitamin D. Nearly all cells have the ability to synthesize cholesterol, with endogenous production accounting for 70 to 80% of total body cholesterol. Data suggests that endogenous production is more than sufficient to meet bodily needs, without evidence of benefit from dietary ingestion. In fact,

Table 2: **Fat Soluble Vitamins**[3,4,16-20]

Vitamin A and the Carotenoids	**Daily RNI/RDA/DRI*:** Male=**1000 RE**, Female=**800 RE**
	*1 retinol equivalent (RE) = 1 µg retinol
	                              = 6 µg beta-carotene
	                              = 3.3 IU retinol
	                              = 9.9 IU beta-carotene
	Daily dose not recommended to exceed 1000 RE
	Therapeutic Dose: Chronic intestinal malabsorption: ages > 8 yrs: 3000-15 000 RE/day
	Xerophthalmia: ages 1-8: 1500-3000 RE/kg orally × 5 days or until recovery; ages > 8 yrs: 150 000 RE orally × 3 days, then 15 000 RE daily × 2 wks then 3000-6000 RE daily × 2 mos.
	Deficiency without corneal changes: ages < 1 yr: 3000 RE/kg/day × 5 days then 2250-4500 RE/day × 10 days; ages 1-8 yrs: 1500-3000 RE/kg/day × 5 days then 5100-10 500 RE/day × 10 days; ages > 8: 30 000 RE daily × 3 days then 7500-15 000 RE daily for 14 days
	Source: Preformed (retinol) from fish, eggs, dairy, liver; carotenoids from dark green leafy vegetables, orange and yellow fruits and vegetables
	Function: Prevention of night blindness, integrity of the epithelia and mucosa, cell-mediated and antibody immunity, role in reproduction
	Deficiency: Night blindness, xerophthalmia (keratinization of ocular tissue), dry rough skin, loss of appetite and diarrhea, reduced resistance to infection
	Excess: Toxic dose: > 10 000 RE/day chronically
	       Acute symptoms: headache, blurred vision, anorexia, vertigo
	       Chronic: bone pain, calcification of ligaments and tendons, skin peeling, neuritis

Vitamin D	**Daily RNI/RDA/DRI:** Male=**200-400 IU**, Female=**200-400 IU**, Pregnancy=**200 IU**
	40 IU vitamin D is equivalent to 1 µg **ergocalciferol** (vitamin D2) or **cholecalciferol** (vitamin D3)
	Cholecalciferol is synthesized in the skin through exposure to UV radiation; it is also present in fish liver oils. Ergocalciferol is produced by irradiation of ergosterol, a provitamin D sterol. Both are metabolized to calcifediol in the liver then hydroxylated in the kidney to **calcitriol**, considered to be the most active of the metabolites.
	Vitamin D is considered a threshold nutrient in terms of ensuring maximum absorption of calcium; with intake of less than 200 IU/day (equivalent to 500 mL of fluid milk) ensure adequate sun exposure equivalent to 15 min of noontime sunlight 2-3 times weekly to hands, arms and face.
	Daily intake should not exceed 2000 IU
	Therapeutic Dose: Breastfed infants: 400 IU daily
	Prevention of primary or steroid-induced osteoporosis: 400-800 IU daily
	Treatment of deficiency in adults: ergocalciferol 5000 IU (125 µg) daily until response.
	For vitamin D-resistant rickets, 12 000 to 500 000 IU (0.3-12.5 mg) daily; for hypoparathyroidism, 50 000 to 200 000 IU (1.25-5 mg) daily
	For management of hypocalcemia and osteodystrophy in patients with chronic renal failure on dialysis: calcitriol 0.25 µg daily to start, increasing by 0.25 µg every 4-8 wks as necessary. Typical maintenance dose is 0.5-1 µg daily; some patients may respond adequately to 0.25 µg every other day.
	Source: Ultraviolet irradiation from the skin; animal sources include dairy (fortified milk), fish liver oils, butter, egg yolk, liver
	Function: Absorption of calcium and phosphorous, proper bone growth and mineralization, calcium resorption, differentiation of epidermis without proliferation
	Deficiency: Children: rickets (bone deformation)
	           Adults: impaired bone remineralization, osteomalacia, osteoporosis
	Excess: Infants: anorexia, vomiting, failure to thrive
	       Adults: soft tissue calcification, hypercalcemia (anorexia, vomiting, polyuria)

Vitamin E (α-tocopherol)	**Daily RNI/RDA/DRI*:** Male=**22 IU**, Female=**22 IU**, Pregnancy=**22 IU** *IU reflect *RRR*-α-tocopherol (natural or *d*-α-tocopherol) vs. *all-rac*-α-tocopherol (synthetic or *dl*-α-tocopherol). IU of the two forms are no longer considered equivalent: e.g., 15 mg (22 IU) of *RRR*-α-tocopherol converts to 30 mg (67 IU) of *all-rac*-α-tocopherol Daily intake not recommended to exceed 1000 mg of either natural or synthetic form **Therapeutic Dose:** Treatment of deficiency in adults: 60-75 IU daily **Source:** Plant oils, legumes, cereal grains, fish oils Note: Vitamin E consists of two families, the **tocopherols** and the **tocotrienols**, each with four naturally occurring compounds designated alpha, beta, gamma and delta respectively. **Alpha tocopherol** is considered the vitamin of main nutritional value and therefore used as reference.

(cont'd)

Table 2: **Fat Soluble Vitamins**[3,4,16-20] *(cont'd)*

Vitamin E **(α-tocopherol)** *(cont'd)*	**Function:** Intracellular antioxidant, free radical scavenger in biological tissues, cellular membrane integrity **Deficiency:** Retinal degeneration, hemolytic anemia, muscle weakness, neurological damage **Excess:** Enzyme interference, antiplatelet activity in high doses (potentially through interference with vitamin K metabolism) with risk of hemorrhage
Vitamin K **(phylloquinone)**	**Source:** Primarily leafy, green vegetables and legumes; synthesis by intestinal bacteria **Therapeutic Dose:** Hemorrhagic Disease of the Newborn: Prophylaxis: 0.5 mg IM for birthweight < 1.5 kg, 1.0 mg for birthweight > 1.5 kg; alternatively oral dose=2 mg at first feeding, repeated at 2-4 wks and 6-8 wks, for a total of 3 doses. Anticoagulant-induced hypoprothrombinemia: Adults: 2.5 to 10 mg IM or SC repeated in 6-8 hours as needed. Children: 2.5-10 mg IM or SC repeated in 6-8 h as needed; infants 1-2 mg IM or SC, repeated in 4-8 h as needed **Function:** Facilitates normal blood coagulation **Deficiency:** Supplementation required for all newborns; hemorrhage, osteoporosis **Excess:** Relatively nontoxic; risk of jaundice with high doses of synthetic
Essential **fatty acids** (omega-3 and omega-6 polyunsaturated fatty acids)	**Daily RNI/RDA/DRI:** Omega-3: Male=**1.5 g**, Female=**1.1 g**, Pregnancy=**1.25 g** Omega-6: Male=**9 g**, Female=**7 g**, Pregnancy=**8 g** **Therapeutic Dose:** N/A **Source:** Vegetable seed oils (corn, safflower, sunflower), flax, marine fish oils **Function:** Precursors of prostaglandins, leukotrienes, prostacyclins, thromboxanes and hydroxy fatty acids, membrane structure **Deficiency:** Growth cessation, dermatosis, water loss, peripheral neuropathy

excess intake is associated with higher cardiovascular risk.[15] The North American diet is typically high in both saturated fat and cholesterol, with a high incidence of associated coronary artery disease. Dietary strategies that incorporate a reduction of both these factors remain a key intervention for reducing cardiovascular risk.[13] Accumulated evidence suggests an intake of less than 300 mg per day in the general population and less than 200 mg per day is the desired limit in those with cardiovascular risk factors.[28]

Created in the processing of unsaturated fats, trans fatty acids have recently been associated with cardio-vascular disease risk.[10] High consumption of partially hydrogenated vegetable oils/trans fatty acids (e.g., margarine, commercially baked goods, snack foods) can raise LDL cholesterol similar to saturated fats. They can also decrease the concentration of HDL cholesterol, an effect not attributed to saturated fat.[7] Guidelines suggest that current levels of trans fatty acids in the diet not be increased.[3]

Pathophysiology[22,29]

A number of methods are used to evaluate nutrient intake, both at the individual and population level. To optimally evaluate nutritional status, combine dietary information with biochemical data such as nutrient blood levels or tissue function tests, clinical data such as physical signs and symptoms, and laboratory testing or anthropometric data such as the BMI.

Goals of Therapy[18,19]

- Prevent or treat nutritional deficiency
- Prevent or treat nondeficiency conditions in which nutrients may impact outcome

Patient Assessment

Healthy individuals with deficiencies in dietary intake, malabsorption or increased nutritional needs, may benefit from specific supplementation. Those who are ill may require supplementation for the following indications: clinical deficiency, maldigestion/malab-sorption, nutrient-responsive nondeficiency diseases or metabolic abnormalities.[30]

Prevention

Dietary sources of nutrients are advocated over sup-plements for ensuring optimum nutrition; however, in

Table 3: **Water-Soluble Vitamins**[3,4,16,18,21]

Vitamin B$_1$ (Thiamine)	**Daily RNI/RDA/DRI:** Male=**1.2 mg**, Female=**1.1 mg**, Pregnancy=**1.4 mg** **Therapeutic Dose:** Treatment of deficiency in adults: 5-30 mg orally daily, as a single dose or in 3 divided doses Treatment of severe alcohol withdrawal: 50-100 mg PO, IV or IM daily. **Source:** Pork, organ meat, sunflower seeds, legumes, whole grains **Function:** Coenzyme in carbohydrate metabolism; nerve and myocardial function **Deficiency:** Beriberi (peripheral neuropathy, edema, heart failure), Wernicke-Korsakoff syndrome, muscle weakness, anorexia **Excess:** Serious adverse events such as gastrointestinal bleeding and hypotension have occurred following repeat IV administration
Vitamin B$_2$ (Riboflavin)	**Daily RNI/RDA/DRI:** Male=**1.3 mg**, Female=**1.1 mg**, Pregnancy=**1.4 mg** **Therapeutic Dose:** Treatment of deficiency in adults: 5-30 mg orally daily in divided doses; children: 3-10 mg orally daily in divided doses **Source:** Widely distributed especially in liver, meats, dairy, mushrooms, oysters **Function:** Coenzyme in energy and protein metabolism; mucous membrane integrity **Deficiency:** Cheilosis, reddened lips, cracks at mouth corners, edema of pharyngeal and oral mucous membranes **Excess:** None known
Vitamin B$_3$ (Niacin)	**Daily RNI/RDA/DRI:** Male=**16 mg**, Female=**14 mg**, Pregnancy=**18 mg** **Therapeutic Dose:** Treatment of deficiency (pellagra) in adults: 300-500 mg daily in divided doses; children: 100-300 mg daily in divided doses Hyperlipidemia: 100 mg orally 3 times daily with meals, increasing by 300 mg daily every 4-7 days to 6 g per daily if necessary **Source:** Fish, liver, lean meats, whole grains, legumes (can be formed from tryptophan) **Function:** Coenzyme in redox reactions, carbohydrate metabolism **Deficiency**: Pellagra (skin and gastrointestinal lesions, nervousness, mental confusion or dementia) **Excess:** Flushing, burning and tingling of face, neck, hands
Vitamin B$_6$ (Pyridoxine)	**Daily RNI/RDA/DRI:** Male=**1.7 mg**, Female=**1.5 mg**, Pregnancy=**1.9 mg** **Therapeutic Dose:** Treatment of deficiency in adults: 2.5-10 mg daily until symptoms resolve then 2-5 mg daily for several weeks Prevention of isoniazid-induced neurotoxicity: 10-50 mg orally daily **Source:** Meats, legumes, potatoes, bananas, salmon, whole grains **Function:** Coenzyme in protein, glycogen and linoleic acid metabolism, factor in hemoglobin formation. **Deficiency:** Irritability, convulsions, muscular twitching, dermatitis, kidney stones **Excess:** Peripheral neuropathy
Folate	**Daily RNI/RDA/DRI:** Male=**400 μg**, Female=**400 μg**, Pregnancy=**600 μg*** *for women capable of becoming pregnant, recommendation is for supplementation with 400 μg of synthetic folate in addition to dietary intake **Therapeutic Dose:** Treatment of deficiency: Children > 8 yrs: typically started at 0.25-1 mg daily followed by 0.4 mg daily; 0.3 mg in children up to 4 yrs, 0.1 mg in infants; higher dosage may be required in some individuals Tropical sprue: 3-15 mg daily **Source:** Legumes, green vegetables, whole wheat products **Function:** Coenzyme in DNA synthesis and amino acid metabolism, red blood cell development **Deficiency:** Megaloblastic anemia, fatigue, GI disturbances, confusion, depression **Excess:** Doses > 1 mg/day can mask vitamin B$_{12}$ deficiency
Pantothenic Acid	**Daily RNI/RDA/DRI:** Male=**5 mg**, Female=**5 mg**, Pregnancy=**6 mg** **Source:** Widespread in food especially egg yolk, liver, kidney, yeast **Function:** Essential to energy metabolism as constituent to coenzyme A **Deficiency:** Impaired sleep, numbness and tingling of hands and feet, fatigue, impaired coordination **Excess:** None reported

(cont'd)

Table 3: **Water-Soluble Vitamins**[3,4,16,18,21] *(cont'd)*

Vitamin B$_{12}$ (Cyanocobalamin)	**Daily RNI/RDA/DRI:** Male=**2.4 µg**, Female=**2.4 µg**, Pregnancy=**2.6 µg** **Therapeutic Dose:** Treatment of deficiency in adults: 30-100 µg IM or SC daily × 5-10 days then 100-200 µg monthly; alternatively oral doses of up to 1000 µg daily may be used; children:100 µg IM or SC daily until total dose of 1-5 mg is given, followed by maintenance dose of 60 µg monthly **Source:** Liver, meat, eggs, dairy, fish **Function:** Coenzyme in DNA synthesis, maturation of red blood cell **Deficiency:** Pernicious anemia, neurologic disorders **Excess:** None reported
Biotin	**Daily RNI/RDA/DRI:** Male=**30 µg**, Female=**30 µg**, Pregnancy=**30 µg** **Source:** Synthesis by digestive tract microflora; organ meats, legumes, vegetables **Function:** Coenzyme in amino acid and fatty acid metabolism; glycogen synthesis **Deficiency:** Rare; fatigue, depression, anorexia, nausea, dermatitis, muscular pains **Excess:** None reported
Vitamin C (Ascorbate)	**Daily RNI/RDA/DRI:** Male=**90 mg**, Female=**75 mg**, Pregnancy=**85 mg** **Therapeutic Dose:** Treatment of scurvy in adults: 100-250 mg orally or parenterally once or twice daily for 2 days to 3 wks; children: 100-300 mg daily in divided doses, orally or parenterally. **Source:** Citrus fruit, tomatoes, strawberries, broccoli, potatoes, green peppers **Function:** Antioxidant, collagen and norepinephrine synthesis, wound healing, cartilage and bone formation. **Deficiency:** Scurvy (degeneration of skin, teeth, blood vessels, bone) anorexia, fatigue, impaired wound healing; smoking has been shown to increase loss of vitamin C, possibly through increased oxidative stress, by approximately 35 mg/day **Excess:** Doses > 1 g may cause GI symptoms; avoidance of high doses recommended in iron storage disease, history of kidney stones, renal disease

certain situations preventive supplementation may be recommended.[3] *Preventive supplements* are defined as vitamin or vitamin/mineral supplements formulated to compensate for inadequacies in the diet of normal persons. In addition, they may be beneficial if there is evidence of increased requirement, mild malabsorption or increased nutrient losses. Traditionally, these products contained 50 to 150% of the RDA for most of the constituents.[19] Table 6 illustrates a number of situations where preventive supplementation may be beneficial. For information regarding available supplements see the *Compendium of Self-Care Products*, published annually by the Canadian Pharmacists Association.

Pharmacologic Therapy

Therapeutic supplements are defined as those which offer 5 to 50 times the RDA/RNI of specific vitamins for therapeutic or pharmacologic purposes.[19]

Current evidence for nutritional intervention in relation to disease is summarized in Table 7.

Supplementation

The need for daily multivitamin supplementation continues to be a controversial topic in nutrition. Guidelines continue to stress the importance of a balanced diet in the maintenance of health rather than focusing on individual nutrients.[3,50] Advocacy for supplementation is compounded by concerns about genetically modified foods, soil contamination and depletion of minerals and other vital nutrients.[51] Increasing popularity of fad diets and caloric restriction can pose further risk, as the intake of less than 1800 kcal per day increases the opportunity for nutritional deficiencies. Evidence supporting supplementation continues to mount when a variety of age groups and situations are examined.[52,53]

Calcium Supplementation

Supplementation continues to be advocated for prevention and treatment of bone loss. A number of salts are used, which vary both in terms of solubility and rate of absorption. To maximize absorption, supplements should be taken in doses of 500 mg or less, ideally with meals.[54] (See Chapter 34.)

Table 4: **Major and Trace Minerals**[3,4,16,18,22,23]

Calcium (Ca)	**Daily RNI/RDA/DRI:** Male=**1000-1200 mg**, Female=**1000-1300 mg** Either through diet or supplementation in divided doses not exceeding 500 mg/dose to maximize absorption **Source:** Milk, cheese, dark green vegetables, dried legumes **Function:** Bone and tooth formation; blood clotting; nerve transmission; muscle contractility **Deficiency:** Stunted growth; rickets, osteoporosis, convulsions **Excess:** Hypercalcemia, renal failure, psychosis
Chloride (Cl)	**Daily RNI/RDA/DRI:=750 mg** **Source:** Wide food distribution **Function:** Acid-base balance, osmotic pressure **Deficiency:** Hypochloremic, hypokalemic alkalosis **Excess:** Hypertension
Magnesium (Mg)	**Daily RNI/RDA/DRI:** Male=**420 mg**, Female=**320 mg**, Pregnancy=**350-400 mg** **Source:** Whole grains, green leafy vegetables, nuts, seafood **Function:** Muscle contraction, enzyme activation, bone and teeth formation **Deficiency:** Growth failure, neuromuscular irritability, potassium loss **Excess:** Diarrhea, hypotension, cardiac disturbances
Phosphorous (P)	**Daily RNI/RDA/DRI: 1000 mg** **Source:** Milk and dairy, meat, poultry, grains, fish **Function:** Bone and tooth formation, acid-base balance, energy production **Deficiency:** Weakness, bone demineralization, calcium loss **Excess:** Hyperphosphatemia in renal disease, jaw erosion
Potassium (K)	**Daily RNI/RDA/DRI: 2000 mg** **Source:** Leafy greens, cantaloupe, bananas, prunes, potatoes, milk, coffee, tea **Function:** Fluid balance, nerve transmission, acid-base balance **Deficiency:** Can be fatal; muscle cramps, cardiac arrhythmia, mental confusion, anorexia **Excess:** Accumulation in impaired kidney function can lead to cardiac arrhythmias
Sodium (Na)	**Daily RNI/RDA/DRI:** N/A **Source:** Table salt, cheese, olives, meat, sardines **Function:** Acid-base and water balance, nerve function **Deficiency:** Muscle cramps, mental apathy, reduced appetite **Excess:** Elevated blood pressure, confusion
Iron (Fe)	**Daily RNI/RDA/DRI:** Male=**9 mg**, Female=**13 mg**, Pregnancy=**18 mg** **Source:** Eggs, lean meats, legumes, grains, leafy greens **Function:** Constituent of hemoglobin and enzymes in energy metabolism **Deficiency:** Iron deficiency anemia (weakness, reduced resistance to infection) **Excess:** Liver cirrhosis, skin pigmentation
Iodine (I)	**Daily RNI/RDA/DRI:** Male=**160 µg**, Female=**160 µg**, Pregnancy=**185 µg** **Source:** Fish, shellfish, dairy, iodized salt **Function:** Constituent of thyroid hormones **Deficiency:** Goiter (enlarged thyroid) **Excess:** Depressed thyroid function
Zinc (Zn)	**Daily RNI/RDA/DRI:** Male=**12 mg**, Female=**9 mg**, Pregnancy=**15 mg** **Source:** Oysters, wheat germ, beef, poultry, whole grains **Function:** Digestive enzyme constituent, skin integrity, wound healing, growth **Deficiency:** Impaired healing, reproductive development and taste/smell acuity **Excess:** Fever, nausea, vomiting, diarrhea

(cont'd)

Table 4: **Major and Trace Minerals**[3,4,16,18,22,23] (cont'd)

Copper (Cu)	**Daily RNI/RDA/DRI: 2 mg** **Source:** Meats, nuts, oysters, drinking water **Function:** Enzyme component in iron metabolism **Deficiency:** Rare; anemia, bone changes **Excess:** Wilson's disease
Fluoride (F)	**Daily RNI/RDA/DRI:** Male=**4 mg**, Female=**3 mg** **Source:** Drinking water, tea, seafood **Function:** Bone and tooth formation **Deficiency:** Predisposition to dental caries **Excess:** Teeth mottling, neurologic disturbances
Selenium (Se)	**Daily RNI/RDA/DRI:** Male=**55 μg**, Female=**55 μg**, Pregnancy=**60 μg** **Source:** Seafood, meat, grains **Function:** Facilitates vitamin E activity (free radical scavenger) **Deficiency:** Anemia (rare) **Excess:** GI disorders, lung irritation
Chromium (Cr)	**Daily RNI/RDA/DRI:** Male=**30 μg**, Female=**20 μg** **Source:** Legumes, cereals, organ meats, fats, vegetable oils, whole grains **Function:** Component of glucose tolerance factor (GTF), potentiates insulin **Deficiency:** Impaired glucose metabolism **Excess:** Enzyme inhibition
Manganese (Mn)	**Daily RNI/RDA/DRI: 3.5 mg** **Source:** Whole grain cereals, leafy greens, nuts, tea **Function:** Enzyme cofactor in multiple reactions **Deficiency:** Impaired growth, skeletal abnormalities
Sulfur (S)	**Source:** Wide protein distribution (meat, fish, eggs, dairy, legumes, nuts) **Function:** Acid-base balance, component of amino acids **Deficiency:** Unknown **Excess:** Unknown
Molybdenum (Mo)	**Daily RNI/RDA/DRI: 45 μg** **Source:** Milk, beans, bread, cereals, legumes **Function:** Component of multiple enzymes **Deficiency:** Tachycardia, headache, confusion

Table 5: **Caffeine Content of Common Foods**[13]

Per 175 mL (6 oz)	Caffeine in mg per serving
Coffee, filter drip	108-180
Coffee, instant	60-90
Coffee, instant decaffeinated	< 6
Tea, brewed strong	78-108
Hot cocoa	6-30
Per 355 mL (12 oz)	
Tea, canned ice	22-36
Cola and other caffeine containing soft drinks	36-90
Per 56 g (2 oz)	
Dark chocolate	40-50
Milk chocolate	3-20

Table 6: **Preventive Supplementation**

Application	Nutrient(s)	Rationale
Food intolerance/avoidance e.g., vegetarianism	Complementary protein, calcium, iron, vitamin B_{12}	B_{12} supplementation equivalent to 2 µg/day recommended for all vegan and lacto-ovo-vegetarians; calcium and iron supplementation should be suggested on a case by case basis.[19] A variety of complementary grains and legumes must be consumed to ensure adequate intake of essential amino acids.
Risk of deficient intake/malabsorption e.g., calorie-reduced or low-fat diet	Fat soluble vitamins, beta-carotene	20 g of dietary fat daily is required to ensure adequate levels of fat soluble nutrients such as vitamins A, D, E, calcium, magnesium and essential fatty acids. Dietary lipid is also believed essential for absorption of beta-carotene from plant sources.[30]
Reduced metabolic function e.g., aging	Vitamin B_{12}	Recommendations for all persons over 50 to consume 2 µg synthetic vitamin B_{12} daily through enriched foods or as supplements.[19]
Pregnancy	Multivitamin with folic acid, iron	Folic acid prior to conception and continued throughout pregnancy at 0.4 mg/day.[3] Increase to 5 mg/day if history of neural tube defect in pregnancy.[19] Moderately increased iron intake recommended during 2nd & 3rd trimesters.[19] Evidence of decreased congenital anomalies specifically cardiac defects with periconceptional use of folic acid.[31]
Prolonged illness/post-op recovery	Multiple nutrients	Evidence for perioperative nutritional support to reduce complications after major surgery.[32]
Drug/Nutrient interaction	Multiple nutrients	Anticoagulants: Effects can be increased by vitamin E, decreased/attenuated by vitamin K. Anticonvulsants: Increases risk of folic acid and vitamin D deficiency.[19] Consider preventive supplementation. Fluoroquinolones/bisphosphonates: Absorption impaired by co-administration with Mg, Ca, Fe or Zn; recommendation to avoid any vitamin/mineral supplementation within 2–4 h.[33,34] Methotrexate: Supplementation with folic acid (1–5 mg/day) to minimize risk of GI and liver toxicity.[19] Orlistat, mineral oil: Risk of fat malabsorption; supplementation with fat-soluble vitamins and beta-carotene is advisable.[19] Systemic glucocorticoids: Ensure adequate calcium and vitamin D intake depending on patient age to minimize risk for negative effects on bone density.[35]

Table 7: **Therapeutic Supplementation and Disease**

Disease	Nutrient(s)	Rationale
Alcoholism	Thiamine, fat-soluble vitamins	Alcoholics may suffer thiamine deficiency because of low intake and impaired absorption and storage, possibly leading to Wernicke-Korsakoff syndrome. Chronic liver disease predisposes to multiple nutrient deficiencies, in particular thiamine and the fat-soluble vitamins A, D and K.[36]
Alzheimer's disease	Folate, B_{12} and B_6	Evidence that oxidative stress and accumulation of free radicals may be involved in disease pathophysiology. In addition, correlation between cognitive skills and serum levels of folate, vitamin B_{12} and B_6 and more recently, homocysteine.[37]
Atherosclerosis	High fibre, low saturated fat diet	Recommendations encourage increased complex carbohydrates (and thereby soluble fibre) primarily through cereals, vegetables, fruits at the expense of fat, specifically saturated fat and cholesterol.[3]
Cancer	High fibre, low saturated fat diet, antioxidant-rich foods; decreased meat and high-fat dairy	Current evidence suggests a 35% reduction in incidence of cancers through dietary intervention with a focus on high fibre content from grains, vegetables, legumes and fruit and low animal fat. Recommendations also include modification of other lifestyle factors such as exercise, alcohol and tobacco use.[14] Energy imbalances, either associated with obesity or underweight, correlate strongly with the incidence of certain cancers, including the breast, colon and prostate.[12] Evidence that regular fish consumption correlates with risk reduction, especially cancers of the digestive tract.[38] Primary role for antioxidants (vitamins A, E and C): Increased consumption of carotenoids in green and yellow vegetables suggest decreased risk of cancer in epithelial tissues; evidence supporting vitamin E supplementation above present recommendations due to protective role against potentially mutagenic products of lipid peroxidation; evidence of ascorbic acid role in reducing formation of nitrosamines (oral carcinogens) from nitrates in food.[39]
Cardiovascular disease	Folate, B_{12} and B_6	Recent evidence of beneficial effects of B_6 and B_{12} (10 mg each daily) along with folate (0.4 mg daily) on reducing elevated homocysteine levels, a vascular toxin associated with coronary artery disease, stroke and deep vein thrombosis.[40,41] This combination also decreases the rate of restenosis and the need for revascularization after coronary angioplasty.[42] Omega-3 fatty acids may have significant effects in prevention of coronary heart disease. Risk reduction in clinical trials with fish oils compared to that seen with lipid-lowering medications used in secondary prevention.[11]
Dental caries	Fluoride	Preventive strategies that focus on optimum fluoride levels (primarily through fluoridated water to a level of 1 mg/L), adequate oral hygiene as well as type and frequency of carbohydrate consumption, especially sucrose.[3]
Depression	B vitamins	Supplementation with thiamine, folate and vitamin B_{12} may be useful in nonresponsive antidepressant therapy where folic acid status may be marginal/deficient.[19,43]

Hypertension	Restricted sodium and alcohol intake	Recommend sodium restriction to a range of 90-130 mmol/day (< 3-7g/day, 2.4 g elemental sodium = 6 g NaCl = 1 tsp table salt) from all sources and alcohol intake not exceeding 14 standard drinks per week (e.g., 720 mL beer, 300 mL wine , 90 mL liquor) for men and nine standard drinks per week for women.[25] A diet rich in vegetables, fruits and low fat dairy products (DASH diet) combined with a reduction of sodium intake to levels below 100 mmol/day (below 6 g/day) have recently been shown to lower mean systolic blood pressure by 11.5 mmHg in patients with hypertension.[44] (See Nutrition Appendix 1.) A systematic review suggests a permanent reduction of dietary saturated fat and partial replacement by unsaturates may lead to a small but important reduction in cardio-vascular risk in trials longer than two years in both high and lower risk groups.[45]
Osteoporosis	Calcium and vitamin D along with other bone supportive nutrients. Restrict intake of refined carbohydrates, caffeine, nicotine	Recommendations stress adequate calcium and vitamin D intake throughout lifetime, particularly during skeletal development. Current guidelines recommend the following daily intakes: 9-12 yrs: 1300 mg; 19-50 yrs: 1000 mg; > 50 yrs: 1000-1500 mg, either through diet or supplementation in divided doses not exceeding 500 mg/dose to maximize absorption. In postmenopausal women using estrogen therapy, 1000 mg is considered sufficient. Vitamin D through diet, sun exposure or daily supplementation equivalent to: 19-50 yrs: 200 IU; 50-70 yrs: 400 IU; > 70 yrs: 600 IU. Evidence that Western diet is typically nutrient deficient through ingestion of significant amounts of refined carbohydrates, fat and canned foods may play a role in development of osteoporosis; studies show supplementation with a variety of bone supporting micronutrients (e.g., magnesium, manganese, boron) in addi-tion to calcium, reduced bone loss to a significant degree compared to calcium alone.[46]
Type 2 diabetes	High complex carbohy-drate, omega-3 fish oils	A diet containing carbohydrates from whole grains, fruits, vegetables and low-fat milk is recommended. The total amount of carbohydrate in meals is more important than the source.[47] Omega-3 fish oil supplementation in type 2 diabetic patients show improvement in both lipid levels and blood pressure control, both significant risk factors for cardiovascular disease in this population.[48] This is believed to outweigh any minor deterioration in glycemic control shown in earlier studies.[49]

Remind consumers that adequate vitamin D levels are needed to ensure optimum calcium absorption. In addition, a number of dietary factors can influence calcium absorption including total intake, excessive dietary fibre, alcohol consumption and physical activity.[55] As well, high levels of caffeine (300 to 400 mg per day), protein or salt may lower retention rates. Consumers should take supplements in divided doses, remote from caffeine intake. Excessive calcium intake should be discouraged due to interference with iron absorption and risk of milk-alkali syndrome, a condition associated with irreversible soft tissue calcification and renal impairment. Excess calcium (above 2500 mg per day) can also cause constipation or gastric irritation.

Fibre Supplementation

In general, dietary fibre intake of 20 to 35 g per day, in a ratio of 3:1 water-insoluble to soluble fibre, is recommended for adequate health benefits. Statistics suggest, however, that average fibre intake levels in North America are closer to 12 g per day.[7] Avoiding fruit, vegetables and legumes, caloric restriction or specific dietary regimens such as wheat avoidance in gluten-free diets, may predispose one to dietary deficiencies. Querying an individual's intake of typical high fibre foods can assist in determining whether supplementation may be warranted. In certain cases, excess fibre intake may be a concern, particularly in individuals with poor nutrition, as this can potentially interfere with absorption of minerals such as calcium, iron and magnesium, as well as a number of trace minerals. See Chapter 21, Constipation, for fibre content of various foods.

Iron Supplementation

A number of factors can contribute to iron deficiency: increased requirements such as pregnancy, infancy or adolescence; decreased intake such as vegetarian diet; diminished absorption as in the elderly, or excessive or regular blood loss seen in menstruating women. Chronic deficiency can lead to anemia, excessive menstrual blood loss, impaired immune function and decreased energy levels.

In treatment of iron deficiency anemia, oral iron replacement therapy is often recommended. Dietary *heme* iron (ferrous from animal sources) is preferable to *non-heme* (ferric from plant) due to higher absorption rates.

Studies show extra meat servings are more effective in maintaining iron status in exercising women than commercially prepared supplements.[4] Additionally, presence of heme iron can increase absorption of iron from non-heme sources. Vitamin C can also improve non-heme iron absorption by improving its solubility in the alkaline pH of the intestine i.e., including one glass of orange juice with a meal can stimulate a threefold increase in absorption.

Should supplementation be warranted, a number of oral iron salts are available, providing a range of elemental iron content. Approximately 30 mg of elemental iron is absorbed from a 180 mg dose of elemental iron per day.

Iron salt	mg/tablet	mg elemental iron/tablet
Ferrous sulfate	300	60
Ferrous gluconate	300	35
Ferrous fumarate	200	66
Ferrous ascorbate	275	33

Generally, nonenteric-coated salts are recommended due to concerns with the effectiveness of enteric-coated and time-release preparations in releasing iron in the gastric environment. In patients with poor tolerance, a polysaccharide-iron complex may be better absorbed and tolerated.[56]

Chelates

Mineral salts such as sulfates and carbonates may have limited absorption. To increase bioavailability, amino acid chelates have been formulated which are minerals bonded to amino acids. Chelation may assist with the mineral transport involved in digestion; limited supportive clinical evidence has been published.[57] If digestion is a concern, however, it may be prudent to address potential absorption issues such as deficiencies in digestive factors, (e.g., betain hydrochloride and pepsin) to ensure proper assimilation of all nutrients from both food and supplement sources.

Health care professionals should continue to advocate the intake of a balanced, nutrient-dense diet while providing information and tools to assist patients to understand and recognize the potential impact of lifestyle issues on overall health.

Suggested Readings

American Dietetic Association/Dietitians of Canada. Appendix 12: Efficacy and safety summary table for dietary supplements. In: *Manual of Clinical Dietetics*. 6th ed. Chicago; 2000:841-852.

Beers MH, Berkow R, eds. *The Merck Manual*. 17th ed. New Jersey: Merck Research Laboratories; 1999. chap 1-5.

Dietitians of Canada. *The ABCs of Healthy Eating. 2002 National Nutrition Month Resource Manual for Health Professionals*. Fall 2001.

Health Canada. *Canada's Food Guide Facts for Healthy Eating*. Ottawa: Ministry of Public Works and Government Services Canada; 2000.

Health Canada. *Nutrition Recommendations, The Report of the Scientific Review Committee*. Ottawa: Health Canada; 1990.

Vitamin supplements. *Med Lett Drugs Ther* 1998;49 (1032).

References

1. Garrison RH Jr, Somer E. Introduction to dietary factors. In: *The Nutrition Desk Reference*. Connecticut: Keats Publishing; 1990:3-12.
2. Garrison RH Jr, Somer E. The macronutreints. In: *The Nutrition Desk Reference*. Connecticut: Keats Publishing; 1990: 13-35.
3. Health Canada. *Nutrition Recommendations, The Report of the Scientific Review Committee*. Ottawa: Health Canada; 1990. Update Food Guide Facts: *Caffeine in Moderation*.
4. McKardle W, Katch F, Katch V. Vitamins, minerals and water. In: *Exercise Physiology*. 4th ed. Maryland: Williams and Wilkins; 1996:35-59.
5. American Dietetic Association/Dietitians of Canada. *Manual of Clinical Dietetics*. 6th ed. Chicago: 2000.
6. Joubert G. Dehydration in children. In: Gray J, ed. *Therapeutic Choices*. 3rd ed. Ottawa: Canadian Pharmacists Association; 2000:648-54.
7. McKardle W, Katch F, Katch V. Carbohydrates, lipids and protein. In: *Exercise Physiology*. 4th ed. Maryland: Williams and Wilkins; 1996:5-33.
8. Voet D, Voet J, Pratt C. *Fundamentals of Biochemistry*. New York: John Wiley & Sons; 1999.
9. Groff JL, Gropper SS. Carbohydrates. In: *Advanced Nutrition and Human Metabolism*. 3rd ed. California: Wadsworth Publishing; 2000:70-105.
10. Groff JL, Gropper SS. Lipids/Proteins. In: *Advanced Nutrition and Human Metabolism*. 3rd ed. California: Wadsworth Publishing; 2000:123-219.
11. Harper CR, Jacobson TA. The fats of life. *Arch Intern Med* 2001;161(8):2185-92.
12. Health Canada. *The Nature and Dimension of Nutrition and Diet-Related Problems*. Country Paper Canada Supplement. Ministry of Public Works and Government Services Canada.
Available at: www.hc-sc.gc.ca/hppb/nutrition/pube/cpcs/cpc4.htm.
13. Health Canada. *Canada's Food Guide Facts for Healthy Eating*. Ottawa: Ministry of Public Works and Government Services Canada; 2000.
14. Williams GM, Williams CL, Weisburger JH. Diet and cancer prevention: the fiber first diet. *Toxicol Sci* 1999;52 (2 suppl): 72-86.
15. Fodor J, Frohlich J, Genest J, McPherson R, for the Working Group on Hypercholesterolemia and Other Dyslipidemias. Recommendations for the management and treatment of dyslipidemia. *CMAJ* 2000:162(10).
16. Food and Nutrition Board, Institute of Medicine-National Academy of Sciences. *Dietary Reference Intakes*. Available at: http://www.nap.edu/openbook/0309071836.
17. Groff JL, Gropper SS. The fat-soluble vitamins. In: *Advanced Nutrition and Human Metabolism*. 3rd ed. California: Wadsworth Publishing; 2000:316-70.
18. Beers MH, Berkow R, eds. *The Merck Manual*. 17th ed. New Jersey: Merck Research Laboratories; 1999.
19. Hoffer LJ. Nutritional supplements for adults. In: Gray J, ed. *Therapeutic Choices*. 3rd ed. Ottawa: Canadian Pharmacists Association; 2000:822-6.
20. Repchinsky C, ed. *Compendium of Pharmaceuticals and Specialties*. 36th ed. Ottawa: Canadian Pharmacists Association; 2001.
21. Groff JL, Gropper SS. The water-soluble vitamins. In: *Advanced Nutrition and Human Metabolism*. 3rd ed. California: Wadsworth Publishing; 2000:245-315.
22. Groff JL, Gropper SS. Macrominerals. In: *Advanced Nutrition and Human Metabolism*. 3rd ed. California: Wadsworth Publishing; 2000:371-400.
23. Groff JL, Gropper SS. Microminerals. In: *Advanced Nutrition and Human Metabolism*. 3rd ed. California: Wadsworth Publishing; 2000:401-70.
24. Sharpe PC, Young IS, Evans AE. Effect of moderate alcohol consumption on lp(a) lipoprotein concentrations. Reduction is supported by other studies. *BMJ* 1998;316(7145):1675.
25. Lifestyle modifications to prevent and control hypertension. *CMAJ* 1999;160:S29.
26. Health Canada. It's your health: *Aluminum and Human Health*. Available at: www.hc-sc.gc.ca Accessed Feb 20, 2002.
27. Groff JL, Gropper SS. Nutrition and the central nervous system. In: *Advanced Nutrition and Human Metabolism*. 3rd ed. California: Wadsworth Publishing; 2000:536-51.
28. Expert Panel on Detection, Evaluation, and Treatment of High Blood Cholesterol in Adults. Summary of the Second Report of the National Cholesterol Education Program (NCEP) Expert Panel on Detection, Evaluation, and Treatment of High Blood Cholesterol in Adults (Adult Treatment Panel II). *JAMA* 1993;269:3015-23.
29. Gibson RS. *Principles of Nutritional Assessment*. New York: Oxford University Press; 1990.
30. Zlotkin S. Minerals and vitamins. In: Gray J, ed. *Therapeutic Choices*. 1st ed. Ottawa: Canadian Pharmacists Association; 1995:694.
31. Hall J, Solehdin F. Folic acid for the prevention of congenital anomalies. *Eur J Pediatr* 1998;157(6):445-50.
32. Fan ST, Lo CM, Lai E et al. Perioperative nutritional support in patients undergoing hepatectomy for hepatocellular carcinoma. *N Engl J Med* 1994;331(23):1547-52.

33. Pronsky Z. *Food Medication Interactions*. 11th ed. Pennsylvania: 2000.

34. Tatro D, Borgsdorf K, Cada D, Hartshorn E, Hussar D. *Drug Interaction Facts*. Update Jan 2001 St. Louis; Facts and Comparisons; 2001.

35. SOGC Canadian Consensus Conference on Menopause and Osteoporosis. *SOCG J* 1998;(5)22-30.

36. Swain M. Chronic liver disease. In: Gray J, ed. *Therapeutic Choices*. 3rd ed. Ottawa: Canadian Pharmacists Association; 2000:354.

37. Nourhashemi F, Gillette-Guyonnet S, Andrieu S, et al. Alzheimer Disease: Protective Factors. *Am J Clin Nutr* 2000;71(2):643S-649S.

38. Fernandez E, Chatenoud L, La Vecchia C, et al. Fish consumption and cancer risk. *Am J Clin Nutr* 1999;70(1):85-90.

39. Levine M, Rumsey S, Daruwala R, et al. Criteria and recommendations for vitamin C intake. *JAMA* 1999;281(15):1415-1423.

40. Rimm EB, Willet WC, Hu FB et al. Folate and vitamin B_6 from diet and supplements in relation to risk of coronary heart disease among women. *JAMA* 1998;279:359-364.

41. Tice JA, Ross E, Coxson PG et al. Cost-effectiveness of vitamin therapy to lower plasma homocysteine levels for the prevention of coronary heart disease. *JAMA* 2001;286(8):936-43.

42. Schnyder G, Roffi M, Pin R et al. Decreased rate of coronary restenosis after lowering of plasma homocysteine levels. *N Engl J Med* 2001;345(22):1593-600.

43. Coppen A, Bailey J. Enhancement of the antidepressant action of fluoxetine by folic acid: a randomized, placebo controlled trial. *J Affect Disord* 2000;60(2):121-30.

44. Sacks FM, Svetkey LP, Vollmer WM et al. Effects on blood pressure of reduced dietary sodium and the dietary approaches to stop hypertension (DASH) diet. *N Engl J Med* 2001;344(1):3-10.

45. Hooper L, Summerbell CD, Higgins JPT et al. Reduced or modified dietary fat for preventing cardiovascular disease (Cochrane Review). In: *The Cochrane Library*. 3. Update Software. Oxford; 2001.

46. Gaby A, Wright J. *Nutrients and Bone Health*. Baltimore, MA: Wright Gaby Nutrition Institute; 1998.

47. Franz MJ, Bantle JP, Beebe CA et al. Evidence-based nutrition principles and recommendations for the treatment and prevention of diabetes and related complications. *Diabetes Care* 2002;1(25):148-98.

48. Connor WE. Diabetes, fish oil and vascular disease. *Ann Intern Med* 1995;123(12):950-951.

49. Lackey V. Omega-3 fatty acid supplementation in non-insulin-dependent diabetes. *Ann Pharmacother* 1990;24(3):258-60.

50. Vitamin supplements. *Med Let Drug Ther* 1998;49(1032).

51. Sugimura T. Nutrition and dietary carcinogens. *Carcinogenesis* 2000;21(3):387-95.

52. Fiatarone MA, O'Neill EF, Ryan ND et al. Exercise training and nutritional supplementation for physical frailty in very elderly people. *N Engl J Med* 1994;330:1759-75.

53. Mascarenhas MR, Tershakove AM, Stettle N. Nutrition intervention in childhood for the prevention of chronic diseases in adulthood. *Curr Opin Pediatr* 1999;11(6):598-604.

54. North American Menopause Society. Consensus opinion: the role of calcium in peri- and postmenopausal women. *J North Am Menopause Soc* 2001;(8)2:84-95.

55. Wolf R, Cauley J, Baker C. Factors associated with calcium absorption efficiency in pre- and perimenopausal women. *Am J Clin Nutr* 2000;72:446-71.

56. Whittemore NB. Common anemias. In: Gray J, ed. *Therapeutic Choices*. 3rd ed. Ottawa: Canadian Pharmacists Association; 2000:644.

57. Pineda O et al. Effectiveness of iron amino acid chelate on the treatment of iron deficiency anemia in adolescents. *J Appl Nutr* 1994;46:1-13.

58. MacGregor GA. Nutrition and blood pressure. *Nutr Metab Cardiovasc Dis* 1999;9(4 suppl):6-15.

59. Health Canada. *Nutrition Labels, Nutrient Content Claims*. Ottawa: Ministry of Public Works and Government Services Canada 2000. Available at: www.hc-sc.gc/hppb/nutrition/labels/e-press.html.

Basic Nutrition—Patient Information

A healthy diet can not only improve quality of life but also can help you live longer.[58] Health Canada produces *Canada's Food Guide to Healthy Eating* to assist in making food choices to ensure optimum food intake. (See attached.) Key to this is a new focus called *total diet approach*, emphasizing that foods are no longer labeled good or bad, but that the overall *pattern* of eating is important for long-term health. Issues such as energy balance, fat content, starch and fibre content, along with moderated intake of salt, alcohol, refined sugar and caffeine, are also addressed and highlighted in five key messages that define *healthy eating*:

- Enjoy a variety of foods.
- Emphasize cereals, breads and other grain products, vegetables and fruits.
- Choose lower-fat dairy products, leaner meats and foods prepared with little or no fat.
- Achieve and maintain healthy body weight by enjoying regular physical activity and healthy eating.
- Limit salt, alcohol and caffeine.

Table 8 highlights sources of key nutrients in each of the four food groups.

The Healthy Eating Scoreboard can be used by individuals to "check off" daily food choices against the recommendations. This tool can help identify eating habits that may need improvement or provide assistance to individuals making dietary changes.

Food Labels

A common challenge in making healthy food choices is a lack of consistency in food labels. Examples of common terms:[59]

- **Serving Size:** indicates both the measure of one serving and how many servings per container per package.
- **Calories:** includes both total calories per serving and fat calories per serving.
- **Percentage of Daily Values:** shows both grams per serving of specific nutrients and the percentage of daily value, usually based on daily intake of 2000 kcal.
- **Common Nutrient Content Terms:**
  - *Reduced or less fat:* at least 25% less fat per serving than the "regular" food cited on the label
  - *Low fat:* less than three grams of fat per serving
  - *Fat free:* less than 0.5 g of fat per serving
  - *Light* or *lite:* at least 50% less fat or one-third fewer calories per serving than the "regular" food cited on the label
  - *Reduced* or *less sodium:* at least 25% less sodium per serving than the "regular" food cited on the label
  - *Source of fibre:* at least 2 g of fibre per serving

Table 8: **Key Nutrients in Canada's Food Guide to Healthy Eating**

Each group is essential because it provides its own set of nutrients

Grain products +	Vegetables and fruits +	Milk products +	Meat and alternatives =	The Food Guide
Protein	—	Protein	Protein	Protein
—	—	Fat	Fat	Fat
Carbohydrate	Carbohydrate	—	—	Carbohydrate
Fibre	Fibre	—	—	Fibre
Thiamine	Thiamine	—	Thiamine	Thiamine
Riboflavin	—	Riboflavin	Riboflavin	Riboflavin
Niacin	—	—	Niacin	Niacin
Folate	Folate	—	Folate	Folate
—	—	Vitamin B_{12}	Vitamin B_{12}	Vitamin B_{12}
—	Vitamin C	—	—	Vitamin C
—	Vitamin A	Vitamin A	—	Vitamin A
—	—	Vitamin D	—	Vitamin D
—	—	Calcium	—	Calcium
Iron	Iron	—	Iron	Iron
Zinc	—	Zinc	Zinc	Zinc
Magnesium	Magnesium	Magnesium	Magnesium	Magnesium

Adapted from: *Canada's Food Guide to Healthy Eating.*

Health Santé
Canada Canada

Canada

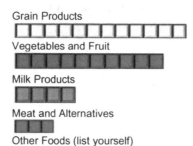

Your Healthy Eating Scorecard

Check off your food choices in the boxes below as you eat them throughout the day. On the bar side of the Food Guide you'll see what makes up 1 serving from each food group. If you like, make copies of this chart and use it over a longer period of time to check your progress.

FOODS

Grain Products

Vegetables and Fruit

Milk Products

Meat and Alternatives

Other Foods (list yourself)

What are serving sizes?

The bar side of the Food Guide explains serving sizes for different foods. For example, in Grain Products, 1 slice of bread equals 1 serving, while 1 bagel, pita or bun equals 2 servings.

The size of servings can vary within the Meat & Alternatives group. For example, 50-100 grams (g) of meat, poultry or fish equals 1 serving. That way, a child may choose a smaller portion size while an adult may choose a larger portion size to get 1 serving.

The Food Guide uses both metric and household measures. That's because you usually buy or prepare foods using either of these measures.

If you don't eat a lot, it's important to choose your food wisely. For example, women should choose foods high in iron such as beef or game meat, whole grain and enriched cereals, peas, beans and lentils. Let the statements on the rainbow side of the Food Guide help you make your choices. People who choose the lower number of servings but are still hungry or losing weight may need more servings from the 4 food groups and other foods.

Energy = Calories

You need food for energy. Energy is measured in Calories, kilocalories (kcal) or Kilojoules (kJ). So more Calories give you more energy. If you follow the Food Guide, you will get between 1800 and 3200 Calories each day.

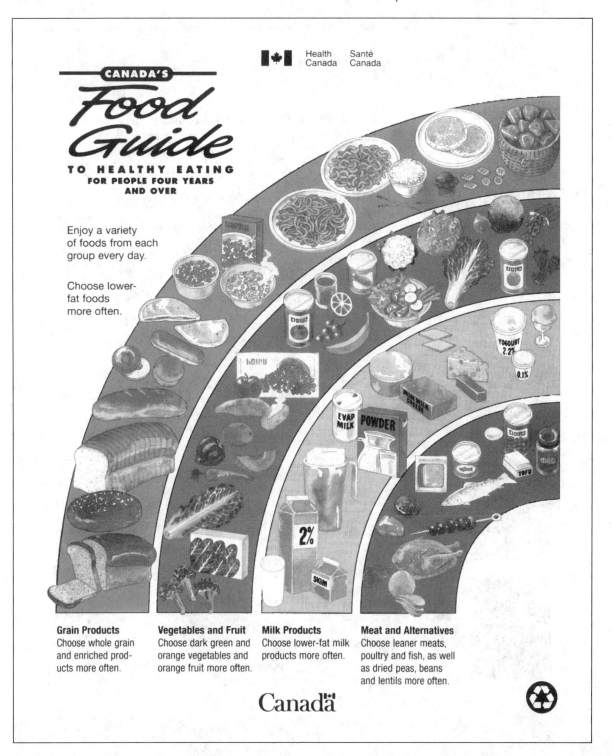

Health Canada   Santé Canada

CANADA'S Food Guide

TO HEALTHY EATING
FOR PEOPLE FOUR YEARS
AND OVER

Enjoy a variety
of foods from each
group every day.

Choose lower-
fat foods
more often.

Grain Products
Choose whole grain
and enriched prod-
ucts more often.

Vegetables and Fruit
Choose dark green and
orange vegetables and
orange fruit more often.

Milk Products
Choose lower-fat milk
products more often.

Meat and Alternatives
Choose leaner meats,
poultry and fish, as well
as dried peas, beans
and lentils more often.

Canada

Reproduced with permission from *Canada's Food Guide to Healthy Eating for People Four Years and Over*, Health Canada.

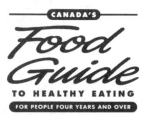

Different People Need Different Amounts of Food

The amount of food you need every day from the 4 food groups and other foods depends on your age, body size, activity level, whether you are male or female and if you are pregnant or breast-feeding. That's why the Food Guide gives a lower and higher number of servings for each food group. For example, young children can choose the lower number of servings, while male teenagers can go to the higher number. Most other people can choose servings somewhere in between.

Grain Products
5–12
SERVINGS PER DAY

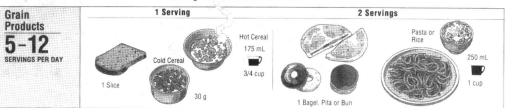

1 Serving

1 Slice

Cold Cereal
30 g

Hot Cereal
175 mL
3/4 cup

2 Servings

1 Bagel, Pita or Bun

Pasta or Rice
250 mL
1 cup

Vegetables & Fruit
5–10
SERVINGS PER DAY

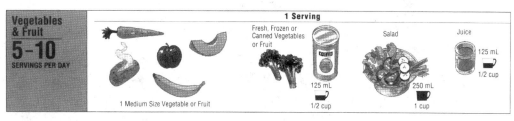

1 Serving

1 Medium Size Vegetable or Fruit

Fresh, Frozen or Canned Vegetables or Fruit
125 mL
1/2 cup

Salad
250 mL
1 cup

Juice
125 mL
1/2 cup

Milk Products
SERVINGS PER DAY
Children 4–9 years: 2–3
Youth 10–16 years: 3–4
Adults: 2–4
Pregnant & Breast-feeding
Women: 3–4

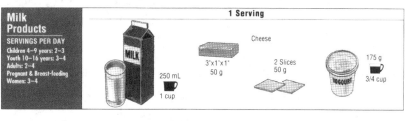

1 Serving

MILK
250 mL
1 cup

Cheese
3"x1"x1"
50 g

2 Slices
50 g

175 g
3/4 cup

Meat & Alternatives
2–3
SERVINGS PER DAY

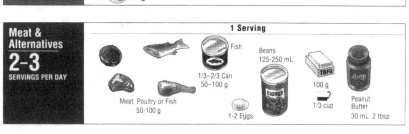

1 Serving

Meat, Poultry or Fish
50–100 g

Fish
1/3–2/3 Can
50–100 g

1–2 Eggs

Beans
125–250 mL

TOFU
100 g
1/3 cup

Peanut Butter
30 mL 2 tbsp

Other Foods

Taste and enjoyment can also come from other foods and beverages that are not part of the 4 food groups. Some of these foods are higher in fat or Calories, so use these foods in moderation.

Chapter 32

Infant Nutrition

Jennifer Peddlesden, BScPharm, IBCLC

Breastfeeding

Exclusive breastfeeding of infants* (as defined by WHO/UNICEF as only breast milk and no other liquids or solids with the exception of drops or syrups consisting of vitamins, mineral supplements, or medicines) is recommended to four to six months by Health Canada, the Canadian Paediatric Society, and Dietitians of Canada.[1] The World Health Organization (WHO) has reaffirmed exclusive breastfeeding to six months.[2] Changes in Canadian recommendations may follow. However, the international consensus is that breastfeeding continues to be an important nutritional, emotional, and immunological contribution to the child at least up to two years of age.[2] Canadian surveys in the mid-1990s showed an average of 77% of Canadian mothers begin breastfeeding and only 23% are still breastfeeding at six months.[3] The province of Quebec has released goals for breastfeeding to 2007 that would see 85% of infants being breastfed at hospital discharge and 50% at six months of age.[4] With breastfeeding initiation rates very low in some provinces and with duration rates below ideal across Canada, health care professionals have a role to play in promotion of this important preventive health measure.

Peer support groups provide information, practical assistance and emotional support for breastfeeding families using a mother-to-mother approach.[5] These include local La Leche League Canada groups or breastfeeding classes. Health care professionals can augment this support by ensuring that therapeutic or other interventions, when and wherever possible, allow a mother to maintain her breastfeeding relationship with her baby.[6] Problems encountered by women that may compromise continuation of breastfeeding should be addressed by *breastfeeding experts*, who may be public health nurses, dietitians, the mother's physician, La Leche League Canada Leaders, or International Board Certified Lactation Consultants (IBCLCs).

Physiology of Breastfeeding

During puberty estrogen and progesterone cause growth of ducts and buds in the breasts that will become the *alveoli*. These alveolar sacs that fill with milk are located at the end point of the ducts. Further growth of breasts takes place up to age 35. Readiness for milk production is completed during pregnancy with increased development of alveoli under the influence of higher levels of hormones. After birth, the rapid decline in the levels of estrogen, and particularly progesterone, trigger milk production. The high level of circulating placental progesterone during pregnancy suppresses action of *prolactin* on the milk-producing cells of the alveoli, although some mothers may notice that they can express drops of *colostrum* from about the fourth month of pregnancy. With the expulsion of the placenta and drop in progesterone, prolactin acts on the cells of the alveoli to produce milk that collects in the lumen of the alveoli. When the baby suckles at the mother's breast or when she sees or senses the baby, *oxytocin* is secreted from the posterior pituitary. Oxytocin causes contraction of the myoepithelium surrounding the alveoli to cause the *milk let-down*, which is the movement of milk out of the alveolar sacs, down the ducts and to the baby via numerous openings in the nipple. Levels of prolactin

---

*Infant is used in this document to refer to a child up to 24 months old unless otherwise specified.

increase tenfold in response to suckling and early in lactation it is this rise which stimulates the cells of the alveoli to produce milk. Colostrum, the yellowish milk produced in the first day or two is high in nutrients and immunoglobulins. Because this substance is small in quantity, the baby is stimulated to nurse frequently which establishes an appropriate milk supply. On day three or four postpartum the milk *comes in* as the colostrum changes to mature milk. Milk supply then increases to the individualized quantity required by the baby or babies in the case of twins or triplets.

As the mother continues to produce milk, oxytocin is secreted each time the infant comes to the breast. Let-downs may occur once or more during a nursing session at which time the mother may notice a tingling sensation or tightness in the breast. Although there continue to be spikes of prolactin each time the baby comes to breast, when the baby is about three months old autocrine control replaces endocrine control as the mother's circulating prolactin levels begin to return to pre-pregnancy values. At this point, removal of milk which contains a protein that acts as a *feed-back inhibitor of lactation*, stimulates further milk production. Hence, milk in the breasts acts to inhibit production of more milk i.e., removal of milk increases supply. (See photo on page PS-5.)[7]

Contraindications

Contraindications to breastfeeding in the mother are few and occur rarely. Breastfeeding might be contraindicated when the mother:[8,9]

- Has HIV/AIDS
- Has breast cancer
- Is taking a contraindicated drug (Table 1)

Note: A mother being treated for active tuberculosis can breastfeed.

Breastfeeding is contraindicated when the baby has:

- Galactosemia, an inborn error of metabolism where the capability of breaking down galactose is absent and the baby cannot tolerate breast milk

Challenges
Societal

A mother may encounter challenges to successful breastfeeding due to lack of support;[16] inappropriate, poor or no information; or birth interventions that interrupt the breastfeeding initiation and process. The Baby-Friendly™ Hospital Initiative encourages and recognizes hospitals, maternity facilities, and community health services that offer an optimal level of care for mothers and infants. A Baby-Friendly™ hospital or maternity centre, through the evidence-based Ten Steps to Successful Breastfeeding (Table 2), helps women to successfully initiate and continue to breastfeed. A randomized trial of breastfeeding promotion demonstrated that infants from "intervention" hospitals were more likely than controls to be breastfed at six months (7.9% vs 0.6%).[19]

Physical (mother)

Women born with the rare condition of insufficient glandular tissue may have difficulty fully breastfeeding.[9] Women who have had breast surgery (e.g.,

---

Table 1: **Drugs Contraindicated or Used with Caution in Breastfeeding**[10-15]

Drugs contraindicated
Antineoplastics
Selected anticonvulsants which may cause sedation in infant such as phenobarbital
Drugs of abuse
Ergot alkaloids in dosages for migraine headaches and related drugs which cause lactation suppression (e.g., cabergoline, bromocriptine)
Radiopharmaceuticals (breastfeeding may have to be interrupted) such as strontium-89, thallium-201

Drugs to use with caution while monitoring the infant
Amiodarone: Monitor drug levels in breast milk and infant plasma and infant thyroid function.
Cyclosporine: Monitor maternal drug levels and levels in infant serum. Monitor infant for signs of immunosuppressant effects (e.g., infections, abnormal blood counts).
Azathioprine: Monitor maternal plasma levels; observe infant for immunosuppressant effects (e.g., infections, abnormal blood counts).
Lithium: Monitor maternal drug level in plasma and milk and infant plasma drug levels; ensure infant hydration is adequate.
Oral contraceptives containing estrogen: Monitor infant weight to ensure sufficient milk supply.

Table 2: **The Baby-Friendly™ Hospital Initiative (BFHI) and the WHO/UNICEF Ten Steps to Successful Breastfeeding**[17,18]

1. Have a written breastfeeding policy that is routinely communicated to all health care staff.
2. Train all health care staff in skills necessary to implement this policy.
3. Inform all pregnant women about the benefits and management of breastfeeding.
4. Help mothers to initiate breastfeeding within a half-hour of birth.
5. Show mothers how to breastfeed and how to maintain lactation even if they should be separated from their infants.
6. Give newborn infants no food or drink other than breast milk, unless medically indicated.
7. Practice rooming-in, allow mothers and infants to remain together 24 hours a day.
8. Encourage breastfeeding on demand.
9. Give no artificial teats or pacifiers (also called dummies or soothers) to breastfeeding infants.
10. Foster the establishment of breastfeeding support groups and refer mothers to them on discharge from the hospital or clinic.

Reproduced with permission from the *World Health Organization*.

lump/cyst removal, breast augmentation or reduction), cancer or central nervous system disorders (e.g., spinal cord injury, multiple sclerosis, stroke) can provide a full or partial supply of breast milk for their babies.[20-22]

Physical (baby)

Multiple births, clefts of the lip and palate, cystic fibrosis, neurological impairment, and Down syndrome are challenges but *not* contraindications to breastfeeding. Babies born with other inborn errors of metabolism may be fed breast milk plus a formula specialized to the condition [e.g., phenylketonuria (PKU), maple syrup urine disease, urea cycle disorders, homocystinuria, tyrosinemia].[8,21,23] Refer these mothers to a breastfeeding expert.

Benefits

Whether to breastfeed should be an informed choice based on health considerations, rather than a lifestyle choice.[6] The benefits of breastfeeding for babies are numerous, according to research from developed countries among predominantly middle-class populations. Although not exhaustive, the following are examples of infant health benefits of breastfeeding. One study of infants 12 months old or less demonstrated that formula-fed babies had twice the incidence of diarrhea as breastfed infants.[24] Of 776 Canadian babies, 44 who were bottle-fed compared to 10 who where breastfed suffered gastrointestinal illness.[25] Although necrotizing enterocolitis (NEC) is rare in breastfed babies, confirmed NEC was 6 to 10 times

more common in exclusively formula-fed babies than in those fed breast milk alone; it was three times more common than in those who received formula plus breast milk.[26] In terms of respiratory illness, 329 bottle-fed babies presented with disease compared to 93 breastfed babies in the study with 776 participants.[25]

Breastfeeding may decrease allergies and asthma. Wheezing was reported in a lower number of breastfed than nonbreastfed children (59% vs 74%).[27] Children younger than four months who received any milk other than breast milk were 25% more likely to be diagnosed with allergies. Extended duration breastfeeding (greater than four months) was associated with less asthma and allergy in this large study.[28] In a separate trial, atopic eczema was reduced (3.3% in breastfed babies vs 6.3% in formula-fed babies).[19]

Research also shows that early cow's milk exposure may be an important determinant of subsequent type 1 diabetes, possibly increasing the risk approximately 1.5 times.[29] Breastfeeding is associated with a 3.16 higher IQ score compared with formula feeding.[30]

For mothers, breastfeeding increases oxytocin leading to less postpartum bleeding and more rapid uterine involution. Lactational amenorrhea causes less menstrual blood loss over the months after delivery; this also results in delayed resumption of ovulation with increased child spacing. As well, lactating women may have an earlier return to pre-pregnancy weight. This also depends on exclusivity and length of total breastfeeding, gestational weight gain, postpartum smoking, and maternal birthplace.[31,32] Breastfeeding women were closer to their pre-pregnancy weight at one month after childbirth than formula-feeding mothers.[33]

Breastfeeding may offer protection for some women against breast cancer.[34,35] The risk of premenopausal breast cancer was slightly reduced in those who had breastfed and those who had children but did not breastfeed (relative risk = 0.78).[36] A nonsignificant reduction in risk of ovarian cancer was seen with both short- and long-term lactation, perhaps because of ovulation suppression associated with lactation.[37]

Risks of not breastfeeding: Bottle-feeding formula or other breast milk substitutes has been associated with some risks.[38,39] For example, in children studied at 18 to 34 months, 2.4% of those fed cow's milk formula presented with allergic manifestations to cow's milk versus 1.7% fed human milk.[40] Infant formulas may contain bacterial contaminants. There is also potential for contamination during mixing/storage by parents or caregivers. Infant formula is more expensive than breastfeeding. According to a 1997 Canadian survey, it costs $540 to $955 for a six-month supply of ready-to-use formula.[41-43] And finally, although the exact role of polyunsaturated fatty acids is not fully known, they have demonstrated a role in visual acuity and cognitive development.[44] Formula or other substitutes lack polyunsaturated fatty acids and immunoglobulins.

Establishment of Breastfeeding
Milk Supply
In the early weeks a baby will come to the breast 10 to 12 times in 24 hours with some feeds clustered together and at least one longer sleep time. Breastfed babies nurse for both food and comfort. When babies are breastfed on cue they self-regulate the quantity and quality of the milk at each feeding. Breastfed babies may seem to be more wakeful, feeding more frequently, because of the components in human milk which are easily and readily digested. Inappropriate use of pacifiers (soothers) and supplements may interfere with milk supply. Pacification of the breastfed baby at the breast keeps the mother's milk supply adequate. It may also prevent *nipple confusion* which is characterized as differences, both mechanical and dynamic, between suckling at the breast and on an artificial nipple. This problem can lead some infants to refuse to take the breast.[8,21]

Adequate milk supply is determined by increases in the baby's weight, length and head circumference, output and behavior. A mother should drink to satisfy thirst, have pale, odorless urine, and eat according to *Canada's Food Guide to Healthy Eating*. A mother who perceives her milk supply has changed should consult a breastfeeding expert.

Hydration and Output[8,21]
Once the mother's milk supply comes in on day three or four postpartum, a well-hydrated healthy baby will have six to eight wet cloth diapers (five to six disposables), and pale, odorless urine. Brick-colored crystals in the baby's diaper indicate the infant is not receiving appropriate amounts of fluid and necessitates referral, especially if the child is under six weeks of age. Once the baby's first stool, called *meconium,* has passed in the first several days, the breastfed baby will have two to five loose, unformed yellow/green/tan bowel movements per day. After six weeks of age the number of bowel movements and wet diapers may become less frequent. Healthy breastfed infants require no extra water, even in hot weather, as long as breastfeeding is readily available to the infant.

Growth Spurts
At three weeks, six weeks and three months, it is normal for babies to nurse more frequently for a few days to increase milk supply to meet their growing needs. By reviewing signs of adequate milk supply as above, health care professionals can help a mother differentiate a growth spurt from a change in milk supply.[8,21]

Sore Nipples
Nipple pain is not normal, although tenderness during the early days is common. The most common cause of nipple pain is improper *latch* of the baby to the breast. Proper latch is attachment of the baby to the mother's breast which causes no overt pain and maximizes transfer of mother's milk to baby. Advise a mother with nipple pain to contact a breastfeeding expert to check the baby's position on the breast.

Thrush (yeast infection) is another common cause of nipple and breast pain, usually occurring later in the course of breastfeeding. Burning or stabbing pain as well as red, shiny skin on the nipple and areola are characteristic signs. Prior treatment with antibiotics predisposes mothers to yeast infections on the breast.[45,46] If the mother is diagnosed with thrush on the breast, both mother and baby must be treated, whether or not the baby has signs of oral thrush. **Antifungal creams** (e.g., nystatin, clotrimazole) should be applied until well absorbed on the dry nipple and areolar areas after each feed. Therapy for a minimum of 14 days is usually recommended. Some experts recommend continuing antifungal therapy for 2 to 14 days after symptoms disappear to prevent recurrence.[47-49] Alternately, **gentian violet** 0.5% aqueous solution may be applied once daily for a maximum of four days. Verify that the formulation does not contain methanol. Nystatin and clotrimazole creams, or gentian violet 0.5% aqueous do not need to be washed off before the baby feeds. Some clinicians may add treatment with oral **fluconazole**, which is considered safe during breastfeeding. Mothers should practice good hygiene to prevent infecting or re-infecting the baby, or infecting herself with a vaginal yeast infection.

If nipple soreness is not due to yeast or poor latch, and other causes have been ruled out (e.g., eczema, psoriasis, herpes, impetigo, contact dermatitis, Paget's disease, tongue tie in the baby)[45] then a USP-modified **lanolin** may be recommended. Other OTC breast creams are not generally recommended as they may obstruct the *Montgomery glands* of the areola. These oil producing glands provide lubrication and secrete lysozyme, which inhibits bacteria on the breast. The contents of vitamin E capsules are also not recommended as the minimum dose of vitamin E for infants is not known. It may also cause skin irritation.[21]

Sore Breasts

Mastitis is a painful inflammatory condition of the breast usually resulting from a plugged duct or a breast infection. A plugged duct occurs when a milk duct is not drained properly and becomes inflamed causing soreness, redness and sometimes a lump. Fever and flu-like symptoms may be present as a result of the inflammation, but may also indicate the presence of an infection.[21] When a plugged duct is not resolved within 24 hours by increased breastfeeding on the affected side, locally applied heat, massage and rest, and an infection ensues, a physician may prescribe an oral antibiotic. Most antibiotics are safe to use during breastfeeding. Mothers with recurring mastitis should be referred to a breastfeeding expert.

Fussy, Colicky Baby

Breastfed babies may be fussy for a number of reasons, such as hunger, the need to be near the mother, colic (see Chapter 26), an oversupply of breast milk or an overactive milk ejection reflex.[8,21] The latter occur when the mother has a generous milk supply and the baby gets an overabundance of foremilk (higher in lactose) that overwhelms the intestinal lactase. Consider this condition if a thriving infant presents with excessive crying, gas and explosive, loose, watery stools. A breastfeeding expert can provide management techniques. This is not an indication for use of lactose-free infant formula. Although foods the mother eats may appear in her milk, fussiness or colic in the baby is seldom the result of the mother's diet.[1]

Gastroesophageal Reflux (GER)

GER is the return of stomach contents into the esophagus. Reflux is a medical condition, not a feeding problem. Overactive milk-ejection reflex and oversupply can be confused with reflux as they share many symptoms. Breastfeeding may continue when the baby has been diagnosed with reflux. Placing the baby in an upright position during feeds as well as for 30 minutes after feeding can help prevent milk from refluxing. Burping and small frequent feeds may also be helpful.[21]

Oral/Diaper Thrush

Babies commonly develop yeast infections in the mouth. These present as white patches on the gums which bleed if scraped, and/or "mother of pearl" look to saliva. As well, the diaper area may present with a bright red diaper rash that is persistent. Infants who have recently taken antibiotics are more susceptible to yeast infections. *Oral* thrush is commonly treated with **nystatin** drops. Caregivers should administer the dosage after feeding and after wiping residual milk from baby's mouth with a gauze pad. The required dose is placed in a medicine cup then applied to the interior surface of baby's mouth with a clean cotton-tipped swab. Using a swab prevents contamination of the dropper and contents of the bottle. Baby should drink any remaining solution left in the cup after application. Some experts recommend that to prevent recurrence, treatment for oral thrush continue 2 to 14 days beyond disappearance of symptoms.[45,48] Use of a soother is a local factor in the colonization and proliferation of yeast in the mouth.[50] As discussed previously, the mother of a baby with oral or diaper yeast may develop this same infection on her breast. If *diaper yeast* is present, advise parents to wash baby's bottom with warm, soapy water, rinse and dry well. Exposure to air is beneficial. Apply **antifungal cream** (e.g., nystatin, clotrimazole) after each diaper change followed by a **zinc-based diaper cream**. Wash cloth diapers in a 10% bleach solution and use one cup of household vinegar in the rinse water, then dry diapers in a hot dryer or in the sun.[45,49] (See Chapter 41)

Stopping Milk Production

Ideally weaning from the breast is done gradually for both mother and baby. However, factors such as abrupt weaning, late miscarriage or stillbirth may result in *engorgement*, and tips on stopping milk production will be necessary.[51] Engorgement is a pathophysiologic condition in which lymphatic, vascular, and interstitial congestion are associated with a rise in milk tension. Milk can be removed to improve comfort by use of a breast pump to take away just enough to be comfortable but not stimulate milk production, or by sitting in a warm bath/shower and leaning over to allow the milk to leak out. Gentle stroking from the chest wall toward the nipple may encourage milk to flow. Cold compresses can reduce engorgement, and an **antiinflammatory analgesic** such as ibuprofen may be helpful for the first 24 hours.

Human Milk Bank

For Canadian infants who are unable to breastfeed due to medical conditions in themselves or their mothers and who require human milk, banked human milk may be available from the BC Children's and Women's Hospital Milk Bank, in Vancouver, British Columbia. After collection, milk is heat-processed to kill bacteria and viruses for prevention of disease transmission. Milk is then frozen and stored according to the guidelines of the Human Milk Banking Association of North America.

Drugs and Breastfeeding

Important predictors of the appearance of a drug in breast milk are the mother's plasma level of the drug representing her total dose and its plasma protein binding. Predictors of low drug levels in breast milk are: high plasma protein binding, low lipid solubility, high molecular weight, short half-life, lack of oral bioavailability, low volume of distribution and single or short-term dosing in the mother. Methods of administering drugs that deliver low levels to the mother's plasma are preferred, such as inhaled or topical medications when available. As the level of the medication in the mother's plasma rises, the amount in her milk rises. When the maternal plasma level falls, the milk level soon falls as well. The practice of "pumping and dumping" breast milk will not remove any more drug from the milk than letting nature take its course and allowing the mother's body to remove the drug via her urine or feces. Most medications and herbals do not reach a breastfed baby in quantities over 1% of the mother's dose[10] (Table 1).

Should a mother be prescribed a contraindicated medication, she may wish to pump milk beforehand or use an appropriate infant formula. To maintain a milk supply she should pump on a nursing schedule, discarding the milk collected during her therapy. After five half-lives following her last dose about 98% of the drug will have left her body and nursing is considered safe.[10]

Homeopathy During Breastfeeding

Many homeopathic remedies have been safely used by breastfeeding mothers as adjunctive treatment for conditions such as low milk supply, oversupply, yeast infections and mastitis.[52]

Social Drug Use

Breastfeeding mothers may consume an occasional social drink of alcohol[10,12] (Table 3). Cigarette smoking is not recommended in breastfeeding mothers. Caregivers should refrain from smoking in the same room as the baby. As well, mothers who choose to smoke should do so after a breastfeeding session. Encourage mothers to reduce cigarette use or use **nicotine replacements** (nicotine patches should be removed at night to reduce infant exposure); nicotine gum should be chewed according to directions for moderate blood levels and mothers should refrain from breastfeeding for two to three hours after using the gum. Use of cannabis by breastfeeding mothers is not recommended. Urine tests of infants exposed to cannabis will test positive for two to three weeks[10] (Table 1).

Table 3: **Time (h:min) From Alcohol Consumption Until the Amount of Alcohol in Milk Reaches Zero for Women of Different Body Weights**[53]

Maternal weight		Number of drinks			
kg	lb	1	2	3	4
40.8	90	2:50	5:40	8:30	11:20
43.1	95	2:46	5:32	8:19	11:05
45.4	100	2:42	5:25	8:08	10:51
47.6	105	2:39	5:19	7:58	10:38
49.9	110	2:36	5:12	7:49	10:25
52.2	115	2:33	5:06	7:39	10:12
54.4	120	2:30	5:00	7:30	10:00
56.7	125	2:27	4:54	7:22	9:49
59.0	130	2:24	4:49	7:13	9:38
61.2	135	2:21	4:43	7:05	9:27
63.5	140	2:19	4:38	6:58	9:17
65.8	145	2:16	4:33	6:50	9:07
68.0	150	2:14	4:29	6:43	8:58
70.3	155	2:12	4:24	6:36	8:48
72.6	160	2:10	4:20	6:30	8:40
74.8	165	2:07	4:15	6:23	8:31
77.1	170	2:05	4:11	6:17	8:23
79.3	175	2:03	4:07	6:11	8:14
81.6	180	2:01	4:03	6:05	8:07
83.9	185	1:59	3:59	5:59	7:59
86.2	190	1:58	3:56	5:54	7:52
88.5	195	1:56	3:52	5:48	7:44
90.7	200	1:54	3:49	5:43	7:38
93.0	205	1:52	3:45	5:38	7:31
95.3	210	1:51	3:42	5:33	7:24

Time is calculated from the beginning of drinking. Assumptions made: alcohol metabolism is constant at 15 mg/dL; height of the women is 162.56 cm (5 feet, 4 inches). 1 drink=340 g (12 oz) of 5% beer or 141.75 g (5 oz) of 11% wine or 42.53 g (1.5 oz) of 40% liquor. Example 1: for a 40.8 kg (90 lb) woman who consumed 3 drinks in 1 h, it would take 8h30 min for there to be no alcohol in her breast milk, but for a 95.3 kg (210 lb) woman drinking the same amount, it would take 5h33 min.
Reprinted with permission from Ho, E et al., Alcohol and Breastfeeding: Calculation of Time to Zero Level in Milk. *Biology of the Neonate* 2001;80:219-222, S. Karger AG., Medical and Scientific Publishers.

Ancillary Breastfeeding Products[8,21]

Mothers benefit from printed information on pump use, milk collection and storage, milk supply, and phone numbers for local breastfeeding support with each pump sale or rental. La Leche League Canada and breast pump manufacturers produce guides for mothers on hand expression, pumping, and storage of breast milk (Resource Tips). Table 4 lists several resources for breast pump sales and rentals.

Reusable, washable, cotton **breast pads** are recommended as disposable pads with plastic or occlusive liners promote dampness and the possibility of a yeast (candida) infection on the breast (Figure 1). Breast pads should be changed with each feeding. Mothers should not use cut-up disposable baby diapers, as the water-retaining beads in the diapers can be harmful to the baby if accidentally ingested. Once breastfeeding is established, after six to eight weeks, leaking is not usually a problem.

Silicone nipple shields are worn over sore or abraded nipples while the baby nurses, to overcome latch problems or to aid infants with physical challenges or impaired suck mechanisms. Over time the use of a nipple shield may lower a mother's milk supply.[21,54] These are best used on the recommendation of a breastfeeding expert.

Breast shells are firm, plastic, cup-shaped devices that can be worn inside the bra *between feeds* to provide air flow during healing of an abraded nipple, or to shape the nipple between feeds for easier latch of the baby (Figure 2). Wearing the shells inside the bra for several hours per day for 6 to 12 weeks before delivery may draw out flat or inverted nipples.[8,21] An estimated 10% of women have nipples that retract rather than protrude when the areola is compressed. However, proper latch of the baby after birth may overcome this problem.[55] Breast shells are not to be used to collect milk or in place of breast pads. Constant pressure on the ducts interferes with natural control mechanisms for leaking.

Supplementary nursing systems allow continued breastfeeding while providing supplemental calories from expressed breast milk or infant formula. The device includes a tiny flexible tube that is taped alongside the mother's nipple, connected to a supply of expressed breast milk or infant formula (Table 4). The mother is able to maintain or increase her milk supply through stimulation by the baby's suckling yet give nourishment without use of an artificial nipple.

Breast Pumps

A mother may use a breast pump to express and store milk when breastfeeding is not possible. With practice, hand expression is easily learned and there are many types of electric or manual breast pumps.[21] Manufacturers can supply a selection of funnel (flange)

sizes as one size will not suit all mothers. Pharmacies should stock only breast pumps from manufacturers whose sales departments provide ready access to replacement parts and service (Figure 3).

Figure 2: **Breast Shell**

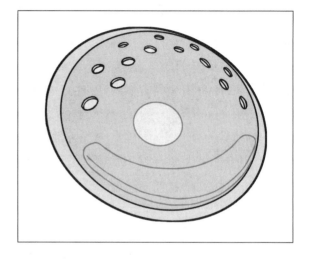

Figure 3: **Breast Pump**

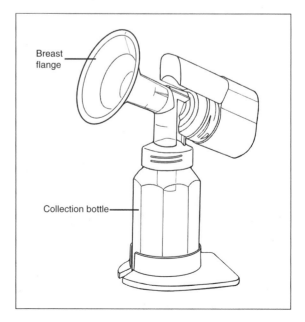

Breast flange

Collection bottle

Figure 1: **Breast Pad**

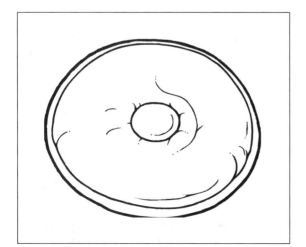

Table 4: **Suppliers of Breast Pumps (Sales/Rental) and Supplementary Nursing System Information**

Hollister 1-800-263-7400 (complete line of pumps and ancillary products)
Medela 1-800-435-8316 (complete line of pumps and ancillary products including a supplemental nursing system)
Both of the above resources provide specially sized pump flanges (funnels) for mothers with large breasts

---

Lact-Aid® International – (423) 744-9090 (supplemental nursing system only)

Full-/Mid-Size Electric Piston Pumps

These pumps are the type rented at breast pump depots. They are most effective and are recommended when mother is separated from a hospitalized baby, when the mother must remove milk quickly and efficiently or when the baby is unable to nurse (i.e., when the mother's breasts are engorged). Most electric piston pumps have adapter kits that allow mothers to pump both breasts at the same time. This increases stimulation, which in turn increases her milk supply and facilitates removal of milk. The kits can often be turned into manual cylinder or handle-squeeze pumps with the purchase of adapter parts.

Battery Operated/Electric Hand Pumps

These stepped-up versions of the manually operated pump are more expensive. The motors create noise and there is the added cost of batteries if the unit does not come with an AC adaptor. Pumps may be supplied in special carry cases that include ice packs for storage of pumped milk as well as bottles and milk containers.

Manual Breast Pumps

Usually a good quality hand-operated pump will suffice for the occasional feed when breastfeeding is not possible. Bicycle horn type pumps are not recommended as lack of control on suction may bruise the breast, and milk can collect and contaminate the bulb.

Report any instances where breast pumps have caused damage or injured a mother during use to Health Canada at 1-800-267-9675.

Infant Formula

Health care professionals should be aware of The International Code of Marketing of Breast milk Substitutes and subsequent WHA Resolutions.[56]

The choice of infant formula is based on the baby's health, risk of allergy in the family, and the components of the formula (Figure 4).

Infant formula manufacturers attempt to parallel breast milk in the proportion of fat, protein and carbohydrate. Most formulas are 0.67 to 0.68 calories per milliliter. The proteins in these formulas commonly are bovine milk protein or bovine whey protein (soluble protein) and/or bovine casein (an insoluble protein which accounts for the white color of cow's milk), or soy-protein isolate. For more information on infant formula composition see the *Compendium of Self-Care Products*, published annually by the Canadian Pharmacists Association.

Twenty-two per cent of adult Canadians have serious problems dealing with printed materials, according to the ABC Canada Literacy Foundation.[57] Mistakes where parents or caregivers inadvertently feed over-diluted or concentrated formula to babies are not uncommon.[58] Feeding of undiluted concentrate can result in serious dehydration and solute overload of the infant's kidneys, whereas overdilution by using ready-to-use instead of concentrate can result in caloric deprivation and failure to thrive. It is very important for parents to understand that concentrated formula is mixed with equal parts of clean water; also, powdered concentrates should be measured using *only* the accompanying measuring tool for that manufacturer.

Cow's milk, protein-based formulas with lactose should be used unless the infant has galactosemia or diagnosed allergy to cow's milk protein. Other reasons are cultural or religious (e.g., vegetarian lifestyle). Lactose is important in facilitating infant brain growth and iron absorption. Primary lactose intolerance due to lactase deficiency is very rare. Lactose-free formula should be used only under supervision of a health care professional trained in nutrition such as a peditrician. To prevent iron deficiency anemia, a source of iron should be started at four months in formula-fed babies who receive no breast milk.[1,20] Alternatives are iron-fortified formula or iron supplement drops (Figure 4).

Cow's milk, protein-based lactose-free formula, contains glucose polymers from corn syrup that are

substituted for lactose. They are suitable for infants with lactose intolerance but because they may contain residual galactose, they are not recommended for infants with galactosemia.

Cow's milk, protein hydrolysate formulas undergo hydrolysation, a process that predigests the milk

---

Figure 4: **Choosing Infant Formula**

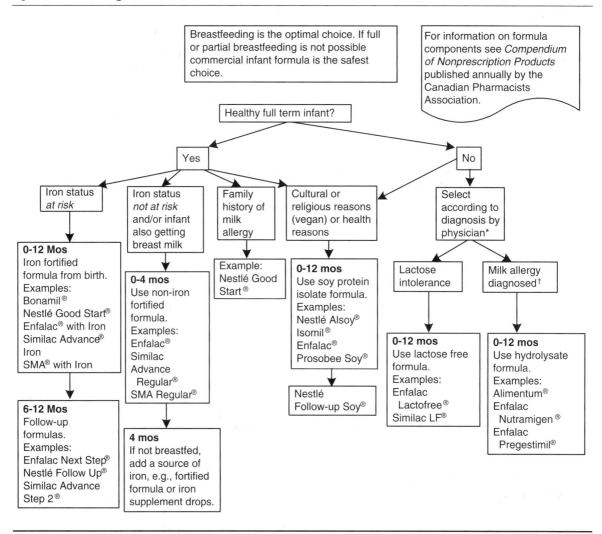

Brand names are examples only.
*Some conditions allow partial breastfeeding (see Breastfeeding: Contraindications and Challenges).
†Swelling/itching of lips, mouth/throat, gastrointestinal symptoms, hives, itching, nasal symptoms, anaphylactic reaction.
Adapted with permission from *Nutrition Assessment Manual for Healthy Full-Term Infants and Children.* Public Health Nutritionists of Saskatchewan, 1999.

protein. Whey-based formulas are less extensively hydrolyzed and can be used for infants at hereditary risk for atopy or for healthy term infants who are not breastfed or partially breastfed. Casein-based formulas, which are more extensively hydrolyzed, are indicated for feeding infants who have diagnosed cow's milk protein or soy protein allergy. They should, however, be used with caution as some infants may be reactive despite the hydrolysation of the protein.

Soy protein isolate formulas have limited indications for use. Soy-based formulas, which are all lactose-free, are not a routine alternative to cow's milk-based formulas. Appropriate uses include infants fed vegan diets and infants with galactosemia. Using soy protein-based formula in management and prevention of proven cow's milk allergy or prevention of atopy is controversial.

Infants allergic to cow's milk protein can also become allergic to soy protein. Soy isolate formula has a lower protein efficiency ratio, a high allergy potential, and a higher content of aluminum than breast milk or cow's milk-based formula.[1,59] Because of concerns about phytoestrogen content,[1] failure to achieve equivalent growth rates and reduced bone mineralization, soy protein-based formulas should not be fed to low birth weight preterm infants.[59]

Follow-up formulas are not superior to starter formulas. Starter formulas or follow-up formulas are a preferred alternative to cow's milk after six months for those infants eating solid foods who are not breastfed or are partially breastfed.[1]

Other specialized formulas are useful in the small number of infants who cannot tolerate formulas based on cow's milk protein or soy protein. Most specialized formulas are iron-fortified and the choice is based on the specific health problem of the infant.

Infant Formula for the Breastfed Baby

Breastfed babies are given infant formula for a number of reasons, such as supplementation of an actual or perceived low breast milk supply or to replace mother's milk when breastfeeding is not possible. Should a healthy breastfed baby require supplementation, it should be on the advice of a health professional knowledgeable in nutrition such as a pediatrician and should be non-iron fortified cow's milk-based formula. Lactoferrin is a bacteriostatic iron-binding protein found in the whey portion of human milk that withholds iron from iron-requiring bacteria. The extra iron in iron-fortified formula may overwhelm the iron-binding capacity of protective lactoferrin in breast milk. This may allow free iron for growth of harmful bacteria.[60-66]

Concentrate, Ready-to-Use or Powder Formula

Ready-to-use formula is the most expensive, but easiest to use. Concentrate must be mixed with equal parts water. Powdered formula may be useful when preparing small quantities as needed. To prevent mixing errors, measuring devices for different brands of powdered formula should not be interchanged. Prepared formula must be refrigerated and used within 24 to 48 hours. Opened cans of ready-to-use or concentrate must be refrigerated and used within 24 to 48 hours. A bottle of formula should not be kept at room temperature for more than one hour.[67]

Alternate Milks

Pasteurized whole cow's milk may be introduced towards the end of the first year of life. Skimmed, partly skimmed 1% and 2% milk are not recommended in the first two years due to the low fat content and the high renal solute load (two times higher than breast milk). Pasteurized goat's milk is not appropriate for infants before the end of the first year. Goat's milk is low in vitamin D, iron, vitamin B_{12} and folate. In the first two years of life, soy beverages (except soy isolate infant formulas), rice or other vegetarian beverages are inappropriate alternatives to breast milk, formula, or pasteurized whole cow's milk. Homemade formulas based on evaporated milk prepared in an attempt to save money[1] provide inappropriate nutrition even when oils and vitamins are added. The cost can be as high as commercial formula.

Bottle-feeding Formula or Breast Milk

Bottles, Nipples, Soothers and Pacifiers

To avoid nipple confusion in the early weeks, cup feeding is an option for supplemental feeding in the breastfed baby.[18,21,68] No one type of bottle or nipple is superior to another, but nipples should allow approximately one drop per second to escape when the bottle is inverted. It has been suggested that plastic nurser bag systems deliver less ingested air than hard plastic or glass formula bottles. All babies benefit emotionally from being held during bottle feedings. Bottles should be avoided during sleep time or as a pacifier to reduce the incidence of infant dental caries.[1] Breastfed babies may accept a bottle feeding more readily if the bottle nipple is warmed and if the caregiver is holding or wearing a piece of the mother's clothing.

Soothers and **pacifiers** should be used with caution in the breastfed baby (especially before six weeks of age) to avoid nipple confusion and interference with the mother's milk supply.[68] A breastfed baby is soothed by having ready access to the breast. Soothers and pacifiers used by a baby being treated for an oral yeast (thrush) infection should be replaced or sterilized regularly during the course of treatment. The same precaution should be taken when topical yeast is being treated on a mother's breast.[50]

Health care professionals must report to Health Canada Consumer Product Safety any infant feeding bottles, nipples, or soothers/pacifiers which, through normal use, deteriorate or become damaged and pose a danger to an infant.

Water for Infant Formula

Only water from the cold water tap should be used for formula. Hot water is likely to contain more lead and other metals.[2] Water should be free of bacterial and chemical contamination. For infants under four months, or older if any question of bacterial or parasitic contamination is present, water should be brought to a rolling boil for two minutes.[1] Boiled water can be stored in a sterilized, tightly closed container for two to three days in the refrigerator or for 24 hours at room temperature.[1,69] Carbonated or mineral waters are not suitable for infant feeding due to mineral content. If well water is used it must be tested for high concentrations of nitrates, nitrites, arsenic, fluoride, lead, or other heavy metals. Health Canada has fact sheets on water contaminants. (Resource Tips)

Vitamin and Mineral Supplementation of Infants

Vitamin D

While it is acknowledged that some babies are at risk for vitamin D deficiency, controversy revolves around whether all breastfed babies should receive supplementation. Those at risk for whom supplementation would be appropriate include dark-skinned infants of dark-skinned women, who both have limited sun exposure, who live in the far north, and whose cultural practices prevent sun exposure to the skin, or those who live in inner city areas and have low vitamin D in their diets. Maternal vitamin D status during pregnancy and breastfeeding affects the vitamin D status of an infant at birth and during breastfeeding, so adequate maternal dietary intake and exposure to ultraviolet light is also important. The Canadian Paediatric Society recommends supplementation for breastfed infants of vitamin D (10 μg or 400 IU) daily until weaned in order to prevent rickets in both healthy and at-risk populations. Formula-fed infants receive vitamin D via commercial infant formula.[1,6,20]

Vitamins A and C

Breastfed infants do not need supplementation of vitamins A and C. Infant formulas include these vitamins.

Fluoride

Fluoride supplements are generally not recommended before eruption of the first permanent tooth. When, on an individual basis, the benefit of supplemental fluoride outweighs the risk of dental fluorosis, practitioners may use these supplements at appropriate dosages in younger children. According to the Canadian Dental Association, the total daily fluoride intake from all sources should not exceed 0.05-0.07 mg fluoride/kg body weight to minimize risk of dental fluorosis.[70] For a further discussion of fluoride, see Chapter 58.

Iron

Healthy, full-term, breastfed infants do not need extra iron until six months, at which time the iron in complementary foods provides appropriate intake.[1,20,21] Iron levels in breast milk are not affected by supplementing the mother's iron intake.[71] Healthy, full-term infants who are not breastfed will need a source of added iron at four months of age, e.g., iron fortified formula or iron supplement drops (Figure 1).

Weaning and Transition to Solid Food

Cultural expectations about weaning vary. When all human cultures are taken into account, two to four years of breastfeeding is considered normal.[21] Weaning begins around the middle of the first year of life[3] when baby starts to take anything other than breast milk, or formula in formula-fed babies. Readiness signs for complementary foods include the ability to sit up, fading of tongue thrust reflex, readiness to chew and maturation of digestive capability, and the ability to pick up and put food in the mouth. First foods should be smooth in texture, moving to coarser foods as baby develops teeth.[72] First foods for breast- or formula-fed babies will depend on the family's cultural practices. As complementary foods displace breast milk or formula, they should be dense in nutrients, and started in small quantities. Infants should be given milk first, and started with a teaspoon of a new food. To allow for recognition of allergies, new foods should be introduced at one week intervals. Wheezing, diarrhea, skin rashes or stomach pain may be signs of food allergy.[67]

Studies found no difference in the sleep patterns of breastfed babies aged five weeks or four months who received solid foods when compared to babies who were not fed solid foods before bedtime.[73,74]

When iron deficiency is a risk, a hemoglobin test can determine whether iron-rich foods such as iron fortified cereals or meats should be started first. Infants totally weaned from the breast before nine months of age should receive iron fortified infant formula.[1]

Breast milk remains an important part of a child's diet up to and beyond two years of age. The same level of immune factors are maintained even as weaning proceeds.[21]

Resource Tips

Breastfeeding Resources

La Leche League International—articles on all aspects of breastfeeding: www.lalecheleague.org. A search-able database for health professionals is found at the Centre for Breastfeeding Information which has the most complete worldwide database on breastfeeding—www.lalecheleague.org/cbi/CBI.html.

Breastfeeding Practice Interest Network for Pharmacists—e-mail bpeddles@cadvision.com or phone/FAX (403) 272-3764.

Distance education courses on breastfeeding for health professionals:
Grant MacEwan College (AB), Mohawk College (ON), Douglas College (BC).

Sources of information for mothers:
www.lalecheleaguecanada.ca or 1-800-665-4324 referral line.
www.promom.org, www.breastfeeding.com.

A lactation consultant—for the nearest IBLCE-certified lactation consultant phone (250) 477-6685 or check www.clca-accl.ca.

Health Canada has fact sheets on water contaminants at www.hc-sc.gc.ca.

The Breastfeeding Committee for Canada at www.geocities.com/HotSprings/Falls/1136.

The International Code of Marketing of Breast milk Substitutes and subsequent WHA resolutions can be found www.ibfan.org.

For information on the BC Children's and Women's Hospital Milk Bank call (604) 875-2282 or e-mail fanne@unixg.abc.ca or www.hmbana.org for the Human Milk Banking Association of North America.

Suggested Readings

Australian Government's National Breastfeeding Strategy. Available at http://www.health.gov.au/pubhlth/strateg/brfeed/. (click on Pharmacy Continuing Education Module).

Canadian Paediatric Society, Dietitians of Canada and Health Canada. *Nutrition for Healthy Term Infants.* Ottawa, Canada: Minister of Public Works and Government Services Canada; 1998. Available at: www.hc-sc.gc.ca (click on Food & Nutrition, then Infants; see also updates and corrections under "Practical Questions for Practitioners").

Canadian Pharmacists Association. *Position Statement on Breastfeeding and Infant Feeding 2001.*

Available at: www. pharmacists.ca (click on News and Views, then Newsroom, then Position Statements).

Hale T. *Medications and Mothers' Milk* 10th ed. Amarillo, TX: Pharmasoft Medical Publishing; 2002.

Health Canada. *Family-centred Maternity and Newborn Care: National Guidelines*. Ottawa: Minister of Public Works and Government Services; 2000. Available at: www.hc-sc.gc.ca (Chapter 7 on Breastfeeding, p 7-1 to 7-33).

Moretti M, Lee A, Ito S. Which drugs are contraindicated during breastfeeding? *Motherisk Update*. Sept 2000. Available at: www.motherisk.org (click on 'Breastfeeding and drugs').

Ozsoyla S. A warm chain for breastfeeding. *Lancet* 1994;344(5):1239-40.

References

1. Canadian Paediatric Society, Dietitians of Canada and Health Canada. *Nutrition for Healthy Term Infants*. Ottawa: Minister of Public Works and Government Services Canada; 1998. Available at: www.hc-sc.gc.ca (click on Food & Nutrition, then Infants; see also updates and corrections under "Practical Questions for Practitioners").

2. World Health Organization. *Global Strategy for Infant and Young Child Feeding: The Optimal Duration of Exclusive Breastfeeding*. 54th World Health Assembly; 2001 May 1; Geneva. Available at: http://www.who.int/wha-1998/EB_WHA/PDF/WHA54/ea54id4.pdf.

3. Health Canada. *Breastfeeding Canada: A Review and Update*. Ottawa: Minister of Public Works and Government Services; 1999. Available at: www.hc-sc.gc.ca.

4. Ministère de la santé et des services sociaux (2001). *L'allaitement maternel au Québec. Lignes directrices*. Québec; p 75. Available at: www.msss.gouv.qc.ca/f/(Publications-Nouveautés).

5. Leite A, Puccini R, Atallah A, Cunha A, Machado M, Capipberibe A et al. Impact of breastfeeding practices promoted by lay counselors: a randomized and controlled clinical trial. In: Feinstein AR, Vandenbrouke JP, eds. Abstracts of the Inclen 15th global meeting of the International Clinical Epidemiology Network. Queretaro, Mexico, *J Clin Epidemiol* 1998;51(suppl 1):10S.

6. Health Canada. *Family-centered Maternity and Newborn Care: National Guidelines*. Ottawa: Minister of Public Works and Government Services; 2000. Available at: www.hc-sc.gc.ca.

7. Lauwers J, Schinskie D. *Counseling the Nursing Mother. A Lactation Consultant's Guide*. 3rd ed. Sudbury, MA: Jones and Bartlett; 2000.

8. Canadian Institute of Child Health. *National Breastfeeding Guidelines for Health Care Providers*. 2nd ed. Ottawa: The Institute; 1996.

9. Akre J, ed. Infant feeding: the physiological basis. *Bull WHO* 1989;67(suppl).

10. Hale T. *Medications and Mothers' Milk*. 10th ed. Amarillo, TX: Pharmasoft Publishing; 2002.

11. Ito S, Matsui D. Drug exposure during lactation. In: Repchinsky C, ed. *Compendium of Pharmaceuticals and Specialties*. Ottawa: Canadian Pharmacists Association; 2002: L19-21.

12. American Academy of Pediatrics Committee on Drugs. The transfer of drugs and other chemicals into human milk. *Pediatrics* 2001;108(3):776-89.

13. Moretti M, Lee A, Ito S. Which drugs are contraindicated during breastfeeding? *Motherisk Update*. Sept 2000. Available at: www.motherisk.org (click on "breastfeeding and drugs").

14. Ito S. Drug therapy for breast-feeding women. *N Engl J Med* 2000;343(2)118-26.

15. Spencer JP, Gonzalez III L, Barnhart D. Medications in the breast-feeding mother. *Am Fam Physician* 2001;64:119-26.

16. Sikorski J, Renfrew MJ. Support for breastfeeding mothers. Cochrane Review. In: *The Cochrane Library*. 1. Update Software. Oxford; 2001.

17. Jones W, Brown D. The pharmacist's contribution to primary care support for lactating mothers requiring medication. *J Soc Admin Pharm* 2000;17(2):88-98.

18. World Health Organization. Family and Reproductive Health. Division of Child Health and Development. *Evidence for the Ten Steps to Successful Breastfeeding*. Geneva: The Organization; 1998.WHO/CHD/98.9.

19. Kramer MS, Chalmers B, Hodnett ED et al. Promotion of breastfeeding intervention trial (PROBIT): a randomized trial in the Republic of Belarus. *JAMA* 2000;285:413-20.

20. Health Canada. *Canadian Perinatal Health Report*. Ottawa: Minister of Public Works and Government Services Canada; 2000.

21. Mohrbacher N, Stock J. *The Breastfeeding Answer Book*. Rev ed. Schaumburg, IL: La Leche League International; 1997.

22. Halbert L. Breastfeeding in the woman with a compromised nervous system. *J Hum Lact* 1998;14(4):327-31.

23. Lawrence RA, Lawrence RM. *Breastfeeding: a Guide for the Medical Profession*. 5th ed. St. Louis, Missouri: Mosby; 1999.

24. Dewey KG, Heinig MJ, Nommsen-Rivers LA. Differences in morbidity between breast-fed and formula-fed infants. *J Pediatr* 1995 May;126(5 pt 1):696-702.

25. Beaudry M, Dufour R, Marcoux S. Relation between infant feeding and infections during the first six months of life. *J Pediatr* 1995;126:191-7.

26. Lucas A, Cole TJ. Breast milk and neonatal necrotising enterocolitis. *Lancet* 1990;336:1519-23.

27. Burr ML, Limb ES, Maguire MJ et al. Infant feeding, wheezing, and allergy: a prospective study. *Arch Dis Child* 1993 Jun;68(6):724-8.

28. Oddy W, Holt PG, Sly PD et al. Association between breast-feeding and asthma in 6 year old children: findings of a prospective birth cohort study. *BMJ* 1999;319(7213):815-19.

29. Gerstein HC. Cow's milk exposure and type I diabetes mellitus. A critical overview of the clinical literature. *Diabetes Care* 1994 Jan;17(1):13-9.

30. Anderson EW, Johnstone BM, Remax DT. Breastfeeding and cognitive development: a meta-analysis. *Am J Clin Nutr* 1999;70:525-33.

31. Haiek LN, Kramer MS, Ciampi A, Tirado R. Postpartum weight loss and infant feeding. *Am Board Fam Pract* 2001 Mar;14(2):85-94.

32. Dewey KG, Heinig MJ, Nommsen LA. Maternal weight-loss patterns during prolonged lactation. *Am J Clin Nutr* 1993 Aug;58(2):162-6.

33. Kramer F. Breastfeeding reduces maternal lower body fat. *J Am Diet* Assoc 1993;93(4):429-33.

34. Tryggvadottir L, Tulinius H, Eyfjord JE, Sigurvinsson T. Breastfeeding and reduced risk of breast cancer in an Icelandic cohort study. *Am J Epidemiol* 2001;154(1):37-42.

35. Newcomb PA, Egan KM, Titus-Ernstoff L et al. Lactation in relation to postmenopausal breast cancer. *J Epidemiol* 1999;150(2):174-82.

36. Newcomb PA, Storer BE, Longnecker MP et al. Lactation and a reduced risk of premenopausal breast cancer. *N Engl J Med* 1994;330(2):81-7.

37. Rosenblatt KLA, Thomas DB. Lactation and the risk of epithelial ovarian cancer. The WHO Collaborative Study of Neoplasia and Steroid Contraceptives. *Int J Epidemiol* 1993; 22:192-97.

38. International Lactation Consultant Association. *Summary of the Hazards of Infant Formula.* Chicago: 1992.

39. International Lactation Consultant Association. *Summary of the Hazards of Infant Formula.* Part 2. Chicago: 1998.

40. Saarinen KM, Juntunen-Backman K, Jarvenpaa AL et al. Breast-feeding and the development of cows' milk protein allergy. *Adv Exp Med Biol* 2000;478:121-30.

41. Weimer J. *The Economic Benefits of Breastfeeding: a Review and Analysis.* Washington, DC: Department of Agriculture (US), Economic Research Service; 2001 Mar Report No. 13: 20.

42. INFACT Canada. The cost of formula and infant feeding security. *INFACT Newsl* 1997;Fall:3.

43. Ball T, Wright A. Health care costs of formula-feeding in the first year of life. *Pediatrics* 1999;103(4):870-76.

44. Heird WC. The role of polyunsaturated fatty acids in term and preterm infants and breastfeeding mothers. *Pediatr Clin North Am* 2001;48(1):173-88.

45. Amir L, Hoover K, Mulford C. *Candidiasis and Breast-feeding.* Lactation Consultant Series #18. Schaumburg, IL: La Leche League International; 1995.

46. Zeretzke K. Yeast infections and the breastfeeding family. *LEAVEN* 1998;34(5):91-96.

47. Auerbach K, Riordan J. Breast-related problems. In: Riordan J, Auerbach K, eds. *Breastfeeding and Human Lactation.* Sudbury, MA:Jones and Bartlett Publishers; 1999:488-92.

48. Newman J. Pitman T. *Dr. Jack Newman's Guide to Breast-feeding.* Toronto: Harper Collins; 2000.

49. Butler R, Koch K. *Treating Thrush in the Breastfeeding Family.* Schaumburg, IL: La Leche League International; 1999.

50. Mattos-Graner RO, de Moraes AB, Rontani RM, Birman EG. Relation of oral yeast infection in Brazilian infants and use of a pacifier. *ASDC J Dent Child* 2001;68(1):33-36.

51. Stoneman L. When the worst happens: helping a mother who has lost a baby. *LEAVEN* 2000;36(1):6-7.

52. Tayler R. *Homeopathy for Pregnancy and Childbirth.* Ottawa: Ottawa School of Homeopathy; 2000.

53. Ho E, Collantes A, Kapur BM, Moretti M, Koren G. Alcohol and breastfeeding: calculation of time to zero level in milk. *Biol Neonate* 2001;80(3):219-22.

54. Parkes K. Nipple shields...friend or foe? *LEAVEN* 2000; 36(31):39-41.

55. Alexander JM, Grant AM, Campbell MJ. Randomized controlled trial of breast shells and Hoffman's exercises for inverted and non-protractile nipples. *BMJ* 1992;304:1030-3.

56. Sokol E, Allain A. *Complying with the Code? A manufacturers' and Distributors' Guide to the Code.* Penang, Malaysia: International Baby Food Action Network (IBFAN); 1998.

57. ABC Literacy Foundation. Available at: www.abc-Canada. org.

58. Potur AH, Kalmaz N. An investigation into feeding errors of 0-4 month old infants. *J Trop Ped* 1996;42(3):173-5.

59. American Academy of Pediatrics. Soy protein based formulas. Recommendations for use in infant feeding. *Pediatrics* 1998;101(1):148-53.

60. Nuijens JH, van Berkel PH, Schanbacher FL. Structure and biological action of lactoferrin. *J Mammary Gland Biol Neoplasia* 1996;1(3):285.

61. Sanchez L, Calvo M, Brock J. Biological role of lactoferrin. *Arch Dis Child* 1992;67:657.

62. Reddy V, Bhaskaram C, Raghuramulu N, Jagadeesan V. Antimicrobial factors in human milk. *Acta Paediatr Scand* 1977;66:229-32.

63. Lonnerdal B, Hernell O. Iron, zinc, copper and selenium status of breastfed infants and infants fed trace element fortified milk-based infant formula. *Acta Pediatr* 1994;83(4):367-73.

64. Persson LA, Lundstrom M, Lonnerdal B, Hernell O. Are weaning foods causing impaired iron and zinc status in 1-year old Swedish infants? A cohort study. *Acta Paediatr* 1998 Jun;87(6):618-22.

65. Barry DM, Reeve AW. Increased incidence of gram-negative neonatal sepsis with intramuscular iron administration. *Pediatrics* 1977;60:908-12.

66. Becroft DM, Dix MR, Faemer K. Intramuscular iron-dextran and susceptibility of neonates to bacterial infections: in vitro studies. *Arch Dis Child* 1977;52:778-81.

67. Capital Health Community Care and Public Health. *Healthy Eating for Two.* Edmonton, AB: Capital Health; 1996.

68. Victora CG, Behague DP, Barros FC, Olinto MT, Weiderpass E. Pacifier use and short breastfeeding duration: cause, consequence or coincidence? *Pediatrics* 1997;99(3):445-53.

69. Centre for Science in the Public Interest. Water, water everywhere... but is it safe to drink? *Nutr Action Health Lett* 2000;27(5):3-7. Available at: www.cspinet.org.

70. Canadian Dental Association. Available at: www.cda-adc.ca.

71. Vuori E, Makinen SM, Kara R, Kuitunen P. The effects of the dietary intakes of copper, iron, manganese, and zinc on the trace element content of human milk. *Am J Clin Nutr* 1980;33:227-31.

72. Naylor A, ed. Morrow A, co-ed. Developmental readiness of normal full term infants to progress from exclusive breast-feeding to the introduction of complementary foods: reviews of the relevant literature concerning infant immunologic, gastrointestinal, oral motor and maternal reproductive and lactational development. Washington, DC. Wellstart International and the LINKAGES Project/Academy for Educational Development; 2001. Available at: http://linkagesproject. org.

73. Keane V, Charney E, Straus J, Roberts K. Do solids help baby sleep through the night? *Am J Dis Child* 1988;142:404-5.

74. Macknin M, Medendorp SV, Maier MC. Infant sleep and bedtime cereal. *Am J Dis Child* 1989;143:1066-8.

With thanks to Linda Gilmour-Kessler P.Dt.

Infant Feeding (Bottle and Breast)—Caregiver Information

Cleaning Equipment, Nipples and Soothers

- Before initial use of a breast pump, breast pump kit, infant feeding bottles, nipples or soothers, sterilize parts that will be in contact with the milk or baby by boiling in a deep pot of water for five to seven minutes. Thereafter, clean by washing in hot soapy water and rinsing with hot water and air-drying. Using a dishwasher with a heat dry cycle is also appropriate.
- For infants who are ill or hospitalized, more frequent sterilization or cleaning may help. Check with your nurse, doctor or hospital.
- For babies with oral thrush (yeast) infections, sterilize bottles, nipples and soothers regularly. Replace worn nipples and soothers as yeast may collect in tiny cracks and re-infect baby.
- *Do not* squeeze liquid dish soap into breast pump parts, bottles, or nipples, as residue can cause contamination.

Collecting/Pumping Breast milk for Your Baby

- If collecting milk while separated from baby, apply warm moist cloths to the breast and massage to aid let-down of milk. Pump six to eight times a day, approximately 20 minutes per session for a daily total of about 120 minutes, switching sides twice during each session. It is not necessary to switch if using a double-pumping system.
- If collecting milk for the occasional feed, pump after baby has breastfed (morning may work best). Do not be discouraged if you get a few drops the first time as it may take several days of regular pumping or hand expression for your supply to increase to provide extra milk for storage. Pump for approximately 20 minutes, switching sides twice if using a single-pumping system. Plan ahead for times when you will need stored milk. Taper pumping sessions before absence from baby to allow supply to return to normal and avoid breast milk leakage.
- Wash hands. Moisten the funnel (flange) of the breast pump with milk or water before beginning to pump. Centre the funnel on the breast.

- A gentle rhythmic pattern of pumping or hand expression works best. Set pumps at the lowest setting to start. If using a hand piston pump, grasp piston from underneath to prevent strain on wrists.
- If using an electric pump turn pump setting to low and turn pump off before removing from breast.
- If pumping is uncomfortable or unproductive after several attempts and checking technique, contact a breastfeeding expert for advice or choice of another pump—each pump differs slightly.
- For information on hand expression of breast milk contact a La Leche League Leader near you at 1-800-665-4324. Hand expression is economical and easily learned.

Storing Breast milk

- Breast milk may be kept at room temperature (19-22° C) for up to 10 hours.
- Refrigerated breast milk (0 to 4° C) may be kept up to 8 days.
- It is not known whether human milk left in the bottle after a feeding can be safely kept until the next feeding.
- Frozen milk may be stored in a freezer (inside a fridge) for two weeks, in a self-contained freezer unit of a fridge 3 to 4 months, or in a deep freezer at a constant minus –19°C for six months or longer. All milk should be labeled and dated.
- Cooled fresh milk may be added to frozen milk.
- Freeze in quantities of 60 to 100 mL. Date each container.
- Store frozen milk in hard plastic or glass containers, or plastic bags specially designed to store breast milk. Disposable bottle liners and freezer bags are inexpensive and do not require washing, but valuable fat may adhere to these bags.
- Breast milk that is collected away from home should be stored in a fridge or cooler until it is transported home sandwiched between frozen cool packs in a small, insulated lunch bag or picnic cooler.*
- Thaw frozen milk by running under warm water and swirling to mix. Thawing in a microwave may

---

*Pryor, G – *Nursing mother, working mother: the essential guide for breastfeeding and staying close to your baby after you return to work.* Boston: Harvard Common Press; 1997.

cause hot spots and high temperatures can destroy valuable components. Previously frozen milk that has thawed can be kept in the refrigerator for 24 hours. Do not refreeze thawed milk.

Tips on Bottle-feeding a Normally Breastfed Baby

- Have someone other than mother bottle-feed the breastfed baby.
- Feed before baby becomes over-hungry and upset. A calm breastfed baby will more readily take an alternate method of feeding.
- Hold the breastfed baby in other than the breast-feeding position when giving the feed.
- All babies benefit emotionally from being held during bottle feedings.
- Have caregiver who gives feeding hold or wear a piece of the mother's clothing near baby.
- If using a bottle and nipple warm the nipple before presenting to the baby. Use a nipple with a small hole (one drop per second or less). Breastfed babies have a strong suck and may be overwhelmed by the fast flow of milk from a nipple with a large hole. If baby refuses one type of nipple, try another.
- Avoid use of a bottle during sleep time or as a pacifier to reduce the incidence of infant caries.
- Use a small cup, a tiny spoon or eyedropper to feed a breastfed baby who refuses to use an artificial nipple.

Mixing and Feeding Infant Formula

- Use only water from the cold water tap. Hot water is likely to contain more lead and other metals and softened water contains higher sodium (salt). Do not use carbonated or mineral waters. Use a water source that is safe and has been tested for bacterial contamination and safe levels of fluoride and other components. For infants under four months, or at any age where there is question of bacterial or parasitic contamination, bring water to a rolling boil for two minutes. Boiled water can be stored in a sterilized, tightly closed container for two to three days in the refrigerator or for 24 hours at room temperature. Test well water for high concentrations of fluoride, nitrates, nitrites, arsenic, lead, or other metals.
- Pour boiling water over tops of cans of ready-to-use or liquid concentrate before opening.
- Mix liquid concentrate with equal parts of water prepared as above.
- Use only the brand-specific measuring spoons provided with cans of powdered concentrate.
- Prepared formula must be refrigerated and used within 24 to 48 hours. Refrigerate opened cans of ready-to-use or concentrate and use within 24 to 48 hours. Prepared formula kept at room temperature must be used within 1 hour.
- Use cans of powdered concentrate within 30 days of opening.
- To feed baby, warm prepared infant formula in a pan of hot water or use a commercial warmer. Microwave heating can cause hot spots that can burn baby. Shake the formula well before testing temperature.

Chapter 33

Weight Management

Shirley Heschuk, BScPharm, MSc

Definition of Obesity

Obesity is a chronic condition (disease) characterized by an accumulation of body fat in adipose tissue resulting from excessive caloric intake and inadequate caloric loss. Various methods are used for objective measurement of obesity. The body mass index (BMI) is the most commonly used clinical measurement and is calculated by dividing the person's weight in kilograms by the person's height in meters squared (kg/m^2).

The Canadian Guidelines for Healthy Weights were released in 1988 and define the BMI categories as:[1,2]
- Zone A: underweight (BMI < 20.0) – may be associated with health problems for some people
- Zone B: acceptable weight (BMI 20.0 to 24.9) – good weight for most people
- Zone C: possibly overweight (BMI 25.0 to 27.0) – may lead to health problems in some people
- Zone D: overweight or obese (BMI > 27.0) – increased risk of developing health problems

The lower end of the ranges given is for the small-framed person with less muscle and the higher end of the range is for a large-framed person, or one who carries more muscle. BMI measurements are useful for ages 20 to 65. It does not apply to infants, children, adolescents, pregnant or breastfeeding women, and adults over 65 years of age. For ages 2 to 20, it is suggested to use the NHANES percentile weight for height, age and gender charts.

The National Institutes of Health (NIH) guidelines, established by the World Health Organization (WHO) in 1995, differs slightly from the Canadian guidelines and defines underweight as a BMI < 18.5, normal weight as a BMI 18.5 to 24.9, overweight as a BMI of 25.0 to 29.9, and obesity as a BMI > 30. They have incorporated central body fat distribution, or abdominal fatness, as an additional measure of obesity-related health risk and morbidity.[3] Waist circumference (WC) is an indirect measure of abdominal fatness. A measure of greater than 88 cm for women and greater than 102 cm for men, indicates an elevated health risk.[3] (Table 1)

Health Canada has established an Expert Working Group on Healthy Weight Guidelines and anticipates release of updated guidelines for the fall of 2002.

Pathophysiology

A recent Canadian Health Survey found that 35% of men and 27% of women have a BMI > 27 and these numbers are climbing steadily.[4] Obesity rates in children are also increasing.[4] There has been an epidemic increase in childhood overweight in the US between 1986 and 1998.[5] Well-designed studies of obesity interventions are required.[6]

The prevalence of obesity, in both men and women, increases with age.[7] Prevalence is also affected by socioeconomic status and ethnic or cultural differences. Poverty and lower educational attainment are associated with higher than average rates of female obesity and affect proportionately more persons in minority populations (e.g., Blacks, Hispanics, and Natives) than in white populations. These differences may be due to the fact that diabetes mellitus and certain other obesity-related conditions, and high-risk body fat distribution (upper body or central obesity) all occur to a greater extent in some minority populations.[7]

There is an inverse relationship between level of physical activity and development of obesity. Obesity is more prevalent in persons with sedentary lifestyles or a physical handicap that restricts activity.[8]

Table 1: **Classification of Overweight and Obesity by Body Mass Index (BMI), Waist Circumference, and Associated Disease Risk**[*2]

	BMI (kg/m²)	Obesity class	Disease risk* (Relative to normal weight and waist circumference)	
			Men ≤ 40 in (≤ 102 cm) Women ≤ 35 in (≤ 88 cm)	> 40 in (> 102 cm) > 35 in (> 88 cm)
Underweight	< 18.5			
Normal[†]	18.5-24.9			
Overweight	25.0-29.9		Increased	High
Obesity	30.0-34.9	I	High	Very high
	35.0-39.9	II	Very high	Very high
Extreme Obesity	≥ 40	III	Extremely high	Extremely high

*Disease risk for type 2 diabetes, hypertension, and cardiovascular disease.
[†]Increased waist circumference can also be a marker for increased risk even in persons of normal weight.
Adapted with permission from the National Heart, Lung and Blood Institute, "Preventing and Managing the Global Epidemic of Obesity. Report of the World Health Organization Consultation of Obesity." WHO, Geneva, June 1997.

Obesity is a chronic disease developing from interactive influences of numerous factors: organic, hereditary (genetics), physiological, metabolic (set-point theory), medications, psychological (social, cultural, behavioral), and environmental.

An identifiable *organic* cause can only be found in a small percentage of people. Weight gain in excess of 1 kg per day invariably implies fluid retention and is frequently a sign of a cardiovascular, renal or hepatic disorder. Other causes may be endocrinopathies such as insulinoma, Cushing's disease or thyroid dysfunction.

The role of *heredity* is not easily assessed, as environmental factors pertaining to food intake greatly confound this issue. If both parents are of normal weight, the incidence of having an obese child is approximately 9%. If one of the parents is obese, the rate increases to 50% and if both of the parents are obese, the rate is 80%.[9]

Adipose tissue grows through an increase in both size and number of cells. It can be stated that fat infants have a higher chance of being obese in adulthood than do lean infants but that obesity is not inevitable for those in the high percentiles of weight for height, age, and gender in the early years.[10] Childhood obesity accounts for only a minority of cases of obesity in adults.[11,12]

Many physiologic factors may affect obesity, such as neurotransmitters, neuropeptides and hormones. The hypothalamus receives input from peripheral satiety sites, leptin (a hormone produced by fat cells), and the indoleamine neurotransmitter system in the brain, all of which are thought to play a role in obesity.

Concerning metabolic influences, proponents of the set-point theory argue that the body has an internal control mechanism, a set-point, probably located in the hypothalamus, that drives the body to maintain a particular level of body fat. Exercise can lower the particular setting, whereas dieting has no effect. Each time we manage to reduce our fat level below our "natural" set-point, the body makes internal adjustments to resist this change and conserve or replenish body fat, making it difficult to lose weight. There is little evidence in support of adaptive metabolic changes as an explanation for the tendency of weight-reduced persons to regain weight.[13]

Weight gain is also a common side effect of certain medications (Table 2).

Psychologically, many of our eating habits are instilled at an early age by social, cultural and environmental influences. In anxiety or depression, food may substitute for satisfaction missed from other sources.

Of the modifiable causes of obesity, dietary intake and physical activity are the major contributors. The

Table 2: **Medications Associated with Weight Gain**[14]

Class	Drugs	Mechanism	Typical weight gain
Psychotropic agents	**Antidepressants** (tricyclic antidepressants)	Unclear. May attenuate serotonin-mediated signal transduction, can produce a reduction in the basal metabolic rate (BMR).	Varies from -0.4 kg/mo to 4.14 kg/mo of therapy and appears to be related to the particular TCA used, and the dose and duration of therapy
	MAOIs	Unclear. Increased hunger and craving for sweets	Less profound than with TCAs
	Antipsychotic drugs	Block dopamine D_2 and serotonin receptors to cause increased appetite	Clozapine – average 12 kg varying over 16 wks of therapy Loxapine – 9 kg in 36 wks
	Lithium	Produces polydipsia, causes sodium and water retention, reduces BMR, inhibits synthesis of thyroid hormone, blocks dopamine receptors inducing feeding, increases GABA functions, which stimulate carbohydrate intake and reduces BMR.	10 kg or more in 6-10 yrs, up to 28 kg has been reported
Anticonvulsant agents	**Valproic acid**	Unclear. Enhances GABA-functions (see above)	15-20 kg over variable lengths of treatment
	Carbamazepine	Water retention – mechanism unclear. Possible antidiuretic hormone involvement. Possible norepinephrine or serotonin effect	Up to 15 kg during a 3-mo treatment course
Steroids/Hormones	**Corticosteroids**	Stimulate food intake, causes hyperinsulinemia which promotes fat deposition	Prednisone – average of 2 kg during a 6 mo daily course of therapy
	Estrogen, progesterone, testosterone or other anabolic/androgenic steroids	Unclear. Possible increased appetite or body fat	Variable
Diabetic agents	**Insulin**	Elimination of glycosuria results in increase in fat mass.	Up to 8 kg during an intensive 3-mo course of therapy
	Oral hypoglycemic agents	Unclear	Up to 5 kg during 3-12 mos of treatment
Antineoplastic agents	**Tamoxifen**	Unclear	Average 2.5-6 kg, up to 10 kg or more
Migraine prophylaxis agents	**Flunarizine**	Possible increased appetite – dopamine effect	4 kg at dose of 10 mg per day for 60 days of treatment
	Pizotifen	Unclear – possible serotonin effect	2-10.5 kg in 8 wks of treatment

combination of the increased availability of low-cost, very palatable, high-energy-density foods, and a great decrease in physical activity, have caused waist girth and weight to rise dramatically in modernized societies.

Health Risks of Obesity[8,15-17]

- Cardiovascular disease: Obesity is an independent risk factor for cardiovascular disease.[18] It is associated with premature acute myocardial infarction[19] and causes a 3.3-fold increase in cardiovascular disease in American women with a BMI > 29 kg/m^2 compared with BMI < 21 kg/m^2.[20]
- Hypertension: Incidence of hypertension is three times higher in obese patients. In the Framingham study, hypertension developed 10 times more often in persons who were 20% or more overweight than in those of normal weight.[21]
- Blood lipids: Obesity is associated with low HDL cholesterol, high triglycerides and possibly high LDL cholesterol. In the Framingham study, every 10% increase in relative weight was associated with an increase in plasma cholesterol of 0.3 mmol/L.[21]
- Insulin resistance: The enlarged fat cell is less sensitive to the antilipolytic and lipogenic actions of insulin.
- Diabetes: Mildly obese persons have a twofold risk, moderately obese, a fivefold risk and severely obese, a tenfold risk of developing type 2 diabetes. In the US, 85% of patients with type 2 diabetes are obese.
- Cancer: The American Cancer Society found that the mortality ratio (actual deaths compared to expected deaths) for cancer in men who are 40% or more overweight is 1.33; the corresponding figure for women is 1.55. Overweight men have significantly higher mortality ratios for colorectal and prostate cancers, and overweight women have significantly higher rates of endometrial, gallbladder, cervical, ovarian and breast cancers.[22]
- Sleep apnea: Obstruction by local accumulation of fat leads to hypoventilation and hypoxia.
- Venous circulatory disease: Varicose veins, venous stasis and pulmonary embolism are more common in obese patients.
- Osteoarthritis: With weight increase, prevalence increases from 0.75% to 1.45% in men and from 0.4% to 1.45% in women.[17]

- Gout: The Canadian Health Survey found that the percentage of men with uric acid levels greater than 416 μmol/L increased from 7% to 31% as the BMI increased from 21 to 31. Women were not affected until they reached a BMI greater than 31, when the percentage prevalence was 7%.[23]
- Gallbladder disease: Gallstones occur three or four times more often in obese than in non-obese persons.
- Skin: Stretch marks (striae), fungal and yeast infections are more common in the obese population.
- Psychological: Poor self-image and impaired social relationships, depression and anxiety are all worsened by obesity.
- Mortality: 1.67 × increase in mortality in subjects with BMI > 26 kg/m^2 than those with BMI < 22.5 kg/m^2.[24]
- Endocrine: (rare, < 1%) Hypothalamic, pituitary, thyroid, adrenal, ovarian, and pancreatic syndromes as well as irregular menses, reduction of fertility, and risk of toxemia all occur in obese patients.

Goals of Therapy

- Refocus from weight change alone, which is aimed at appearance, to weight management, achieving the best weight possible in the context of overall health
- Reduce body weight or at least prevent further gain – for initial weight loss, a realistic goal of 10% weight reduction should be set (approximately 1 kg weight loss per week over six months)
- Abate the complications associated with obesity and underweight
- Achieve and maintain a healthy weight range (BMI between 20 and 24.9 for Canadian guidelines; BMI between 18.5 and 24.9 for NIH guidelines) long term

Patient Assessment

Obesity is very difficult to treat. Assess the patient for readiness and motivation to lose weight. This includes:

- Reasons and motivation for weight loss
- Approach and results of previous attempts at weight loss
- Support expected from family and friends
- Understanding of risks and benefits

- Attitudes toward physical activity
- Time availability
- Potential barriers to the patient's adoption of change

The first step is to assess the individual's weight status and risk factors (Table 3). The approaches include diet, exercise, behavioral modification, drugs, and surgery. In Canada, weight reduction is recommended to overweight (obese) adults (BMI > 27) with obesity-related diseases.[2] In the US model (NIH guidelines), weight loss is recommended for obese (BMI ≥ 30) and for overweight (BMI 25.0 to 29.9) individuals with at least two other risk factors or an elevated WC.[3] Individuals with lesser risk should be counseled to make effective lifestyle changes to prevent weight gain. An assessment tool for patients with weight-related complaints is presented in Figure 1.[2]

Table 3: **Factors that Increase Morbidity in Obese Patients**[2]

Established heart disease
Presence of other atherosclerotic diseases
Type 2 diabetes
Sleep apnea
Cigarette smoking
Hypertension
High LDL cholesterol
Low HDL cholesterol
Impaired fasting glucose
Family history of premature coronary heart disease
Age ≥ 45 yrs for men or age ≥ 55 yrs for women
  (or postmenopausal)

Underweight: When energy consumption is < 1800 kcal/day, it becomes difficult to meet the recommended nutrient requirements. Those with a BMI < 20 (Canadian guidelines) or BMI < 18.5 (NIH guidelines) are considered underweight. Physical, physiological and psychological factors all play a role. The elderly are particularly prone to being malnourished, as are those suffering from eating disorders (anorexia nervosa, bulimia nervosa, bingeing,) chronic diseases such as AIDS/HIV, and those with poor eating habits.

Some of the causes of malnutrition include:
- Poverty

- Diseases that reduce appetite, decrease absorption or utilization of nutrients or increase requirements for nutrients
- Drugs that cause nausea and vomiting and/or affect absorption, utilization or excretion of nutrients. (See Chapter 20)
- Ignorance about good nutrition or food preparation
- Dental problems
- Depression or mental problems
- Decreased physical ability to buy food or prepare a meal
- Alcoholism
- Eating disorders[25]

Eating Disorders

Anorexia nervosa is a self-imposed starvation syndrome characterized by extreme loss of weight, excessive exercise, body image disturbance, and an intense fear of becoming overweight, despite being grossly underweight.[26]

Bulimia nervosa is characterized by recurrent episodes of compulsive gorging or binge eating and then purging to prevent weight gain from occurring. Unlike the anorexic, who is excessively thin, the bulimic is usually of normal weight but weight fluctuates.[27,28]

Binge-eating disorder is characterized by chronic consumption of massive quantities of food. Diagnosis is based on having an average of two binge-eating episodes per week for six months, triggered by emotions such as frustration, anger, depression, and anxiety.[29]

Table 4: **Warning Signs of Anorexia and Bulimia**[30]

Anorexia:	Bulimia:
Loss of significant amount of weight.	Bingeing, or eating uncontrollably.
Continuing to diet (although thin).	Purging by strict dieting, fasting, vigorous exercise, vomiting, or abusing laxatives or diuretics in an attempt to lose weight.
Feeling fat, even after losing weight.	
Fear of weight gain.	Using the bathroom frequently after meals.
Cessation of monthly menstrual periods.	Preoccupation with body weight.

(cont'd)

Figure 1: **Assessment of Obese and Underweight Patients**

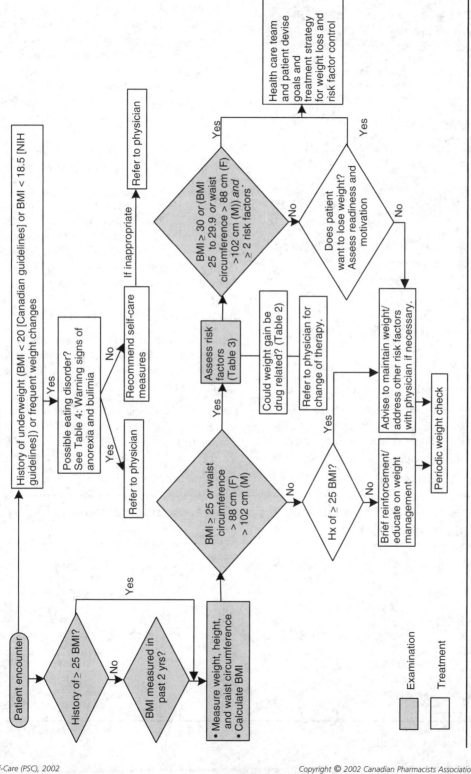

This algorithm applies only to the assessment for overweight and obesity and subsequent decisions based on that assessment. It does not include any initial overall assessment for cardiovascular risk factors or diseases that are indicated.

Note: Canadian Guidelines: Weight reduction measures if BMI ≥ 27 with obesity-related risk factors[1,2] (Table 3).

Adapted with permission from National Institutes of Health/National Heart, Lung, and Blood Institute. Clinical guidelines on the identification, evaluation, and treatment of over-weight and obesity in adults: the evidence report. June 17, 1998:1-228.

Table 4: **Warning Signs of Anorexia and Bulimia**[30] *(cont'd)*

Preoccupation with food, calories, nutrition, and/or cooking.	Depression or mood swings. Irregular menstrual periods.
Preferring to eat in isolation.	Dental problems, swollen cheeks or glands, heartburn or bloating
Exercising compulsively.	
Bingeing and purging	

Health professionals should lead efforts to prevent eating disorders by learning to promote self-esteem in their patients and teaching patients that people can be healthy at every size. Warn patients of the potential dangers of inappropriate methods of weight loss including medications (see Inappropriate Medication for Weight Loss).

Nonpharmacologic Therapy

Diet Therapy

Calorie Restriction

There is strong evidence that low-calorie diets consisting of approximately 1000 to 1200 kcal per day can reduce body weight by an average of 8% over 3 to 12 months.[31] If caloric intake is reduced by 500 kcal per day, it will result in weight loss of approximately 0.5 kg per week. The diet must be nutritionally adequate (diets under 1100 kcal per day do not contain adequate amounts of vitamins and minerals, therefore supplementation may be recommended). A balanced diet can be obtained by following *Canada's Food Guide to Healthy Eating* (CFGHE) and ensuring that the fat content of the diet is below 30% of total calories, which helps to lower the caloric content of the diet.[23] (See Chapter 31.) A reduction of fat without reducing total caloric intake is generally not sufficient for weight loss. The typical North American diet is generally too high in fat, especially saturated fat (Table 5).

Increasing dietary fibre may facilitate weight loss.[38] Both soluble fibre (e.g., pectins, gums, psyllium, oat-bran) and insoluble fibre (e.g., cellulose, lignins) promote satiety by delaying gastric emptying and causing a feeling of fullness.[39] Insoluble fibre adds bulk and increases water in the stool, which speeds the passage of food through the intestinal tract, allowing less time for absorption of nutrients.[40]

Meal replacement products are available as a substitute for one to two meals. They should be followed by at least one regular meal per day to make a total of about 1500 calories per day.

Eating less than 1000 kcal per day long term is not recommended as compliance is difficult. It may cause a reduction in resting metabolic rate, promoting weight regain upon cessation of energy restriction.[16]

Table 5: **Comparison of Nutrient Content of Canada's Food Guide to Healthy Eating (CFGHE) to other diets**[2,31-37]

Diet	Calories	Fat (%)	Saturated fat (%)	Protein (%)	CHO (%)	Fibre (g)
CFGHE	1800	30	10	15	55	30
Typical American Diet	2200	35	16	15	50	9
Weight Watchers	1462	25	6	20	56	26
Dr. Atkins (New-Rev.)*	1800	60	18	30	10	10
The Zone*	1000	30	8	30	40	10
CHO Addicts*	1476	54	24	23	24	8
Sugar Busters*	1521	28	7	33	39	25
Dr. Ornish†	1273	9	2	15	81	38

*High-protein diet.
†High-carbohydrate diet.

Very-Low-Calorie Diets (VLCD)

These are usually liquid diets supplying about 400 to 800 kcal per day and produce rapid weight loss while minimizing the protein losses of starvation.[41] They are recommended only for obese clients (BMI ≥ 30) and must be administered under close medical supervision. These diets appear to be safe and effective in promoting short-term weight loss but the long-term maintenance is poor and no better than other methods of weight reduction.[8] Examples of such diets are the Cambridge® and the Optifast® diets.

Popular (Fad) Diets[32,42]

These diets promise miracle cures for losing weight, many with little effort. They often lack nutritional balance and promote high protein, high fat or low carbohydrate intakes, or even elimination of certain foods or food groups. The weight loss is usually short-lived and is often the result of short-term calorie restriction and/or water loss (diuresis), which is quickly regained upon cessation of the diet.

Examples of these diets include *food-specific diets* which make the unfounded claim that some foods have special properties than can cause weight loss. Eventually boredom sets in and one stops eating the allowed food, or at least enough of the allowed food to maintain weight. Examples include Eat Right 4 Your Type® and The New Hollywood Diet®.

Another example of a fad diet are the current *high-protein, low-carbohydrate diets* which are based on the idea that by limiting the amount of carbohydrate, the body is forced to use the fat already stored. There is no scientific evidence for this. High-protein diets may increase calcium loss from bone.[32] These diets can also trigger ketosis, which could lead to dehydration, gout, orthostatic hypotension and electrolyte imbalance, and possibly result in kidney and liver damage.[16] Weight loss induced by high-protein, low-carbohydrate diets is largely attributable to the loss of water, glycogen, and lean tissue. Examples include The Montignac Diet®, The Carbohydrate Addict's Life-Span Program®, Dr. Atkins New Diet Revolution®, Protein Power®, Sugar Busters®, and The Zone®.[32-36]

Finally, *high-fibre, low-calorie diets* promote weight loss through consumption of large amounts of fibre. Eating a large amount of fibre will not cause weight loss; only eating fewer calories will. Examples include:

Dr. Ornish's Eat More, Weigh Less®, Dr. Bob Arnot's Revolutionary Weight Control Program®.[32,37]

Low-fat, low-calorie diets are most successful in maintaining weight loss. A diet high in vegetables, fruits, complex carbohydrates (whole grains and legumes), and low-fat dairy is a moderate-fat, low-calorie diet that prevents weight gain, results in weight loss and weight maintenance[2] (Table 6).

Fat Substitutes

Fat substitutes are carbohydrate-, protein- or lipid-based. The carbohydrate- and protein-based products provide less than the 9 kcal per gram of fat. They allow incorporation of extra water into foods by binding to it, which decreases the calories per serving. They have a moist, thick, texture, which mimics the richness of fat. The fatty acids in lipid-based fat substitutes are arranged on the glycerol molecule in order to inhibit absorption. Olestra is a carbohydrate-based product available in the US.

"Low-fat foods" should not be confused with "low-calorie foods"; the calories saved by eating low-fat foods are often negligible, especially if more is eaten.[16,42]

Artificial Sweeteners

Nutritive sweeteners include sorbitol, mannitol, and xylitol, which are sugar alcohols. They have about half the calories of sugar because the body absorbs them more slowly and incompletely. The side effect of this slow absorption is diarrhea.

The *non-nutritive sweeteners* are saccharin, aspartame, acesulfame potassium (acesulfame K), sucralose, cyclamate, and the herbal, stevia. They are so intensely sweet that tiny amounts can be used, so the calories they provide are undetectable (Table 7). Saccharin is classified in Schedule III and requires a safety warning due to risk of carcinogenesis in rats. Studies assessing the risk have shown conflicting results.[44]

Fasting

Fasting to cleanse the body and jump-start a weight-loss diet has been used traditionally. But fasting deprives the body of nutrients and results in low energy, weakness, and lightheadedness, not real weight loss. Any weight loss is water and muscle, not fat, and weight will be regained when eating is started again. It does not clear toxins from the body, rather

Table 6: **Dietary Recommendation for Weight Loss: Low-Calorie Step I & Step II Diets**[2]

Step I Diet

Nutrient	Recommended intake
Calories	Approximately 500 to 1000 kcal per day reduction from usual intake
Total Fat	30% or less of total calories
Saturated Fatty Acids	8 to 10% of total calories
Monounsaturated Fatty Acids	Up to 15% of total calories
Polyunsaturated Fatty Acids	Up to 10% of total calories
Cholesterol	< 300 mg per day
Protein	Approximately 15% of total calories
Carbohydrate	55% or more of total calories
Sodium Chloride	No more than 100 mmol per day (approximately 2.4 g of sodium or approximately 6 g of sodium chloride)
Calcium	1000 to 1500 mg
Fibre	20 to 30 g

Step II Diet: For Patients With High Blood Cholesterol Levels

Saturated fats	< 7% of total calories
Cholesterol levels	< 200 mg per day
All of the other nutrients are the same as Step I.	

Reproduced with permission from National Institutes of Health/National Heart, Lung and Blood Institute, *Clinical guidelines on the identification, evaluation, and treatment of overweight and obesity in adults: the evidence report.* June, 1998:1-228.

ketones can build up when carbohydrates are not available for energy.[16]

Physical Activity/Exercise

Regular aerobic exercise increases energy expenditure, favors the mobilization of adipose tissue and is helpful in weight maintenance. The Canadian Society for Exercise Physiology and Health Canada established an overall goal for individual Canadians to accumulate at least 60 minutes of physical activity every day (in periods of at least 10 minutes each) to stay healthy or to improve health.[16] Aerobic exercise (e.g., walking) is the most effective for burning fat. Physical activity plus diet produces more weight loss than either diet or physical activity alone.[1] The moderately-to-severely obese are often poor candidates for exercise, and any regimen should be preceded by a thorough medical evaluation.

Behavioral Modification

The goal of behavioral modification is to reduce, change, or eradicate lifestyle habits that have caused or contributed to weight gain. Through maintenance of a diary, patients become aware of what and how

much they eat as a background for changing that behavior. The aim is to break learned associations between environmental cues and food intake.

Interventions that incorporate these strategies produce gradual and moderate weight loss.[45] With systematic manipulation of all factors associated with eating and exercise patterns, there is evidence that with an average length of 18 weeks of treatment, an average weight loss of 9.9 kg is obtained.[46] Patients are able to maintain, on average, about two-thirds of their initial weight loss 9 to 10 months after behavioral counseling ends.[47]

Size Acceptance[16]

It is important to help people realize that there is no ideal body size, shape, or weight for an individual and that people of all sizes and shapes can reduce their risk of poor health by adopting a healthy lifestyle.

Weight Maintenance and Prevention of Weight Regain

The maintenance of a reduced body weight is difficult. After six months of weight loss, the rate of weight loss usually declines and plateaus.[2] Successful weight

Table 7: **Artificial Sweeteners**[15,43]

Product	Calories/g	Sweetness compared to sugar	Heat stable (can be used in cooking)	Comments
Acesulfame K	0	200x	Yes	Caution if sulfa allergy. Contains potassium-caution in potassium restricted diets
Aspartame	4 kcal/g (so sweet that very little is used)	160-220x	No	Contraindicated in patients with phenylketonuria. Allergy possible. No adverse effects normally associated with ingestion of less than 50 mg/kg/per day.
Cyclamate	0	30x	Yes	Acceptable daily intake is up to 4 mg. Large doses cause diarrhea. Photosensitivity has been reported.[39]
Sucralose	0	600x	Yes	Used to replace sugar g for g in baking. Passes through the body intact
Xylitol, sorbitol, and mannitol	Approximately 2 kcal/g but very little is absorbed, therefore virtually no calories	Approximately 1/2x as sweet as sugar		Not readily absorbed and can cause osmotic diarrhea

maintenance is defined as a weight regain of < 3 kg in two years and a sustained reduction in waist circumference of at least 4 cm. Patients on a reducing diet experience a 15 to 20% drop in metabolic rate.[48] This reduced metabolic rate may also make it easier to regain weight on returning to a more normal diet. After a patient has achieved the goals of weight loss, dietary therapy, physical activity, and behavior therapy should be continued indefinitely; otherwise, excess weight likely will be regained.[2]

Weight Loss Programs

There are a number of self-help programs such as Weight Watchers®, NutriSystem®, Overeaters Anonymous®, and Take Off Pounds Sensibly® (TOPS) for support and motivation (see also Resource Tips).

Surgery

Bariatric or weight-reduction surgery is considered for people with a BMI ≥ 40 or with BMI 35 to 40 who have high-risk comorbid conditions and whose obesity is refractory to other approaches.[2]

Surgical treatment of obesity is based on one of two principles:
—A short bowel is created to produce malabsorption of ingested calories (gastric bypass), and
—A small stomach is created to prevent much caloric intake at any one time (gastroplasty – stapling of the stomach).

Success has been variable. These patients are likely to need life-long medical supervision.[49] Surgical therapy for obesity, such as gastric bypass, has been shown to maintain a weight loss of approximately 33% of body weight for more than 10 years.[50]

Liposuction, a cosmetic surgical procedure, removes fat to reshape the body. It removes some fat cells, but a compensatory hypertrophy of remaining adipose tissue after lipectomy has been demonstrated.[49] There are risks such as blood clots, perforation injuries, and skin and nerve damage. Liposuction does not foster good eating habits.

Underweight

Patients who are underweight can increase nutrient intake by eating at mealtime; increasing the number and size of servings; increasing nutrient density by adding extra protein, carbohydrate and fat and by feeding more frequently. Restricting physical exercise so there is a positive energy balance can be beneficial, as can behavior modification.

Pharmacologic Therapy

Use of *nonprescription drugs* for weight loss is limited and drug therapy must be monitored both for safety and efficacy (Table 8). **Caffeine** has been used to facilitate weight loss; however, any loss is mainly due to diuretic effect. At the same time, caffeine increases heart rate, blood pressure and muscle stimulation. As such, it is not recommended in the treatment of obesity.[51]

Although studies suggest effects are small and contradictory, **chromium** has been claimed to increase lean body mass and decrease weight.[52] Adverse effects have included chronic renal failure with doses of 1200 µg daily for several months.[53]

Several *alternative therapies* have been used to assist patients in achieving weight loss with varying levels of evidence for clinical efficacy.

Apple cider vinegar is fermented juice from crushed apples containing pectin, vitamins and minerals; it may act as a bulk-forming agent. Clinical trials are needed to assess efficacy.

Pyruvate promotes transport of glucose into muscle cells and is claimed to increase metabolism and fat utilization. Human studies showed a reduction of weight but the participants consumed low calorie diets (500-1000 kcal/day) and used doses of pyruvate five to seven times the daily recommended dose.[54] Safety and efficacy have not been established.

Chitosan binds to fat, decreasing its absorption as well as acting as a fibre to increase feelings of satiety. It has not been shown to be more effective than placebo.[55] It may even block the absorption of fat-soluble vitamins and increase calcium excretion. In spite of this information if a patients chooses chitosan, make them aware it is derived from shellfish and should be avoided if the patient is allergic.

Garcinia cambogia, also known as hydroxycitric acid or hydroxycitrate, has been used in weight control but studies have shown no significant weight loss or fat mass loss beyond that observed with placebo.[56]

Table 8: **Nonprescription Weight Loss Products**[15,16]

Product	Mechanism of action	Suggested dose	Side effects	Comments
Benzocaine	Local anesthetic numbs the oral cavity to decrease taste sensation	3-4 mg in gum, lozenge, or tablets; chew gum or suck tablets 30 min before meals.	Numbs oral cavity and gastric mucosa. Topical anesthesia may impair swallowing and increase risk of aspiration. Numbness of tongue may increase risk of biting trauma.	Clinical trials needed to assess efficacy.
Bulk-Forming Agents (fibre, methylcellulose, psyllium)	Delayed gastric emptying creates a feeling of fullness and satiety	10 g/daily in divided doses	Cramping, bloating, flatulence, blockage of esophagus, intestine, or fecal impaction if not taken with sufficient fluid. Allergy to psyllium	Clinical trials needed to evaluate efficacy. Similar effect may be obtained by eating high-fibre vegetables and fruits.

Prescription Drugs

These drugs are recommended only for obese patients with BMI ≥ 30 or BMI ≥ 27 with co-morbidities who have not responded adequately to an appropriate weight-reducing diet alone. They should be used as adjunctive therapy within a weight management program.

Anorectic Drugs

These medications act centrally, on the appetite centre, through brain catecholamines, dopamine, or serotonin pathways. Amphetamine-like drugs not only decrease appetite, they also elevate mood and increase arousal, probably by making norepinephrine and dopamine more abundant at synapses. Amphetamines are no longer used due to addictive properties.

Fenfluramine and dexfenfluramine have been removed from the market following reports of valvular heart disease and primary pulmonary hypertension.

Sibutramine is both a serotonin and norepinephrine reuptake inhibitor (SNRI) which reduces food intake (by enhancing satiety) and increases energy expenditure (by inducing thermogenesis through activation of the β_3-system). Weight loss tends to plateau after one year, with some people reporting a loss of about 10% of starting weight. The safety and effectiveness of sibutramine beyond one year has not been established.[57]

Lipase Inhibitors[58]

Orlistat inhibits fat absorption in the intestine by blocking pancreatic lipase. As a result, about 30% of ingested fat is passed in the stool. Side effects include loose and oily stools (especially if a low fat diet is not consumed), fecal incontinence, abdominal cramping, and nausea. In comparison to placebo, there is a modest increase in weight reduction (about an additional 4 to 5%).

Inappropriate Medications for Weight Loss

Syrup of Ipecac: People with eating disorders use syrup of ipecac to induce vomiting. Repeated use can cause cardiotoxicity and dental erosion from acidic stomach contents.

Laxatives: Laxatives are used to speed up the passage of food through the gastrointestinal tract to decrease the absorption of calories. However, they have little or no effect on reducing weight, as the ingested calories have already been absorbed by the time the laxative takes effect. Prolonged use of laxatives causes electrolyte imbalance, and suppresses the natural urge to have a bowel movement, leading to constipation.

Diuretics: An initial weight loss is due to dehydration but continued use causes electrolyte imbalances.

Ephedra (Ma Huang): The Federal Drug Administration and Health Canada have issued warnings about the use of ephedra in weight loss, body building or increasing energy.[59] Ephedrine increases the release of norepinephrine which suppresses appetite, enhances thermogenesis and speeds metabolism. Side effects include insomnia, nervousness, seizures, stroke, heart attack and even death. Ephedra is authorized by Health Canada for use only as a nasal decongestant in cold products. These products have smaller dosages and are less likely to be abused.[59]

Thermogenic Agents

Thyroid hormone is advocated for the treatment of obesity because of its thermogenic properties. However, very substantial doses are required (390 to 910 mg) to even slightly increase basal metabolic rate (BMR) and this can cause cardiovascular effects. Thyroid hormones should be avoided unless there is a thyroid deficiency.[15]

Monitoring of Therapy

- Evaluate at *six months* to determine success and assess further need for additional weight loss. If necessary, refer to a dietitian, exercise physiologist, psychologist, and/or physician, if there is no success in weight reduction.
- Assess if patient has been able to reach and maintain a healthy weight range (BMI from 18.5 to 24.9).
- If patient is on medications for obesity, assess tolerance as well as whether the patient is sustaining improved diet and activity patterns.

Resource Tips

Calculation of BMI

http://www.hc-sc.ca/hppb/nutrition/bmi/chart_java.html

Obesity

American Obesity Association
www.obesity.org

Canada's Food Guide to Healthy Eating
http://www.hc-sc.gc.ca/hppb/nutrition/pube/food guid/foodguide.html

Canada's Physical Activity Guide to Healthy Active Living
www.paguide.com
http://www.hc-sc.gc.ca/hppb/paguide/main.html

Healthy Weight Network
www.healthyweightnetwork.com

National Center for Overcoming Overeating
www.overcomingovereating.com

Eating Disorders

National Eating Disorder Information Center
www.nedic.ca
(416) 340-4156; fax (416) 340-4736

The National Eating Disorders Association
www.edap.org or www.NationalEatingDisorders.org

Suggested Readings

ADA Reports: Position of the American Dietetic Association: Nutrition intervention in the treatment of anorexia nervosa, bulimia nervosa, and binge eating. *J Am Diet Assoc* 1991;94:902-11.

Continuing Education Monograph from the American Pharmaceutical Association. *Concepts in Comprehensive Weight Management – Managing Obesity as a Chronic Disease* Available at: www.aphanet.org/education/specialrpts/obesity/pdf.

Dickerson LM, Clarke PJ. Drug therapy for obesity. *Am Fam Physician* 2000;61:2131-8;2143.

Douketis JD, Feightner JW, Attia J, Feldman WF, with the Canadian Task Force on Preventive Health Care. Periodic health examination, 1999 update: 1. Detection, prevention and treatment of obesity. *CMAJ* 1999;160(4):513-25.

Freedman HR, King J, Kennedy E. Popular diets: a scientific review. *Obesity Res* 2001;9(suppl 1):1S-40S.

National Institutes of Health/National Heart, Lung and Blood Institute. *Clinical Guidelines on the Identification, Evaluation, and Treatment of Overweight and Obesity in Adults: the Evidence Report.* June 1998: 1-228. Available at: http://www.nhlbi.nih.gov/guidelines/obesity/ob_home.htm.

National Institutes of Health/National Heart, Lung, and Blood Institute. North American Association for the Study of Obesity. *The Practical Guide: Identification, Evaluation, and Treatment of Overweight and Obesity in Adults.* Oct 2000.

References

1. *Canadian Guidelines for Healthy Weights: Report of an expert group convened by Health Promotion Directorate, Health Services and Promotion Branch.* Ottawa: Health Promotion Directorate, Department of National Health and Welfare; 1988.
2. Douketis JD, Feightner JW, Attia J, Feldman WF, with the Canadian Task Force on Preventive Health Care. Periodic health examination, 1999 update: 1. Detection, prevention and treatment of obesity. *CMAJ* 1999;160(4):513-25.
3. National Institutes of Health/National Heart, Lung and Blood Institute. *Clinical guidelines on the identification, evaluation, and treatment of overweight and obesity in adults: the evidence report.* June, 1998:1-228. http://www.nhlbi.nih.gov/guidelines/obesity/ob_home.htm.
4. Macdonald SM, Reeder BA, Chen Y, Despres JP, and the Canadian Heart Health Surveys Research Group. Obesity in Canada: a descriptive analysis. *CMAJ* 1997;157(1Suppl):S3-S9.
5. Strauss RS, Pollack HA. Epidemic increase in childhood overweight, 1986-1998. *JAMA* 2001;286(22):2845-48.
6. Campbell K, Waters E, O'Meara S, Summerbell C. Interventions for preventing obesity in children (Cochrane Review). In: *The Cochrane Library.* 3. Oxford: Update Software; 2001
7. Williamson MS. Descriptive epidemiology of body weight and weight change in U.S. adults. *Ann Intern Med* 1993; 119(7 pt 2):646-9.
8. Mandl DL, Jason IL. Obesity and eating disorders. In: *Textbook of Therapeutics: Drug and Disease Management.* 7th ed. Herfindal ET, Gourley DR, eds. Baltimore, MD: Lippincott Williams & Wilkins; 2000:1271-88.
9. Price RA, Cadoret RJ, Stunkard AJ, Troughton E. Genetic contributions to human fatness: an adoption study. *Am J Psychiatry* 1987;144:1003-8.
10. Black D, James WPI, Besser GM. Obesity. *J R Coll Physicians Lond* 1983;17:5-65.
11. Dietz WH. Critical periods in childhood for the development of obesity. *Am J Clin Nutr* 1994;59:955-9.
12. Laitinen J, Power C, Jarvelin MR. Family social class, maternal body mass index, childhood body mass index, and age at menarche as predictors of adult obesity. *Am J Clin Nutr* 2001;74(3):287-94.

13. Weinsier RL, Nagy TR, Hunter GR, Darnell BE, Hensrud DD, Weiss HL. Do adaptive changes in metabolic rate favor weight regain in weight-reduced individuals? An examination of the set-point theory. *Am J Clin Nutr* 2000 72(5): 1088-94.

14. Pijl H, Meinders AE. Bodyweight change as an adverse effect of drug treatment. Mechanisms and management. *Drug Safety* 1996;14:329-42.

15. Insel P, Turner RE, Ross D: Energy balance, body composition, and weight management. In: *Nutrition*. 1st ed. Insel P, ed. Sudbury, MA: Jones and Bartlett Publishers; 2001: 283-325.

16. American Dietetic Association/Dietitians of Canada. *Manual of Clinical Dietetics*. 6th ed. Chicago: 2000:365-86.

17. Pi-Sunyer FX. Medical Hazards of Obesity. *Ann Intern Med* 1993;119(7pt2):655-60.

18. Eckel RH, Krauss RM. American Heart Association Call to Action: Obesity as a major risk factor for coronary heart disease. *Circulation* 1998;97:2099-100.

19. Suwaidi JA, Wright RS, Grill JP et al. Obesity is associated with premature occurrence of acute myocardial infarction. *Clin Cardiol* 2001;24:542-7.

20. Manson JE, Willet WC, Stampfer MJ. Body weight and mortality among women. *N Engl J Med* 1995;333:677-85.

21. Kannek WB, Brand N, Skinner JJ Jr, Dawber TR, McNamara PM. The relation of adiposity to blood pressure and development of hypertension. The Framingham Study. *Ann Intern Med* 1967;67:48-59.

22. Garfinkel L. Overweight and cancer. *Ann Intern Med* 1985;103:1-36.

23. Health and Welfare Canada. *Using the Food Guide: Canada's Food Guide to Healthy Eating*. Ottawa, ON; 1992.

24. Lee L, Paffenbarger RS. Change in body weight and longevity. *JAMA* 1992;268:2045-9.

25. Roland DA. Nutrition in adulthood and the later years. In: Krause MV, Mahan LK, eds. *Food, Nutrition and Diet Therapy*. 7th ed. Philadelphia: WB Saunders; 1984:324.

26. Beresin EV. Anorexia nervosa. *Compr Ther* 1997;23:664-71.

27. Muscari ME. Primary care of adolescents with bulimia nervosa. *J Pediatr Health Care* 1996;10:17-23.

28. Mehkr PS. Eating disorders: bulimia nervosa. *Hosp Pract* 1996;31(2):107-14,120,123,126.

29. Fairburn CG, Welch SL, Hay PJ. The classification of recurrent overeating: the "binge eating disorder" proposal. *Int J Eat Disord* 1993;13(2):155-9.

30. Insel P, Turner RE, Ross D. Eating disorders. In: Insel P, ed. *Nutrition*. Sudbury, MA: Jones and Bartlett Publishers; 2001.

31. Rolls B, Bell EA. Dietary approaches to the treatment of obesity. *Med Clin North Am Obesity* 2000;84(2):401-18.

32. Freedman HR, King J, Kennedy E. Popular diets: a scientific review. *Obesity Res* 2001;9(suppl 1):1S-40S.

33. Anon. The Atkins Diet. *Med Lett Drugs Ther* 2000;52:42 (1080).

34. Atkins RC. *Dr. Atkin's New Diet Revolution*. Avon Books; 1992.

35. Sears B. *Enter The Zone*. Harper Collins; 1995.

36. Stewart HL, Morrison CB, Andrews SS, Balart LA. *Sugar Busters*. Ballantine Books; 1998.

37. Ornish D. *Eat More, Weigh Less*. New York: Harper Paperbooks; 1993.

38. Ludwig DS, Pereira MA, Kroenke CH et al. Dietary fibre, weight gain, and cardiovascular disease risk factors in young adults. *JAMA* 1999; 282:1539-46.

39. Rolls B. Carbohydrates, fats and satiety. *Am J Clin Nutr* 1995;61(4suppl):S960-S967.

40. Burton-Freeman B. Dietary fiber and energy regulation. *J Nutr* 2000;130:272S-275S.

41. Pi-Sunyer FX. The role of very-low-calorie diets in obesity. *Am J Clin Nutr* 1992;56(suppl):S240-S243.

42. Are reduced-fat foods keeping Americans healthier? *Tufts U Health Nutr Lett* 1998;16(1):4-5.

43. Jellin JM, Gregory P, Batz F et al. Stevia In: *Pharmacist's Letter/Prescriber's Letter Natural Medicine's Comprehensive Database*. 3rd ed. Stockton, CA: Therapeutic Research Faculty; 2000:990-1.

44. Saccharin: ref: Saccharin. In: Reynolds JEF, ed. *Martindale: The Extra Pharmacopoeia*. 28th ed. London: Pharmaceutical Press; 1982:429.

45. Foreyt JP, Poston II WSC. The role of the behaviorial counselor in obesity treatment. *J Am Diet Assoc* 1998;98 (10suppl2):527-30.

46. Forety JP, Goodrick GK. Evidence for success of behavior modification in weight loss and control. *Ann Intern Med* 1993;119(7pt2):698-701.

47. Wing RR. Behavioral approaches to the treatment of obesity. In: Bray GA, Bouchard C, James WPT, eds. *Handbook of Obesity*. New York: Marcel Dekker; 1998:855-73.

48. Apfelbaum M, Bostsarron T, Lucatis D. Effect of caloric restriction and excessive caloric intake on energy expenditure. *Am J Clin Nutr* 1971;24:1405-9.

49. Greenway FL. Surgery for obesity. *Endocrinol Metab Clin North Am* 1996;25(4):1005-27.

50. Long SD, O'Brien K, MacDonald KG Jr, et al. Weight loss in severely obese subjects prevents the progression of impaired glucose tolerance to type II diabetes: a longitudinal interventional study. *Diabetes Care* 1994;17:372-5.

51. Toubro S, Astrup, AV, Breum L et al. Safety and efficacy of long-term treatment with ephedrine, caffeine and an ephedrine/caffeine mixture. *Int J Obes Relat Metab Discord* 1993;17(suppl 1):S69-72.

52. Wasser WG, Feldman NS, D'Agati VD. Chronic renal failure after ingestion of over-the-counter chromium picolinate [letter]. *Ann Intern Med* 1997;126:410.

53. Amato P, Morales AJ, Yen SS. Effects of chromium picolinate supplementation on insulin sensitivity, serum lipids, and body composition in healthy, non-obese, older men and women. *J Gerontol A Biol Sci Med Sci* 2000;5:M260-M263.

54. Stanko RT, Reynolds HR, Hoyson R, Janosky JE, Wolf R. Pyruvate supplementation of a low-cholesterol, low-fat diet: effects on plasma lipid concentrations and body composition in hyperlipidemic patients. *Am J Clin Nutr* 1994;59(2):423-7.

55. Pittler MH, Abbot NC, Harkness Ef, Ernst E. Randomized, double-blind trial of chitosan for body weight reduction. *Eur J Clin Nutr* 1999;53:379-81.

56. Heymsfield SB, Allison DB, Vasselli JR, Pietrobelli A, Greenfield D, Nunez C. Garcinia cambogia (hydroxycitric acid) as a potential antiobesity agent: a randomized controlled trial. *JAMA* 1998;280(18):1596-600.

57. Anon. *MERIDIA Product Monograph*. Markham, ON: Knoll Pharma; 2001.

58. Anon. Orlistat for Obesity. *Med Lett Drugs Ther* 1999; 41(1055):55-6.

59. Anon. FDA proposes constraints on ephedrine dietary supplements. *Am J Health Syst Pharm* 1997;54:1578.

Weight Management—Patient Information

- Set short-term, achievable goals. If you need to lose 25 kg, first set a goal of losing 2.5 to 5 kg. Losing 0.5 to 1 kg per week over six months is reasonable (2.2 lbs=1 kg).
- Don't go on a crash diet. Think long-term. Change your eating habits so that meals and snacks are balanced with a variety of healthy foods. Consult *Canada's Food Guide to Healthy Eating* to follow a balanced diet.
- Increase your activity. Pick an exercise routine that suits your lifestyle. Use the stairs rather than the elevator. Park so that you have to walk farther. Try to obtain 30 minutes of aerobic exercise, like walking, at least three times per week.
- Don't give up. After losing a few pounds you may plateau. Don't cut back further on calories, your body may need to adjust to the new fat and calorie levels.
- Give yourself a break. If you overeat one day, just get back on the plan the following day.
- See your doctor if necessary. If you are 30% or more above normal weight for you, your doctor may recommend a medically supervised very-low-calorie diet or drug therapy.
- Social support: identify a friend or family member who can provide social support and reinforcement for behavior change. Community support groups or web sites are available.

Special Diets[1]

Shirley Heschuk, BScPharm, MSc

Some patients require diets, which are either restricted or enhanced in certain nutrients, for health reasons. The following describes some of these special diets. An appropriate assessment is necessary to determine whether a special diet would benefit a specific patient.

Sodium-Restricted Diet

Purpose

Prevent accumulation of fluid and/or promote a net loss of excess body water.

Indications for Use

- Essential hypertension: There is a correlation between a moderately reduced sodium intake and blood pressure reduction.[2,3]
- Congestive heart failure (CHF): Sodium restriction is the primary diet therapy in treating CHF. For mild to moderate heart failure a sodium restriction of 3 g (130 mmol) per day is recommended; if unresponsive to this measure or in severe CHF, sodium should be further restricted to 2 g (87 mmol) per day. Persons receiving 80 mg of furosemide or more for greater than 3 months may require a 2 g (87 mmol) per day restriction to increase the effectiveness of diuretic therapy.[4]
- Renal disease: Sodium intake should be modified to facilitate blood pressure control, to maintain normal hydration status, and to help prevent congestive heart failure and pulmonary edema. Fluid status and appropriateness of sodium intake can be monitored through blood pressure, interdialytic weight gains, signs of edema, and thirst. Generally, the recommended intake of sodium is 2 to 3 g per day (87 to 130 mmol).[1]
- Liver disease: Fluid and electrolyte status must be monitored. Sodium restriction may be required.

Amount of Nutrient Allowed

Note: 2.4 g elemental sodium = 6 g NaCl = 1 tsp table salt.

Severe: 0.5 g (22 mmol) per day
Strict: 1 g (44 mmol) per day
Mild/Moderate: 2 to 3 g (87-130 mmol) per day
No added salt: 4 g (174 mmol) per day

Comments

Reduce intake of high-sodium processed foods, beverages, and condiments (fast foods; smoked, salted meats; regular canned foods; snack foods; salad dressings). Use salt substitutes (KCl). Most salt substitutes contain less than 1 mmol of sodium per teaspoon but large amounts of potassium (30 to 50 mmol per teaspoon). Patients with renal disease should not use salt substitutes, as ingestion of additional potassium could result in hyperkalemia.

Potassium-Modified Diet

Purpose

Maintain normal potassium levels in hypo- and hyperkalemic patients.

Note: normal plasma potassium level is 3.5 to 5 mmol/L.

High Potassium—Indications

During use of certain medications such as potassium-wasting thiazide-type diuretics; antibiotics, e.g., gentamicin.

Amount of Nutrient Suggested

Two to four grams (50 to 100 mmol) per day in addition to consumption in the current diet. With planning this can be accomplished with diet alone, without potassium supplementation.

Dietary sources of potassium include potatoes, bananas, melons, spinach, fresh meat, milk and salt substitutes containing potassium chloride (KCl). Pharmacologic choices are potassium supplements and potassium-sparing diuretics.

Low Potassium—Indications
Impaired renal function; during use of ACE inhibitors.

Amount of Nutrient Allowed
Restricted to a maximum of 2 to 2.5 g (50 to 65 mmol) potassium per day. At levels less than 1.6 g (40 mmol) per day, the diet can be deficient in calcium, iron, vitamin C, folate, and B vitamins.

Low-potassium in diet: Restrict fruits and vegetables high in potassium content (see above).

Fat-Restricted Diet

Purpose
Prevent symptoms of intolerance (diarrhea, flatulence, abdominal pain) to high intakes of dietary fat, and control nutrient losses caused by malabsorptive disorders.

Indications
Bile salt deficiency; pancreatic insufficiency; defects in the absorptive capability of the intestinal mucosa.

Fat Restriction
Mild: 30 to 35% total kcal per day as fat.
Moderate: 25% total kcal per day as fat.
Severe: 10 to 15% total kcal per day as fat.
< 50 g fat per day is considered a low-fat diet.

Comments
Those with malabsorption syndromes may be deficient in fat soluble vitamins and other micronutrients. Supplementing with vitamins A, D, E and K is suggested. Water-miscible forms of the fat-soluble vitamins are available.

In severe fat restriction, protein may need to be supplemented.

Lactose-Restricted Diet

Purpose
Prevent or reduce gastrointestinal symptoms of bloating, flatulence, cramping, nausea and diarrhea associated with consumption of the disaccharide lactose.

Indications
"Lactose-intolerant" individuals vary in the ability to digest lactose and the amount of lactase in their system. Total lactose avoidance is usually not necessary except in galactosemia. True lactase deficiency can be clinically diagnosed with a breath hydrogen test, which measures hydrogen produced by colonic bacteria in the presence of unabsorbed sugars.

Comments
The three main types of lactase deficiency are: congenital, secondary, and primary.
- Congenital: Extremely rare and requires a lifelong lactose-free or very low-lactose diet.
- Secondary: Transient in nature and develops secondary to illness or disease involving mucosal injury.
- Primary: The most prevalent type, presents with a late onset. It usually occurs with increasing age and individuals exhibit tolerance to various levels of lactose.

The goals of the diet for the lactose-intolerant patient are:
- To reduce lactose intake to a level that will not cause intestinal symptoms, and
- To provide for adequate nutrient intake.

If dairy products cannot be tolerated at all, supplementation with calcium and vitamin D may be required.

Enzymatic lactase products break down lactose into digestible sugars — glucose and galactose. Normally three to four drops are taken with milk or dairy products.

Note: It is important to read ingredient lists on food and drug labels, as many fillers contain lactose. For lactose-containing pharmaceuticals see the *Compendium of Pharmaceuticals and Specialties* published annually by the Canadian Pharmacists Association.

Gluten-Restricted Diet

Purpose

Prevent the gastrointestinal symptoms of gluten intolerance (cramps and diarrhea).

Indications

For patients with celiac disease, or who cannot tolerate gluten, which is contained in wheat, rye, oat, barley, and triticale protein.

Amount of Nutrient Allowed

Any product entering the digestive system must be gluten-free. Careful review of ingredient lists on food and drug labels to determine if gluten-containing ingredients are present is important. Avoid all gluten products: wheat, rye, oat, barley, and triticale protein. Substitute corn, rice, potato flour, tapioca, sago and arrowroot. Resources include the Canadian Celiac Association (www.celiac.ca) and Gluten Intolerance Group of North America (www.gluten.ca). For information on gluten-containing pharmaceuticals as well as gluten-free manufacturers see the *Compendium of Pharmaceuticals and Specialties*, published annually by the Canadian Pharmacists Association.

Fibre-Restricted Diet

Purpose

Reduce the frequency and volume of fecal output while prolonging intestinal transit time, and prevent blockage of stenosed gastrointestinal tract.

Indications

Ulcerative colitis; Crohn's disease; diverticulitis; stenosis of the intestine. During an acute episode of inflammatory bowel disease (ulcerative colitis, Crohn's disease), bowel rest and/or a low fibre diet are recommended to limit the pain and frequency of stools and to prevent obstruction when the lumen of the colon is narrowed or stenosed.[5]

Amount of Nutrient Allowed

Reduce indigestible carbohydrate intake by limiting amounts of well-cooked or canned vegetables and canned, cooked or very ripe fruit products. Replace whole-grain breads and cereals with refined products.

Limit fibre intake to < 10 g per day. Foods that contain < 2 g fibre per serving include: ½ english muffin,

¾ cup Cheerios®, ½ cup cooked rice, ½ grapefruit, ½ cup celery, 2 tbsp walnuts.

Note: Fibre is a substance found in plant that cannot be hydrolyzed by the digestive system. Fibre can be divided into soluble and insoluble based on physiochemical properties. *Soluble* fibre occurs as pectins (e.g., bananas, apples), mucilage (e.g., psyllium) and gum (e.g., oatmeal, legumes). *Insoluble* fibre includes cellulose (e.g., wheat bran, apples), hemicellulose (e.g., whole wheat) and lignin (e.g., potatoes).

Soluble fibre is permitted on this diet.

High-Fibre Diet

Purpose

Increase fecal bulk and promote regularity; normalize serum lipid levels; blunt postprandial blood glucose response.

Indications

- Inflammatory bowel disease: When the disease is in remission or under control, a high fiber diet (as tolerated) is recommended to stimulate peristalsis and improve the tone of the muscular wall of the gastrointestinal tract, especially the colon.[5]
- Hypercholesterolemia: Small but significant decreases in total and LDL cholesterol are seen with various soluble fibres.[6,7]
- Diabetes: Soluble fibre has a small effect on inhibiting blood glucose absorption from the small intestine.[8]
- Colon cancer: There is no evidence that a high-fibre diet reduces the recurrence of colorectal polyps, which can develop into colorectal cancers. High-fibre intakes do increase stool weight and decrease transit time, and greater stool weights have been correlated with lower risk of cancer.[9]

Amount of Nutrient Suggested

25 to 30 g of fibre per day is recommended. Emphasis is on fibre-rich foods such as fruits, legumes, vegetables, and whole-grain breads and cereals. Adequate amounts of non-caffeinated liquid (eight 8-oz glasses or 2 L per day) are required to prevent dehydration. Increase fibre content gradually to minimize abdominal distress, bloating, flatulence, cramps, and diarrhea. Examples of high fibre (5+ g per serving) foods include: ⅓ cup 100% bran cereal, ½ cup cooked

barley, ½ cup peas, 1 medium raw apple with skin, 1 oz almonds.

High-Calorie, High-Protein Diet

Purpose

Provide energy and nutrients in excess of usual requirements; prevent malnutrition; promote weight gain; meet need for increased nutrients; optimise an individual's ability to respond to medical treatment.

Indications

For patients with poor intake, e.g., cancer, HIV/AIDS, chronic GI problems, burns, wounds, trauma, renal dialysis, failure to thrive, preparation for planned surgery.

Amount of Nutrient Suggested

Calorie-dense and protein-dense foods, e.g., milk, peanut butter, nuts, seeds, beef, chicken, fish, pork, and eggs.

Meal replacement products are not generally nutritionally complete and require at least one regular meal daily to meet required nutrients, [e.g., complete (Ensure®); incomplete (Boost®, Carnation Instant Breakfast®)].

Oral supplements: Formulated liquid diets are nutritionally complete for oral or feeding-tube use. Some are modified for specific disease states. A multitude of nutritionally complete formulated liquid diets are available for oral use (e.g., Isocal®) or tube feeding (e.g., Jevity®). Elemental liquid formulas are useful for patients with difficulties in digestion and absorption as they are readily absorbed (e.g., Vital HN®). More specialized formulated liquid diets have been designed to fulfill the nutrition requirements of patients suffering from certain diseases (e.g., Pulmocare® for COPD; Oxepa® for ventilated patients). For a listing of adult nutrition products see the *Compendium of Self-Care Products* published annually by the Canadian Pharmacists Association.

Purine-Restricted Diet

Purpose

Decrease elevated blood and urinary uric acid levels.

Indications

Used in conjunction with medication for patients with hyperuricemia, gouty arthritis and urinary uric acid lithiasis.

Amount of Nutrient Allowed

Limit protein to 10 to 15% of total calories per day. Avoid animal products except dairy products and eggs. Avoid alcohol. Follow *Canada's Food Guide to Healthy Eating* (see Chapter 31). Drink 2 to 3 L or 8 to 12 cups of fluid daily. This helps to dilute urinary uric acid.

Tyramine-Controlled Diet

Purpose

Prevent the adverse reactions associated with consuming foods containing tyramine and other amines while on MAOI therapy.

Indications

Prevent hypertensive crisis in patients receiving MAOIs.

Amount of Nutrient Allowed

Avoid tyramine-containing foods such as aged, mature cheeses; dry fermented sausages (salami); smoked or pickled fish; non-fresh meat or poultry; leftovers containing meat, fish, or poultry; red wine, overripe, spoiled, moldy, or fermented fruit or vegetables.

Comments

Cottage cheese and processed cheese are allowed. Heat does not destroy tyramine.

References

1. American Dietetic Association/Dietitians of Canada. *Manual of Clinical Dietetics.* 6th ed. Chicago; 2000.
2. Cutler JA, Follmann D, Allender PS. Randomized trials of sodium reduction: an overview. *Am J Clin Nutr* 1997;65 (suppl):643S-651S.
3. Midgly JP, Matthew AC, Greenwood CMT, Logan AT. Effect of reduced dietary sodium on blood pressure: a meta-analysis of randomized controlled trials. *JAMA* 1996;275:1590-7.
4. Dracup K, Baker DW, Dunbar SB, et al. Management of heart failure: counseling, education, and lifestyle modifications. *JAMA* 1994;272:1442-6.
5. O'Sullivan A, O'Movain A. Nutrition therapy in Crohn's Disease. *Inflammatory Bowel Dis* 1998;4:45-53.

6. Position of the American Dietetic Association: health implications of dietary fiber. *J Am Diet Assoc* 1993;93:1446.

7. Brown L, Rosner B, Willett WW, Sacks FM. Cholesterol-lowering effects of dietary as fiber: a meta-analysis. *Am J Clin Nutr* 1999;69:30-42.

8. Frans MJ, Horton ES, Bantle JP et al. Nutrition principles for the management of diabetes and related complications. *Diabetes Care* 1994;17:490-518.

9. Cummings JH, Bingham S, Heaton KW et al. Fecal weight, colon cancer risk, and dietary intake of nonstarch polysaccharides (dietary fiber). *Gastroenterology* 1992;103:1783-9.

Sports Nutrition

Shirley Heschuk, BScPharm, MSc

Dietary goals for athletes are quantitative values for macronutrient intakes relative to total energy intakes. They are similar to those developed for the general population (Table 1).[1]

Table 1: **Dietary Goals for Athletes (% of Total Energy in Diet)**

Nutrient	% of total energy/day
Protein	10-15
Total fat	< 30
Total carbohydrate	60-70 (for endurance athletes) 55-65 (for recreational athletes)

For optimal performance, energy consumption must be sufficient to match that expended. The amount of energy intake required depends on the basal metabolic rate (BMR), the energy expended in physical activity, and the thermic effect of food.

The Competitive Athlete

Competitive athletes need an adequate energy intake for athletic performance, and to maintain or increase lean body mass. They must consume enough calories to meet this energy demand. Some athletes require > 5000 calories per day.[2]

Carbohydrate

Carbohydrate-rich diets can help maximize muscle and liver glycogen stores before exercise and promote faster recovery of stores after exercise. A minimum of 60% of total calories should be from carbohydrate. Complex carbohydrates (e.g., starch, dextrin) are preferred because they supply a sustained release of energy, being digested slowly compared to simple sugars. They also provide fibre, iron (if enriched) and many of the B vitamins necessary for energy metabolism.

Suggested carbohydrate intakes are:[2]

- Before intense training or competition: 1 to 4.5 g carbohydrate per kilogram body weight, one to four hours before exercise.
- During exercise or competition: 30 to 60 g of carbohydrate every hour.
- After intense exercise or competition: 1 to 1.5 g carbohydrate per kilogram body weight for the first 30 minutes, then every two hours. The total carbohydrate intake over the next 24 hours should be about 7 to 9 g/kg or 500 to 600 g.[3] Timing of intake is important. If carbohydrate consumption is delayed more than four hours after exercising, the rate of glycogen synthesis is one-half that of consumption during the first two hours after exercising. Providing a carbohydrate supplement soon after exercise seems to enhance muscle glycogen recovery process by ensuring there is an adequate supply of carbohydrate to prevent hypoglycemia and the development of insulin resistance.[4]

Carbohydrate loading is recommended for athletes who compete in events that last 90 minutes or longer, such as marathons, triathlons and cross-country skiing. The athlete consumes 60 to 70% of calories from carbohydrate along with a decrease in exercise intensity and duration prior to competition. Athletes who follow this regimen for up to a week before competition can double the glycogen content of exercised muscles. The downside is that for every gram of glycogen stored in muscle tissue, the body also stores 2.7 g of water. This causes weight gain and a feeling of sluggishness.[2]

Fat

Sports nutritionists recommend that athletes consume 15 to 25% of calories as dietary fat. Extreme fat restriction limits food choices and sources of protein, iron, zinc and essential fatty acids. For those athletes requiring a high caloric intake (> 5000 cal per day), it is still recommended to get no more than 30% of calories from fat.[2] A high-fat diet is associated with impairment in exercise capacity,[5] and an increased risk of cardiovascular disease.[6]

Protein

Canada's Food Guide for Healthy Eating recommends an intake of 0.8 g protein/kg body weight per day for the sedentary person. People who engage in low-intensity exercise do not need additional protein.[7]

Athletes who engage in vigorous activities have slightly higher protein needs:[8]
- Strength athlete: 1.6 to 1.7 g/kg body weight per day.
- Endurance athlete: 1.2 to 1.4 g/kg body weight per day.

The maximum usable amount for adults is 2.0 g/kg body weight per day.

Athletes usually do not have difficulty consuming enough protein by adhering to the recommendation to consume 10 to 15% of total energy as protein, unless they are on a restrictive diet. Meeting this increased amount of protein does not require the use of protein or amino acid supplements. The best way to obtain protein is to consume high-quality protein foods, including low-fat dairy products, egg whites, legumes, lean beef and pork, chicken, turkey, and fish.

Contrary to what many athletes believe, excess dietary protein does not have an anabolic effect and any excess will be oxidized for energy production.

There are, in general, few side effects arising from daily protein intakes under 2.0 g/kg in healthy people. Some of the concerns of high protein intake include:
- Diets high in protein are often high in fat.
- Excessive protein intake enhances diuresis, thus increasing the risk for dehydration, as the body attempts to excrete excess nitrogen.
- Acceleration of the progression of pre-existing renal disease.[9]

- Increased urinary calcium excretion resulting in adverse affects on bone (osteoporosis).[10]

High intakes of single amino acids may impair absorption of other amino acids. The safety and quality of amino acid supplements are questionable. They are expensive and their efficacy has not been established.[11]

Vitamin and Mineral Requirements of the Athlete[2]

B vitamins are essential for energy metabolism and are adequately supplied in the diet if adequate calories and plenty of complex carbohydrates, fruit and vegetables are part of the diet. Vegetarians may need a vitamin B_{12} supplement.

Calcium helps to protect against stress fractures and, coupled with exercise, delays the onset of osteoporosis. Intake of 1300 mg of elemental calcium per day is recommended.

Iron is needed to carry oxygen to active muscle cells. Female athletes are at higher risk for iron deficiency as a result of menstrual losses. However, mild iron deficiency has little effect on performance.[12] Any concern of iron deficiency should be assessed by a physician.

Other Trace Minerals

Strenuous exercise can lower the body's reserve of **copper** (essential for red blood cell synthesis) and **zinc** (important in many enzymes related to energy production). This may cause marginal deficiencies, but does not necessarily require supplementation. High-dose supplements of iron, copper or zinc can interfere with the normal absorption of these and other minerals, so an excess of one mineral can cause a deficiency of others.[2] A dietitian can suggest a training diet that would meet an athlete's needs for vitamins and minerals through food, which is preferable to taking supplements.

Fluid Needs During Exercise

Exercise generates body heat, which is lost through evaporation of fluid (sweat) from the skin. Some elite athletes lose as much as one to two litres of fluid per hour and therefore, without fluid replacement, dehydration can occur quickly.[2]

Water can replace fluid loss in sweat but may not be adequate for rehydration because it does not contain energy (calories) or electrolytes.

Optimal sports drinks provide energy (from glucose, glucose polymers, sucrose) and electrolytes that promote rapid absorption. Beverages containing 6 to 10% glucose or sucrose are absorbed as rapidly as water and provide energy needed for prolonged exercise.[13] Electrolytes replace sodium, chloride and potassium lost and enhance the palatability of the beverage. Sodium and chloride help ensure an adequate intake of fluid and stimulate greater rehydration after exercise.

Fruit juices and soft drinks are concentrated sources of carbohydrates (> 10% carbohydrate concentration) that may deter fluid replacement and cause gastrointestinal discomfort[13] (Table 2).

Nutritional Supplements and Ergogenic Aids (Performance Enhancers)

Nutritional supplements are unnecessary for athletes who select a variety of foods to meet their energy needs. Female athletes may require iron and calcium supplements if their diets are low in these nutrients.

Liquid supplements and sports bars that contain carbohydrates, protein and fat provide an easy way to increase energy intake. Athletes should read labels in order to incorporate these into their daily diet. Sports drinks can contribute to needed fluids and carbohydrates before, during and after exercise. Some of these products may contain other components believed to be ergogenic (e.g., chromium, amino acids, ginseng), which increase the cost.

Most dietary supplements are marketed as ergogenic aids (performance enhancers) and lack vigorous clinical trials to evaluate efficacy (see Sports Appendix).

Arginine, lysine or **ornithine** used in high doses may cause transient increases in human growth hormone levels, but their effect is not sustained enough to increase muscle mass or decrease body fat.[14] As well, large doses may cause diarrhea and nausea while inhibiting the absorption of other amino acids. High protein foods should be recommended rather than amino acids as supplements.

Table 2: **Fluid Replacement Comparisons**[13]

Product	Carbohydrate source	Carbohydrate concentration %	Sodium content mEq/L	Potassium content mEq/L	Osmolality[‡] mOsm/kg (refers to concentration)
Recommended	Glucose, glucose polymer, sucrose	6-10%	10-20	2.5-5.0	250-360
Gatorade®*	Sucrose, glucose, fructose	6.3-9.3	18.3-29.1	2.9	280-360
PowerAde®*	Sucrose, glucose, fructose	8.8	5.4	2.9	381
AllSport®*	Glucose, fructose, sucrose	8.5-8.7	8.6-10.8	3.3	516
Coca-Cola®†	High fructose, sucrose	11.3	1.1	trace	600-715

*These products are available in a variety of flavors that vary in composition.
†Contains caffeine.
‡Osmolality (mOsm/kg) of a formula is usually higher than osmolarity (mOsm/L), but the two are often used interchangeably. Osmolality of normal body fluids is 300 mOsm/kg which is isotonic. Fluids closest to this osmolality are best tolerated.
Reprinted with permission from Marriage B, Schnurr H, Carter-Erdman KA, Reading K. *Sports Nutrition Resource Manual* 2nd ed. Sports Medicine Council of Alberta. Revised June 1999.

Although commonly used, **chromium** does not enhance muscle strength, size or lean body mass.[15] There have been case reports of severe side effects such as anemia, liver dysfunction and kidney failure.

Creatine in maintenance doses of 3 g per day for up to 28 days may increase muscular strength for sports such as weight lifting, but is ineffective in endurance sports.[16] It causes muscle cramps, dehydration and possible weight gain, liver or kidney problems.[17]

Like the majority of these dietary supplements, **DHEA** (dehydroepiandrosterone) has not been thoroughly studied, but it does not promote weight reduction as claimed. It is associated with possible serious adverse effects such as insulin resistance, liver damage and increased risk of breast, endometrial and prostate cancers.[11]

HMB (beta-hydroxy-beta-methylbutyrate) in doses of 1.5 to 3 g daily, is thought to increase muscle strength and lean body mass. However, evidence in humans is preliminary and long-term data is lacking.[18]

Although promoted for improving aerobic and anaerobic exercise performance and decreasing body fat, current studies do not support any ergogenic effect of **L-Carnitine**.[19]

Studies of **ginseng** also show no effect on athletic performance or delaying fatigue.[20,21]

Phosphate salts in doses of 4 g per day for several days before competition are believed to act as buffers of metabolic acids, thereby delaying fatigue and enhancing physical power during aerobic and anaerobic exercise. No proof exists, however, that it improves anaerobic exercise performance. It may aid in the capacity to use oxygen during exercise. High doses may cause cramps, nausea and diarrhea.

Resource Tips

Sport, Cardiovascular and Wellness Nutritionists (practice group of the American Dietetic Association): www.nutrifit.org

Sportscience is a peer-reviewed site for sport reserach. www.sportsci.org

NIH Office of Dietary Supplements at http://dietary-supplements.info.nih.gov

Suggested Readings

Berning JR, Steen SN. *Nutrition for Sport and Exercise.* 2nd ed. Gauthersburg, MD: Aspen Publishers; 1998.

Jellin JM. *Pharmacist's Letter Continuing Education Booklet: Sports Supplements* Stockton, CA: Pharmacist's Letter; 1999;99(2).

Marriage B, Schnurr H, Carter-Erdman KA, Reading K. *Sports Nutrition Resource Manual.* 2nd ed. Sports Medicine Council of Alberta; Rev June 1999.

Rosenbloom CA. *Sports Nutrition.* 3rd ed. Chicago: American Dietetic Association; 2000.

Sarubin A. *The Health Professional's Guide to Popular Dietary Supplements.* Chicago: American Dietetic Association; 2000.

References

1. Deakin V. Measuring nutritional status of athletes: clinical and research perspectives. In: Burke L, Deakin V, eds. *Clinical Sports Nutrition.* 2nd ed. Australia: McGraw-Hill; 2000.
2. Insel P, Turner RE, Ross D. Sports nutrition. In: Insel P, ed. *Nutrition.* Sudbury, MA: Jones and Bartlett Publishers; 2001:480-521.
3. Coyle E. Substrate utilization during exercise in active people. *Am J Clin Nutr* 1995;61(suppl):968S-979S.
4. Ivy JL. Role of carbohydrate in physical aActivity. *Clin Sports Med* 1999;18(3):469-84.
5. Hawley JA, Brouns F, Jeukendrup AE. Strategies to enhance fat utilisation during exercise. *Sports Med* 1998;25:241-57.
6. Sarno S, Kaprio J. Life expectancy of former athletes. *Sports Med* 1994;17:149-51.
7. Carroll C. Protein and exercise. In: Rosenbloom CA, ed. *Sports Nutrition.* 3rd ed. Chicago: American Dietetic Association; 2000.
8. Lemon PW. Dietary protein requirements in athletes. *J Nutr Biochem* 1997;8:52.
9. Brenner BM, Meter TW, Hosteler D. Protein intake and the progressive nature of kidney disease: the role of hemodynamically mediated glomerular sclerosis in aging, renal ablation, and intrinsic renal disease. *N Engl J Med* 1982; 307:652-7.
10. Barzel US, Massey LK. Excess dietary protein can adversely affect bone. *J Nutr* 1998;128:1051-3.
11. Slavin JL, Lanners G, Engstrom MA. Amino acid supplements: beneficial or risky? *Phys Sportsmed* 1988;16(3):221-4.
12. Zhu YI, Haas JD. Iron depletion without anemia and physical performance in young women. *Am J Clin Nutr* 1997;66:334-1.
13. Marriage B, Schnurr H, Carter-Erdman KA, Reading K. *Sports Nutrition Resource Manual.* 2nd ed. Sports Medicine Council of Alberta; Rev June 1999.
14. Susminski RR, Robertson RJ, Gross Fl, Arslanian S, Kang J, DaSilva S et al. Acute effect of amino acid ingestion and resistance exercise on human growth hormone concentration in young men. *Int J Sport Nutr* 1997;7:48-60.

15. Lukaski HC, Bolonchuk WW, Siders WA et al. Chromium supplementation and resistance training: effects on body composition, strength and trace element status of men. *Am J Clin Nutr* 1996;63:954-65.

16. Harris RC, Soderlund K, Hultman E. Elevation of creatine in resting and exercised muscle of normal subjects by creatine supplementation. *Clin Sci* 1992;83:367-4.

17. Pritchard NR, Kairn PA. Renal dysfunction accompanying oral creatine supplements. *Lancet* 1998;351:1252-3.

18. Nissen S, Sharp R, Ray M, Rathmacher D, Rice D, Fuller JC et al. Effect of leucine metabolite beta-hydroxy-beta-methyl-butyrate on muscle metabolism during resistance-training. *J Appl Physiol* 1996;81:2095-04.

19. Colombani P, Wenk C, Kunz I, Krahenbuhl S, Kuhart M, Arnold M et al. Effects of L-carnitine supplementation on physical performance and energy metabolism of endurance-trained athletes: a double-blind crossover field study. *Eur J Appl Physiol Occup Physiol* 1996;73:434-9.

20. Allen JD, McLung J, Nelson AG, Welsch M. Ginseng supplementation does not enhance healthy young adults' peak aerobic exercise performance. *J Am Coll Nutr* 1998;17:462-6.

21. Morris AC, Jacobs I, McLellan TM, Klugerman A, Wang LCH, Zamecni KJ. No ergogenic effect of ginseng ingestion. *Int J Sports Nutr* 1996;6:263-71.

Nutrition Advice—Information for the Athlete

Optimum athletic performance can be obtained with the following dietary recommendations:

- A high-carbohydrate diet promotes maximal energy storage.
  - —60 to 70% of total energy for endurance athletes.
  - —55 to 65% of total energy for recreational athletes.
  - —Increase the number of servings from the grain products, and the vegetables and fruit groups.
- A low-fat intake providing 25 to 30% of energy with no more than 10% of energy from saturated fats.
  - —Choose lower-fat dairy products (skim, 1% milk, cheese with < 20% milk fat, yogurt < 2% milk fat).
  - —Choose lean cuts of meat (lean ground beef, sirloin, and flank steaks).
  - —Bake or broil foods, rather than frying.
- Adequate (not excessive) protein is required to provide muscle maintenance and repair, and production of antibodies to fight infection. Protein requirements are:
  - —0.8 g/kg body weight per day – sedentary, or recreational athlete.
  - —1.2 to 1.4 g/kg body weight per day – endurance athlete.
  - —1.6 to 1.7 g/kg body weight per day – strength athlete.
  - —2.0 g/kg body weight per day – maximum usable amount for adults.

These requirements are easily met when 15% of the total energy is provided by protein in the diet.

- If a variety of foods are included in the diet, vitamin and mineral supplementation is not required.
- Adequate fluid levels are required to maintain proper hydration:
  - —600 mL – two hours pre-game.
  - —250-500 mL – 15 to 30 minutes pre-game.
  - —90-150 mL – every 15 minutes during game.
  - —For exercise < 3 hours duration: water is best.
  - —For exercise > 3 hours duration: dilute glucose and electrolyte solutions.

Musculoskeletal Conditions
Section Highlights

Chapter 34: **Osteoporosis**

    Assessment of risk factors
    Drug causes
    Prevention
    Calcium intake
    Calcium food sources
    Lifestyle changes

Chapter 35: **Low Back Pain**

    Nonpharmacologic Therapy
    Acetaminophen
    NSAIDs
    Muscle relaxants
    Alternative therapy

Chapter 36: **Osteoarthritis**

    Osteoarthritis versus rheumatoid arthritis
    Acetaminophen
    NSAIDs
    Topical counterirritants

Chapter 37: **Sports Injuries**

    Bursitis
    Sprains and strains
    Plantar fasciitis
    Shin splints
    Stress fractures
    Tendonitis
    Selected injuries requiring immediate medical attention
    Oral analgesics
    Muscle relaxants
    External analgesics
    Corticosteroids
    Vapocoolants

Sports Appendix: **Drug Use and Abuse in Sports**

Common ergogenic aids found in nonprescription products

Common ergogenic aids found in prescription products

    Anabolic steroids

Recreational drugs

Nutritional supplements, natural or herbal products

    Creatine

    DHEA

Banned/restricted substances

Chapter 34

Osteoporosis

Lalitha Raman-Wilms, PharmD, FCSHP

Pathophysiology

Definition

Osteoporosis is a skeletal disease characterized by bone mass that is low enough to cause the skeleton to be fragile and vulnerable to fractures. The World Health Organization has established guidelines for the diagnosis of osteoporosis based on the bone mineral density (BMD) readings at the lumbar spine and femoral neck. Osteoporosis is defined as a BMD of more than 2.5 standard deviations (SD) below the mean for young adult white women. A BMD between –1.0 and –2.5 signifies osteopenia.[1] Diagnosis is usually confirmed by measuring the individual's BMD using dual energy X-ray absorptiometry (DEXA), which is considered the gold standard. In those who have sustained fractures, an X-ray is usually used to confirm the fracture.

Bone Physiology

Bone is constantly renewed. The bone-remodeling unit consists of osteoblasts (cells that lay down new bone) and osteoclasts (cells that resorb bone). The coupling of this process ensures that early in life, more bone is laid down as the child grows. Around the third decade of life, this coupling process reaches a plateau, when the amount of bone broken down is balanced by the amount of new bone formed. At this point, which is usually attained between the ages of 25 and 35, the BMD is referred to as the peak bone mass and is the highest BMD that the individual will attain. After the third decade, age-related changes favor resorption, resulting in a gradual loss of 0.3 to 0.5% of bone mass per year. In women, lack of estrogen at menopause leads to accelerated bone loss of 2 to 3% per year; this loss continues for the first 5 to 10 years after menopause. Women, in general, have a lower peak bone mass compared to men, further increasing their risk for osteoporosis.

Most of the body's calcium is stored in bone. Calcium is essential for functions such as muscle contraction and nerve conduction. With insufficient calcium intake, parathyroid hormone (PTH) is released, leading to calcium resorption from bone, coupled with an increase in calcium absorption from the GI tract. There is also an increase in vitamin D activation by the kidneys. This feedback normally helps maintain an adequate serum calcium level. Deficiency in vitamin D can result in secondary hyperparathyroidism and an increase in calcium resorption from bone.

Clinical Presentation

Clinically, osteoporosis may present with fractures and/or pain associated with fractures. Common sites for fracture include the wrist, spine and hip. Wrist and spinal compression fractures are seen earlier in the disease, while hip fractures usually occur in the seventh or eighth decade of life. Many patients may go undiagnosed, as often the only symptom they report is nonspecific chronic back pain. The main indicator of osteoporosis is a low BMD. However, BMD is presently not indicated as a general screening tool for all individuals. Hence, identification of risk factors for this disease is important in assessing an individual's risk. Along with age-related bone loss, major risk factors include postmenopausal status, family history and diet-related factors (Table 1).[2] In addition to these well-established risk factors, conditions such as anorexia nervosa, bulimia, liver disease, renal disease, malabsorption syndromes and pituitary abnormalities can increase the risk for osteoporosis.[3] Also, several drugs have been associated with the development of osteoporosis (Table 2)[4,5] and patients on these medications should be monitored closely.

Factors that can increase the risk for falls (and therefore fractures) should also be examined. In the elderly, this may include poor eyesight, poor lighting in hallways and loose rugs. Ensuring that non-slip mats are placed in bathtubs and avoiding the use of bath oils in the tub can prevent falls. Drugs such as benzodiazepines, tricyclic antidepressants and antipsychotic agents have been associated with an increased risk for falls.[6,7]

Prevalence

Osteoporosis affects about one in four women and one in eight men in Canada.[2] Individuals with osteoporosis can suffer from chronic disabling pain from vertebral fractures. In severe cases, kyphosis (curvature of the spine – hunching) can cause shortness of breath and dysphagia. In individuals who have sustained a hip fracture, the mortality in the first year has been reported to be as high as 20%.[8] Hip fracture is one of the leading causes of institutionalization in the elderly. A fear of falling and decreased functioning can lead to social isolation, anxiety and depression. Additionally, the annual cost of acute care management associated with osteoporosis is estimated at about 1.3 billion dollars in Canada.[2]

Table 1: **Risk Factors for Osteoporosis**[2]

Nonmodifiable
- Postmenopausal female (not on estrogen therapy)
- Premature menopause (< 45 yrs)
- Family history (e.g., mother)
- Caucasian or Eurasian ancestry
- Thin and small-boned

Modifiable
- Low calcium intake (< 1000 mg elemental calcium per day)
- Inadequate sunlight exposure
- Sedentary lifestyle
- Cigarette smoking
- Alcohol
- Caffeine-containing beverages

Goals of Therapy

- Prevent osteoporosis by maximizing and/or maintaining existing BMD
- Minimize adverse outcomes of osteoporosis by maximizing BMD and preventing fractures
- Minimize the risk of falls

Table 2: **Drugs Associated with Development of Osteoporosis**[4,5]

Corticosteroids (e.g., prednisone)
Levothyroxine (in excessive doses)
Anticonvulsants (e.g., phenytoin)
Heparin (with long-term therapy)
Antineoplastics
Aluminum-containing antacids

Patient Assessment (Figures 1,2)

In assessing patients for their risk for osteoporosis, consider their age, family history, medical conditions, diet, smoking, alcohol use and lifestyle factors. Rule out drug-induced causes of osteoporosis (Table 2) in patients presenting with fractures and/or low bone density. Individuals who have sustained a fracture, have multiple risk factors and/or are postmenopausal women not on estrogen therapy, should be referred to their physician for possible determination of their BMD and consideration of prescription therapy.[2]

Prevention

Strategies for preventing osteoporosis should be considered at a young age. In children, adolescents and young adults, ensuring adequate calcium intake and exercise will help maximize peak bone mass. In middle-aged and older adults, in addition to these strategies, ensuring adequate vitamin D intake can help maintain bone mass. The best source of calcium and vitamin D is the diet. Recommend calcium and/or vitamin D supplementation for those whose diet is inadequate.

Nonpharmacologic Therapy

Adequate dietary calcium and vitamin D intake, regular exercise and lifestyle changes such as minimizing caffeine and alcohol intake are all important in maintaining bone mass. For those with osteoporosis, strategies to prevent falls should be implemented. In the elderly with osteoporosis, a referral to an occupational therapist for a home safety visit may be beneficial (see Appendix A).

Figure 1: **Assessment Tool for Determining Risk for Osteoporosis**[2]

Use the following checklist as a guide in determining an individual's risk for developing osteoporosis:

Yes	No	
		Non-modifiable
☐	☐	Postmenopausal female (not on estrogen therapy)
☐	☐	Caucasian or Eurasian ancestry
☐	☐	Thin and "small-boned"
☐	☐	Family history of osteoporosis (e.g., mother)
		Modifiable
☐	☐	Daily calcium intake (through diet and supplements) is less than 1000 mg
☐	☐	Inadequate sunlight exposure (less than 20 min, 3-4 times weekly)
☐	☐	Sedentary lifestyle – exercises (e.g., a 20-min walk) less than 3-5 times a week
☐	☐	Current cigarette smoker
☐	☐	Consumes ≥ 2 alcoholic drinks per day
☐	☐	Consumes ≥ 3-4 cups of caffeine-containing beverages per day
☐	☐	Takes one or more of these medications long-term: corticosteroids, thyroid supplement, anticonvulsants, heparin, immunosuppressants

If a patient has multiple risk factors (≥ 3) or has a drug-induced cause, refer them to their physician for an assessment. Additionally, anyone over the age of 50 years who has low BMD and/or has sustained a fracture should be evaluated by their physician for possible osteoporosis therapy.

Dietary Measures

Adequate intake of calcium and vitamin D are essential to help increase peak bone mass in the early years and to help maintain bone mass later in life. Calcium requirements vary by age and gender (Table 3).[9,10] Vitamin D requirements in older adults and in those with osteoporosis are between 400 and 800 IU per day.[10] New guidelines to be released in 2002 by The Osteoporosis Society of Canada are consistent with these previous recommendations.[11]

Daily calcium needs are best met by dietary management. There are many foods that are high in calcium (Table 4).[10] In Canada, milk and some breads are fortified with vitamin D. Additionally, exposure to the sun (about 20 minutes, three to four times per week) is important for the skin to synthesize vitamin D.

Exercise

Weight-bearing exercise in the young can help increase peak bone mass. In older individuals (postmenopausal), regular weight-bearing exercise such as walking or jogging can help maintain bone mass.

Swimming, although an excellent cardiovascular exercise, is not weight-bearing. Additional benefits of exercising regularly include increased muscle strength and flexibility, which can minimize the risk for falls.

Table 3: **Recommended Dietary Intake of Calcium**[9,10]

Age, years	Recommended intake of elemental calcium (mg per day)
7-9	700
10-12 (boys)	900
10-12 (girls)	1200-1400
13-16	1200-1400
17-18	1200
19-49	1000
50-65 (women)	1000-1500
50-65 (men)	1000
postmenopausal women taking estrogen	1000
> 65 (men and women)	1500

Figure 2: **Assessment of Patients with Osteoporosis**

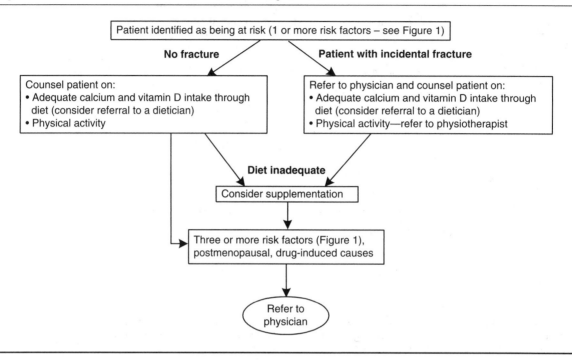

Lifestyle Changes

Consider cigarette smoking cessation and minimizing alcohol and caffeine intake[2] when identifying strategies to decrease the risk for osteoporosis. Smoking cessation has other health benefits, such as a decrease in risk for heart disease and cancer. Limiting the amount of caffeine-containing beverages (cola, hot chocolate, coffee, tea) to no more than three servings daily can help minimize calcium loss. Excess alcohol consumption can impact on bone formation and the ability of the body to absorb calcium. For general good health, no more than two alcoholic drinks per day is recommended.

Nonprescription Therapy

Calcium Supplements

If an individual's diet is not sufficient to meet the daily calcium requirements, consider supplementation. Calcium supplements are available in various salt forms.[2] Commonly used forms are the carbonate and citrate salts. Calcium carbonate is most often recom-

mended as it is inexpensive and is available in many dosage forms. The carbonate salt usually requires an acidic environment for proper absorption. Individuals who may have decreased acid secretion, such as those on H_2-antagonists or proton pump inhibitors, should consider supplementation with calcium citrate, as its absorption is not affected by these agents. Calcium carbonate is available from natural sources such as oyster shells, or is synthetically produced. Both sources are equally effective. With many brands available, it is important to ensure that the chosen product undergoes proper dissolution and absorption.

There is concern regarding lead content of natural calcium supplements. Investigators assessed 17 different calcium carbonate products for their lead content.[12] Although the amount of lead was variable among products, when doses used in osteoporosis were considered, the lead content did not pose a risk to the patient. In individuals taking calcium at much higher doses (e.g., as a phosphate binder in renal disease), consideration of lead content in these products may be more important.[8]

Table 4: **Dietary Sources of Calcium**[11]

Food item	Serving size	mg elemental calcium
Cheese	50 g	350-480
Macaroni and cheese	1 cup	380
Milkshake	300 mL	350
Yogurt	175 mL	250-330
Milk (2%, 1%, skim, chocolate)	250 mL	300-320
Sardines, with bones	84 g	320
Salmon, with bones	125 mL	270
Almonds, dry-roasted	125 mL	210
Soybeans, cooked	250 mL	190
Tofu, with calcium sulfate	100 g	150
Broccoli, raw	125 mL	38
Banana, medium-sized	175 g	10
Figs, dried	10	270
Soup, made with milk	250 mL	189

Clinical Efficacy

Several controlled studies have demonstrated that supplemental calcium can significantly slow the rate of bone loss in postmenopausal women.[13,14] However, calcium is not as effective as estrogen replacement therapy and there is an added benefit in bone density when both are administered.[14,15] Calcium in conjunction with exercise improves bone mass significantly, as compared to exercise alone. Some studies indicate that calcium may have more effect on forearm (cortical) bone than on vertebral bone. Based on the evidence, the Osteoporosis Society of Canada and the Society of Obstetricians and Gynecologists of Canada recommend that calcium intake should be optimized in all individuals for preventing and treating osteoporosis.[2,11]

Administration

If the amount of daily supplementation required is more than 500 mg of elemental calcium, the total amount should be divided into two or three doses, taken with or after meals. Counsel patients selecting a product on the amount of elemental calcium available per tablet, depending on the salt form (Table 5). Calcium supplements are available as tablets, chewables, effervescent and liquid formulations. For information on available calcium supplements, see the *Compendium of Self-Care Products*, published annually by the Canadian Pharmacists Association.

Calcium can decrease the absorption of many drugs such as tetracycline, ciprofloxacin and bisphosphonates. Calcium should not be taken within three hours of these and other drugs, to avoid this possible interaction.

Adverse Effects

Side effects of calcium include constipation, flatulence, nausea and rarely, renal stones.

Vitamin D Analogs

Vitamin D is essential for normal calcium absorption and good bone health. With vitamin D deficiency, less than 10% of calcium is absorbed. Vitamin D is produced in the body usually through exposure to sunlight and is absorbed from the diet. Milk is the best food source of vitamin D. For individuals over 65 years of age, and for those who are home bound

Table 5: **Elemental Calcium Content of Calcium Salts**

Calcium salt	Percentage elemental calcium
Calcium carbonate	40%
Calcium citrate	21%
Calcium gluconate	9.3%
Calcium lactate	13%

or institutionalized, daily vitamin D supplementation is recommended.[2,11] In addition, individuals who use a sunscreen on a regular basis may be unable to synthesize vitamin D, and will benefit from supplementation.

Clinical Efficacy

Vitamin D at 800 IU daily, when given with adequate calcium supplementation, has resulted in a moderate increase in bone mass[16] and a decrease in fracture risk in elderly men and women.[17] Adequate calcium intake (Table 3) should be ensured when supplementing with vitamin D. The current recommendation for those $\geq$ 65 years of age is 400 to 800 IU of vitamin D daily and 800 IU daily for those with osteoporosis.[11]

Administration

Vitamin D is available in various forms. Cholecalciferol (vitamin D_3) or ergocalciferol (vitamin D_2) may be used. Calcitriol, which is an active form of vitamin D, is usually not required unless the patient has renal or hepatic impairment and is not able to activate vitamin D. Most multivitamins contain 400 IU of vitamin D. Vitamin D is also present in fish oils (in conjunction with vitamin A). Mineral oil can impair the absorption of vitamin D and other fat-soluble vitamins.

Adverse Effects

Side effects from vitamin D may be seen with high doses and include hypercalciuria, hypercalcemia, renal calcification and renal stones.

Sodium Fluoride

Sodium fluoride increases bone formation by stimulating osteoblasts. Initial trials using immediate-release sodium fluoride resulted in an increase in bone density. However, no reduction in vertebral fractures was observed in these patients and in fact, there was a suggestion of an increase in peripheral fractures. The likely cause is thought to be the abnormal development of new bone in these individuals. Later studies using lower doses of slow-release fluoride (25 mg twice daily) in conjunction with supplemental calcium have shown promising results.[18] Larger controlled trials are needed to further clarify fluoride's efficacy and safety. At present, fluoride cannot be considered an option in the treatment of osteoporosis.

Prescription Therapy

Prescription therapy for osteoporosis has undergone a dramatic shift. Recommendations for the *treatment* of osteoporosis, based on a review of published studies and evidence based medicine, have changed.[19]

Hormone replacement therapy (HRT) was the gold standard for the prevention and treatment of postmenopausal osteoporosis; however, this is no longer true. The evidence that HRT was useful in the treatment of osteoporosis was primarily based on epidemiological data, but there are no well-designed randomized controlled trials that demonstrate HRT reduces vertebral or hip fractures.

There are, however, large randomized controlled trials to show that both **alendronate** and **risedronate** decrease vertebral and hip fractures. Therefore, these two bisphosphonates have become the gold standard for the treatment of osteoporosis.

Raloxifene and **calcitonin** have been shown to decrease vertebral fractures in randomized, controlled trials. Estrogen and **etidronate** appear to reduce vertebral fractures; however, these trials were not as well-designed.

In men, in addition to bisphosphonates and calcitonin, **testosterone** may be considered in those who are hypogonadal.[20]

Prevention of bone loss has been demonstrated with HRT, raloxifene and the bisphosphonates; therefore, any of these therapies may be used in individuals with osteopenia.[19]

Combination therapy with a bisposphonate and HRT has been shown to have synergistic effects on bone compared to either agent alone; however, because no reduction in fractures has been shown, this therapy should be only used in individuals not responding to a single agent.[19]

Herbal Remedies

Isoflavones such as genistein and daidzein have been considered for their potential effect on bone mass. It has been observed that the rate of osteoporosis in Japanese women is much less than North American women, even though the former have a slighter build. A possible reason is that the diet of Japanese women is high in products that contain isoflavones, such as soybeans.

Isoflavones belong to a group of compounds called flavonoids which are commonly found in photosynthesizing cells of plants. There are over 4000 flavonoids identified to date. **Ipriflavone** (Ostivone®) is a synthetic isoflavone derivative. Flavonoids appear to have estrogenic, antiestrogenic or aromatase inhibitory activity. There is some indication that ipriflavone may have a similar effect to estrogens on bone mineralization, without having a direct estrogen-like activity.[21]

In animal studies, ipriflavone has been shown to inhibit osteoclast function. It may also be able to promote bone formation through osteoblast stimulation.

Review of Evidence[21-25]

Fifteen randomized, placebo-controlled studies have examined the use of ipriflavone for prevention of postmenopausal bone loss. Active treatment included ipriflavone 600 mg daily (given 200 mg three times daily) and all subjects were given supplemental calcium (500 mg to 1 g daily).

The primary endpoint was BMD as measured by DEXA. All study subjects were postmenopausal women aged 47 to 85 years of age with a BMD of 1 to > 2 SD below age-matched females. The trials ranged in duration from six months to three years. Nine of the 15 trials were able to demonstrate a significant difference between the ipriflavone and placebo groups. The differences ranged from 0 to 7.1% increase in BMD with ipriflavone compared to 0 to −3% decrease with placebo. Three of the studies reported no difference between active treatment and placebo and the remaining three did not report results between the groups.

Adverse Effects

The most common side effects were abdominal pain, nausea, diarrhea and constipation, with no significant difference between ipriflavone and placebo in most trials. In one study,[25] women treated with ipriflavone experienced a significant decrease in lymphocyte concentration, which was not observed in the placebo group. The decrease in lymphocytes occurred after six months and returned to normal in most patients within 24 months of discontinuation. The clinical significance of this event is not known and the trial subjects did not present with clinical symptoms related to it.

Drug Interactions

The interactions between ipriflavone and other medications have not been well-studied. Ipriflavone and its metabolites can inhibit cytochrome P450 enzymes, hence, there is a potential for interaction with drugs such as theophylline, tolbutamide, phenytoin, warfarin and nifedipine.

Place in Therapy[26]

Ipriflavone appears to maintain or increase bone mineral density in the radius and spine of postmenopausal women. There are no studies that have considered its effect on fractures. Also, its long-term safety is unclear, including the significance of lymphocytopenia reported in a recent trial. Before recommending this agent in the prevention of bone loss, many of these issues need to be clarified.

Administration

In clinical trials, ipriflavone has been administered as 200 mg, three times daily. It is preferable to take it with meals. As ipriflavone and its metabolites are excreted in the urine, adjustments in dosage may be required with renal impairment.

Monitoring of Therapy

Table 6 lists some measures to reduce modifiable risks and how to monitor their success.

Resource Tips

Osteoporosis Society of Canada:
http://www.osteoporosis.ca

Suggested Readings

Canadian consensus conference on menopause and osteoporosis. *Journal SOGC* 1998; 20(13): 22-30 and 47-54.

O'Connell MB. Prevention and treatment of osteoporosis in the elderly. *Pharmacotherapy* 1999; 19(1pt2):7S-20S.

Table 6: **Monitoring Outcome of Modifiable Risk Reduction Measures**

Risk factor	Recommendation	Expected outcome	Considerations
Low calcium intake	Ensure diet is adequate (may refer to dietician). Add supplements to meet total daily requirements (Table 3).	If baseline BMD available, maintain BMD. With osteoporosis, want to see no further loss in BMD, no fractures	If supplements recommended, counsel patient on proper administration and prevention of constipation and drug interactions. Calculate appropriate number of tablets based on salt form (Table 5).
Sedentary lifestyle	If osteoporosis is not diagnosed, recommend weight-bearing exercises, such as walking. If patient has significant cardiovascular disease or osteoporosis, refer to physician and physiotherapist.		Exercise should be started gradually and tailored according to the individual's health status (e.g., consider conditions such as cardiovascular or respiratory disease)
Inadequate vitamin D intake or > 65 years of age	If > 65 yrs of age, recommend 800 IU of vitamin D daily.		If patient is taking a multivitamin, check for amount of vitamin D.

Osteoporosis Society of Canada. Clinical Practice Guidelines for the diagnosis and management of osteoporosis. *CMAJ* 1996;155(8):1113-33 (new guidelines to be published in 2002).

Osteoporosis Society of Canada web site: http://www.osteoporosis.ca

Watts NB. Focus on primary care: postmenopausal osteoporosis. *Obstet Gynecol Surv* 1999; 54(8):532-8.

References

1. Kanis JA, Melton LJ, Christiansen C. The diagnosis of osteoporosis. *J Bone Miner Res* 1994;9:1137-41.
2. Yuen CK, Kendler D, Khan A, et al. Canadian consensus on menopause and osteoporosis. *J Obstet Gynecol* 2001;23:979-88.
3. Taxel P. Osteoporosis: detection, prevention, and treatment in primary care. *Geriatrics* 1998;53(8):22-40.
4. Tannirandorn P, Epstein S. Drug-induced bone loss. *Osteoporos Int* 2000;11(8):637-59.
5. Bohannon AD, Lyles KW. Drug-induced bone disease. *Clin Geriatr Med* 1994;10(4):611-23.
6. Ray WA, Griffin MR, Schaffner W, Baugh DK, Melton LJ. Psychotropic drug use and the risk of hip fracture. N *Engl J Med* 1987;316:363-9.
7. Cummings SR, Nevitt MC, Browner WS, et al. Risk factors for hip fracture in white women. *N Engl J Med* 1995;332:767-73.
8. NIH Consensus Development Panel on Osteoporosis, Prevention, Diagnosis, and Therapy. Osteoporosis prevention, diagnosis, and therapy. *JAMA* 2001;285(6):785-95.
9. Osteoporosis Society of Canada. *Daily Calcium Intake Guide*, Toronto, Ontario, Canada.
10. Murray TM. Prevention and management of osteoporosis: Consensus statements from the Scientific Advisory Board of the Osteoporosis Society of Canada. 4. Calcium nutrition and osteoporosis. *CMAJ* 1996;155(7):935-9.
11. Osteoporosis Society of Canada, Toronto, Ontario, Canada.
12. Edward R, Szabo NJ and Tebbett IR. Lead content of calcium supplements. *JAMA* 2000;284(11):1425-9.
13. Reid IR, Ames RW, Evans MC, Gamble GD, Sharpe SJ. Effect of calcium supplementation on bone loss in postmenopausal women. *N Engl J Med* 1993;328:460-4.
14. Aloia JF, Vaswani A, Yeh JK, Ross PL, Flaster E, Dilmanian FA. Calcium supplementation with and without hormone replacement therapy to prevent postmenopausal bone loss. *Ann Intern Med* 1994;120:97-103.
15. Prince RL, Smith M, Dick IM, et al. Prevention of postmenopausal osteoporosis. *N Engl J Med* 1991;325:1189-95.
16. Dawson-Hughes B, Harris SS, Krall EA, Dallal GE. Effect of calcium and vitamin D supplementation on bone density in men and women 65 years of age or older. *N Engl J Med* 1997;337:670-6.
17. Chapuy MC, Arlot ME, Duboeuf F, et al. Vitamin D3 and calcium to prevent hip fractures in elderly women. *N Engl J Med* 1992;327:1637-42.
18. Pak CYC, Sakhaee K, Adams-Huet B, et al. Treatment of postmenopausal osteoporosis with slow-release sodium fluoride. *Ann Intern Med* 1995;123:401-8.
19. Smith T, Contestabile E. Executive summary, Canadian consensus on menopause and osteoporosis. *J Obstet Gynecol* 2001;23:829-35.
20. Behre HM, Kliesch S, Leifke E, Link TM, Nieschlage E. Long-term effect of testosterone therapy on bone mineral density in hypogonadal men. *J Clin Endocrinol Metab* 1997;82:2386-90.

21. Melis GB, Paoletti AM, Cagnacci A, et al. Lack of any estrogenic effect of ipriflavone in postmenopausal women. *J Endocrinol Invest* 1992;15:755-61.
22. Kovacs AB. Efficacy of ipriflavone in the prevention and treatment of postmenopausal osteoporosis. *Agents Action* 1994;41:86-7.
23. Adami S, Bufalino L, Cervetti R, et al. *Osteoporosis Int* 1997;7:119-25.
24. Gennari C, Adami S, Agnusdei D, et al. Effect of chronic treatment with ipriflavone in postmenopausal women with low bone mass. *Calcif Tissue Int* 1997;61:S19-22.
25. Alexandersen P, Toussaint A, Christiansen C, et al. Ipriflavone in the treatment of postmenopausal osteoporosis. *JAMA* 2001;285:482-8.
26. Osteoporosis Society of Canada. *Position Statement on Ipriflavone.* Toronto, Ontario, Canada: 2000.

Osteoporosis—Patient Information

Osteoporosis is a condition where the bones are thin and can easily break. Even if you do not have osteoporosis, you can do a lot to prevent this condition. Your pharmacist or doctor can help you identify any risks you may have for this disease.

Women are at higher risk for this condition. Other factors that may increase your risk include a family history of osteoporosis, if you are a postmenopausal woman, and certain medications. By taking steps early, you can help prevent osteoporosis.

Ensuring that you have an adequate daily calcium and vitamin D intake is important for your bones. Also, regular exercise, such as walking, can help prevent further bone loss. If you already have osteoporosis, check with your doctor or physiotherapist before deciding to do exercises.

The best way to get your daily calcium and vitamin D is through your diet. If you are not able to get enough calcium and vitamin D from your diet, your pharmacist can recommend supplements for you.

Recommended Dietary Calcium Intake

Age, years	Recommended intake of elemental calcium (mg per day)
7-9	700
10-12 (boys)	900
10-12 (girls)	1200-1400
13-16	1200-1400
17-18	1200
19-49	1000
50-65 (women)	1000-1500
50-65 (men)	1000
post-menopausal women taking estrogen	1000
> 65 (men and women)	1500

Dietary Sources of Calcium

Food item	Serving size	mg elemental calcium
Cheese	50 g	350-480
Macaroni and cheese	1 cup	380
Milkshake	300 mL	350
Yogurt	175 mL	250-330
Milk (2%, 1%, skim, chocolate)	250 mL	300-320
Sardines, with bones	84 g	320
Salmon, with bones	125 mL	270
Almonds, dry-roasted	125 mL	210
Soybeans, cooked	250 mL	190
Tofu, with calcium sulfate	100 g	150
Broccoli, raw	125 mL	38
Banana, medium size	175 g	10
Figs, dried	10	270
Soup, made with milk	250 mL	189

In addition to calcium and vitamin D, many medication options are now available to help make your bones stronger. You can discuss these with your doctor to see if you would benefit from these.

For more information on osteoporosis, contact the Osteoporosis Society of Canada at: http://www.osteoporosis.ca or 1-800-463-6842.

Chapter 35

Low Back Pain

Debora Kwan, BScPhm, MSc and Christine Papoushek, PharmD

Pathophysiology

Low back pain is defined as spinal and paraspinal symptoms in the lumbosacral region that can extend to the gluteal muscles, hips and lower extremities.[1,2] Of the various musculoskeletal disorders, it is the condition that is most responsible for physician assessment and utilization of medication. In the United States, low back pain ranks as the second most common symptomatic reason for seeking physician assessment and the fifth most common reason overall for physician visits.[1-3] Given this, the annual individual (10 to 20%) and lifetime individual prevalence (60 to 85%) are not surprising statistics. Unfortunately, this high prevalence is associated with significant direct and indirect costs on the health care system due to direct medical care, disability, decreased productivity and time lost from work.[1-4]

The causes of low back pain are typically separated into two categories, mechanical and nonmechanical (Table 1).[1,2,4,5] Mechanical back pain may be further subdivided in order to separate sciatica from muscular-ligamentous injuries. Sciatica may be due to many nonmuscular-nonligamentous mechanical causes of low back pain. It is a syndrome characterized by pain that radiates to the buttocks and down the posterior-lateral aspect of the leg. It may be described as a "shooting pain" originating in the lumbar region (sciatic nerve).

Muscular-ligamentous injuries of the low back such as strains and sprains are the most common cause of low back pain, resulting in approximately 70% of occurrences. The symptoms, similar to those experienced with other muscle, ligament and tendon disorders, include localized pain of varying severity, spasm, inflammation and immobility. The second most common mechanical cause of low back pain is degenerative disease of the disks and facet joints (located between the vertebrae) of the spine.

Nonmechanical low back pain typically results from more severe etiologies (Table 1) and is associated with atypical symptoms that require urgent assessment and management.

Low back pain is differentiated into acute and chronic phases depending on the duration of the symptoms: 2 to 4 weeks (acute); 4 to 12 weeks (sub-acute); > 12 weeks (chronic). Earlier studies on low back pain suggest that symptoms are self-limiting and resolve within the first four weeks in approximately 90% of individuals. More recent evidence suggests that pain and disability one year after the first episode of acute low back pain is present in approximately 75% of individuals.[6] This finding is further supported by the recurrent nature of the disease, with approximately 25 to 50% of individuals experiencing recurrent low back pain within the first year.[2,6] In addition, up to 10% of individuals will progress to chronic symptoms resulting in significant time away from work.[3] To summarize, low back pain may be described as an intermittent disease that is associated with acute exacerbations and remissions.

Factors that can increase the risk for low back pain include heavy lifting or twisting, prolonged standing or sitting without position changes, intense physical activity or movement without proper warm-up or stretching of the muscles, obesity, poor posture and conditioning, and smoking.[1,4]

Goals of Therapy

- Relieve symptoms
- Maintain or improve mobility
- Prevent or minimize re-injury

Table 1: **Causes of Low Back Pain**[1,2,4,5]

Mechanical	Nonmechanical
Muscular/ligamentous strain and sprain	Cancer
Facet joint syndrome/degenerative disease*	Infection
Sacroiliac syndromes	Inflammatory arthritis (e.g., anklylosing spondylitis)
Segmental dysfunction	Visceral disease
Somatic dysfunction	–Pelvic organs (e.g., prostatitis, endometriosis)
Myofascial syndrome	–Renal disease (e.g., pyelonephritis)
Herniated disk	–Vascular disease (e.g., abdominal aortic aneurysm)
Spinal stenosis	–Gastrointestinal disease (e.g., pancreatitis)
Osteoporosis with compression fracture	
Spondylolysis (breakdown of vertebrae)	
Spondylolisthesis (anterior displacement of one vertebra over the one beneath it)	
Fractures	
Congenital disease (kyphosis, scoliosis)	
Paget's disease	

Facet joint syndrome = degenerative disease of the facet joints.

- Minimize functional disability and improve physical functioning
- Educate patients and caregivers to assist them to understand the condition and make informed decisions about which therapies to choose
- Minimize immobility

Patient Assessment

The most important aspect of assessing low back pain is ruling out potential serious etiologies that require immediate evaluation by a physician. Chronic, non-mechanical or sciatic conditions should be ruled out prior to patient self-management. Figure 1 shows an algorithm for assessing patients with low back pain.

General Principles of Therapy

Current pharmacologic therapies for low back pain provide symptomatic relief but are not curative. Therefore, the choice of agent is based on a combination of risk versus benefit, cost and patient preference. Pharmacologic therapy should always be initiated in combination with nonpharmacologic modalities. If tolerated, pharmacologic therapies should be tried for at least two to four weeks in order to allow the patient to fully assess effectiveness.

Numerous approaches with various levels of evidence have been evaluated in the management of low back pain (Table 2). Overall, the available evidence lacks

rigor with respect to trial methodologies, including sample size, randomization, blinding, confounding variables, population variances (e.g., acute, chronic, +/- pain radiation) and published treatment comparisons. Nonetheless, systematic reviews and guidelines of such therapies lend adequate support to current recommendations for treating low back pain.[5,7-9]

Nonpharmacologic Therapy

In acute low back pain (< 12 weeks), the primary recommendation is to maintain usual activity, and avoid bedrest or potentially aggravating activities (e.g., heavy lifting, twisting, high impact exercise) which may exacerbate the pain or worsen the injury. Although historically bedrest for two to seven days was a general recommendation, this has not been shown to be effective with respect to pain relief, functional status or decreasing time lost from work, and may contribute to delayed recovery and debilitation.[5,7,9,10] A recent trial of patients with acute low back pain demonstrated that continuing ordinary activities within the limits permitted by the pain leads to a more rapid recovery than either bed-rest or back mobilizing activities when evaluated over 12 weeks.[10]

Other nonpharmacologic therapies such as back manipulation and physical therapy exercises may be of limited value in the management of acute back pain (< 4 weeks). Back exercises and spinal manipulation in acute episodes are no more effective than other modalities such as usual care, manual therapy (massage, mobilization or soft-tissue techniques), back school (a structured program where individuals are taught how to maximize recovery and minimize recurrences of low back pain) or NSAIDs.[8,11] A study comparing chiropractic manipulation, physical ther-

---

Figure 1: **Assessment of Patients with Low Back Pain**[1,2,5,7]

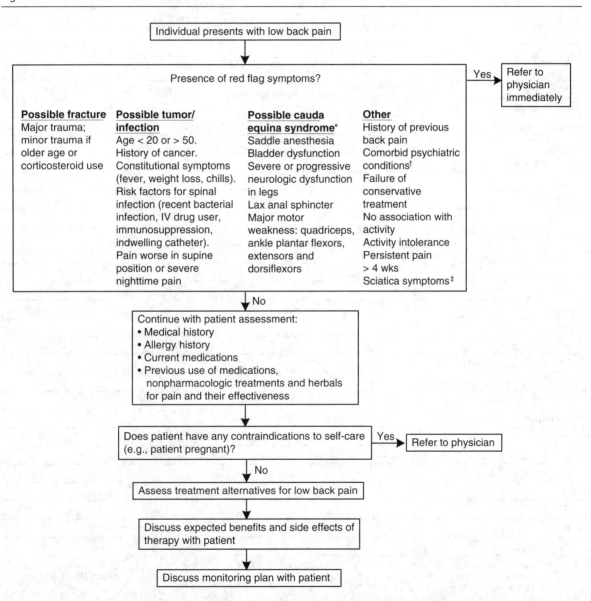

Cauda equina syndrome: a rare clinical syndrome characterized by dull pain in the lower back and upper buttock region, analgesia in the buttocks, genitalia or thigh, accompanied by a disturbance of bowel and bladder function.
†*History of depression, psychological distress or substance abuse can increase likelihood of persistent back pain.*
‡*Sharp/burning pain radiating down posterior-lateral aspect of one or both legs. Symptoms worsen with change of position.*

Table 2: **Conservative Treatments for Low Back Pain**[2]

Treatment	Strength of evidence*
Oral drugs	
Nonnarcotic analgesics[†]	
Acetaminophen	C
Aspirin	B
NSAIDs	B
Narcotic analgesics[‡]	C
Muscle relaxants[‡]	C
Antidepressants[π]	C
Corticosteroids	C
Physical measures	
Bed rest	B
Activity modification[†]	D
Exercise[†#]	C
Manipulation[†]	B
Local heat	
Superficial (hot packs)	C
Deep (ultrasound or diathermy)	C
Local cold	C
Massage, mobilization, and other soft-tissue techniques	C
Corsets	D
Traction	B
Injection drugs	
Anesthetics (epidural and facet joint)	(D,C)
Corticosteroids (epidural and facet joint)	(D,C)
Intradiskal chymopapain	
Stimulation	
Acupuncture	D
Transcutaneous electrical nerve stimulation (TENS)[π]	C
Implanted neurostimulators[π]	C
Other	
Biofeedback[π]	C
Back school[π]	C
Behavioral therapy[π]	

*Research-based evidence rating system from acute low back pain expert panel: A, strong (multiple relevant and high-quality scientific studies); B, moderate (1 relevant, high-quality scientific study or multiple adequate scientific studies); C, limited (at least 1 adequate scientific study); D, no study meeting panel inclusion criteria.
[†]Recommended treatments for acute low back pain.
[‡]In selected patients, may be considered as appropriate treatments for acute low back pain.
[π]Generally reserved for chronic low back pain.
[#]Exercise is not recommended during the acute phase, only after the acute symptoms subside.
Reproduced with permission from Atlas et al. Evaluating and managing acute low back pain in the primary care setting. *J Gen Intern Med* 2001;16:120-31.

apy exercise and education showed no difference between the former two and only marginal improvement over the use of an educational booklet after four weeks of intervention.[12] This study validates the discussion on whether the cost of these treatment strategies in the short-term is justified given the minimal benefit seen with the acute patient. On the other hand, patients who experience persistent, chronic pain may benefit from these therapies. Exercises, without demonstrated predominance of one over another, have been shown to be superior to usual care in patients experiencing chronic pain.[11] Other modalities such as lumbar supports, corsets, shoe lifts and insoles have shown little promise in the acute patient. However, in the management of chronic low back pain, these alternatives may provide some preventive relief. Of note, shoe lifts are not recommended when lower limb length difference is $\leq$ 2 cm.[5]

Surgical therapy is considered in individuals with unresolved sciatica, cauda equina syndrome, spinal stenosis with persistent and disabling symptoms or spondylolisthesis.[4]

Finally, the evidence pertaining to behavioral therapy is weak. A recent systematic review suggests that the use of behavioral therapy may produce small to moderate benefit in improving general functional status and pain intensity only when compared to no treatment for chronic low back pain. In contrast, there is no demonstrated benefit when compared against or in conjunction with other forms of therapy. Furthermore, there appears to be no benefit of one form of therapy over another.[13] Due to numerous limitations on the quality of this data and the need for stronger evidence, behavioral therapy for chronic low back pain should be incorporated on an individual basis and under the care of a qualified professional.

In summary, the current recommendation is to reserve the use of physical therapy exercises and spinal manipulation for individuals who fail to improve over the acute episode (> 3 to 4 weeks).[4,7] Encourage patients to maintain ordinary activity and increase their level of activity based on pain tolerance. In addition, preventive strategies such as weight loss, abdominal, back and leg strengthening, smoking cessation, ergonomic adjustments and avoidance of prolonged sitting or standing should be considered for the long-term management and prevention of chronic back pain.[1,2,4,14]

Pharmacologic Therapy[5,7,8,15]

(Table 3)

The natural course of acute back pain (isolated episodes versus chronic pain) leads to gradual improvement in symptoms in 75 to 90% of individuals over four weeks[6] and there is no cure for acute, non-specific, mechanical pain. Therefore, drug therapy is primarily intended to relieve pain and discomfort in the short term and facilitate activity.[2] Long-term therapy with prescription medications may be required in individuals who experience chronic back pain.

The agents evaluated to some degree include acetaminophen, various NSAIDs, opioid analgesics and muscle relaxants in various doses, formulations (injection, topical gel, oral) and duration (majority: 14 days; range: 1 to 42 days).[8] **NSAIDs** may result in global improvement of back pain when compared to placebo with no demonstrated superiority of one specific NSAID.[7,8] Although there are no placebo-controlled trials with **acetaminophen**, small trials comparing NSAIDs to acetaminophen suggest that these agents produce similar outcomes with respect to pain relief. Since the safety profile for acetaminophen tends to be better than for NSAIDs, it may be considered a first line option in alleviating symptoms associated with back pain.[5,7] Small, comparative trials of opioid analgesics to NSAIDs report conflicting results and thus opioids may be reserved for individuals who do not respond to acetaminophen or NSAIDs.[7,8] Since combination products containing **acetaminophen**, **caffeine** and **codeine** (8 mg) are available without a prescription, they may be reasonable options for non-responsive individuals in the short-term.

Muscle relaxants, as a class, are generally not recommended for the management of acute or chronic low back pain. Evidence suggests that these agents provide similar benefit to NSAIDs and do not result in additive benefit when used in combination.[8] In addition, the side effect profile and potential for long-term abuse render these agents undesirable. In low back pain, as with other muscular strain disorders, the complexity of spasm physiology makes it difficult to determine the extent to which spasm is contributing to the injury or symptoms. Therefore, the benefit of OTC "muscle relaxants" which possess little direct muscular relaxing effects are minimal. Situations in which muscle relaxants may be used in the management of low

Table 3: **Nonprescription Products for Low Back Pain**[7,16-21]

Drug	Usual dose	Expected clinical benefit (time frame)	Adverse effects/ Precautions	Clinically significant drug interactions	Comments
Oral analgesics:					
Acetaminophen	325-1000 mg q4-6 h SR: 650 mg q8h (max 4 g per day)	Maximal onset of pain relief within 24-48 h	Hepatotoxicity: increased risk in patients with excessive alcohol intake (> 3 drinks per day), malnourishment or pre-existing hepatic disease. Baseline LFTs should be measured in high-risk patients.	Alcohol (see precautions). Warfarin (with regular use of > 2 g per day acetaminophen). Phenytoin (may increase metabolism of acetaminophen and formation of toxic metabolite thereby increasing the risk of hepatotoxicity; risk may be higher in patients taking high therapeutic doses of acetaminophen and phenytoin chronically. Interaction has not been well-documented).	Lower doses may be required in patients with severe hepatic and renal disease. Caution with concurrent use of acetaminophen-containing OTC products (do not exceed 4 g per day). Continuous therapy should be considered in individuals with pain persisting throughout the day. PRN dosing is acceptable for episodic pain of short duration.
NSAIDs: ASA Ibuprofen	Ibuprofen: 200-400 mg q6-8h; usual maximum daily dose: 3200 mg per day. ASA: 325-650 mg q6-8h; usual maximum daily dose: 3900 mg per day (not recommended for use if CrCl <10 mL/min)		Local GI effects (dyspepsia, diarrhea), GI complications (ulceration/ upper GI bleed). CHF may be exacerbated. Renal effects: more likely in the elderly or patients with pre-existing renal disease or comorbid conditions that may affect renal function (e.g., diabetes, CHF, hypertension). ↑LFTs: transient; hepatotoxicity is rare; more likely to occur in patients with pre-existing hepatic disease or in patients with excessive alcohol intake (> 3 drinks per day).	Warfarin (↑ bleeding risk via antiplatelet effects and GI complications); monitor INR more frequently during initial period after NSAID started and watch for signs of bleeding. ↑Lithium levels – monitor levels. ↑Methotrexate levels (rare) – monitor for toxicity. Antihypertensives (e.g., beta-blockers, diuretics, ACEI): possible ↓ in antihypertensive effects); measure baseline BP, remeasure 1-2 wks after starting NSAID and adjust antihypertensive therapy as required.	NSAIDs are not a substitute for ASA being taken for MI or stroke prophylaxis. Avoid concurrent use of NSAID-containing OTC products (increased risk of GI-related side effects). Continuous therapy should be considered in individuals with pain persisting throughout the day. PRN dosing is acceptable for episodic pain of short duration. Consider prophylaxis with misoprostol or proton pump inhibitor in high risk patients (Table 5). Avoid NSAIDs in patients with ASA or ibuprofen hypersensitivity.

Agent	Dosage	Onset	Adverse effects	Drug interactions	Comments
Acetaminophen + caffeine + codeine 8 mg	1-2 tablets q4-6h (maximum 4 g acetaminophen per day)		See acetaminophen. Sedation, nausea, vomiting, constipation.	See acetaminophen. Concurrent use of other sedating or constipating medications.	Recommended for short-term use (e.g., 2-3 days). Elderly are at increased risk for adverse effects.
Skeletal muscle relaxants:					
Chlorzoxazone Methocarbamol Orphenadrine	Chlorzoxazone: 250-750mg TID-QID. Methocarbamol: 400-1000 mg QID. Orphenadrine: 50-100 mg BID-TID	Maximal onset within 12-24 h (> 24 h for orphenadrine)	Sedation, dizziness, light-headedness, nausea. Anticholinergic effects: hallucinations, agitation, dry mouth, constipation, urinary retention, blurred vision (orphenadrine). Orphenadrine is con-traindicated with angle closure glaucoma, BPH, bladder obstruction, achalasia, myasthenia gravis. Hepatotoxicity has been associated with chlorzoxa-zone.	Other CNS sedating medications. Anticholinergics	No agent has demonstrated superior efficacy. Although effective compared to placebo, use of these agents gener-ally *not recommended* due to side effect profile. If utilized, use only in the short-term (2-3 days). Elderly are at increased risk for adverse effects.
Herbals:					
White willow bark	240 mg per day	Onset: 1-3 wks	Minimal adverse effects reported with oral use. One case of hypersensitiv-ity reported in clinical trial. Theoretical (but unproven) risks associated with tan-nins include kidney and liver damage, GI intoler-ance.	Theoretical drug interaction with tannin-containing herbs. Significance of other interactions are unknown due to the lack of informa-tion pertaining to the exact salicylate content.	Long-term efficacy and toxicity are unknown. Lack of product standardization may result in inter- and intra-product variability. Has only been studied in *chronic* low back pain. Constituents include tannins, flavo-noids and salicylates (metabolite). Exact mechanism of action unknown, but may possess antiinflammatory activity. Avoid in patients with history of salicylate hypersensitivity.

SR=sustained release.

Table 4: **Monitoring Therapy for Low Back Pain**

Parameter	Degree	Timeframe	Action/Comments
Pain relief	Elimination or improvement toward predefined goals as set by patient at the beginning of therapy	**Patient or care provider:** assess daily **Pharmacist:** phone call day 3, 7, 14 and 28	Refer to physician if symptoms not relieved after adequate trial of at least 2 analgesics or if new or worsening pain symptoms develop during therapy. Considerations: • Use visual analog scale or other individual measure to quantify and characterize pain (e.g., ADLs – walking, gardening). • Trial each analgesic for 2-4 wks at optimal doses in order for patient to fully assess impact on daily activities and functioning. • Considerations in timing of medications: –Around-the-clock vs. PRN. –Take dose of analgesic at least 1 h prior to activities that may exacerbate pain.
Nausea, dyspepsia, abdominal discomfort	Minimal or none during therapy	**Patient or care provider:** monitor daily **Pharmacist:** phone call on day 3 and 7	Change therapy if symptoms severe or intolerable. Minimize development by advising to take with food or milk. Assess risk of GI complications (Table 5). If high risk, refer to physician. Otherwise, consider antacids or OTC H_2RAs to treat dyspepsia.
Hematemesis, melena, hematochezia	None during therapy	**Patient or care provider:** monitor daily on an ongoing basis **Pharmacist:** phone call on day 3 and 7	Patient should seek medical attention if these signs or symptoms develop. Discontinue therapy immediately.
Renal function and signs of fluid retention (i.e. weight gain or edema) in high risk patients (Table 3—ASA or ibuprofen)	No significant change in renal function	Serum creatinine and Na+, K+ at baseline, q1-2 week × 3 then periodically afterwards. Patient to monitor for signs of fluid retention on an ongoing basis (e.g., edema; patients with severe CHF should measure their weight daily).	Discontinue NSAID if significant change in serum creatinine, electrolytes or signs of fluid retention occur.
Recurrent low back injury.	Avoid or minimize	**Patient:** Ongoing	Patient to seek medical attention if develop recurrent episodes in an effort to identify and implement potential nonpharmacologic strategies for management and prevention.
Functional ability after acute injury	Avoid immobilization. Perform usual activity to tolerable pain level. Patient able to perform ADLs	**Patient:** daily **Pharmacist:** Phone call on day 3 and 7	Refer to physician if unable to perform ADLs.

ADL = activities of daily living; H_2RA = H_2-receptor antagonist.

back pain include when patients have contraindications, failure with all other treatment modalities, or have been diagnosed as having a neurologic, spastic component to their disease. However, in the latter case, these patients require management with agents possessing more specific muscle relaxing activity that are available only by prescription (e.g., tizanidine, baclofen).[14]

Table 5: **Risk Factors for the Development of Upper GI Adverse Events**[23,24]

Established:
Age ≥ 65 yrs
History of ulcer
Concomitant use of corticosteroids, anticoagulants
Use of higher doses of NSAIDs
Use of more than one NSAID
Presence of multiple systemic disorders

Possible:
Concomitant infection with *Helicobacter pylori*
Cigarette smoking
Regular alcohol consumption

Alternative Therapy

There have been numerous claims that agents such as **D-phenylalanine**, **devil's claw**, **ginger**, **tumeric** and **white willow bark** are effective in managing symptoms of low back pain. Aside from white willow bark, there is no evidence to demonstrate any positive effects for low back pain.

A randomized, placebo-controlled, double-blind study in chronic low back pain demonstrated an increased percentage of patients who were pain-free at four weeks with high dose white willow bark (39% vs. 21% vs. 6% for 240 mg vs. 120 mg vs. placebo, respectively).[21,22] Note that the quantity of active ingredient was standardized for this study and this cannot be expected with the products currently available in Canada.

Monitoring of Therapy

Table 4 provides a monitoring plan for patients with low back pain.

Advice for the Patient

Counsel patients on:
- The importance of using nondrug measures concurrently with medication;
- The importance of maintaining ordinary activities and increasing level of activity based on pain tolerance;
- Expected benefits of treatment;
- Possible side effects and their management (Table 3);
- When to contact a physician.

Resource Tips

For more information on low back pain, contact:
The North American Chronic Pain Association
of Canada
60 Lorne Avenue
Dartmouth, Nova Scotia
B2Y 3E7
http://www.chronicpaincanada.org

Suggested Readings

Atlas SJ, Deyo RA. Evaluating and managing acute low back pain in the primary care setting. *J Gen Intern Med* 2001;16:120-31.

Chen SW, Gong WC. Rheumatic disorders. In: Koda-Kimble M, Young LY, eds. *Applied Therapeutics: the Clinical Use of Drugs*. 7th ed. Baltimore, MD: Lippincott Williams and Wilkins, 2001:41-1 to 41-41.

Deyo RA, Weinstein JN. Low back pain. *N Engl J Med* 2001;344(5):363-70.

References

1. Kaufmann JA. Low back pain: diagnosis and management in primary care. *Primary Care Practice* 1999;3(4):376-93.
2. Atlas SJ, Deyo RA. Evaluating and managing acute low back pain in the primary care setting. *J Gen Intern Med* 2001;16: 120-31.
3. Andersson GB. Epidemiological features of chronic low-back pain. *Lancet* 1999;354:581-5.
4. Deyo RA, Weinstein JN. Low back pain. *N Engl J Med* 2001; 344(5):363-70.
5. Anonymous. Acute lower back problems in adults. Clinical Practice Guidelines 14. AHCPR Publication No. 95-0642: December 1994.
6. Croft PR, Macfarlane GJ, Papageorgiou AC, Thomas E, Silman AJ. Outcome of low back pain in general practice: a prospective study. *BMJ* 1998;316:1356-9.

7. Ontario Program for Optimal Therapeutics (OPOT). *Ontario Treatment Guidelines for Osteoarthiris, Rheumatoid Arthritis, and Acute Musculoskeletal Injury.* 1st ed. Toronto, ON: Queen's Printer of Ontario, 2000.

8. van Tulder MW, Scholten RJ, Koes BW, Deyo RA. Non-steroidal anti-inflammatory drugs for low back pain: a systematic review within the framework of the Cochrane Collaboration Back Review Group. *Spine* 2000;25:2501-13.

9. van Tulder MW, Koes BW, Bouter LM. Conservative treatment of acute and chronic nonspecific low back pain: a systematic review of randomized controlled trials of the most common interventions. *Spine* 1997;22:2128-56.

10. Malmivaara A, Hakkinen U, Heinrichs M, et al. The treatment of acute low back pain – bed rest, exercises, or ordinary activity? *N Engl J Med* 1995;332:351-5.

11. van Tulder MW, Malmivaara A, Esmail R, Koes B. Exercise therapy for low back pain: a systematic review within the framework of the Cochrane Collaboration Back Review Group. *Spine* 2000;25:2784-96.

12. Cherkin DC, Deyo RA, Battie M et al. A comparison of physical therapy, chiropractic manipulation, and provision of an educational booklet for the treatment of patients with low back pain. *N Engl J Med* 1998;339:1021-9.

13. van Tulder MW, Ostelo R, Vlaeyen JWS, Linton SJ, Morley SJ, Assendelft WJ. Behavioral treatment for chronic low back pain: a systematic review within the framework of the Cochrane Back Review Group. *Spine* 2000;25(20):2688-99.

14. Deyo RA. Drug therapy for back pain. Which drugs help which patients? *Spine* 1996;21(24):2840-50.

15. Koes BW, Scholten RJ, Mens JM, Bouter LM. Efficacy of non-steroidal anti-inflammatory drugs for low back pain: a systematic review of randomised clinical trials. *Ann Rheum Dis* 1997;56:214-23.

16. Allen LV, Berardi RR, DeSimone EM, Engle JP, Popovich NG, Rosenthal WM, Tietze KJ, eds. *Handbook of Nonprescription Drugs.* 12th ed. Washington DC: American Pharmaceutical Association, 2000.

17. Micromedex Healthcare Series Vol. 108. Expiry December, 2001.

18. Elenbaas J. Centrally acting oral skeletal muscle relaxants. *Am J Hosp Pharm* 1980;37:1313-23.

19. Balano KB. Anti-inflammatory drugs and myorelaxants. *Orthopedics* 1996;23(2):329-34.

20. Hawkey CJ, Karrasch JA, Szczepanski L, et al. Omeprazole compared with misoprostol for ulcers associated with non-steroidal antiinflammatory drugs. *N Engl J Med* 1998;338:727-34.

21. Natural Medicines Comprehensive Database. Available at: www.naturaldatabase.com. Accessed December 7, 2001.

22. Chrubasik S, Eisenberg E, Balan E, Weinberger T, Luzzati R, Conradt C. Treatment of low back pain exacerbations with willow bark: a randomized, double-blind study. *Am J Med* 2000;109(1):9-14.

23. Wolfe MM, Lichtenstein DR, Singh G. Gastrointestinal toxicity of nonsteroidal antiinflammatory drugs. *N Engl J Med* 1999;340(24):1888-99.

24. American College of Rheumatology Subcommittee on Osteoarthritis Guidelines. Recommendations for the medical management of osteoarthritis of the hip and knee: 2000 update. *Arthritis Rheum* 2000;43(9):1905-15.

Low Back Pain—Patient Information

Why do so many people have low back pain?

Low back pain is a very common problem because the lower back carries most of your weight. Four out of five adults have back pain at some time in their life.

What are the most common causes of low back pain?

The most common cause of low back pain involves pulled muscles and spasms, usually as a result of sports or work-related injury. However, any type of improper, excess lifting or twisting can cause stress on the lower back causing strains or sprains of the muscles.

Other common causes include sciatica or osteoarthritis of the spine. Osteoarthritis causes a loss of cushioning between the disks in your spine which then may cause the bones to harden and stiffen. This leads to pain and discomfort.

Sciatica is caused by a squeezing of a nerve within your spinal column. This can happen when a disk slips out of its spot between your backbones. Your nerve becomes inflamed and causes pain which may travel from your back down into your leg.

What usually happens when someone has back pain?

The majority of individuals who experience back pain will see a gradual improvement in symptoms over a few weeks. This is similar to what is expected when other muscles or ligaments are injured.

In the beginning of the painful episode, you will be asked specific questions by your doctor or other health care provider to rule out any potential serious causes of low back pain. Although these causes are extremely rare, it is important that these are excluded before treatment is chosen.

What warning signs should I look for with low back pain?

Contact your doctor if you have back pain plus any of the following conditions:
• Fever

• Past use of steroids, like prednisone
• Unexplained weight loss
• Pain that worsens or does not get better when you stop moving and rest
• Previous history of back injury
• Problems with your bladder or bowel
• Weakness in your legs
• Severe pain restricting complete mobility
• A history of cancer

How is back pain treated?

Most of the time, back pain gets better in two to four weeks with very little treatment. This treatment usually consists of:
• Maintaining usual activity
• Minimizing bed rest since it may slow the healing process
• Taking over-the-counter pain medications
• Applying ice in the first one to three days.

If symptoms don't improve within three to four weeks, your doctor may send you to a therapist to receive special exercises.

How can I prevent back pain?

It is common for back pain to recur. Therefore, it is important to follow simple prevention measures to avoid chronic pain.
• If related to a work injury, discuss preventive measures with your supervisor or occupational health staff.
• Use correct lifting and moving techniques (bend your knees, use leg muscles to lift, tighten stomach, avoid bending when lifting).
• Exercise regularly to keep your back muscles strong and flexible.
• Don't slouch; poor posture puts a strain on your lower back.
• Maintain your proper body weight to avoid straining your back muscles.
• Maintain a positive attitude about your personal and professional life. Studies have shown an increased tendency for low back problems in people who are unhappy with their personal life.

Chapter 36

Osteoarthritis

Debora Kwan, BScPhm, MSc and Christine Papoushek, PharmD

Pathophysiology

Osteoarthritis (OA) is the most common form of arthritis. There is no universally accepted definition of OA, but it is characterized by abnormalities in the synthesis and degradation of articular cartilage in synovial joints. It is estimated to affect 1 in 10 Canadian adults.[1] In the elderly, it ranks second to cardiovascular disease in terms of causing chronic disability.[2]

OA results from damage and destabilization of synovial joints. Synovial joints are structures in which the opposing bony surfaces are covered with a layer of cartilage. There is also a joint cavity containing synovial fluid and lined with synovial membrane.[3] Cartilage acts as a shock absorber and, with synovial fluid, provides a smooth, low-friction surface for movement. Surrounding the joints is the articular capsule, ligaments, muscles and tendons, all of which act to stabilize and protect the joint.

Synovial joints are present in fingers, wrists, ankles, knees and hips. In a normal joint, cartilage is in a continuous process of formation and degradation. In OA, two processes occur which lead to joint destruction. First, there is progressive cartilage breakdown without adequate formation, leading to thinning of the articular cartilage and instability of the joint. Second, *osteophytes* or bony outgrowths appear. These represent new bone formation in areas away from the area of cartilage destruction. Although the role of osteophytes is unclear, they may act in part as stabilizers in response to joint destruction.

The most significant risk factor for OA is advancing age. Other risk factors include obesity, quadriceps muscle weakness, genetic susceptibility, major trauma and joint overuse or injury associated with certain sports and occupations.[4]

It is estimated that by age 65, up to 70% of people will have radiographic evidence of OA. However, only one-third of them will complain of symptoms.

Goals of Therapy

- Relieve symptoms
- Maintain or improve mobility
- Minimize functional disability and improve physical functioning
- Educate patients and caregivers to assist them to understand their condition and make informed decisions about which therapies to choose

Patient Assessment

Joint pain is the most common symptom of OA. The pain does not arise from the damaged cartilage itself, but is the result of the various stresses placed on the muscles, ligaments and tendons in the areas surrounding the cartilage as a result of the damage. Stiffness after inactivity and limited range of motion are other common symptoms. Inflammation may or may not be present. Crepitus may be present with joint movement. Table 1 lists the signs and symptoms of OA.

Rheumatoid arthritis is a systemic inflammatory disease that often presents with joint pain as one of many symptoms. The scope of this chapter does not include the management of rheumatoid arthritis; however, symptom recognition is important so that patients with suspected rheumatoid arthritis can be referred to a physician for a full work-up and appropriate therapy to control inflammation and delay disease progression (Table 1).

Since joint pain can have a number of causes, it is important that more serious conditions requiring medical intervention be ruled out. In particular, recent history of significant trauma, hot, swollen joints and signs and symptoms of infection should prompt a physician referral.

Reports of arthralgia have occurred with numerous drugs; however, the numbers are small and often a cause and effect relationship cannot be clearly established. There are also a number of medications that have been implicated in drug-induced systemic lupus erythematosus (SLE), of which arthalgia is often a presenting symptom. Medications associated with SLE include: acebutolol, carbamazepine, chlorpromazine, hydralazine, isoniazid, methyldopa, minocycline, penicillamine, procainamide, quinidine and sulfasalazine.[6] Fortunately, these arthalgias usually resolve with discontinuation of the offending agent.

Figure 1 shows an algorithm for assessing patients with joint pain.

General Principles of Therapy

Current pharmacologic therapies for OA provide symptomatic relief but are not curative. Therefore, the choice of agent is based on a combination of risk versus benefit, cost and patient preference. Pharmacologic therapy should always be initiated in combination with nonpharmacologic modalities. If tolerated, pharmacologic therapies (except localized therapy) should be tried for at least two to four weeks in order to allow the patient to fully assess its effectiveness.

Nonpharmacologic Therapy

Nonpharmacologic therapy (Table 2) should always be initiated first or started concurrently with drug therapy. The quality of published evidence supporting these modalities is varied. There is reasonably good evidence to support the use of exercise,[8] exercise plus physiotherapy,[22] TENS[19] and patient education for self-management and social support.[11-14]

Surgery is usually reserved as a last resort for patients with severe, painful and activity-limiting OA who have tried other pharmacologic and nonpharmacologic modalities.[17]

Table 1: **Clinical Features of Osteoarthritis versus Rheumatoid Arthritis[5]**

Feature	Osteoarthritis	Rheumatoid arthritis
Symptoms:		
Stiffness	Morning or after periods of inactivity; usually lasts < 30 min	Significant, prolonged (> 60 min) in the morning
Symptoms localized	Yes – limited to affected joints	No
Pain	Worsens with activity or after prolonged use (especially with weight bearing activity).	Worsens after prolonged inactivity; usually improves with activity.
Signs:		
Symmetry	Occasional	Common
Tenderness	Unusual	Over entire exposed joint spaces.
Inflammation	Unusual	Common
Instability	Occasional; buckling or joint instability can result in decreased range of movement and falls.	Uncommon
Multisystem disease	No	Often feel systemically unwell (e.g., can have one or more of fatigue, fever, chills, weight loss, hair loss, dry mouth or dry eyes)

Figure 1: **Assessment of Patients with Joint Pain**[3,7]

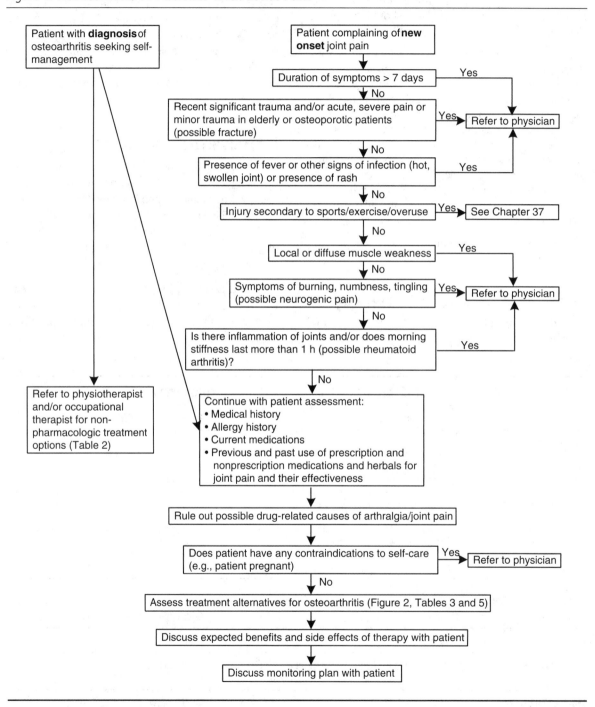

Table 2: **Nonpharmacologic Therapy for Osteoarthritis**

Modalities supported by evidence	Purpose/Benefits
Strength training and aerobic exercise[8,9,10]	• Reduce pain • Preserve flexibility • Improve range of motion and strength • Decrease need for analgesic medication and decrease physician visits
Patient education for self-management[11]	• Reduce pain • Decrease frequency of physician visits • Overall improvement in quality of life
Social support (e.g., telephone follow-up);[12,13] education of family members and caregivers[14]	• Improve pain and functional status
Use of ambulation aids and assistive devices (e.g., canes, grab bar, raised toilet seat)[15,16]	• Improve functional status and ambulation • Facilitate carrying out activities of daily living
Joint protection (e.g., splints, braces) and energy conservation (e.g., avoidance of stair climbing, take short rest periods, pace activities)[17]	• Minimize pain • Improve joint function
Weight loss in obesity (i.e., reduction in body fat)[18]	• Decrease load on weight bearing joints • Improvement in symptoms in OA of knee
Corrective footwear[17]	• To correct abnormal biomechanics secondary to OA knee
Surgery[17]	• Indicated in patients with severe symptomatic OA who have failed nonsurgical strategies and continue to have significant limitations in activities of daily living
TENS (transcutaneous electrical nerve stimulation)[19]	• Pain control in OA knee
Acupuncture[20]	• May improve pain, not function in OA knee
Lack of evidence to support use of these modalities	
Heat, cold, massage	• Lack of well-designed randomized controlled trials • Anecdotal evidence suggests alleviation of pain • Massage produces counterirritation
Low level laser[21]	• Lack of evidence and inconsistencies between trials to recommend use in OA

Pharmacologic Therapy

Nonprescription Agents (Table 3)

Acetaminophen

The American College of Rheumatology recommends acetaminophen as the initial drug of choice for symptomatic relief of OA.[17] The rationale for using acetaminophen is largely based on the fact that it is relatively safe, well tolerated and easily accessible. Acetaminophen and NSAIDs are comparable in their ability to provide pain relief in mild to moderate OA of the knee.[26,27] There are no published trials of acetaminophen in OA of the hip.

Maximum therapeutic doses should be tried for an adequate period (two to three weeks) in order to assess efficacy. Conditions such as chronic alcohol abuse and liver disease preclude the long-term use of maximum therapeutic doses and should be investigated prior to beginning therapy.

Table 3: **Nonprescription Therapy of Osteoarthritis**[3,7,23,25,26]

Drug	Therapeutic effects and usual dose	Onset of action	Adverse effects/ Precautions	Clinically significant drug interactions	Comments
Oral analgesics:					
Acetaminophen	325-1000 mg q4-6h SR: 650 mg q8h (max 4 g per day)	Maximal onset of pain relief within 24-48 h	Hepatotoxicity – increased risk in patients with excessive alcohol intake (> 3 drinks per day), malnourishment or pre-existing hepatic disease. Baseline LFTs should be measured in high-risk patients.	Alcohol (see precautions). Warfarin (with regular use of > 2 g per day acetaminophen). Phenytoin (may increase metabolism of acetaminophen and formation of toxic metabolite thereby increasing the risk of hepatotoxicity; risk may be higher in patients taking high thera-peutic doses of acetaminophen and phenytoin chronically. Interaction has not been well-documented).	Lower doses may be required in patients with severe hepatic and renal disease. Caution with concurrent use of acetaminophen-containing OTC products (do not exceed 4 g per day). Continuous therapy should be considered in individuals with pain persisting throughout the day. PRN dosing is acceptable for episodic pain of short duration.
NSAIDs: ASA Ibuprofen	Ibuprofen: 200-400 mg q6-8h; usual maximum daily dose: 3200 mg per day. ASA: 325-650 mg q6-8h; usual maximum daily dose: 3900 mg per day (not recom-mended for use if CrCl < 10 mL/min)		Local GI effects: dyspepsia, diarrhea. GI complications: ulcera-tion/upper GI bleed. CHF may be exacerbated by use of NSAIDs. Renal effects: more likely in elderly or patients with pre-existing renal disease or comorbid conditions that may affect renal func-tion (e.g., diabetes, CHF, hypertension). ↑ LFTs: transient; hepato-toxicity is rare; more likely to occur in patients with pre-existing hepatic dis-ease or in patients with excessive alcohol intake (> 3 drinks per day).	Warfarin (↑ bleeding risk); monitor INR more frequently during initial period after NSAID started and watch for signs of bleeding. ↑ Lithium levels – monitor levels. ↑ Methotrexate levels (rare) – monitor for toxicity. Antihypertensives (e.g., beta-blockers, diuretics, ACEI): possible ↓ in antihypertensive effects. Measure baseline BP, then remeasure in 1-2 wk and adjust antihypertensive therapy as required.	NSAIDs are not a substitute for ASA being taken for MI or stroke prophy-laxis. Avoid concurrent use of NSAID-containing OTC products (increased risk of GI-related side effects). Continuous therapy should be considered in individuals with pain persisting throughout the day. PRN dosing is acceptable for episodic pain of short duration. Consider prophylaxis with misoprostol or proton pump inhibitor in high risk patients (Table 4). Avoid NSAIDs in patients with ASA or ibuprofen hypersensitivity.

Acetaminophen + caffeine + codeine 8 mg	1-2 tablets q4-6h (maximum 4 g acetaminophen per day)	See acetaminophen. Sedation, nausea, vomiting, constipation	See acetaminophen. Concurrent use of other sedating or constipating medications	Recommended for short-term use only (e.g., 2-3 days). Elderly are at increased risk for adverse effects.
Alternative therapies:			
Glucosamine sulfate Glucosamine HCl Chondroitin sulfate	Glucosamine sulfate 500 mg TID (more extensively studied than HCl product). Chondroitin 400 mg TID Onset: 1-3 wks	Nausea, dyspepsia, diarrhea. Glucosamine products derived from marine exoskeletons might cause allergic reactions in people with shellfish allergies. To date, no such reactions have been documented.		Long term efficacy and toxicity are unknown. Lack of product standardization may result in inter- and intra- product variation. Less evidence for efficacy of chondroitin compared to glucosamine. Awaiting results of study sponsored by National Institute of Health (NIH) comparing monotherapy of each and combination therapy.

SR = sustained release

NSAIDs

Only ibuprofen and ASA are available without a prescription in Canada. Both the American College of Rheumatology[17] and the American Geriatrics Society[28] recommend NSAIDs as second-line therapy after failure of acetaminophen in management of OA pain. Although acetaminophen is superior in terms of safety, NSAIDs are preferred by OA patients due to better pain relief.[29,30] Not surprisingly, patients who discontinue NSAID use due to toxicity are less willing to resume therapy with another NSAID.[29]

In terms of which NSAID is the most efficacious or safest in OA, there are no definitive data to indicate the superiority of one over another. Systematic reviews have consistently identified lack of standardization in case definition of OA, outcome assessments[31] and failure to use therapeutically equivalent doses[32] as limitations to being able to draw any conclusions.

GI complications are the side effects of greatest concern with NSAID therapy.

Common local GI effects such as nausea and dyspepsia occur in approximately 10 to 20% of NSAID users and are relatively minor in clinical significance. More serious GI complications such as perforated ulcers and hemorrhage have been estimated to occur in OA patients at an incidence of less than 1% per year.[33] Although the incidence appears low, because NSAIDs are one of the most commonly prescribed drug classes, a relatively large number of patients is affected. Unfortunately, the presence of local GI symptoms such as dyspepsia is not a predictor for serious GI complications and vice versa. There is also no definitive evidence to show that one NSAID has an advantage over another in terms of causing GI complications. However, there are several factors that increase a patient's risk for the development of upper GI adverse events (Table 4).

Prior to starting NSAID therapy, patients at risk of developing serious NSAID-related GI complications should be identified and preventive measures taken. H_2RAs and antacids provide relief from dyspeptic symptoms, but not against more serious GI complications. Misoprostol and proton pump inhibitors such as omeprazole are both appropriate options for preventing serious GI complications such as gastric ulcer, perforation, gastric outlet obstruction or bleeding.[25,34,35]

Table 4: **Risk Factors for the Development of Upper GI Adverse Events**[17,33]

Established:
Age ≥ 65 yrs
History of ulcer
Concomitant use of corticosteroids, anticoagulants
Use of higher doses of NSAIDs
Use of more than one NSAID
Presence of multiple systemic disorders

Possible:
Concomitant infection with *Helicobacter pylori*
Cigarette smoking
Regular alcohol consumption

Combination Products

Numerous combination analgesic products containing codeine 8 mg are available OTC. The effectiveness of using low-dose combination codeine products compared with single ingredient products (e.g., NSAIDs, acetaminophen) for OA has not been adequately studied.

Topical Counterirritants (Table 5)

Although there is little evidence to support their use in OA, topical agents are a reasonable alternative for patients who cannot tolerate or are reluctant to use systemic agents. They may also be tried as an adjunct to systemic agents where pain relief is not adequate.

Methyl salicylate and **trolamine salicyate** act as counterirritants and analgesics. Methyl salicylate has not been shown to improve symptoms in osteoarthritis. One study found trolamine salicylate was significantly better than placebo in improving pain and stiffness in patients with OA of the hands.[36] Since they are readily available OTC, the potential exists for overuse of these products leading to salicylate toxicity.[37]

The evidence for using **capsaicin** in OA is limited to a few small, short-term studies[38-40] and one meta-analysis.[41] Compared with placebo, capsaicin has been shown to decrease pain symptoms over a 4 to 12 week period in patients with OA of the hand[40] or knee.[38,39] In these studies, concomitant use of acetaminophen[38] or NSAIDs[39,40] was permitted. Capsaicin's role in OA management may be more as adjuvant therapy after unsatisfactory trials of acetaminophen or NSAIDs. Unfortunately, the tingling and burning sensation caused by capsaicin often prevents an adequate trial of this medication.

Alternative Agents

Glucosamine and **chondroitin** are endogenous substances that are responsible for maintaining the integrity of cartilage within a joint. Exogenous formulations (i.e., glucosamine sulfate, glucosamine hydrochloride, chondroitin sulfate) have been evaluated in the treatment of OA primarily for their pharmacologic effect that mimics their physiologic effect on cartilage tissue. The proposed mechanisms of action are to stimulate the production of cartilage, prevent cartilage destruction by inhibiting inflammatory mediators and/or enzymes, and maintain viscosity of the joint.[42,43] This may result in positive outcomes such as a decrease in pain and an increase in function. In addition, preliminary studies suggest these agents may possess chondroprotective effects resulting in a decrease in joint space narrowing.[44] However, this finding needs to be further validated and quantified in larger studies.[45]

Evidence suggests that these agents *may* be beneficial in decreasing pain and increasing mobility in the short-term.[46,47] However, limitations with respect to study design, publication bias, long-term efficacy and safety, and product variation may influence the individual results seen with these agents.[17] As a result, these agents should not be recommended as first-line therapy.

Prescription Medications

COX-2 Inhibitors

Celecoxib and **rofecoxib** are as effective as NSAIDs for pain control in OA of the hip and knee[48] and are

Table 5: **Nonprescription Topical Counterirritants for Osteoarthritis**[3,23]

Drug	Dose and onset	Adverse effects/ Precautions	Drug interactions (clinically significant)	Comments
Methyl salicylate Trolamine salicylate	For all products: Apply up to 3-4 times per day. Onset of maximal effect: 2-4 wks (with continuous usage)	Avoid in ASA allergic patients. Use with caution in patients with conditions associated with ASA sensitivity (i.e., severe asthma or nasal polyps). Salicylate toxicity may occur if applied over large surface area or on broken skin.	Warfarin: Potentiation of anticoagulant effects; monitor INR more frequently and watch for signs of bleeding if ongoing concurrent use (especially if topical product is being applied over a large area).	For all products: Do not apply near mucous membranes or on broken skin. Do not cover with tight or occlusive dressing. Do not place heating devices (e.g., hot water bottle, heating pad) on skin after application of product.
Menthol		Discontinue if hypersensitivity occurs (signs include irritation, rash, burning, stinging, swelling or infection).		
Capsaicin	Capsaicin should be applied 3-4 times per day continuously for 2-4 wks to achieve maximum therapeutic effect	Apply with gloves and wash hands thoroughly after application to avoid irritation of other areas. Tingling, burning or redness will occur in the majority of patients. Usually decreases within 72 h with repeated use; if effect is bothersome, pre-treatment with topical lidocaine or EMLA® cream may help.		

associated with a lower incidence of gastroduodenal ulcers compared to NSAIDs.[49,50] The comparative safety of COX-2 inhibitors versus NSAIDs plus cytoprotection has not been evaluated. Similar to NSAIDs, COX-2 inhibitors can exacerbate pre-existing renal disease. Baseline and periodic monitoring of creatinine clearance and electrolytes should be carried out in high-risk patients.

Localized Therapy

The use of **intra-articular corticosteroids** in OA is limited to acute knee pain and patients who have local signs of inflammation and joint effusion. If joints are painful and swollen, aspiration of fluid followed by intra-articular injection of a glucocorticoid (e.g., triamcinolone hexacetonide) is effective in temporarily (i.e., four to six weeks) decreasing pain and increasing quadriceps strength.[7] It is often used in combination with other therapies, although it can be used as monotherapy. Repeated injections may damage cartilage. As such, it is recommended that the same site not be injected more than three to four times per year.[7,17]

The efficacy of intra-articular corticosteroids for hip OA has not been studied and use is not routinely recommended because of the risk of cartilage damage through repeated injections.[15]

Hyaluronan is a linear polysaccharide found in synovial fluid. Three to five weekly injections have modest pain relieving effects in patients with mild to moderate OA of the knee.[7] The onset of pain relief is slower than with corticosteroids, although the effect may last longer. The effect of repeated courses of hyaluronan injections is unknown. The injections are expensive, costing over $200 for three injections. The use of these products is usually reserved for those patients who have failed other therapies.

Narcotic Analgesics

In patients who do not respond to other analgesics or experience acute exacerbations of OA pain, a narcotic analgesic used alone or in combination with acetaminophen or NSAIDs may be useful.[17] However, side effects such as sedation, constipation, tolerance and dependence limit the long-term use of these agents.

Figure 2 summarizes various osteoarthritis treatment options.

Figure 2: **Algorithm for Treatment of Osteoarthritis**

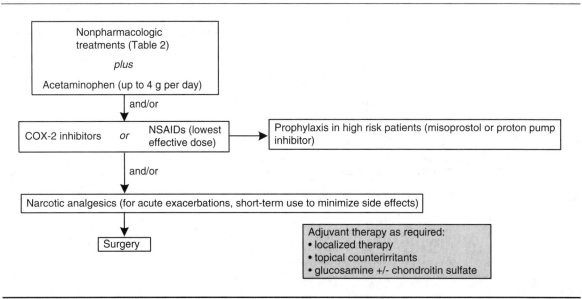

Monitoring of Therapy

Table 6 provides a monitoring plan for patients with osteoarthritis.

Advice for the Patient

Counsel patients on:

- The importance of using nondrug measures concurrently with medication therapy;
- Expected benefits of therapy;
- Possible side effects and their management;
- When to contact a physician.

Resource Tips

For more information on OA contact:
The Arthritis Society (National Office)
393 University Avenue, Suite 1700
Toronto, Ontario M5G 1E6
Canada
Tel.: 1-800-321-1433
Web site: www.arthritis.ca

Table 6: **Monitoring Therapy of Osteoarthritis**

Parameter	Degree	Timeframe	Action/Comments

Pain relief	Elimination or improvement toward predefined goals as set by patient	**Patient:** assess daily
		Pharmacist: phone call on days 3, 7, 14 and 28
			Refer to physician if not receiving symptom relief after adequate trial of at least two analgesics or on development of new or worsening pain during therapy.
			Considerations:
			• Use visual analog scale or other individual measure to quantify and characterize pain (e.g., ADLs – walking, gardening)
			• Establish acceptable level of pain control and functioning with the patient at the beginning of therapy
			•Considerations in timing of medications:
			  –Around-the-clock vs. PRN
			  –Take dose of analgesic at least 1 h prior to activities that may exacerbate pain.

Nausea, dyspepsia, abdominal discomfort	Minimal or none during therapy	**Patient:** monitor daily **Pharmacist:** phone call on days 3 and 7	Change therapy if symptoms severe or intolerable. Minimize development by advising to take with food or milk. Assess risk of GI complications (Table 4). If high risk, refer to physician. Otherwise, consider antacids or OTC H$_2$RAs to treat dyspepsia.
Hematemesis, melena, hematochezia	None during therapy	**Patient:** monitor daily on an ongoing basis **Pharmacist:** phone call on days 3 and 7	Patient should seek medical attention if these signs or symptoms develop. Discontinue therapy immediately.
Renal function and signs of fluid retention (e.g., weight gain or edema) in high risk patients (ASA or ibuprofen—see Table 3)	No significant change in renal function	**Physician:** Serum creatinine and Na+, K+ at baseline, q1-2 week × 3 then periodically afterwards. Patient to monitor for signs of fluid retention on an ongoing basis (e.g., edema; patients with severe CHF should measure their weight daily).	Discontinue NSAID if significant change in serum creatinine or electrolytes or signs of fluid retention.

ADL=activities of daily living; H$_2$RA = H$_2$-receptor antagonist

Suggested Readings

American College of Rheumatology Subcommittee on Osteoarthritis Guidelines. Recommendations for the medical management of osteoarthritis of the hip and knee: 2000 update. *Arthritis Rheum* 2000;43(9): 1905-15.

Chen SW, Gong WC. Rheumatic Disorders in: Koda-Kimble M, Young LY editors. *Applied Therapeutics: the Clinical Use of Drugs.* 7th edition. Lippincott Williams and Wilkins, 2001.

Clark BM. Rheumatology: 9. Physical and occupational therapy in the management of arthritis. *CMAJ* 2000; 163(8):999-1005.

Ontario Program for Optimal Therapeutics (OPOT). *Ontario Treatment Guidelines for Osteoarthritis, Rheumatoid Arthritis, and Acute Musculoskeletal Injury.* 1st ed. Toronto, ON: Queen's Printer of Ontario, 2000.

References

1. The Arthritis Society. Available at: www.arthritis.ca. Accessed on December 7, 2001.
2. Hawker G. Epidemiology of arthritis and osteoporosis. In: Williams J, Badley EM, eds. *Patterns of Health Care in Ontario: Arthritis and Related Conditions.* Toronto: ICES, 1998:1-10.
3. Allen LV, Berardi RR, DeSimone EM, Engle JP, Popovich NG, Rosenthal WM, Tietze KJ, eds. *Handbook of Nonprescription Drugs.* 12th ed. Washington DC: American Pharmaceutical Association, 2000.
4. Creamer P, Hochberg MC. Osteoarthritis. *Lancet* 1997;350: 503-9.
5. American College of Rheumatology Ad Hoc Committee on Clinical Guidelines. Guidelines for the initial evaluation of the adult patient with acute musculoskeletal symptoms. *Arthritis Rheum* 1996;39(1):1-8.
6. Vergne P, Bertin P, Bonnet C, Scotto C, Treves R. Drug-induced rheumatic disorders. *Drug Safety* 2000;23(4):279-93.
7. Ontario Program for Optimal Therapeutics (OPOT). *Ontario Treatment Guidelines for Osteoarthritis, Rheumatoid Arthritis, and Acute Musculoskeletal Injury.* 1st ed. Toronto, ON: Queen's Printer of Ontario, 2000.
8. Van Baar M, Assendelft WJJ, Dekker J, Oostendorp RA, Bijlsma JW. Effectiveness of exercise therapy in patients with osteoarthritis of the hip or knee: a systematic review of randomized clinical trials. *Arthritis Rheum* 1999;42:1361-9.
9. Ettinger WH Jr, Burns R, Messier SP, et al. A randomized trial comparing aerobic exercise and resistance exercise with a health education program in older adults with knee osteoarthritis: the Fitness Arthritis and Seniors Trial (FAST). *JAMA* 1997;277:25-31.
10. Van Baar ME, Dekker J, Oostendorp RAB, et al. The effectiveness of exercise therapy in patients with osteoarthritis of the hip or knee: a randomized clinical trial. *J Rheumatol* 1998;25:2432-9.
11. Superio-Cabuslay E, Ward MM, Lorig KR. Patient education interventions in osteoarthritis and rheumatoid arthritis: a meta-analytic comparison with nonsteroidal antiinflammatory drug treatment. *Arthritis Care Res* 1996;9:292-301
12. Weinberger M, Tierney WM, Cowper PA, Katz BP, Booher PA. Cost-effectiveness of increased telephone contact for patients with osteoarthritis. *Arthritis Rheum* 1993;36(2): 243-6.
13. Weinberger M, Tierney WM, Booher P, Katz BP. Can the provision of information to patients with osteoarthritis improve functional status? *Arthritis Rheum* 1989;32(12): 1577-83.
14. Keefe FJ, Caldwell DS, Baucom D, Salley A, Robinson E, Timmons K, et al. Spouse-assisted coping skills training in the management of osteoarthritic knee pain. *Arthritis Care Res* 1996;9:279-91.
15. Hochberg MC, Altman RD, Brandt KD, et al. Guidelines for the medical management of osteoarthritis. Part I. Osteoarthritis of the hip. American College of Rheumatology. *Arthritis Rheum* 1995;38:1535-40.
16. Hochberg MC, Altman RD, Brandt KD, et al. Guidelines for the medication management of osteoarthritis. Part II. Osteoarthritis of the knee. American College of Rheumatology. *Arthritis Rheum* 1995;38:1541-6.
17. American College of Rheumatology Subcommittee on Osteoarthritis Guidelines. Recommendations for the medical management of osteoarthritis of the hip and knee: 2000 update. *Arthritis Rheum* 2000;43(9):1905-15.
18. Toda Y, Toda T, Takemura S, Wada T, Morimoto T, Ogawa R. Change in body fat, but not body weight or metabolic correlates of obesity, is related to symptomatic relief of obese patients with knee osteoarthritis after a weight control program. *J Rheumatol* 1998;25:2181-6.
19. Osiri M, Welch V, Brosseau L, et al. Transcutaneous electrical nerve stimulation for knee osteoarthritis (Cochrane Review). In: *The Cochrane Library,* Issue 2, 2001. Oxford: Update Software.
20. Ezzo J, Hadhazy V, Birch S, et al. Acupuncture for osteoarthritis of the knee. *Arthritis Rheum* 2001;44(4):819-25.
21. Brosseau L, Welch V, Wells G, et al. Low level laser therapy (Classes I, II and III) for treating osteoarthritis (Cochrane Review). In: *The Cochrane Library,* Issue 2, 2001. Oxford: Update Software.
22. Deyle GD, Henderson NE, Matekel RL, Ryder MG, Garber MB, Allison SC. Effectiveness of manual physical therapy and exercise in osteoarthritis of the knee. *Ann Intern Med* 1999;132:173-81.
23. Micromedex Healthcare Series Vol. 108. Expiry December, 2001.
24. Balano, KB. Antiinflammatory drugs and myorelaxants. *Orthopedics* 1996;23(2):329-34.
25. Hawkey CJ, Karrasch JA, Szczepanski L, et al. Omeprazole compared with misoprostol for ulcers associated with nonsteroidal antiinflammatory drugs. *N Engl J Med* 1998;338:727-34.
26. Williams HJ, Ward JR, Egger MJ, et. al. Comparison of naproxen and acetaminophen in a two-year study of treatment of osteoarthritis of the knee. *Arthritis Rheum* 1993;36:1196-206.
27. Bradley JD, Brandt KD, Katz BP, Kalasinski LA, Ryan SI. Comparison of an antiinflammatory dose of ibuprofen, an analgesic dose of ibuprofen and acetaminophen in the treatment of patients with osteoarthritis of the knee. *N Engl J Med* 1991;325:87-91.

28. AGS Panel on Chronic Pain in Older Persons. The management of chronic pain in older persons. *J Am Geriatr Soc* 1998;46(5):635-51.

29. Pincus T, Swearingen C, Cummins P, Callahan LF. Preference for nonsteroidal antiinflammatory drugs versus acetaminophen and concomitant use of both types of drugs in patients with osteoarthritis. *J Rheumatol* 2000;27:1020-7.

30. Wolfe F, Zhao S, Lane N. Preference for nonsteroidal antiinflammatory drugs over acetaminophen by rheumatic disease patients. *Arthritis Rheum* 2000;43(2):378-85.

31. Towheed T, Shea B, Wells G, Hochberg M. Analgesia and non-aspirin, non-steroidal antiinflammatory drugs for osteoarthritis of the hip (Cochrane Review). In: *The Cochrane Library*, Issue 2, 2001. Oxford: Update Software.

32. Watson MC, Brookes ST, Kirwan JR, Faulkner A. Non-aspirin, non-steroidal antiinflammatory drugs for treating osteoarthritis of the knee (Cochrane Review). In: *The Cochrane Library*, Issue 2, 2001. Oxford: Update Software.

33. Wolfe MM, Lichtenstein DR, Singh G. Gastrointestinal toxicity of nonsteroidal antiinflammatory drugs. *N Engl J Med* 1999;340(24):1888-99.

34. Silverstein FE, Graham DY, Senior JR, et al. Misoprostol reduced serious gastrointestinal complications in patients with rheumatoid arthritis receiving nonsteroidal antiinflammatory drugs. *Ann Intern Med* 1995;123:241-9.

35. Raskin JB, White RH, Jackson JE, et al. Misoprostol dosage in the prevention of nonsteroidal antiinflammatory drug-induced gastric and duodenal ulcers: a comparison of three regimens. *Ann Intern Med* 1995;123:344-50.

36. Rothacker DQ, Lee I, Littlejohn TW. Topical NSAIDs for musculoskeletal conditions. A review of the literature effectiveness of a single topical application of 10% trolamine salicylate cream in the symptomatic treatment of osteoarthritis. *J Clin Rheumatol* 1998;4:6-12.

37. Joss JD, LeBlond RF. Potentiation of warfarin anticoagulation associated with topical methyl salicylate. *Ann Pharmacother* 2000;34:729-33.

38. Altman RD, Aven A, Holmburg CE, Pfeifer LM, Sack M, Young GT. Capsaicin cream 0.025% as monotherapy for osteoarthritis: a double-blind study. *Sem Arthritis Rheum* 1994;23(6):Suppl 3:25-33.

39. Deal CL, Schnitzer TJ, Lipstein E, Seibold JR, Stevens RM, Levy MD. Treatment of arthritis with topical capsaicin: a double-blind trial. *Clin Ther* 1991;13(3):383-95.

40. McCarthy GM, McCarty DJ. Effect of topical capsaicin in the therapy of painful osteoarthritis of the hands. *J Rheumatol* 1992;19:604-7.

41. Zhang WY, Po AL. The effectiveness of topically applied capsaicin. *Eur J Clin Pharmacol* 1994;46:517-22.

42. Da Camara CC, Dowless GV. Glucosamine sulfate for osteoarthritis. *Ann Pharmacother* 1998;32:580-7.

43. Deal CL, Moskowitz RW. Nutraceuticals as therapuetic agents in osteoarthritis. *Osteoarthritis* 1999;25(2):379-94.

44. Reginster JY, Deroisy R, Rovati LC, et al. Long-term effects of glucosamine sulfate on osteoarthritis progression: a randomised placebo-controlled clinical trial. *Lancet* 2001;357:251-56.

45. Lippiello L, Woodward J, Karpman R, Hammad TA. In vivo chondroprotection and metabolic synergy of glucosamine and chondroitin sulfate. *Clin Orthop* 2000;381:229-40.

46. Towheed TE, Anastassiades TP, Shea B, Houpt J, Welch V, Hochberg MC. Glucosamine therapy for treating osteoarthritis (Cochrane Review). In: *The Cochrane Library*, Issue 2, 2001. Oxford: Update Software.

47. McAlindon TE, LaValley MP, Gulin JP, Felson DT. Glucosamine and chondroitin for treatment of osteoarthritis: a systematic quality assessment and meta-analysis. *JAMA* 2000;283(11):1469-75.

48. Tannenbaum H, Peloso PMJ, Russell AS, Marlow B. An evidence-based approach to prescribing NSAIDs in the treatment of osteoarthritis and rheumatoid arthritis: the second Canadian consensus conference. *Can J Clin Pharmacol* 2000;7:suppl A.

49. Bombardier C, Laine L, Reicin A, et. al. Comparison of upper gastrointestinal toxicity of rofecoxib and naproxen in patients with rheumatoid arthritis. *N Engl J Med* 2000;343(21):1520-8.

50. Silverstein FE, Faich G, Goldstein JL, et. al. Gastrointestinal toxicity with celecoxib vs. nonsteroidal antiinflammatory drugs for osteoarthritis and rheumatoid arthritis. *JAMA* 2000;284(10):1247-55.

Osteoarthritis—Patient Information

What is osteoarthritis?

Osteoarthritis (OA) is also known as degenerative joint disease. It is the most common kind of arthritis. It usually affects the joints of the neck, lower back, knees, hips and fingers of middle-aged and older people.

What causes osteoarthritis?

OA results from breakdown of joint cartilage. This can happen for many reasons. Some kinds of OA are passed from one generation to the next. In most people, OA occurs when the cartilage that normally cushions and protects the joints becomes worn down or works less efficiently. The wear and tear on the joints may also occur in joints that have suffered previous injury or been subjected to prolonged heavy use.

What are the signs and symptoms of osteoarthritis?

People with OA experience pain, stiffness and poor function in or around the joint. Sometimes a grating sound can be heard when moving the joint.

OA can be diagnosed by your doctor using a combination of X-rays, physical examination and ruling out other types of arthritis.

The goals of treatment are to:

- Decrease pain and discomfort so that you can continue to carry out your usual daily activities;
- Protect your joints.

Always try non-drug measures first and combine them with drugs if needed.

Non-drug measures:

- Consult a physiotherapist and/or occupational therapist for tips on exercises and devices to reduce pain, strengthen and protect the affected joints.
- Consider weight loss if you are overweight to relieve stress on your joints.
- Learn as much as you can about OA to improve your knowledge about how best to manage pain and protect your joints.

Nonprescription medications:

There are several types of medications available for helping with OA pain. If you need to use pain medication for more than seven days in a row, talk to your doctor to see if this is the best treatment for you.

Chapter 37

Sports Injuries

Lily Lum, BScPharm

Pathophysiology

Participation in sports activities and exercise programs is increasing as people become more health conscious. Although commonly associated with health benefits, sport and exercise can also cause injuries.[1,2] Individuals in all age groups benefit from regular exercise when it is performed properly. In people over 45 years of age, the benefits of exercise (e.g., prevention of coronary heart disease and osteoporosis) outweigh the risk of sports-related injuries. However, younger individuals appear to derive less benefit from exercise in terms of disease prevention and may be involved in exercise or sports activities that carry a relatively high risk of injury.[3,4]

The types of sports-related injuries that can occur in athletes or individuals are varied. Sports-related injuries can be caused by trauma, overuse of specific parts of the body such as muscles or joints, and environmental factors.[4] Acute injuries such as ligament sprains and muscle strains are usually caused by sudden trauma and are more likely to occur in contact sports. Overuse or chronic injuries are more subtle and are most commonly associated with sports that involve repetitive movements. The acronym of the **3Fs** or the **terrible toos** – too fast, too far and too frequent – is often used to describe the cause of overuse injuries.[1] Some of the more common sports-related injuries such as strains and sprains, overuse injuries (e.g., Achilles tendinitis, bursitis, plantar fasciitis, shin splints, and tennis elbow), and stress fractures are defined in the following section.[1,4-6]

Bursitis

Bursitis is the inflammation of a bursa. Bursa are tiny, fluid-containing sac-like structures that are located wherever there might be friction, such as between bones and the muscles and tendons near joints

(Figure 1). When they become inflamed, movement or pressure is painful. The most common areas where bursitis occurs are the elbow, knee and shoulder.

Sprain

A sprain is an injury to a ligament caused by over-stretching or twisting. In the ankle, a common area for sprains, it is mainly the lateral ligaments of the joint that tear. Symptoms include pain, swelling and tenderness, with later bruising around the injury. Symptomatically, severe sprains may be difficult to differentiate from fractures and an X-ray may be needed to make a firm diagnosis.[1,4]

Strain

A strain is an injury to a muscle and is also referred to as a torn or pulled muscle. It is usually caused by overstretching and is characterized by pain and swelling. Muscle strains vary in severity, from damage to the fibers with the muscle sheath left intact, to complete rupture of the muscle.[1,6]

Plantar Fasciitis

A common condition causing heel pain, plantar fasciitis involves inflammation of the plantar fascia, the tough, fibrous band of tissue that runs along the sole of the foot. Inflammation usually occurs following increased or repetitive activity such as jogging.[6,7]

Shin Splints

Shin pain resulting from damage to the muscles along the shin is known as shin splints.[5]

Stress Fractures

Tiny cracks in bones that often result from repeated, excessive impact are stress fractures.[6] Any bone can suffer a stress fracture but they usually happen in the feet, ankle, and legs. An individual may not even notice when a stress fracture initially occurs. The pain decreases with rest and increases with activity. The pain increases over time and gets worse when pressure is applied. Pain starts progressively earlier in the workout and may become so severe that it prohibits exercise and persists even during rest. The area may or may not show signs of tenderness and swelling. Athletes required to jump repetitively (e.g., gymnasts, basketball players) often get stress fractures.[8] They can be mistaken for shin splints because both can cause mid-calf discomfort. However, stress fractures are more serious than shin splints, the pain lasts longer, and the injury takes longer to heal.

Tendonitis

Tendonitis is the inflammation of a tendon, a thick fibrous cord that attaches muscle to bone. Two common examples of tendonitis are Achilles tendonitis and tennis elbow. *Achilles tendonitis* is inflammation of the Achilles tendon (tendon which connects the heel to the calf muscle).[5] The patient with Achilles tendonitis experiences pain and tenderness just above the heel.

Tennis elbow, also known as lateral epicondylitis, is an inflammation of the tendons attached to the outside, or lateral side, of the elbow at the bony prominence of the arm bone.[6] It commonly occurs in racquet sports and activities that require repetitive, one-sided movements (such as tennis). The patient experiences pain and tenderness outside of the area at and below the elbow joint.

Sports injuries can also be caused by environmental factors. Disorders such as heat stroke can occur in athletes or individuals participating in outdoor sports activities during hot temperatures.[1] For further information on heat-related illness, see Chapter 10.

Goals of Therapy

- Provide relief of symptoms
- Promote healing of the injury
- Prevent re-injury or aggravation of the injury

Patient Assessment

An assessment plan for patients suffering from musculoskeletal sports injuries is illustrated in Figure 2.

Figure 1: **Knee Joint—Sagital Section**

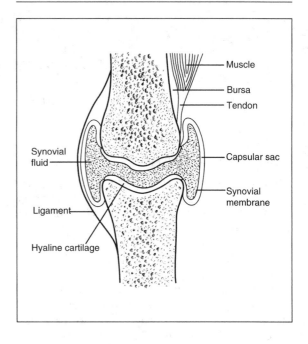

Symptoms of selected non-soft tissue injuries that require immediate medical attention are described in Table 1.

Prevention

Proper conditioning and training prevent many sports-related injuries. Muscle pain and stiffness commonly occur 24 hours after unaccustomed intense physical activity.[6] Appropriate warm-up exercises, stretching and cooling down (gradually slowing down before stopping the exercise) should be routinely performed. Warmed up muscles are more pliable and less likely to tear. Stretching allows the muscles to lengthen so that they can contract and perform more effectively. Cooling down can prevent dizziness and fainting. In a person who exercises vigorously and suddenly stops, blood can pool in the dilated leg veins causing dizziness and fainting. Cooling down maintains the increased circulation and helps clear the build-up of lactic acid in the bloodstream.[5] A gradual increase in the intensity and duration of workouts and adequate fluid replacement are also important preventive measures.

Figure 2: **Assessment of Patients with Musculoskeletal Sports Injuries**

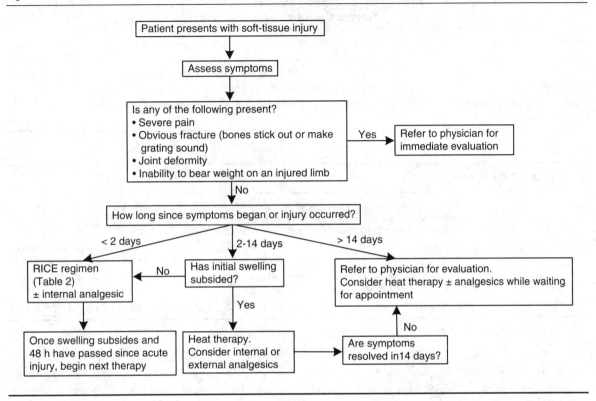

RICE = Rest, Ice, Compression, Elevation

Warning signs of impending injury include extreme fatigue, pain and lack of enthusiasm for training.[1] Protective equipment (e.g., helmet, eye protection, mouth guard, knee and wrist pads) and proper footwear are essential for those participating in sports with a high risk of falls (e.g., in-line skating) or those requiring direct contact with playing equipment or other players (e.g., boxing, football).[4,13] Note that eyeglasses cannot be relied upon for eye protection.

Nonpharmacologic Therapy

The four essentials of early management of soft-tissue injuries can be remembered by the acronym **RICE**: **R**est, **I**ce, **C**ompression, **E**levation (Table 2).[1,4,5]

After 48 hours have passed and the initial swelling has subsided, the RICE regimen may be replaced by heat, massage and/or rehabilitation with physical therapy if necessary.[5]

Heat Versus Cold Therapy

Should patients apply heat or cold therapy to a sports injury? As a general rule, the application of cold is the preferred immediate treatment (i.e., first 24 to 48 hours) for most acute musculoskeletal injuries.[14] Sources of cold therapy include ice bags (putting crushed ice in a thick plastic bag), commercial cold gel packs, or simply bags of frozen peas or corn.[15] The application time for cold therapy varies depending on the body part and comfort but usually ranges from 10 to 30 minutes. Apply cold at regular intervals throughout the waking hours of the day, allowing a few hours between treatments. Areas with little body fat (bony areas such as the knee, ankle and elbow) do not tolerate cold as well as fatty areas (such as thigh and buttocks). For bony areas, application time should be kept to the lower end (10 minutes); double the time when applying to fatty areas. Applying too much cold for too long can cause frostbite and tissue damage. A

Table 1: **Selected Injuries Requiring Immediate Medical Attention**[6,8-12]

Injury	Symptoms that warrant immediate medical attention
Eye injury	Blurred vision, loss of vision, moderate to severe eye discomfort or pain.
Head injury	Confusion, amnesia, headache, loss of consciousness after injury, tinnitus, drowsiness, dizziness, nausea, vomiting, convulsions, unusual eye movements or slurred speech.
Nosebleed	Bleeding lasting longer than 20 min.
Tympanic membrane perforation (ruptured eardrum)	Earache, partial hearing loss, slight bleeding or discharge from ear.

Table 2: **RICE Regimen**

Rest	Immobilization is recommended for at least the first 24 h to avoid aggravation of the injury. If long term rest is indicated, the unaffected joint(s) should be exercised to prevent tissue atrophy and loss of coordination. Rest for a prolonged period of time is usually discouraged for muscle injuries.
Ice	The application of cold (*cryotherapy*) to an injury reduces local blood flow by constricting blood vessels, limiting the swelling. Apply cold therapy at regular intervals allowing a few hours between treatments.
Compression	An elasticized bandage applied to an injured area for at least the first 24 h can reduce swelling, support a weak joint or provide a protective layer for wounds.
Elevation	The injured area should be raised above the level of the heart to help drain fluid and reduce swelling.

thin towel can be placed between the ice bag and skin to prevent frostbite. Cold therapy should be used with caution by patients with poor circulation such as those with diabetes or Raynaud's disease since these patients already have reduced local blood flow.[15]

Heat therapy is recommended after the first 48 hours, when the swelling has subsided, and during the chronic rehabilitative phases of the injury.[16] Local heat possesses a number of properties: it produces analgesia through its effect on free nerve endings, decreases the incidence of painful muscle spasm by relaxing muscles and reduces joint stiffness by decreasing synovial fluid viscosity. Heat causes vasodilation producing increased blood flow, which in turn helps provide a greater local supply of nutrients, oxygen, antibodies, leukocytes and enzymes to the injured area. Waste products from the inflammatory process are transported away with the increased blood circulation.[14] Heat may be applied for 20 to 30 minutes, every two to four hours as needed. Contraindications to the use of local heat therapy include patients who are unconscious, those with impaired skin sensitivity, poor circulation or open wounds.[14,16] Sources of local heat therapy include hot water bottles, electric heating pads, commercial heat packs and infrared heat lamps.[14] Care should be taken to avoid burns from the use of heat therapy products. Hot water bottles and heat packs can be wrapped with a towel or cloth for comfort and safety. Heating pads and heat lamps should be kept on low to moderate settings.[16]

Pharmacologic Therapy
Oral Analgesics
Oral analgesics such as acetaminophen and NSAIDs can provide effective relief of musculoskeletal pain.[1,4,5,17] They may be useful in acute as well as chronic injuries. Advise patients to take the lowest dose that is effective for relieving their pain and inflammation. Acetaminophen or NSAIDs can be given concurrently with opioids for an additive analgesic effect. Thus, codeine can be found in combination products for the treatment of moderate or moderately severe pain. When taken alone in usual doses (e.g., 15 to 30 mg), **codeine** is no more effective than ASA or acetaminophen.[18] Codeine is regarded as second-line therapy for management of sports injuries. Opioids, in general, may be drugs of choice in severe, acute pain or cancer pain but have

limited use for most sports injuries. With injuries such as bone fractures, which are often extremely painful, short-term use of acetaminophen and codeine combinations may be warranted.[17]

Muscle Relaxants

Nonprescription muscle relaxants (e.g., methocarbamol, chlorzoxazone) generally are intended to provide pain relief when muscle spasm is a component of an acute injury. However, muscle relaxants are not routinely recommended and are not considered first line therapy in acute musculoskeletal injuries because of their limited effectiveness in providing pain relief.[19]

Table 3 lists the most common oral pharmacologic agents used in sports injuries.

External Analgesics

External analgesics (e.g., methyl salicylate, menthol, camphor, capsaicin) have been traditional remedies for the treatment of general aches and pains. Although of limited value, they may be useful during rehabilitation as cooling or heating rubs or as accompaniments to massage therapy.[1] Although most physicians do not prescribe external analgesics, patients frequently purchase these products for self-treatment.[17]

Some patients may experience skin sensitivity to these products, such as rash or blisters. External analgesics should not be applied to acute injuries where there is bleeding, under dressings or on open wounds, since they may further irritate the wound area.[1] They should not be used more than three or four times a day. It is also advisable not to use external analgesics concurrently with thermotherapy devices since burns may result.[22]

Topical NSAIDs

Although the role of oral NSAIDs is well established in reducing pain, swelling and inflammation resulting from sports injuries, the use of topical NSAIDs is not well established.[23-25] It is theorized that topical application minimizes the risk of side effects associ-

ated with systemic therapy (e.g., gastrointestinal toxicity). In Canada, no topical NSAIDs are currently marketed for the treatment of acute soft tissue injuries. Pharmacists can extemporaneously compound these products. Special commercial bases (e.g., Phlogel®, Diffusimax®) are available for extemporaneous compounding of topical NSAIDs. Some NSAIDs commonly incorporated into topical formulations include diclofenac and ketoprofen.[26-28] A meta-analysis of 86 randomized, placebo-controlled trials of transdermal NSAIDs involving 10 160 patients concluded that topical NSAIDs are effective in relieving pain in acute and chronic conditions.[29]

Corticosteroid Injections

Many painful conditions involving tendonitis improve with local corticosteroid injection therapy. Several precautions should be taken when considering such therapy. For example, the number of injections in any area or joint should be limited to three per year because of concerns about the risk of tendon rupture and osteoporosis.[30,31]

Vapocoolants

Some topical anesthetic preparations, known as vapocoolants or refrigerants (e.g., ethyl chloride, Fluori-Methane®), may be useful when applied topically to control the pain associated with injuries such as sprained ankles and bursitis. Side effects appear to be minimal, although cutaneous sensitization may occur. The product Fluori-Methane® (dichlorofluoromethane 15%/trichloromonofluoromethane 85%) utilizes the "spray and stretch" technique — the product is sprayed onto the injured area, blocking pain impulses so the muscle can be stretched to its normal length in a pain-free state.[32,33]

Monitoring of Therapy

Table 4 provides a monitoring plan framework for soft tissue sports injuries which should be individualized.

Table 3: **Nonprescription Drug Therapy for Sports Injuries**[20,21]

Drug	Dosing schedule	Side effects	Drug interactions	Comments
Oral Analgesics				
Acetaminophen	325-500 mg q3h PRN or 325-650 mg q4h PRN or 650 mg – 1000 mg q6h PRN. Maximum daily dose 4 g.	Hepatotoxicity associated with chronic use, especially at high doses.	Isoniazid, phenytoin, warfarin, zidovudine	
ASA	325-500 mg q3h PRN or 325-650 mg q4h PRN or 650 mg – 1 g q6h PRN	GI bleeding; hypersensitivity; tinnitus (may indicate salicylate toxicity)	Anticoagulants, sulfonylureas, methotrexate, probenecid	Avoid use in pregnancy near term. Do not use in children because of association with Reye's syndrome. May require discontinuation prior to surgery to avoid bleeding. Best avoided in patients at risk of peptic ulcer and asthma.
Combination codeine products	1-2 tablets q4h PRN	Dizziness, drowsiness, nausea, vomiting, constipation	Alcohol, CNS depressants	Use of opioids for a long time or in high doses can be habit forming (causing mental or physical dependency); stopping the drug abruptly may lead to withdrawal symptoms.
Ibuprofen	200-400 mg q4-6h PRN; maximum daily dose 1200 mg for self-medication	Abdominal discomfort, epigastric pain, nausea, diarrhea, dizziness, drowsiness	Anticoagulants, digitalis, lithium, methotrexate, phenytoin	Caution in ASA-sensitive patients. Avoid use in pregnancy near term. Best avoided in patients at risk of peptic ulcer.
Muscle Relaxants				
Chlorzoxazone	500 mg TID – QID	Blurred vision, dizziness, drowsiness, lightheadedness, reddish-orange urine discoloration. Fatal hepatotoxicity reported.	Alcohol, CNS depressants	**Not recommended for routine use.** If utilized, only recommend short-term use (2-3 days).
Methocarbamol	500 mg – 1.5 g QID	Blurred vision, dizziness, drowsiness, lightheadedness	Alcohol, CNS depressants	**Not recommended for routine use.** If utilized, only recommend short-term use (2-3 days).
Orphenadrine	50-100 mg BID-TID	Anticholinergic effects (hallucinations, agitation, dry mouth, constipation, urinary retention, blurred vision). Drowsiness, dizziness, lightheadedness	Alcohol, CNS depressants, anticholinergics	Contraindicated with angle closure glaucoma, BPH, bladder obstruction, myasthenia gravis, achalasia. **Not recommended for routine use.** If utilized, only recommend short-term use (2-3 days).

Table 4: **Monitoring Therapy for Soft Tissue Sports Injuries**

Symptoms	Monitoring	Endpoint of therapy	Actions
Pain and swelling from muscle sprain or strain and overuse injuries.	**Patient:** daily **Pharmacist or health care provider:** after 14 days of therapy	Decrease in pain and swelling over a 14-day period. Gradually, the injured area can be used with minimal discomfort and eventually daily activities can be performed without pain.	If pain symptoms have not improved after 14 days of self-care, refer to a physician. If pain is worsening despite drug therapy, refer to a physician immediately.

Suggested Readings

John Hopkins University and Health System. Department of Orthopaedic Surgery Web page. *Sports medicine and shoulder surgery patient guides.* Available at: http://www.hopkinsmedicine. org/orthopedicsurgery/sports/guides.html.

Harries M, Williams C, Stannish WD, Micheli LJ, eds. *Oxford Textbook of Sports Medicine.* Oxford, UK: Oxford University Press, 1998.

Kayne S. Sport and exercise. In: Harman RJ, ed. *Handbook of Pharmacy Health Education.* 2nd ed. London, UK: Pharmaceutical Press, 1998:191-232.

Sallis RE, Massimino F. *ACSM's Essentials of Sports Medicine.* St. Louis, MI: Mosby, 1997.

References

1. Nykamp D. Sports Injuries. *US Pharm* 1992;17(4):34-55.
2. Balancing sport risk and health benefits (editorial). *The Physician and Sportsmedicine* 1999;27(6):1-2.
3. Sport for all – is it cost effective? (editorial). *Drug Ther Perspect* 1994;3(9):14-6.
4. Kayne S. Sport and exercise. In: Harman RJ, ed: *Handbook of Pharmacy Health Education.* 2nd ed. London: The Pharmaceutical Press, 1998:191-232.
5. Sports injuries. In: Berkow R, ed: *The Merck Manual of Medical Information.* New York: Merck & Co., Inc, 1997: 286-302.
6. John Hopkins Department of Orthopaedic Surgery. *Sports medicine and shoulder surgery patient guides.* Http://www. med.jhu.edu/ortho/sports/guides.html.
7. Edwards C, Stilman P. Musculoskeletal disorders. *Pharm J* 1993;251:733-8.
8. Medlineplus Medical Encyclopedia. Eye emergencies. Available at: http://www.nlm.nih.gov/medlineplus/ency/ article/000054.htm. Accessed March 1, 2002.
9. Mayo Clinic. Disease & Conditions A-Z: Concussion. Available at: http://www.mayoclinic.com/findinformation/ diseasesandconditions.htm. Accessed March 1, 2002.
10. Harvey R. Managing sprains and strains. *Pharm J* 1997; 259(6957):292-4.
11. Medlineplus Medical Encyclopedia. Nosebleed—injury. Available at: http://www.nlm.nih.gov/medlineplus/ency/ article/000020.htm. Accessed March 1, 2002.
12. Mayo Clinic. Ears and hearing: ruptured eardrum. Available at: http://www.mayoclinic.com/findinformation/ conditioncenters. Accessed March 1, 2002.
13. Roberts WO. Keeping sports safe: physicians should take the lead. *The Physician and Sportsmedicine* 1998;26(5):25-30.
14. Sherman M. A primer on use of hot or cold therapy. *US Pharm* 1987;12:72-81.
15. Stamford B. Giving injuries the cold treatment. *The Physician and Sportsmedicine* 1996;24(3):99-102.
16. Pray WS. Use of local heat for minor injuries. *US Pharm* 1993;18(10):39-45.
17. Thornton JS. Pain relief for acute soft-tissue injuries. *The Physician and Sportsmedicine* 1997;25(10):108-21.
18. Drugs for pain. *Med Lett Drugs Ther* 1998;40(1033):79-80.
19. Ontario Musculoskeletal Therapeutics Review Panel. *Ontario Treatment Guidelenes for Osteoarthritis, Rheumatoid Arthritis, and Acute Musculoskeletal Injury.* 1st ed. Toronto, ON: Queen's Printer of Ontario; 2000.
20. Chlorzoxazone hepatotoxicity. *Med Lett Drugs Ther* 1996; 38(974):46.
21. McEvoy GK, ed. *AHFS 2001 Drug Information.* 43rd ed. Bethesda, MD: American Society of Health-System Pharmacists, 2001.
22. Injuries to muscles, ligaments, and tendons. In: Pray WS: *Nonprescription Product Therapeutics.* Lippincott Williams & Wilkins, 1999:295-309.
23. Heyneman CA. Topical nonsteroidal anti-inflammatory drugs for acute soft tissue injuries. *Ann Pharmacother* 1995;29: 780-2.
24. Herxheimer A (ed). More topical NSAIDS: worth the rub? *Drug Ther Bull* 1990;28(7):27-8.
25. Buchanan NMM. Is there a place for topical NSAIDS? *Pharm J* 1997;259(6957):294-5.
26. Hudson S. Compounding for athletes: successful sports compounds. *Int J Pharm Compound* 1999;3(5):382-3.
27. What is Diffusimax®? Drug Information and Research Centre – New Drugs/Drug News 1999;17(6):3.
28. Allen LV. Ketoprofen gel. *US Pharm* 1993;18(11):98-100.
29. Moore RA, Tramer MR, Carroll D, Wiffen PJ, McQuay HJ. Quantitive systematic review of topically applied nonsteroidal anti-inflammatory drugs. *BMJ* 1998;316:333-8.
30. Pfenninger JL. Injections of joints and soft tissue: part I. General guidelines. *Am Fam Physician* 1991;44:1196-202.
31. Sherman M. Health-care team provides support for tennis elbow. *Can Pharm J* 1982;115:351-3.
32. Drugdex editorial staff. Fluorimethane spray availability (drug consult). In: Conner CR, Rumack BH, eds. Drugdex Information System. Denver, Colorado: Micromedex (edition expired 2/28/97).
33. Fluori-Methane® product monograph. Cleveland, OH: Gebauer Company, 1994.

Sports Injuries—Patient Information

Participation in sports and exercise is associated with health benefits but can also lead to sports injuries.

Some Common Sports Injuries

Achilles tendonitis: Painful inflammation of the Achilles tendon (which connects the heel to the calf muscle).

Muscle strains: Torn or pulled muscles.

Plantar fasciitis: Heel pain.

Shin splints: Sore, stiff areas along the shin bones above the ankles.

How To Prevent Sport Injuries

Keep sports activities and exercise safe. The following tips can help prevent injuries:

- Do warm-up exercises and stretching before any sport or exercise program.
- Slowly increase the intensity and duration of your work out.
- Drink enough fluids.
- Wear appropriate clothing and protective equipment, especially in high-risk sports activities.

What To Do If You Have A Sports Injury

Following sudden sports injuries, remember **RICE** – Rest, Ice, Compression and Elevation. Use **RICE** for the first two days after an injury or until the swelling goes away.

Rest: Rest the injured area to prevent worsening the injury.

Ice: Apply ice every few hours to reduce the swelling. If a bony area like the knee has been hurt, only keep the ice on for 10 minutes; otherwise keep it on for 20 minutes. Remember to keep a towel between the ice bag and your skin to prevent frostbite.

Compression: Bandage the injury to reduce swelling, support a joint or protect the wound.

Elevation: Raise the injury above the level of the heart to allow the fluid to drain and reduce swelling.

If you think you may need medication for pain and swelling, talk to your pharmacist or doctor.

If a sports injury does not get better in two weeks or if the pain gets worse despite treatment, see your doctor.

Drug Use and Abuse in Sports

Lily Lum, BScPharm

Introduction

Olympic athletes of ancient Greece are believed to have used herbs and mushrooms to improve athletic performance.[1,2] Now, in the age of the modern Olympic games, athletes continue to take substances that are not officially permitted (i.e., banned substances) to boost their performance and give them an advantage to win.

Ergogenic (performance-enhancing) drug use or doping is defined as "the administration of or use by a competing athlete of any substance foreign to the body or of any physiological substance taken in abnormal quantity or taken by an abnormal route of entry into the body with the sole intention of increasing in an artificial manner his/her performance in competition."[1] Sports organizations have developed anti-doping policies and drug testing programs in order to protect the health of the athletes and to keep competition fair and drug free.[3] Although drugs carry potential adverse effects, most athletes who use them view the risk to benefit ratio as favorable.[4] Ergogenic aids come from many sources and the list often appears endless as access to such products is easy, especially with use of the Internet. Ergogenic aids may be prescription or nonprescription drugs, recreational drugs such as alcohol and marijuana, nutritional supplements and herbal or natural products.

Nonprescription Drugs

A number of agents found in nonprescription products are used as ergogenic aids (Table 1).

Table 1: **Common Ergogenic Aids Found in Nonprescription Products**[1-6]

Drug/Drug class	Reason for abuse	Adverse effects	Comments
Caffeine	Increased alertness; reduced perception of fatigue; increased endurance	Nervousness, insomnia, tremors, diuresis	I — Found in many nonprescription sleep aids and stimulants.
Codeine	Treatment of pain allows athlete to participate while injured but has potential to further aggravate injury	Dizziness, lightheadedness, drowsiness, nausea or vomiting, constipation	I — Found in nonprescription combination analgesic products.
Creatine	Muscle-performance enhancer	Dizziness, diarrhea; liver and kidney toxicity at high doses	E
Cyproheptadine	Promotes appetite and weight gain	Drowsiness	N
Sympathomimetics (e.g., phenylephrine, pseudoephedrine)	Increased subjective energy ("energizing" effect), decreased appetite and increased metabolism	Restlessness, nervousness, tachycardia, arrhythmias, hypertension	N — Found in many nonprescription cold preparations.

E = Evidence to support; I = Inconclusive or conflicting evidence; N = No evidence or theoretical, based on pharmacologic actions.

Prescription Drugs

Many prescription drugs are also used as ergogenic aids (Table 2). **Anabolic steroids** are the best known. They are synthetic derivatives of the male sex hormone testosterone.[1] Individuals use anabolic steroids primarily to increase muscle mass and strength. Athletes who take anabolic steroids employ unusual dosing regimens in an attempt to increase the effects of the drugs, prevent detection or decrease the occurrence of drug-related adverse effects. *Stacking* is a technique where several different anabolic agents

Table 2: **Common Ergogenic Aids Found in Prescription Products**[1-6]

Drug/Drug class	Reason for abuse	Adverse effects	Comments
Anabolic steroids	Increase muscle mass and strength	Liver toxicity; acne; gynecomastia in males; masculinization in females; premature closure of the growth centers of long bones (adolescents); psychiatric effects such as psychosis, aggression, euphoria, depression	E
Beta-blockers	Reduce anxiety, hand tremor and heart rate	Dizziness or lightheadedness; unusual tiredness or weakness; sexual dysfunction	N
Beta$_2$-agonists	Anabolic effects	Dizziness, lightheadedness, nervousness, tremor, nausea, increased heart rate	I (No evidence with inhaled formulations.)
Diuretics	Promote excretion of banned substances	Dizziness or lightheadedness; photosensitivity (with thiazides)	N
Peptide hormones/ analogues 1. Erythropoietin	Increases red blood cell production, thus increasing aerobic capacity	Chest pain; shortness of breath; increased blood pressure	E
2. Human growth hormone	Anabolic effects	If growth hormone is given to children or adults with normal growth, who do not need growth hormone, serious unwanted effects may occur because levels in the body become too high. These effects include the development of diabetes; abnormal growth of bones and internal organs such as the heart, kidneys, and liver; atherosclerosis and hypertension	I
Probenecid	Promotes urinary excretion of a banned substance	Headache; joint pain, redness, or swelling; loss of appetite; nausea	N
Tamoxifen	Reverses gynecomastia caused by steroids	Hot flushes, weight gain in females; sexual dysfunction in males.	N

E = Evidence to support; I = Inconclusive or conflicting evidence; N = No evidence or theoretical, based on pharmacologic actions.

Table 3: **Banned/Restricted Substances**[12]

Banned/Restricted	Examples	Comments
Anabolic agents	Androstenedione Dehydroepiandrosterone Fluoxymesterone Nandrolone Stanozolol Testosterone	Banned
Beta$_2$-agonists	Clenbuterol	When given orally or by injection, beta$_2$-agonists may have anabolic effects. Salbutamol, salmeterol and terbutaline by inhalation are permitted but must be declared.
Beta-blockers	Acebutolol Atenolol Metoprolol Propranolol	All beta blockers are banned; there are no exceptions.
Caffeine		A urine specimen will be considered positive if the concentration of caffeine exceeds 12 mcg/mL. The normal ingestion of coffee, tea, or colas will not cause this limit to be exceeded or even remotely approached.
Diuretics	Acetazolamide Furosemide Hydrochlorothiazide Spironolactone Triamterene	Diuretics are banned because they are used to promote urinary excretion of a banned substance.
Glucocorticoids	Fluticasone Hydrocortisone Methylprednisolone Prednisone	The use of glucocorticoids is banned except for topical use, by inhalation, and by intra-articular or local injection.
Local anesthetics	Bupivacaine Lidocaine Procaine	Local or intra-articular injections of local anesthetics are permitted if they are medically justified.
Narcotics	Hydrocodone Hydromorphone Meperidine Morphine	Some narcotics such as codeine, dextromethorphan, diphenoxylate and propoxyphene are permitted for medical use but must be declared.
Peptide hormones and analogues	Chorionic gonadotrophin (HCG) Growth hormone Erythropoietin Insulin Tamoxifen	Insulin is permitted only to treat athletes with certified insulin-dependent diabetes.
Stimulants	Ephedrine Phenylephrine Pseudoephedrine	The use of decongestant nasal sprays is permitted.
Substances that alter the integrity of urine samples	Bicarbonate loading Probenecid	Banned

(oral and injectable) are used concomitantly in order to produce a synergistic effect. *Cycling* is a dosing technique with on and off periods of drug use. *Pyramiding* is another dosing technique where low doses are initiated, increased to a plateau sometimes 10 to 100 times the recommended therapeutic dose and then tapered down to the original level.[1,4,7] Much of what is known about the side effects of anabolic steroids involves patients receiving therapeutic doses for treatment of disease.

Recreational Drugs

Alcohol and marijuana may be abused by athletes with the misconception that these recreational drugs can reduce anxiety. In sports requiring precision, such as riflery events, alcohol in low doses may reduce essential tremor and may be banned. On the other hand, alcohol and marijuana can actually impair athletic performance.[1,3]

Nutritional Supplements, Herbals or Natural Products

There are countless products described as nutritional supplements, herbals or natural products with claims of possessing anabolic properties (e.g., chromium picolinate, creatine) or other ergogenic effects.[6,8] Because of the well-known toxicity associated with anabolic steroids, natural products are perceived as less or not harmful. Natural products are also more accessible to the public. Herbal or natural products are often promoted in a misleading fashion and usually have no scientific evidence to support their claims of anabolic or performance-enhancing effects.[8]

Creatine is widely used as an ergogenic aid. It is a naturally occurring compound produced by the liver, kidneys and pancreas from the amino acids glycine, arginine and methionine. Most individuals also consume 1-2 g exogenous creatine daily, primarily from meat and fish.[9]

Creatine is promoted as improving muscle strength and appearance. Studies on its effectiveness are conflicting. It may improve performance in power sports (e.g., weight lifting, sprinting) but has not demonstrated any benefit in endurance sports (e.g., cycling, cross-country running).[9,10]

Side effects are usually minimal and include nausea, vomiting, diarrhea, muscle cramps and weight gain (the latter is thought to be due to water retention). The effects of long-term use are unknown but there are concerns regarding renal and hepatic damage.[9,10]

Androstenedione is a precursor of testosterone and estrone. There is some evidence that it may elevate testosterone levels and increase strength and muscle mass during resistance training.[9] Information on the side effects of long-term use is not available but these are expected to be similar to those of anabolic steroids.[9,11] Though it is illegal in Canada, some athletes may obtain supplies from the United States or over the Internet.

Chromium is a popular sports supplement. It is discussed in Nutrition Appendix 2: Sports Nutrition.

Banned/Restricted Substances

Banned substances are not permitted for use by the athlete because they are believed to enhance performance. Restricted substances may be permitted for use by the athlete for specified medical conditions and may require declaration by the athlete. Table 3 lists categories of drugs that may be considered banned substances in amateur sports.

The list of banned and restricted substances varies between different sport organizations and is constantly changing. The Canadian Centre for Ethics in Sport (CCES) publishes a booklet with a listing of banned and restricted doping classes and methods (see Resource Tips).

Resource Tips

Canadian Centre for Ethics in Sport (CCES)
http://www.cces.ca
1-800-672-7775

Suggested Readings

Ahrendt DM. Ergogenic aids: counseling the athlete. *Am Fam Physician* 2001;63:913-22.

Anabolic Steroid Abuse. National Institute on Drug Abuse (NIDA) Research Report Series. NIH Publication No. 00-3721 April 2000. (www.nida.nih.gov/ResearchReports/Steroids/AnabolicSteroids.html).

Barron RL, Vanscoy GJ. Natural products and the athlete: facts and folklore. *Ann Pharmacother* 1993;27(5):607-15.

Catlin DH, Murray TH. Performance-enhancing drugs, fair competition, and Olympic sport. *JAMA* 1996;276(3):231-7.

Kayne S. Creatine: the athlete's wonder supplement? *Pharm J* 1999;263:906-8.

References

1. Wagner JC. Enhancement of athletic performance with drugs – an overview. *Sports Med* 1991;12(4):250-65.
2. Merchant WF. Medications and athletes – increasing your sports medicine knowledge. *Am Drug* 1992;206(5):6-13.
3. Catlin DH, Murray TH. Performance-enhancing drugs, fair competition, and Olympic sport. *JAMA* 1996;276(3):231-7.
4. Goldwire MA, Price KO. Sports pharmacy: counseling athletes about banned drugs. *Am Pharmacy* 1995;NS35(5):24-30.
5. Woolley BH. The latest fads to increase muscle mass and energy. *Postgrad Med* 1991;89(2):197-205.
6. Ahrendt DM. Ergogenic aids: counseling the athlete. *Am Fam Physician* 2001;63:913-22.
7. Nykamp D. Sports injuries. *US Pharm* 1992;17(4):34-55.
8. Barron RL, Vanscoy GJ. Natural products and the athlete: facts and folklore. *Ann Pharmacother* 1993;27(5):607-15.
9. Barnes CL, Kushner JM. Use of creatine and androstenedione to enhance athletic performance. *US Pharm* 2001;26(8):47-9.
10. Levien T. Creatine. Pharmacist's Letter document #130706. Stockton, CA: Therapeutic Research Center; 1997.
11. Tatro DS. Sports diets and supplements. *Facts and Comparisons DrugLink* 1999;3(2):12-15.
12. Canadian Centre for Ethics in Sport (CCES). *Achieving Drug-free Sport*. Available at: http://www.cces.ca/pdfs/drug-class.pdf. Accessed March 22, 2002.

Drugs and Sport—Information for the Athlete

Athletes or individuals may want to take drugs or substances they think will improve their sports ability or improve their body image. You may have been told that steroids will build more muscle. Perhaps you have been told that some drugs make you faster, lose fat, or less tired. Be cautious and avoid such products. They may be harmful, not effective, and/or not allowed in sport.

Are they safe?
Steroids are well known to cause serious side effects such as liver problems, mood changes, abnormal breast enlargement (in males) and masculinization (in females). For reliable information on side effects of other drugs or substances used in sports, ask your pharmacist. It is best to avoid products in which little is known about their side effects.

Are they banned?
For a list of banned substances in sports, check with your national or local sport organization. Different sport organizations may ban different substances. Carefully check the name of the ingredients of any medication you are taking. Some medications have similar brand names; one may contain a banned substance while the other not. For example, Robitussin contains guaifenesin and is permitted but Robitussin-PE contains pseudoephedrine, a banned substance. If you have any questions regarding your medications, consult your pharmacist.

Are they legal?
The majority of drugs require a prescription from your doctor. Some drugs may be obtained illegally.

What if I am taking drugs for an illness?
Some drugs can be taken for an illness or medical condition provided they are declared. Information on this process can be obtained from the Canadian Centre for Ethics in Sport (1-800-672-7775 or www.cces.ca).

Foot Conditions Section Highlights

Foot Symptom Assessment

Chapter 38: **Athlete's Foot**

      Morphologic variants of athlete's foot
      Nonprescription products for treatment of athlete's foot

Chapter 39: **Corns, Calluses, Bunions and Ingrown Toenails**

      Proper shoe fit
      Nonprescription products for treatment of corns and calluses

Chapter 40: **Plantar Warts**

      Nonprescription products for treatment of plantar warts

Foot Symptom Assessment[1-5]

Anne Mallin, BScPhm

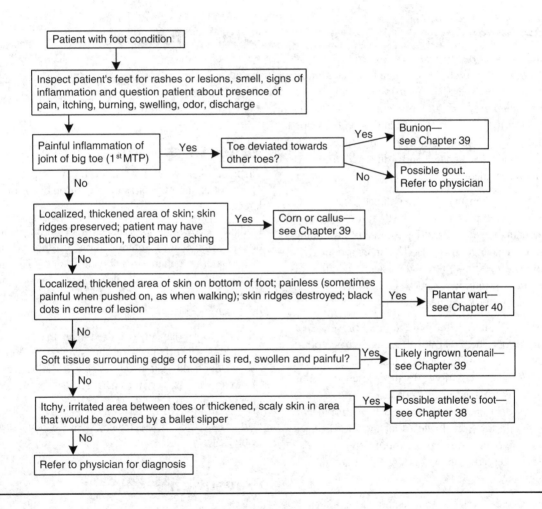

Patient with foot condition

Inspect patient's feet for rashes or lesions, smell, signs of inflammation and question patient about presence of pain, itching, burning, swelling, odor, discharge

Painful inflammation of joint of big toe (1st MTP) — Yes → Toe deviated towards other toes? — Yes → Bunion—see Chapter 39 / No → Possible gout. Refer to physician

No

Localized, thickened area of skin; skin ridges preserved; patient may have burning sensation, foot pain or aching — Yes → Corn or callus—see Chapter 39

No

Localized, thickened area of skin on bottom of foot; painless (sometimes painful when pushed on, as when walking); skin ridges destroyed; black dots in centre of lesion — Yes → Plantar wart—see Chapter 40

No

Soft tissue surrounding edge of toenail is red, swollen and painful? — Yes → Likely ingrown toenail—see Chapter 39

No

Itchy, irritated area between toes or thickened, scaly skin in area that would be covered by a ballet slipper — Yes → Possible athlete's foot—see Chapter 38

No

Refer to physician for diagnosis

References

1. Edwards C, Stillman P. *Minor Illness or Major Disease?* 3rd ed. London, UK: Pharmaceutical Press, 2000.
2. American Podiatric Medical Association. *Your podiatric physician talks about warts*. Available at: http://www.apma.org/topics/Warts/htm. Accessed July 27, 2001.
3. Baxter J. Feet not just there to keep your socks on. *New Zealand Pharmacy* 1996 (Dec): 10-12.
4. Nork SE, Couglin RR. How to examine a foot and what to do with a bunion. *Primary Care* 1996;23(2): 281-97.
5. Singh D, Bentley G, Trevino SG. Callosities, corns and calluses. *BMJ* 1996; 312: 1403-6.

Chapter 38

Athlete's Foot

Anne Mallin, BScPhm

Pathophysiology

Athlete's foot (*tinea pedis*) is a superficial fungal infection of the feet.[1] The fungal species most commonly involved are *Trichophyton rubrum*, *Trichophyton mentagrophytes* and *Epidermophyton floccosum*.[2-4] Up to 70% of the population will acquire this infection at some point in their lives.[5] It is most common in teenage and adult males and is uncommon in children.[1,3]

Tinea pedis is transmitted either directly via contact with an infected person or indirectly through contact with contaminated surfaces (e.g., floors of swimming pools, gym change rooms).[5] The infection can be spread to other parts of the body, usually the groin or underarms, by autoinoculation (i.e., touching feet, then touching self elsewhere).[6]

Hyperhidrosis may contribute to the presence of athlete's foot. The creation of warm, dark, poorly ventilated, moist environments, which promote fungal growth may also contribute to the presence of this condition. The regular wearing of shoes, with or without socks or hosiery, can create such environments. Other risk factors for athlete's foot include diabetes mellitus, immunosuppression, peripheral vascular disease, occluded skin, poor hygiene, malnutrition and trauma.[4]

Tinea pedis may progress to ulceration if the infection extends into the dermis. Complications may also include secondary bacterial infections that may be localized or spreading (e.g., cellulitis, lymphangitis). Patients with diabetes or those who have had saphenous vein grafts for coronary artery bypass are especially prone to secondary bacterial infections.[1]

Goals of Therapy[7]

- Control symptoms
- Cure infection
- Prevent recurrence
- Prevent transmission to others

Patient Assessment

Tinea pedis may present in several ways (Table 1). The most common presentation is chronic interdigital infection.

Evidence of blisters, pruritic lesions, burning sensations, redness and inflammation in the favored locations or in a characteristic pattern on the feet may indicate the presence of athlete's foot. The skin may appear macerated and an odor may be present. See photo on page PS-1.

Athlete's foot may be confused with the following conditions: disturbances of the sweat mechanism; contact dermatitis, often due to dyes or adhesives in footwear; eczema; erythrasma; psoriasis or bacterial infections.[8]

Figure 1 depicts an approach to assessing and managing athlete's foot.

Prevention[2,5]

All individuals should
- Change socks daily (more frequently if feet are sweaty)
- Allow shoes to dry completely before being worn again. This may take two or three days; it may be necessary to alternate pairs of shoes on different days.

Table 1: **Morphologic Variants of Tinea Pedis**

Variant	Lesion morphology	Typical location	Special considerations
Chronic interdigital infection	Fissures, scaling or maceration in the interdigital spaces	Very often, the infection is found on the lateral toe webs usually between the fourth and fifth or third and fourth toes. From this area, the infection often spreads to the instep or sole of the foot.	Humidity and warmth worsen this condition. Therefore, patients whose feet are prone to excessive sweating should be encouraged to treat their hyperhidrosis along with the fungal infection.
Mocassin-type infection	Chronic, papulosqua-mous pattern	Generally found on both feet, it is characterized by a mild inflammation and diffuse scaling on the soles of the feet. Often the toenails are affected (i.e., onychomycosis).	Involvement of the toenails perpetuates the infection such that the toenail infection must be treated by oral antifungal therapy or surgically removed in order to successfully treat the tinea pedis.
Vesicular	Small vesicles	Near the instep and on the midanterior plantar surface. Skin scaling is also observed in this area and on the toe webs.	Often caused by *T. mentagrophytes*. More prevalent in the summer.
Acute ulcerative disease	Macerated, denuded, weeping lesions	Sole of the foot	Very often, hyperkeratosis and a pungent odor are present. This infection may be complicated by an overgrowth of opportunistic, gram-negative bacteria such as *Proteus* or *Pseudomonas* and for this reason is often referred to as gram-negative athlete's foot or dermatophytosis complex.

Adapted from Miller B. Foot care products. In: Carruthers-Czyzewski P, ed. *Nonprescription Drug Reference for Health Professionals.* Ottawa, ON: Canadian Pharmaceutical Association, 1996:262.

- Dry feet thoroughly, paying special attention to areas between the toes.
- Do not go barefoot in public facilities such as pools or gym change rooms.
- Wear socks made of natural materials (e.g., cotton, wool).

An antiperspirant can also be applied to the feet to decrease sweating.

In addition to the above measures, individuals with a history of athlete's foot may dust an antifungal powder on their feet to prevent further recurrences. Antifungal powder should not be placed in shoes as coagulation of powder and moisture create an unfavorable environment.

Nonpharmacologic Treatment

Individuals with tinea pedis should follow the guidelines described under Prevention as adjuncts to pharmacologic treatment. Unless these measures are followed so that moist, humid conditions do not exist, recurrence is almost 100%.[2]

Separating the toes with a cotton ball also aids in absorption of moisture and decreases moisture build-up.

Pharmacologic Treatment[1,4,13,15]

Information on the relative efficacy of **chlorophenesin** is lacking. Other agents are effective in providing symptom relief and curing infection. Medication should be applied twice daily to a clean, dry foot for two to four weeks, including one week after the lesion has disappeared. These agents are generally well tolerated. The most common adverse reactions are minor local symptoms (e.g., burning, stinging). Occasionally, local allergic reactions may occur.

The nonprescription agents used to treat athlete's foot are described in Table 2.

The selection of dosage form is based on individual preference. Generally, ointments remain in contact with the affected area for a longer period of time than creams; however, there is the danger of creating an occlusive barrier, which promotes skin maceration and retards wound healing. Powders may be either nonmedicated or medicated and are also absorbent. Solutions, sprays or foams applied directly to the skin should be allowed to air dry.

Table 2: **Nonprescription Products for Treatment of Athlete's Foot**[15]

Drug	Dose	Adverse effects	Comments
Imidazole derivative azole antifungals			
Clotrimazole 1%	Thin layer, twice daily (morning and evening)	For all imidazoles: Local skin irritation or hypersensitivity (e.g., burning, erythema, itching, rash, stinging)	Available as cream. Not to be used on children < 2 yrs of age unless directed by physician. Avoid contact with eyes.
Miconazole nitrate 2%	Thin layer, twice daily (morning and evening)		Available as cream, spray powder. Not to be used on children < 2 yrs of age unless directed by physician. Avoid contact with eyes. Do not inhale powder.
Oxiconazole 1%	Twice daily (morning and evening)		Available as cream, lotion. Not to be used on children < 12 yrs of age unless directed by physician. Avoid contact with eyes, nose, mouth and mucous membranes.
Tioconazole 1%	Thin layer, twice daily (morning and evening)		Available as cream. Not to be used on children < 2 yrs of age unless directed by physician. Use on children < 12 yrs of age should be supervised. Avoid contact with eyes.
Miscellaneous antifungals			
Butenafine HCl 1%	Once daily (thin layer)	Symptoms of local skin irritation or hypersensitivity (e.g., burning, erythema, itching, rash, stinging)	Available as cream. Not to be used on children < 12 yrs of age. Avoid contact with eyes and mucous membranes.
Chlorophenesin 1%	Apply after bathing and drying affected area	None reported	Available as cream. Not to be used on children < 3 yrs of age.
Tolnaftate 1%	Twice daily (morning and evening)	Possible symptoms of local skin irritation or hypersensitivity (e.g., burning, erythema, itching, rash, stinging)	Available as cream, gel, liquid, powder, spray powder. Not to be used on children < 2 yrs of age unless directed by physician. Avoid contact with eyes.
Undecylenic acid +/– undecylenate salts (total concentrations 10-25%)	Twice daily (morning and evening)	Symptoms of local skin irritation or hypersensitivity (e.g., burning, erythema, itching, rash, stinging)	Available as liquid, ointment, powder, spray (aerosol). Not to be used on children < 2 yrs of age unless directed by physician. Avoid contact with eyes and mucous membranes. Avoid inhaling powder preparations.

Figure 1: **Assessment and Treatment of Patients with Athlete's Foot**[1,3-5,7-14]

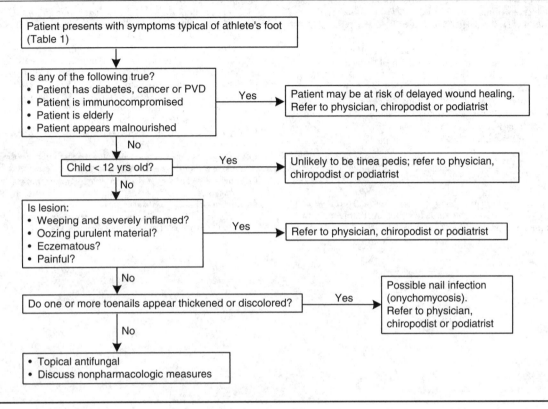

PVD = peripheral vascular disease.

Topical terbinafine is available by prescription and produces similar cure rates as nonprescription topical agents, but requires only one week of therapy. Other prescription agents include oral terbinafine, ketoconazole, itraconazole and griseofulvin. These may be indicated for infections of the nail or infections that are resistant to topical treatment.

Monitoring of Therapy[5,6]

Subsequent rash during therapy may indicate an allergic reaction to the product. The patient should discontinue use of the product and consult a physician, chiropodist or podiatrist.

If no improvement is seen within two weeks, or if symptoms have not completely disappeared within six weeks of treatment, refer the patient to a physician, chiropodist or podiatrist.

Advice for the Patient

- Emphasize the importance of finishing the recommended course to prevent recurrence, even though symptoms may improve before the treatment course is complete.[5]
- Instruct patients to dry the feet last after showering or bathing and use a clean towel every day, to prevent autoinoculation.
- Tell patients to not go barefoot around the home or in public areas until the infection is cured to prevent transmission to others.

References

1. Fitzpatrick TB, Johnson RA, Wolff K, Suurmond D. Fungal infections of the skin & hair. In: *Color Atlas and Synopsis of Clinical Dermatology.* 4th ed. New York. McGraw-Hill: 2001: 684-725.

2. Donaldson R. Athlete's foot. *Can Pharm J* 1998 Apr: 33.

3. Canadian Paediatric Society. Antifungal agents for common paediatric infections. *Paediatr Child Health* 2000;5(8): 477-82.

4. DeSimone II EM, Maag P. Common superficial fungal infections. *US Pharm* 1999;24(4). Available at: http://www. uspharmacist.com/Newlook/DisplayArticle. cfm? item_num= 358. Accessed Jan 29, 2002.

5. Stafford VE. Patient consult: athlete's foot. *US Pharm* 2000;25(3). Available at: http://www.uspharmacist.com/ Newlook/DisplayArticle. cfm? item_num=491. Accessed July 27, 2001.

6. American Podiatric Medical Association. *Your podiatric physician talks about athlete's foot.* Available at http:// apma.org/topics/athfoot.htm. Accessed July 27, 2001.

7. Crawford F, Hart R, Bell-Syer SEM, Torgerson DJ, Young P, Russell J. Athlete's foot and fungally infected toenails. *BMJ* 2001;322:288-9.

8. Beers M, Berkow R, eds. *The Merck Manual of Diagnosis and Therapy.* 17th ed. Whitehouse Station, NJ: Merck Research Laboratories, 1999.

9. Bélanger D. Athlete's foot. *Can Pharm J* 2000 Nov: 19.

10. Miller B. Foot care products. In: Carruthers-Czyzewski P, ed. *Nonprescription Drug Reference for Health Professionals.* Ottawa: Canadian Pharmaceutical Association; 1996:261-274.

11. American Diabetes Association clinical practice recommendations. Foot care in patients with diabetes mellitus. *Diabetes Care* 1997;20(Suppl 1):S31.

12. Anonymous. May I see the pharmacist? *Aus Pharm* 1997; 16(4):223.

13. Bedinghaus JM, Niedfeldt MW. Over-the-counter foot remedies. *Am Fam Physician* 2001;64:791-6.

14. American Academy of Dermatology. *Patient information – athlete's foot.* Available at: http://www.aad.org/pamphlets/ Athletfoot.html. Accessed January 30, 2002.

15. Repchinsky C, ed. *Compendium of Nonprescription Products.* Ottawa, ON: Canadian Pharmacists Association, 2001.

Athlete's Foot—Patient Information

Athlete's foot is a fungal infection of the skin of the feet. The symptoms range from redness and itchiness on the soles of the feet, to peeling and scaling in between the third, fourth or fifth toes of the foot. These symptoms can sometimes be mistaken for other foot conditions like bacterial infections, eczema, contact dermatitis or psoriasis.

If you have athlete's foot, strict attention to good foot hygiene is important to help cure it.

- Wash feet daily in lukewarm water with a mild, nondeodorant soap.
- Rinse feet well and dry carefully with a soft towel, especially between the toes.
- Do not soak your feet longer than 10 minutes.
- Do not go barefoot in places where you could catch athlete's foot again or spread it to other people. Wear sandals in pool or shower areas.
- Change your shoes and socks daily.
- Wear socks made of natural materials like cotton or wool.

- Wear shoes that provide good ventilation (for example, made from leather or canvas), so moisture will escape from the shoe and allow the feet to breathe.
- Do not share personal items such as towels.
- Use a nonabsorbent bath mat that can be disinfected.

Products that kill the fungus that causes athlete's foot are available without a prescription as creams, gels, lotions, ointments, powders and sprays. Your pharmacist can help you choose the one that is best for you. These products can be applied twice daily for at least two weeks.

See your doctor, podiatrist or chiropodist if:
- You do not see any improvement in your symptoms within two weeks;
- Your symptoms are not completely gone in six weeks.

If nonprescription products do not work, your doctor may prescribe medication you take by mouth to treat the infection.

Chapter 39

Corns, Calluses, Bunions and Ingrown Toenails

Anne Mallin, BScPhm

Pathophysiology

Corns and Calluses[1-4]

Corns (*clavus, heloma*) and calluses (*tyloma*) occur when keratinization becomes overactive in an attempt to protect the foot from excessive friction or pressure from the skin rubbing against bony areas of the foot.

Poorly fitting footwear can lead to the presence of corns and calluses by placing pressure on bony areas or causing excess friction. Calluses may also form as a result of weight gain, abnormal gait or foot structure (e.g., bunion, hammertoe). Corns and calluses are not contagious and are observed in most age groups.

Bunion[3,5]

A bunion (*hallux valgus*) is a deformed big toe joint (first metatarsophalangeal or MTP joint), where the joint is angled outward with the big toe angled toward the other toes (Figure 1). When the joint of the little toe is involved it is called a *bunionette*.

Heredity of foot type, abnormal gait, constant abnormal joint motion and pressure and the wearing of tight-fitting shoes may all contribute to the presence of bunions. They are 10 times more common in women than men, likely due to the wearing of narrow, pointed-toe shoes.

Goals of Therapy[1]

- Relieve symptoms
- Remove the cause of the lesion so that it may regress (or not progress in the case of bunions)
- Prevent recurrences

Figure 1: **Bunion**

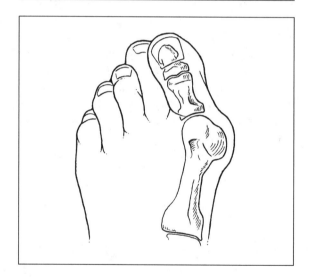

Patient Assessment[1,3,6]

When possible, inspect the patient's foot and footwear. Note the presence of lesions, rashes or obvious abnormalities in foot structure such as bunions or hammertoes. Check the fit of the shoe (see Proper Shoe Fit), paying special attention to its length and the width and depth of the toe box.

Corns and Calluses

The appearance of corns is that of tough layers of compacted, dead skin cells, which may have a central cone (*radix*) over the bony area or spur. The radix is triangular in shape and points inward. The affected area may also be yellowed in color. "Hard corns" favor the areas over the fifth toe joint and on the soles of the feet, while "soft corns" are found between the toes, especially between the fourth and fifth. A soft corn is essentially a hard corn that has absorbed moisture from sweat, becoming macerated. Corns are rarely found under a toenail. See photo of a typical corn on page PS-1.

Calluses have a similar appearance to corns and tend to be well defined. They are of relatively even thickness and do not have a radix. They tend to occur on the soles of the feet, especially on the ball or heel of the foot.

A burning sensation and pain when the corn or callus is compressed may indicate the presence of corns or calluses. Corns may also become inflamed or infected.

Hard corns may be confused with plantar warts. However, when the top layer of skin cells is removed, pinpoint bleeding is observed with plantar warts. In addition, skin ridges pass through corns but around plantar warts.

Soft corns are often confused with athlete's foot. However, soft corns are often quite painful, whereas athlete's foot tends to be itchy and usually not painful.

Bunions

A bunion looks like a bump on the outside edge of the affected foot. Its distinctive appearance, along with swelling, pain and redness are characteristic of this foot condition. Refer individuals with a bunion to a physician, podiatrist or chiropodist in order to receive early treatment to stabilize the joint and therefore reduce arthritic development.

Figure 2 depicts the assessment and management of corns, calluses and bunions.

Nonpharmacologic Therapy[1-3,5-6]

Identifying and removing the cause of the lesion is the most important step in the treatment of corns, calluses or bunions. The most common intervention is a change in footwear and this is often the only treatment required. See Proper Shoe Fit below.

Debridement of a corn or callus using a pumice stone can be accomplished after soaking the area in warm

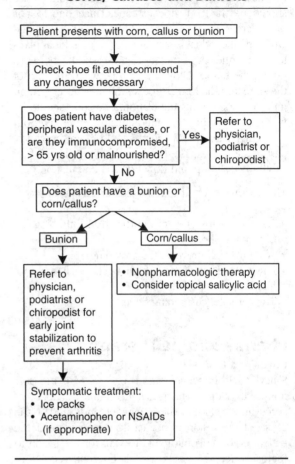

Figure 2: **Assessment of Patients with Corns, Calluses and Bunions**[1,3,6,7]

water for about 10 minutes. A foot file (emery board) can be used on a dry foot.

Devices such as cushions, felt pads and latex foam can be used to protect a corn, callus or bunion. These are available in a variety of shapes and sizes to accommodate the various lesions. Custom pads can be constructed from moleskin and lambswool. Placing lambswool between the toes affected by a soft corn decreases the pain. Orthotic devices may be inserted into footwear to provide arch support and to distribute body weight more equitably so that excess pressure is removed from the affected area of the foot. Orthotic devices may also be used to stabilize the MTP joint in the case of a bunion. Surgery (bunionectomy) may be used as a last resort.

Proper Shoe Fit[5,6,8,9]

If possible, shoes should be purchased at the end of the day when feet are most swollen. Both shoes should be tried on, not just one, since one foot is often larger than the other. Shoes should be fitted while the individual is standing. If the individual plans to wear orthotics in the shoe, these should be worn during the fitting. Allow 1.25 cm between the end of the shoe and the longest toe so the toes do not bump into the shoe during ambulation. The shoe should be wide enough to accommodate the toes without crowding. The first MTP joint should be in the widest part of the toebox. The heel should fit snugly; the foot should not slip up and down during ambulation.

The following are desirable characteristics of footwear:
- Lace up: helps prevent the toes from bumping the end of the shoe.
- Wide toebox: prevents toe crowding.
- Lower heels (< 5 cm): high heels push the foot forward, crowding the toes.
- Thicker sole: cushioning effect.

Pharmacologic Therapy

Corns and Calluses

Salicylic acid in concentrations up to 40% is the only nonprescription agent available for the treatment of corns and calluses. These may be indicated if the cause of the lesion is not easily corrected or if the patient is too uncomfortable to wait for the lesion to regress once the cause has been removed. Nonprescription products are described in Table 1.

Plasters and pads tend to adhere to the lesion better than liquid dosage forms. Salicylic acid will damage normal skin, so it is important it not be applied outside the edge of the corn or callus. Plasters and medicated disks should be trimmed to the size and shape of the lesion. When liquid preparations are used, the normal skin surrounding the lesion can be protected with an occlusive application of petrolatum or a mechanical occlusion, such as a bandage with an aperture for application of the product. Products should be applied to a clean, dry foot. Liquid collodion vehicles should not be used by the elderly with potentially poor vision, or by children with the potential for poisoning by ingestion or by inhalation.

Bunions[5]

Ice packs and the use of usual doses of acetaminophen or NSAIDs are used to reduce pain and swelling of an inflamed bunion. If conservative therapy is inadequate, intra-articular corticosteroids may be administered for pain reduction.

Monitoring of Therapy

Corns and Calluses

Clinical improvement should be evident in 10 to 14 days. The patient should inspect the affected area at least twice weekly until healing is complete. If no improvement is noted, refer the patient to a physician, podiatrist or chiropodist. If normal skin surrounding the lesion is damaged by incorrect use of salicylic acid preparations, the patient should discontinue use of the product until the normal skin is healed. If the lesion

---

Table 1: **Nonprescription Products for Treatment of Corns and Calluses**[10]

Drug	Dose	Adverse effects	Comments
Salicylic acid 12.6% or 17.6%	Once or twice daily	Excessive burning or irritation	Available as liquid. Not to be used by individuals with diabetes, peripheral vascular disease or impaired circulation. Highly flammable; store away from fire or flame. Avoid inhaling fumes. Do not apply to broken, infected or irritated skin.
Salicylic acid 40%	Every 24-48 h	Excessive burning or irritation	Available as pads, plasters. Not to be used by individuals with diabetes, peripheral vascular disease or impaired circulation. Do not apply to broken, infected or irritated skin.

---

becomes red or inflamed or drains purulent material, refer the patient to a physician, chiropodist or podiatrist.

Ingrown Toenails[11,12]

Ingrown toenails have nail edges that curve and grow into the soft tissue surrounding the toenails, usually that of the big toes. The soft tissue that has been penetrated by the nail edge becomes irritated and often appears red and inflamed.

The individual will probably experience pain, generated by the penetration and irritation of the soft tissue surrounding the toenail. Tenderness of the immediate area and abscess formation may also be present.

The incidence of ingrown toenails in males is double that of females and is predominant between the ages of 10 and 30 years.

Heredity, the improper trimming of toenails, trauma and toe crowding all may contribute to the development of ingrown toenails. To prevent toenails from becoming ingrown, trim them straight across and do not round the corners. The corners of nails should project beyond the skin (Figure 3).

Refer patients with ingrown toenails to a physician, chiropodist or podiatrist. A topical antibiotic cream or ointment can be applied and the toe bandaged for protection in the interim. The offending nail edge often must be surgically removed. Depending upon the presence and extent of infection, systemic antibiotics may be required.

Local anesthetics, such as **benzocaine** 20% solution, have been used as analgesics.

Hypertonic saline or magnesium sulfate footbath solutions reduce inflammation if the area is infected.

Polyurethane foam toecaps are useful as a protective device.

Determining optimum shoe fit and altering footwear to remove pressure points may prevent recurrences of ingrown toenails. See Proper Shoe Fit.

Advice for the Patient

Counsel the patient regarding:
- Proper fit of footwear;
- Strategies for preventing future occurrences;
- Nonpharmacologic treatment;
- Proper use of protective devices;
- Proper use of a salicylic acid product, if indicated, and
- When to seek medical attention.

Figure 3: **Trimming of Ingrown Toenails**

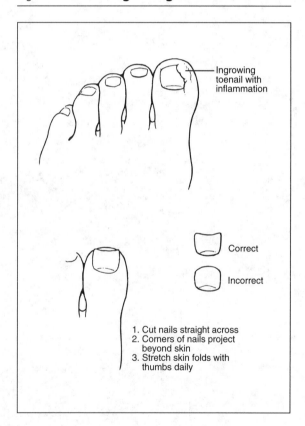

Ingrowing toenail with inflammation

Correct

Incorrect

1. Cut nails straight across
2. Corners of nails project beyond skin
3. Stretch skin folds with thumbs daily

Suggested Readings

Nork SE, Coughlin RR. How to examine a foot and what to do with a bunion. *Primary Care* 1996;23 (2):281-97.

Singh D, Bentley G, Trevino SG. Callosities, corns, and calluses. *BMJ* 1996;312:1403-6.

References

1. Singh D, Bentley G, Trevino SG. Callosities, corns, and calluses. *BMJ* 1996;312:1403-6.

2. Knight AL. Selected disorders of the skin. In: Taylor RB, ed. *Family Medicine Principles and Practice*. 4th ed. New York, NY: Springer-Verlag, 1994:952-3.

3. Silverskiöld JP. Common foot problems: relieving the pain of bunions, keratoses, corns, and calluses. *Postgrad Med* 1991; 89(5):183-8.

4. Donaldson R. Corns – a common foot problem. *Can Pharm J* 1998 May: 54.

5. American Podiatric Medical Association. *Your podiatric physician talks about bunions*. Available at http://www.apma.org/topics/bunions.htm. Accessed July 27, 2001.

6. Nork SE, Coughlin RR. How to examine a foot and what to do with a bunion. *Primary Care* 1996;23(2):281-97.

7. Edwards C, Stillman P. *Minor Illness or Major Disease*. 3rd ed. London, UK: Pharmaceutical Press, 2000.

8. Bedinghaus JM, Niedfeldt MW. Over-the-counter foot remedies. *Am Fam Physician* 2001;64:791-6.

9. Richards RN. Calluses, corns and shoes. *Semin Dermatol* 1991;10(2):112-4.

10. Repchinsky C, ed. *Compendium of Nonprescription Products*. Ottawa, ON: Canadian Pharmacists Association, 2001.

11. American Podiatric Medical Association. *Your podiatric physician talks about nail problems*. Available at: http://www.apma.org/topics/nail.htm. Accessed July 27, 2001.

12. Hensman L. Foot care. In: Carruthers-Czyzewski P, ed. *Self Medication: Reference for Health Care Professionals*. Ottawa, ON: Canadian Pharmacists Association, 1992: 337-48.

Corns and Calluses—Patient Information

Corns and calluses are caused by friction or pressure from the skin rubbing against the bony areas of the feet. They look like thick, tough layers of skin. Corns are usually found on or between the toes. Calluses are found on the soles of the feet. Symptoms may include burning or red, painful feet.

Here are some things you can do that may help:
• Make sure your shoes fit properly. They should not crowd the toes or allow your foot to slip around in the heel. They should also leave at least 1.25 cm (1/2 inch) space between the tip of your longest toe and the front of the shoe.

• Apply a felt pad with a hole in the centre over a corn to reduce pressure on the area.
• Put a latex foam insole into your shoe or apply moleskin to the affected area to cushion and protect your foot.
• Try a pumice stone on a wet foot or callus file on a dry foot to remove dry skin build-up.
• Never cut a corn or callus yourself with any instrument.

Nonprescription products are available to help remove the corn or callus. Talk to your pharmacist to see if one is right for you.

Bunions—Patient Information

A bunion looks like a bump on the outside edge of the foot. It is caused by a deformed big toe joint that causes the big toe to point towards the other toes of the foot. If you are experiencing pain or discomfort, consult a podiatrist, physician or chiropodist.

It is important to relieve pressure on the bunion to reduce pain and keep the deformity from getting worse, thereby avoiding surgery.

Here are some things you can do that may help:
• Avoid wearing narrow-fitting shoes or shoes with heels over 5 cm (2 inches) high.

• Use felt pads (moleskin) or latex foam to cushion the bunion to relieve the pressure points and eliminate friction.
• Apply ice packs to the bunion throughout the day if it becomes painful or swollen.
• Nonprescription pain relievers such as ibuprofen may help with pain and swelling. Talk to your pharmacist for help in choosing a pain reliever.

If icepacks and nonprescription pain relievers do not work, your doctor may inject cortisone into the joint. Eventually some people need surgery to correct the problem.

Chapter 40

Plantar Warts

Anne Mallin, BScPhm

Pathophysiology[1-7]

Warts found on the soles of the feet are called plantar warts (*verrucae plantaris*).

Warts are benign tumors caused by the human papillomavirus (HPV).[1] The virus infects the upper epidermis and causes squamous epithelial cells to proliferate.[2] The infection exists only in humans and is transmitted via contact with another lesion or contaminated surfaces.[3] Infection usually occurs through small cuts or microabrasions.[4,5] While infection may become clinically evident through the appearance of warts, it may also remain latent or cause subclinical infection where the change in the skin surface is not evident to the naked eye.[1] The incubation period between initial infection and the appearance of warty lesions varies from one to eight months.[6] Up to 30% of warts spontaneously regress within six months due to cell-mediated immunity, but those that do not frequently proliferate. Regression is more likely in children and with warts of short duration.

Plantar warts may occur singly or in clusters (*mosaic warts*). They are uncommon in infancy and are most common in children and young adults. The peak incidence of warts occurs between 12 and 16 years of age.

Risk factors for plantar warts include immunosuppression and exposure to environments where the virus may contaminate surfaces (e.g., swimming pool decks, communal showers).

Goals of Therapy[5]

- Alleviate or prevent pain due to the wart
- Eradicate lesions and prevent their proliferation
- Prevent recurrence
- Prevent transmission to others

Patient Assessment[2,4,5,8,9]

Most warts are harmless. However, depending upon their size, number and location, they can cause pain and may be a source of embarrassment to the patient.

Plantar warts are often symptomless, producing pain only upon pressure. This pain is usually greater on lateral compression (i.e., when the lesion is pinched from the sides) than with direct pressure. They are usually rough, firm hyperkeratoses that, unlike common warts on the hands, grow inwards due to pressure from walking. Warts are often gray or brown in color. Thrombosed capillaries may appear as black dots in the centre of the lesion, or these may only be evident as pinpoint bleeding that occurs if the lesion is pared by a physician. Unlike corns, skin striations tend to run around the wart, as opposed to through it. Plantar warts tend to arise on the heel or the ball of the foot where microabrasions are more likely to occur and allow inoculation. (See photo on page PS-1.)

Figure 1 depicts the assessment of the patient with a plantar wart.

Prevention[4]

Give patients the following instructions:
- Avoid walking barefoot. Take special care to keep feet covered when in areas where transmission may be more common (e.g., swimming pool decks, gym showers and change rooms).
- Change shoes and socks every day.
- Keep feet clean and dry.

Figure 1: **Assessment of Plantar Warts**

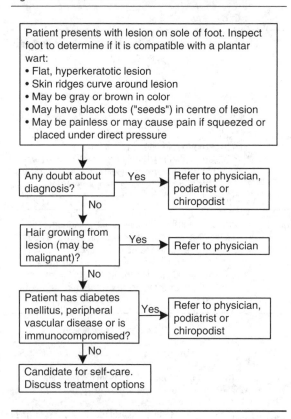

Patient presents with lesion on sole of foot. Inspect foot to determine if it is compatible with a plantar wart:
- Flat, hyperkeratotic lesion
- Skin ridges curve around lesion
- May be gray or brown in color
- May have black dots ("seeds") in centre of lesion
- May be painless or may cause pain if squeezed or placed under direct pressure

Any doubt about diagnosis? — Yes → Refer to physician, podiatrist or chiropodist

No

Hair growing from lesion (may be malignant)? — Yes → Refer to physician

No

Patient has diabetes mellitus, peripheral vascular disease or is immunocompromised? — Yes → Refer to physician, podiatrist or chiropodist

No

Candidate for self-care. Discuss treatment options

- Avoid touching warts on someone else or on another part of your body.

Pharmacologic Therapy[5]

Table 1 describes preparations available for self-treatment of plantar warts. The ingredient common to all products is **salicylic acid** in concentrations of 11 to 40%. The advantages of salicylic acid include minimal discomfort and a low risk of scarring. Disadvantages include the length of treatment.[5]

Cantharidin 0.7% is a vesicant available without a prescription but that must be applied by a physician, podiatrist or chiropodist. After application the lesion is kept occluded for three to seven days. During this time a blister is formed and the wart becomes necrotic. Treatment may need to be repeated. In some patients, pain may interfere with ambulation.

A medical device containing **dimethylether** and **propane** is available without a prescription. Based on the liquid nitrogen method, the product freezes the wart and causes a blister to form under it, resulting in the wart falling off approximately 10 days after treatment.[11] Efficacy in inducing cell temperatures adequate for cell necrosis may be lower than that achieved by liquid nitrogen because of its higher temperature (–57°C as opposed to –196°C).[3] Its role in self-care is yet to be determined.

Other treatment options available through a physician, podiatrist or chiropodist include cryotherapy with liquid nitrogen, electrosurgery and curettage.[1]

A systematic review concluded that topical treatments with salicylic acid are both safe and effective. In addition, there is no clear evidence that other treatments (e.g., cryotherapy with liquid nitrogen) offer any advantage with regard to either cure rate or adverse effects.[7]

Cure rates with any method of treatment are in the 60 to 70% range. Cure rates are higher in children, immunocompetent hosts and when the duration of infection is short. They are lower if the wart has failed to respond to any other type of treatment. Mosaic warts are also more resistant to treatment than single lesions.[3,7] Even when treatment appears to have been successful, warts may recur. This may be due to failure to remove tissue in which the virus has caused only latent or subclinical infection.

Monitoring of Therapy[9]

Check with the patient every four weeks to see if any improvement has been noted and to encourage compliance. If the lesion persists after 12 weeks of self-treatment, refer the patient to a physician, podiatrist or chiropodist.

If normal skin is damaged and becomes painful or inflamed or drains purulent material, refer the patient to a physician, podiatrist or chiropodist.

Advice for the Patient

Counsel patients on:
- Keeping the wart covered to prevent transmission to other people;

Table 1: **Nonprescription Products for Treatment of Plantar Warts**[10]

Drug	Dose	Adverse effects	Comments
Formalin 5%/ Lactic acid 10%/ Salicylic acid 25%	Once daily	Excessive burning/irritation	Available as ointment. Not to be used by individuals with diabetes, peripheral vascular disease or impaired circulation. Wash hands thoroughly after applying. Should not be used without the advice of a health professional. Do not use if the affected area becomes red, irritated or inflamed.
Lactic acid 16.7%/ Salicylic acid 16.7%	Once daily	Excessive burning/irritation	Available as liquid. Not to be used by individuals with diabetes, peripheral vascular disease or impaired circulation. Highly flammable; store away from fire or flame. Avoid inhaling fumes. Do not use if the affected area becomes red, irritated or inflamed.
Salicylic acid 11-40%	Gel/liquid: once or twice daily Pads/plasters: every 48 h	Excessive burning/irritation	Various strengths available as gel, liquid, pads, plasters. Not to be used by individuals with diabetes, peripheral vascular disease or impaired circulation. Liquid form highly flammable; store away from fire or flame. Avoid inhaling fumes of liquid form. Do not use if the affected area becomes red, irritated or inflamed.

- The importance of not trying "bathroom surgery" to remove the wart themselves;
- Proper use of the preparation chosen;
- Possible adverse effects and how to prevent and manage them (Table 1), and
- Maximum period of self-treatment (12 weeks).

Suggested Readings

Landsman MJ, Mancuso JE, Abramow SP. Diagnosis, pathophysiology and treatment of plantar verruca. *Clin Podiatric Med Surg* 1996;13(1): 55-71.

Sterling JC, Handfield-Jones S, Hudson PM. Guidelines for the management of cutaneous warts. *Brit J Dermatol* 2001;144:4-11.

References

1. Drake LA, Ceilley RI, Cornelison RL et al. Guidelines of care for warts: human papillomavirus. *J Am Acad Dermatol* 1995; 32:98-103.
2. Verbov J. How to manage warts. *Arch Dis Child* 1999;80: 97-9.
3. Sterling JC, Handfield-Jones S, Hudson PM. Guidelines for the management of cutaneous warts. *Brit J Dermatol* 2001; 144:4-11.
4. American Podiatric Medical Association. *Your podiatric physician talks about warts.* Available at: www.apma.org/topics/Warts.htm. Accessed July 27, 2001.
5. Landsman MJ, Mancuso JE, Abramow SP. Diagnosis, pathophysiology and treatment of plantar verruca. *Clin Podiatric Med Surg* 1996;13(1):55-71.
6. Bolton RA. Nongenital warts: classification and treatment options. *Am Fam Physician* 1991;43(6):2049-56.
7. Gibbs S, Harvey I, Sterling JC, Stark R. Local treatments for cutaneous warts (Cochrane Review). In: *The Cochrane Library*, Issue 3, 2001. Oxford: Update Software.
8. Baxter J. Feet not just there to keep your socks on. *New Zealand Pharmacy* 1996 Dec: 10-12.
9. Popovich NG, Newton GD. Minor foot disorders. In: Allen LV Jr., Berardi RR, DeSimone EM et al, eds. *Handbook of Nonprescription Drugs.* 12th ed. Washington, DC: American Pharmaceutical Association; 2000:781-818.
10. Repchinsky C, ed. *Compendium of Nonprescription Products.* Ottawa, ON: Canadian Pharmacists Association; 2001.
11. Anonymous. Information Leaflet Wartner®. Toronto, ON: Aurium Pharma Inc; 2002.

Plantar Warts—Patient Information

What is a plantar wart?

A plantar wart is a wart on the bottom of the foot. They are caused by a viral infection of the skin. They are usually harmless but are sometimes painful.

Where does the virus come from?

You catch the virus by touching someone else's wart or touching a surface with the virus on it. Common places where the virus can be found are swimming pool decks and gym or dormitory showers.

How can I prevent plantar warts?

- Do not go barefoot in public places. Wear shower or pool shoes when necessary.
- Try not to touch another person's warts.
- Keep your feet clean and dry.
- Change your shoes and socks every day.

How are plantar warts treated?

There are a number of wart removal products available without a prescription. These should not be used by people with diabetes, poor circulation or weak immune systems. Most contain a type of acid that, over time, eats away the wart. These can take up to 12 weeks to work. There are also treatments available from your doctor. Talk to your pharmacist about the treatment that is best for you.

Correct Use of Topical Salicylic Acid Products

- Soak the affected area in warm water for 10 minutes, then gently rub away loose tissue with a pumice stone or rough washcloth.
- If using a liquid preparation, protect healthy skin with a thin layer of petroleum jelly. Apply the wart remover one drop at a time until the affected area is covered, let air dry, then cover with waterproof adhesive tape. If the preparation touches healthy skin, immediately wash it off with soap and water.
- If using a plaster, trim it to the size and shape of the wart before application.
- If using a disk with a pad, choose a disk of the proper size, apply, then cover with the pad supplied.
- Do not apply to skin that is red, broken or swollen.
- Do not use the product more often than recommended.
- Do not use for more than 12 weeks.

See your doctor or a foot specialist if the wart is not gone after 12 weeks of treatment, or if the healthy skin around the wart becomes broken, red or irritated.

Dermatologic Conditions Section Highlights

Summary of Common Skin Conditions

Chapter 41: **Dermatitis**

    Atopic dermatitis/contact dermatitis/stasis dermatitis
        Differentiating features of eczematous dermatitis
        Suggested approaches for treating atopic/contact dermatitis
    Diaper dermatitis
        Prevention
        Differential diagnosis of diaper dermatitis
        Suggested approach for treating diaper dermatitis

Chapter 42: **Dandruff, Seborrhea and Psoriasis**

    Characteristics, differential diagnosis and management
    Comparisons among dandruff, seborrhea and psoriasis
    Suggested approaches for treating dandruff, scalp seborrhea and psoriasis

Chapter 43: **Acne**

    Differential diagnosis of acne
    Severity grading of acne lesions
    Suggested approach for treating acne with nonprescription medication

Chapter 44: **Cosmetic Dermatology**

    Perspiration and body odor
    Hair care and hair growth concerns
        Drugs associated with hair loss
        Hair care and styling products
    Dry skin and sun-induced skin damage
        Radiation effects and sunscreen coverage
        Sunscreen ingredients

Chapter 45: **Viral Skin Rashes**

    Characteristics of Selected Viral Skin Rashes
    Prevention

Summary of **Common Skin Conditions**[1-4] by Penny F. Miller

Condition	Signs and symptoms	Location(s)	Management
Scalp			
Tinea capitis	Bald patch(es) with round, scaling lesions;itchy. May be inflamed boggy nodule.	Scalp (usually in children)	Refer to physician
Head lice	White spots (nits) clinging to base of hair that are not easily removed; itchy.	Scalp especially sides and posterior aspects (commonly in children).	Self-care
Psoriasis	Silver scales on an elevated erythematous base (plaques). Pin-point bleeding spots are evident when scales are scratched off. Symmetric distribution is common.	Posterior scalp	Refer to physician for diagnosis; OTC management depending on severity at diagnosis
Dandruff	Diffuse,white flakes without redness; mildly itchy.	Scalp	Self-care
Shingles	Unilateral, painful, grouped blisters with eventual crusts. The lesions are arranged in a linear (dermatomal) pattern along a sensory nerve.	Scalp, forehead and face	Refer to physician.
Seborrheic dermatitis	Mildly red patches with yellowish, greasy scale. Ill-defined borders.	Scalp,eyebrows and nasolabial folds.	Self-care; refer to physician if severe
Trunk			
Shingles (Herpes zoster)	Painful vesicles in a unilateral dermatomal distribution with eventual crusting	Dermatomal distribution – linear from back to chest or abdomen	Refer to physician
Tinea corporis	Round, red, scaly patches with well-defined raised edges; central clearing and itchy	Trunk, limbs	Self-care
Photosensitivity reaction – Phototoxic reaction	Exaggerated sunburn (may be blistered if severe)	Sun-exposed areas	Self-care
Photosensitivity reaction – Photoallergic reaction	Red, itchy papules with no sharp borders	Any skin area	Self-care
Pityriasis versicolor	Light-colored patches on tanned skin or darker–colored patches on untanned skin; fine scale	Chest, back	Self-care

(cont'd)

Summary of Common Skin Conditions[1-4] *(cont'd)*

Condition	Signs and symptoms	Location(s)	Management
Face			
Acne	Comedones, papules, pustules and cysts. Commonly in adolescents.	Face	Self-care if mild; refer to physician if moderate-severe
Acne rosacea	Papules, pustules (no comedones); flushing in blush areas.	Face	Refer to physician
Perioral dermatitis	Discrete red or flesh-colored papules and pustules. May be pruritic and burning.	Around mouth and nasolabial folds	Refer to physician
Folliculitis	Small red pustules surrounding hair follicles.	Bearded (hairy) areas	Self-care
Furuncles	Painful, red, raised lump (nodules) with pus-filled centre around hair follicle.	Bearded (hairy) areas, back of neck	Self-care
Carbuncles	Large, painful, red, raised nodules with pus-filled center around multiple hair follicles; fever, malaise, adenopathy.	Bearded (hairy) areas, back of neck	Refer to physician
Cold sores (Herpes simplex)	Tingling sensation progessing to tiny painful, grouped blisters, then crusts.	Lips	Self-care; refer to physician if genital involvement or immunocompromised
Impetigo	Weeping vesicles with honey-colored crusts. Erythema surrounds lesion. Adenopathy is common.	Around nose and mouth (usually)	Self-care if a few small lesions; otherwise, refer to physician
Photosensitivity reaction – Phototoxic reaction	Exaggerated sunburn	Sun-exposed skin areas	Self-care unless severe; refer to physician for reassessment of drug therapy if necessary
Photosensitivity reaction – Photoallergic reaction	Red itchy vesicles	Any skin area	Self-care unless severe; refer to physician for reassessment of drug therapy if necessary
Contact dermatitis	Localized, itchy, red vesicles	Any skin area in contact with allergen	Self-care unless severe
Atopic dermatitis	Red, itchy ,weeping vesicles; eventually see chronic changes – lichenified dry skin (thickened, accentuated skin markings)	Infants: face (cheeks) Adolescents and young adults: sides of neck	Refer to physician

Limbs

	Description	Location	Recommendation
Contact dermatitis	Localized, itchy red vesicles	Hands, wrists or any area exposed to contact allergen	Self-care unless severe
Common warts	Skin-colored, well-defined, small, round, rough-surfaced papules. May see black dots on surface	Hands, fingers, around nails	Self-care
Flat warts	Multiple smooth, flat or slightly elevated reddish papules	Hands	Refer to physician
Psoriasis	Red plaques with a silvery scale	Knees, elbows	Refer to physician for diagnosis; OTC management depending on severity at diagnosis
Scabies	Red lesions possibly with thin gray lines; itching that increases at night	Finger webs and wrists; armpits	Refer for diagnosis; self-care management
Atopic dermatitis	Red, itchy vesicles	Extensor areas in infants; flexural area in adolescents and adults	Refer to physician
Cellulitis	Red, hot, hard, painful skin area with systemic symptoms of fever and malaise	Often at site of trauma	Refer to physician immediately
Stasis dermatitis	Red, itchy vesicles, edema followed by brownish, scaly, thickened skin; pain	Lower legs, ankles (in older adults)	Refer to physician

Genitals

	Description	Location	Recommendation
Pubic lice	Crab lice and eggs detectable; very itchy	Genital area; other hairy areas	Self-care
Candidiasis	Red, moist rash with irregular edges and satellite lesions (papules outside the edge of the rash); itchy and sore	Skin folds such as groin (gluteal fold), under breasts, axillae	Self-care
Tinea cruris	Red-brown, bilateral, well-demarcated rash; itchy	Inner aspect of thighs and pubic area; scrotum and penis is spared in males. Often associated with tinea pedis	Self-care

(cont'd)

Summary of Common Skin Conditions[1-4] *(cont'd)*

Condition	Signs and symptoms	Location(s)	Management
Genitals *(cont'd)*			
Psoriasis	Bilateral, red, sharply demarcated plaques (scales are absent in intertriginous areas)	Intergluteal folds (groin), axillae	Refer to physician for diagnosis; OTC management depending on severity at diagnosis

Only the most common signs and symptoms, presentations and locations are listed; not inclusive.
Systemic symptoms accompanying these rashes should be referred.
Any conditions not responding to self-care management should be referred.
Viral exanthems, foot and nail conditions not included.

References

1. Hooper BJ, Goldman MP. *Primary Dermatologic Care.* St. Louis, MI: Mosby, Inc; 1999.
2. Goldstein BG, Goldstein AO. *Practical Dermatology* 2nd ed. 1997:71-7.
3. Lookingbill DP, Marks JG. *Principles of Dermatology* 3rd ed. Philadelphia, PA: WB Saunders. 2000.
4. Edwards C, Stillman P. *Minor Illness or Major Disease? Responding to symptoms in the pharmacy.* 3rd ed. London: Pharmaceutical Press; 2000.

Chapter 41

Dermatitis

Debra Sibbald, BScPhm, MA (Adult Education)

Atopic, Contact and Stasis Dermatitis

Pathophysiology

The most important function of the skin is serving as a two-way barrier. It prevents loss of water and electrolytes while retarding entry of foreign materials, chemical poisons and radiation. The barrier function of the stratum corneum is provided through three mechanisms. The lipid component of the semiperme- able cell membrane stores lipid-soluble substances, and resists physical and chemical insults. Removal of lipid content destroys this regulatory function. Keratin absorbs and retains water and regulates skin hydration. Intercellular spaces contain hygroscopic substances which absorb moisture and permit passage of water-soluble drugs (Figure 1).

Figure 1: **Epidermis**

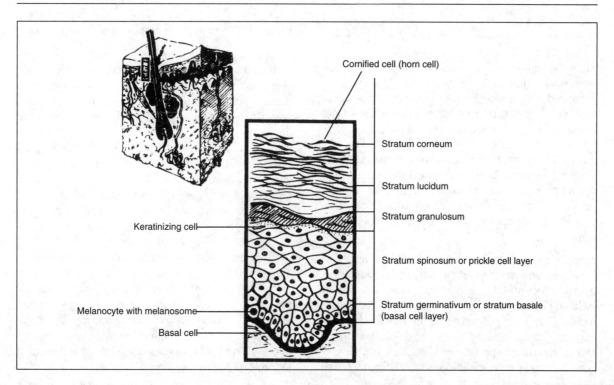

Cornified cell (horn cell)

Stratum corneum

Stratum lucidum

Stratum granulosum

Keratinizing cell

Stratum spinosum or prickle cell layer

Stratum germinativum or stratum basale (basal cell layer)

Melanocyte with melanosome

Basal cell

Skin hydration is normally 10 to 20% water by weight. When hydration drops below 10%, the corneum becomes brittle and cracks easily, allowing irritants to penetrate. This leads to mild inflammation and impairs cell maturation. Chapping results. Factors decreasing skin hydration include low ambient humidity, extremes of temperature, overuse of surface active agents (e.g., soaps), physical and chemical trauma, age, body site, and occlusion which diminishes skin resistance to foreign substances.

Barrier efficiency will begin to regenerate within 24 hours of damage by forming a temporary barrier of parakeratotic cells and dried exudate, reforming the horny layer over 12 to 25 days.[1]

> Dermatitis is a nonspecific term describing both acute and chronic skin reactions with corresponding clinical patterns and history. Although the word *eczema* (boiling over) has been used synonymously with *atopic dermatitis*, most dermatologists use the term to describe an acute, nonspecific skin reaction that exhibits erythema, scaling, vesicles and crusts. It does not describe dry, lichenified chronic lesions. The term dermatitis is less specific and describes both acute and chronic skin reactions.

Atopy is defined as a sensitivity of skin and mucous membranes toward environmental factors with enhanced IgE synthesis and/or altered nonspecific reactivity.[2] Eighty to 85% of patients with *atopic dermatitis* have high levels of total IgE which correlate with the severity of clinical disease. The IgE causes an eczema-type reaction rather than a classic urticarial reaction. Eosinophils are involved in producing proinflammatory products in the skin. Twenty per cent of patients show normal IgE levels and lack specific sensitization against inhalant and food allergens.

Atopic individuals have an increased family history of hay fever, asthma and chronic rhinitis. In addition to genetic predisposition, exogenous provoking factors including natural substances such as house dust mites, molds, furry pets, pollen, penicillin and foods influence the manifestation, course and localization of atopic dermatitis. The seasonal variation has several contributing factors: environmental allergens cause relapses in summer, while climatic influences may cause clearing in summer sun and worsening in the dry, cold air of winter. Heat and sweating will worsen the skin condition. Stress also contributes.[2] Controversy has existed for many years about the role of diet as an aggravating factor. In selected infants and children, food allergens may play a role in disease progression. Five foods are identified as frequent culprits, in the following order: eggs, milk, peanuts, soy and wheat.[3] Irritants such as disinfectants, solvents and allergens in skin care products play an important role. Intolerance to wool is a hallmark of atopy. Atopic patients have an increased propensity for cutaneous viral infections, including herpes simplex, molluscum contagiosum, and warts; fungal infections such as dermatophytosis, pityriasis (tinea) versicolor, and candidiasis; and bacterial infections such as *S. aureus*.[3]

Atopic dermatitis begins in infancy, but is rarely present at birth, and decreases in intensity with age. In approximately 80% of cases of atopic dermatitis, the problem develops during the first year of life, and in up to 90% of cases the onset occurs before five years of age.[4] Atopic dermatitis affects 10 to 20% of the population. The disease is genetically predetermined, with a risk of 70% if both parents are involved, and a higher risk of inheritance from mother than father.

Allergic contact dermatitis is a delayed or cell-mediated hypersensitivity reaction induced by previously sensitized lymphocytes resulting from exposure of sensitized individuals to contact allergens. Allergenic substances must be processed within the epidermis by the Langerhans cells that conjugate them with proteins. These are presented to the lymphocytes, initiating a sequence of cytokine-mediated events and inflammatory response. Most of these cellular reactions produce sensitization in only a small percentage of those exposed. The incubation period after initial sensitization is 5 to 21 days and 12 to 48 hours after subsequent re-exposure, but the reaction may continue to develop for several weeks.[4] The predisposition to develop allergic contact dermatitis is genetic. The most common contact allergens include plants of the *Rhus* genus, nickel, rubber, ethylenediamine (a stabilizer in many topical preparations) and paraphenylenediamine (ingredient in black hair dye and industrial chemicals).[5] A list is presented in Table 1. Nearly any chemical can produce contact dermatitis. Small molecules are most likely to be sensitizers since they penetrate the epidermis more readily. The possibility of cross-sensitization with other chemicals is very important. The most notable are listed in Table 2. Cross-sensitization may prohibit use of critically important systemically administered drugs.[4]

Primary irritant contact dermatitis is a nonallergic reaction that can be produced by exposure to any substance, including chemical, physical and biological agents, if the concentration and duration of contact are sufficient. Mild irritants such as soaps, detergents and most solvents require repeated or sustained contact to produce inflammation. Strong irritants such as acids and alkalis may injure the skin immediately. Irritant effects may be considerably enhanced by occlusion.

In *hand dermatitis*, frequent washing of the hands damages the skin through a combination of mechanisms: increased skin permeability from alkali-induced

Table 1: **Common Causes of Contact Dermatitis**

Allergic Contact Dermatitis

Substance	Source
Rhus genus	Poison ivy, poison oak, mangos
Nickel	Metal alloys, hairpins, jewelry, zippers, hair dyes
Ethylenediamine	Dyes, fungicides, medications
Rubber accelerators (Mercapto/carba/thiuram)	Rubber products (ostomy products, bandages, latex products, toys, condoms, diaphragms, goggles, pacifiers)
Paraphenylenediamine	Hair and clothing dyes, chemical photographic use
Potassium dichromate	Cement, leather, household cleansers, bleaches
Neomycin	Topical antibiotic creams, eye and ear preparations
Latex	Rubber products, e.g., gloves, catheters, balloons, plants
Bacitracin	Topical antibiotic creams, eye and ear preparations
Benzocaine	Topical antibiotic creams, eye and ear preparations
Lanolin	Topical medications, bath oils and cosmetics
Fragrances	Topical medications, baby products and cosmetics
Cetylsteryl alcohols	Topical medications, cosmetics, paste bandages
Quaternium 15	Preservative in topical medications and cosmetics
Topical antihistamines	Topical medications
Aloe vera	Topical medications and cosmetics

Irritant Contact Dermatitis

Acids	Oxidants
Alkalis	Solvents
Enzymes	Surfactants

Table 2: **Cross-sensitizers with Common Contact Allergens**

Sensitizer	Cross-sensitizers
Ethylenediamine	Aminophylline, ethylenediamine antihistamine products
Latex	Bananas, kiwi, pineapple, chestnuts, avocados, apricots, cherries, grapes, passion fruit, potatoes, peaches, tomatoes
Local anesthetics (ester type, e.g., benzocaine)	Para-amino containing-compounds (widely used in topicals): parabens, some oral hypoglycemics, sulfonamides, thiazide diuretics
Neomycin	Aminoglycosides (gentamicin, tobramcyin), framycetin
Rhus	Lacquers, mangos, cashews and ginkgo

damage to the keratin; removal of lipids and amino acids from the skin; and alteration of the skin's buffering capacity. Intensification may also be produced by irritants such as waxes, polishes and turpentine as well as through excoriation or rubbing.[4] Hand dermatitis may affect one in nine adults in any given year, predominating in females with a ratio of greater than 5:1.[6]

Aggravating factors play a large role in contact dermatitis since the extent and severity varies with the frequency and duration of exposure; presence of infected, inflamed or burned skin; degree of allergic sensitivity and mechanical factors such as pressure, friction and excessive perspiration, which may intensify the dermatitis.[4] Secondary infection with bacteria or fungi is more likely in dermatitic skin, and extremes in temperature, humidity, sweating and occlusion can lower the threshold for irritation.[7] Allergic contact dermatitis decreases with age. The skin of elderly people over the age of 65 is less reactive to allergens in particular, due to diminished immune function that occurs with age, while lower incidence rates among children are due to limited exposure to allergens.[8] Risk is reduced with impairment of cell-mediated immunity, such as AIDS, lymphomas, or atopic dermatitis. The incidence of contact dermatitis in Caucasians is greater than in African-Americans due to their greater skin reactivity. Caucasians have a looser packing of skin layers and fewer intercellular lipids, making their skin more permeable to irritants and allergens.[9]

Individuals at risk for contact dermatitis are often those who are exposed to these substances occupationally or as part of their daily routine. Although women develop contact dermatitis more often than men, it is primarily because women are more frequently exposed to irritants, allergens and wet work, and not because of differences in skin reactivity.[9] Hand dermatitis is often seen in housewives, health care professionals, hairdressers and dishwashers, especially in those who have atopic dermatitis. Susceptibility is greater among younger people. Seasonal variation occurs with increased prevalence during winter months and exposure to cold, dry air.[6] Latex allergy is common in health care providers. *Rhus* dermatitis is seen less often in dark-skinned individuals, more commonly in younger persons, and is a hazard for outdoor workers and enthusiasts.

Stasis dermatitis is commonly seen in middle-aged or elderly patients and in women more frequently than in men. Approximately a third of patients have a previous history of deep vein thrombophlebitis related to trauma, pregnancy, surgery or prolonged illness.[4]

Eczematous eruptions can also occur with many drugs given either externally or internally and cross-sensitivity may exist to structurally-related drugs given by either route of administration. Common orally administered sensitizers include antibiotics, phenothiazines, and the ester group of anesthetics. As a rule, the eruption starts shortly after the administration of the drug, if previous sensitization has occurred. Patch testing with the responsible drug will give positive results. Table 3 lists drugs which commonly evoke eczematous reactions.[10]

Table 3: **Drugs Which Commonly Cause Eczematous Eruptions**[10]

Group	Drug
Antibiotics	Chloramphenicol
	Clioquinol
	Gentamicin
	Kanamycin
	Neomycin
	Penicillin
	Streptomycin
	Sulfonamides
Antihistamines	Promethazine
Beta-blockers	Metoprolol
	Oxprenolol
	Propranolol
	Timolol
Diuretics	Thiazide diuretics
Sulfonylureas	Tolbutamide
	Chlorpropamide
Tranquilizers	Chlorpromazine and related phenothiazines
Miscellaneous	Aminophylline
	Carbamazepine
	Chloral hydrate
	Cyanocobalamin
	Fluorouracil
	Idoxuridine
	Minoxidil
	Nitroglycerin
	Nystatin
	Procainamide
	Quinine
	Quinidine

Goals of Therapy

- Eliminate individual trigger factors or contact exposure to irritants and allergens
- Provide symptomatic relief while decreasing skin lesions
- Implement preventive measures focusing on decreasing the number of episodic flares, lengthening symptom-free periods, and prevention of excoriations
- Develop coping strategies and expectations for patients/caregivers

Patient Assessment

Skin changes in dermatitis reflect the pattern of inflammatory response. They appear much the same in all forms of dermatitis according to the time frame of occurrence of the reaction, regardless of cause.

When the reaction is acute, the earliest and mildest changes are erythema (redness) caused by engorgement and dilatation of the small blood vessels and, usually, swelling (edema) resulting from leakage of fluid from blood vessels and accumulation in tissues. If swelling is severe, skin cells form vesicles that fill with edema fluid; this process is called vesiculation or blistering. Breakage of blisters results in oozing or weeping and evaporation of this fluid causes crusting and scaling.

Dermatitis may progress to a chronic stage. The skin becomes dry, fissured and cracked. With prolonged itching and scratching, it thickens, and the normal skin markings become more prominent. This process is called lichenification. The skin may show damage from scratching (linear or punctate scarring) and hyperpigmentation or hypopigmentation.[11]

The pattern of dermatitis and its trigger factors influence the clinical classification and therapy. Table 4 outlines the differentiating features of the types of eczematous dermatitis described in this chapter. An approach for assessment of patients with dermatitis is shown in Figure 2.

Atopic dermatitis presents as an intensely pruritic acute, subacute and chronic eruption seen in characteristic patterns in infants, children and adults. The symptoms and signs of atopic dermatitis are numerous, but usually nonspecific. Atopic dermatitis has no

primary skin lesion and the clinical presentation of eczematous skin lesions represents skin changes induced by constant scratching and excoriations.[12] The skin is typically dry and the lesions scaly, though they may be vesicular, weeping or oozing in the acute stage. The pruritus may be focal or generalized if skin is dry and may be most intense during evening and nights. It is usually intermittent and leads to vigorous itch-scratch cycles, with consequently common secondary bacterial infection of excoriated lesions.[4]

Distribution of lesions depends on the age of the patient, with infantile, childhood and adolescent phases. Redness and chapping of a baby's cheeks can be the earliest signs of atopic dermatitis. This chapping usually begins at two to three months of age and persists for two years. An infantile eruption shows all the features of acute eczema, with scalp, neck and diaper area involvement generally limited to infants.

A remission usually occurs between two and four years of age. Subsequently, a chronically relapsing dermatitis begins. Visual signs of chronic atopic dermatitis include less redness, increased dryness and early lichenification with thickened skin, hyperpigmentation and accentuation of skin furrows due to repeated rubbing and scratching. Involvement of the back of the arms and the front of the legs is seen first and later a transition occurs to the elbows and knee folds. Frictional areas such as wrists and ankles are regular sites, and localization may occur to the toes. With occlusive footwear there may be excessive sweating and drying of the feet. As the child reaches adulthood, recurrent outbreaks diminish or disappear. In adolescents and adults, the involvement may be generalized, but flexural accentuation is the hallmark of clinical disease.

Other minor features exhibited by atopic patients include recurrent conjunctivitis, cheilitis, infraorbital folds (Dennie-Morgan lines), recurrent infections, especially viral, and impaired cell-mediated immunity.[12] (See photo on page PS-1)

The clinical appearance of *contact dermatitis* is determined by the severity and acuteness of the inflammation. The area involved usually reflects the pattern of the contacting substance and may have sharp linear margins or unusual geographic shapes. It may spread to distant sites through lymphocytes. Contact

Figure 2: **Assessment of Patients with Dermatitis**

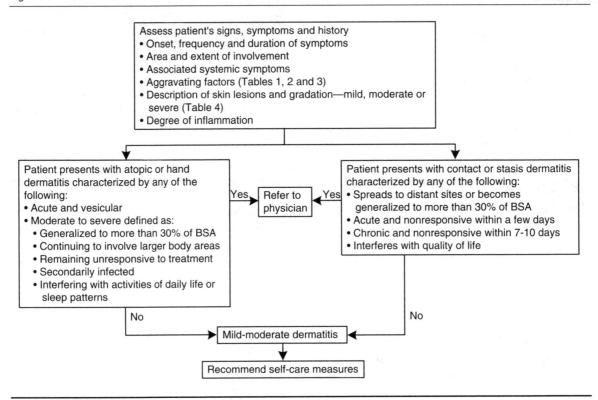

Assess patient's signs, symptoms and history
- Onset, frequency and duration of symptoms
- Area and extent of involvement
- Associated systemic symptoms
- Aggravating factors (Tables 1, 2 and 3)
- Description of skin lesions and gradation—mild, moderate or severe (Table 4)
- Degree of inflammation

Patient presents with atopic or hand dermatitis characterized by any of the following:
- Acute and vesicular
- Moderate to severe defined as:
  - Generalized to more than 30% of BSA
  - Continuing to involve larger body areas
  - Remaining unresponsive to treatment
  - Secondarily infected
  - Interfering with activities of daily life or sleep patterns

Yes → Refer to physician ← Yes

Patient presents with contact or stasis dermatitis characterized by any of the following:
- Spreads to distant sites or becomes generalized to more than 30% of BSA
- Acute and nonresponsive within a few days
- Chronic and nonresponsive within 7-10 days
- Interferes with quality of life

No → Mild-moderate dermatitis ← No

Recommend self-care measures

---

substances may be transferred from the primary site by touch to involved distant areas, especially the eyelids and neck which are very reactive sites. The face may display reaction to substances applied to the scalp. Scalp, palms and sole areas are more resistant.

Acute reactions are often red, edematous papules in the early phase, which become vesicles and bullae that ooze if the reaction is severe enough. Chronic reactions produce an entirely different clinical picture in which primary lesions are minimal and secondary changes such as dryness, lichenification, pigment changes, hyperkeratosis or thickening, excoriation and fissuring predominate. As with other forms of acute and chronic dermatitis, itching is the primary symptom.[13]

The most frequently encountered form of *allergic contact dermatitis* is *Rhus* (poison ivy) dermatitis, characterized by redness, papules, vesicles and bullae with a linear streaking distribution. Pruritus and

edema are key features.[4] Latex dermatitis is becoming a critically important occupational disease in health care workers.

Hand dermatitis occurs principally on the fingers, web spaces, and dorsa of the hand. Palms are spared and dryness, erythema and scaling are early features. It often begins on the fourth finger, beneath a ring.[4]

Stasis dermatitis, which occurs due to venous insufficiency, is seen on the lower leg. Acute changes consist of inflammation, edema, pigmentation and ulceration. The eruption may be erythematous and oozing, with marked inflammation. Chronic stasis results in scaling, discoloration and lichenification and is accompanied by edema due to venous disease. This may result in fibrosis producing hardening and induration of soft tissue. Pigmentation is invariably present in the early stages due to dermal extravasation of red blood cells following small venule rupture. Superficial ulceration may result from acute inflamma-

Table 4: **Differentiating Features of Eczematous Dermatitis**

Condition	Duration/Location	Description	Trigger factors	Aims of therapy
Atopic dermatitis	2 mos: chest, face, neck, diaper area. 2 yrs: scalp, neck, extremities. 4–10 yrs: scattered – neck, wrist, elbow, knee. 12–20 yrs: flexor areas, hands.	Cycles of itching and scratching. Red, raised blisters with oozing, dry skin Less acute and oozing – dry papules, thickening, peri-orbital edema and erythema Dry, thickened, hyperpigmented plaques	Extreme heat or cold, rapid temperature changes, sweating, irritant or occlusive clothing (wool or nylon), soaps and detergents, greases, environmental allergens, anxiety, infections.	Decrease trigger factors and pruritus Suppress inflammation Lubricate skin Alleviate anxiety
Contact dermatitis (irritant and allergic)	Irritant/allergic: in contact area Allergic: may generalize	Unusual patterns resembling contacting substance Acute: red, blisters, oozing, may erode Chronic: dry, thick, fissured	Irritant: time and concentration of irritant Allergic: sensitization to allergen	Decrease contact exposure to irritants and allergens If dry, wet it If wet, dry it
Dry skin	Lower legs (shins), dorsa of hands, forearms	Mild to moderate: dry skin with fine scale; diffuse or round patches Severe: cracks and fissures in diamond pattern with redness	Increasing age, decreased humidity, increased indoor heat, cold dry winter air, contact with soaps and irritants, hypothyroidism	Replace water in the skin and the environment
Hand dermatitis	Irritant: sides of the fingers, less often throughout palms Allergic: back of the hands	Redness, dryness, chapping; small vesicles; excess sweating	Repeated contact with primary irritants, soap and water, solvents and detergents Family history of atopic dermatitis or psoriasis	Decrease contact exposure
Stasis dermatitis	Lower leg, proximal to medial malleolus	Acute: inflammation, edema, pigmentation and ulceration Chronic: scaling, discoloration, lichenification	Venous insufficiency, and edema, upright posture, hot, humid environment, sensitizers	Decrease triggers, bed rest and elevation, compression of leg

tion and may heal or progress to deeper ulcers. Superficial venous varicosities may also be present.[4]

Table 5 outlines the other conditions which should be considered in the differential diagnosis of eczematous dermatitis.

Refer patients with atopic dermatitis to a physician for treatment if the dermatitis is acute and vesicular, moderate to severe defined as: generalized to more than 30% of the body surface area (BSA), continues to involve larger body areas; remains unresponsive, secondarily infected or interferes with activities of daily life or sleep patterns.

Refer patients with contact or stasis dermatitis if the dermatitis spreads to distant sites or becomes generalized to more than 30% of BSA, is acute and nonresponsive within a few days, edema persists or increases within a few days, is chronic and nonresponsive within 7 to 10 days, or interferes with quality of life.

Nonpharmacologic Therapy

An algorithm for the treatment of atopic dermatitis is shown in Figure 3, and for contact dermatitis in Figure 4.

Atopic Dermatitis

Control of trigger factors and anxiety is a major strategy. Control of exposure to environmental inhaled allergens is important. Direct contact with allergens and irritants should be reduced. Choose corduroy or cotton clothing because wool or nylon irritate and increase sweating and itch. Avoid fabric softener and bleach. Limit soap cleansing to axillae and groin, using mild soaps, creams or soapless cleansers (Table 6), restricting baths or showers to once weekly, if possible. Water temperature should be warm, not hot.

Temperature and humidity control will reduce problems related to heat and perspiration. Air conditioning in the summer and a cool air humidifier in the winter may be helpful. Swimming may be a better tolerated sport than those involving intense perspiration or physical contact.

Wearing cotton gloves or mittens to prevent scratching and secondary infections allows healing of affected hands. Keeping fingernails clean and short is essential.

Diet intervention is only indicated in about 10 to 15% of children, when the disease is of sufficient severity, and the provocation by certain food is of sufficient probability. Restrictions in diet should not have greater impact on quality of life than the disease. Risks of dietary restriction must be kept in mind: such diets may lead to malnutrition and deficiencies, carry the risk of anaphylactic reactions upon rechallenge to a restricted food, and challenge the psychological and social well-being of the child.[2]

Contact Dermatitis

The primary recommendation in contact dermatitis is to decrease contact exposure to irritants and allergens. A thorough history is essential in identifying the cause, especially any previous treatments that may have exacerbated symptoms or cross-reacted with the irritant or allergen. Protect the damaged skin against secondary infection until the acute stage subsides. Do not allow debris due to oozing, scaling and crusting to accumulate.

Patients with irritant contact dermatitis should avoid such irritants as soaps, detergents, bleaches and moist vegetables (for example, onions or garlic). Rings should be removed while working. Hands can be protected with plastic or vinyl gloves worn with cotton liners, but rubber gloves should be avoided. In

---

Table 5: **Differential Diagnosis of Eczematous Dermatitis**

Immunodeficiencies
Papulosquamous conditions
    Psoriasis
    Seborrhea
Metabolic diseases
    Fatty acid deficiencies
Infections and Infestations
    Scabies
    Candidiasis
    Herpes
    Tinea
    Staphylococcus aureus infections (impetigo)
Neoplasms
    Cutaneous T-cell lymphoma
Photosensitivity

Figure 3: **Suggested Approach for Treating Atopic Dermatitis**

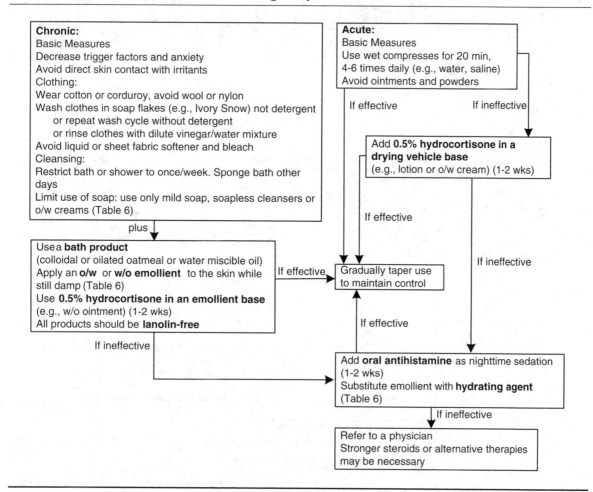

hand dermatitis, activity that involves friction, pressure, squeezing or twisting should be avoided.

In acute allergic or irritant dermatitis, the area should be washed immediately and thoroughly. If wet or oozing, compresses with saline or tap water can be applied for 20 to 30 minutes, four to six times daily.

Solutions for **wet dressings** used in atopic and contact dermatitis may include ordinary tap water and saline, in addition to astringent and antiseptic compounds. The action of a wet dressing is primarily physical, and thus water or physiological saline are generally the solutions of choice as they are convenient, inexpensive and pose no problems of

sensitivity or damage to healing wounds. It is very important to note that the technique used in applying wet dressings determines one of two opposing effects on the skin: used as compresses, they are drying, whereas used as soaks, they are hydrating.

Applied as **compresses**, wet dressings cool and dry the skin through evaporation. They reduce inflammatory blood flow, cleanse the skin of exudates, crusts and debris, and help maintain drainage of infected areas through vasoconstriction. They are indicated in acute eczematous conditions with oozing and crusting. The solution should be tepid or room temperature, although cold solution is effective to

Figure 4: **Suggested Approach for Treating Contact Dermatitis**

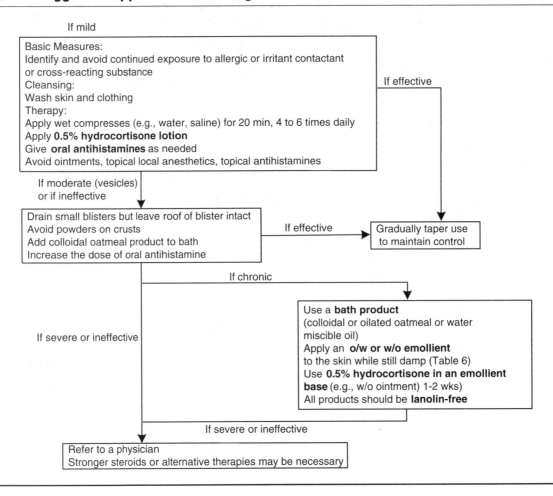

If mild

Basic Measures:
Identify and avoid continued exposure to allergic or irritant contactant
or cross-reacting substance
Cleansing:
Wash skin and clothing
Therapy:
Apply wet compresses (e.g., water, saline) for 20 min, 4 to 6 times daily
Apply **0.5% hydrocortisone lotion**
Give **oral antihistamines** as needed
Avoid ointments, topical local anesthetics, topical antihistamines

If effective

If moderate (vesicles)
or if ineffective

Drain small blisters but leave roof of blister intact
Avoid powders on crusts
Add colloidal oatmeal product to bath
Increase the dose of oral antihistamine

If effective

Gradually taper use
to maintain control

If chronic

If severe or ineffective

Use a **bath product**
(colloidal or oilated oatmeal or water
miscible oil)
Apply an **o/w or w/o emollient**
to the skin while still damp (Table 6)
Use **0.5% hydrocortisone in an emollient
base** (e.g., w/o ointment) 1-2 wks)
All products should be **lanolin-free**

If severe or ineffective

Refer to a physician
Stronger steroids or alternative therapies may be necessary

relieve itch in skin that is otherwise nonsymptomatic. A nonirritating gauze or thin cloth is soaked with solution, then wrung gently so it remains wet but not dripping. The compress is applied to the skin, removed, remoistened and reapplied every few minutes for 20- to 30-minute periods, four to six times daily. After removal, a lotion may be applied to the skin, but occlusion with an ointment should be avoided. Powders are not applied to any exudative lesion as they crust, causing bleeding on removal and increased risk of infection.

Applied as **soaks**, wet dressings soften hardened crusts in scaling conditions, and can hydrate the skin. To apply a soak, saturate the cloth and apply to the area for 15 to 20 minutes without removal. This procedure occludes and breaks down underlying tissue. Soaks are never used for acute, exudating dermatitis as they may macerate the skin, further damaging barrier function. Chronic contact dermatitis that is dry or fissured should be soaked for five minutes rather than compressed before application of an occlusive emollient.

Aluminum acetate (Burow's solution) contains approximately 5% aluminum acetate and is diluted 1:10 to 1:40 for use. It is easy to use, comes in tablets or powders, and is drying, soothing and mildly antiseptic. There is no evidence that it has a clinical advantage over saline or tap water.

Table 6: **Pharmacologic Alternatives for Dermatitis**

Drug	Dosing	Onset/duration	Side effects	Dosage forms	Comments
Bath products					
Bath oils	Apply at the end of the bath or after the bath 5 mL of oil/ 50 mL water with a cotton swab while the skin is still damp.	Onset: immediate Duration: effective until oil removed with towel	Allergic sensitization may occur due to lanolin, fragrance and other contact sensitizers. May make the bathtub slippery.	Oil with or without surfactants. Capsules	Acts as a barrier to reduce water loss. Soothes irritated skin
Oatmeal products	Must be properly dispersed in water to be effective.	Onset: immediate Duration: effective until removed with towel	Can clump and clog drain.	Dry powder, plain or oilated	Colloidal Provides relief for itching skin May contain oils and can act as an emollient
Mild soaps					
Opaque: Examples: Lowila® Petrophyllic®	Rinse well after washing. In atopics, restrict to axillae and groin.	Onset: immediate Duration: effective until washed and wiped off	Drying	Bar	May contain moisturizers
Transparent soaps: Examples: Pears® Neutrogena®	Rinse well after washing. In atopics, restrict to axillae and groin.	Onset: immediate Duration: effective until washed and wiped off	May be less drying than opaque soaps.	Bar	More water soluble but not as effective as other cleansers
Soapless cleansers Examples: Prevex Cleanser® Spectro Jel®	Apply and rinse	Onset: immediate Duration: effective until washed or wiped off	Minor irritation seldom seen.	Lotion, gel	Thin layer of product is left on skin allowing for retention of water.
Emollients					
Examples: Aquaderm® Aquatain® Glaxal Base® Keri Lotion® Lubriderm® Moisturel® Neutrogena Cream®	Apply PRN several times daily preferably while skin is damp.	Onset: immediate Duration: intermediate (6-8 h)	Allergic sensitization may occur if contains lanolin, selected preservatives, fragrance and other contact sensitizers.	o/w creams and lotion	Retards evaporation of water As oil content increases becomes more occlusive

(cont'd)

Table 6: **Pharmacologic Alternatives for Dermatitis** *(cont'd)*

Drug	Dosing	Onset/duration	Side effects	Dosage forms	Comments
Emollients *(cont'd)*					
Prevex Hand Protective Cream®		Onset: immediate Duration: intermediate (6-8 h)			Used to protect against irritants such as chemicals, detergents, polishes and water. For prevention and treatment of occupational hand eczema
Hydrating agents					
Examples: Complex 15® Dermal Therapy® Lachydrin® Lacticare® Neostrata® Uremol®	Apply PRN several times daily preferably while skin is damp.	Onset: quick Duration: intermediate (6-8 h)	Allergic sensitization may occur if contains lanolin, selected preservatives, fragrance and other contact sensitizers.	o/w creams and lotions	Emollient base prevents water evaporation and hydrating agents (urea, alpha-hydroxy acids) attract water to skin.
Antiinflammatory					
Hydrocortisone	Apply thin layer sparingly 2-3 times daily PRN.	Onset: quick. Duration: under 10 h	Allergic sensitization may occur if contains lanolin, selected preservatives, fragrance and other contact sensitizers.	Lotion, cream, ointment. 0.5% is OTC	Temporary relief of redness, pain, swelling and itch
Antihistamines					
Oral 1st generation most effective i.e., ethanolamine (diphenhydramine). 2nd generation not effective for itch.	Not to be used for more than 2 wks	Onset: immediate to 1 h Duration: 4-6 h	Drowsiness: caution if used during day or while operating machinery.	Tablets, capsules, liquid	Decrease pruritus due to inhibition of histamine only. Primary effect is sedation. Avoid topicals – contact sensitizers and ineffective

Stasis Dermatitis

The reduction of edema is important and achieved through bed rest and elevation of the extremity. After edema subsides, compressive support in the form of an elastic bandage should be applied. After healing of the dermatitis, advise the life-long use of elastic compression stockings.[4]

Pharmacologic Therapy

In most dermatitis conditions, a degree of dryness at some stage initiates or exacerbates the symptoms. The primary means of correcting dryness is to add water to the skin and then to apply a hydrophobic substance to keep it there. Pharmacologic alternatives for eczematous conditions are found in Table 6.

Bath Products

Bath oils applied during or after bathing help to reduce the rate of water loss through the epidermis. They help control dry skin symptoms but are less effective than lotions and creams applied directly to wet skin, since they are diluted with water, are in contact with the skin for a short time period, and most of the deposited oil is wiped off when towel drying. If added at the beginning of the bath, they may prevent rather than enhance hydration and thus should be added near the end of the bath to trap water in the skin.

Most bath oils combine mineral or vegetable oils with surfactants that disperse oil through the bath. Concentrations of surfactants (e.g., sodium lauryl sulfate) above 4% reduce the affinity of oil for the skin. Products with fragrance and lanolin should be avoided. Oil used as a single ingredient will float on top of the water. Bath oil capsules enclose small amounts of oil in soft, flexible gelatin capsules that dissolve in hot water. They may necessitate a higher water temperature than desirable and often contain a higher percentage of fragrance.

Bath salts should be avoided. They are highly fragranced, and soften water by raising the alkalinity. This may cause itching or redness to sensitive skin. Detergent bubble baths should be avoided in dry or itchy skin.

Colloidal oatmeal preparations contain starch and protein and are effective antipruritics for itch. For dry skin, they are not as effective as oils in trapping water to maintain hydration unless the oilated versions are used.

Soaps are made from animal or vegetable fat and alkali. Fatty acid plus sodium or potassium hydroxide produce a water-soluble soap. Toilet soaps are usually made from palmitic, stearic or oleic acids. Hard sodium soaps are suitable for bars, flakes and powders while more soluble potassium soaps are used for liquid preparations.

Excessive washing may remove lipids and water that normally keep the stratum corneum soft and pliable. Avoid deodorant, germicidal or fragranced soaps which irritate eczematic skin. There is little difference in the drying effects of various toilet soaps. No well-substantiated evidence demonstrates that addition of neutral fats or cold cream counteracts the drying effect. It is improbable that a simple cleansing agent can achieve two opposed tasks at one time: removal of soil from the skin and deposition of fat on the skin, especially since the soap is rinsed off.

Softer and more water-soluble, **transparent** soaps (or glycerin soaps) do not last long nor lather well. They claim to be less drying or irritating than alkaline **opaque** soaps. However, objective clinical evaluations are lacking. **Soapless cleansers** lack lipid and are available in lotion and gel forms. Lotions can be applied liberally and have a foaming action. Removed gently, they leave a thin film on the skin to aid in water retention.

Choice of soap depends on the type of dermatitis. In acute atopic or contact dermatitis, soap should be avoided. For chronic dermatitis, and for dry skin, a mild, nonalkaline soap, an aqueous cream, or a soap-free cleanser can be used alternately (Table 6). Soap is applied only to intact skin, without rubbing or massaging. Sufficient water should be used to rinse away all traces of soap.

Emollients

Emollients or moisturizers are semi-solid bases designed to control dryness. They cannot keep skin soft and flexible without the required concentration of water in the skin. Very little water from emollients is absorbed by the skin: most water evaporates when the emollient is applied. This emphasizes the need to apply them while the skin is still damp from bathing.

They leave an oily film on the surface which retards evaporation of moisture and maintains hydration and flexibility.

There is a wide selection of emollients including lotions, creams and ointments. Most are oil-in-water or water-in-oil emulsions. The greater the oil content, the greater the occlusion and the less drying through evaporation. Users are often intolerant of oil or water-in-oil products because the greasy texture increases discomfort. Greasy applications are unsuitable for acute oozing dermatitis. In contrast, evaporating water from oil-in-water creams or more liquid oil-in-water lotions produces a cooling effect which alleviates pruritus. A smaller amount of oil content is left as a residual film to protect hydration.

Petrolatum is a derivative of petroleum. It provides an occlusive effect but is cosmetically unacceptable as it feels greasy and does not wash off easily. It has the tendency to irritate, particularly erythematous or sensitized skin. It is best avoided in atopic and contact dermatitis, but is discussed further as an alternative for diaper dermatitis.

The emollient should be scrutinized for other ingredients, as some preservatives, emulsifiers and fragrances may aggravate atopic dermatitis or an allergic dermatitis through their sensitization potential (e.g., lanolin, parabens, cresols, sodium lauryl sulfate, cetylsteryl alcohols and fragrance). It should be chosen for its drying or lubricating properties as suitable for the stage of dermatitis. For an acute, wet dermatitis that has been compressed, a lotion should be applied after oozing stops, to facilitate dryness. In less acute, drier dermatitis, an oil-in-water emulsion base is appropriate. In chronic, very dry or scaly dermatitis, a water-in-oil emulsion gives maximum lubrication. Hairy areas may require gels or lotions.

Hydrating Agents

Hydrating agents are emollients to which **humectants** have been added. These ingredients have hygroscopic (water-attracting) properties, enabling them to attract water into the stratum corneum and hydrate the skin. Examples include glycerin, propylene glycol, urea, alpha-hydroxy acids and phospholipids. Some ingredients such as urea also soften keratin. Because they draw water and hydrate the skin, they are more efficacious for dry skin than emollients, which merely trap water present on the skin.

Glycerin is a humectant that helps keep the product moist and facilitates spreading. In optimal concentrations of 50% or less, glycerin helps retard water evaporation, keeping it in close contact with the skin. There is no evidence that glycerin is absorbed through the skin.

Propylene glycol is a viscous, colorless, odorless, hygroscopic liquid used as a solvent and vehicle for water-insoluble or unstable compounds. The pH may vary from 4 to 8 with these products and an acid pH may result in an irritant reaction. A small percentage of patients may be hypersensitive to propylene glycol.

Phospholipid products contain lecithin, which hydrolyzes to yield oleic, palmitic and stearic fatty acids. Lecithin is a water-binding agent that occurs naturally in the skin. Each phospholipid molecule forms a complex with 15 molecules of water. Water is drawn to and kept in the skin for hydration, keeping it soft and resilient. These preparations may also contain mineral oil, glycerin and lanolin.

Urea's main effect is to draw water into the stratum corneum, although there are claims for keratolytic, antifungal, antipruritic, anesthetic and antiinfective properties.

The concentration of urea determines its effect. Concentrations of 10% hydrate dry skin and 15% accelerate fibrin digestion. Concentrations of 20 to 30% are antipruritic, break down keratin, decrease the thickness of the stratum corneum and are used in scaling conditions such as ichthyosis. Concentrations of 40% are proteolytic and may be used to dissolve and peel dystrophic nails. Urea is sometimes combined with other active ingredients, such as corticosteroids, anthralin and benzoyl peroxide, to accelerate skin penetration. Combinations with hydrocortisone are useful for the dry itching skin of atopic dermatitis.[14]

Alpha-hydroxy acids (e.g., lactic, citric, glycolic, malic, pyruvic and glucuronic acids) may increase biosynthesis of mucopolysaccharides, contributing to the natural control of keratinization. Concentrations of 2 to 5% applied twice daily are best for use on larger areas or on the whole body as these compounds may produce irritation at concentrations of 10% or higher.[15]

Topical Corticosteroids

Hydrocortisone is indicated in mild, acute or chronic atopic dermatitis or contact dermatitis, due to its nonspecific antiinflammatory action. Hydrocortisone provides a good clinical response in suppressing reactive symptoms and underlying mechanisms in atopic dermatitis, allergic and irritant contact dermatitis, the inflammatory phase of dry skin and stasis dermatitis. Hydrocortisone lacks the antiproliferative effects of stronger steroids that give rise to both increased efficacy and increased side effects such as skin thinning, striae, telangiectasia, purpura and acne. Therapy should not exceed a two-week course. Tolerance or lack of response to hydrocortisone may require use of stronger corticosteroids; however, they should not be used on the face and in skin folds, where hydrocortisone remains the steroid of choice.[16,17]

Antihistamines

Oral **antihistamines** act by blocking H_1-receptors thereby reducing pruritus caused by histamine. However, pruritus associated with atopic dermatitis is thought to be caused by mediators other than histamine. There is no evidence that second generation antihistamines such as cetirizine are helpful in relieving pruritus due to atopic dermatitis.[18] The main effect of antihistamines comes from their side effects. First generation antihistamines cause drowsiness and this effect may help patients with atopic or contact dermatitis (adults and children) by promoting sleep in the presence of pruritus. In these situations, first generation antihistamines should be used before going to sleep.

Alternative Therapy

Some alternative therapies have been tested in patients with dermatitis. The disturbed epidermal barrier function of atopic dermatitis has been linked to altered metabolism of unsaturated fatty acids. This is the theoretical rationale for the treatment with **essential fatty acids** such as dihomogamma linolenic acid, or evening primrose oil. Use is characterized by a low incidence of side effects but also low efficacy in adults, with results in children no better than placebo. Two potential problems associated with its use are its high cost and the lack of standardization; adulterated brands may simply contain corn oil. Its use is clinically unsubstantiated and should not be recommended.[2,19]

The antieczematous efficacy of traditional Chinese herbal medicines has been confirmed by one study.[20] However, some preparations have been reported to cause toxic reactions resulting in fatality, and adulteration with other substances such as corticosteroids.[21,22] **Borage oil** has been used in atopic eczema, although efficacy has not been proven.[23] These natural remedies are not harmless and should not be recommended over traditional, standardized and proven therapies.

Prescription medications including more **potent corticosteroids** are sometimes necessary. A reasonable approach is to use low potency steroids and emollients twice weekly for maintenance of chronic dry lesions and mid- or high-potency steroids intermittently in short periods for acute exacerbations. Because dermatitis may rebound when topical corticosteroids are withdrawn, apply steroids in intermittent courses rather than as continuous treatment. Switching to an alternate steroid after a rest period may elicit clinical response again. Topical steroids need to be supplemented or substituted with steroid-sparing agents such as bath oils, emollients, hydrating agents and oral antihistamines. Steroid-sparing strategies can be tried either alone or alternating.[12] It is possible to develop an allergic sensitivity to steroid preparations. Refer patients with any dermatitis that does not improve or deteriorates after administration to a physician, and discontinue steroid administration.

The use of **immunosuppressant drugs** such as low dose oral cyclosporine in short courses is considered a third-line treatment for severe atopic dermatitis in adults where previous treatment with corticosteroids is ineffective.[24] An analogue, topical tacrolimus, shows high efficacy for recalcitrant cases and low side effects after one year of use. Longer-term studies are not yet available. These drugs and a similar investigational drug, topical or oral ascomycin, may be important future developments.[2,25,26]

Antiinfectives may be necessary as skin infections are common in patients with atopic dermatitis and can provoke exacerbation or relapses of symptoms. However, these products should not be used on a long-term basis as they have no preventive effects.

Antibiotics should be as specific as possible to limit the development of bacterial resistance.

Stasis Dermatitis

Local treatment of stasis dermatitis varies with the state of inflammation. Only those topical medications considered essential should be applied as patients with stasis dermatitis are readily sensitized; 80% of chronic patients are at risk for contact dermatitis. Ointment bases are the most common inciting agents.[27]

Monitoring of Therapy

Table 7 provides a monitoring plan which should be individualized. Patients should use a diary to monitor parameters. Changes in symptoms due to treatment can be correlated with alterations in trigger factors, such as irritants and foods. Stress, anxiety or depression levels should be tracked if they are suspected aggravating factors, and may lessen as skin symptoms improve.

Table 7: **Monitoring Therapy for Dermatitis**

Monitoring	**Patient:** daily while on drug therapy **Pharmacist/Physician:** acute dermatitis: after 7-10 days of therapy or next visit; chronic dermatitis: after 2-3 wks or next visit	
Positive endpoints (dermatitis resolution/control; relief of symptoms)		
Acute	Time frame/Degree of change	Actions
Inflammation (redness, swelling, pain, warmth)	Decrease by 50% within 7-10 days	Taper therapy in response to resolution: if endpoints not achieved, refer to a physician for further therapy.
Surface area involved	No progression	
Extension to other sites or generalization	None	
Blister formation	No new blisters after 1-2 days	
Itch/scratching	Control to tolerable level within 7-10 days	
Disruption of sleep or daily activities	Restoration of normal patterns within 2-3 wks	
Stress, anxiety, depression	Re-establish normal pattern within 2-3 wks	
Chronic		
Changes in inflammation, scaling, dryness, itch, scratching	Control by 4-8 wks	If endpoints not achieved, refer to a physician for further therapy.
Progression of severity	No progression of severity	
Recurrent episodes	Lengthening of symptom-free periods throughout therapy	
Lichenification	No further lichenification throughout therapy	
Negative endpoints (treatment side effects)		
Allergic reactions	None	If occur – discontinue therapy.
Severe dryness, irritation (redness, inflammation, stinging, etc.)	Minimal Should disappear, diminish or be controlled with continued use.	If severe, decrease dose, concentration or frequency of use. If still no improvement, refer to physician for further treatment.

Diaper Dermatitis

Pathophysiology

The peak incidence of diaper dermatitis (diaper rash, nappy rash) has been reported as age 8 to 12 months, although a survey of 12 000 parents of newborns reported 25% incidence at four weeks.[1,2] It is estimated that 7 to 35%, on average 10%, of infants are affected.[3] Two-thirds of all infants have mild symptoms at some time and one-fourth to one-third will progress to moderate to severe episodes. The decrease in incidence of moderate-severe diaper rash to 2% in the last 30 years, while the prevalence has remained constant, is attributed to the accessibility of disposable diapers since the 1970s.[4]

Both reusable and disposable diapers create a warm and humid environment in the diaper area, trapping urine and feces against the skin surface. If the wearer is not changed immediately when wet or soiled, the covered skin, the cutaneous and gut flora, and excreta interact with the diaper to produce dermatitis.[1] Because of immature skin appendages, scanty sweating, incompletely organized superficial vasculature and inactive sebaceous glands, an infant's skin is susceptible to drying and chapping.[5]

Moisture and the Diaper

Urination decreases in frequency from 20 times daily in the newborn to eight times daily after two months whereas defecation, initially three to six times daily in the newborn, decreases as autonomic and muscular control develops at around 8 months. The average infant excretes 400 to 600 mL of urine and usually excretes feces one to three times during a 24-hour period. The diaper acts as a barrier to diminish or prevent evaporation. The resultant edema of the stratum corneum alters the epidermal barrier, making the skin more susceptible to other factors. Skin exposed to water for 24 hours is more likely to manifest erosions following friction. Maceration promotes overgrowth of bacteria and yeast.[6,7]

Controversy persists about whether cloth or disposable diapers better minimize diaper dermatitis, because variables such as duration of wetness and frequency of diaper change are not controlled in many studies. Reusable cloth diapers may contribute to dermatitis if not adequately washed and rinsed of harsh cleansing chemicals. Airtight plastic occlusion to prevent leakage of urine and stool increases the chances for excessive hydration and maceration of skin due to decreased evaporation of moisture. Newer disposable diapers minimize this by wicking urine and water away from the skin surface to outer diaper layers. Prolonged wearing of any diaper promotes damage to the skin. Infants may need six diaper changes daily.[7]

Friction and Contact Irritation

A primary causative factor is repeated friction as the infant or immobilized patient shifts in the bed or chair. Excessive body folds increase areas of skin-to-skin contact. More frictional injury occurs if the skin is wet, producing chafing and shiny erythema, and allowing other irritants to harm the skin.[7]

Urine and Ammonia

Experiments verify that the level of ammonia, a known skin irritant, in infant urine is not sufficient to cause or initiate diaper dermatitis but may aggravate an existing inflammatory process. Damaged skin is more susceptible to irritating effects of ammonia, which is liberated by urease enzymes from cutaneous or colonic bacteria.[6] Urine hydrates the skin and makes it more vulnerable to frictional injury.[7]

Feces and Alkaline pH

Lipases and proteolytic enzymes present in feces may induce contact irritant dermatitis by attacking the epidermis and raising the surface pH to alkaline range. Ammonia also raises the pH of the skin, making it more susceptible to damage or infection. Loose and watery stools, common in infants, contribute to excessive hydration and frictional forces.[7] Breastfed infants, whose feces are less copious, less alkaline and less caustic, may have less diaper rash than bottle-fed infants. Foods that increase the urinary and fecal pH, such as high protein diets, may contribute to diaper rash.

Microorganisms

The GI tract is an important reservoir for *C. albicans*, a secondary invader of dermatitic skin, present in 70 to 80% of patients with diaper dermatitis, as opposed to 10 to 12.5% in those without diaper dermatitis.[7-9] Candida is most frequently found in the periphery of intense diaper dermatitis, particularly in pustules. It instigates some forms of diaper dermatitis and specific treatment is often warranted. Colonization of dermatitic skin by *S. aureus* can occur frequently, and can be suspected in a severely inflamed dermatitis with follicular pustules.

Onset of diaper dermatitis is gradual but may not be clinically apparent until an abrupt appearance of observable skin changes appear in the few hours between diaper changes.

Infants with atopic or seborrheic dermatitis, psoriasis, the incontinent immobilized patient, and the incontinent elderly are at greater risk for the development of diaper dermatitis.[10] Diaper rash can also be a manifestation of other diseases such as Kawasaki's syndrome, granuloma gluteale infantum, and cytomegalovirus. Unusual manifestations of diaper rash may occur in infants born to immunocompromised mothers. Frequent vigorous cleansing with detergents or soaps can actually induce contact dermatitis and can easily aggravate already inflamed, damaged skin. Untreated or infected diaper dermatitis can progress to skin ulceration, infection of the penis or vulva, and urinary tract infections.

The risk of drug-induced diaper dermatitis, which may be allergic or irritant contact dermatitis, is greater in infants than in other patients due to the thin epidermis, the high surface-to-volume ratio and the differences in systemic metabolism and detoxification in very young children, particularly those with inflamed skin. Elderly diapered patients with atrophic skin are similarly more susceptible to injury from topical agents.[5] In addition to the topical medications listed in Tables 8(a) and 8(b) which directly cause contact dermatitis, medications can contribute to diaper dermatitis through secondary effects. Oral medications can affect the motility and flora of the GI tract (e.g., antibiotics) or the autonomic control of urination and defecation, especially if given frequently. Some foods, such as caffeine and citrus juices, are irritating when eliminated from the body.

Goals of Therapy

- Relief of symptoms
- Resolution of dermatitis
- Prevention of complications and recurrences

Patient Assessment

Diaper dermatitis is a "geographic" diagnosis, occurring in patients of any age who wear diapers. The location of diaper rash is the area covered by the specific boundaries of the diaper, circumferenced around the lower abdomen and the lumbar back at about the level of the umbilicus, and below, around the upper thighs, encompassing the genitalia, perineum, and buttocks.[1] It may be more extensive on the front or back if the diaper wearer lies primarily in

Table 8(a): **Substances Which may Cause Contact Dermatitis in the Diaper Area**[5]

Ethylenediamine	Penicillin
Lanolin	Peruvian Balsam
Neomycin	Sulfonamides
PABA derivatives (e.g., benzocaine)	Thimerosol
Parabens	Topical antihistamines

Table 8 (b): **Substances to Avoid in the Diaper Area**[5]

Sensitizer or toxin	Effect
Alcohol	Dehydration
Benzocaine and resorcinol	Contact sensitivity, methemoglobinemia
Camphor	Seizures
Potent topical corticosteroids	Cushing's syndrome, atrophic changes, acne, superinfections
Topical salicylates (methyl salicylate)	Salicylate intoxication, metabolic acidosis

one position. Primary diaper dermatitis is an irritant contact dermatitis or chafing rash. Clinically, diaper dermatitis appears as erythematous, often shiny patches over the convex surfaces of the diaper area, usually sparing the inguinal skin folds. It may appear dusky purple on darker skin. The spectrum of severity ranges from mild, with erythema, to severe, with vesicles, oozing and widespread erosions.[2] The infant may be asymptomatic. It may resolve spontaneously or wax and wane, but is commonly treated. Candida diaper dermatitis is characterized by early maceration of the anal mucosa and perianal skin, progressing over days to confluent tomato-red plaques, papules, pustules, peripheral scale and satellite papules, which are most likely to culture positive for Candida. It almost always involves the inguinal creases. Pustules may not be seen due to maceration under the diaper.[1,2]

An approach to the patient with diaper dermatitis can be found in Figure 5. A summary of the possible differential diagnoses related to diaper dermatitis is provided in Table 9.

Refer the patient to a physician for investigation of other possibilities, including a contact sensitivity, infection or alternate diagnosis, when:
- The rash has been identified correctly but fails to improve after a week of recommended treatment;
- Pain, inflammation or itching has increased;
- There are oozing blisters or pus;
- The dermatitis has not healed in 7 to 10 days;
- The dermatitis has an acute onset;
- The dermatitis is chronic or recurs frequently;
- There is a complicated secondary infection, a urinary tract infection or infection of the penis or vulva;
- There are systemic symptoms (e.g., fever, diarrhea, nausea, vomiting, rash or skin lesions elsewhere);
- There are signs of immunodeficiency, deep ulceration or signs of abuse or neglect;
- The dermatitis is associated with another disease state;
- There are behavioral changes in the patient.

Prevention

Prevention (and treatment) of diaper dermatitis is important for the duration of time the patient is exposed to the wearing of diapers. Factors involved

Figure 5: **Assessment of Diaper Dermatitis**

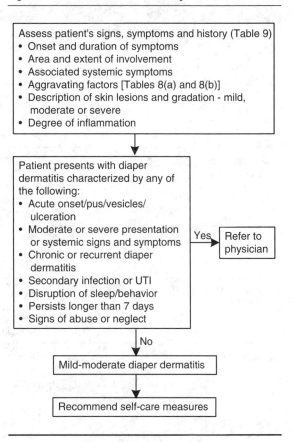

can be thought of in terms of an acronym which combines both nonpharmacologic and pharmacologic measures:

A   air, absorptives, antifungals, antiinflammatories
B   barriers
C   cleansing
D   diaper
E   education

Nonpharmacologic Therapy

The first step is to discontinue any of the aggravating factors previously discussed.

Air: It is important to allow "air" drying to diminish the damaging effects of occlusion and maceration, by removing the diaper for as long as is practical during cleansing, treatment and changes. Avoid practices that

Table 9: **Differential Diagnosis of Diaper Dermatitis**

Diagnosis	Symptoms
Primary irritant diaper dermatitis	Erythematous, often shiny patches over the convex surfaces of the diaper area, usually sparing the inguinal skin folds.
Candida diaper dermatitis	Early maceration of the anal mucosa and perianal skin, progressing over days to confluent tomato-red plaques, papules, pustules, peripheral scale and satellite papules, almost always involving the inguinal creases. Lack of sebum by age 4 months, or oral antibiotic therapy for otitis media may be factors. May have thrush in oral cavity.
Miliaria rubra (prickly heat, heat rash)	Clear superficial vesicles without inflammation in newborns, or in older infants, tiny red papules and papulovesicles, sometimes pruritic due to eccrine sweat duct occlusion. Also found in overlapping skin folds in infants, especially neck and axillary folds. May be caused by occlusion from plastic outer coverings of diapers.
Allergic contact dermatitis	More common in infants over 12 mos. Failure to respond to treatment for irritant dermatitis. Allergy to component of topical preparation. More severe in flexural areas since topical agent may concentrate in folds.
Seborrheic dermatitis	Well-circumscribed, erythematous, greasy scaly plaques with flexural accentuation, typically asymptomatic. May involve scalp, neck, face, axilla and retroauricular areas as well. Occurs in the first 6 months of life and extremely common in the aged.
Atopic dermatitis	Usually not in the groin, but atopics are more susceptible to irritant dermatitis, which may present as acute dermatitis or chronic lichenification. History of pruritus, eczema, especially in flexural areas, asthma, or allergic rhinitis. Later onset (after 2 mos) and family history of atopy.
Psoriasis	Less common. Brilliant erythematous plaques in the diaper area, lack of silvery scale due to hydrating effect of diapers. Family history of psoriasis and typical lesions elsewhere on the body. Lack of response to topical steroids and anti-yeast medications.
Scabies	Excoriations and ill-defined papular eruptions in the diaper area. Burrows on palms, soles, axillary and genital areas, nipples, umbilicus and finger webs. Itching persists 3-4 wks after treatment.
Bullous impetigo	Large flaccid bullae filled with straw-colored liquid in the first few weeks of life. Ruptured bullae leave red, denuded areas and honey coloured crusts.
Histiocytosis	Very rare. Recalcitrant diaper dermatitis with erythematous papules surmounted by scale, may be hemorrhagic. Involvement of scalp and retroauricular areas. Systemic symptoms of hepatosplenomegaly, anemia, and lymphadenopathy.
Acrodermatitis enteropathica	Disorder of zinc metabolism leading to perioral, perineal, and sacral skin erosions and erythematous, well-demarcated scaly plaques. Infants may also have alopecia, growth failure, diarrhea and irritability.
Congenital syphilis	Copper-colored erythematous macules and papules and moist erosions in the diaper region, denuded sacral areas. May have anemia, hepatosplenomegaly, jaundice, bone involvement.

may cause chapping and burns, such as drying of the skin of the buttocks with a hair dryer, even on the lowest setting, or exposure to infrared lamps.

Barriers: **Powders** are potentially dangerous and best avoided. **Cornstarch** reduces friction. It may absorb some moisture, although inefficiently compared to pastes, and it does not wick moisture away from the skin surface. It arguably may serve as a culture medium for *C. albicans*; authors debate whether this will promote or aggravate diaper dermatitis.[11] **Talc** is a finely milled form of hydrous magnesium silicate which is more a lubricant than an absorbent. It reduces friction, and adheres well to the skin. Notwithstanding, respiratory problems may develop from aspiration of cornstarch or talc, unless applied to a cotton puff, or the hands, and dabbed on.[12] Metabolic alkalosis has been reported in an infant whose diaper rash was treated with baking soda.[13] When powders are applied to broken or oozing skin they can form a crust which may lead to infection.

Cleansing should be gentle, and the frequency of washing should be decreased. Rinsing with water is sufficient to remove urine and mild soaps (Table 6) should be used for feces removal. This is especially important for the atopic child whose skin is further irritated by frequent washing with soap and water. The area should be blotted dry. Commercial diaper wipes should be avoided if they contain chemicals such as alcohol, soap, fragrance and lanolin, especially if they add to skin irritation. Most wipes are recommended to be discontinued if the skin is broken. If there is oozing and crusting with acute inflammation, compressing with wet dressings (tap water, normal saline, astringents) or oatmeal baths have been recommended. However, there are no studies comparing astringents such as aluminum acetate to plain tap water or normal saline, the body's natural fluid, and these have less risk of further damage to the skin. (See Dermatitis-Wet dressings.[1]) Oilated or non-oilated oatmeal baths may be soothing to diaper dermatitis. Irritant contact dermatitis has been reported from overuse of acid pH cleansers.[14]

Diapers: As a barrier and an absorptive device, an appropriately chosen diaper can prevent and ameliorate diaper dermatitis. Diapers inappropriately chosen or used may exacerbate this condition. Diapers should be changed as frequently as is practical to reduce occlusion, decrease contact time of urine and feces with skin, reduce mechanical irritation and trauma and discourage onset of secondary infection. Discourage double-diapering to lengthen intervals between changes. The visually unsoiled part of the diaper should never be used to wipe or clean the diaper area. Plastic pants should be avoided with cloth diapers. Choice of diaper is highly personal and surrounded by controversy. Some consider cloth more economical, comfortable and environmentally friendly. Others prefer the convenience of disposable diapers. Disposable diapers with absorbent gelling material in their core (superabsorbent) have been shown to decrease the amount of moisture on the skin better than cloth diapers[15] and produce fewer diaper rashes of less severity than cloth[16] or nongel-lined diapers.[17,18] These diapers wick moisture vertically, reducing maceration and mixing of urine with feces. Some newer disposable diapers may contain protectants. The diaper may also be therapeutic for atopic children, as the "tropical" environment may effectively rehydrate dry, atopic skin.[18]

Care of Cloth Diapers: If cloth diapers are used, they should be washed with mild detergent, avoiding water softeners or harsh soaps, and may be rinsed of bleach by running through an additional rinse cycle. A cup of vinegar in the final rinse water lowers the pH of the diapers. Commercial diaper services rinse diapers of harsh chemicals, sterilize them, and iron them to kill bacteria, fungi and yeasts.

Education: Patients and caregivers must understand both prevention and treatment of diaper dermatitis (see Diaper Dermatitis—Patient Information).

Pharmacologic Therapy

An approach to treating diaper dermatitis is presented in Figure 6. Pharmacologic alternatives for diaper dermatitis are summarized in Table 10.

Barrier bases are the mainstay of topical diaper dermatitis therapy and can be of two types: those that provide a water-impermeable barrier only, and those that are both barrier and water-absorptive in nature. In addition to their respective effects on moisture, both types physically shield the skin from outside irritants, protect surfaces that are healing, and lubricate against maceration and friction. Such products usually contain a mixture of ingredients including zinc oxide, petrolatum, mineral oil, eucerin, lanolin, or a silicone base in

Figure 6: **Suggested Approach for Treating Diaper Dermatitis**

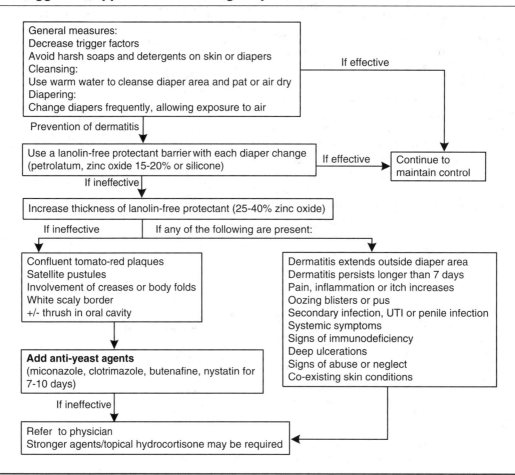

the vehicle, with or without absorptive ingredients such as talc, cornstarch or kaolin. Some may also contain astringents such as hamamelis (witch hazel), which may be a sensitizer, or vitamins such as A, or D and A in the form of cod liver oil. Preservative and fragrance may be present. Some of these added constituents are of dubious value, or may be contact sensitizers. First aid products not approved for diaper dermatitis should be avoided as they may contain other harmful ingredients, such as an unnecessary antibiotic or a sensitizing anesthetic.

The use of barriers is recommended as both prevention and treatment of diaper dermatitis. Use will help prevent dermatitis in all diaper wearers with risk

factors present, and especially in newborns with frequent urination and defecation, those with sensitive skin, or patients with coexisting conditions. Thicker, absorptive barriers are suggested for treatment of an existing dermatitis.

Barrier-only products that are suitable for use in diaper dermatitis are either oleaginous hydrocarbon bases, absorption bases, or silicone bases. **Petrolatum**, yellow or decolorized white, is a translucent oil-phase greasy preparation with no capacity to absorb moisture. It traps moisture present on the skin surface underneath it and may lead to maceration if applied to overhydrated skin. As a mineral-derived product, it may be irritating to inflamed skin.

Table 10: **Pharmacologic Alternatives for Diaper Dermatitis**

Drug	Dosing	Onset/Duration	Side effects	Dosage forms	Comments
Barrier products					
Zinc Oxide Examples: 15% and lanolin free: Desitin Creamy Ointment® > 25% pastes and lanolin free: Triple Care EPC®	Reapply every few hours in a thick layer. Remove with mineral oil or water	Immediate onset. Lasts for about 3 h	Not irritating. Formulations which contain additives such as lanolin, preservative, fragrance, may be sensitizing.	Cream, ointment, paste, powder	Astringent and antiseptic actions as well as absorbent and protectant properties. Effective preventive measure at lower concentrations (15%) Very effective treatment measure at concentrations above 25%
Silicone-based products (dimethicone or dimethylpolysiloxane) Example: No Sting Barrier®	Reapply every few hours in a thick layer. Remove with mineral oil or water	Immediate onset. Lasts for about 3 h	Not irritating. Formulations which contain additives such as lanolin, preservatives, fragrance, may be sensitizing.	Cream	Water-repellent only. Soothe by protecting against irritants
Anti-yeast agents					
Imidazoles: Clotrimazole Miconazole	Thin layer reapplied every 12 h	Clinical improvement and relief of pruritus within 1 wk. Duration of treatment is 1-2 wks.	Skin blistering, irritation, burning, pruritus, stinging. Cross-sensitivity to other azole derivatives.	Cream/spray	Inhibits ergosterol synthesis resulting in increased cellular permeability, causing leakage of cellular contents, some antiinflammatory and G+ antibacterial action.
Nystatin	Applied to affected area 2-3 times a day	Onset within 24-72 h after initiation of therapy. 2 wks sufficient for therapy	Skin irritation (rash, urticaria) primarily due to preservatives (parabens) in some formulations. May stain clothing.	Cream and ointment	Effective only against Candida
Antiinflammatory agents					
Hydrocortisone	Must be reapplied throughout the day (up to 3 times). Should not be used for more than 1 wk	Onset in terms of pruritus is immediate, inflammation takes about 2 days.	Mild to severe skin irritations. Hypersensitivity in small population.	Cream, lotion and ointment form. Powder form should be used for extemporaneous mixtures.	Effective antiinflammatory agent

Anhydrous lanolin, a sheep wool fat product, and **anhydrous Eucerin®**, a wool fat alcohol extraction which is less sticky and has less odor, are two translucent oil-phase "absorption" bases. However, these wool-derived substances are strong contact allergens and should be avoided in patients who have an allergic contact dermatitis, open or inflamed skin, or atopic dermatitis. Lanolin-like products may be components of commercial combination bases, wipes or oils for diaper dermatitis and the labels should be scrutinized carefully when selecting products for patients who could be potentially sensitized. Absorption bases are therefore less widely suitable and less appropriate than oleaginous bases for diaper dermatitis. Silicone-based products containing **dimethicone** or **dimethylpolysiloxane**, are synthetic bases which are water-repellent only, and soothe by protecting against irritants.

Bases which are both *barrier* and *absorptive* are usually creams or pastes with various percentages of **zinc oxide**. Zinc oxide, a mild antiseptic, is both astringent in nature and functions as an absorptive powder as concentrations increase. Moderate concentrations of zinc oxide (e.g., 15%) are usually creams, easy to spread, and good for daily maintenance to prevent diaper dermatitis. Higher concentrations, up to 40%, are very stiff, have enhanced absorptive and astringent properties and are suitable for treatment of diaper dermatitis. Pastes are especially useful for diaper dermatitis associated with diarrhea or increased stool output.[19] They may need to be spread gently with a tongue depressor or spatula, and removed with mineral oil. Although zinc absorption through the skin has been reported in a child with acrodermatitis enteropathica, zinc is a naturally occurring essential mineral and part of daily dietary requirements.[20] Zinc gluconate has been given orally in a double-blind, placebo-controlled study during the first four months of infancy with a reported decrease in incidence of diaper rash. Zinc levels were not measured.[21] Zinc oxide paste is often used as a protectant for stasis dermatitis. A plain zinc oxide barrier is preferable to those which may sensitize due to the presence of other constituents, such as aloe vera. Vitamins are popular additives to diaper rash barrier products, but no benefit has been demonstrated compared to zinc oxide, lanolin and petrolatum alone.[22]

Topical anti-yeast preparations may be necessary in a diaper dermatitis that has been ongoing for more than three days since it is likely colonized with Candida and may need preventive anti-yeast therapy. A diaper dermatitis which is beefy red with a lacy, scaly border and satellite pustules, involving the creases, is probably actively infected with Candida, requiring specific treatment. Topical imidazoles are a primary choice. Topical **miconazole 1%** or **clotrimazole 2%** are nonprescription antifungal preparations that can be used twice daily for one week. They are generally 70 to 90% effective against Candida. Antifungal preparations are supplied in creamy, opaque polyethylene glycol bases that are water-soluble. They contain no oil or water phases, nor do they require preservatives, but function to keep the antifungal at the skin surface, where it can release the medication to attack the yeast in the stratum corneum. They should be applied first, followed by the barrier cream.

Topical **butenafine** is an OTC butyl-amine, marketed for athlete's foot, but also effective against Candida. It can be applied once daily and efficacy is approximately 80%.

Topical **nystatin** is also an OTC anti-yeast preparation with efficacy slightly less than the imidazoles, around 70%. It typically requires longer, about two weeks, for symptoms to resolve. Nystatin is known to cause staining.

Once the inflammation has subsided, the anti-yeast preparation should be discontinued, and treatment with the barrier cream continued.

Topical **hydrocortisone** 0.5% can be applied to the occluded area under the diaper. With the exception of topical 1% hydrocortisone, more potent steroids will be absorbed due to heat and moisture and can cause serious side effects. Do not recommend hydrocortisone for use in children under two years of age without the supervision of a physician. Hydrocortisone can be added to the regimen for short periods of one to two weeks only, if severe inflammation exists. It can be used with a barrier cream only if the diaper dermatitis is an irritant dermatitis, or with an anti-yeast preparation as well, in the case of prevention or treatment of Candida. If used as a cream or ointment with an anti-yeast cream in a polyethylene glycol base, the steroid should be applied first.

The only prescription steroid that should be applied to diaper dermatitis is 1% hydrocortisone. Hydrocortisone 1% is sometimes added as a powder to commercial antifungal preparations as an extemporaneous mixture to facilitate compliance. Equal parts of hydrocortisone and antifungal creams should not be mixed as the resultant product contains half the required concentration of each active agent, and half the required concentration of preservative. This may lead to a lack of therapeutic response, and the possibility of resistance arising with continued use. Once inflammation subsides, the steroid should be discontinued.

The success of therapy for diaper dermatitis depends as much on the choice of the *vehicle* as on the choice of the pharmacologically active agent. In general, compresses of wet dressings cleanse, soften and cool the skin; powders, either loose or incorporated into pastes, protect the skin mechanically, absorb fluid, and decrease friction; lotions and emulsions cool and protect mechanically; ointments protect, soften and lubricate; and pastes combine the properties of both powders (absorb, protect, decrease friction) and the ointment bases (soften, lubricate) into which they are incorporated.

Herbals for diaper dermatitis include such concoctions as oils of sandalwood, peppermint, and lavender mixed together; calendula cream; chickweed root, powdered comfrey root, goldenseal root powder, sweet almond oil, and beeswax to be heated in a cast-iron pan and strained through cheesecloth before applying to the diaper rash.[23] They are sold over-the-counter with few instructions, no regulation as to purity or potential toxicity, and should not be recommended.[24]

Monitoring of Therapy

Taper therapy in response to improvement or resolution. Also monitor the side effects of drug therapy. If allergic reactions occur, discontinue therapy. If the condition worsens due to irritation, alter therapy. Severe inflammation should be minimal, and disappear after continued use. (See Table 11)

Suggested Readings (Dermatitis)

Klaus MV, Wieselthier JS. Contact dermatitis. *Am Fam Physician* 1993;48(4):629-32.

Sampson HA. Atopic dermatitis. *Ann Allergy* 1992; (69):469-81.

Sidbury R, Hanifin JM. Old, new and emerging therapies for atopic dermatitis. *Dermatol Clin* 2000; 18(1):1-11.

Sternbach G, Callen JP. Dermatitis. *Emerg Med Clin North Am* 1985;3(4):677-92.

Zug KA, McKay M. Eczematous dermatitis: a practical review. *Am Fam Physician* 1996;54(4):1243-50.

Suggested Readings (Diaper Dermatitis)

Boiko S. Treatment of diaper dermatitis. *Dermatol Clin* 1999;17(1):235-40.

Leyden JJ. Diaper dermatitis. *Dermatol Clin* 1986; 4(1):23-7.

References (Dermatitis)

1. Fox SI. *Human Physiology*. 6th ed. Toronto: McGraw Hill; 1999:16-19.
2. Ruzicka T. Atopic eczema between rationality and irrationality. *Arch Dermatol* 1998;134(11):1462-69.
3. Sampson H, Scaon S. Natural history of food hypersensitivity in children with atopic dermatitis. *J Pediatr* 1989;115: 23-27.
4. Sternbach G, Callen JP. Dermatitis. *Emerg Med Clin North Am* 1985;3(4):677-92.
5. Klaus MV, Wieselthier JS. Contact dermatitis. *Am Fam Physician* 1993;48(4):629-32.
6. Landow K. Hand dermatitis: the perennial scourge. *Postgrad Med* 1998;103(1):141-52.
7. Zug KA, McKay M. Eczematous dermatitis: a practical review. *Am Fam Physician* 1996;54(4):1243-50.
8. Belsito DV. The diagnostic evaluation, treatment, and prevention of allergic contact dermatitis in the new millennium. *J Allergy Clin Immunol* 2000;105(3):409-20.
9. Robinson MK. Population differences in skin structure and physiology and the susceptibility to irritant and allergic contact dermatitis: implications for skin safety testing and risk assessment. *Contact Dermatitis* 1999;41:65-79.
10. Bruinsma W. *A Guide to Drug Eruptions*. 5th ed. File of Medicines. Oosthuizen, the Netherlands: European Book Service; 1990:6,30-31.
11. Mitchell W, Lynh P. *Principles and Practice of Dermatology*. 2nd ed. New York: Churchill Livingstone; 1996:419-26.
12. Charlesworth EN. Allergic skin disease: atopic dermatitis as a prototype. *Allergy Immunol* 1998;25(4):775-90.
13. Pariser RJ. Allergic and reactive dermatoses: How to identify and treat them. *Postgrad Med* 1991;89(8):75-85.
14. Farber EM, South DA. Urea ointment in the nonsurgical avulsion of nail dystrophies. *Cutis* 1978;22:689-92.

Table 11: **Monitoring Therapy for Diaper Dermatitis**

| Monitoring | **Patient or caregiver:** daily while on drug therapy. |
| | **Pharmacist/Health care provider:** after 1-2 wks of therapy or next visit. |

Positive endpoints (dermatitis resolution/control; relief of symptoms)

Short-term	Time frame/Degree of change	Actions
Inflammation (redness, swelling, pain, warmth)	Decrease by 80% within 1-2 wks.	Taper therapy in response to resolution; if endpoints not achieved, refer to a physician for further therapy.
Surface area involved	No progression	
Extension to body folds, other sites or generalization	None	
Blister formation and oozing	No new blisters, cessation of oozing after 1-2 days	
Appearance of border scale or satellite pustules	None	
Disruption of sleep behavior	Restoration of normal pattern within 2-3 wks.	
Long-term		
Progression of severity	No progression of severity	If endpoints not achieved, refer to a physician for further therapy.
Recurrent episodes	Lengthening of symptom-free periods throughout therapy	

Negative endpoints (treatment side effects)

Allergic reactions	None	If occur – discontinue therapy.
Severe dryness, irritation (redness, inflammation, stinging, etc.)	Minimal. Should disappear, diminish or be controlled with continued use.	If severe, decrease dose, concentration or frequency of use. If still no improvement, refer to physician for further treatment.

15. Van Scott EJ, Yu RJ. Control of keratinization with alphahydroxy acids and related compounds. *Arch Dermatol* 1974; 110:586-90.
16. Snell ES. The pharmacological properties of corticosteroids. *Br J Dermatol* 1976;94(suppl):15-23.
17. Sneddon IB. Clinical use of topical corticosteroids. *Drugs* 1976;11:193-9.
18. Ainley-Walker PF, Patel L, David TJ. Side to side comparison of topical treatment in atopic dermatitis. *Arch Dis Child* 1998;79:149-52.
19. Leung DYM. Atopic dermatitis: immunobiology and treatment with immune modulators. *Clin Exp Immunol* 1997; 107(suppl):25-30.
20. Sheehan MP, Atherton DJ. A controlled trial of traditional Chinese medicinal plants in widepread non-exudative atopic eczema. *Br J Dermatol* 1992;126:179-84.
21. Ferguson JE, Chalmers RJG, Rowlands J. Reversible dilated cardiomyopathy following treatment of atopic eczema with Chinese herbal medicine *Br J Dermatol* 1997;136: 592-93.
22. Chan TYK, Chan JCN, Tomlinson B, Critchley JAJH. Chinese herbal medicines revisited: a Hong Kong perspective. *Lancet* 1993;32:1532-34.
23. Henz BM, Jablonska S, van de Kerkhof PC et al. Double blind, multicentre analysis of the efficacy of borage oil in patients with atopic eczema. *Br J Dermatol* 1999;140:685-8.
24. Harper JI, Ahmed I, Barclay G et al. Cyclosporin for severe childhood atopic dermatitis: short course versus continuous therapy. *Br J Dermatol* 2000;142:52-8.
25. Sugiura H. Long-term efficacy of tacrolimus ointment for recalcitrant facial erythema resistant to topical corticosteroids in adult patients with atopic dermatitis. *Arch Dermatol* 2000; 136:1062-3.

26. Reitamo S, Rusicka T, Jablonska S. Safety and efficacy of 1 year of tacrolimus ointment monotherapy in adults with atopic dermatitis. *Arch Dermatol* 2000;136:999-1006.

27. Ryan TJ. The management of the consequences of chronic venous stasis. *Clin Exp Dermatol* 1982;7:423-8.

References (Diaper Dermatitis)

1. Boiko S. Treatment of diaper dermatitis. *Dermatol Clin* 1999; 17(1):235-40.

2. Sires UI, Mallory SB. Diaper dermatitis. *Postgrad Med* 1995; 98(6):79-86.

3. Hansen RC, Krafchick BR et al. Diaper dermatitis. Supplement to *Contemporary Pediatrics*. Montvale, NJ: Medical Economics; 1998:8.

4. Weston WI, Lane AT, Weston JA. Diaper dermatitis: current concepts. *Pediatrics* 1980;66(4):532-6.

5. Schanzer MC, Wilkin JK. Diaper dermatitis. *Am Fam Physician* 1982;25(4):127-32.

6. Honig PJ. Diaper dermatitis: factors to consider in diagnosis and treatment. *Postgrad Med* 1983;74(6):79-88.

7. Leyden JJ. Diaper dermatitis. *Dermatol Clin* 1986;4(1):23-27.

8. de Wet PM, Rode H, van Dyk A, Millar A. Perianal candidosis – a comparative study with mupirocin and nystatin. *Int J Dermatol* 1999;38:618-22.

9. Mentes LF, Pittillo RF, Hunt D et al. Micro flora of infant's skin: comparison of types of micro-organisms between normal skin and diaper dermatitis. *Arch Dermatol* 1971;103:400-6.

10. Makrides HC, MacFarlane TN. An investigation of the factors involved in increased adherence of C. albicans to epithelial cells mediated by E. coli. *Microbios* 1983;38:177-85.

11. Belsito DV. The diagnostic evaluation, treatment, and prevention of allergic contact dermatitis in the new millennium. *J Allergy Clin Immunol* 2000;105(3):409-20.

12. Mifenson HC, Greensher J, DiTommaso R. Baby powder – a hazard! *Pediatrics* 1981;68(7):82-6.

13. Gonzales J, Hogg RJ. Metabolic alkalosis secondary to baking soda treatment of a diaper rash. *Pediatrics* 1981;67(6):820-2.

14. Patrizi A, Neri I, Marzaduri S et al. Pigmented and hyperkeratotic napkin dermatitis: a liquid detergent irritant dermatitis. *Dermatology* 1996;193:36.

15. Singalavanija S, Frieden IJ. Diaper dermatitis. *Pediatr Rev* 1995;16(4):142-7.

16. Charlesworth EN. Allergic skin disease: atopic dermatitis as a prototype. *Allergy Immunol* 1998;25(4):775-90.

17. Janniger CK, Thomas I. Diaper dermatitis: an approach to prevention employing effective diaper care. *Cutis* 1993;52 (3):153-5.

18. Wong DL, Brantly D, Clutter LB et al. Diapering choices: a critical review of the issues. *Pediatr Nurs* 1992;18:41.

19. Kramer D, Honig PJ. Diaper dermatitis in the hospitalized child. *J Enterostom Ther* 1988;15:167.

20. Parra CA, Smalik AV. Percutaneous absorption of zinc in acrodermatitis enteropathica. *Dermatologica* 1981;163:413.

21. Collipp PJ. Effects of oral zinc supplements on diaper rash in normal infants. *J Med Assoc Ga* 1989;78:621.

22. Bosch-Banyeras JM, Catala M, Mas P et al. Diaper dermatitis: value of vitamin A topically applied. *Clin Pediatr* 1988; 27:448.

23. *Web MD Health*. Available at: http://my.webmd.com.

24. Van D. The herbal medicine boom: understanding what patients are taking. *Cleve Clin J Med* 1998;65:129.

Atopic or Contact Dermatitis—Patient Information

Atopic dermatitis is an unpredictable condition in which the skin is dry, itchy and sensitive. Contact dermatitis is associated with an itchy rash that is caused by something to which an irritation or allergy develops.
- The goal of treatment is to relieve itch, dryness and irritation.
- Treat as soon as symptoms appear to avoid complications or spreading.

General measures:
—Decrease known trigger factors.
—Avoid direct skin contact with irritants.
—Wear cotton or corduroy, avoid wool or nylon.
—Wash clothes in soap flakes (e.g., Ivory Snow®) not detergent, or repeat wash cycle without detergent, or rinse clothes with dilute vinegar/water mixture
—Avoid liquid or sheet fabric softener, and bleach.
—Use a cool air humidifier.
—Keep nails short.
—Stop scratching or rubbing – use worry beads, pet rock or bean bag.
—Small children can use cotton socks or mittens at night to decrease scratching.

- Eat a healthy, balanced diet, unless foods have been identified as aggravating factors.
- Use plastic or vinyl gloves with cotton liners for any wet work. Avoid latex products.

- Be aware that stress may aggravate skin symptoms. Try to minimize its effect through relaxation or exercise.

Cleansing:
- Restrict bath to once/week. Sponge bath or quick shower other days.
  —Use warm, not hot, water.
  —Limit use of soap, use only mild soap or soapless cleansers
- All products should be lanolin-free.
- Use a bath product: colloidal or oilated oatmeal or water miscible oil
- Apply an emollient to the skin while still damp
  —if not effective for dryness, substitute emollient with hydrating agent containing urea, lactic acid, alpha-hydroxy acids, phospholipids

Your pharmacist can help you select an appropriate product.

- Use 0.5% hydrocortisone in an emollient base.
- Try an oral antihistamine as nighttime sedation for a one-week period if itch is severe.
- Continue proper skin care on a daily basis to control symptoms.
- See your physician if the rash fails to improve after a week of recommended treatment, pain, inflammation or itching has increased, there are oozing blisters, fever or diarrhea, or the rash recurs frequently.

Diaper Dermatitis—Patient/Caregiver Information

The goal of treatment is to relieve inflammation and prevent infection.

Treat as soon as symptoms appear to avoid complications or spreading.

General Measures:
- Decrease trigger factors.
- Avoid harsh soaps and detergents on skin or diapers.
- Avoid direct skin contact with irritants.
- Wash diapers in soap flakes (e.g., Ivory Snow®) not detergent, or repeat wash cycle without detergent, or rinse clothes with dilute vinegar/water mixture.
  — Avoid liquid or sheet fabric softener and bleach.

Cleansing:
- Change diapers frequently, allowing exposure to air.
- Never double-diaper or use plastic pants.
- Avoid wiping the diaper area with any part of a soiled diaper.
- Use warm water to cleanse diaper area and pat or air dry.
- Avoid use of perfumed or lanolin-containing diaper wipes.

- Limit use of soap; use only mild soap or soapless cleansers
- All products should be lanolin-free.
- Avoid powders. If inhaled, they may cause serious breathing problems.
- Apply a lanolin-free barrier cream to the skin with each diaper change: petrolatum, zinc oxide 15-20% or silicone.
- If ineffective, use a thicker lanolin-free barrier paste with each diaper change: 25 to 40% zinc oxide.
  Your pharmacist can help you to select an appropriate product.
- Avoid foods that provoke diarrhea.
- Try to avoid irritants (caffeine, citrus or spicy foods) in mother's diet in breastfed infants.
- Eat a healthy balanced diet.
- Continue proper skin care on a daily basis to control symptoms.

Consult a pharmacist or doctor if the rash:
  —Persists for longer than one week;
  —Becomes more painful, inflamed or itchy;
  —Spreads to other areas;
  —Develops blisters, pus-filled spots, open sores, a scaly border, or extends into the body folds.

Chapter 42

Dandruff, Seborrhea and Psoriasis

Debra Sibbald, BScPhm, MA (Adult Education)

Pathophysiology

Dandruff, seborrhea and psoriasis belong to the group of papulosquamous cutaneous disorders, which are the most commonly encountered skin problems. They are characterized by palpable, usually erythematous eruptions that typically all have a variable degree of scaling.[1] They may be difficult to distinguish from one another.

Dandruff and Seborrhea

Uncommon in childhood, dandruff usually begins to be apparent between ages 10 and 20, and affects up to 40% of men and women over age 30.[2]

Seborrhea is found in about 3% of the population, affecting persons of all ages.[2] It occurs more frequently in infants within the first three months of life and in adults 30 to 60 years of age. In the latter group it tends to affect men more than women, probably because androgens control sebaceous gland activity. In adolescents and adults, it is commonly manifested as "dandruff" or as an erythema of the nasolabial folds, ranging in intensity from barely perceptible to marked, waxing and waning from teens throughout adulthood.[3] The incidence in patients with HIV may be as high as 85%.[4]

Dandruff is primarily a cosmetic problem. Turnover rate of skin cells may be twice the normal rate. It is associated with a dry environment but *Pityrosporum ovale* may be present in some cases and play an inflammatory role. Although a relatively stable condition, it may be exacerbated by poor hygiene or a dry winter environment. Patients who develop itching may decrease shampooing due to the drying effects. This allows further scale accumulation.

The etiology of seborrheic dermatitis remains unknown. Hormonal factors have been implicated.

The occurrence of seborrhea in the neonatal period and remission by 6 to 12 months suggests a response to maternal androgen stimulation; the reoccurrence postpuberty is further evidence of a response to androgen stimulation.[4] It has been suggested that seborrheic dermatitis is an inflammatory response to *Pityrosporum ovale*, a lipophilic yeast of the Malassezia genus.[5] This remains unproven, although strongly substantiated by the response of seborrhea to some antifungal medications.[4,6,7]

Environmental factors such as low humidity and temperature, as well as stress, may provoke flares of seborrhea.[1] Bright light suppresses melatonin while UVA and UVB light inhibit the growth of *P. ovale* and many patients report improvement in seborrhea during the summer.[8] Genetics, as well as other co-morbid diseases, may predispose specific populations to seborrheic dermatitis. HIV-infected patients are more prone to an atypical explosive onset of seborrhea, with more severe and generalized involvement. The exact reason for this is unknown. Patients with CNS disorders (e.g., Parkinson's disease, cranial nerve palsies, major truncal paralyses) also appear to be prone to the development of seborrheic dermatitis, tend to develop more extensive disease and are frequently refractory to treatment. It has been postulated that immobility in these patients results in increased pooling of sebum permitting overgrowth of *P. ovale*.[9] Metals such as gold and arsenic have been reported to produce seborrheic eruptions.[1] Danazol, an androgen, and penicillamine also produce seborrhea frequently and may require treatment.[10-12] A more detailed list of drugs inducing seborrhea and psoriasis is found in Table 1.

Psoriasis

Psoriasis is a common medical condition in which psychosocial issues create a significant burden. One to three per cent of the population have psoriasis, and although the onset is seen at any age, there are two incidence peaks: age 16 to 22 for the more severe, type I psoriasis, and age 57 to 60 for the less severe, type II psoriasis. Men and women are affected in equal numbers. It has no known cure, and may be symptomatic throughout life, deteriorate with age, or wax and wane in severity.[13-16]

Psoriasis is probably inherited in most individuals by a multifactorial rather than a simple gene pattern. Genetic and environmental factors determine the clinical manifestations. About 30% of patients with psoriasis have a positive family history. If both parents are psoriasis sufferers, there is a 70% chance of contracting the disorder. Although family history is more closely associated with earlier onset psoriasis, it will not predict the age of onset, severity of disease, or coexistence of psoriatic arthritis.

Immunological factors are important in the expression of psoriasis, and involve antigen-dependent activation. In a susceptible, primed individual, local epidermal cells become activated, proliferate and release cytokines. These cause vasodilation and recruit cellular and humoral immune factors to the skin, reversing the normal CD_4/CD_8 lymphocyte ratios in the epidermis. The dividing epidermal cell cycle is shortened from 163 hours to 37 hours and epidermal transit from the basal layer, which usually takes 18 to 26 days, accelerates to three to four days. The skin becomes thickened with immature keratin on the surface, exhibiting the characteristic silvery scale. Leukocyte chemotaxis may lead to local pustule formation and a generalized inflammatory response results in erythroderma.[13,17] Psoriasis resolves without scarring, but may leave temporary hypopigmentation. It is a disease of control rather than cure, with relapses occurring unpredictably after weeks or months of remission.

A wide variety of environmental triggers may precipitate the first psoriatic skin lesions in a genetically susceptible individual, or induce flares in patients in remission. These include excessive alcohol ingestion, obesity, stress, pregnancy, infections (beta-hemolytic streptococcus, viral, HIV) or trauma. The Koebner phenomenon is the appearance of psoriatic lesions within 10 to 14 days after localized trauma. While most psoriasis patients improve with ultraviolet light, a small percentage (approximately 10%) are worse in the summer and relapses may be triggered paradoxically by ultraviolet light exposure.

Table 1: **Drugs Known to Trigger Seborrhea and Psoriasis**[12]

Drugs known to trigger seborrhea

Auranofin	Cimetidine	Haloperidol	Penicillamine
Aurothioglucose	Danazol	Interferons, alpha	Phenothiazines
Buspirone	Gold	Lithium	Psoralens
Chlorpromazine	Griseofulvin	Methyldopa	Thiothixene

Drugs known to trigger psoriasis

ACE inhibitors	Chloroquine	Glyburide	Penicillamine
Acebutolol	Chlorthalidone	Gold	Phenylbutazone
Amiodarone	Cimetidine	Hydroxychloroquine	Pindolol
Amoxicillin	Clomipramine	Ibuprofen	Propranolol
Ampicillin	Clonidine	Indomethacin	Pyrazolones
Arsenic	Co-trimoxazole	Interferons, alpha	Sotalol
Aspirin	Cyclosporine	Ketoprofen	Sulfonamides
Atenolol	Diclofenac	Labetalol	Tacrine
Auranofin	Digoxin	Levamisole	Terbinafine
Aurothioglucose	Dipyridamole	Lithium	Tetracycline
Beta-blockers	Enalapril	Metoprolol	Timolol
Bisoprolol	Fluoxetine	Nadolol	Trazodone
Captopril	Gemfibrozil	NSAIDs	
Chlorambucil	Glipizide	Omeprazole	

Psychosocial problems plague the psoriatic patient, who has very visible signs and symptoms which can have a profound effect on quality of life. There is a high rate of alcoholism in some studies of psoriatic patients. Patients are very self-conscious in public places, refusing to participate in health clubs or sporting activities. Clothes have to be chosen carefully so they will not allow shedding scale to be detected. Psoriasis may also inhibit intimate relationships and sexual activity.

Drugs aggravating psoriasis include beta-blockers, lithium, oral steroids, antimalarials, alcohol and NSAIDs; beta-blockers have been implicated in stimulating an initial episode[14,17,18] (Table 1).

Patient Assessment

A systematic approach to the assessment of dandruff, seborrhea and psoriasis consists of assessing a patient's signs, symptoms and history for the following (consider Tables 2 and 3):

- Onset, frequency and duration of symptoms
- Area and extent of involvement
- Associated systemic symptoms
- Aggravating factors
- Description of skin lesions
- Attempted treatments

Dandruff

Dandruff (*pityriasis simplex capitis*) is a noninflammatory increased shedding of small flakes of scale from an otherwise normal scalp. The scales are silver-grey, in patches or diffuse, and may separate fully or become detached only after combing. Dandruff is usually asymptomatic, although itching may develop. It is usually symmetrical, and absent in the bald area of male pattern baldness. There is no evidence of other skin disease on the scalp or elsewhere.[2,19,20] Dandruff does not present with scalp erythema. The characteristic scale is easy to diagnose yet often confused with other scaling conditions of the scalp such as seborrhea, tinea capitis and psoriasis.[2] A summary of differential diagnosis and management is provided in Table 2, and a comparison of dandruff, seborrhea and psoriasis in Table 3.

Seborrhea

Seborrhea is an inflammatory, erythematous, greasy, scaling eruption often confused with dandruff. (See photo on page PS-5.) In adolescents and adults, seborrheic dermatitis typically affects symmetric areas of the skin rich in sebaceous glands, including hairy areas of the head, such as scalp, scalp margin, eyebrows, eyelashes, mustache and beard. Other common sites are the forehead, nasolabial folds, external ear canals and postauricular creases. Seborrhea of the trunk may appear in the presternal area and in infants, in body folds, including the axillae, navel, groin, inframammary and anogenital areas.[4]

Seborrheic dermatitis typically presents as mild, greasy scaling of the scalp, which may be thick and accumulate, with erythematous plaques and scaling of the nasolabial folds and behind the ears and elsewhere in the above distribution. It begins in small patches, rapidly spreading, with diffuse fine scale that can be white, off-white or yellow, with no signs of acute dermatitis, such as oozing or weeping.[3] It typically flares and resolves in a cyclic or seasonal fashion, often in response to stress. Pruritus varies, and is more frequent in scalp and ear canal involvement.[1]

Profuse powdery scale of the eyebrows may compromise wearing of contact lenses. The eyelids alone may be affected, developing honey-colored crusting called *marginal blepharitis*. Paranasal involvement is typically seen in young women, who may lack dandruff, while the commonest type of facial seborrhea in males is a follicular erythematous form involving upper lips, beard, scalp, back, flanks and abdomen. Sometimes, plaques present with thick, adherent silvery scale as seen with psoriasis which usually spares the face, called *sebopsoriasis*.[1] Ear involvement is called *otitis externa*. On the trunk, two forms may appear, follicular (more common) or macular (rare). In infants, the entire scalp may be covered with thick, dry adherent yellowish-brown scale overlying erythema called "cradle cap." This appears in the third or fourth week, and may also involve the central face, forehead and ears. A widespread erythema with cheesy exudate sometimes presents in the flexural folds, manifesting as diaper dermatitis in infants or an intertriginous genital eruption in adults. These may generalize.[3]

In both children and adults, persistent generalized seborrheic dermatitis may be associated with human immunodeficiency virus (HIV) infection. There is a predominance of inflammatory and hyperkeratotic lesions, with involvement of trunk, groin and extremities, and occasionally erythroderma, alopecia, and hyper- or hypopigmentation.[3]

Table 2: **Characteristics, Differential Diagnosis and Management of Dandruff, Seborrhea and Psoriasis**

Form	Characteristics	Differential diagnosis	Action
Dandruff			
Scalp	Dry, white scale scattered diffusely over scalp	Seborrhea Psoriasis Atopic dermatitis Tinea capitis	Self-care management
Seborrhea			
Scalp	Greasy, yellowish scale over erythematous patches	Dandruff Psoriasis Atopic dermatitis Tinea capitis	Self-care management. Refer to physician if moderate-severe
Facial	Greasy, yellowish scale over erythematous patches, involvement of nasolabial folds, eyebrows, eyelashes, lips, retroauricular areas	Atopic dermatitis (infants) Rosacea Systemic lupus erythematosus Contact dermatitis	Refer to physician
Groin	Bilaterally symmetric, with reddish-brown fine scaling patches, in infants	Atopic dermatitis (infants) Dermatophytosis Psoriasis Candidiasis	Refer to physician
Psoriasis			
Chronic forms of psoriasis			
Plaque	Classic form: sharply defined erythematous papules which coalesce, covered with distinctive silver scale when untreated. Auspitz sign – punctate bleeding points when scale removed. Localized: extensors (arms and legs), scalp, ears, palms, soles. Generalized: (face, trunk, flexures) or one site with/without nails, nail pits – loss of color, thickening, distal destruction	Nummular eczema Atopic dermatitis Drug reactions T-Cell lymphoma	Refer to physician for diagnosis. Self-care management if mild

(cont'd)

Table 2: **Characteristics, Differential Diagnosis and Management of Dandruff, Seborrhea and Psoriasis** (cont'd)

Form	Characteristics	Differential diagnosis	Action
Psoriasis (cont'd)			
Flexural	In body folds and flexures No scale Demarcated erythema	Intertrigo areas: Tinea in males (active border) Candida in females (satellite pustules) Contact dermatitis – allergic or irritant (location of contact)	Refer to physician
Scalp	Silvery scale, discrete margins, extends beyond the scalp margins; may accompany any form or may be the only visible sign	Seborrhea	Refer to physician for diagnosis Self-care management if mild
Acute and subacute forms of psoriasis			
Guttate	Small, discrete, erythematous papular lesions; appears suddenly after upper respiratory tract infection (streptococcal) in children or young adults; may be the initial presentation; takes months to resolve	Pityriasis rosea Secondary syphilis Pityriasis lichenoides	Refer to physician
Pustular	Local (palms and soles): chronic in women who smoke, stable but troublesome. Systemic: uncommon but serious, starts with systemic signs and symptoms such as fever, leukocytosis, general malaise, followed by pustules (2-3 mm) on erythematous skin; may generalize and require hospitalization, steroids are contraindicated	Chronic dyshydrotic eczema – itch is predominant vs pain in psoriasis	Refer to physician
Erythrodermic	Generalized erythema without any characteristic lesions	Atopic dermatitis Drug reactions can present as severe skin disorders	Refer to physician

Table 3: **Comparisons Among Dandruff, Seborrhea and Psoriasis**

Disorder	Dandruff	Seborrhea	Psoriasis
Lesions	On nonerythematous base with fine, diffuse scale	Erythema with mild greasy yellow scale, plaques with indistinct margins	Annular well-demarcated silvery scaly plaques, with erythematous base, bleed easily
Common sites	Scalp	Central face, scalp, mid-chest	Scalp, elbows, knees, sacrum
Palms and Soles	No	No	Common
Nails	No	No	Pitting, thickening, dystrophy
Hair and Scalp	Yes	Yes, hair may thin.	Thick scale common
Intertrigo	No	Inverse type, glans penis, mostly infants	Common
Pruritus	Due to dryness	Rarely	Sometimes
Associated systemic symptoms	None	None (worse in AIDS); infants may generalize	May generalize, psoriatic arthritis.

The diagnosis of seborrhea can sometimes be obvious. Failure to respond to therapy may indicate coexisting diseases such as fungal infections, psoriasis or AIDS. Scalp seborrhea must be distinguished from atopic dermatitis, tinea capitis and psoriasis. Atopic dermatitis in adults tends to affect the antecubital (inner elbow) and popliteal (behind the knee) fossae. In infants atopic dermatitis has the same sites of predilection as seborrhea: face, diaper areas and extensor limbs, but seborrhea may have axillary involvement, lack of scratching and absence of oozing and weeping. The distinction between seborrhea and psoriasis may be clarified by psoriasiform lesions elsewhere on the body or pitting of the nails. Facial seborrhea can be confused with rosacea, which displays central facial erythema, or forehead only, or systemic lupus erythematosus, which exhibits a butterfly-like rash. Seborrhea of the groin may resemble dermatophytosis, psoriasis and candidiasis; seborrhea tends to be bilaterally symmetric, with reddish-brown patches that respond quickly to therapy. A very rare condition confused with seborrhea in infants is histiocytosis X, associated with systemic signs such as fever[3] (Table 2).

Refer patients to a dermatologist if the diagnosis is in doubt, sudden onset in a young patient in which HIV is suspected or the patient is not responding to treatment. They should also be referred if the condition is widespread or generalized.

Psoriasis

Psoriasis is a chronic, inflammatory hyperproliferative disease of the skin and nails, with periods of remission and relapse. It presents in various clinical forms: chronic plaque psoriasis is most common, and guttate, erythrodermic and pustular psorasis are less common, acute or subacute variants. *Chronic plaque psoriasis* presents with the classic lesion, a well-demarcated, thickened, red plaque with an adherent immature silvery-white scale, which tends to become confluent. It occurs typically on the extensor surface of the arms and legs, elbows, knees, sacrum, buttocks and scalp, but the ears, extremities, palms and soles are also common sites. Patients with generalized psoriasis may also have facial, trunk or flexural involvement. Lesions in the flexures (axillae, groin) may lack scale, and exhibit only well-demarcated red patches. The initial presentation of psoriasis may be localized to a single site. Often nails are affected, and careful total skin examination may reveal nail pits or distal destruction of a nail with loss of color and thickening.[13]

Guttate psoriasis, named for its drop-like appearance, presents as a sudden eruption of pinpoint, dark red, and subsequently scaling lesions on the trunk and limbs, often preceded by a viral or streptococcal infection in children or young adults. It may occur characteristically as an initial presentation of psoriasis in genetically susceptible patients. Diagnosis may be confirmed by a throat swab and an ASOT even in unrecognized or asymptomatic cases. Despite treatment of the initial symptomatic streptococcal infection, guttate psoriasis may take many months to resolve, and recurrent upper respiratory infections may induce flares.[21,22]

Pustular psoriasis may be generalized (acute) or localized (subacute). In the generalized form, patients with or without a previous history develop systemic symptoms including fever, leukocytosis and general malaise. Pregnancy may be a trigger. The pustules often start in localized plaques and may generalize quickly without systemic treatment. Individual lesions often are painful erythematous plaques with rows or clusters of tender, bright yellow, non-follicular pustules. This is an acute emergency requiring systemic therapy and may be very resistant to treatment.[21] The localized pustular form of psoriasis is often seen on the trunk and proximal extremities. It may respond to topical treatment but systemic agents are often necessary. Chronic pustular psoriasis limited to the palms and soles is more common in women who smoke. Deep painful pustules, clustered in erythematous plaques, extend from the palms and soles around the sides of the hands and feet to the dorsal surface.[13,23]

Erythrodermic psoriasis presents as a nonspecific, fiery erythema over 75% of the body with desquamation and edema. This unstable acute form may develop from chronic forms of psoriasis and may be associated with serious systemic illness. Provoking factors include sudden withdrawal of potent therapies (especially systemic steroids), trauma or illness.

The prevalence of coexisting psoriatic arthritis in psoriatic patients ranges from 5 to more than 10%. Although the ESR is often elevated, the generalized subtype may be distinguishable from rheumatoid arthritis in lacking rheumatoid factors or other autoantibodies. Psoriasis in HIV-positive patients has a high incidence of psoriatic arthritis or Reiter's syndrome and is often difficult to control.

Diagnosis is usually based on the typical appearance, and history of the lesions. The Auspitz sign, punctate bleeding at the site of scale removal, is diagnostic. A positive family history, detection of lesions in characteristic sites undetected by the patient, or presence of nail changes and psoriatic arthritis may also assist diagnostically. Nonplaque forms of psoriasis may be more difficult to diagnose.

Assessment of Psoriasis

Treatment objectives are based upon two components: the patient's own perception of disability and need for treatment, and an objective assessment of the extent and severity of body involvement. Measures such as body mapping and the *psoriasis area and severity index* (PASI score) are used by physicians and may serve as a rough guide of objective improvement with treatment. A PASI score measures scale, erythema and infiltration, each on a 1 to 4 scale and multiplies this quotient times the percentage of the body region measured (e.g., head, limb, trunk). However, such scores equate severity with involvement of similar surface areas and do not reflect different degrees of disability and distress created by certain sites, such as trunk and hands. Thus, the patient's view of desirable outcomes must be considered in determining therapeutic choices based on risk to benefit ratios. Many patients choose to live with some aspects of their condition.[12,16]

Only chronic forms of plaque and scalp psoriasis can be managed with self-care after an appropriate diagnosis. Refer all other types of psoriasis to a physician for both diagnosis and management (Table 2).

Goals of Therapy

Dandruff:
- Reduce or eliminate scale and flaking
- Prevent recurrence by improving scalp hygiene
- Avoid environmental triggers

Seborrhea:
- Reduce fungus and the resulting scaling and inflammation
- Relieve symptoms such as pruritus
- Educate on the importance of control through good hygiene
- Eliminate or reduce environmental triggers

Psoriasis:
- Minimize the extent and severity of psoriasis and the resulting disruption of quality of life
- Relieve associated symptoms
- Eliminate or reduce trigger factors

Prevention of Psoriasis

Measures to prevent and control psoriasis require recognition of environmental components to limit progress at any stage, and to reduce frequency and severity of relapses. Patients must be aware of triggers such as streptococcal infections, drugs, injury, low humidity and emotional stress. The "Three-P Concept" of management of psoriasis evolved from a study of severely affected patients, and includes:
- Prevention of injury
- Persistence in avoiding overtreatment
- Pauses or rest periods in treatment with anti-anxiety measures, emollients, and humidification[24]

Educate patients about their disease and encourage them to take responsibility for self-care to decrease morbidity.

Dandruff and Seborrhea Nonpharmacologic Therapy

Dandruff may improve in a moist environment. Encourage use of a cool air humidifier. The main measure to remove scale and ease itching is the use of daily cleansing with a regular shampoo. Figure 1 provides a suggested approach for the treatment of dandruff and seborrhea.

For seborrhea the first steps are to discontinue aggravating factors and control stress. Seborrhea often improves in the summer months and in sunlight.[25] Irritating soaps, heavy gels, hairsprays and greasy creams should be avoided. Excessive hot water may dry out the skin. Because dry air can provoke symptoms, placing a cool air humidifier or dish of water in the room provides moisture.[26]

Patients should use a nonmedicated shampoo at least three times per week to help eliminate dirt and oil. Those with surfactants (e.g., sodium lauryl sulfate) and detergents are better able to remove unsightly scales and will lead to clinical improvement and decreased scaling for about four days.[27] To be

effective, the shampoo must be massaged into the scalp for four to five minutes, rinsed thoroughly and

Figure 1: **Treatment of Dandruff and Scalp Seborrhea**

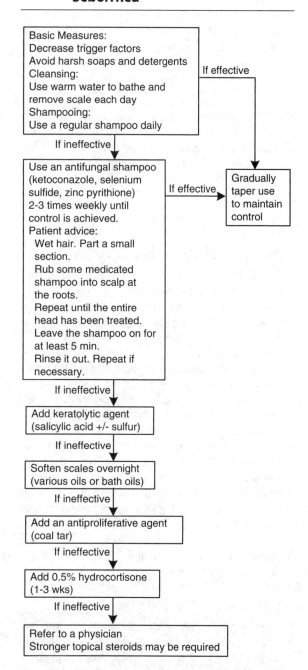

repeated. Frequency of shampooing can be decreased or increased according to the patient's response. Once-weekly shampooing may be more reasonable for institutionalized patients.[4] Patients may also cut their hair shorter or trim their beards to decrease symptoms.[25] If the scalp is covered with diffuse, dense scale, the scale may be removed prior to using a medicated shampoo by applying warm oil (mineral or olive), or a much more easily rinsed surfactant-containing bath oil to the scalp for several hours or overnight and then rinsing. Affected eyelids can be compressed with warm water to remove scale.

Cradle cap is self-limiting and a conservative approach should be taken. A mild, nonmedicated shampoo should be used initially for frequent washing. Scale may be softened with a surfactant-containing bath oil, gently brushed free with a baby brush and washed clear. If this is not helpful, refer to a physician.

Pharmacologic Therapy

Effective therapy is based on antifungal action, with associated antiinflammatory and keratolytic action. Antiseptic activity is much less important.[7] Antifungal preparations which decrease colonization by lipophilic yeast include azole agents, selenium sulfide, and zinc pyrithione. Topical steroids are effective antiinflammatory agents. For severe disease, keratolytics such as salicylic acid or coal tar preparations may be used to remove dense scale, then topical steroids applied. Other options for removing adherent scale involve applying any of a variety of oils to soften the area overnight, followed by use of a detergent or coal tar shampoo.[4] Pharmacologic treatment options for dandruff include a variety of OTC antipytrosporal shampoos (discussed with treatment of scalp seborrhea). Table 4 describes nonprescription choices for the treatment of dandruff, seborrhea and psoriasis.

Treatment of Scalp and Beard Areas

Treat dandruff by daily shampooing with a regular shampoo. If this is ineffective, an antifungal shampoo can be used as for scalp seborrhea.

Seborrhea can be controlled by daily or alternate day shampooing with an antifungal shampoo. Instruct patients to part their hair in small sections, and apply and massage the medicated shampoo or scalp treatment into the scalp at the hair roots. This should be repeated until the entire scalp has been treated. Medicated therapies should be left in contact with the scalp or beard 2 to 20 minutes depending on the product used. For more severe cases, they can be left overnight under a shower cap, before rinsing, in order for the treatment to interact with the skin of the scalp. Moisturizing, nonmedicated shampoos or conditioners can be used afterward to prevent dessication of the hair.[4]

Antifungals

Ketoconazole is the most effective antimycotic imidazole against *P. ovale*, due to greater effects on 5-lipoxygenase and leukotriene-B4 production, suppressing inflammation more readily.[28] At therapeutic concentrations, ketoconazole is fungistatic; higher fungicidal concentrations are not used in vivo.[29] Ketoconazole exhibits stronger in vitro inhibition of Pityrosporum and superior clinical results in animal models compared to selenium sulfide and zinc pyrithione.[30] As a cytostatic, it also slows cell turnover.[25] Ketoconazole 2% shampoo showed equal clinical efficacy to selenium sulfide 2.5% with better patient tolerance in a trial of 246 patients with moderate to severe scalp symptoms.[31] Ketoconazole is available as a prescription agent, and as a nonprescription shampoo for scalp application two to four times weekly, with three days in between shampoos. Five to ten millilitres of shampoo should be worked into lather, left on for 5 to 10 minutes and rinsed. Approximately 80% of patients have good symptomatic response within four weeks. Maintenance therapy is used once every one to two weeks.[7]

The FDA has classified **selenium sulfide** as a keratolytic, slowing down scale production and epidermal proliferation, but a fungicidal effect against numerous strains of Pityrosporum has been shown in the laboratory[32] and it may have fungistatic action on the scalp.[20] Although the use of 2.5% selenium sulfide shampoo in seborrheic dermatitis of the scalp has been shown to improve dandruff, folliculitis, pain and dryness, symptomatic seborrhea recurred in more than 50% of patients.[33] It should be used no more than twice weekly as excessive use could cause oily hair and hair loss.[20] All jewelry should be removed before application. The hair should be wet with lukewarm water and enough medication applied to the scalp to work up lather. The lather should remain on the scalp

Table 4: **Nonprescription Therapies for Dandruff, Seborrhea and Psoriasis**

Drug	Dosing	Onset/Duration	Side effects	Interactions	Dosage forms/Convenience	Comments
Scalp treatments for dandruff, seborrhea and psoriasis						
Antifungal agents						
Ketoconazole	Shampoo: 2-4 times weekly. Can apply topically to scalp, beard, face and body. Prophylaxis-one treatment every 1 or 2 wks.	Requires 2-4 wks to see effect. Follow by interval necessary to keep the condition under control.	Avoid eye areas. Safe with < 1% absorption. Less irritating than selenium sulfide. Minimal scalp and skin irritation, greasy or dry hair or scalp, itching or stinging.	May rebound when used with steroid: continue steroid at the onset of ketoconazole shampoo treatment, and withdraw the corticosteroid in 2-3 weeks.	2% shampoo is OTC. Oral tablets 200 mg and 2% cream are prescription	
Selenium sulfide	2.5%: Shampoo, rinse and repeat. 2 applications per week for 2 wks and afterwards use at less frequent intervals; do not use more than 3 times per week.	Requires 2-4 wks to see effect. Follow by interval necessary to keep the condition under control.	Excessive use may cause oily hair and hair loss. Will sting if applied to broken skin.	May discolor bleached, tinted or permanent-waved hair. Avoid use of these hair products within 2 days of treatment with selenium sulfide. Remove all jewelry.	1-2.5% shampoos, liquids	Cannot be used on damaged or inflamed skin. Avoid eye area
Zinc pyrithione	Shampoo: Shampoo twice; use a regular shampoo first before using the treatment; leave shampoo on for at least 5 min before rinsing.	Requires 2-4 wks to see effect. Follow by interval necessary to keep the condition under control.	Safe to use even after hair tints or perm solutions.	May discolor hair if metal-based tints are used.	Bar, cream, lotion, lotion shampoo	
Keratolytic Agents						
Salicylic acid and sulfur	Use on scalp at least 2 times a week massaging thoroughly into scalp area.	Requires 2-4 wks to see effect. Follow by interval necessary to keep the condition under control.	Irritation, redness or peeling. Irritating to mucous membranes and eyes.	Salicylic acid enhances penetration of topical agents through stratum corneum.	OTC. Bar, cleansing lotion and shampoo	Although approved for single use, most OTC products contain sulfur in combination with salicylic acid, and often with coal tar also.
Coal tar	Tar is more effective with prolonged contact time.		Folliculitis (especially of hairy regions), acne, contact dermatitis, photosensitivity, unappealing odor, stains skin and hair.	Additive antimitotic activity with UVA and B.	Gels, creams, ointments and shampoos. Crude coal tar and tar distillates (1/5 to 1/10 the potency of crude coal tar)	

(cont'd)

Table 4: **Nonprescription Therapies for Dandruff, Seborrhea and Psoriasis** *(cont'd)*

Drug	Dosing	Onset/Duration	Side effects	Interactions	Dosage forms/ Convenience	Comments
Psoriasis topical therapy						
Steroids	BID – TID Ointments are most effective, but creams more acceptable in folds and lotions for the scalp.	Quick onset. Short remission. Limit repeats – 2-3 wks of therapy with steroid-sparing agents and measures to provide steroid-free periods.	Tachyphylaxis occurs with moderate to potent steroids. Ointments are less cosmetically acceptable. Absorption greatest for creases and genitals, least from palms and soles. Use occlusion with caution.		Prescription – lotions, gels, creams. OTC – hydrocortisone 0.5% (not antiproliferative)	Potent topical steroids contraindicated for rosacea, acne vulgaris, perioral dermatitis or perianal and genital pruritus.
Anthralins	Daily (intermittently for 15-30 min) or overnight	Chronic requires 4-12 wks. Long remission.	Local staining and irritation – can be removed with salicylic acid. Too strong with tar or keratolytics	With UVB = Ingram routine	OTC Pastes 0.025% to 0.2% Creams-0.1%,0.2%, 0.4%,1-2%	Preparations should be used over at least 3-4 wks – ring with plain topical; alternate with steroid paste.
Tars	Daily. Soaks for scale removal start with 5% and increase as tolerated – soak 5-10 min. Overnight to soften scale apply prior to steroids	4 wks for full effect. Sustained results with continued application	Messy and odorous. Cover with cotton/gloves. Apply in linear direction of hair growth to avoid folliculitis – do not rub in circular motion.	With UVB = Goeckerman routine. Added to steroid creams – one month expiry date	OTC crude coal tar (4%), liquid coal tar extracts (5-20%)	Contraindicated for diffuse, acutely inflamed, or open wounds

for 2 to 3 minutes before rinsing. Apply the medicine again and rinse well. Hands should be washed thoroughly after use.[27] The hair should be rinsed well for at least 5 minutes after using selenium sulfide if used on light blond, gray, or chemically treated (bleached, tinted or permanent-waved) hair. This will lessen the chance of the hair becoming discolored. It should not be used within two days of hair coloring or perming.[27] This product should not be applied to damaged or inflamed skin because this will increase the absorption of the drug and cause stinging.

Zinc pyrithione is also classified as keratolytic, but effects on membrane transport, macromolecular synthesis, cell structure and function have been demonstrated.[34] It has cytostatic properties and reduces counts of Pityrosporum.[7,20] Weekly shampooing with 1% zinc pyrithione significantly reduced dandruff in one study, but resolution of symptoms was not complete after nine treatments.[7] It is supplied in bar, cream and shampoo dosage forms which are available without prescription in 1 to 2% concentrations. Zinc pyrithione has few reported side effects,[27] and has not been shown to cause problems during pregnancy or nursing. The shampoo should be applied to wet hair, lathered, left on for several minutes, rinsed, with a repeat if desired. It can be applied to scalp, beard, face and body. Its effectiveness may be destroyed by oxidizers and reducers, as well as heavy metal ions contained in hair dyes applied as shampoos to change white or gray hair to a more natural color.

Antiinflammatory Agents

Corticosteroids decrease pruritus and inflammation, producing clinical improvement in seborrheic dermatitis and dandruff. Topical corticosteroids are intended for temporary use. Long-term use of potent agents is discouraged for controlling seborrhea since relapse rates are often high,[35] and it may lead to undesirable side effects such as atrophy, telangiectasia, poor wound healing, perioral dermatitis and pustular acne. Topical 0.5% hydrocortisone could be used once or twice daily for one to three weeks to reduce inflammation, with judicious use of other steroid-sparing agents. It should be discontinued when itching and erythema disappear. This regimen can be repeated after a rest period. Maintenance with an antidandruff shampoo should then be adequate.[4] Patients should be referred to a physician if more potent steroid use

is warranted. Topical hydrocortisone 0.5% is available in cream, ointment or lotion form; stronger steroids are also available as solutions. The form selected is determined by the patient and the treatment site. Ointments are preferred for use on areas that are resistant to absorption or dry or scaly, due to their occlusive nature. Avoid ointments if acne is a problem. Creams are used in moist areas due to their drying effect, while lotions and solutions are best for the scalp and hairy areas or for large areas that require a minimal application. A scalp solution is generally preferred by Caucasian and Asian patients but may be too drying for Black patients, who may prefer ointments. The potency of the same steroid is affected by the vehicle: ointment > cream > lotion.[4] Figure 2 illustrates the amount of cream required for topical therapy.

Keratolytic Agents

Salicylic acid and sulfur: These agents have minimal antifungal activity but are mildly effective because of their keratolytic and antiseptic activities. They are either used alone or combined with other active ingredients. Salicylic acid provides a keratolytic effect by loosening the bonds between keratinocytes in the skin, which helps detach flakes and increases the penetration of other drugs.[1,7] Products containing salicylic acid and sulfur are more potent, but are proportionally more irritating and require some precautions when used.[20] They are available without prescription and the bar, cleansing lotion and shampoo forms include salicylic acid 2 to 3% and sulfur 3 to 5%. All products should be lathered into the scalp with continued rubbing for at least five minutes and rinsed thoroughly. Young children may be at increased risk of unwanted side effects because of increased absorption of salicylic acid through the skin. It should not be applied to large areas of the body or used for long periods of time in this population.[27] Other drying preparations such as cosmetics, soaps or alcohol-containing preparations should be discontinued. Generally, products containing salicylic acid and sulfur should be used no more than twice a week unless otherwise directed by a physician.

Coal tar is mildly effective for seborrhea because it reduces local swelling and inflammation, relieves itching and is keratolytic and antiseptic. However, it has minimal antifungal activity.[7] It is available in shampoo, ointment, lotion, gel and bath forms. Coal

Figure 2: **Amount of Cream Required for TID Application × 10 days**

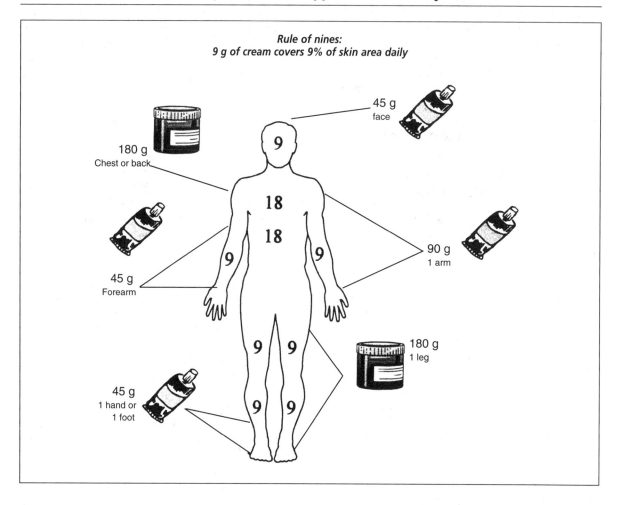

Rule of nines:
9 g of cream covers 9% of skin area daily

45 g
face

180 g
Chest or back

90 g
1 arm

45 g
Forearm

180 g
1 leg

45 g
1 hand or
1 foot

tar products are messy, can stain blond or gray hair and clothing, have an unpleasant odor and could possibly cause tar acne, contact dermatitis,[27] and photosensitivity.[26] They are used once daily to once weekly on the beard, face, body or scalp. As they are irritating, the eye area should be avoided and a sunblock applied when outdoors. Irritation generally subsides following discontinuation or when the frequency of use is reduced. Coal tar preparations may also contain alcohol that will cause burning and irritation of acutely inflamed skin.

Comparative Clinical Studies
Selenium sulfide, zinc pyrithione and coal tar shampoos have been compared in the treatment of dandruff, with twice weekly shampooing producing complete clearance in 32, 15 and 10% of each group, respectively.[7] A second crossover study resulted in freedom from symptoms in 80% of patients after four weeks' therapy, with no difference between selenium sulfide 2.5% and purified coal tar 2% shampoos.[33] Ketoconazole has demonstrated clinical superiority over hydrocortisone, zinc pyrithione and selenium sulfide.[7] Overall, ketoconazole and hydrocortisone have better clinical responses in the treatment of seborrhea and dandruff compared with other agents. Ketoconazole is more effective against Pityrosporum on the skin with fewer adverse effects compared to hydrocortisone. With respect to comparative efficacy,

these compounds can be ranked as ketoconazole = hydrocortisone > selenium sulfide > zinc pyrithione > coal tar.[7]

Treatment of the Face and Body

Seborrhea of the face may be washed three to four times daily if necessary with effective shampoos, as detailed previously. Alternatively, ketoconazole 2% cream (prescription) may be applied once or twice daily to affected areas. Often, 0.5 to 1.0% hydrocortisone will be added once or twice daily to affected areas until inflammation resolves. Refer patients unresponsive to these routines for more potent combinations or steroid pulse therapies.[4]

Herbal Therapy

Viola tricolor (Heartsease) and *Avenae stramentum* (Oat Straw) are herbal formulations that claim to be effective for mild cases of seborrhea. *Viola tricolor* is applied externally as a poultice or in an infusion to the area at a dose of 15 mL three times daily. *Avenae stramentum* is administered in a bath soak (100 g). **Tea tree oil** (*Melaleuca alternifolia*) leaves contain terpinen-4-ol, which has shown some in vitro activity against the lipophilic yeast *M. furfur*. Five to 10% solutions are used as external antifungals.[36] There is no compelling evidence to show these herbals are efficacious. Further, the use of herbal preparations which are non-standardized should be discouraged in favor of traditional quality-controlled preparations.[37]

Prescription therapies for seborrhea include stronger steroids, although these should not be used on the face. Sodium sulfacetamide 10% lotion is sometimes used in these cases. There are no comparative trials for the use of this agent. Prescription ketoconazole 2% cream is another available choice.

Psoriasis
Nonpharmacologic Therapy

Advise patients to avoid triggers and skin irritants, such as soap. Bathing as well as use of a cool air humidifier can be beneficial. Aqueous creams can serve as cleansers and emollients as skin should stay moist. Caution patients about removing scale, which could trigger a flare.

Pharmacologic Therapy

Topical treatments are first line therapy for patients with mild to moderate plaque psoriasis, and are primarily directed toward altering the immune mechanism of the disease, with secondary attention to reduction and removal of scale, inflammation and dryness. Choices include emollients, antiinflammatory agents, antimitotic and immune modulating agents. Systemic therapy is warranted for severe, extensive psoriasis, or where topical therapy is ineffective or needs supplementation.[16] Rotation of therapies is important in managing the capricious nature of psoriasis. It is best to use a step-wise approach to treatment, moving ahead if there is no response or if the response decreases. Figure 3 is a suggested approach for the treatment of psoriasis.

Penetration

The vehicles in which active topical ingredients are applied may have considerable influence on therapy. Enhancement of penetration of active drug can be accomplished in three ways: an occlusive base may enhance penetration of active drug and inhibit cell division in its own right, or occlusion with plastic wrap can also be used; keratolytics such as salicylic acid or sulfur may remove the scale that is limiting penetration; and specific agents such as urea or propylene glycol may assist penetration.[38] Topical agents may be designed to promote retention of active agents within the epidermis. Gels provide drying and cooling effects, are cosmetically acceptable, diffuse throughout and remove easily from the scalp while concentrating drug delivery by evaporation.

Chronic Plaque Psoriasis
Trunk and Extremities

Topical steroids are an integral component of psoriasis treatment because they are antiinflammatory, inhibit epidermal proliferation and alter immune reactions. Nonprescription **hydrocortisone** is only antiinflammatory and lacks the antiproliferative effects of stronger steroids that give rise to both increased efficacy and increased side effects such as skin thinning, striae, telangiectasia, purpura and acne. As a result, plaques of psoriasis on the trunk and extremities are often treated with mid-potency topical prescription steroids. Combined with these therapies are nonprescription steroid-sparing agents.

Figure 3: **Suggested Approach for Treating Psoriasis**

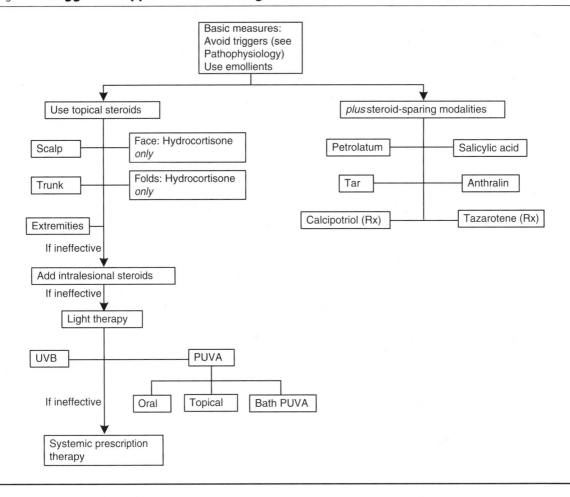

One of the simplest steroid-sparing agents is **petrolatum**. It can be used for one out of every four applications initially. As psoriasis improves, after two to six weeks, gradually increase the number of applications until it almost completely replaces topical steroids. Petrolatum is antiproliferative for epidermal cells, will decrease or help diminish surrounding skin irritation from steroid-sparing agents by ringing psoriatic plaques, and helps prevent steroid tachyphylaxis.

Since **salicylic acid** breaks down keratin topically, it increases percutaneous absorption of topical steroids. It can be added to most topical steroids in concentrations of 3 to 5%, affixing a one month expiry date to cream formulations. Salicylic acid is also available as

an ointment (10% urea/5% salicylic acid) as a steroid-sparing alternative.

Crude coal tar is a key nonprescription agent for psoriasis due to its antimitotic and antipruritic effects. It is a frequently used, safe and effective topical preparation, producing clearing with long remissions. Concentrations of 0.5 to 1% increased to a maximum of 10%, are used. Modified tar extracts incorporated into solutions and gels are less effective, although cosmetically superior. Four per cent crude coal tar is equivalent to 10 to 20% of the tar distillate, liquor carbonis detergens (LCD). This product can be added in 5 to 10% quantities to steroid ointments and creams if a one month expiry date is affixed. Though tar is extremely effective, psoriatic patients may find it difficult to adhere to treatment due to its side effects and prolonged treatment durations of two to four weeks. Application in circular motions may cause inflammation of the hair follicles, that can be diminished by applying the tar in linear strokes in the direction hairs sit flat against the skin. The photosensitizing action of tar enhances its efficacy in psoriasis: pretreatment for two hours is followed by ultraviolet B light treatments in ambulatory clinics (Goeckerman routine).[39,40] If a patient does not have a drug plan, it may be more economical to apply topical tar creams or gels prior to the application of a topical steroid.

Anthralin (dithranol) is also antimitotic, useful for thick plaques and can induce prolonged remissions. Salicylic acid must be added to stabilize against oxidation to anthrone, especially in zinc oxide bases, and some preparations include chloroform as a dispersing agent.[38] New application strategies to reduce side effects include a daily short contact method of 15 to 30 minutes for strong applications of 1% to 2% in stiff pastes or cream formulations of 0.1%, 0.2% and 0.4%. Lesions can be ringed with paste or petrolatum to protect surrounding skin. Problems with anthralin include burning, staining of skin and clothes, and discoloration of blond hair. It is contraindicated in flexures or on the genitals, where irritation is excessive. It should not be compounded or used with tar but may be alternated with topical steroids. Four weeks should be allowed for an early response. Ambulatory clinic patients may sometimes have effects increased through the addition of ultraviolet light (Ingram routine).[39]

Flexures, Face and Scalp Regions

Absorption of topical steroid through the skin is greatly increased in flexure areas and the face, and these areas should be limited to use of **hydrocortisone**. If psoriatic lesions in the flexures become superimposed with tinea or candida, 1% hydrocortisone powder can be added to topical **imidazole** creams, or two creams used in succession. Imidazoles have antiinflammatory, antifungal and some gram-positive antibacterial effects.

Scalp treatments include tar preparations, with or without salicylic acid, anthralin, steroids or prescription calcipotriol solution or tazarotene gel. Water-washable vehicles are preferred. Keratolytics which decrease scale should be left on a minimum of 5 to 10 minutes, or overnight, covered with a shower cap. After rinsing, steroid lotions or gels can be applied, reserving higher potencies for pulse therapies of two weeks in resistant cases. Antifungal preparations which are cytostatic such as ketoconazole, selenium sulfide and zinc pyrithione are not suitable for treatment of psoriatic scalps.

Alternative Therapy

Herbal and alternative therapies such as aloe vera, beta-carotene, zinc, selenium, vitamin B complex, flax seed oil, yellow dock, horsetail, lavender and ginger (in the bath), acupuncture, ayurveda (see Appendix C), and magnets have been advised in the general media or on Internet sites. Since these treatments lack controlled studies of their efficacy, side effects or interactions with recommended treatments, they should not be considered. Psoriasis sufferers, due to distress over their condition, may turn in desperation to the Internet and other nonregulated sources of information. For example, one product which is advertised on the Internet contains banana extracts and 1% coal tar. However, since it has not been approved as a drug, product identification (i.e., labeling) and ingredients are not monitored or regulated. "Miracle cures" touted on the Internet may in fact worsen a patient's condition.

Prescription Therapy

Stronger topical corticosteroids such as those 9 to 12 times more potent than hydrocortisone may be necessary for shorter periods (e.g., two-week intervals) on the palms and soles. Steroids such as clobetasone 17-butyrate have less antiproliferative side effects while maintaining adequate potency. Ultrapotent steroids may increase the risk of adrenal suppression. Apply the steroid in a thin layer, since only that which touches the skin is absorbed. Initially apply the steroid more often, two or three times daily, and once the condition begins to respond, limit the daily frequency to the least number of applications necessary to maintain control. Other agents such as tar liquids and salicylic acid are frequently extemporaneously compounded with commercial preparations of steroids. The addition of liquid tar, strong electrolytes, acids, such as salicylic acid, and alkalis will diminish the stability of cream preparations causing cracking, which becomes apparent over a one-month period.

Also, with these additions, the valerate salt of betamethasone transfers over 30 days, from the 17- to the 21-carbon position, diminishing the clinical potency of this steroid up to 20-fold. This *transesterification* will not happen with a dipropionate preparation, which has ester groups attached at both 17- and 21-carbon positions.

Topical corticosteroids seldom produce long remissions and psoriasis tends to rebound promptly when they are withdrawn. Moreover, steroid action, especially with more potent agents, may peak in the first two weeks of therapy and subsequently lose therapeutic effectiveness (tachyphylaxis) due to fatigue of steroid receptors on the superficial dermal blood vessels. Topical steroids should be supplemented or substituted with steroid-sparing agents such as plain petrolatum, salicylic acid, tar, anthralin, calcipotriol or tazarotene. Steroid-sparing strategies can be tried either alone or alternately.

Calcipotriol is a vitamin D3 analog, which enhances keratinocyte differentiation and inhibits proliferation and cytokines. Available as a cream, ointment or scalp solution, it is used either as a single agent twice daily or alternatively with topical steroids on a morning and evening schedule. Remissions are shorter than with anthralin, but for acute treatment, it has been shown to be equal to betamethasone and more effective than anthralin, or 15% tar in aqueous cream. For scalp lesions, it is less effective than steroids but more effective than tar, and is primarily used as a steroid-sparing agent rather than monotherapy in this area. It can be used in children and pregnancy. Its effect is increased with occlusion.[41]

Tazarotene is the first of a new generation of receptor-selective retinoids for topical treatment of psoriasis. It is a useful steroid-sparing agent which appears to inhibit keratinocyte proliferation, regulate differentiation and modify inflammatory infiltration.

Fluocinonide, a potent topical steroid, is available in an oil base for scalp psoriasis. It is applied to a moistened scalp under a shower cap overnight for 10 days for induction of control and then twice weekly for maintenance. This can facilitate clearing of difficult scalp psoriasis unresponsive to other topical regimens. Extemporaneous mixtures often include tar, salicylic acid and a steroid in a surfactant-containing oil.

Intralesional injections of **triamcinolone** are occasionally used for resistant plaques, to a maximum of 20 mg every three to six weeks.

Ultraviolet radiation, which inhibits epidermal mitosis, can be very useful in more severe, extensive (> 30%) or resistant cases of psoriasis, in addition to topical therapy, such as tar or anthralin. Oral or topical **psoralens** are used as photosensitisers combined with ultraviolet A therapy (PUVA = psoralen + UVA). Side effects of phototherapy include acute burns, usually with improper dosage, increase in chronic precancerous or skin cancer changes, atypical pigmentation and photoaging.

Acitretin is an oral retinoid used in pustular or erythrodermic psoriasis. Its effect is partly due to inhibition of leukocyte migration. It is a teratogen stored in the body long-term and should never be administered to a female of childbearing potential without appropriate birth control.

Sulfasalazine is an antimicrobial active in the colon which may be useful in treating psoriasis, and in controlling psoriatic arthritis, in about 50% of patients. The mechanism is undetermined.

Methotrexate, a folic acid antagonist, is useful for acute psoriasis particularly accompanied by psoriatic arthritis.

Cyclosporine selectively inhibits T-helper cells (CD_4 cells), monocytes and Langerhans cells and can be useful in severe psoriasis. It is very effective as monotherapy, and has a different side effect profile from other treatments.

Monitoring of Therapy

Table 5 presents a monitoring framework for patients with dandruff, seborrhea or psoriasis. The parameters should be monitored by the patient, in a diary. Scale will improve quite quickly with cosmetic treatment and hygiene control; thickness of scale will improve more slowly and erythema will take longest to respond.

The side effects of drug therapy should also be monitored. If allergic reactions occur, therapy should be discontinued. If the condition worsens due to irritation, therapy should be altered. Failure to meet the listed endpoints should result in alteration of

Table 5: **Monitoring Therapy for Dandruff, Seborrhea and Psoriasis**

Monitoring	**Patient:** daily while on drug therapy **Health care provider:** after 2-3 wks or next visit	
Parameter	**Time frame/Degree of change**	**Actions**
Positive endpoints (symptom resolution/control)		
Scale	Decrease by 50% within 7-10 days	Taper therapy in response to resolution: if endpoints not achieved, refer to a physician for further therapy.
Thickness of plaque	Decrease by 50% within 6-8 wks and by 75% within 8-12 wks	
Redness	Decrease by 50% within 8-12 wks and by 75% within 12-16 wks	
Surface area involved	Decrease by 50% within 6-8 wks and by 75% within 8-12 wks	
Extension to other sites or generalization	None	
Itch/scratching	Decrease to tolerable level within 1-2 wks	
Disruption of sleep or daily activities	Restoration of normal patterns within 2-3 wks	
Stress, anxiety, depression	Restoration of normal patterns within 2-3 wks.	
Progression of severity	No progression of severity	
Recurrent episodes	Lengthening of symptom-free periods through-out therapy	
Negative endpoints (treatment side effects)		
Allergic reactions	None	If they occur, discontinue therapy.
Severe dryness, irritation (redness, inflam-mation, stinging, etc).	Minimal Should disappear, diminish or be controlled with continued use	If severe, decrease dose, concen-tration or frequency of use. If still no improvement, refer to physician for further treatment.

dosage or drug therapy. Therapy should be appropriately tapered in response to improvement or resolution.

Resource Tips

A number of self-help support groups exist that can be accessed through the Internet. The Psoriasis Association, which is a self-help organization founded in 1968, provides support and information on all aspects of the condition.

The Psoriasis Association: http://www.timewarp.demon.co.uk/psoriasis.html.

The National Psoriasis Foundation: fax: (503) 245-0626 http://www.psoriasis.org

The National Institute of Arthritis and Musculoskeletal and Skin Diseases http://www.nih.gov/niams/health-info/psoriafs.htm

Suggested Readings

Gardner SS, McKay M. Seborrhea, psoriasis and the papulosquamous dermatosis. *Primary Care* 1989; 16(3):739-61.

Hay RJ, Grahman-Brown RA. Dandruff and seborrhoeic dermatitis: causes and management. *Clin Exp Dermatol* 1997;22:3-6.

Janniger CK, Schwartz RA. Seborrheic dermatitis. *Am Fam Physician* 1995;52(1):149-55.

Johnson BA, Nunley JR. Treatment of seborrheic dermatitis. *Am Fam Physician* 2000;61(9):2703-10.

Tooley P. Dandruff: an irritating problem. *Practitioner* 1990;29:594-6.

Weller PA. Psoriasis. *Med J Aust* 1996;165(4):216-21.

References

1. Gardner SS, McKay M. Seborrhea, psoriasis and the papulosquamous dermatosis. *Primary Care* 1989;16(3):739-61.
2. Shuster S. The aetiology of dandruff and the mode of action of therapeutic agents. *Br J Dermatol* 1984;111:235-42.
3. Janniger CK, Schwartz RA. Seborrheic dermatitis. *Am Fam Physician* 1995;52(1):149-55.
4. Johnson BA, Nunley JR. Treatment of seborrheic dermatitis. *Am Fam Physician* 2000;61(9):2703-10.
5. Hay RJ, Grahman-Brown RA. Dandruff and seborrhoeic dermatitis: causes and management. *Clin Exp Dermatol* 1997;22:3-6.
6. Parry ME, Sharpe GR. Seborrheic dermatitis is not caused by an altered immune response to Malassezia yeast. *Br J Dermatol* 1998;139:254-63.
7. McGrath JM, Murphy GM. The control of seborrhoeic dermatitis and dandruff by antipityrosporal drugs. *Drugs* 1991;41(2):178-84.
8. Maieta G, Rongioletti R, Rebora A. Seborrheic dermatitis and daylight. *Acta Derm Venereol (Stock)* 1991;71:538-9.
9. Cowley NC, Farr PM, Shuster S. The permissive effect of sebum in seborrhoeic dermatitis: an explanation of the rash in neurological disorders. *Br J Dermatol* 1990;122:71-6.
10. Zone J, Ward J, Boyce E, Schupback C. Penicillamine-induced pemphigus. *JAMA* 1982;247(19):2705-7.
11. Greenberg RD. Acne vulgaris associated with antigonadotropic (Danazol) therapy. *Cutis* 1979;24(4):431-3.
12. Litt JZ, Pawlak WA. *Drug Eruption Reference Manual.* 4th ed. Cleveland: Wal-Zac Enterprises; 1995:1-13.
13. Weller PA. Psoriasis. *Med J Aust* 1996;165(4):216-21.
14. Young DW, Downey DJ. Psoriasis: therapeutic aspects. *NZ Med J* 1993;106(950):63-4.
15. Stern RS. Epidemiology of psoriasis. *Derm Clin* 1995;13(4):717-22.
16. Ashcroft DM, Li Wan Po A, Griffiths CEM. Therapeutic strategies for psoriasis. *J Clin Pharm Ther* 2000;25:1-10.
17. Kadunce DP, Krueger, GG. Pathogenesis of psoriasis: current concepts. *Derm Clin* 1995;13(4):723-37.
18. Williams REA. Guidelines for management of patients with psoriasis. *BMJ* 1991;303:829-35.
19. Rigoni C, Toffolo P, Cantu A, Beretta D, Terenzio C. 1% econazole hair shampoo in the treatment of pityriasis captitis; a comparative study versus zinc pyrithione shampoo. *Dermatol Venereol* 1989;124(11-12): LXVII-LXX.
20. Tooley P. Dandruff: an irritating problem. *Practitioner* 1990;29:594-6.
21. Lauritz B. The management of psoriasis. *Aust Fam Physician* 1982;11(9):704-12.
22. Christophers E, Kiene P. Guttate and plaque psoriasis. *Derm Clin* 1995;13(4):751-6.
23. Prytowsky JH, Cohen PR. Pustular and erythrodermic psoriasis. *Derm Clin* 1995;13(4):757-70.
24. Farber EM, Nal L. An appraisal of measures to prevent and control psoriasis. *J Am Acad Dermatol* 1984;10: 511-17.
25. Amit G, Pandya MD. Seborrheic dermatitis or tinea capitis: don't be fooled. *Int J Dermatol* 1998;37:827-8.
26. Arndt KA, Wintaub BU, Robinson JK, Leboit PE. *Primary Care Dermatology.* Boston: WB Saunders; 1997.
27. Arndt KA. *Manual of Dermatologic Therapeutics.* 5th ed. Boston: Little Brown & Company; 1995.
28. Cauwenbergh G. International experience with ketoconazole shampoo in the treatment of seborrhoeic dermatitis and dandruff. In: Shuster S, Blatchford N, eds. *Seborrhoeic Dermatitits and Dandruff: A Fungal Disease.* Royal Society of Medicine International Congress and Symposium Series No. 132;35-42, Royal Society of Medicine Services Ltd; 1988.
29. Borges M. Ultrastructural correlates of antimycotic treatment. *Curr Top Med Mycol* 1986;2:1.
30. Van Cutsem J, van Gerven F, Fransen J, Schrooten P, Janssen PA. The in vitro antifungal activity of ketoconazole, zinc pyrithione and selenium sulfide against pityrosporum and their efficacy as a shampoo in the treatment of experimental pityrosporesis in guinea pigs. *J Am Acad Dermatol* 1990;22(6t1):993-8.
31. Danby FW, Maddin WS, Margesson LJ, Rosethal D. A randomized, double-blind, placebo-controlled trial of ketoconazole 2% shampoo versus selenium sulfide 2.5% shampoo in the treatment of moderate to severe dandruff. *J Am Acad Dermatol* 1993;29(6):1008-12.
32. Butterfield W. Sensitivities of Pityrosporum sp to selected commercial shampoos. *Br J Dermatol* 1987;116:233-5.
33. Frederickson T. Controlled comparison of Clinitar shampoo and Selsun shampoo in the treatment of seborrheic dermatitis of the scalp. *Br J Clin Pract* 1985;29:25-8.
34. Chandler CJ, Segel IH. Mechanism of the antimicrobial action of pyrithione: effects on membrane transport. ATP levels, and protein synthesis. *Antimicrob Agents Chemother* 1978;14:60-8.
35. Faergemann J. Seborrhoeic dermatitis and Pityrosporum orbiculare: treatment of seborrhoeic dermatitis of the scalp with miconazole-hydrocortione, miconazole and hydrocortisone. *Br J Dermatol* 1986;114:695-700.
36. Nenoff P, Haustein UF, Brandt W. Antifungal activity of the essential oil of Melaleuca alternifolia (tea tree oil) against pathogenic fungi in vitro. *Skin Pharmacol* 1996;9(6):388-94.
37. Gruenwald J, Brendler T, Jaenicke C et al, eds. *PDR for Herbal Medicines.* 1st ed. Montvale, NJ: Medical Economics Company; 1998.
38. Hodge L, Comaish JS. Psoriasis: current concepts in management. *Drugs* 1977;13:288-96.
39. Silverman A, Menter A, Hairston JL. Tars and anthralins. *Dermatol Clin* 1995;13(4):817-33.
40. Muller SA, Perry HO. The Goeckerman treatment in psoriasis: six decades of experience of the Mayo Clinic. *Cutis* 1984;34(3):265-8,270.
41. Murdoch D, Clissold SP. Calcipitriol. *Drugs* 1992;43(3):415-29.

Seborrhea—Patient Information

About Seborrhea

Seborrhea is a common skin problem which appears as a red rash and greasy scales on the scalp, face, eyebrows and eyelids, and mid-chest. Infants may have seborrhea on the scalp ("cradle cap"), body folds or in the diaper area, which goes away after about six months. Seborrhea is common in men, the elderly, and persons with oily skin, Parkinson's disease or AIDS. A number of factors cause seborrhea, including yeast, hormones and stress.

Cleansing

- Treatment helps keep seborrhea under control. It's important to keep your body clean.
- Use warm, not hot or cold, water to bathe or shower each day to help remove scale.
- Avoid use of harsh soaps on your skin or strong detergents on your clothes.

Shampooing

- You may use a regular shampoo daily to remove scale. Having scale does not mean that your hair is too dry. Scales appear because you need to wash your hair more often.
- Medicated shampoos: Wet your hair. Part a small section. Rub some medicated shampoo into your scalp at the roots. Repeat until the entire head has been treated. Leave the shampoo on for at least five minutes. Rinse it out. Repeat if necessary.
- Use the medicated shampoo, two to three times a week or as directed to keep seborrhea under control.

- Cradle Cap: First try a mild, nonmedicated baby shampoo. If that doesn't work, try a mild dandruff shampoo. If scales are thick, soften first by rubbing on warm oil or bath oil. Gently brush with a baby hairbrush. Then use shampoo, and rinse well.

Moisturizing

- Keep skin well-lubricated at all times to reduce dryness and scratching.
- An emollient cream can be used as a cleanser and a moisturizer.
- Apply creams smoothly in the direction hairs lie flat.
- Use a sunscreen: it will protect your skin from sun damage and keep it moist.

Triggers

- Reduce or control factors which may aggravate seborrhea, such as sweating, high temperatures and depression.
- Use a cool air humidifier.
- Maintain a healthy diet, with moderate exercise and sufficient rest.
- Reduce stress by pursuing hobbies, and increasing leisure or vacation time.

Medications

- Ask your pharmacist or doctor about medications which may make seborrhea worse.
- Ask your pharmacist or doctor about cosmetics, herbals, over-the-counter products, or alternative therapies before trying them.
- Do not stop taking your prescribed medications without checking with your pharmacist or doctor.

Psoriasis—Patient Information

About Psoriasis

Psoriasis is a common, chronic condition that has periods of clearing and relapse. It appears in various forms. The most common is formation of scaling, elevated red patches on the scalp, arms, legs and trunk. It may also involve disfigurement of the nails. A number of factors trigger psoriasis, including heredity, stress, environmental factors, alcohol, obesity and trauma.

Cleansing

- Use warm, not hot or cold, water to bathe or shower each day.
- Avoid use of harsh soaps on your skin or strong detergents on your clothes.

Moisturizing

- Keep your skin well-lubricated at all times to reduce dryness and scratching.
- An emollient cream can serve as a cleanser and a moisturizer.
- Apply creams smoothly in the direction hairs lie flat.
- Use a sunscreen: it will protect your skin from sun damage and keep it moist.

Itch

- Keep nails short and avoid scratching.
- Avoid liquid or sheet fabric softeners.
- Avoid tight, restrictive clothing; loose-fitting garments will reduce friction.
- Avoid rough synthetics, nylon or wool fabrics; substitute cotton or corduroy.
- Use a cool air humidifier.

Triggers

- Reduce or control factors which may trigger or worsen a flare: alcohol, smoking, increased weight, physical trauma, sunburn.
- Maintain a healthy diet and moderate exercise.
- Reduce stress by pursuing hobbies, and increasing leisure or vacation time.

Medications

- Ask your pharmacist or doctor about medications which may make psoriasis worse:
  —beta-blockers
  —lithium
  —antimalarials
  —oral steroids
  —nonsteroidal antiinflammatory drugs
- Ask your pharmacist or doctor about cosmetics, herbals, over-the-counter products, or alternative therapies before trying them.
- Do not stop taking your prescribed medications without checking with your pharmacist or doctor.

Other Problems

- Ask your doctor about treatment for nail changes or joint pain.

Chapter 43

Acne

Debra Sibbald, BScPhm, MA (Adult Education)

Pathophysiology

Acne vulgaris, or acne, is a common, multifactorial, self-limiting skin disorder. Although perceived as benign, acne is associated with important physical and psychological problems. Acne vulgaris is present in about 80% of people between the ages of 11 and 30. It is not limited to teenagers, can begin as early as the neonatal period, and is present in 20 to 30% of individuals aged 20 to 40. The intensity and duration varies for each individual, becoming less active in most cases as adolescence ends. It is often more severe in males, but more persistent in females, who may have periodic premenstrual flares until menopause.[1]

The pathogenesis of acne progresses through four major stages:
1. Increased follicular keratinization
2. Increased sebum production
3. Bacterial lipolysis of sebum triglycerides to free fatty acids
4. Inflammation

Acne is the result of the development of an obstructed sebaceous follicle, called a microcomedone. Sebaceous glands (Figure 1) increase their size and activity in response to circulating androgens while the infrainfundibulum increases its keratinization of cells. The cells adhere to each other in an expanding mass, which forms a dense keratinous plug. Sebum, produced in increasing amounts by the active gland, becomes trapped behind the keratin plug, contributing to comedone formation.

Acne usually begins in the prepubertal period, when the adrenal glands mature, and progresses as androgen production and sebaceous gland activity increase with gonad development. Most patients with acne have sebaceous glands that are hyperresponsive to

Figure 1: **The Skin**

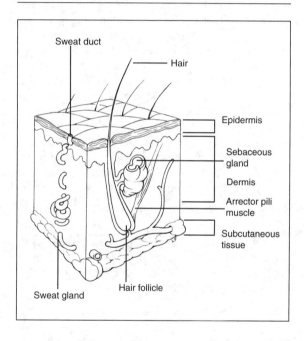

androgens, rather than an overproduction of androgens, with some exceptions.[2]

The comedone, filled with lipid substrate, provides ideal conditions for overgrowth of the anaerobe *P. acnes*, which produces a lipase that can hydrolyze sebum triglycerides into free fatty acids. These free fatty acids may trigger the changes that lead to the increase in keratinization and microcomedone formation.[3,4] This closed comedone, or whitehead, is the first clinically visible lesion of acne and takes approximately five months to develop. The closed comedone is almost completely obstructed to drainage and has a tendency to rupture.[5-7]

As the plug extends to the upper canal and dilates its opening, an open comedone, or blackhead, is formed. Its dark color is not due to dirt but to either oxidized lipid and melanin or to the impacted mass of horny cells. The cylindrically-shaped, open comedone is very stable and may persist for a long time as soluble substances and liquid sebum escape more easily. Acne that is characterized by open and closed comedones is called noninflammatory acne.

P. acnes also produces enzymes which increase the permeability of the follicular wall, causing it to rupture, releasing keratin, hair and lipids and irritating free fatty acids into the dermis. Several different types of inflammatory lesions may form. A superficial aggregation of neutrophils forms a *pustule*, a raised white lesion filled with pus, usually less than 5 mm in diameter. Superficial pustules usually resolve within a few days without scarring. A deeper, dermal, inflammatory infiltration will produce a *nodule*, the most severe variant of acne. They are warm, tender, firm lesions, with a diameter of 5 mm or greater. They may be suppurative or hemorrhagic within the dermis, may involve adjacent follicles and sometimes extend down to fat. Suppurative nodules can be called cysts because they resemble inflamed epidermal cysts. The cascade of the pathogenesis of acne is shown in Figure 2.

Hyperpigmentation and scarring are two sequelae of acne. A time delay of up to three years between acne onset and adequate treatment correlates to degrees of scarring and emphasizes the need for earlier therapy.[8,9]

Acne can either be caused or exacerbated by a variety of factors. Newborns or two- to three-month-old infants may develop papules, pustules and less commonly closed or open comedones, primarily on the cheeks, due to placental transfer of maternal androgens (*neonatal acne*). The acne subsides within a few months with regular maturation. Boys are affected more often than girls because of a transient increase in testosterone secretion during the third and fourth month of intrauterine life. Resolution occurs without therapy.[10]

Acneform eruptions may be provoked by *hormonal changes* such as androgenic and anti-estrogenic progestogens, found in oral contraceptives. Hormonal changes in pregnancy may also change the appearance of acne. Seventy per cent of females may complain of premenstrual flares. The pilosebaceous duct opening is significantly smaller between days 15 to 20 of the menstrual cycle, causing duct obstruction which impedes sebum flow, and changes in keratin hydration.[11,12]

The application of some topical agents may promote the formation of acne (*contact acne*). This can be due to the use of cosmetics or topical medications or to occupational hazards. Comedone formation through mechanically occluded follicles (*pomade acne*) may occur with the use of oil-based scalp preparations on the forehead and temples, oily lubricants in infants and children, and the application of topical tar products. Tar folliculitis can be minimized by applying the tar in the direction the hair grows out at the skin surface, leaving the angle beneath the hair free of tar to allow secretion of duct contents. In some postadolescent women, acne can be caused or made worse by the liberal use of oily cosmetics (*cosmetic acne*). This commonly occurs in a perioral distribution with a clear zone around the lips; acne due to application of hairspray may develop around the hair margins.[13] Closed comedones, papules, pustules and nodules may be induced by contact with occupational materials including acnegenic industrial agents such as coal tar, pitch, mineral oil and petroleum oil (*occupational acne*). Ingestion, inhalation or transcutaneous penetration of halogenated aromatic hydrocarbons, including the polychlorobiphenyls in paint, varnishes, lacquers, fungicides, insecticides, herbicides, wood preservatives and various oils, produce a distinct form of occupational acne (*chloracne*). Within a few months of sufficient exposure, open and closed comedones appear on the chest, temples and behind the ears. Inflammatory lesions may follow.[14]

Physical pressure from headbands, violins, chin straps, sports helmets, guitar straps and orthopedic braces have induced localized acne (*acne mechanica*). Mechanical friction should be eliminated or reduced. Wool or other rough textured fabrics and occlusive clothing may also be irritants.

Acne patients manipulate their comedones and pustules with finger pressure by picking, excoriating or pinching in an attempt to drain lesions, often subconsciously or during sleep (*acne excoriée*). Crusting erosions, scarring and hyperpigmentation may result from the ensuing rupture and inflammation.

Figure 2: **Pathogenesis of Acne Cascade**

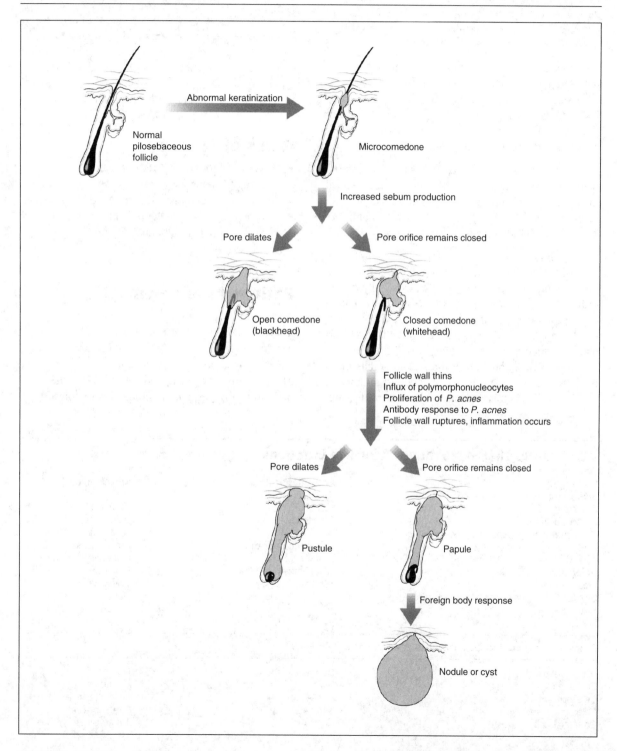

Acne is uninfluenced by diet, but a balanced diet should be advised for overall health. Some patients wish to restrict certain foods they perceive exacerbate acne (chocolate, cola drinks, milk and milk products).[15,16]

Environmental factors including heat and humidity may induce comedones, while pressure, friction and excessive scrubbing or washing can exacerbate existing acne by causing microcomedones to rupture. Hair styles low on the forehead or neck may cause excess sweating and occlusion and make acne worse.[17]

Emotions such as intense anger and stress can exacerbate acne, causing flares or increasing mechanical manipulation. Two-thirds of affected teenagers wish that they could speak with their physician about acne, but only one-third actually do.[18]

Certain drugs may cause acneform eruptions (*drug-induced acne*). Systemic corticosteroids can cause a pustular inflammatory form of acne, especially on the trunk. Onset is abrupt, two to six weeks after initiation of therapy. Acne has also been associated with most of the potent topical steroids, but not with hydrocortisone, which lacks the ability to inhibit protein synthesis. Discontinuation of the steroid results in an initial worsening of the appearance due to removal of the antiinflammatory action of the steroid itself.

Caution patients about this reaction, which can be subdued through judicious use of topical hydrocortisone.[19-21]

Halogens, especially an excess of iodide in seafood, salt and health foods, can worsen acne. Other drugs that may induce acne include heavy metals (lithium and cobalt in vitamin B_{12}), antiepileptics and tuberculostatics.[22] A more detailed list is found in Table 1.

Goals of Therapy

- Alleviate symptoms by reducing the number and severity of lesions
- Limit disease duration and recurrence
- Prevent long-term disfigurement associated with scarring and hyperpigmentation
- Avoid psychological suffering

Patient Assessment

An assessment plan for patients with acne is presented in Figure 3. The patient history must include drug or nondrug measures used for acne currently and in the past, as well as outcomes with these therapies. Allergy, particularly to ingredients of OTC acne products, and atopy are important features to consider.

Table 1: **Drugs That May Produce Acne-like Eruptions**[23]

Hormones:	**Antiepileptic drugs:**	**Miscellaneous:**
Androgenic hormones in women	Hydantoin derivatives	Cyclosporine
Corticosteroids	Phenobarbital	Cyanocobalamin
Corticotropin (ACTH)	Trimethadione	Dantrolene
Oral contraceptives (especially those with high		Gold salts
progestin component)	**Tuberculostatic drugs:**	Lithium salts
	Ethambutol	Maprotiline
Halogens:	Ethionamide	Psoralens
Bromides	Isoniazid	Quinidine
Chlorides		Quinine
Halothane		Topical coal tar
Iodides		

Drugs that may produce papular/pustular eruptions or folliculitis

Carbamazepine	Dactinomycin	Norfloxacin
Cephalexin	Diltiazem	Piperazine
Cefazolin	Furosemide	Pyrimethamine
Chloramphenicol	Isoniazid	Streptomycin
Co-trimoxazole	Naproxen	Tetracyclines

Figure 3: **Assessment of Patients with Acne**

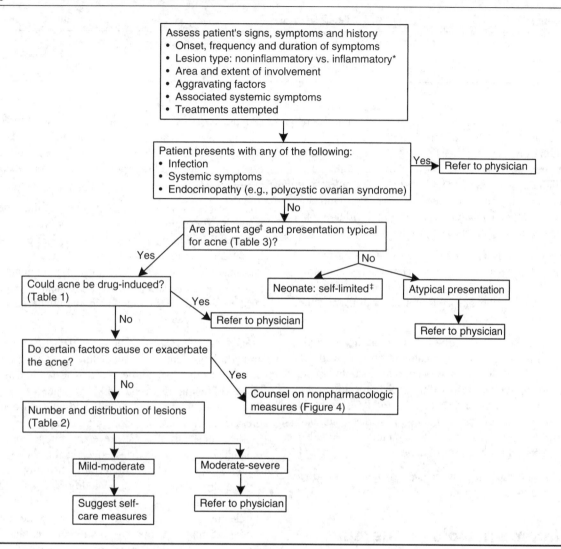

*Noninflammatory (open/closed comedones)/Inflammatory (papules, pustules, nodules/cysts).
†Typical ages 12-25 years; onset after puberty may signal acne rosacea.
‡Baby oil should be avoided as it may aggravate follicular occlusion.[24]

Acne vulgaris can be noninflammatory or inflammatory. Noninflammatory acne is characterized by open and closed comedones. Inflammatory acne is traditionally characterized as having papulo-pustular and/or nodular lesions. The severity grading is based on lesion count approximations, as shown in Table 2. Lesions are usually located on the face, back, neck and chest, and may extend to buttocks or extremities.

Often resolution of these lesions leaves erythematous or pigmented macules that can persist for months or longer, especially in dark-skinned individuals.

Acne vulgaris is rarely misdiagnosed. The most commonly mistaken conditions include rosacea, perioral dermatitis, gram-negative folliculitis and drug-induced acne.[26]

Table 2: **Severity Grading of Inflammatory Acne Lesions**[25]

Severity	Papules/Pustules	Nodules
Mild	Few to several	None
Moderate	Several to many	Few to several
Severe	Numerous and/or extensive	Many

Acne rosacea is a chronic relapsing condition, occurring after age 30, in fair-complexioned persons, commonly Celtic. The first sign is easy flushing (redness or erythema), followed by development of inflammatory lesions with edema, papules and pustules, appearing on the nose, cheeks, chin and forehead, with telangiectasia as the condition progresses. Refer patients to a physician for treatment.[27]

Perioral dermatitis occurs primarily in young women and adolescents and is characterized by erythema, scaling, and papulo-pustular lesions commonly clustered around the nasolabial folds, mouth, and chin. The cause is unknown.[26]

Gram-negative folliculitis may complicate acne, occurring after long-term treatment of acne with oral antibiotics. Folliculitis may occur due to staphylococci. There is a sudden onset of superficial pustules around the nose, chin, and cheeks. Patients should be referred to a physician.[26] Table 3 provides a summary and includes conditions less commonly included in the differential diagnosis of acne.

Table 4 summarizes when acne patients should be referred to a physician.

Nonpharmacologic Therapy

Washing: Patients should wash no more than twice daily with a mild soap or soapless cleanser (see Chapter 41, Table 6). Acne patients wash too frequently, attempting to remove surface oils. There is no evidence this is helpful since surface lipids do not affect acne.[28] Contributory lipids are deep in the follicle and not removed through washing. Antiseptic cleansers, while producing a clean, refreshed feeling, remove only surface dirt, oil, and aerobic bacteria. They do not affect *P. acnes*. There is no evidence that one washing regimen is superior. Scrubbing should be minimized to prevent follicular rupture. Soaps produce a drying effect on the skin due to detergent action. As medicated cleansers require increased contact time, this drying action is pronounced, especially with peeling agents. Avoid cream-based cleansers.

Shaving: Males should try both electric and safety razors to determine which is more comfortable for shaving. When using a safety razor, the beard should be softened with soap and warm water or shaving gel. Shaving should be done as lightly and infrequently as possible, using a sharp blade avoiding nicking lesions. Strokes should be in the direction of hair growth, shaving each area only once.

Comedone extraction: Comedone extraction, useful and painless, results in immediate cosmetic improvement although it has not been widely tested in clinical trials. Following cleansing with hot water, a comedone extractor is placed over the lesion and gentle pressure applied until the contents are expressed. This removes unsightly lesions, preventing progression to inflammation. A correctly sized extractor allows the central keratin plug to extrude through the opening. The small end of a plastic eye dropper, with bulb removed, may also be used. These instruments should be cleaned with alcohol after each use. Some initial reddening may be apparent. If the contents are not expressed with modest pressure, patients should not continue since improper extraction may further irritate the skin. A physician should be consulted if this technique is too difficult for the patient to manage. Since the follicle is difficult to remove completely, comedones may recur between 25 and 50 days following expression.

Ultraviolet light: Although ultraviolet light was recommended in the past for desquamation, it is no longer advised since the carcinogenic and photoaging effects of ultraviolet exposure are well-established. Moreover, inflamed skin is more susceptible to the damaging

Table 3: **Differential Diagnosis**

Kinds of acne

Acne variant	Comedones Open	Closed	Pustules	Papules	Nodules	Other
Vulgaris	X	X	X	X	X	
Drug-induced		+/–	X	X		
Neonatal		X	X	+/–		
Conglobata			X	XX	XX	Cysts, abscesses, sinus tracts
Fulminans			X	XX	XX	Ulcerating cysts
Contact:						
—Pomade		XX	X			
—Cosmetic	X	XX	XX	X		
—Occupational (oil)		XX	X	X		
—Chloracne	XX	XX	X	X		
Endocrine			XX	X	X	
Excoriated			X	X		Crusts, scars, erosions, hyperpigmentation
Mechanical		XX	XX	X		
Rosacea			X	X	+/–	Erythema, edema, telangiectasia

Other conditions

Milia

Folliculitis—gram-negative, staphylococcal, candida

Warts

Dental sinuses or epidermoid cysts

Table 4: **When to Refer an Acne Patient to a Physician**

Some patients may require further investigation, prescription therapy or other modalities.

If the etiology of the acne is drug-induced or an endocrinopathy

If acne is moderate to severe

Patients who are nonresponsive to nonprescription therapy

Patients who experience scarring, especially if moderate to severe

effects of ultraviolet light. Acne patients should apply sunscreens (SPF ≥ 15) in alcohol or oil-free bases and avoid using the acnegenic benzophenones (see Chapter 44). The sunscreen should be applied as the first product.

Encourage patients with acne to discontinue or avoid any aggravating factors, maintain a balanced diet and control stress. Evidence shows that by being empathetic and informative during counseling, the health professional may motivate the patient to continue long-term therapy.[29-32]

Prevention

Persistent low-grade acne in women after their mid-twenties is frequently caused by heavy cosmetic use. Adolescent acne in younger women may be exacerbated with makeup overuse. The problem is perpetuated when the resultant blemishes are concealed with more cosmetics.

Advise patients to stop using oil-containing cosmetics and avoid cosmetic programs that advocate applying multiple layers of cream-based cleansers and cover-ups. Various creams and cosmetics used during a beauty salon facial may precipitate acne in such patients. The patient should wash twice daily with a mild soap, and restrict cosmetic use to products labeled oil-free rather than water-based, including makeup, moisturizers or sunscreens. Since the spread time of oil-free makeup is decreased, best results are achieved if applied to one-quarter of the face at a time. Topical medication should be applied after gentle cleansing, and a foundation lotion may be used, sparingly, as a concealer.[33]

Water-based cosmetics may contain significant amounts of oil in the form of undiluted vegetable oils, lanolin, fatty acid esters (butyl stearate, isopropyl myristate), fatty acids (stearic acid), fatty acid alcohols, cocoa butter, coconut oil, red veterinary petrolatum, and sunscreens containing benzophenones. Flesh-tone tinted acne formulations may be recommended.[34,35]

Oil-free makeups are well-tolerated and lipstick, eye shadow, eyeliner, eyebrow pencils and loose face powders are relatively innocuous. Heavier, oil-based preparations, particularly moisturizers and hairsprays, clog pores and accelerate comedone formation.[36]

Coverup cosmetics for acne are available in several skin tones, in lotion and cream forms. They may be applied as cosmetics two or three times daily, over the entire face or to individual lesions. They are usually water-based, nongreasy preparations, often containing peeling agents, antibacterials or hydroquinone. Most contain sulfur. However, nonmedicated, *oil-free* makeups are preferable to water-based products. Water-based products, containing small amounts of oil, are more likely than oil-free to contribute to pore-blockage. The term "noncomedogenic" may refer to either water-based vehicles or products that are free of substances known to induce comedones. They are not necessarily oil-free.

Since the action of most therapeutic acne agents is to dry the skin, the use of moisturizers is counterproductive. Patients with acne should be restricted to oil-free products unless absolutely necessary because of treatment with strong drying agents or isotretinoin. Examples of moisturizers considered noncomedogenic include Keri-Lyte®, Moisturel® and Neutrogena®.[12]

Pharmacologic Therapy

Figure 4 provides an approach for treating acne with nonprescription medication.

Medicated Soaps and Washes

Medicated soaps and washes may contain topical antiseptics, or peeling agents such as salicylic acid, sulfur or benzoyl peroxide, alone or in combination. Most washes should remain on the skin from 15 seconds to 5 minutes followed by thorough rinsing. This limits the amount of time the active ingredient is in contact with the skin. Other cleansers are applied after washing and left on the skin without rinsing. Quaternary ammonium compounds are cationic detergents that are inactivated quickly in the presence of organic material, such as sebum. The duration of action of these products is short.

Bacteriostatic soaps, such as hexachlorophene, carbanilides and salicylanilides (halogenated hydroxyphenols), have been found to be acnegenic.[28] Few ordinary soaps induce acne. However, acne patients are particularly susceptible to comedogenic contactants, and if these soaps are applied several times daily for long periods, they may become troublesome. Soaps containing coal tar, which can induce folliculitis, are not indicated for acne.

Chlorhexidine inhibits in vitro growth of *P. acnes.*[37] A 4% chlorhexidine gluconate preparation in a detergent base has been shown to be as effective as benzoyl peroxide washes in patients with mild acne, and both preparations reduced the number of inflammatory and noninflammatory lesions after 8 and 12 weeks, compared to vehicle alone.[38]

Polyester cleansing sponges (e.g., Buf-Puf®) are synthetics that abrade the skin surface, removing superficial debris. They are unlikely to unseat comedones, considering the structure of these lesions. The sponges are available in soft or coarse textures, with or without soap. Caution patients against using a circular or rubbing motion that will increase irritation, and instruct them to use single, gentle, continuous strokes on each side of the face, from the midline out towards the ears.

Alcohol-detergent medicated pads, impregnated with salicylic acid 0.5%, have reduced inflammatory lesions and open comedones in mild to moderate acne. This type of medication is less abrasive, not rinsed off and convenient.[39]

Cationic (C) bond strips that become activated by water are now available. The dirt/oil in the pores is anionic. As the strip dries, the C-bond binds the anionic dirt and removes it when the strip is peeled off.

Abrasives consist of finely divided particles of fused aluminum or plastic together with cleansing and wetting agents. Abrasives peel and remove surface debris and may assist resorption of papules and pustules. Despite vigorous rubbing, removal of comedones is not accomplished. Particles, such as sodium tetraborate decahydrate, dissolve on use and their abrasiveness is limited.[40] The effectiveness of an abrasive cleanser containing polyethylene granules and the same cleansing agent without the abrasive granules has been compared in patients with mild to moderate acne. No significant difference was noted. These products are not indicated in most cases but may be used in a patient who responds empirically.[41]

Vehicles

Nongreasy solutions, gels, lotions and creams should be selected as bases for topical acne preparations. Many contain ethanol or isopropyl alcohol, which is more lipid-soluble and may be preferred. Propylene glycol is sometimes present in small amounts to add viscosity and lessen the drying effects of strong peeling agents. Solutions are used mainly with topical antibiotics, which are often dissolved in alcohol. An 8% **glycolic acid** solution is available for use alone or for incorporation in topical antibiotic preparations. Solutions and washes can be more easily applied to large areas such as the back.[42] Gels are drying but may cause a burning irritation in some patients and may prevent certain kinds of cosmetics from adhering to the skin.[43] Propylene glycol gels are easy to apply and dry without a visible or sticky film. Nonalcoholic gels may be as effective and less drying than alcoholic solutions. Alcoholic or acetone gels are usually more drying and provide better penetration of the active ingredient. Lotions are slightly less drying and creams are more emollient. Discourage moisturizers and oil-based products.

Consider the patient's skin type and preferences in the choice of vehicle for topical agents: patients with oily skin often prefer vehicles with higher proportions of alcohol (solutions and gels) while those with dry or sensitive skin prefer non-irritating lotions and creams. Lotions can be used with any skin type, and spread well over hair-bearing skin, but will burn or dry if they contain propylene glycol. Also consider the compatibility of vehicles and agents with cosmetics.

How to Use Topical Preparations

Topical preparations should not be applied to individual lesions but to the whole area affected by acne to prevent new lesions from developing, using care around the eyelid, mouth and neck, which chafe easily. Lotions should be applied with a cotton swab once or twice a day after washing or at bedtime if they leave a visible residue.

Exfoliants (peeling agents)

Exfoliants induce continuous mild drying and peeling by primary irritation, damaging the superficial layers of the skin and inciting inflammation. This stimulates mitosis, thickening the epidermis, and increasing horny cells, scaling and erythema. A decrease in sweating results in a dry, less oily surface and may superficially resolve pustular lesions.

The efficacy of topical exfoliants in retarding comedone formation and accelerating their loss (comedolysis) was studied in a rabbit model. The prescription product retinoic acid (tretinoin) was most active compared to benzoyl peroxide and salicylic acid which were less active. Traditional nonprescription exfoliants, including phenol, resorcinol, betanapthol,

Figure 4: **Treating Acne with Nonprescription Medication**

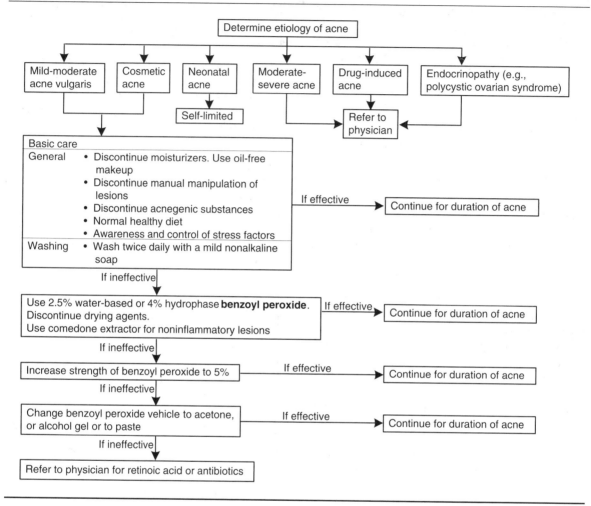

sulfur, Vleminckx's solution and sodium thiosulfate, are weak or ineffective. These agents are not comedolytic as they affect the superficial epidermis rather than the hair canal. They have been supplanted by superior effective agents (Table 5).[44,45]

Resorcinol, a phenol derivative, is less keratolytic than salicylic acid. It is an irritant and sensitizer and is said to be both bactericidal and fungicidal. Products containing resorcinol 1 to 2% have been used for acne, often in combination with other peeling agents, such as sulfur or salicylic acid. The US Food and Drug Administration (FDA) considers resorcinol 2% and resorcinol monoacetate 3%, in combination with

sulfur 3 to 8%, to be safe and effective. However, it is not convinced that resorcinol and resorcinol acetate are safe and effective when used as single ingredients, and has placed such products in Category II (not generally recognized as safe and effective, or misbranded). Although these compounds are inferior to other therapeutic modalities, there are several products containing these single ingredients on the Canadian market.[45]

Salicylic acid (Table 5) has comedolytic activity, although the concentrations in commercial preparations (less than 2 to 3%) are generally low. While concentrations less than 2% may actually increase

Table 5: **Nonprescription Agents Used to Treat Acne**

Drug	Dosing	Onset/Duration	Side effects	Interactions	Dosage forms
Exfoliants (peeling agents)					
Benzoyl peroxide	Daily or BID	Must be used for 8-12 wks before noted improvement. Duration of treatment is long-term. Dosing schedules adjusted PRN for chronic control. Taper off until natural resolution.	Produces mild irritant dermatitis. Dryness and peeling appear after a few days. Contact allergic dermatitis and cross-reactions with other sensitizers May bleach hair. Odor remains on clothing and bed sheets.	Chemically incompatible with retinoic acid Cross reactions with other sensitizers, such as Peruvian balsam, cinnamon and other benzoic acid derivatives (topical anesthetics)	Topical –lotion, alcohol or acetone gels, water-based vehicles, hydrophase gel, pastes, and washes. OTC: 2.5%, 4%, 5% Rx: 8% and 10%
Salicylic acid	Daily or BID		Initial irritation 3-6% is keratolytic causing softening of horny layer	Increases penetration of active ingredients	Gels, lotions, toners, cleansers, sticks, pads, washes and astringents
Antibacterials					
Benzoyl peroxide	Daily or BID	Onset: Rapid – the number of inflamed lesions could decrease within 5 days. Duration: Bactericidal effect lasts for at least 48 h. Therapy may continue for as long as the condition exists.	See above	See above	See above

keratinization, concentrations between 3 and 6% are keratolytic, softening the horny layer and shedding scales. Lower concentrations are sometimes combined with sulfur to produce an additive keratolytic effect. Concentrations of up to 5 to 10% can be used for acne, beginning with a low concentration and increasing as tolerance to the irritation develops. It is an effective agent, although as a peeling agent, slightly less potent than equal strength benzoyl peroxide. It may have antiinflammatory properties that help dry inflammatory lesions.[26] Its keratolytic effect may enhance the absorption of other agents. Although the FDA recognizes salicylic acid as safe and effective, it offers no advantages over more modern topical agents such as benzoyl peroxide.[45-47]

Sulfur is used in the precipitated or colloidal form in concentrations of 2 to 10%. Sulfur compounds (e.g., sulfides, thioglycolates, sulfites, thiols, cysteines and thioacetates) are also available and somewhat weaker. Sulfur helps resolve comedones by its exfoliant action. Its popularity is due to its ability to quickly resolve pustules and papules, mask and conceal lesions (similar to a thick foundation lotion), produce irritation leading to skin peeling and mild antibacterial action. Although it is often combined with salicylic acid or resorcinol to increase its effect, its use is limited by its offensive odor and the availability of more effective agents.[48]

It has met the criteria of the FDA Advisory Review Panel for OTC topical acne products, but its antibacterial effects were not recognized. Sodium thiosulfate, zinc sulfate, and zinc sulfide were not considered safe and effective.

Antibacterials

Choices for antibacterial therapy include benzoyl peroxide, as well as prescription topical and systemic antibiotics, and combination products. These drugs kill *P. acnes* and inhibit the production of pro-inflammatory mediators by organisms that are not killed.[3]

Benzoyl peroxide (Table 5) preparations are the single most useful group of topical nonprescription agents and agents of first choice for most patients with acne vulgaris. Benzoyl peroxide has three principle actions useful in both noninflammatory and inflammatory acne. It produces powerful anaerobic antibacterial activity due to slow release of oxygen,

comedolysis and depression of sebum production. It has a rapid (within two hours) bactericidal effect that lasts at least 48 hours. As a result, it may decrease the number of inflamed lesions within five days. Its anti-acne effect is augmented by increased blood flow, dermal irritation, local anesthetic properties and promotion of healing.[49-52] Since the primary effect of benzoyl peroxide is antibacterial, it is most effective for inflammatory acne. Many patients with noninflammatory comedonal acne will respond to its peeling action.

Cleansers containing benzoyl peroxide are available as nonprescription liquid washes and solid bars of various strengths. The desquamative and antibacterial effectiveness in a soap or wash is minimized by limited contact time and removal with proper rinsing. Stable lotions are available in 2.5, 5 and 10%. Alcohol and acetone gels facilitate bioavailability and may be more effective, while water-based vehicles are less irritating and better tolerated. A 4% hydrophase gel (Solugel®) is available that suspends crystals of benzoyl peroxide in a dimethylisosorbide solvent as the water in the base evaporates. The resulting solution is absorbed by the skin, leaving no film. The manufacturer claims the resulting efficacy is equal to 10% benzoyl peroxide with the minimal irritation of a 2.5% aqueous base gel. This may be an alternative for the patient with easily irritated skin who requires additional potency. This vehicle is easily combined with prepackaged clindamycin or erythromycin powders. Paste vehicles are stiffer and more drying than ointments or creams, facilitate absorption and allow the active ingredients to stay localized.

Concentrations of 2.5, 5 and 10% in a water-based gel have been compared with the vehicle alone. The 2.5% formulation is equivalent to the 5 and 10% formulation in reducing the number of inflammatory lesions. The lower strength is not as effective a peeler compared to higher strengths. Irritant side effects with the 2.5% gel are less frequent than with the 10% gel but equivalent to the 5% gel. The lowest concentration of benzoyl peroxide should be used for treating patients with easily irritated skin and may lessen irritation when used in combination topical therapy with comedolytic agents.

Benzoyl peroxide may bleach hair and clothing. It produces a mild primary irritant dermatitis that settles over continued use and is more likely to occur with fair complexions, those with a tendency to irritancy or who easily sunburn. There are rare reports of contact allergic dermatitis. Cross-reactions with other sensitizers, notably Peruvian balsam and cinnamon, are well established. It may cross-sensitize to other benzoic acid derivatives such as topical anesthetics. Concomitant use of an abrasive cleanser may initiate or enhance sensitization.[53] Another side effect is body odor from breakdown of the benzoyl peroxide that remains on clothing and bed sheets. Although links have been made in mice experiments, there is no indication that the normal use of benzoyl peroxide in the treatment of acne is associated with an increased risk of facial skin cancer. Overall the cutaneous use of benzoyl peroxide is relatively safe.[54-57]

Benzoyl peroxide has been used in combination with other anti-acne medications, such as sulfur and chlorhydroxyquinoline, or in formulations with urea to facilitate drug delivery. No significant improvement has been demonstrated.

Preparations of benzoyl peroxide are available without prescription in concentrations up to 5%. Recommend the weakest concentration (2.5%) in a water-based formulation or the 4% hydrophase, for anyone with a history of skin irritation, or who must use combination therapy.[58] There are many suggested routines to initiate therapy. One is to gently cleanse the skin and apply the preparation for 15 minutes the first evening, avoiding the eyes and mucous membranes. A mild stinging and reddening will appear. Each evening the time should be doubled until left on for four hours and subsequently all night. Dryness and peeling will appear after a few days. Once tolerance is achieved, the strength may be increased to 5% or the base changed to the acetone or alcohol gels, or paste. Alternatively, benzoyl peroxide can be applied for two hours for four nights, four hours for four nights, and then left on all night. It is important to wash the product off in the morning. Other drying agents should be discontinued. A sunscreen is recommended if benzoyl peroxide is used. To avoid interactions, apply the sunscreen during the day and the benzoyl peroxide at night.

Other Agents

To control pigmentation, **hydroquinone**, which reversibly damages melanocytes, is used as a nonprescription hypopigmenting agent in concentrations of 2 to 4%. Preparations are available as clear or tinted gels, which are more drying, and as vanishing or opaque, flesh-tinted creams. These products may also contain alpha-hydroxy acids or sunscreens. Epidermal but not dermal pigmentation will fade. Onset of response is usually three to four weeks, and the depigmentation lasts for two to six months but is reversible.

For some patients with mild scarring, nonprescription alpha-hydroxy acids may be used, while severe scarring may be corrected with other treatment modalities that require a dermatologist consultation. Dermabrasion, local excision, collagen implants, chemical peels (e.g., 70% glycolic acid) and laser therapy have been used to improve scarring. Usually the scar is not completely removed, but a more cosmetically acceptable result is achieved.[12]

Alternative Therapy

Tea tree oil contains terpinen-4-ol which appears responsible for some antimicrobial activity. In a study comparing 5% tea tree oil gel to 5% benzoyl peroxide lotion, both reduced the number of inflamed and noninflamed lesions. A systematic review of randomized clinical trials concludes there is no compelling evidence to show tea tree oil is effective in any dermatologic condition.[59] Further, the use of herbal preparations which are nonstandardized should be discouraged in favor of traditional quality-controlled preparations that have evidence of efficacy.[60]

Prescription Agents

Exfoliants: Keratinization is controlled with peeling agents that prevent or eliminate comedones. Peeling is the best treatment for most forms of acne, especially milder cases, and even severe forms will benefit noticeably. The most powerful peeling agents are prescription medications. Retinoic acid (vitamin A acid or tretinoin) slows the desquamation process, reducing numbers of both microcomedones and comedones.[3] It is a powerful exfoliant and is not to be used in pregnant women because of risk to the fetus.

Adapalene has shown clinical benefits for noninflammatory acne similar to those of topical tretinoin and causes less local irritation.[61] It is better at reducing inflammatory lesions and total lesion count.[43]

Tazarotene reduces both noninflammatory and inflammatory lesions. It is as effective as adapalene in reducing noninflammatory and inflammatory lesion counts when applied half as frequently. Compared with tretinoin it is as effective for comedonal and more effective for inflammatory lesions when applied once daily.[43,62,63]

Systemic isotretinoin exerts a primary effect on comedogenesis, causing a decrease in size and reduction in formation of new comedones.[3]

Antibacterials: Erythromycin, clindamycin and tetracycline are all available as single ingredient topical preparations. Clindamycin is preferred because of potent action, lack of absorption and limited systemic indications due to associated pseudomembranous colitis. It can also be combined with benzoyl peroxide. Erythromycin is available alone and in combination with retinoic acid or benzoyl peroxide. Some topical antibiotic-benzoyl peroxide combinations require refrigeration.

Systemic antibiotics including tetracycline, minocycline and erythromycin are often most convenient for the patient. Tetracycline is the drug of choice based on fewest side effects, widest acceptance, and a direct antiinflammatory action.[64] Oral antibiotics are often combined with topical agents, and the antibiotic may be discontinued after six months of therapy.[65] Prolonged oral administration may cause overgrowth of gram-negative organisms, producing a refractory folliculitis and necessitating discontinuation.

Antisebum agents: No topical agents directly influence the production of sebum. Systemic drugs that influence sebum production include high dose estrogens, antiandrogens (cyproterone acetate), spironolactone and the retinoid isotretinoin.

Isotretinoin, a natural metabolite of vitamin A, should be reserved for unresponsive, severe, nodulo-cystic acne. Because of teratogenicity, contraceptive measures must be started one month before and continue one month after therapy, normally for four months. Drying agents must be discontinued, and moisturizers used.

Monitoring of Therapy

Table 6 provides a monitoring framework for patients with acne. Parameters should be monitored by the patient, in a diary. Therapy should be appropriately tapered in response to improvement or resolution.

The health care professional should be responsible for ensuring that the treatment plan remains on schedule, is effective and no adverse effects are occurring. The patient should be contacted within two to three weeks to determine progress.

Suggested Readings

Brown S, Shalita AR. Acne vulgaris. *Lancet* 1998;351: 1871-6.

Healy E, Simpson N. Acne vulgaris. *BMJ* 1994;308: 831-3.

Johnson BA, Nunley JR. Topical therapy for acne vulgaris: How do you choose the best drug for each patient? *Postgrad Med J* 2000;107(3):69-80.

Lever L, Marks R. Current views on the aetiology, pathogenesis and treatment of acne vulgaris. *Drugs* 1990;39(5):681-92.

Leyden JJ. Therapy for acne vulgaris. *N Engl J Med* 1997;336(16):1156-62.

Maddin WS, Landells IDR, Poulin Y et al. Treatment of acne vulgaris and prevention of acne scarring: Canadian Consensus Guidelines. *J Cutan Med Surg* 2000;4(suppl 1):S4-2-S4-13.

Russell JJ. Topical therapy for acne. *Am Fam Physician* 2000;61(2):357-365.

Strasburger VC. Acne: what every pediatrician should know about treatment. *Pediatr Clin North Am* 1997; 44(6):1505-23.

Thiboutot DM. New treatments and therapeutic strategies for acne. *Arch Fam Med* 2000;9(2): 179-87.

References

1. Leyden J, Shalita AR. Rational therapy for acne vulgaris: an update on topical treatment. *J Am Acad Dermatol* 1986;15: 907-14.
2. Leyden JJ. Therapy for acne vulgaris. *N Engl J Med* 1997; 336(16):1156-62.
3. Shalita AR. Genesis of free fatty acids. *J Invest Dermatol* 1974;62:332-5.
4. Tucker SB, Rogers S, Winkleman RK. Inflammation in acne vulgaris: leukocyte attraction and cytotoxicity by comedonal material. *J Invest Dermatol* 1985;74:21-5.
5. Winston MH, Shalita AR. Acne vulgaris. *Pediatr Clin North Am* 1991;38(4):889–903.
6. Plewig G, Kligman AM. The dynamics of primary comedo formation. In: Plewig G, Kligman AM, eds. *Acne: Morphogenesis and Treatment.* New York: Springer-Verlag; 1975: 58-107.
7. Puissegur-Lupo M. Acne vulgaris, treatments and their rationale. *Postgrad Med* 1985;78(7):76–88.

Table 6: **Monitoring Therapy for Acne**

Monitoring	**Patient:** daily while on drug therapy **Pharmacist:** every 4-8 wks of therapy or next pharmacy visit	
Short-term	**Time frame/Degree of change**	**Actions**
Positive endpoints (Acne resolution/control)		
Lesion count	Decrease by 10-25% within 4-8 wks, with control, or more than a 50% decrease within 2-4 mos.	If endpoints not achieved, refer to a physician for further therapy.
Comedones	Resolve by 3-4 mos.	
Inflammatory lesions	Resolve within a few weeks	
Anxiety or depression	Achieve control or improvement within 2-4 mos.	
Long-term		
Progression of severity Recurrent episodes	No progression of severity. Lengthening of acne-free periods throughout therapy.	If endpoints not achieved, refer to a physician for further therapy.
Scarring or pigmentation	No further scarring or pigmentation throughout therapy.	
Negative endpoints (treatment side effects)		
Severe dryness, irritation (redness, inflammation, stinging, etc.)	Minimal. Should disappear, diminish or be controlled with continued use	If severe, decrease dose, concentration or frequency of use. If still no improvement, refer to physician for further treatment.

8. Layton AM, Henderson CA, Cunliffe WJ. A clinical evaluation of acne scarring and its incidence. *Clin Exp Dermatol* 1994; 9:303-8.

9. Thiboutot DM. Acne: an overview of clinical research findings. *Dermatol Clin* 1997;15(1):97-109.

10. Katsambas AD, Katoulis AC, Stavropoulos P. Acne neonatorum: a study of 22 cases. *Int J Dermatol* 1999;38(2)128-30.

11. Williams M, Cunliffe WJ. Explanation for premenstrual acne. *Lancet* 1973;2:1055.

12. Strasburger VC. Acne: what every pediatrician should know about treatment. *Pediatr Clin North Am* 1997;44(6):1505-23.

13. Zatulove A, Konnerth NA. Comedogenicity testing of cosmetics. *Cutis* 1987;39(6):521.

14. Taylor JS. Chloracne: a continuing problem. *Cutis* 1974; 13:585.

15. Rosenberg EW. Acne diet reconsidered. *Arch Dermatol* 1981; 117(4):193-5.

16. Fulton JE, Plewig G, Kligman AM. Effect of chocolate on acne vulgaris. *JAMA* 1969;210:2071.

17. Shalita AR. Acne vulgaris: pathogenesis and treatment. *Cosmet Toiletries* 1983;98:57-60.

18. Malus M, LaChance PA, Lamy L, Macaulay A, Vanasse M. Priorities in adolescent health care: the teenagers' viewpoint. *J Fam Pract* 1987;25:159-62.

19. Kelly AP. Acne and related disorders. In: Sams WM, Lynch PJ, eds: *Principles and Practice of Dermatology.* New York: Churchill Livingstone; 1990:1014.

20. MacDonald Hull S, Sunliffe WJ. The use of a corticosteroid cream for immediate reduction in the clinical signs of acne vulgaris. *Acta Derm Venereol* 1989;69(5):452-3.

21. Brodell RT, O'Brien MR. Topical corticosteroid-induced acne: three treatment strategies to break the 'addiction cycle'. *Postgrad Med* 1999;106(6):225-6,229.

22. Hitch JM. Acneform eruption induced by drugs and chemicals. *JAMA* 1969;200:879.

23. Bruisma W. A *Guide to Drug Eruptions.* 5th ed. Oosthuizen, The Netherlands: European Book Service; 1990:6.

24. Forest MG, Cathiard A, Bertrand JA. Evidence of testicular activity in early infancy. *J Clin Endocrinol Metab* 1973;37:148.

25. Pochi PE, Shalita AR, Straus JC et al. Report of the consensus conference on acne classification. *J Am Acad Dermatol* 1991;24(3):495-500.

26. Johnson BA, Nunley JR. Topical therapy for acne vulgaris: How do you choose the best drug for each patient? *Postgrad Med J* 2000;107(3):69-80.

27. Habif TP. Acne, rosacea, and related disorders. In: Klein EA, Menczer BS, eds. *Clinical Dermatology.* Toronto: Mosby; 1990:756.

28. Plewig G, Kligman AM. Acne detergicans. In: Plewig G, Kligman AM, eds: *Acne: Morphogenesis and Treatment.* New York: Springer-Verlag; 1975:270-325.

29. Feldman W, Hodgson C, Corber S et al. Health concerns and health-related behaviours of adolescents. *Can Med Assoc J* 1986;134:489-493.

30. Koo JYM, Smith LL. Psychologic aspects of acne. *Pediatr Dermatol* 1991;8(3):185-8.

31. Krowchuck DR, Stancin R, Keskinen R, Waler R, Bass J, Anglin TM. The psychosocial effects of acne on adolescents. *Pediatr Dermatol* 1991;8(4):332-8.

32. Klassen AF, Newton JN, Mallon E. Measuring quality of life in people referred for specialist care of acne: comparing generic and disease-specific measures. *J Am Acad Dermatol* 2000;43(2pt1):229-33.

33. Epinette WW, Gresit MC, Osols II. The role of cosmetics in postadolescent acne. *Cutis* 1982;29(5):500-4,514.

34. Plewig G, Kligman AM. Acne cosmetica. In: Plewig G, Kligman AM, eds. *Acne: Morphogenesis and Treatment.* New York: Springer-Verlag; 1975:226-9.

35. Mills OH, Kligman AM. Comedogenicity of sunscreens. experimental observations in rabbits. *Arch Dermatol* 1982; 118(6):417-9.

36. Walzer RA. Acne: some answers to a complexion problem In: Walzer RA, ed. *Skintelligence: How to be Smart About Your Skin.* New York: ACC; 1981:53-69.

37. Stoughton RB. Comparative in vitro bioassay of skin penetration and activity of chlorhexidine preparations and other topical agents against *P. acnes*: an assessment of their potential use in the treatment of acne vulgaris. ICI: American Inc. Research report on file, CLR-120, Mar 1979.

38. Stoughton RB, Leyden JJ. Efficacy of 4 percent chlorhexidine gluconate skin cleanser in the treatment of acne vulgaris. *Cutis* 1987;39(6):551-3.

39. Shalita AR. Treatment of mild and moderate acne vulgaris with salicylic acid in an alcohol-detergent vehicle. *Cutis* 1982;28(11):556-8.

40. Arndt KA. Acne. In: Arndt KA, ed. *Manual of Dermatologic Therapeutics.* 4th ed. Toronto: Little, Brown; 1989: 3-13.

41. Fulgha CC, Caltalano PM, Childers RC et al. Abrasive cleansing in the management of acne vulgaris. *Arch Dermatol* 1982;118(9):658-9.

42. Thiboutot DM. New treatments and therapeutic strategies for acne. *Arch Fam Med* 2000;9(2):179-87.

43. Russell JJ. Topical therapy for acne. *Am Fam Physician* 2000; 61(2):357-65.

44. Brown S. Therapeutic potpourri. *Dermatol Clin* 1989; 7(1):71-4.

45. Sykes NL, Webster GF. Acne: a review of optimum treatment. *Drugs* 1994;48(1):59-70.

46. Zander E, Weisman S. Treatment of acne vulgaris with salicylic acid pads. *Clin Ther* 1992;14:247-53.

47. Shalita AR. Comparison of a salicylic acid cleanser and a benzoyl peroxide wash in the treatment of acne vulgaris. *Clin Ther* 1989;11:264-7.

48. Lin AN, Reimer RJ, Carter DM. Sulfur revisited. *J Am Acad Dermatol* 1988;18:553-8.

49. Cotterill JA. Benzoyl peroxide. *Acta Derm Venereol (Stock)* 1980;89(suppl):57-63.

50. Cunliffe WJ, Holland KT. The effect of benzoyl peroxide on acne. *Acta Derm Venereol (Stock)* 1981;61(3):267-9.

51. Lassus A. Local treatment of acne. A clinical study and evaluation of the effect of different concentrations of benzoyl peroxide gel. *Curr Med Res Opin* 1981;7(6):370-3.

52. Cunliffe WJ, Dodman B, Eady R. Benzoyl peroxide in acne. *Practitioner* 1978;220(3):470-82.

53. Maddin S. Benzoyl peroxide. *Can J Dermatol* 1989;1(4):92.

54. Report of the Expert Advisory Committee on Dermatology. The carcinogenic activity of benzoyl peroxide. *Information Letter* Ottawa: Health Protection Branch (Canada); 1987; 711:1-9.

55. Cunliffe WJ, Burke B. Benzoyl peroxide: lack of sensitization. *Acta Derm Venereol (Stock)* 1982;62(5):458-9.

56. Tkach JR. Allergic contact urticaria to benzoyl peroxide. *Cutis* 1982;29(2)187-8.

57. Rietschel RL, Duncan SH. Benzoyl peroxide reactions in an acne study group. *Contact Dermatitis* 1982;8:323-6.

58. Mills OH, Kligman AM, Pochi P, Comite H. Comparing 2.5% 5% and 10% benzoyl peroxide on inflammatory acne vulgaris. *Int J Dermatol* 1986;25(12):664-7.

59. Ernst E, Huntley A. Tea tree oil: a systematic review of randomized clinical trials. *Forsh-Komplementarmed* 2000;7(1): 17-20.

60. Combest, W. Tea tree oil. *US Pharm* 1999(April):35-38.

61. Verschoore M, Langner A, Wolska M, Jablonska S, Czernielewski J, Schaefer H. Vehicle controlled study of CD 271 lotion in the topical treatment of acne vulgaris. *J Invest Dermatol* 1993;100:221.

62. Gibson JR. Rationale for the development of new topical treatments for acne vulgaris. *Cutis* 1996;57:13-19.

63. Kakita L. Tazarotene versus tretinoin or adapalene in the treatment of acne vulgaris. *J Am Acad Dermatol* 2000;43 (2pt3):851-4.

64. Dalzeil K, Dykes PJ, Marks R. The effect of tetracycline and erythromycin in a model of acne-type inflammation. *Br J Exp Pathol* 1987;68:67-70.

65. Hughes BR, Murphy CE, Barnett J, Cunliffe WJ. Strategy of acne therapy with long-term antibiotics. *Br J Dermatol* 1989;121:623-8.

Acne—Patient Information

Acne is a common skin disorder that affects most adolescents and some adults. It generally appears as pimples, or larger pustules on the face, chest, back and upper arms. Although it tends to disappear in adulthood, acne may cause scarring and emotional difficulties as the disease progresses.

- The goal of acne treatment is to stop the formation of new pimples. Unfortunately, that takes time. Although this is a difficult period, try not to be discouraged!
- Treat acne as soon as it appears to avoid complications such as scarring.
- Allow six to eight weeks of treatment before assessing improvement. Some medications cause initial reddening or worsening that subsides with treatment. These may need to be introduced gradually. If acne does not improve with an adequate course of nonprescription medication, consult a physician.
- Do not use greasy cosmetics, coversticks, moisturizers, hair pomades, scalp oils, eye creams or hairspray. Even one application of a greasy cosmetic can perpetuate acne for months.
- Do not use makeup regularly. If necessary, use an oil-free preparation with the words "noncomedogenic" or "nonacnegenic" on the label and remove carefully at bedtime.
- Discuss any current medications for acne, other conditions, or any materials you may contact at work with the health professional who is advising you about treatment. Some substances may cause acne.
- Acne is not caused by dirt. Washing your face too often can irritate your skin and may make your acne worse. Wash your skin gently twice daily with water alone or a mild, non-alkaline soap or soapless cleanser. Do not rub or scrub your skin.
- Shampoo hair regularly; if it is oily, wash it more frequently. Keep your hair off your face as much as possible and tie it back during sleep.

- Do not manipulate acne lesions; avoid picking, scratching, popping or squeezing. Keeping a daily diary of the number of times you touch your skin may help to decrease this habit. Discuss with your health care provider if a comedone extractor may be used.
- Eliminate friction from objects such as headbands, violins, chin straps, sports helmets, guitar straps and orthopedic braces.
- Males with acne who shave should try both an electric and a safety razor to determine comfort. If using a safety razor, soften your beard thoroughly with soap and warm water. Shave as lightly and as seldom as possible and always use a sharp blade. Stroke over each area only once in the direction of hair growth.
- Eat a healthy, balanced diet. Foods are usually not aggravating factors.
- Be aware that stress may aggravate acne. Try to minimize its effect through relaxation or exercise.
- Apply acne medication to the entire affected area. In most cases, it is best not to spot-treat lesions. Use a clean swab for each application and discard.
- A tan can hide acne, but tanning can also damage your skin. To prevent this, use an oil-free sunscreen with a sun protection factor (SPF) of at least 15, in an alcohol lotion or gel form. Apply the sunscreen after cleansing and before acne medication. If using benzoyl peroxide, apply the sunscreen during the day and the benzoyl peroxide at night.
- Continue necessary skin care measures to avoid outbreaks until the tendency to have acne has passed.
- See a physician if acne is moderate to severe, is caused by medication or other medical conditions, or is not responsive to nonprescription medication used for a few months.

Chapter 44

Cosmetic Dermatology

Dale Wright, BSP, MSc, MDE

Perspiration and Body Odor

Pathophysiology

The primary function of sweat is to regulate body heat through evaporative cooling of water secreted to the skin's surface.[1] Sweat glands consist of a secretory coil in the dermis and a duct that transports sweat to the skin surface (Figure 1).

There are three types of sweat glands: eccrine, apocrine, and apoeccrine.[2]

- Eccrine sweat glands are primarily responsible for body cooling. They cover the skin surface with the greatest numbers on the palms and soles, then face, head and trunk.

Figure 1: **The Skin**

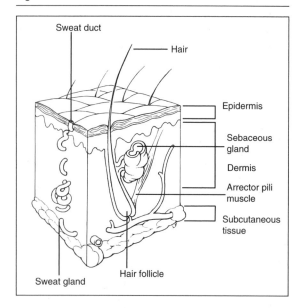

- Apocrine glands are found in the underarm, nipple, and genital areas, and usually open onto hair follicles. They become functional at puberty. Apocrine sweat is a milky, viscid, odorless secretion containing fatty substances. Bacterial breakdown of these chemicals produces body odor.
- Apoeccrine glands have structural features of both eccrine and apocrine glands. They are found only in the underarm area of adults.

Physiologic sweating is a natural reaction to thermal and emotional stimuli. Hot environments, over-clothing and exercise all trigger the hypothalamic sweat centre to increase heat loss through cutaneous vasodilation and generalized sweat production, especially on the face and trunk. Sweating around the lips and forehead is a physiologic response to eating hot or spicy foods. Emotional stimuli such as anxiety, embarrassment, fear, anger, excitement or mental stress can cause sweating from the palms, soles, underarms, and forehead. The cerebral cortex appears to control sweating from the palms and soles by acting on a hypothalamic sweat centre separate from that controlling thermal sweating.[3]

Hyperhidrosis is defined as excessive sweating beyond that required for body cooling. It is estimated to affect between 0.6% and 1% of the general population. It affects both sexes equally, although women may seek treatment more often than men. Hyperhidrosis can be secondary to fever, or an underlying medical condition. It has also been seen in alcohol and drug withdrawal syndromes as well as during menopausal hot flashes.[3] Sweating has been reported as a side effect of acetaminophen, ASA, insulin, antiemetics, morphine, bethanechol, pilocarpine, physostigmine, propranolol, neostigmine, cyclobenzaprine and SSRI antidepressants.[3,4]

The most common form of excess sweating is *primary* (idiopathic, essential) *hyperhidrosis*. Patients often describe profuse sweating in response to emotional stimuli, which is usually localized to the hands, feet, and sometimes the underarm area. Occasionally they will describe continuous excess sweating of these areas during waking hours. Sweating does not occur while sleeping, nor is there a marked increase in thermal sweating.[4] Primary hyperhidrosis usually begins at puberty, but can occur in infants or children. Note that normal, healthy infants and children can sweat around the head while asleep.[3] Primary hyperhidrosis can lead to embarrassment, low self-esteem and social withdrawal. Excessive hand sweating can sometimes interfere with occupational activities.[5] Secondary hyperhidrosis is often generalized, although neurologic lesions can cause a localized or unusual sweating pattern.[4]

Bromhidrosis refers to sweat that has an offensive odor. Sweat is usually odorless, although occasionally excretion of odor-causing chemicals in sweat, like garlic, can produce an odor. Body odor is generally produced by the action of bacteria on fatty substances in apocrine sweat (e.g., underarm odor), or on macerated skin cells in constantly damp areas, like feet in individuals with hyperhidrosis. Predisposing factors to bromhidrosis include hyperhidrosis, obesity, intertrigo and poor body hygiene.[1] Armpit hair is not a causative factor, but can contribute by increasing the surface area available for bacterial action on sweat.[6]

Goals of Therapy

- Control socially undesirable body odor
- Control underarm wetness resulting from normal, physiologic sweating
- Reduce the quantity of sweat excretion in hyperhidrosis to a tolerable level that permits participation in work and social situations
- Prevent complications of hyperhidrosis involving the feet – odor, blisters, infection

Patient Assessment

Concerns about body odor and underarm wetness resulting from normal, physiologic sweating often can

be managed without physician referral. Refer patients with excessive sweating, sweating of recent onset in adults, or sweating in an unusual pattern to a physician for evaluation. An assessment plan for patients with perspiration-related complaints is presented in Figure 2.

Nonpharmacologic Therapy

General Measures
Prevention is sometimes possible with physiologic sweating. A cool environment and low humidity can decrease perspiration. Natural fibres are more breathable than synthetics and cool, porous clothing should be chosen.[3] It might be possible to avoid some activities known to produce excessive sweating, such as certain stressful situations or exercising in hot weather. Water and electrolytes lost through sweating should be replaced regularly. Underarm shields primarily act as barriers, preventing wetness from staining clothing.

Personal Hygiene
To manage body odor, a regular bath or shower with a skin cleanser (soap or synthetic detergent) is essential to prevent build-up of bacteria, sweat and dead skin cells that interact to produce body odor. It has not been proven that antibacterial or deodorant cleansers are more effective than regular skin cleansers for routine personal hygiene.[7] A daily bath or shower may be necessary for some people. When a full bath or shower is not possible, sponging in the underarm and genital areas can help control the major source of body odor. Shaving the armpits can reduce the propagation of body odor by reducing the surface area for bacterial action. Wearing clean clothes will reduce odor from bacterial action on sweat-soaked fibres.[8]

Foot Care
Foot care is important for patients with excessive foot sweating and/or odor. Feet should be washed regularly using a skin cleanser and dried thoroughly. Daily washing may be needed for odor control followed by application of an absorbent foot powder. Non-occlusive footwear made of natural materials, such as leather shoes or sandals, should be worn with cotton or wool socks.

Figure 2: **Assessment of Patients with Perspiration and/or Body Odor Complaints**

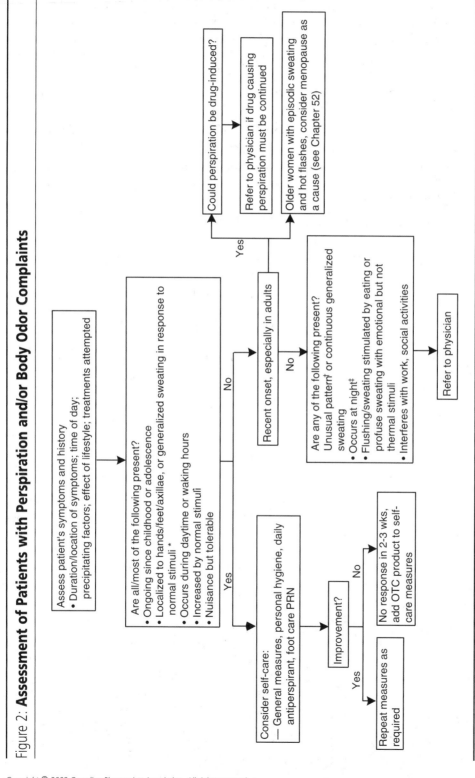

*Heat, exercise, emotional factors.
†Unusual pattern, e.g., whole face, unilateral.
‡Note that episodic sweating at night can occur in menopause; healthy children/infants often sweat on the head at night.

Iontophoresis

Iontophoresis uses a special water bath apparatus to introduce a mild electrical current of soluble ions into the skin. It blocks the sweat duct at the skin surface. Iontophoresis is often used for hyperhidrosis of the hands and feet not responding to conservative therapy.[4] Some patients purchase iontophoresis units for maintenance treatment at home. Side effects are minor. For prevention of tingling and burning in areas of broken skin, petrolatum should be applied for protection. Skin erythema can be managed with topical 0.5% hydrocortisone ointment. Excessive drying and cracking of the skin is treated with moisturizers and reduced frequency of treatments.

Pharmacologic Therapy

The most common nonprescription agents used to manage perspiration and body odor problems are described in Table 1. The mainstay of treatment is daily use of antiperspirants as part of a personal hygiene regimen. Antiperspirants reduce sweating by mechanically obstructing sweat gland pores. They also have a deodorant action by reducing the amount of sweat available for bacterial action, and by mild antibacterial effects. They are more effective for odor control than deodorants alone, which may contain antibacterial chemicals or perfumes to mask odors.[8]

Antiperspirants can be applied to the feet and hands for profuse sweating experienced in primary hyperhidrosis. The more potent and irritating **aluminum chloride** formulations should be reserved for patients with primary hyperhidrosis not responding adequately to daily use of a high-concentration roll-on formulation of **aluminum zirconium tetrachlorohydrate**. Antiperspirant foot powders and astringent soaks can be tried for hand and foot sweating,[8] but are less likely to be effective because of their low concentration of aluminum salts.

Absorption of aluminum from antiperspirants is minimal, and is not considered a significant contribution to the body burden of aluminum.[9] Evidence does not support an association between exposure to aluminum through regular use of aluminum-containing antiperspirants and development of dementia or Alzheimer's disease in people with healthy kidneys.[10]

Aluminum-containing deodorant stones are claimed to inhibit bacterial growth, but comparative efficacy with conventional antiperspirants is unknown. Formaldehyde, glutaraldehyde and tannic acid were once used to treat palmar-plantar hyperhidrosis. They are rarely used now because side effects of skin discoloration, irritation, and sensitization in the case of formaldehyde outweigh the benefits.[4,5] None are available in commercial formulations to treat hyperhidrosis.

Methenamine hydrolyzes on the skin to form formaldehyde and ammonia.[5] It is available in Canada in a cream formulation. **Tannic acid** in combination with **triclosan** is available in an aerosol product.

Prescription systemic drug therapy is sometimes suggested for debilitating hyperhidrosis not responding to topical therapy. Systemic anticholinergics such as glycopyrrolate 2 mg three or four times a day are helpful, but the side effects of dry mouth, blurred vision, constipation and urinary retention are poorly tolerated.[3,4] A variety of drugs have been anecdotally reported to improve hyperhidrosis in individual patients, including oxybutynin, benztropine, indomethacin, diltiazem, and clonidine.[4] Recently, local injections of botulinum toxin have been shown useful to treat palmar and axillary hyperhidrosis. Clinical usefulness of this treatment is limited by the need for multiple injections at each site, repeated at 4- to 12-month intervals.[4]

Monitoring of Therapy

Table 2 provides a monitoring plan framework which should be individualized.

Table 1: **Nonprescription Management of Perspiration and Body Odor**

Product	Action	Uses	Comments
Skin cleanser – soap (alkali salts of fatty acids), synthetic detergents[7]	Surfactants aid in removal of dirt and oils from skin. Added skin conditioners (e.g., superfatting agents, glycerin, polymers, petrolatum) make skin feel soft, smooth.	Use during bathing as part of a personal hygiene regimen to remove odor-producing substances.	Soaps, synthetic detergents are equally effective. However, soaps may be less effective, more irritating in hard water. Contact allergies to product additives can occur.
Antibacterial deodorants[7] (e.g., benzethonium chloride, triclosan)	Inhibit growth of odor-producing bacteria. Products may also contain odor-masking chemicals such as perfumes.	Use as part of a personal hygiene regimen.	Available in Canada only in deodorant or antibacterial body washes. Deodorants are not as effective as antiperspirants in controlling body odor. Irritation and contact allergies are possible.
Aluminum or aluminum-zirconium chlorohydrate salts and related compounds, 15-25%[4-6]	Blocks sweat gland pores to reduce sweat secretion. Controls odor by reducing the amount of sweat available to bacterial action, by suppressing bacterial growth, and by binding odor-producing chemicals. Alcohol in the formulation contributes to antibacterial effects.	Apply to underarms daily as part of a personal hygiene regimen. Apply to palms, soles as needed to control sweating in primary hyperhidrosis.	Lotions, roll-ons are more effective than sticks or sprays. Roll-ons with aluminum tetrachlorohydrate are most effective. If irritation occurs, try a different brand, different active ingredient, or lower concentration of ingredients. Avoid applying to freshly shaved or abraded skin. Zirconium-containing products are more irritating.
Aluminum chlorohydrate 4% foot powder	As above	Apply to feet as needed to help control local sweating.	Low concentration limits efficacy.
Aluminum acetate or aluminum sulfate astringent solutions[7]	Astringent action can help dry hands and feet.	Soak hands or feet as needed to encourage dryness in mild, local hyperhidrosis.	Low concentration of aluminum limits efficacy.
Aluminum chloride in anhydrous alcohol[3,4,6]	May block sweat gland pores and/or cause atrophy of the secretory apparatus. Deodorant action as above for aluminum salts.	Use on underarms, hands or feet in hyperhidrosis not responding to conventional antiperspirants. Apply daily until sweating is reduced, then once or twice weekly as required. May be used with daily application of conventional antiperspirants for odor control.	Very irritating, especially in the presence of water. To minimize irritation, apply only to dry skin. Apply at bedtime, wash off in the morning. Relieve irritation by reducing frequency of use or with hydrocortisone cream. Start with the low concentration (6.25%). Use the high concentration (20%) only on hands/feet if tolerated. Occlusion with plastic wrap may be required in resistant cases.

Table 2: **Monitoring Therapy for Perspiration and Body Odor**

Symptom	Monitoring	Endpoint	Actions
Underarm wetness	**Patient:** daily **Pharmacist:** next visit. If a 2-3 wk trial of general measures and a daily personal hygiene routine that includes a conventional antiperspirant is ineffective, add 6.25% aluminum chloride. Response may take up to 4 wks.	Dry axillae in resting, non-stressed state at comfortable room temperature after 4 wks of intervention.	If patient cannot tolerate aluminum chloride or is not responding after a 4-wk trial, refer to a physician. If aluminum chloride effective, reduce frequency to level required to maintain effect.
Hand sweating	**Patient:** daily **Pharmacist:** next visit. If daily astringent soaks and/or daily use of conventional antiperspirants for 1-2 wks is ineffective, try aluminum chloride. Response may take up to 4 wks.	Hand sweating reduced to a tolerable level after 4 wks of intervention.	If hand sweating interferes with social or occupational activities, refer to a physician. If patient cannot tolerate aluminum chloride or is not responding after a 4-wk trial, refer to a physician.
Foot sweating	**Patient:** daily **Pharmacist:** next visit. Treatment plan as for hand sweating. Also, ensure patient has a good foot care routine (see Nonpharmacologic Therapy).	Foot sweating reduced to a tolerable level after 4 wks of intervention.	If patient cannot tolerate aluminum chloride or is not responding after a 4-wk trial, refer to a physician.
Body odor	**Patient/family:** daily **Pharmacist:** next visit. Ensure daily personal hygiene routine includes washing with a cleansing agent, clean clothes, use of aluminum-containing antiperspirant.	Offensive body odor eliminated after 1-2 wks of intervention.	If personal hygiene measures and antiperspirants are ineffective after 1-2 wks, refer to physician.
Skin irritation from antiperspirants	**Patient:** daily **Pharmacist:** next visit, or have patient call. Ensure correct use. Try different brand, lower concentration, or zirconium-free product. Treat symptomatically with 0.5% hydrocortisone cream.	Antiperspirant tolerated with minimal or no irritation.	If irritation continues, stop antiperspirant and refer to physician.

Hair Care and Hair Growth

Pathophysiology

Visible hair is dead protein, formed from keratinization of cells arising from the hair follicle bulb deep in the dermis.[1] The outer cuticle of the hair shaft protects and holds the inner cortex together.[1] Vellus hairs cover most of the body. Terminal hair, which grows on the head, beard (males), pubic and underarm areas at puberty, is longer, coarser and more pigmented. Androgens are important in regulating hair growth in these areas.[2] Hair growth is cyclical. The active growing phase (anagen) is followed by a transitional phase (catagen) before the final resting phase (telogen), at the end of which the hair is shed. Normally about 100 scalp hairs are shed each day. Longer hairs in the scalp and beard areas have a long growing phase (two to six years), while hairs in other areas, such as on the arms, have a long resting phase.[3] Usually more than 85% of hairs are in the growing phase. The average growth rate of scalp hair is six inches per year.[1]

Hair loss (alopecia) has a variety of causes:

- The *natural aging* process results in a slow, steady, diffuse thinning of scalp hair in both men and women, most noticeable after age 50. With age, hair becomes finer, drier and duller. Less pigment is produced resulting in gray hair. Women with a marked increase in hair thinning after menopause probably have androgenic alopecia.[4]
- *Androgenic alopecia* (androgenetic alopecia, male-pattern baldness, female-pattern baldness), a hereditary form of androgen-induced diffuse hair loss, accounts for 95% of cases of accelerated hair loss.[5] Hair loss begins between puberty and age 40, and approximately 50% of men and 40% of women will exhibit this trait before age 50.[5] Under the influence of androgens, hair follicles in susceptible areas (frontal and temple areas in men, and crown of both men and women) gradually become smaller and the growing phase shortens resulting in smaller, finer hairs that cover the scalp poorly.[1]
- In *telogen effluvium* an abnormal number of hairs enter the resting phase. Excessive hair shedding and thinning occurs in the scalp, pubic and underarm areas about three to four months later. Causes include hormonal changes in pregnancy, severe psychological stress, injury or stress from infections, serious illness or major surgery, endocrine disorders and drug therapy. Chemotherapy causes *anagen effluvium*, abruptly stopping hair growth in the anagen phase. Hair loss is usually sudden and severe, affecting most scalp hairs simultaneously.[6] Normal hair growth is usually restored once the underlying cause is removed. Some drug-related causes of hair loss are listed in Table 3.
- Patchy hair loss can be caused by skin diseases, or by *alopecia areata*, an autoimmune disease affecting about 2% of the population. Alopecia areata may involve patchy areas on the scalp, the entire scalp, or all body hair may be lost. Hair breakage from blow drying with excessive heat, or use of harsh chemicals on hair (e.g., bleaching, coloring or straightening agents) can contribute to patchy hair loss.[4]

Hirsutism is the production of excessive terminal hair in a male-pattern distribution in women. It is usually a consequence of increased androgen activity. It can be caused by an underlying medical problem or by drugs with androgenic side effects (e.g., danazol, corticosteroids, cyclosporine, anabolic steroids and androgenic progestagens).[2] *Hypertrichosis* is an

---

Table 3: **Drugs Associated with Hair Loss**[6,7]

Androgens	Beta-blockers – metoprolol, nadolol, propranolol
Anticoagulants – heparin, heparinoids, coumarins, indandiones	Clofibrate
	Colchicine
Anticonvulsants – carbamazepine, hydantoins, valproic acid	Interferons
Antineoplastics	Lithium
Antithyroids – iodine, thiouracil, carbimazole	Nonsteroidal antiinflammatories – ibuprofen, indomethacin, salicylates
Antidepressants – desipramine, fluoxetine, imipramine, maprotiline	Oral contraceptives
	Oral retinoids – etretinate, isotretinoin

---

apparent increase in vellus hair.[3] It has been reported with cyclosporine, erythropoietin, calcium channel blockers and tretinoin. The mechanism(s) of abnormal hair growth with these drugs is not established.[6]

Goals of Therapy

- Maintain healthy-appearing scalp hair
- Control unwanted body hair
- In androgenic alopecia, retard hair thinning and increase scalp coverage

Patient Assessment

Because effective nonprescription options for management of hair loss and hirsutism are limited, the assessment process is an opportunity to inform patients about the various factors that contribute to hair growth changes. Refer patients with unusual changes in hair growth and/or significant concerns about their hair changes to a physician for further investigation. An approach to the patient with hair-related concerns is presented in Figure 3.

Nonpharmacologic Therapy

There is a broad spectrum of what is considered "healthy, normal hair," since hair color, texture, body and curliness is genetically determined. For example, straight hair reflects light better than curly, and may appear more shiny. Fine hair may more readily appear greasy from the effects of normal scalp oil. When the cuticle is damaged, hair can appear dull and feel rough and brittle. To maintain healthy hair and minimize damage:

- Minimize exposure to sun, chlorine, and harsh chemical treatments such as permanents, dyes, bleaches and straighteners.[8]
- Avoid excessive brushing. Use a brush with natural, round-ended bristles, and brush gently. Use a wide-toothed comb to detangle or comb wet hair.
- Avoid excess heat. Use a lower setting on a blow dryer, and use a diffuser to blow dry chemical-treated hair. Avoid overuse of heated styling tools such as curling irons and rollers.[9]

Regular washing of hair and scalp removes oily build-up, dead skin cells, microorganisms, cosmetics and dirt that can all contribute to dull, lifeless-appearing hair. The optimum frequency of hair washing depends on the individual, but daily shampooing is not harmful and may be necessary in those with oily hair.[9] A special shampoo is not needed, since all detergents remove oil well. Moisturizing conditioners, which may include oils to increase lubrication, are best avoided on oily hair. People with dry-feeling hair will benefit from washing their hair every two or three days to allow normal scalp oils to lubricate the hair. A mild shampoo will avoid drying the hair further, followed by a moisturizing or lubricating conditioner.[8] Damaged hair may benefit from a mild shampoo, or an acid pH shampoo, which makes the hair feel more normal.[9] Dandruff control may require a special shampoo (see Chapter 42).

Various hair care products can be used to cosmetically enhance the hair's appearance (Table 4). Use of hair styling products and permanents to make hair appear fuller in age-related and androgenic alopecia is encouraged.[1] Applying powdered eye shadow to the scalp provides a darker background that can disguise thin hair. Hair weaving and bonding are styling techniques that fix hairpieces to remaining scalp hair to increase hair density.[8]

Excess hair can be controlled with physical removal by shaving, waxing or sugaring, plucking or electrolysis. *Shaving* removes hair at the skin level and is suitable for most areas, but the hair grows back quickly. It does not change hair quality, texture, or quantity, nor does it affect the rate of hair growth.[9] Sub-surface removal with waxing, sugaring or plucking can be painful for large areas, but the effect lasts three to six weeks.[9] *Sugaring* may be less painful than waxing, because the sugaring compound adheres to the hair, not the skin as wax does. *Cold waxing* involves application of wax-impregnated strips that are pressed on the skin then pulled off in the direction opposite to hair growth. No information is available on the relative efficacy of these different methods of hair removal. Because infection is a possible sequela of sub-surface hair removal, this type of removal is not recommended for people with diabetes or skin infections. In *electrolysis*, an electrical current passed through a fine needle inserted into the hair follicle is used to destroy the hair bulb. It is a slow, painful, expensive process most suitable for small areas. Scarring and pigmentation are possible.[3] Laser hair removal can treat larger areas more quickly than

Figure 3: **Assessment of Patients with Hair Loss/Hair Growth**

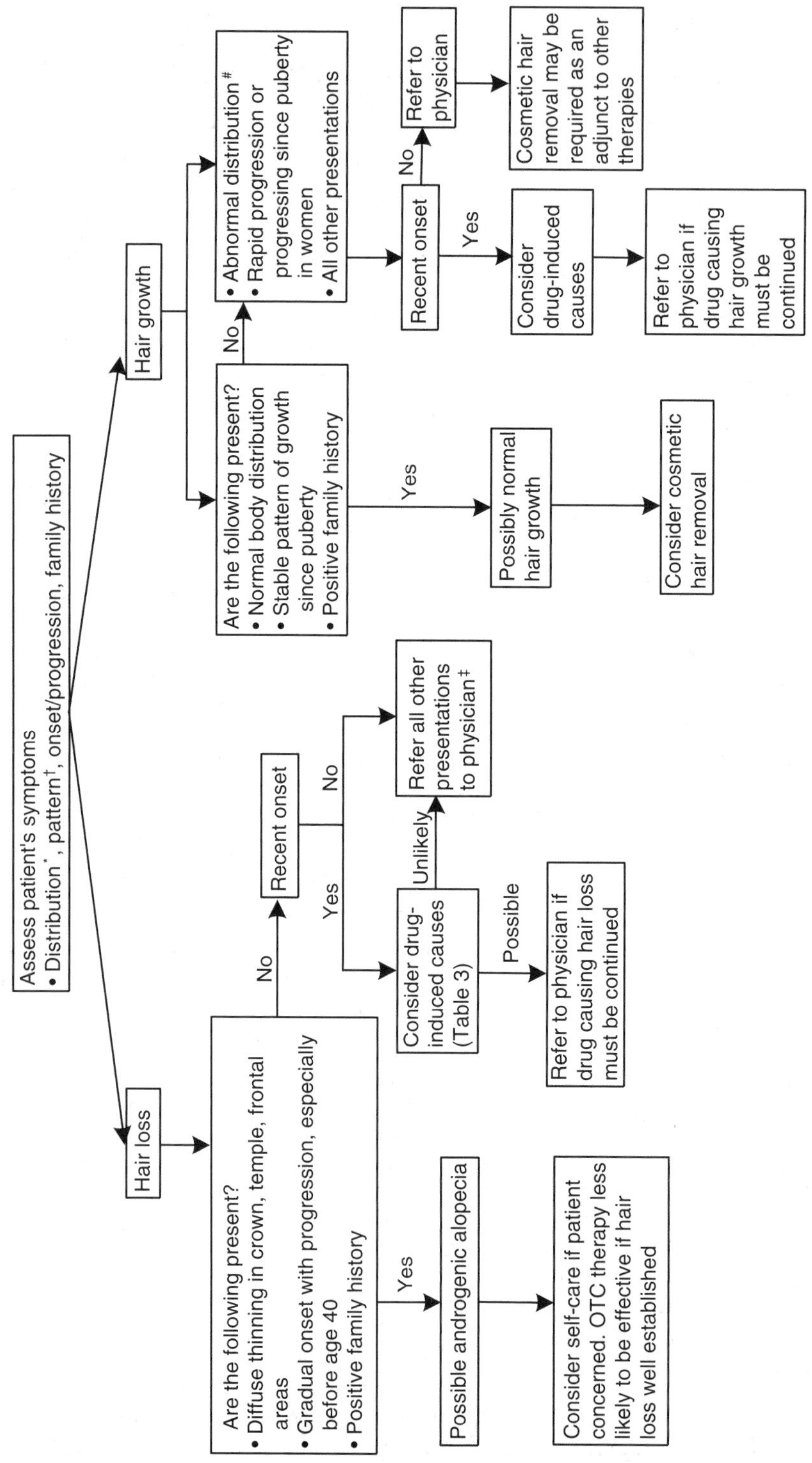

Assess patient's symptoms
- Distribution*, pattern†, onset/progression, family history

Hair loss

Are the following present?
- Diffuse thinning in crown, temple, frontal areas
- Gradual onset with progression, especially before age 40
- Positive family history

Yes → Possible androgenic alopecia → Consider self-care if patient concerned. OTC therapy less likely to be effective if hair loss well established

No → Recent onset

Recent onset — No → Refer all other presentations to physician‡

Recent onset — Yes → Consider drug-induced causes (Table 3)

Consider drug-induced causes (Table 3) — Unlikely → Refer all other presentations to physician‡

Consider drug-induced causes (Table 3) — Possible → Refer to physician if drug causing hair loss must be continued

Hair growth

Are the following present?
- Normal body distribution
- Stable pattern of growth since puberty
- Positive family history

Yes → Possibly normal hair growth → Consider cosmetic hair removal

No → Abnormal distribution #
- Rapid progression or progressing since puberty in women
- All other presentations

Recent onset — No → Refer to physician → Cosmetic hair removal may be required as an adjunct to other therapies

Recent onset — Yes → Consider drug-induced causes → Refer to physician if drug causing hair growth must be continued

*Distribution of hair loss: all over or patchy.
†Pattern of hair loss: visible shedding, clumps falling out.
‡e.g., patchy hair loss or thinning all over, noticeable shedding or hair falling out in clumps, abrupt onset.
#Women with excess hair growth on face/chest/back.

Table 4: **Hair Care and Styling Products**[6,8]

Product	Action	Uses	Comments
Shampoo	Detergent component helps remove oil, dirt. Baby shampoos contain amphoteric detergents that are less irritating to eyes. Products for damaged hair have a lower pH. Volumizing shampoos contain proteins to coat hair.	Routine use as part of a personal hygiene regimen	Daily use is not harmful. Oily scalps do not need a special shampoo. Low pH shampoos do not provide extra benefit, but damaged hair may feel more normal.
Conditioner	Contains cationic polymers or oils that coat the hair shaft. Lubricates, reduces damage from brushing, helps dispel static from removal of oil. Hair may appear shinier. Addition of oils increases lubrication, may help damaged hair.	Improves appearance and manageability of hair. More effective to use a separate conditioner than a conditioning shampoo	Oil-containing products can make fine or oily hair appear dull and greasy.
Styling sprays, mousses, gels	Contain large molecular weight polymers, proteins, and/or resins to hold hair in place or coat hair, adding thickness and texture. Silicone-containing products smooth the hair shaft, increase shine, manageability.	Improve appearance and manageability of hair. May be useful for those with thinning hair	May build up with regular use, especially silicone products. Hair may feel sticky, rubbery, dull, hard-to-style. Remove with weekly use of build-up remover.
Hair dyes	Temporary color and henna coat the cuticle only. Semipermanent color penetrates cuticle and cortex, lasting through about 6 shampoos. Permanent color deeply penetrates cortex and can lighten or darken hair. Color-restorers coat cuticle and contain metals that oxidize to a brownish tint.	Alter the appearance of hair	Temporary dyes are safe, gentle, wash out easily. Henna stains, dries, stiffens, damages hair. Avoid regular use. Allergic reactions possible with aniline dyes. Permanent dyes with ammonia and/or peroxide can damage hair.
Permanents, straighteners	Changes chemical structure of hair shaft, altering natural shape of hair.	Alter the appearance of hair	May damage hair if too strong, left on too long, used too often. Treated hair susceptible to damage from sun, chemicals, heat.

electrolysis. The various lasers available use melanin within the hair follicle as a light-absorbing compound. Large, well-designed trials of efficacy have not been performed. Side effects are mild to moderate pain with blistering in about ten per cent of patients.[10]

Pharmacologic Therapy

Topical **minoxidil** is the only nonprescription drug treatment proven to promote hair growth in alopecia of various causes, including androgenic alopecia (Table 5).[1] It is the only drug available to promote hair growth in women. It is not effective in normal age-related hair thinning, and will be less effective in cases of advanced hair loss.[4] A minimum trial of four to six months is recommended. If the patient is satisfied with the results, continued use is necessary to maintain the new hair growth.

Women with excess facial hair often disguise it by bleaching. **Bleaching** is simple, inexpensive and painless, but occasionally irritating.[8] It is most effective for fine hair or hair that is not thick or long. Hair bleaching products contain two components which must be mixed immediately before use: hydrogen peroxide (bleaching agent) and ammonium hydroxide (activator). To maintain the effect, bleaching must be repeated every few weeks. Bleach should be left on the face a maximum of 15 minutes with patch testing before use. It should not be applied to inflamed skin, newly plucked areas or skin treated with retinoids, glycolic acid or alpha-hydroxy acids.

Chemical depilatories containing thioglycolates are an alternative to physical removal of unwanted hair. They break down and dissolve hair just below the skin surface by hydrolyzing disulfide bonds. These products are irritating, so should be confined to use on the legs only.[8] Lower concentration products are available for use in the groin area. Application of a mild topical steroid cream before use can help decrease irritation.[9] To reduce absorption of the chemical, avoid use immediately after a hot bath or shower.[8]

Alternative Therapies

A variety of herbal and other treatments that are promoted to control hair loss have not been proven effective using standard testing methods. Oral **herbal** treatments include saw palmetto (*Serenoa repens*), maiden hair, horsetail, Fabao D® and Formula 101®.[11] Topical herbals (e.g., arnica, black bryony, essential oils) have also been used in the treatment of hair loss, but significant side effects, as well as lack of proven efficacy, limit their use.[11] **Nutritional supplements** such as zinc, biotin, folic acid and amino acids may also be useful in hair loss in those with severe nutritional deficiencies. With a normal diet, nutritional supplements are not helpful. These products are of questionable benefit and can be expensive.

Nonprescription products claiming to slow the growth rate of hair contain assorted herbal ingredients. No data exists to substantiate claims that they slow or stop hair growth.

Prescription Treatments

Minoxidil 5% solution is available on prescription and is slightly more effective than the nonprescription 2% solution in men but not women.[11] Finasteride 1 mg daily is the only other drug approved to treat androgenic alopecia in men. Finasteride does not appear to be effective in men over 60 years of age or postmenopausal women.[2,4] Treatment of androgenic alopecia in women is unsatisfactory. It usually involves combination therapy with antiandrogens (e.g., estrogen, progesterone, spironolactone, cyproterone acetate, flutamide, cimetidine).[12] Alopecia areata is typically treated with immunomodulating therapies such as oral or intradermal glucocorticoids or topical anthralin. Topical immunotherapy with the chemical diphencyprone[2] (diphenylcyclopropenone, DPCP), a contact allergen, is an unapproved treatment for alopecia areata.[5] Treatment stimulates hair growth but does not prevent hair loss, and is most effective in mild cases.

Eflornithine 13.9% is a prescription cream used to reduce the growth rate of facial hair in some women with excess facial hair. In clinical trials, some improvement was seen in 58% of women after eight weeks, with marked improvement in 32%.[13] *Antiandrogens* are also used to treat hirsutism in women.[3]

Monitoring of Therapy

Table 6 provides a framework for monitoring therapy for hair conditions.

Table 5: **Nonprescription Management of Hair Loss**

Product	Dose/Use	Effects	Side Effects	Comments
Minoxidil solution 2%*[1]	1 mL twice daily. Apply to dry scalp, spread lightly with a finger. Apply at least 4 h before bedtime to minimize losses on pillows/sheets.	Increases hair counts, hair shaft diameter, slows hair loss. Mechanism unknown.	Scalp dryness, scaling, itching, redness in 7%. Allergic dermatitis possible. Facial hypertrichosis in 5% of women. Temporary increased shedding may occur at 10-12 wks. No systemic effects with usual dose.	Spray application limits scalp access so is not recommended. All benefits/new growth are lost when stopped.

Only nonprescription treatment with proven efficacy.

Table 6: **Monitoring Therapy for Hair Conditions**

Symptom	Monitoring	Endpoint	Actions
Hair thinning	**Patient:** monthly **Pharmacist/Physician:** Minimum of 6-12 mos required to assess benefit.	Reduced thinning, improved scalp coverage. Note that full restoration of hair is not seen	Continue therapy indefinitely if patient satisfied with results. Patient must weigh benefits vs. cost of continuing.
Excess hair shedding	**Patient:** weekly **Pharmacist/Physician:** Shedding can take 4 mos or longer to improve.	Normal rate of hair loss (about 100 hairs per day) within 4-6 mos	Refer if shedding does not resolve in 4-6 mos after removal of trigger.
Excess hair growth	**Patient:** monthly **Pharmacist/Physician:** Assess adequacy of cosmetic methods after 2-3 wks. Minimum of 6 mos required to assess benefit of prescribed therapy in reducing hair growth.	Cosmetically acceptable appearance	Cosmetic management of excess hair is usually required.
Skin irritation from topical agents	**Patient:** daily **Pharmacist/Physician:** Inquire at next visit or have patient call. Redness or irritation usually seen in 1 to 2 days.	Minimal to no skin irritation	Stop using product. Treat symptomatically with topical 0.5% hydrocortisone.

Dry Skin and Sun-induced Skin Damage

Pathophysiology

The skin and its appendages (e.g., sweat glands, sebaceous glands, hair follicles) serve several important functions. They protect against minor injury, help control body temperature and water loss, prevent invasion by microorganisms, and prevent radiation damage from sun exposure. The skin is composed of three main layers: epidermis which includes the stratum corneum, dermis, and subcutaneous layer[1] (Figure 1).

The term "dry skin" is commonly used to describe skin that feels rough, brittle and scaly, and sometimes appears to be flaky. Although the word "dry" implies lack of water in the skin, skin water content is not a factor in most cases, nor will adding water to superficial skin layers correct the problem.[2] The underlying problem appears to be abnormal structure, cohesion, and organization of superficial cells in the stratum corneum. Turnover of stratum corneum cells is slowed. Damage to the stratum corneum can enhance dermal water loss and worsen the problem. In more advanced cases, fissures, inflammation and secondary infection can occur.[3] Rough, dry-appearing skin has many causes, some of which are listed in Table 7.

Ultraviolet radiation from sun exposure causes both acute and chronic changes in the epidermis, dermis, and connective tissue (Figure 4). Acutely, sunburn and immune suppression occur, while chronic sun exposure can cause *photoaging* and *skin cancer*.[4]

- Ultrashort wave ultraviolet C radiation (200-290 nm) is the most carcinogenic of the sun's rays, but is trapped by the earth's ozone layer.[5]
- Shortwave ultraviolet B radiation (290 to 320 nm) damages the stratum corneum and epidermal layers, and plays a role in both skin cancer and photoaging.[5] Acute exposure increases blood flow to the skin and activates inflammatory pathways, resulting in reddened skin and sunburn. However, even at doses too low to cause skin reddening, UVB can still cause local and systemic immunosuppression, direct damage to DNA, and other skin cell abnormalities that increase the risk of skin cancer.[4] Persistent pigmentation following acute sun exposure is due to hyperplasia of melanocytes in the epidermis. It is uncertain whether this protects against further UV-induced damage.[4] The daily UV index measures UVB radiation. UVB is stronger in the summer, at midday (11 am to 3 pm), at high altitudes, and is intensified by wind, humidity, high temperatures and reflective surfaces (e.g., water, sand, snow, concrete).[5] The *sun protection factor* (SPF) of a sunscreen is determined by comparing the amount of UVB energy from an artificial light source required to produce a standard erythema reaction with and without a sunscreen. Note that there is currently no standard SPF system for UVA radiation.

- Longwave ultraviolet A radiation (320 to 400 nm) penetrates the dermis and subcutaneous fat. Together with UVB it is a major factor in photoaging. It contributes 10 to 15% to sunburn erythema. Shortwave UVA (320 to 340 nm) causes direct changes to DNA while longwave UVA (340 to 400 nm) causes indirect DNA damage. Although UVA is a less potent carcinogen than UVB or UVC, it is a significant contributor to skin cancer risk because more reaches the earth than other types of UV radiation.[4,5] UVA is important in phototoxic drug eruptions, because it is absorbed by **photosensitizing drugs** such as the quinolones, tetracycline, sulfonamides, amiodarone, and tricyclic antidepressants.[5] Tanning salons, which use bulbs that primarily emit UVA, are not a safe way to tan.[4]

Photoaging from sun exposure is sometimes referred to as "premature skin aging" because the effects can be seen many years before normal age-related changes are noted in non-sun-exposed areas. The difference between the signs of normal aging and photoaging can readily be seen by comparing non-sun-exposed areas of the body with skin on the face, arms and hands. Signs of "aging" on their face and neck are of most concern to individuals. It is thought that most facial signs of aging are actually due to sun exposure. Much of the damage is often done before the age of 20 if a person spends a lot of time outdoors without sunscreen as a child or young person.[5,10] Smoking accelerates facial signs of photoaging.[6] Skin

Table 7: **Factors Contributing to Dry Skin**[6]

Genetic abnormalities in keratocyte composition or function (e.g., ichthyosis)
Normal skin aging
Low humidity (e.g., cold climates with winter winds)
Medical conditions (e.g., hypothyroidism, chronic renal failure)
Exposure to UV radiation or chemicals (e.g., sun)
Abrasion
Certain skin conditions (e.g., atopic dermatitis)
Drugs known to cause dry skin (e.g., vitamin A, retinoids, anticholinergics, niacin and other cholesterol-lowering agents)

Figure 4: **UV Radiation Effects and Sunscreen Coverage**[4,5,7-9]

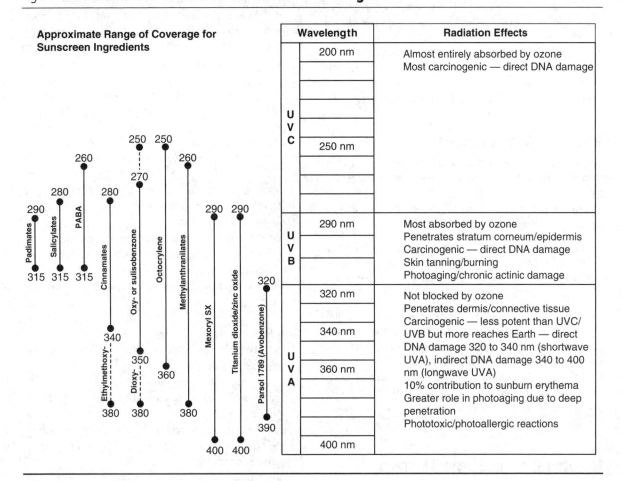

Approximate Range of Coverage for Sunscreen Ingredients

Wavelength		Radiation Effects
U V C	200 nm	Almost entirely absorbed by ozone Most carcinogenic — direct DNA damage
	250 nm	
U V B	290 nm	Most absorbed by ozone Penetrates stratum corneum/epidermis Carcinogenic — direct DNA damage Skin tanning/burning Photoaging/chronic actinic damage
U V A	320 nm	Not blocked by ozone Penetrates dermis/connective tissue Carcinogenic — less potent than UVC/UVB but more reaches Earth — direct DNA damage 320 to 340 nm (shortwave UVA), indirect DNA damage 340 to 400 nm (longwave UVA) 10% contribution to sunburn erythema Greater role in photoaging due to deep penetration Phototoxic/photoallergic reactions
	340 nm	
	360 nm	
	400 nm	

changes in photoaging differ from those in normal skin aging. In photoaged skin, changes in the stratum corneum and epidermal cells result in rough, coarse, dull-appearing skin with fine and deep wrinkles. In more advanced photoaging, deposition of abnormal elastic fibres, decreased collagen, and pigment changes in the upper dermis results in deeply wrinkled, yellowish skin. Mottled pigmentation and solar lentigines ("liver spots") are secondary to abnormal melanocyte activity. Vascular changes in the dermis can cause telangiectasias and easy bruising. A change in the properties of water-retentive glycosaminoglycan contributes to the dry, rough, leathery appearance of photoaged skin.[11]

Actinic keratosis is a common sun-induced lesion that begins as an area of increased vascularity which feels rough and scaly.[4] (See photo on page PS-2.) In up to 20% of cases it can progress to squamous cell carcinoma, marked by inflammation, oozing, pain or an increase in diameter of the hyperkeratotic area. The relationship between sun exposure and skin cancer is complex. Squamous cell carcinoma risk is related to cumulative lifetime sun exposure, therefore people with visibly photoaged skin are at greater risk. Basal cell carcinoma and melanoma appear to be related to sun exposure in childhood and adolescence.[10] In addition, melanoma is influenced by skin type (most common in fair-skinned people) and genetics.

Goals of Therapy

- Reduce the unpleasant feel of rough, scaly skin
- Facilitate repair of the barrier function of the stratum corneum
- Prevent acute and long-term sun-induced skin damage, including photoaging and some types of skin cancer
- Reduce the visible effects of photoaging on the skin

Patient Assessment

An approach to the patient with concerns about dry skin is presented in Figure 5. Dry skin is usually managed with nonprescription therapy unless advanced damage to the stratum corneum has resulted in inflammation or secondary infection.

If the concern is sun-induced skin damage, determine if the goal is prevention (i.e., selection and use of sunscreens) or treatment. Figure 6 presents an assessment of patients requesting sun protection.

Nonprescription therapies offer only modest benefits to those with visible signs of facial photoaging. In particular, patients with suspicious lesions, such as irregularly shaped moles that are changing, sores that won't heal, or patchy areas of scaly, roughened skin that seem to be growing, should be referred to a physician. An approach to patients with concerns about sun-induced skin damage is presented in Figure 7.

Nonpharmacologic Therapy

Dry Skin

A number of measures can be advised that will reduce the feeling of dry, rough skin.

- Hot water and soap can be drying, therefore advise a short shower with warm water and minimal soap. Suggest reducing bathing to every second day, if possible. Skin should be patted dry after bathing, rather than rubbed vigorously.[3]
- Recommend a mild glycerin soap, a soap with added oils or a soapless cleanser. Suggest avoiding use of soap on driest areas unless required to remove visible oil or dirt.[3]
- For those who like baths, a bath in warm, not hot, water with added bath oils can improve the feel of dry skin. They should avoid the use of bubble bath, which is a detergent and potential irritant for dry skin.

- Advise applying a moisturizer (Table 8) while the skin is still damp to attempt to retain some moisture in the skin. For mild symptoms, suggest an emollient cream or lotion formulation. For greater moisturizing effect, suggest a product containing both occlusive and humectant ingredients.[2,12] Ointments are more occlusive than creams and offer a greater moisturizing effect. Although oil-in-water emulsion formulations are more cosmetically appealing, they are shorter acting and less effective than water-in-oil emulsions.[3] When itching is present, occlusive-containing products alone are preferred.[12]
- In dry climates in the winter, suggest humidifying indoor air. Skin should be protected from the drying effects of cold and wind by using gloves, facemasks and scarves.[3]
- For dry, chapped lips, advise frequent application of a lip balm.[3] Encourage children (and adults) not to lick their lips, because this will make the problem worse and extend chapping to the perioral area.

Sun-induced Skin Damage

To reduce acute and chronic effects of sun exposure, advise patients to:

- Avoid direct sun exposure at midday (11 am to 3 pm) when UVB rays are strongest. They should seek shade as much as possible if they have to be outside. Note that some light energy will penetrate leafy trees and umbrellas, and will be reflected from surfaces outside the shaded area.[5]
- Wear protective clothing if possible (e.g., broad-brimmed hat, sunglasses, long-sleeved shirt, long pants). Special sun-blocking fabrics have been developed and are particularly useful for children. However, even a cotton T-shirt will offer an SPF of 8, a more tightly woven cotton/polyester shirt has an SPF of 15, and a polyester/lycra shirt has an SPF of 35. Note that wet clothing and loosely woven fabrics allow more light penetration.[5]
- Avoid tanning lamps and sun-lamps.
- Avoid cosmetic tanning.

Pharmacologic Therapy

Keratolytics (Table 8) are beneficial in dry skin conditions and to reduce some of the minor effects of photoaging. By promoting turnover of stratum corneum cells, they decrease fine wrinkling, improve skin texture, and make skin feel smoother.[11] They have minimal effects on coarse wrinkling or abnormal pigmentation. Concentration and an acidic formula-

tion are important to the action of alpha-hydroxy acids. Beta-hydroxy acids, such as salicylic acid, are also effective keratolytics in dry skin conditions and reduce fine wrinkles in photoaged skin. They can be

Figure 5: **Assessment of Patients with Dry Skin**

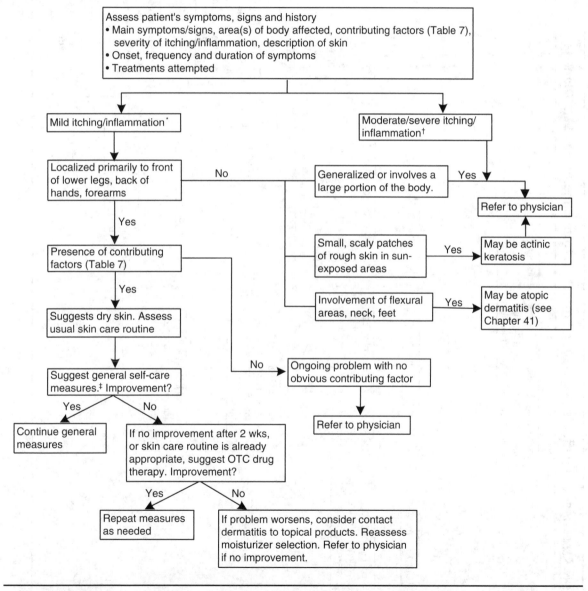

*Rough, harsh, scaly-feeling skin. May be mildly itchy with flaking and redness.
†Symptoms of pain or intense itching. Presence of significant inflammation possibly with rash or scaly plaques, or infection.
‡General self-care measures e.g., bathing, mild soap, moisturizer use.

Figure 6: **Assessment of Patients Requesting Protection from Sun-induced Skin Damage**

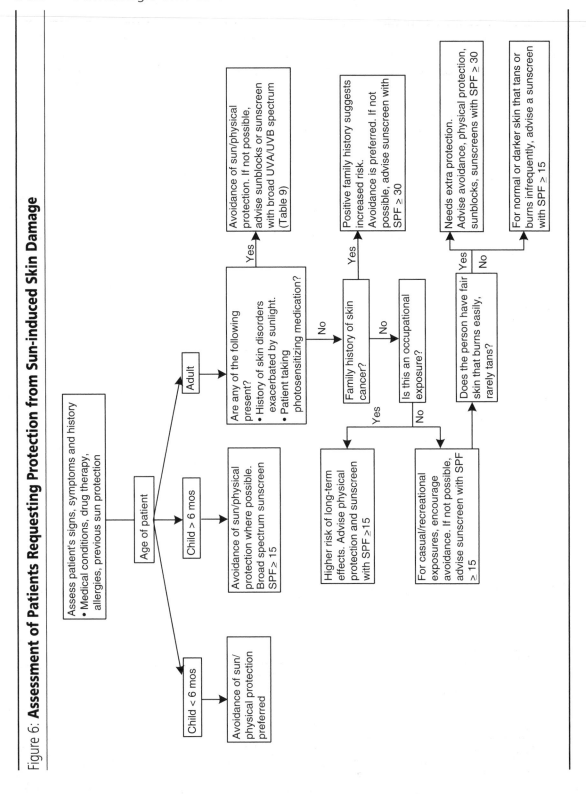

used in combination with alpha-hydroxy acids. Keratolytics can be irritating to the skin, especially at higher concentrations. They should be used carefully around the eyes. Higher concentration products (e.g., alpha-hydroxy acids greater than 10%), and/or those with a pH lower than 3.5 are available on prescription, or used as "peels" by cosmetologists or dermatologists.[2] Peels may improve actinic keratoses and fine wrinkling, but high-concentration peels carry a risk of scarring.

Figure 7: **Assessment of Patients Requesting Treatment for Non-acute Sun-induced Skin Damage**

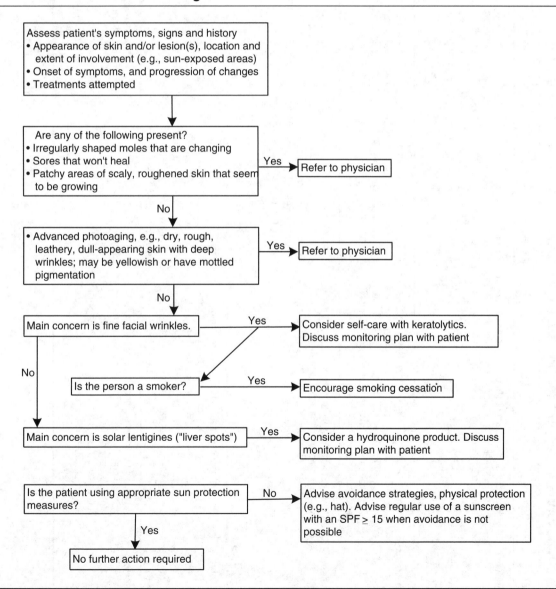

Smoking significantly increases the rate of facial photoaging.

Table 8: **Moisturizer Ingredients for Dry Skin and Photoaging**[2,4,12]

Type	Action	Examples	Comments
Occlusives[2,12]	Physically block surface of stratum corneum to prevent further water loss, which promotes barrier repair. May help trap water in skin if applied to damp skin.	Petrolatum Mineral oil, paraffin, squalene; dimethicone, cyclomethicone; cocoa butter, lanolin, beeswax, carnuba, lecithin; lanolin acid or alcohol, stearic acid, cetyl alcohol, stearyl stearate	Petrolatum is the only effective occlusive. The others act mainly as emollients.[12] They are occlusive only when applied heavily. Lanolin can cause contact hypersensitivity. Silicones often found in "oil-free" products.
Humectants[2,12]	Attract water from lower skin layers to increase water content of stratum corneum. Attract water from the environment if ambient humidity exceeds 70%. Swell to fill holes in stratum corneum, reducing roughness, and plumping up fine wrinkles.	Glycerin, honey, gelatin, urea, sodium lactate, propylene glycol, sorbitol, pyrrolidone carboxilic acid, hyaluronic acid	Never used alone because they will increase water loss. Propylene glycol is also used as a solvent for other ingredients.
Emollients[2,12]	Oily substances that fill crevices between cells in the stratum corneum to make skin feel smoother. Choice of emollient(s) influences product feel and spreadability. No effect on water loss.	*Greasy/Stiff:* castor oil, almond oil, oleyl oleate *Creamy:* caprylic/capric triglyceride, octyl dodecanol, cetearyl isononanoate, oleyl alcohol, decyl oleate, hexyl/octyl laurate *Nongreasy/easy spreading:* dioctyl cyclohexane, isopropyl stearate/myristate/palmitate, dibutyladipate	Stearic acid, stearyl alcohol, cetyl alcohol also function as emulsifiers.
Keratolytics/ exfoliants[2,12]	Dissolve bonds between corneocytes to promote shedding and turnover of stratum corneum. Expose water-binding sites in corneocytes to promote water retention. Improve skin texture, reduce roughness, and decrease the appearance of fine wrinkles.	Urea Alpha-hydroxy acids (AHAs) – glycolic acid, lactic acid (monocarboxylic acids); malic acid (dicarboxylic acid); citric acid (tricarboxylic acid or "triple fruit acid") Beta-hydroxy acids – salicylic acid	Useful in hyperkeratotic conditions to reduce scaliness. "Cocktails" of AHAs are no better than a single ingredient. Irritating, increased sun sensitivity.
Vitamins[2,4]	Antioxidant vitamins claimed to prevent or treat photoaging. More likely effect is as a humectant. Alpha-tocopherol has minor sunscreen activity. Tocopheryl acetate is a good skin conditioner. Small amounts of vitamin A converted to retinol in the skin are less effective than prescription retinoids.	Vitamin A palmitate/retinyl palmitate, retinol Vitamin E – tocopheryl acetate, alpha tocopherol	Conversion of topical retinoids to retinoic acid is minimal, therefore effects on photoaging are limited. Tocopheryl acetate often used as a preservative to prevent oxidation of product.

Nonprescription topical **retinoids** contain retinyl palmitate (vitamin A palmitate) or a stabilized form of retinol, which are less readily oxidized to biologically inactive forms in the presence of light than other retinoids. Both must be converted to active retinoic acid by the skin. Efficacy of these products in treating photoaging is limited because the skin can convert only small amounts to retinoic acid. Prescription retinoids are more effective.[2]

Antioxidants such as vitamins C and E or coenzyme Q10 (ubiquinone) may be found in cosmetics or facial creams that claim to prevent sun damage or treat wrinkles. There is insufficient clinical evidence to confirm they are effective at reducing the effects of sun damage.[13] Anti-wrinkle creams with added **protein** such as collagen, elastin, DNA or enzymes may cause a temporary reduction in the appearance of fine wrinkles because they shrink and stretch the skin when they dry. These substances will not be absorbed through the skin to replace or repair proteins damaged through the skin aging process. There is no evidence to substantiate the claims that they reverse the aging process or reduce wrinkles.[14]

Sunscreens are effective at reducing sun tanning and sunburn. They can also reduce photoaging and development of actinic keratoses, and promote regression of existing actinic keratoses possibly reducing the risk of squamous cell carcinoma. There is little evidence that sunscreens reduce the risk of basal cell carcinoma or malignant melanoma.[10] Sunscreens are an adjunct only, and should be used to protect the skin rather than prolong the time that can be spent in the direct sun.

Physical blockers (Table 9) reflect and scatter all light, while chemical sunscreens absorb UV radiation to prevent its penetration to viable cells of the epidermis.[10] Combinations of two or more chemical agents are required to produce a sunscreen that absorbs UV radiation throughout the UVB and UVA spectrum. To prevent phototoxic or photoallergic reactions from drugs, the sunscreen must provide full-spectrum UVA coverage. Sunscreens work immediately upon application, although applying them at least 30 minutes before swimming ensures penetration of the skin.[10] Repeated application does not extend the duration of sun-protection and is usually not required, especially for those agents with good skin adherence (Table 9). Water-resistant products reduce loss of less adherent

sunscreens during swimming or during activities where there is a lot of sweating. Sunscreens do not significantly reduce vitamin D production.[10]

Under natural light conditions, the effectiveness of sunscreens is less than the labelled sun protection factor (SPF).[10] In addition, the amount of sunscreen applied in typical use is much less than the standard amount used in the laboratory. However, a sunscreen with a labelled SPF of 15 can potentially block 93% of UVB rays when applied in a *sufficient amount*.[10,16] An average size adult should use at least 3 mL for the face and neck, 3 mL for each arm and shoulder, 5 mL for each of front and back of torso, and 5 mL for each leg.[11] Using smaller amounts of sunscreen substantially reduces the protection factor. Sunscreens with an SPF of 30 or more block only 4% more UVB rays, but may be preferred for people with fair skin who burn easily. Sunscreens should not be used in infants less than six months of age. Instead, use clothing, hats and shade to protect infants from sun.

Tanning Agents: Sunless tanning products contain **dihydroxyacetone** (DHA), a dye which imparts an orange-brown color to the stratum corneum when applied topically. The darkness of the color depends on the concentration of the product and the area to which it is applied. Deeper staining will occur in areas with thicker stratum corneum (e.g., palms/soles, roughened areas over knees/elbows). Color change is observed in one hour and is maximal by 8 to 24 hours. Repeated daily applications may be required to achieve the desired depth of color. The agent must be reapplied every few days to maintain an even color. The color is resistant to swimming, washing, and perspiration. To minimize staining of nails and palms, hands should be washed after use. The brown color of DHA on the skin has mild (SPF 3 to 4) sunscreen activity, as well as some protection in the UVA range. However, a conventional sunscreen will still be required for adequate protection from acute sun exposure.[17] Because dihydroxyacetone is considered nontoxic, these products are regulated as cosmetics, not as drugs.

Depigmenting Agents: Most creams that reduce solar lentigines contain **hydroquinone**, although there is at least one on the market that contains the related compound **monobenzone**. These drugs inhibit the production of melanin. They are often formulated with sunscreens, since sun exposure may

Table 9: **Sunscreen Ingredients**

Class	Wavelength	Comments
Physical blocks[7,9] e.g., titanium dioxide, zinc oxide	UVB, UVA (full-spectrum)	Clear formulations of micronized particles are cosmetically more appealing. Some absorption of microfine titanium can occur but significance of this is not known.
PABA (para-aminobenzoic acid) and its esters[9,15] e.g., padimate O (octyl dimethyl PABA), padimate A (amyl dimethyl PABA), ethyl dihydroxy PABA	UVB	May cause contact/photocontact dermatitis. Avoid in individuals with allergy to sulfonamides, thiazides, ester-type anesthetics, saccharin, sodium cyclamate, aniline dyes. May stain fabrics yellow with sun exposure. Adhere well to skin.
Salicylates[9,15] e.g., homosalate, octyl salicylate, triethanolamine salicylate, ethylhexyl salicylate	UVB	Easily removed by abrasion, perspiration or swimming. Rarely causes contact dermatitis.
Cinnamates[9,15] e.g., octyl methoxycinnamate (Parsol MCX), 2-ethoxy p-methoxycinnamate (Cinoxate) ethyl methoxycinnamate, octyl cyanophenylcinnamate (Octocrylene)	UVB – upper UVB/lower UVA (280-340 nm) (octocrylene broadest 250-360 nm)	Easily removed by abrasion, perspiration or swimming. Photostabilizes dibenzoylmethanes, often found in combination. 2-ethylhexyl p-methoxycinnamate weakly mutagenic and increased tumor development in mice exposed to UV radiation. Human effects unknown. Octocrylene: With coverage in low UVA range can make claim of UVB/UVA protection.
Benzophenones[9,15] e.g., hydroxymethoxybenzophenone (oxybenzone, benzophenone-3), dihydroxymethoxybenzophenone (dioxybenzone, benzophenone-8)), hydroxymethoxybenzophenone sulphonic acid (sulisobenzone)	UVB and lower UVA (260-380 nm) (dioxybenzone is broadest – 250-390 nm)	May advertise broad-spectrum UVB/UVA protection, since covers most of UVB plus lower-mid UVA range. May cause contact dermatitis. Photocontact dermatitis possible with oxybenzone. 1-2% oxybenzone absorbed, but toxicity unknown.
Dibenzoylmethanes[9,15] e.g., butyl methoxydibenzoylmethane (avobenzone, Parsol 1789)	UVA	Significant photodegradation occurs. Can be reduced by combining with Mexoryl SX or cinnamates. May accelerate degradation of methoxycinnamate.
Benzylidene camphor derivatives[9,15] e.g., 4-methylbenzylidene camphor, terephthalylidene dicamphor sulfonic acid (Mexoryl SX)	UVB (4-methylbenzylidene camphor – 300 nm) UVA (Mexoryl SX – 400 nm)	Usually combined with another sunscreen. Reduces photodegradation of avobenzone.

reverse the bleaching effect of the chemical. Skin irritation, redness, and allergic or contact dermatitis have been reported as side effects. The effect of monobenzone is unpredictable and irreversible so this product is generally used only for extensive vitiligo under supervision of a dermatologist.[8]

Prescription Treatment
Tretinoin produces both cellular and clinical improvement in photoaged skin.[11] Over 6 to 12 months, skin becomes smoother and less sallow, fine and coarse wrinkles are reduced, and pigment is less mottled.[11]

Chemical peels using high concentrations of glycolic or trichloroacetic acid can improve skin texture, reduce actinic keratoses, and decrease fine wrinkling. Topical 5-fluorouracil has been used for patients with widespread actinic keratoses or severe actinic damage, but is poorly tolerated because the inflammatory phase of the treatment is both uncomfortable and unsightly. Dermabrasion and laser resurfacing are surgical techniques used in moderate to severe photoaging. Other cosmetic surgery options include collagen or lipid injections to fill in deep wrinkles. Botulinum toxin injected into the face reduces wrinkles by paralyzing muscles in the area.

Table 10 provides a plan for monitoring therapy for dry skin and photoaging.

Suggested Readings

Perspiration and Body Odor
Leung AKC, Chan PYH, Choi MCK. Hyperhidrosis. *Int J Dermatol* 1999;38:561-7.

Stolman LP. Treatment of hyperhidrosis. *Dermatol Clin* 1998;16(4):863-7.

Hair Care and Hair Growth
Hock DL, Seifer DE. New treatments of hyperandrogenism and hirsutism. *Obstet Gynecol Clin North Am* 2000;27(3):567-81.

Price VH. Treatment of hair loss. *N Engl J Med* 1999;341(13):965-73.

Sawaya ME, Shapiro J. Androgenetic alopecia: new approved and unapproved treatments. *Dermatol Clin* 2000;18(1):47-61.

Shapiro J, Wiseman M, Lui H. Practical management of hair loss. *Can Fam Physician* 2000;46:1469-77.

Tosti A, Misciali C, Piraccini BM, Peluso AM, Bardazzi F. Drug-induced hair loss and hair growth. Incidence, management, and avoidance. *Drug Safety* 1994;10(4):310-7.

Dry Skin and Sun-induced Skin Damage
Billow JA, Baer RK, Van Riper GC. Combatting dry and aging skin. *US Pharmacist* 2000;25(4):52-4,57-8,60.

Draelos ZD. Therapeutic moisturizers. *Dermatol Clin* 2000;18(4):597-607.

Lawrence N. New and emerging treatments for photoaging. *Dermatol Clin* 2000;18(1):99-112.

McLean DL, Gallagher R. Sunscreens. Use and misuse. *Dermatol Clin* 1998;16(2):219-26.

Sibbald D. Pursuing the fountain of youth. Prevention and treatment of photoaging. *Pharm Pract* 1996; 12:80-2,84-5,88,90-1.

Table 10: **Monitoring Therapy for Dry Skin and Photoaging**

Symptom	Monitoring	Endpoint	Actions
Rough, scaly skin	**Patient:** daily **Pharmacist:** Follow-up after 2 wks. If inadequate response to general measures, try a keratolytic.	Skin feels smoother, no longer red or irritated.	If redness or inflammation persists, add 0.5% hydrocortisone. Refer to a physician if no improvement with hydrocortisone after 7-10 days. If irritation worsens, consider allergy to moisturizer ingredient.
Early photodamage e.g., fine wrinkles, dry skin	**Patient:** 3-6 mos **Pharmacist:** May take 4-6 mos for noticeable effect from keratolytics.	Skin seems softer, smoother, fine wrinkles less apparent.	Switch to higher concentration product if tolerated. Refer to physician if self-management results are inadequate for patient.

References

Perspiration and Body Odor

1. Wenzel FG, Horn TD. Nonneoplastic disorders of the eccrine glands. *J Am Acad Dermatol* 1998;38(1):1-17.
2. Goldsmith LA. Biology of eccrine and apocrine sweat glands. In: Freedberg IM, Eisen AZ, Wolff K et al, eds. *Fitzpatrick's Dermatology in General Medicine*. 5th ed. New York: McGraw-Hill; 1999:155-64.
3. Leung AKC, Chan PYH, Choi MCK. Hyperhidrosis. *Int J Dermatol* 1999;38:561-7.
4. Stolman LP. Treatment of hyperhidrosis. *Dermatol Clin* 1998;16(4):863-7.
5. White JW. Treatment of primary hyperhidrosis. *Mayo Clin Proc* 1986;61:951-6.
6. Turkington CA, Dover JS. *Skin Deep, an A-Z of Skin Disorders, Treatments, and Health*. New York: Facts on File; 1996.
7. Ertel K. Modern skin cleansers. *Dermatol Clin* 2000;18(4):561-75.
8. Boyd S. *The Skin Sourcebook*. Los Angeles: Lowell House; 1998:6
9. Flarend R, Bin T, Elmore D, Hem SL. A preliminary study of the dermal absorption of aluminum from antiperspirants using aluminum-26. *Food Chem Toxicol* 2001;39(2):163-8.
10. Munoz DG. Is exposure to aluminum a risk factor for the development of Alzheimer's disease? No. *Arch Neurol* 1998;55:737-9.

Hair Care and Hair Growth

1. Jackson E. Hair disorders. *Primary Care* 2000;27(2):319-32.
2. Price VH. Treatment of hair loss. *N Engl J Med* 1999;341(13):965-73.
3. Hock DL, Seifer DE. New treatments of hyperandrogenism and hirsutism. *Obstet Gynecol Clin North Am* 2000;27(3):567-81.
4. Sperling LC, Mezebish OS. Hair diseases. *Med Clin North Am* 1998;82(5):1155-69.
5. Shapiro J, Wiseman M, Lui H. Practical management of hair loss. *Can Fam Physician* 2000;46:1469-77.
6. Tosti A, Misciali C, Piraccini BM, Peluso AM, Bardazzi F. Drug-induced hair loss and hair growth. Incidence, management, and avoidance. *Drug Safety* 1994;10(4):310-7.
7. Han NH, Nowakowski PA, West DP. Drug-induced skin reactions. In: DiPiro J, Talbert RL, Yee GC et al, eds. *Pharmacotherapy, a Pathophysiologic Approach*. Stamford: Appleton & Lange; 1999:1509.
8. Turkington CA, Dover JS. *Skin Deep, an A-Z of Skin Disorders, Treatments, and Health*. New York: Facts on File; 1996.
9. Bergfeld WF, Masline SR. *A Woman Doctor's Guide to Skin Care*. New York: Hyperion; 1995.
10. Laser hair removal. *Med Lett* 1999;41(1058):68-9.
11. Sawaya ME, Shapiro J. Androgenetic alopecia: new approved and unapproved treatments. *Dermatol Clin* 2000;18(1):47-61.
12. Bergfeld WF. Androgenetic alopecia: an autosomal dominant disorder. *Am J Med* 1995; 98(suppl 1A):95S-98S.
13. *Product Monograph, Vaniqa*. Bristol-Myers Squibb (USA). July 2000.

Dry Skin and Sun-induced Skin Damage

1. Bond CA. Skin disorders I. In: Koda-Kimble MA, Young LY, eds. *Applied Therapeutics, the Clinical Use of Drugs*. Vancouver, WA: Applied Therapeutics; 1992:64-1-6.
2. Draelos ZD. Therapeutic moisturizers. *Dermatol Clin* 2000;18(4):597-607.
3. Billow JA, Baer RK, Van Riper GC. Combatting dry and aging skin. *US Pharmacist* 2000;25(4):52-4,57-8,60.
4. Lincoln EA. Sun-induced skin changes. *Primary Care* 2000;27(2):435-45.
5. Sibbald D. Pursuing the fountain of youth. Prevention and treatment of photoaging. *Pharm Pract* 1996;12:80-2,84-5,88,90-1.
6. Fitzpatrick TB, Bernhard JD, Cropley TG. The structure of skin lesions and fundamentals of diagnosis. In: Freedberg IM, Eisen AE, Wolff K et al, eds. *Fitzpatrick's Dermatology in General Medicine*. 5th ed. New York: McGraw-Hill; 1999:155-64.
7. McLean DL, Gallagher R. Sunscreens. Use and misuse. *Dermatol Clin* 1998;16(2):219-26.
8. Pellat S. Sunscreen and tanning products. In: Carruthers-Czyzewski P, ed. *Nonprescription Drug Reference for Health Professionals*. Ottawa: Canadian Pharmaceutical Association; 1996:641.
9. Guenther L. Sunburn. In: Gray J, ed. *Therapeutic Choices*. 3rd ed. Ottawa: Canadian Pharmacists Association; 2000:511.
10. Uitto J. Understanding premature skin aging. *N Engl J Med* 1997;337(20):1463-5.
11. Lawrence N. New and emerging treatments for photoaging. *Dermatol Clin* 2000;18(1):99-112.
12. Wehr RF, Krochmal L. Considerations in selecting a moisturizer. *Cutis* 1987;39(6):512-5.
13. Kligman D. Cosmeceuticals. *Dermatol Clin* 2000;18(4):609-15.
14. Turkington CA, Dover JS. *Skin Deep, an A-Z of Skin Disorders, Treatments, and Health*. New York: Facts on File; 1996.
15. West DP, Rumsfield JA. Skin disorders II. In: Koda-Kimble MA, Young LY, eds. *Applied Therapeutics, the Clinical Use of Drugs*. Vancouver, WA: Applied Therapeutics; 1992:65-1-14.
16. Diffey B. Has the sun protection factor had its day? *BMJ* 2000; 320:176-7.
17. Levy S. Tanning preparations. *Dermatol Clin* 2000;18(4):591-6.

Perspiration or Body Odor—Patient Information

- Good personal hygiene is important to prevent body odor:
  - —Have a bath or shower using soap or a soapless skin cleaner regularly to prevent build-up of bacteria, sweat, and dead skin cells. Some people may have to wash each day.
  - —Wear clean clothes to reduce odor.
  - —Apply an antiperspirant to the underarm area each day, even on days you don't bathe.

- If you have problems with sweaty feet and/or foot odor:
  - —Wash feet regularly and dry thoroughly. Some people may need to wash their feet each day.
  - —Use an absorbent foot powder.
  - —Wear breathable footwear, such as leather shoes or sandals and cotton or wool socks.
  - —Avoid wearing shoes or sandals without socks.

  - —Try applying an antiperspirant to the bottoms of your feet if they are very sweaty.

- If you have extremely sweaty hands, feet, or underarms, talk to your pharmacist or doctor about trying a stronger antiperspirant containing aluminum chloride. To reduce irritation from aluminum chloride-containing antiperspirants:
  - —Apply only to dry skin. If needed, use a blow dryer to ensure the area is dry.
  - —Apply it at night and wash it off first thing in the morning before you begin to sweat.
  - —Use a regular antiperspirant for odor-control during the day.
  - —Once your sweating is controlled, try to reduce the use of aluminum chloride to once or twice a week.
  - —Advise your pharmacist and doctor about any serious skin irritation you experience.

Hair Concerns—Patient Information

- Tips to keep your hair looking healthy include:
  —Wash hair regularly to remove dirt, oil, and skin cell build-up. Daily shampooing is not harmful and may be needed for people with oily hair. For people with dry-feeling hair, less frequent washing allows natural scalp oils to condition the hair.
  —It is more effective to use a separate conditioner than a conditioning shampoo. People with oily hair may find moisturizing conditioners make the problem worse. People with dry-feeling or damaged hair should use a mild shampoo and a moisturizing conditioner. Acid pH shampoos can make hair damaged by chemicals feel more normal.
  —Limit hair exposure to sun, chlorine, and harsh chemical treatments such as permanents, dyes, bleaches and straighteners.
  —Brush hair gently using a brush with round-ended bristles. Avoid excessive brushing. Use a wide-toothed comb to detangle or comb wet hair.
  —Reduce the damaging effect of high heat on hair by using a lower setting on your blow dryer, avoiding overuse of heated styling tools such as curling irons and rollers, and using a diffuser to blow dry chemically treated hair.

With age, hair gradually loses its pigment and becomes gray. Hair becomes finer, drier, and duller in appearance. Scalp hair gradually becomes thinner after age 50 in both men and women.

- The most common cause of increased hair thinning is male-pattern/female-pattern baldness. This is a genetic trait caused by increased action of male hormones on hair growth. It is a myth that people with this type of hair loss have too many male hormones in their body. This type of hair loss can start anywhere from your teens to middle age. It is more pronounced in women after menopause.
- It is not harmful to disguise thinning hair by using hair styling products such as hair dyes or permanents or even eye shadow.
- Minoxidil 2% solution is the only nonprescription treatment that might help thinning hair.
  —Use only 1 mL twice a day.
  —Apply it directly to your scalp using your fingers. Wash your hands after using minoxidil. Avoid getting your scalp wet for four hours after applying the minoxidil.
  —It is normal to notice some temporary increased hair shedding after 10 to 12 weeks.
  —Some people experience skin irritation; women might notice an increased growth of fine hair on the face.
  —You must use minoxidil for at least six months before deciding if the effect is adequate. Normal hair growth and density will not be restored.
  —You must continue to use it to maintain any benefits you experience.

Dry Skin—Patient Information

- Dry skin can occur with other skin conditions, or in normal skin as a result of aging, illness, dry climates, wind and cold. It occurs when the outer layer of skin has been damaged. It doesn't always mean that the skin is lacking water.
- Some things you can do to prevent dry skin include:
  —Use a humidifier if you live in a dry climate, especially in the winter.
  —Keep the room temperature at the lowest comfortable level in the winter.
  —Water dries out the skin, so bathe or shower every two to three days using warm, not hot, water.
  —Soap makes dry skin worse, so use a mild soap or one with added moisturizers; avoid using soap on dry skin areas unless you need to remove visible dirt or oil.

- To treat dry skin, try some of the following:
  —Add a bath oil (not bubble bath) to the water in the last five minutes of your bath. Caution: it will make the tub very slippery.

  —Rub a moisturizing lotion or cream into your skin while it is still damp to help hold in moisture.
  —Rub a moisturizing lotion or cream into your skin at least twice a day, morning and night, or more often if the skin feels very rough (e.g., on the hands).
  —Try special dry skin creams containing urea or lactic acid if regular moisturizers don't help. Note that these products can be irritating to cuts or abrasions on your skin.
  —For dry, chapped lips, apply a lip balm frequently. Do not lick your lips, because this will make the problem worse and extend the rough, irritated feeling to skin around the mouth.
  —If your skin is very red or itchy, 0.5% hydrocortisone cream may help. If there is no improvement after 7 to 10 days, see your pharmacist or physician.

Sun-induced Skin Damage—Patient Information

- Sunlight causes damage to the skin that can be seen right away, such as redness or sunburn. It also causes damage that you can't see right away, even when your skin doesn't change color. This can show up many years later as skin cancer, or as signs of aging especially on your face, such as wrinkles, dryness, dullness, yellowing or an uneven skin color.

- Here are some things you can do to help prevent immediate skin damage (e.g., sunburn) and delayed effects of sun exposure (e.g., wrinkles, skin cancer):
  —Avoid direct sun exposure from 11 am to 3 pm when the sun's rays are the strongest. Seek shade if you have to be outside. Some sunlight will go through leafy trees and umbrellas, and will be reflected from surfaces outside the shaded area.
  —If possible, protect your skin with clothing (e.g., broad-brimmed hat, sunglasses, long-sleeved shirt, long pants). Special sun blocking fabrics are available, but even a cotton T-shirt will offer some protection. Wet clothing and loosely woven fabrics allow more light through.
  —Avoid tanning lamps and sun-lamps. These are not a safe way to tan; they still result in wrinkles and put you at risk for skin cancer.
  —Staying in the sun for long periods of time with the intent of tanning increases your risk of skin damage, including wrinkles. A tan does not necessarily protect you from further sun damage.
  —In infants under six months of age, it is best to avoid sun exposure. If you have to be outside, keep the baby in a shaded area or use clothing to protect them from the sun.

- If you have to be in the sun, sunscreens can help protect your skin. They do not completely prevent skin damage from sunlight, however. Here are some tips to help you get the most benefit from your sunscreen:
  —Sunscreens work as soon as you apply them. If you are going swimming, apply it 30 minutes before you go in the water to allow it time to get absorbed into your skin.
  —You do not usually need to reapply sunscreens unless you have been swimming or sweating a lot. Use a water-resistant product if you know you will be swimming or sweating a lot.
  —To get the full effect of the labeled sun protection factor (SPF) you have to use lots of sunscreen. An average-size adult should use at least ½ teaspoon (2.5 mL) for the face and neck, ½ teaspoon (2.5 mL) for each arm and shoulder, ½ to 1 teaspoon (2.5 mL to 5 mL) on your chest and on your back, and 1 teaspoon (5 mL) for each leg.
  —Avoid using chemical sunscreens on children less than six months old. It is safe to use sun blocking creams, such as titanium dioxide or zinc oxide.
  —Sunscreens are very irritating to the eyes. If you are using sunscreen on a child who rubs their eyes a lot, it might help to wash their hands after applying sunscreen. If you get sunscreen in your eye, flush your eye with lots of lukewarm water.

Viral Skin Rashes

Sandra Knowles, BScPhm

Pathophysiology (Table 1)

Rubeola (measles)

The introduction of the measles vaccine in 1963 dramatically changed the epidemiology of rubeola with reported incidence rates now 98% below those of the prevaccine era. Measles virus (paramyxovirus) is spread primarily via respiratory droplets. Koplik spots, which are small gray-blue specks on an erythematous base, appear in the prodromal period. These are found on the buccal mucosa during the prodrome but disappear within 48 hours after the onset of rash. They are generally diagnostic for measles although they may be associated with the human parvovirus B19 (erythema infectiosum). Two to three days after Koplik spots appear, a purplish red, maculopapular eruption appears on the scalp, face and neck that spreads downwards. Complications of measles most often include otitis media and rarely bronchopneumonia, encephalitis, myocarditis and pericarditis.

Rubella (German measles)

Although the prodrome and skin eruption are milder than in typical measles, rubella has devastating effects on the developing fetus if contracted during the first trimester of pregnancy. The rubella virus (RNA togavirus) is spread by respiratory droplets.

Erythema Infectiosum (Fifth disease)

Erythema infectiosum is an exanthem caused by human parvovirus B19 and thought to be spread by respiratory droplet secretions. Over 50% of infections are asymptomatic. There are three stages to the eruption: sudden onset of macular erythema on the face giving a "slapped cheek" appearance; after one day, erythematous macular eruption that can last up to seven days occurs on the extensor extremities; a reticulated or lacy erythema appears on the extensor extremities that can last up to three weeks. The third stage can recur secondary to friction and sun exposure.[1] (See photo on page PS-2.)

Roseola Infantum (Sixth disease)

The mode of transmission of roseola is unknown. After an incubation period of 5 to 15 days, children present with a high fever without an associated illness. The fever lasts three to five days before the skin eruption develops. The rash begins on the chest generalizing into a pink, maculopapular eruption which lasts 24 to 48 hours.

Gianotti-Crosti Syndrome (Papular acrodermatitis of childhood)

The skin eruption is characterized by erythematous, flat-topped papules symmetrically distributed on the face, buttocks and extremities of children. The trunk is usually spared and the lesions are most commonly non-pruritic. The eruption is self-limited, with spontaneous resolution in three weeks. Associated features may include lymphadenopathy, hepatomegaly and occasionally splenomegaly. The eruption is associated with a variety of infectious agents including Epstein-Barr virus, cytomegalovirus and hepatitis B. As well, various immunizations such as influenza, diphtheria and measles have been associated with Gianotti-Crosti syndrome.[2] (See photos on page PS-2.)

Hand-foot-mouth Disease

The incubation period is four to six days with a high rate of contagion. Following an absent or mild prodrome, lesions appear in the oral mucosa and affect the palms and soles. Characteristic grey-white vesiculopustules develop that are often asymptomatic. Hand-foot-mouth disease is caused by enteroviruses, mostly of the coxsackie A16 variety. The virus is

Table 1: Characteristics of Selected Viral Skin Rashes

Disease	Prodromal features	Skin eruption	Incubation period	Infectious period	Differential diagnosis	Prevention	Treatment
Rubeola (measles)	3-4 days of fever, cough, coryza, photophobia, conjunctivitis, Koplik spots	Erythematous macules and papules appear initially behind ears and along hairline and spread downward. Fade by day 5 of eruption	8-12 days	1-2 days before prodrome until 4 days after skin eruption	Morbilliform rash: similar to drug eruptions and viral exanthems; Koplik spots generally diagnostic	Measles vaccine	Supportive care (e.g., antipyretics)
Rubella (German measles)	Children: usually none or mild fever and lymphadenopathy. Adolescents/adults: fever, malaise, sore throat, nausea, painful occipital lymphadenopathy	Starts on face and neck as mild pink erythematous macules and papules, and generalizes over 1-2 days. Lesions fade within 2-3 days	14-21 days	5-7 days prior to eruption until 3-5 days after	Nonspecific viral exanthems. Drug eruptions	Rubella vaccine	Supportive care (e.g., antipyretics)
Erythema infectiosum (Fifth disease)	Children: mild fever, sore throat and malaise. Adults: flu-like symptoms, arthralgias and arthritis	Red erythematous macules on cheeks with "slapped cheek" appearance followed by maculopapular eruption on proximal extremities, which fades from centre out producing reticulated "lacy" pattern. Resolves in 1 week	4-14 days	Prior to onset of eruption (only considered mildly contagious)	Systemic lupus erythematosus (butterfly pattern over the bridge of the nose)	None	Supportive care
Roseola infantum (Sixth disease; human herpes virus 6 infection)	High fever for 3-4 days	Lesions start on chest and rapidly generalize into a pink maculopapular eruption. Fade within 24-48 hours	7-15 days	During illness	Measles, scarlet fever, rubella	None	Supportive care

Disease	Prodrome/symptoms	Lesions	Incubation	Period of communicability	Differential diagnosis	Prevention	Treatment
Gianotti-Crosti syndrome	Upper respiratory infection in 1/3 of patients	Sudden eruption of flat-topped, non-pruritic erythematous papules that are symmetrically distributed over face, buttocks, and extremities. Resolves in 2-8 weeks	Unknown	Unknown	Lichen planus, drug eruption, pityriasis rosea	None	Usually none required
Hand-foot-mouth disease	Absent or mild and occur 1-2 days before lesions. Low-grade fever, anorexia, malaise, sore mouth	Blisters or ulcers surrounded by red halos form in the back of mouth and on tongue, palms, soles, and buttocks	4-6 days	From first appearance until blister-like lesions disappear	Unique disease based on incubation period and distribution of lesions	None	Good oral hydration
Varicella (chickenpox)	None to fever, malaise, cough, sore throat	Erythematous macules which develop central vesicles and 2 days later pustules and crusts. Total healing 16 days	10-21 days	2 days prior to eruption until 5 days after	Insect bites during early stages. Kaposi's varicelliform eruption (*eczema herpeticum*)	Varicella vaccine	Children: supportive care. Adults: antivirals (e.g., acyclovir, famciclovir)
Herpes zoster (shingles)	Children: none. Adults: dull ache up to 1 week prior to eruption	Occur in a dermatomal distribution and consist of grouped vesicles and bullae on an erythematous base. Persist for 10-14 days	Not applicable	Until primary crusts have healed	Insect bites, herpes simplex virus	None	Children: none. Adults: antivirals within 48-72 hours of initial appearance of lesions

See Chapter 46: Drug-induced Skin Reactions, Table 1: Dermatologic Terminology.

spread by direct contact with nose and throat discharges and feces of infected people. (See photo on page PS-2.)

Varicella (chickenpox)

Chickenpox is a highly infectious disease caused by the varicella zoster virus (VZV). It is transmitted via inhalation of respiratory secretions or contact with skin lesions. Lesions, which are intensely pruritic, appear as scattered eruptions which vesiculate, rupture and then crust. The vesicles are often described as looking like "drops of water."[3] Secondary bacterial infection of the lesions and otitis media are the most common complications of varicella occurring in 5 to 10% of children. Healthy children rarely develop the serious side effects such as pneumonitis, encephalitis, cerebellar ataxis and Reye's syndrome. Complications are more common and severe in adults or immuno-compromised individuals (adults or children).[4] As well, the risk of fetal death is between 20 and 30% largely due to pneumonitis and hepatitis in a fetus exposed to a secondary viremia in utero before maternal immunity has developed. (See photo on page PS-2.)

Herpes Zoster (shingles)

Herpes zoster is caused by a reactivation of the varicella zoster virus that has remained latent in the sensory ganglia after a previous primary infection with chickenpox. Herpes zoster is primarily a disease of elderly people but it can occur across all age groups, especially in immunocompromised individuals. It is not known what causes reactivation, although physical trauma, ultraviolet light or stress at a time when the host's immune system is decreased may play a role.[5] Approximately 15% of those who have had the primary infection develop herpes zoster.[6] The dermatomal distribution of herpes zoster can vary although the thoracic area is involved in more than half of all cases. Only one to eight per cent of patients develop recurrences.[7] Individuals who have never had chickenpox may develop herpes zoster varicella if exposed to an individual with acute herpes zoster vesicles. The most common and feared complication of herpes zoster is postherpetic neuralgia; the pain is described as continuous aching, itching or burning.[4] (See photo on page PS-3.)

Goals of Therapy

- Minimize patient discomfort
- Shorten duration of symptoms
- Prevent complications

Patient Assessment

An assessment for pediatric patients with a skin eruption is found in Figure 1. Prior to recommending a product for symptomatic relief, evaluate the severity of the patient's condition. Referral to a physician should be considered when:

- The causative factor/organism is doubtful;
- Initial treatment has not been helpful or the condition is getting worse;
- Fever and/or malaise is associated with the skin eruption, or
- The patient has an underlying condition, such as diabetes, cancer or HIV-infection, or the patient is on chronic corticosteroid therapy.

Note that many other viral-induced eruptions (e.g., herpes simplex, eruptions associated with respiratory and enteric viruses) are not included in Figure 1.

Prevention

Vaccines have been developed for the prevention of measles, rubella and varicella. For current recommendations on immunization schedules for infants and children for the measles, mumps and rubella vaccine, see the *Compendium of Pharmaceuticals and Specialties* published annually by the Canadian Pharmacists Association. The varicella virus vaccine is recommended for primary vaccination of healthy persons 12 months of age who are susceptible to the disease.[8]

High-risk patients, such as patients with cancer or HIV-infection, should avoid exposure to patients with viral-induced skin eruptions. All women of child-bearing age should be tested for rubella antibodies and vaccinated if necessary. As well, pregnant women not previously infected with chickenpox should avoid contact with infected individuals.

Nonpharmacologic Therapy

Minimizing patient discomfort is the key, and often the only, treatment that can be offered to patients with a viral skin eruption.

Figure 1: **Assessment of Pediatric Patients with Skin Eruption**

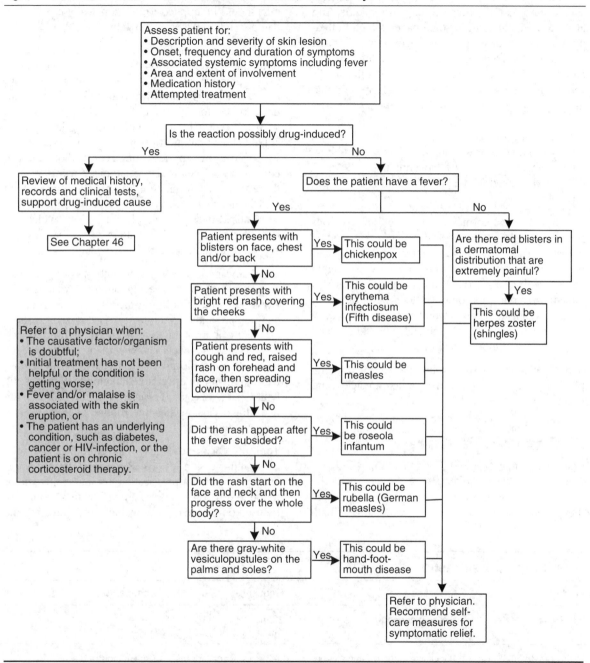

Note: Many other viral-induced eruptions (e.g., herpes simplex, eruption associated with respiratory and enteric viruses) are not included.

Many viral skin eruptions are associated with intense pruritus. Since it is exacerbated by dry skin, using a simple emollient is often helpful. A humidifier can also be used, although in some patients high humidity may also cause pruritus secondary to sweat retention. Good hygiene including gentle cleansing and drying of lesions as well as trimming of fingernails should be observed to prevent bacterial infection that may develop from scratching the pruritic lesions. The sensation of itching is generally increased if the skin is warm. Therefore, cooling the skin by tepid showering or bathing can often bring relief. As well, rubbing an ice cube over the rash or covering the rash with a clean cloth soaked in cold water will provide temporary relief.

Avoiding factors that may enhance pruritus, such as wearing of tight elasticized apparel or coarse woolen fabrics, is also important. Cornstarch or sodium bicarbonate baths have been used to relieve itching in patients with chickenpox. Add two cups of cornstarch mixed with four cups of water to a bathtub full of water. Bathing is recommended once or twice daily for approximately 15 to 20 minutes. The skin should be gently patted, not rubbed, when drying.

Remind patients to stay well-hydrated by drinking plenty of fluids, which can include popsicles and gelatin.

Pharmacologic Therapy

Colloidal oatmeal bath preparations may help to relieve pruritus. To be effective the product should be well dispersed in the bathtub water. For dispersion, the patient should fill a strainer with oatmeal bath preparation and hold under the faucet as water fills the tub. Unscented moisture cream or white petrolatum should be applied to the skin while it is slightly damp to retard water evaporation.

Local agents are useful for relieving pruritus and for reducing bacterial colonization of damaged skin. Cool compresses (e.g., gauze or other thin cloth moistened with **5% aluminum acetate**–Burow's solution) applied for 20 minutes four to six times daily can be used, especially for weeping, oozing lesions (see Table 2 for application of topical agents). **Calamine lotion** can be applied after removal of the wet compresses. Other traditional topical agents include those that contain menthol, camphor and phenol, all of which provide symptomatic relief. Concern has been raised over possible phenol toxicity, which has been described in patients with extensive bullous poison ivy who developed renal toxicity.[9]

Local anesthetics block conduction along axonal membranes, thereby relieving itching as well as pain. However, topical local anesthetics (e.g., benzocaine) are not recommended due to risk of sensitization, especially if applied to broken or fissured skin.[10] Post-herpetic neuralgia has been treated with eutectic lidocaine and prilocaine cream **(EMLA)** with temporary improvement of variable duration.[11] However, the typical large size of the area to be treated and the need for occlusion limit the routine use of EMLA in this situation.

Topical corticosteroids may relieve the itching associated with the skin lesions. **Hydrocortisone 0.5%** is available without a prescription in ointment, cream or lotion. Hydrocortisone-containing products should not be used on bacterial- or fungal-infected skin since the

Table 2: **Topical Treatments**

Product	Application	Frequency	Comments
5% aluminum acetate	Weeping or oozing lesions	20 minutes 4-6 times daily	
Hydrocortisone 0.5% (cream, ointment, lotion)	Noninfected, non-weeping lesions	3-4 times per day for up to 7 days	Cream: moist areas Ointment: dry or scaly lesions Lotion: scalp or other hairy areas
Capsaicin cream	Treatment of post-herpetic neuralgia	3-4 times per day	Adverse effects include local burning, stinging and irritation

corticosteroid may mask the symptoms of the dermatologic infection and allow the infection to progress. For adults and children two years of age and older, hydrocortisone can be applied sparingly, with gentle massage, onto the affected area up to three or four times a day. Since absorption of corticosteroids is enhanced in children under 18 months of age, topical nonprescription corticosteroids are not routinely recommended in this age group. If the skin lesions persist or worsen after more than seven days of hydrocortisone therapy, the patient should seek the advice of a physician.

Capsaicin 0.025% cream is a topical preparation made from the naturally occurring substance found in hot chili peppers. Applied to the affected area at least three to four times daily, it has been shown to be effective in the treatment of post-herpetic neuralgia.[12] Unfortunately, local burning, stinging, and irritation are common although they usually disappear with repeated application.

Antihistamines are effective in the treatment of pruritus. Both traditional H1-blocking anthistamines or newer non-sedative antihistamines are effective.[13] In general, the use of H2-blocking antihistamines is not recommended for the relief of pruritus associated with viral infections. (See Chapter 12 for adult and pediatric doses of nonprescription oral antihistamines.) Topical antihistamines are usually not recommended because of the risk of sensitization resulting in contact dermatitis.[14]

Many viral diseases are associated with a fever, especially in the prodromal stages. **Antipyretics** can be recommended to provide symptomatic relief as well as preventing possible complications such as febrile seizures (e.g., in patients with roseola infantum).

Acetaminophen and **ibuprofen** are recommended as first-line antipyretic agents. (See Chapter 9 for adult and pediatric doses of nonprescription antipyretics.) However, acetaminophen was found to delay the clearance of the varicella zoster virus, as shown by delayed scabbing of the lesions;[15] the clinical significance of this is not known.

Acetylsalicylic acid should be avoided because of the possible association of Reye's syndrome with salicylate administration[16] in children with viral infections, in particular those caused by influenza B and varicella zoster viruses.[17,18] However, some foreign countries still advocate the use of ASA in children. Parents who travel abroad should be warned regarding this potential risk.[19] There are no case reports of Reye's syndrome in patients with herpes zoster receiving ASA for cardiovascular prophylaxis; many clinicians elect to continue ASA during the acute illness. If analgesics are required in these patients, recommend acetaminophen or ibuprofen as there has been no association between these agents and the development of Reye's syndrome.

Mild analgesics (e.g., ASA, nonsteroidal antiinflammatory drugs, acetaminophen) are sometimes recommended for the treatment of acute pain associated with herpes; however, they are often not effective.[20] The pain in acute herpes zoster is frequently moderate to severe and warrants the use of narcotics.

For patients with mouth lesions, recommend warm water rinses or alternatively saline rinses (5 to 15 mL of table salt in 125 to 250 mL of warm tap water.) Hydrogen peroxide (half-strength) has also been used as a mouth rinse. As well, frequent oral hygiene with a soft-bristle tooth brush is recommended. Patients should avoid alcohol and glycerin-based mouthwashes; petrolatum jelly can be applied to lips as needed.

Alternative Therapy
Witch hazel (hamamelis water), an herbal therapy, has been used for centuries as an astringent. The product may be applied as often as necessary to treat minor skin irritations although it can be sensitizing.[21] It is available from various manufacturers as distilled witch hazel.

Prescription antiviral therapy may be used in select patients.
- *Chickenpox:* If initiated within 24 hours of rash onset, acyclovir may decrease the total number of new lesions formed and lower the need for antipruritic and analgesic treatment. In immunocompetent children, acyclovir is not generally recommended. However for immunocompetent adults and all immunocompromised hosts, treatment with acyclovir is suggested.[5, 22] There have been no studies evaluating famciclovir, penciclovir or valacyclovir for patients with chickenpox.
- *Acute herpes zoster:* Antiviral therapy with acyclovir, valacyclovir and famciclovir have been shown to speed resolution of the acute lesional events and

perhaps reduce the risk for prolonged pain. In patients 50 years of age and over or any patient with moderate to severe acute pain, antiviral therapy should be initiated if the duration of the rash is less than 72 hours.[5]

Monitoring of Therapy

A monitoring plan for patients with viral exanthems is outlined in Table 3. Additional advice should be provided regarding:
- Time that patients are considered infectious
- Referral to physician for possible use of antivirals for patients with herpes zoster and varicella (especially adults and those who are immunocompromised)
- Immunization of all children for measles, mumps and rubella, and also for varicella

Suggested Readings

Bialecki C, Feder HM, Grant-Kels JM. The six classic childhood exanthems: a review and update. *J Am Acad Dermatol* 1989;21:891-903.

Bligard CA, Millikan LE. Acute exanthems in children: clues to differential diagnosis of viral disease. *Postgrad Med* 1986;79:150-67.

McCrary ML, Severson J, Tyring SK. Varicella zoster virus. *J Am Acad Dermatol* 1999;41:1-14.

Millikan LE. Pruritus: unapproved treatments or indications. *Clin Dermatol* 2000;18:149-152.

References

1. Gable E, Liu G, Morrell D. Pediatric exanthems. *Primary Care* 2000;27:353-69.
2. Bjorge Nelson J, Seabury Stone M. Update on selected viral exanthems. *Curr Opin Pediatr* 2000;12:359-64.
3. Bligard C, Millikan L. Acute exanthems in children: clues to differential diagnosis of viral disease. *Postgrad Med* 1986;79:150-167.
4. McCrary M, Severson J, Tyring S. Varicella zoster virus. *J Am Acad Dermatol* 1999;41:1-14.
5. Cohen J. Recent advances in varicella zoster virus infection. *Ann Intern Med* 1999;130:922-32.
6. Gershon A. Varicella-zoster virus: prospects for control. *Adv Pediatr Infect Dis* 1995;10:93-124.
7. Mamdani F. Pharmacologic management of herpes zoster and postherpetic neuralgia. *Can Fam Physician* 1994;40:321-32.
8. National Committee on Immunization. Statement on recommended use of varicella virus vaccine. *Can Commun Dis Rep* 1999;25:1-10.
9. Millikan L. Pruritus: unapproved treatments or indications. *Clin Dermatol* 2000;18:149-52.
10. Rietschel R, Fowler J et al, eds. *Fisher's Contact Dermatitis*. Baltimore: Williams & Wilkins; 1995.
11. Milligan K, Atkinson R, Schofield P. Lidocaine-prilocaine cream in postherpetic neuralgia. *BMJ* 1989;298:253.
12. Bernestine J, Korman N, Bickers D, Dahl M, Millikan L. Topical capsaicin treatment of chronic postherpetic neuralgia. *J Am Acad Dermatol* 1989;21:265-70.
13. Ormerod A. Urticaria: recognition, causes and treatment. *Drugs* 1994;48:717-30.

Table 3: **Monitoring Therapy for Viral Skin Rashes**

Symptoms	Monitoring	Endpoint of therapy	Actions
Pruritus associated with skin eruption	**Patient:** daily while on therapy **Pharmacist:** after 2 days of therapy or next pharmacy visit	To decrease itching within 24-48 h	If therapy ineffective after 24-48 h, and treatment still required, refer patient to physician for assessment
Fever	**Patient:** twice daily while on therapy **Pharmacist:** after 2 days or next pharmacy visit	To decrease fever within 4-6 h of therapy	If fever persists for more than 48 h, refer patient to physician
Pain, especially with herpes zoster	**Patient:** daily **Pharmacist:** after 2 days or next pharmacy visit	To decrease pain to acceptable levels for the patient within 24 h	If pain persists despite appropriate nonprescription medication, refer patient to physician
Sedation (due to antihistamine therapy: this may be a desired effect from therapy)	**Patient:** daily **Pharmacist/Physician:** after 3 days or next pharmacy visit	No sedation, especially if patient driving or using heavy machinery	If sedation not desired, recommend a nonsedative antihistamine

14. Anonymous. Rash promises for topical antihistamines. *Drug Ther Bull* 1992;30:49-50.

15. Doran T, De Angelis C, Baumgardner R et al. Acetaminophen: More harm than good for chickenpox? *J Pediatr* 1989;114:1045-8.

16. Starko K, Ray C, Dominguez L, Stromberg W, Woodall D. Reye's syndrome and salicylate use. *Pediatrics* 1980;66: 859-64.

17. Waldman R, Hall W, McGee H, van Amburg G. Aspirin as a risk factor in Reye's syndrome. *JAMA* 1982;247:3089-94.

18. Halpin J, Holtzhauer F, Campbell R et al. Reye's syndrome and medication use. *JAMA* 1982;248:687-91.

19. Donaldson M, Fleming P. Reye's syndrome in children travelling abroad. *Lancet* 1988;2:1073.

20. Wood A. Post-herpetic neuralgia: pathogenesis, treatment and prevention. *N Engl J Med* 1996;4:32-42.

21. Anonymous. Witch hazel. In: Hebel S, ed. *The Review of Natural Products*. St. Louis: Facts and Comparisons; 1997.

22. Snoeck R, Andrei G, De Clercq E. Current pharmacological approaches to the therapy of varicella zoster virus infections. *Drugs* 1999;57:187-206.

Acknowledgement:

Thank you to Dr. Bernice Krafchik, MB, Ch.B, FRCPC, for allowing the use of her photographs and providing thoughtful comments regarding the manuscript.

Shingles—Patient Information

Shingles, also known as herpes zoster, is a viral disease that is caused by the same virus that causes chickenpox. You can only get shingles if you had chickenpox in the past. Shingles is more commonly seen in people over the age of 50 or those with a weak immune system. During the chickenpox infection, the virus is stored in nerve cells in the spinal cord. The virus remains in a resting phase in these nerve cells for years before it is reactivated (during times of stress or illness) and travels down the nerves to the skin to produce shingles (zoster). Patients usually complain of pain, which is followed by a red rash with small fluid-filled blisters. In some patients, the pain may continue long after the rash has cleared.

See your doctor to discuss treatment of shingles with prescription drugs. These medicines work best if you start them in the first three days after you get the rash.

Ways to be more comfortable:

- To stop the itching, use calamine lotion. Cool baths (with or without oatmeal) or showers are also helpful.
- If your itching is particularly bothersome, you can take an antihistamine. Ask your pharmacist or doctor which one is best for you.
- The rash should be kept clean and dry. Trim fingernails to prevent scratching and a bacterial infection of the skin.
- Loose clothing (not woolen) should be worn.
- Acetaminophen or ibuprofen can be used for the treatment of pain and fever. Acetylsalicylic acid (Aspirin®, ASA) is not recommended because of the possible risk of developing Reye's syndrome, a liver problem.
- Tell your doctor immediately if you develop eye problems.

Fifth Disease—Patient Information

Fifth disease is a common childhood viral infection causing a "slapped cheek" appearance and a rash. It most commonly affects young children. The child is generally well, but occasionally has a slight fever and headache. Children develop firm red cheeks, which feel burning hot. A rash follows one to four days later, that can persist for up to six weeks.

Affected children may remain at school as the infectious stage occurs before the rash appears. No specific treatment is needed. However, if the child is feeling uncomfortable then:

- Application of ice-cold compresses can relieve the discomfort of burning hot cheeks. Rubbing an ice cube over the rash or covering the rash with a clean cloth soaked in cold water will provide temporary relief. To avoid skin injury, stop cold treatment when the skin feels numb.
- Acetaminophen or ibuprofen can be used for the treatment of fever. Acetylsalicylic acid (Aspirin®, ASA) is not recommended because of the risk of developing Reye's syndrome, a liver problem.

Chickenpox—Patient Information

Chickenpox is a common highly contagious infection of children caused by the varicella zoster virus. It is spread by direct contact (by touching the blisters) or from an infected person's cough or sneeze. Two to three weeks after exposure, chickenpox spots appear on the body.

Chickenpox usually affects children and starts with a slightly raised temperature, tiredness and an itchy rash with small blisters that dry up and form scabs in two to four days. More severe but rare problems that can occur are pneumonia (especially in adults), skin infection, and blood infection. Chickenpox can be extremely serious for pregnant women who have not had chickenpox before, and people with poor resistance (those who have leukemia, immune suppression or immunodeficiency, including HIV).

People with chickenpox are infectious for two days before the rash appears and remain so until all the blisters have dried up (about five to ten days).

There is a chickenpox (varicella) vaccine. It can be used as a protective measure in all children and adults who have not had chickenpox before.

Antiviral drugs (such as acyclovir) may be used in some healthy children and adults, if started early in the course of the disease. For patients with decreased immune function, antiviral therapy should be started. In most healthy children, no specific treatment is used.

Ways to keep comfortable:
- To stop the itching, use calamine lotion. Cool baths (with or without an oatmeal bath product or half a cup of baking soda) and showers are also helpful.
- If the itching is particularly bothersome, use an antihistamine. Ask your pharmacist or doctor which one is best for you.
- Keep the rash clean and dry. Trim fingernails to prevent scratching which can cause a bacterial infection of the skin.
- Wear loose clothing (not woolen).
- Acetaminophen or ibuprofen can be used for the treatment of fever. Acetylsalicylic acid (Aspirin®, ASA) is not recommended because of the risk of developing Reye's syndrome, a liver problem.
- For mouth sores, rinse with warm water.

Chapter 46

Drug-induced Skin Reactions

Sandra Knowles, BScPhm

Pathophysiology

Drug-induced skin eruptions are the most frequently observed adverse reactions to medications. In the Boston Collaborative Drug Surveillance Program, the prevalence of cutaneous adverse drug reactions (ADRs) in hospitalized patients was 2.2%.[1]

The morphology of cutaneous eruptions (Table 1 and Figure 1) may be broadly classified as exanthematous, urticarial, blistering, or pustular. Within each of these categories, the presence of a fever or other accompanying symptoms other than itch signals a more serious reaction, which requires immediate referral to a physician (Table 2).[2]

Exanthematous Eruptions

Simple Eruptions

Exanthematous eruptions, also known as morbilliform or maculopapular eruptions, are the most common cutaneous ADRs. They usually start as erythematous macules and papules on the trunk, become confluent and later spread symmetrically to the face and limbs; there is no evidence of blistering or pustulation. Resolution occurs with a change in color from bright red to a brownish red. This color change may be followed by scaling or desquamation. Pruritus is a frequent clinical symptom but is not necessarily present. Simple eruptions usually begin within 7 to 10 days of starting therapy and resolve within 7 to 14 days after discontinuation of the drug.

Complex Exanthems

Hypersensitivity syndrome reaction is a complex drug reaction that includes the triad of fever, skin eruption (usually exanthematous) and internal organ involvement such as hepatitis, nephritis or agranulocytosis. The syndrome usually begins with fever at two to three weeks from initial drug exposure, and patients often initially complain of malaise.[3] (See photo on page PS-3.)

Table 1: **Dermatologic Terminology**

Bulla	A vesicle greater than 0.5 cm in diameter
Desquamation	Peeling of the skin
Erythema	Abnormal redness of the skin
Exanthem	An eruptive disease
Macule	A circumscribed, flat lesion less than 1 cm in diameter that differs from surrounding skin because of its color
Morbilliform	Measles-like eruption
Papule	A solid, circumscribed, elevated lesion less than 1 cm diameter
Plaque	An elevated, flat lesion greater than 1 cm in diameter
Purpura	Impalpable (macular) unblanchable purple spots
Pustule	A vesicle or bulla (usually less than 1 cm in diameter) filled with purulent exudates
Urticaria	Hives or an eruption of itching wheals
Vesicle	Blister or a small, circumscribed, elevation of the skin filled with clear fluid
Wheal	A transitory, elevated papule or plaque caused by edema of the skin

Figure 1: Description of Drug Eruptions

	Exanthematous		Urticarial		Blistering		Pustular	
Fever	No → Simple	Yes → Hypersensitivity syndrome reaction	No → Urticaria and/or angioedema	Yes → Serum sickness-like reaction	No → Fixed drug eruption	Yes → SJS, TEN	No → Acneiform	Yes → AGEP
Onset after initial exposure	<7 days	14-21 days	Minutes-hours	7-21 days	Hours to days	7-14 days	1-3 weeks	Days
Clinical features	Rash only	Fever, rash, internal organ involvement (may be asymptomatic)	Urticaria ± angioedema	Fever, rash, arthralgias ± lymphadenopathy	Solitary erythematous macules that recur in the same skin area after readministration of drug	Targets ± epidermal detachment	Atypical areas: arms, legs. No comedones	Many pustules on diffuse erythematous base. Fever. 50% have other cutaneous lesions 25% have mucosal erosions
Common drug causes	β-lactam antibiotics Sulfonamides Anticonvulsant medications[1]	Sulfonamides Anticonvulsants (barbiturates, phenytoin, carbamazepine, lamotrigine)[4] Dapsone Allopurinol[5]	Penicillin Sulfonamides ASA and NSAIDs[6] Narcotic analgesics[7] Radiocontrast media ACE inhibitors[8]	Cefaclor[9] Penicillins Sulfonamides Minocycline[10] Bupropion[11]	Barbiturates NSAIDs Acetaminophen Tetracycline Sulfonamides	Sulfonamides Anticonvulsants (barbiturates, phenytoin, carbamazepine, lamotrigine) NSAIDs (esp. piroxicam) Allopurinol[5]	Isoniazid Anticonvulsants Lithium Androgens Systemic corticosteroids	β-lactam antibiotics Macrolide antibiotics Calcium channel blockers
Treatment	Symptomatic therapy (e.g., antihistamines, soothing baths)	Corticosteroids, symptomatic therapy	Symptomatic relief (e.g., antihistamines); angioedema requires immediate therapy with epinephrine; avoid ASA/NSAIDs since can exacerbate skin lesions	Symptomatic treatment (including antipyretic, antihistamine); short course of oral corticosteroids in patients with severe symptoms	Symptomatic therapy (e.g., moisturizer, topical corticosteroid)	Supportive measures, intravenous immune globulin (IVIG), cyclosporine	Topical tretinoin (if drug cannot be discontinued)	Symptomatic therapy, corticosteroids if severe
Testing	Mononucleosis	CBC, liver enzymes, urinalysis, thyroid function tests	Skin test for penicillin		CBC, liver enzymes, urinalysis, skin biopsy		CBC, skin biopsy	

Table 2: **Clinical Features of Severe Cutaneous Drug Reactions**[2]

- Fever
- Enlarged lymph nodes
- Arthralgias or arthritis
- Shortness of breath, wheezing, hypotension
- Confluent and diffuse erythema
- Facial edema or involvement of central part of face
- Palpable purpura
- Skin tenderness
- Blisters or epidermal detachment
- Mucous membrane erosions
- Angioedema or swelling of tongue

Urticarial Eruptions

Simple Eruptions

Urticaria, characterized by extremely pruritic red raised wheals of varying sizes and shapes, and angioedema, affecting deep dermal and subcutaneous tissues, are reversible types of edema affecting the skin. In general, individual lesions of urticaria last for less than 24 hours, although new lesions continually develop. Although many different medications can cause urticaria, angioedema or both, other causal agents are food, physical factors (e.g., cold, pressure), infections and idiopathic factors. In fact, medications account for only 5 to 10% of urticaria cases.

Complex Eruptions

Serum sickness-like reactions are defined by fever, rash (usually urticarial), and arthralgias occurring one to three weeks after drug initiation. In contrast to true serum sickness, serum sickness-like reactions are not associated with immune complex formation, vasculitis or renal lesions. (See photo on page PS-3.)

Blistering Eruptions

Simple Eruptions

Fixed drug eruptions usually appear as pruritic, erythematous, bright-red or dusky-red macules that may evolve into an edematous plaque. In some patients multiple lesions may be present. Blistering and erosion may occur on mucosal surfaces and some patients may complain of burning or stinging on the affected skin sites. Fixed drug eruptions recur in the same skin area after readministration of the causative medication.[12]

Complex Eruptions

Serious dermatologic eruptions include Stevens-Johnson syndrome (SJS) and toxic epidermal necrolysis (TEN). The typical course of TEN consists of extreme illness with generalized tender or painful erythema of the skin followed by extensive epidermal necrosis and sloughing of any area of skin or mucous membrane leading to marked loss of fluids and electrolytes.[13] It also predisposes the patient to pneumonia and septicemia. Mortality as high as 30% has been reported as a result of these complications. (See photo on page PS-5.)

Pustular Eruptions

Simple Eruptions

Drug-induced acne may appear in atypical areas, such as arms and legs, and comedones are usually absent. (See photo on page PS-5.)

Complex Eruptions

Acute generalized exanthematous pustulosis (AGEP) is characterized by acute onset, with fever and a cutaneous eruption with nonfollicular pustules.[14] Generalized desquamation occurs two weeks after the initial reaction. (See photo on page PS-3.)

Other Skin Eruptions

Photosensitivity

Photosensitivity is an adverse cutaneous response to normally harmless doses of ultraviolet radiation. UVA rays are responsible for the majority of photosensitivity reactions. There are two types of photosensitivity reactions: phototoxicity and photoallergy.

Phototoxicity, the more common type, refers to an increased reactivity of the skin to UV radiation. This can occur on the first exposure to a drug, is dose related and is confined to exposed areas of the skin (e.g., face, neckline, back of the hands, arms, forearms and tops of feet). It generally resembles an exaggerated sunburn. These reactions do not contraindicate continued treatment with the drug, or its reintroduction, as long as effective protection against sunlight is ensured. Drugs associated with phototoxicity include tetracyclines, fluoroquinolones, amiodarone, phenothiazines and methotrexate.

Photoallergic reactions involve the immune system and therefore require prior sensitization to the drug. Photoallergy is delayed, usually occurring within 24 to

48 hours of exposure. Pruritus may occur prior to the onset of the cutaneous eruption. The lesions are often eczematous (e.g., with erythema, vesicles and scaling) and may spread beyond exposed areas.[15,16] NSAIDs, sulfonamides, chloroquine and carbamazepine have been reported to cause photoallergic reactions.

Patient Assessment (Figure 2)

The patient with a drug eruption often requires a referral to a physician. Although the rash may be self-limiting and only require OTC treatment, the patient may require alternative therapy. Many drug eruptions are more complex in that they are also associated with systemic signs. A patient who develops any systemic symptoms such as malaise, fever or shortness of breath, requires immediate referral to a physician since this may signal a more serious reaction.[2]

Since many skin diseases mimic drug reactions, it is important to carefully evaluate other causes of the cutaneous eruption. For example, guttate psoriasis may develop in a person being treated with penicillin for streptococcal infection, but the skin lesions are those of psoriasis and not a drug reaction. Differential diagnoses often include viral exanthems (e.g., infectious mononucleosis, rubella or roseola), bacterial infections, Kawasaki disease, collagen vascular disease and neoplasia. Disease states can also act as cofactors in the development of a cutaneous eruption. For example, patients with infectious mononucleosis who are also taking ampicillin or amoxicillin are at an increased risk for developing an exanthematous eruption compared to other patients (60 to 100% vs. 3 to 7%, respectively).

Cutaneous reactions to drugs frequently occur in complicated clinical scenarios that may include exposure to multiple agents, in which case a timeline should be developed. It is important that a detailed history be obtained for evaluation of an adverse drug reaction. This includes dosage, rechallenge and dechallenge, and onset of reaction. A history of prior exposure to the drug and related compounds is also important. If a patient has become sensitized to a drug they have received previously, on re-exposure to that drug the rash may appear sooner. New drugs initiated within the preceding six weeks are potential causative agents, as are drugs that have been used intermittently, including OTC preparations and herbal and naturopathic remedies.

The final step in the assessment of a patient with a cutaneous eruption is to determine the probability that each possible drug may have caused the reaction. It is, in fact, more common to mislabel a cutaneous eruption as a drug reaction than to diagnose it. This misdiagnosis may unnecessarily limit the future use of a particular medication or any related compound. It is important to document the possible drug reaction in the patient's medical and pharmacy records to ensure that future therapies are not pharmacologically and/or chemically related to the suspect drug.

Goals of Therapy

- Attempt to determine causality of the drug eruption
- Control symptoms associated with the drug eruption (e.g., pruritus)
- Provide patient education about drugs to avoid and those which can be used in the future
- For patients with photosensitivity reactions, provide information regarding preventive measures (e.g., avoiding UV radiation, wearing broad-spectrum sunscreen)
- Report all unexpected or serious ADRs or reactions to recently marketed drugs to the Adverse Drug Reaction Reporting Unit, Continuing Assessment Division, Bureau of Drug Surveillance or to a regional ADR centre

Nonpharmacologic Therapy

Many drug-induced skin eruptions, such as urticaria, are often pruritic. Dry skin and overheating can exacerbate pruritus. Overbathing, hot water, harsh soaps and bubble bath preparations dry and irritate the skin and should be avoided.[17] A simple physical measure is cooling the skin by tepid showering. Four tablespoons of baking soda in the bath may also help to relieve pruritus associated with urticaria. Tap water compresses can be used on blistering lesions. To compress, moisten gauze or other thin cloth in warm tap water and apply for 20 minutes four to six times daily. Alternatively, the compresses can be applied intermittently, one minute on – one minute off for 20 minutes. Oral lesions can be treated with warm water or saline rinses. Avoidance of factors that may enhance pruritus, such as wearing of tight elasticized apparel or coarse woolen fabrics, is also important.

Figure 2: **Assessment of Patients with Drug-induced Skin Reactions**

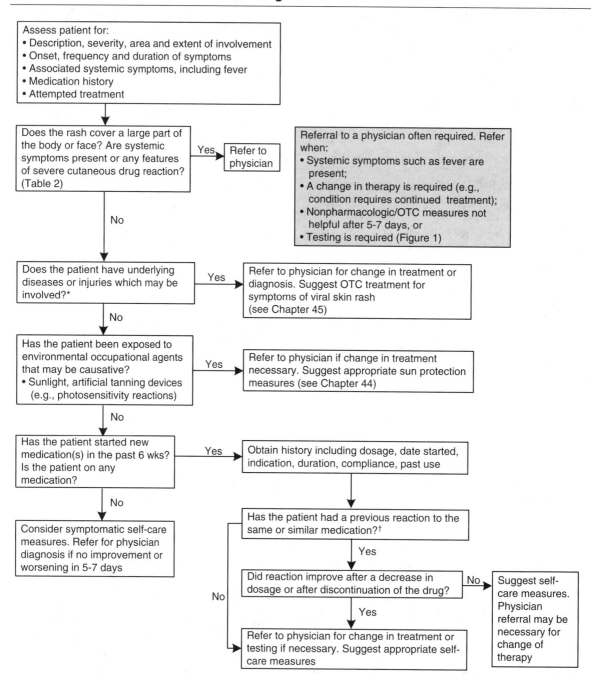

Examples of underlying diseases include infectious mononucleosis and ampicillin-related reactions; HIV and co-trimoxazole; infectious etiologies, e.g., viral skin rash, bacterial infections.
†*At this point, perform a literature search to determine if this reaction has been reported in association with this drug.*

Pharmacologic Therapy

Antihistamines are effective in the treatment of pruritus associated with urticaria and other dermatologic conditions. Both traditional H1-blocking antihistamines and newer nonsedating antihistamines have been shown to be effective in the treatment of pruritus associated with urticaria.[18] (See Chapter 12 for adult and pediatric doses of nonprescription oral antihistamines.) The addition of H2-blocking antihistamines (e.g., rantidine, famotidine) has been used in some patients with chronic urticaria with some initial benefit;[19] patients with acute drug-induced urticaria do not generally require additional therapy with H2-blocking antihistamines. Patients whose symptoms do not improve within five to seven days should be referred to a physician. The use of topical antihistamines, such as those containing diphenhydramine, is not recommended due to risk of allergic contact dermatitis as well as increased systemic absorption when applied to open lesions. Patients with urticarial lesions should avoid NSAIDs or ASA since these agents may exacerbate urticaria; they are common causes of drug-induced urticaria.

> Discontinuation of the offending drug is considered paramount in the management of patients with cutaneous eruptions. However, in some cases the drug may be continued and the reaction "treated through." This decision is influenced by the severity and probable course of the reaction, disease for which the drug was prescribed, ease or difficulty with which the reaction can be managed and the availability of chemically unrelated drugs with similar pharmacologic properties.[20]

Bathing with colloidal oatmeal bath preparations is helpful for pruritus. Unscented moisture cream or white petrolatum should be applied to the skin while it is slightly damp to retard water evaporation. Topical agents may be kept in a refrigerator because the physical cooling enhances their antipruritic effect.

Topical cream or lotion astringents, such as plain **calamine lotion** or **zinc oxide** cream, can also be used. The use of cooling salves such as menthol 0.25 to 0.5% or camphor 0.25 to 0.5% cream may be helpful although they may occasionally be irritating.

Another local treatment is half-strength hydrogen peroxide rinses for oral lesions.

Patients with photosensitivity reactions should be counseled to stay out of the sun until the reaction resolves, or to wear sunscreen and protective clothing. Exposed areas should be covered with a sunscreen that protects in the UVA range with a minimum SPF of 15 to 30. (See Chapter 44 for a further discussion of sunscreens.) Mild to moderate phototoxic reactions can be managed as ordinary sunburn (e.g., oral analgesics, cooling compresses or baths, emollient lotions).[16]

Topical corticosteroids are often used in the management of patients with drug-induced skin eruptions. **Hydrocortisone 0.5%** is available without a prescription in ointment, cream or lotion. Ointments are more occlusive and are preferred for dry or scaly lesions whereas creams are used in moist areas since they are more drying. Lotions are useful for the scalp and other hairy areas or for application to large body areas. Adults and children two years of age and older can apply hydrocortisone sparingly, with gentle massage, onto the affected area up to three or four times a day. If the skin lesions persist or worsen after five to seven days of hydrocortisone therapy, the patient should seek the advice of a physician.

Monitoring of Therapy

Pharmacists can provide symptomatic therapy for patients with drug-induced skin lesions. After discontinuation of the offending medication, most drug-induced cutaneous eruptions will resolve in five to seven days. However, for patients with serious drug-induced reactions, symptoms generally begin to abate within days, but this may vary from weeks to months. Many patients require a referral to a physician; some patients may require a change in therapy, drug testing or follow-up (e.g., measurement of liver function tests). It is recommended that any patient who has a fever or other accompanying symptoms such as malaise seek the advice of a physician.[7]

Advice for the Patient[1]

The patient must be provided with information regarding the adverse drug reaction. This includes the drug involved in the reaction (if known), the patient's predisposition to possible recurrence on exposure to the drug, potential cross-reaction to other drugs (e.g., ASA and NSAIDs) and genetic predisposition of family members, if applicable. No genetic basis has been found for most adverse drug reactions, including penicillin-allergic reactions. However, for serious reactions such as hypersensitivity syndrome reaction, serum sickness-like reactions to cefaclor and serious dermatologic reactions (e.g., SJS and TEN), the risk in first-degree relatives of patients who have had reactions is substantially higher and counseling family members is a crucial part of the management process.[21] In addition, advise the patient to enrol in the Medic Alert program.

Suggested Readings

Drake L, Dinehart S, Farmer R et al. Guidelines of care for cutaneous adverse drug reactions. *J Am Acad Dermatol* 1996;35:458-61.

Knowles S, Shapiro L, Shear NH. Drug eruptions. *Curr Probl Dermatol* 2000;12:58-62.

Roujeau JC, Stern R. Severe adverse cutaneous reactions to drugs. *N Engl J Med* 1994;331:1272-85.

References

1. Bigby M, Jick S, Jick H, Arndt K. Drug-induced cutaneous reactions: a report from the Boston Collaborative Drug Surveillance Program on 15,438 consecutive inpatients, 1975 to 1982. *JAMA* 1986;256:3358-63.
2. Roujeau JC, Stern R. Severe adverse cutaneous reactions to drugs. *N Engl J Med* 1994;331(19):1272-85.
3. Shear N, Spielberg S. In vitro evaluation of a toxic metabolite of sulfadiazine. *Can J Physiol Pharmacol* 1985;63:1370-2.
4. Knowles S, Shapiro L, Shear N. Anticonvulsant hypersensitivity syndrome: incidence, prevention and management. *Drug Safety* 1999;21:489-501.
5. Roujeau J, Kelly J, Naldi L et al. Medication use and the risk of Stevens-Johnson syndrome or toxic epidermal necrolysis. *N Engl J Med* 1995;333:1600-7.
6. Manning M, Stevenson D, Mathison D. Reactions to aspirin and other nonsteroidal anti-inflammatory drugs. *Immun Allergy Clin North Am* 1992;12:611-31.
7. Fisher M, Harle D, Baldo B. Anaphylactoid reactions to narcotic analgesics. *Clin Rev Allergy* 1991;9:309-18.
8. Pracy J, McGlashan J, Walsh R, Gleeson M. Angioedema secondary to angiotensin-converting enzyme inhibitors. *J Laryngol Otol* 1994;108:696-8.
9. Kearns G, Wheeler J, Childress S, Letzig L. Serum sickness-like reactions to cefaclor: role of hepatic metabolism and individual susceptibility. *J Pediatr* 1994;125:805-11.
10. Knowles S, Shapiro L, Shear N. Serious adverse reactions induced by minocycline: a report of 13 patients and review of the literature. *Arch Dermatol* 1996;132:934-9.
11. McCollom R, Elbe D, Ritchie A. Bupropion-induced serum sickness-like reaction. *Ann Pharmacother* 2000;34:471-3.
12. Commens C. Fixed drug eruption. *Aust J Dermatol* 1983;24:1-8.
13. Bastuji-Garin S, Rzany B, Stern R, Shear N, Naldi L, Roujeau J. Clinical classification of cases of toxic epidermal necrolysis, Stevens-Johnson syndrome, and erythema multiforme. *Arch Dermatol* 1993;129:92-6.
14. Beylot C, Doutre M, Beylot-Barry M. Acute generalized exanthematous pustulosis. *Semin Cutaneous Med Surg* 1996;15:244-9.
15. Anonymous. Drug-induced cutaneous photosensitivity. *Prescrire Int* 2000;9:117-22.
16. Pierce S. Drug induced photosensitivity. *Distillate* 1997;23:13-6.
17. Finlayson L. Pruritus. In: Gray J, ed. *Therapeutic Choices.* 3rd ed. Ottawa: Canadian Pharmacists Association; 2000:543.
18. Ormerod A. Urticaria: recognition, causes and treatment. *Drugs* 1994;48:717-30.
19. Cohen S, Monroe E. Combined H1 and H2 antihistamine treatment of chronic urticaria. *J Allergy Clin Immunol* 1980;65:1189-93.
20. Drake L, Dinehart S, Farmer R et al. Guidelines of care for cutaneous adverse drug reactions. *J Am Acad Dermatol* 1996;35:458-61.
21. Shear N, Spielberg S. Anticonvulsant hypersensitivity syndrome, in vitro assessment of risk. *J Clin Invest* 1988;82:1826-32.

Acknowledgement

The author would like to thank John R. Sullivan, MB BS, FACD, for his helpful, insightful and practical comments, as well as the use of his pictorial library.

Drug-induced Skin Reactions—Patient Information

You have a skin rash that may be related to drug therapy. The suspected drug is _____

_____ .

It is important to remember that not all skin rashes are caused by drugs but can be caused by infections or other diseases. Contact your physician and other health care professionals to inform them about your rash since some drugs may cause similar reactions and will need to be avoided in the future. As well, it is recommended that you register in the Medic Alert program.

Many rashes can be treated with simple measures and over-the-counter medications. For rashes that are itchy:

- Cool the skin with lukewarm showers and use a moisturizer when needed.
- Keep your creams and ointments in the refrigerator because the coolness will help control the itch.
- Avoid tight clothing or coarse woolen fabrics.
- Avoid overheating (e.g., don't wear too many clothes).
- An antihistamine can be used to relieve the itching. If your itching is worse at night, choose an antihistamine that causes drowsiness (e.g., diphenhydramine, chlorpheniramine). If your itching is bothersome during the day, choose an antihistamine that does not cause drowsiness (e.g., fexofenadine, loratadine, cetirizine). Check with your pharmacist since some antihistamines may interfere with other medications or medical conditions.
- Use of antihistamines in creams is not recommended.
- Plain calamine lotion or zinc oxide cream can be applied on the lesions, as needed.
- Oatmeal bath preparations or the use of baking soda in the bath (four tablespoons in bathwater) may also be helpful.
- Hydrocortisone 0.5% cream, ointment or lotion is available without a prescription. Ask your doctor or pharmacist how often to apply it and for how long. Only a small amount should be applied to the rash. Ointments can be used for dry areas and creams are recommended for moist areas. Lotions are useful for the scalp and other hairy areas.

Once you have stopped the suspected drug, the rash may continue to get worse for one to two days but then slowly improve in five to seven days. If the rash does not improve or worsens, or if you have a fever or feel like you have the flu (loss of appetite, nausea), see your doctor.

Chapter 47

Skin Infections and Infestations

Penny F. Miller, BSc(Pharm), MA

Bacterial Skin Infections

The skin has a remarkable ability to protect against the external environment. A number of protective mechanisms are involved. The uppermost layer of the epidermis, the stratum corneum, provides a physical barrier to invading organisms and is constantly shed to ward them off. Sebaceous glands secrete oily sebum providing an acidic pH of 5.5 that is unfavorable for microbial growth. The normal flora of the skin compete with potential pathogenic organisms. An effective immune system includes the Langerhans' cells in the epidermis and the mast cells and macrophages in the dermis. Still infections do occur, usually as a result of a break in the integrity of the skin. Other predisposing conditions for microbial invasion include excessive exposure to water through sweating, bathing, occlusion, increasing skin temperature or scrubbing the skin. Common bacterial skin infections include impetigo, furuncles and carbuncles.[1]

Impetigo
Pathophysiology

Impetigo is a very common and highly contagious skin infection involving the uppermost portion of the epidermis. Most cases occur in preschool-aged children but it can affect any age group. The infection is spread through direct contact with the lesions or infected exudates and develops quickly at sites of minor trauma. Crowding, poor personal hygiene and warm, humid conditions promote the spread of impetigo. Predisposing factors for impetigo include varicella, arthropod reaction, burns, scabies, atopic dermatitis, diabetes mellitus, hypogammaglobulinemia and HIV infection. The causative organisms are *S. aureus* either alone or in combination with group A beta-hemolytic streptococci (*S. pyogenes*).[2-7]

There are two distinct clinical presentations of impetigo. *Non-bullous impetigo* presents as small blisters (vesicles) filled with amber fluid that exudes and eventually dries to leave a honey-colored crust. Lesions are often multiple, involve the central face or extremities and may be associated with local adenopathy. The lesions may be tender and slightly itchy. The less common form, *bullous impetigo*, is almost exclusively caused by an exfoliating toxin-producing *S. aureus* phage group II.[8] It presents as very large blisters (bullae) that eventually rupture after three to five days and leave a thin varnish-like crust.[8] Rarely (less than 1% of cases[6]), streptococcal impetigo leads to acute glomerulonephritis as an immunologic response to the presence of a nephritogenic strain of *S. pyogenes*. Topical and/or oral antibiotic treatment of impetigo due to group A streptococcus does not prevent poststreptococcal glomerulonephritis. Other infrequent complications of impetigo include cellulitis, osteomyelitis, septic arthritis, pneumonia and septicemia.[9] Fortunately, rheumatic fever is not a risk following streptococcal impetigo.[4-7] (See photo on page PS-5.)

Goals of Therapy
- Eradicate causative organisms
- Relieve symptoms and resolve lesions
- Prevent the spread of infection

Patient Assessment

Table 1 provides a description and differential diagnosis of impetigo.

When the infection is localized and limited to two or three small areas, topical antibiotic therapy can be used. Refer patients to a physician for consideration of systemic therapy if the condition is widespread; if the patient is immunocompromised or has valvular heart disease; if there are signs of fever or bacteremia; or if there is a lack of improvement after 24 to 48 hours of topical therapy.[12] The toxin produced by the strain of *S. aureus* causing bullous impetigo may spread throughout the blood to cause a serious disorder, generalized staphylococcal scalded skin syndrome. This is more likely to occur in young children, people with renal impairment or who are immunocompromised.[13] Therefore, a physician should be consulted to manage bullous impetigo.[6] Patients with recurrent bouts of impetigo, or an infection of unknown etiology, should also be seen by a physician.

Nonpharmacologic Therapy

Prior to application of a topical antibacterial, impetigo crusts should be removed with warm water or saline compresses or soap and water washes. Compresses applied for 10 to 15 minutes and repeated three to four times daily, using a clean compress for each application, may hasten the healing process.[9-11] Patients should not manipulate the lesions as the infection could spread.

Pharmacologic Therapy

Several nonprescription topical antibiotics are available to treat impetigo that is localized to two or three limited regions. Antibiotic treatment of the affected person may limit the spread to others.[5]

One topical treatment of choice is **mupirocin** 2% ointment applied three times daily for 7 to 10 days or until all lesions have healed.[13] It requires a prescription in most provinces. Antibiotics containing **polymyxin B** and **bacitracin** or **gramicidin** may be initiated where there is a recent, small lesion but there is no scientific evidence of efficacy in impetigo treatment[9-11] (Table 2).

Prescription therapy includes **fusidic acid** 2% cream or ointment applied three times daily for 7 to 10 days or until all lesions have healed.[14-15] Systemic antibiotics active against beta-lactamase producing *S. aureus* and *S. pyogenes* such as cephalexin or cloxacillin are recommended.[5,12,16-18] Recurrent impetigo may occur when there is *S. aureus* carriage in the anterior nares or perineum. Refer these recurrent cases to a physician for culture and if positive, treatment with topical mupirocin or fusidic acid two to three times daily for two to three days should eradicate this carrier state.[12]

Monitoring of Therapy[4-6]

Table 3 presents a monitoring framework for patients with impetigo. Healing of lesions should be apparent within two to three days of therapy and are no longer infectious about 48 hours after the initiation of treatment. Lesions usually heal without scarring.[19] Physician referral is advised if lesions spread, or if fever or other systemic symptoms arise.

Furuncles and Carbuncles
Pathophysiology

Furuncles (boils) and carbuncles are staphylococcal infections located around hair follicles. Often they begin as superficial folliculitis, yellowish pustules at the hair base, then spread to deeper layers of the skin. (See photo on page PS-3.) Furuncles are most common in adolescence and early adulthood; carbuncles occur more often in older males.[7,9,20,21]

Furuncles spread into the dermis to produce a painful and erythematous swelling with a central pustule. Pus often drains spontaneously. Carbuncles penetrate deeper over a larger area than furuncles with involvement of numerous adjacent follicles and extension into the subcutaneous fat. Hairy areas subjected to irritation from perspiration or friction, such as the bearded area of the face, back of neck, buttocks and axillae are common sites of infection[7,9,21] (See Figure 1).

Predisposing factors for these infections include obesity and suppressed immune states as in diabetes mellitus or with corticosteroid use. Close contact with individuals with furunculosis appears to be a risk factor for the development of the infection.[20] Furuncles can progress to become carbuncles or cause a cellulitis.[21] Carbuncles have the potential to cause bacteremia with resultant morbidity or mortality.[7] Recurrent cases can occur especially if *S. aureus* is present in a carrier state in the anterior nares or perineum.[7,21]

Goals of Therapy

- Eradicate causative organisms
- Relieve symptoms and resolve lesions
- Prevent more serious infections

Table 1: **Characteristics and Differential Diagnosis of Selected Bacterial Skin Infections**[9-11]

Condition	Distribution	Lesion	Differential diagnosis
Non-bullous impetigo	Face, arms or legs	Primary lesions are vesicles and pustules. Secondary lesions occurring later are yellow or honey-colored crusts, with erosions and erythema surrounding the lesion.	Ecthyma: a crust but unlike impetigo, it is a deeper infection through the dermis causing ulcers and it is usually found on the lower extremities following a scratch. Tinea corporis: inflammatory pustules but unlike impetigo, has a central clearing and develops more slowly. Herpes simplex, herpes zoster, varicella and other blistering disorders such as contact dermatitis may be misdiagnosed as impetigo. However, unlike impetigo, these conditions have vesicles that are initially clear rather than honey-colored. Contact or atopic dermatitis typically produce marked pruritus. Herpes usually recur in the same location on the skin.
Furuncles and carbuncles	Hairy areas: face, back of neck, buttocks and axillae.	Primary lesions are inflammatory nodules around hair follicles. Secondary lesions are pustular with drainage.	Acne vulgaris: pus-filled nodules and cysts on the face and upper trunk, but other acne lesions such as comedones, papules and pustules are present. Hydradenitis suppurativa: pustules and exudative sinus tracts in the areas of apocrine glands, namely, the axillae and groin of young women after puberty.

Table 2: **Nonprescription Topical Antibacterial Agents**

Active ingredients	Gram-positive spectrum	Gram-negative spectrum	Contact dermatitis	Comments
Mupirocin 2% (Schedule I – prescription in most provinces)	Yes	No	Rare	As effective as systemic antibiotics in impetigo. Apply 3 times daily × 7-10 days. No cross-resistance.
Bacitracin 500 IU/g	Yes	No	Rare	Stable only in petrolatum (ointment). Apply 1-3 times daily.
Polymyxin B sulfate 10,000 IU/g, gramicidin 0.25 mg/g (or Bacitracin 500 IU/g.)	Yes	Yes	Rare	Rarely nephrotoxicity when applied to large denuded areas. Apply 1-3 times daily.

Figure 1: **Folliculitis, Furuncle and Carbuncle**

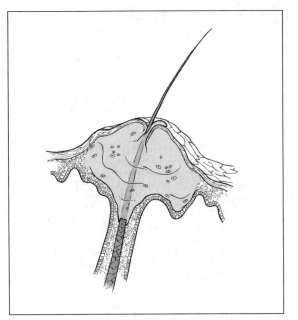

Folliculitis

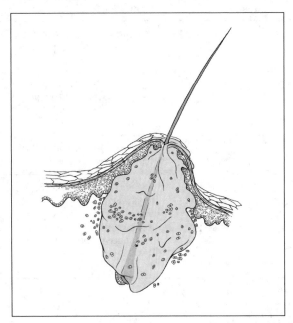

Furuncle

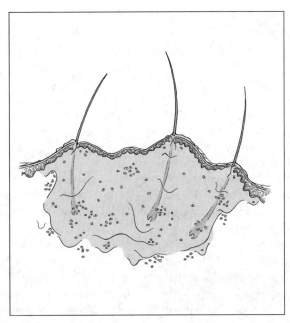

Carbuncle

Table 3: **Monitoring Therapy for Impetigo**[4-6,10]

Symptoms	Monitoring	Endpoint of therapy	Actions
Vesicles and crusts	**Patient:** daily while on therapy	Clearing of all lesions by 7-10 days. Return of normal skin appearance within 2-3 wks.	If no improvement or worsening by day 3, refer patient to physician.
Bullous lesions	**Patient:** daily while on therapy **Pharmacist/Physician:** after 3 days if no improvement with therapy	Clearing of all lesions. Return of normal skin appearance within 2-3 wks.	Refer patient to physician for alternate treatment if no improvement or worsening by day 3.
Hematuria or other urinary tract symptoms	**Patient:** daily while on therapy and for weeks following	No renal problems	Refer patient to physician.
Postinflammatory pigmentary skin change	**Patient:** weekly after therapy is completed	Resolution several months after clearing of initial infection	Refer patient to physician if persisting.
Allergy to topical agents	**Patient:** daily while on therapy **Pharmacist/Physician:** after 1 wk or next pharmacy visit	No allergy	Stop therapy. See physician.
Irritation caused by topical agents		Little to no irritation that subsides with continued use	Stop therapy if no improvement after several doses.

Patient Assessment[9-11]

A description and differential diagnosis of furuncles and carbuncles is found in Table 1. Fever, malaise and local adenopathy are more common in patients with carbuncles than furuncles. Patients who have a fever, recurrent furuncles, carbuncles, or an infection of unknown etiology should be referred to a physician.

Nonpharmacologic Therapy

A furuncle is a fluctuant mass of walled off purulent material that normally ruptures and drains pus spontaneously. Warm water or saline compresses applied for 20 to 30 minutes three or four times daily may promote spontaneous drainage and help relieve discomfort.[9-11] Washing the area with soap and water or chlorhexidine 4% four times daily to reduce the S. aureus colony counts is advised.[22] Lesions should be covered with a sterile dressing and not touched to avoid spreading. Personal items contacting the lesion should be washed daily in hot water and not shared. Furuncles that are large or unresponsive to warm compresses and carbuncles usually require surgical incision and drainage by a physician.[11]

Pharmacologic Therapy

Since carbuncles are deeper and more extensive skin infections, systemic treatment is required. Antimicrobial agents active against beta-lactamase producing S. aureus such as cephalexin or cloxacillin are recommended.[12] If lesions do not resolve, surgical drainage may be required.

Patients with recurrent furuncles or carbuncles who have documented S. aureus of the nasal passageways should apply **mupirocin** 2% ointment to the anterior nares twice daily for five days each month indefinitely.[9,23] If this is unsuccessful, oral rifampin plus cloxacillin added to the mupirocin topical nasal treatment is advised.[16]

Additional suppressive regimens for recurrent furunculosis include **vitamin C** 1000 mg daily for four to six weeks[24] or long-term, low-dose clindamycin 150 mg daily for three months.[25] Although the benefit with vitamin C was demonstrable only in patients with impaired immunity, a trial of vitamin C may be a reasonable approach for any patient with recurrent furuncles since neutrophil function tests are expensive and not readily available to identify this group of immune-impaired individuals.[24]

Monitoring of Therapy

After spontaneous or surgical drainage, healing usually occurs within a week. Large lesions may heal with a scar. Patients with recurrent infections may have underlying systemic illnesses that require investigation and management by a physician. A monitoring framework for patients with furuncles or carbuncles can be found in Table 4.

Table 4: **Monitoring Therapy of Furuncles/Carbuncles**

Symptoms	Monitoring	Endpoint of therapy	Actions
Boils and pus	**Patient:** daily while on therapy	No more drainage of pus and lesions are healed over several weeks.	If no improvement or worsening by day 3, refer patient to a physician.
Fever	**Patient:** daily while on therapy. **Pharmacist:** After 48 hours	Return to normal body temperature.	If no improvement by day 2, refer patient to a physician.
Pain on palpation	**Patient:** daily while on therapy	Relief of pain as the lesion heals.	If no improvement or worsening by day 3, refer patient to a physician.
Recurrent lesions	**Patient:** watch for any new lesions for weeks and months following the initial lesions	No recurrent infections.	Refer patient to a physician for culture of anterior nares and perineum.
Allergy to topical agents	**Patient:** daily while on therapy.	No allergy.	Stop therapy. See physician.
Irritation caused by topical agents	**Pharmacist:** after 1 wk or next pharmacy visit	Little to no irritation that subsides with continued use.	Stop therapy if no improvement after several doses.

Fungal Skin Infections

Superficial fungal infections are very common skin diseases affecting millions of people worldwide. Three genera of dermatophytes namely, Trichophyton, Epidermophyton and Microsporum, as well as yeast-like fungi, Candida or *Malassezia furfur* (previously known as *Pityrosporum orbiculare* or *Pityrosporum ovale*) are responsible for most infections.[26,27]

Dermatophyte Infections
Pathophysiology

Dermatophytes survive on dead keratin, the top layer of the epidermis, and affect the hair, nails and skin. Mucosal tissues are spared as they lack a keratin layer. Infections are transmitted through direct contact with infected persons, or occasionally infected soil or animals. There are many predisposing factors to dermatophyte infections including conditions that increase moisture such as occlusive clothing or shoes and warm humid climates. In addition, conditions of impaired immunity as in diabetes, HIV infection and chemotherapy treatments can contribute to a dermatophyte infection. Dermatophyte infections are commonly called *ringworm* or *tinea* which means fungus. Classification of tinea infections is based on their anatomic location rather than the fungal species.[26,27]

Tinea Corporis
The classic presentation affects the smooth and bare (glabrous) areas of the trunk or legs and begins as a flat, circular, scaly spot with a raised vesicular border that advances circumferentially (outward).[28] (See photo on page PS-4.)

Tinea Cruris

Tinea cruris or "jock itch" involves the groin area (namely the medial and upper parts of the thigh and the pubic area). Occasionally the anal cleft is affected. Unlike yeast infections, the scrotum and penis are spared. The infection occurs most often in men during the summer months. Often a reservoir for the infection is found on the feet.[29] The lesions are usually bilateral, scaly with red-brown centres and a clearly defined raised border. Pruritus is common.

Tinea Manuum

An infrequent infection, tinea manuum may present as the classic pattern of limited erythema and scaling of the palmar surface of the hands. Another form produces diffuse dryness and hyperkeratosis of only one palm and is associated with tinea pedis, referred to as "one hand two feet" presentation.[29]

Tinea Capitis

Tinea capitis is a dermatophyte infection involving the scalp hair follicles and adjacent skin. Children are primarily affected. It often appears as an annular patch of itchy, scaling skin and hair loss. Hairs may break off at the surface to produce black dots. Some patients may develop a boggy inflammatory mass called a kerion that can result in scarring and permanent hair loss.[30]

Tinea pedis/athlete's foot is discussed in Chapter 38.

Goals of Therapy

- Eradicate causative organism
- Resolve the lesion and symptoms
- Prevent spread of the infection
- Prevent secondary complications

Patient Assessment[9,10]

Assess patient's signs, symptoms and history including:

- location and distribution of lesions
- aggravating factors, impact on activities and quality of life
- treatments attempted

If the etiology of the infection is unclear, the patient should be seen by a physician.

Characteristics and differential diagnosis of fungal skin infections can be found in Table 5. Nonprescription topical antifungal treatment is effective for tinea corporis, tinea cruris and tinea pedis.[31] Nonprescription therapy can be attempted for tinea manuum but because of the thickness of palmar skin and frequent association with infected fingernails, systemic therapy is often necessary. Patients with tinea capitis, tinea unguium (i.e., tinea of the nails) and those who respond poorly to topical therapy should see a physician for possible oral antifungal treatment.[32]

Nonpharmacologic Therapy

Skin should be kept clean and dry to discourage fungal proliferation. Using an electric hairdryer on the cool setting will aid in drying the skin; avoid excessive rubbing with towels. Loose fitting cotton clothing that allows adequate ventilation is encouraged. Nonmedicated powders can be used to absorb excess perspiration but cornstarch should be avoided since it may provide nourishment for fungi, thereby delaying resolution. Clothing and linens of the infected person should be laundered separately from other family members.[9-10]

Pharmacologic Therapy

Many nonprescription options are available for the treatment of fungal skin infections. Topical antifungal treatment is effective for tinea corporis, tinea cruris and tinea pedis.[16,31] Liberal use of antifungal powder (e.g., tolnaftate, undecylenic acid) may help to absorb skin perspiration and prevent rubbing. The imidazoles or azoles (e.g., miconazole, clotrimazole) are effective as are undecylenic acid and tolnaftate.[33] No differences in efficacy have been demonstrated between individual allylamines (terbinafine) or individual azoles but the allylamines are more effective than the azoles. The azoles are equally efficacious as undecylenic acid but may be more effective than tolnaftate. The estimated cure rate is 73% for azoles and 80% for allylamines; however, a shorter treatment course, once daily application and longer remission periods are achieved with terbinafine, a prescription allylamine.[33-35] It is important to note that nystatin is ineffective in the treatment of dermatophytosis.[36] Tinea cruris should be treated for two weeks, tinea corporis for four weeks with physician referral if no improvement occurs (Table 6).

Table 5: Characteristics and Differential Diagnosis of Fungal Skin Infections[9-11]

Condition	Distribution	Lesions	Differential diagnosis
Tinea corporis	Exposed areas, namely, trunk, limbs and face	Typically annular (round), erythematous patch, scaly with a vesicular border and central clearing	Psoriasis: thick and silvery scales often in a symmetrical arrangement. Seborrheic dermatitis: yellow, greasy scales affecting face, scalp and central chest. Nummular eczema: smaller lesions usually affecting arms, legs and neck. Lyme disease: an initial erythematous circular lesion (erythema migrans) with a central clearing at the site of the tick bite. It lacks scales. Pityriasis rosea: acute onset of small scaled lesions in a Christmas tree distribution on the trunk. A single salmon-colored patch that can be mistaken for tinea corporis appears on the trunk two weeks preceding this rash.
Tinea cruris	Symmetrically involving the upper inner thigh and groin. The penis and scrotum are usually spared.	Annular, erythematous patch, with scales and central clearing. The borders are well-defined.	Candidiasis: very red with poorly defined borders and has satellite lesions (vesicles, papules) outside the borders of the rash. The scrotum or penis may be involved. Erythrasma: an overgrowth of normal bacterial flora, *Corynebacterium minutissimum*, presents as bilateral, irregular shaped, brown plaques with scales found in intertriginous (skin fold) areas. Psoriasis: symmetrical erythematous patches. Seborrheic dermatitis: usually also involves the scalp, face and central chest.
Tinea manuum	Palmar surface of the hand more often than the back of the hand. Only one hand may be involved if it occurs in conjunction with tinea pedis.	Usually dry, mild diffuse scales on an erythematous base	Allergic or contact dermatitis: acute onset and very pruritic. Atopic dermatitis usually involves other skin areas. Psoriasis: silvery scale. Involved nails are pitted.
Tinea capitis	Scalp	May be quite varied from an irregular shaped scaly patch with broken hairs or a very inflamed soft, swollen mass called a kerion with hair loss	Seborrheic dermatitis: yellow-greasy scales often involves the hairline and face. Impetigo: honey-colored crusts. Psoriasis: symmetric distribution of silvery scales on reddened base. Alopecia areata: small non-scaly patches of sudden hair loss.
Pityriasis versicolor	Back, chest, upper arms	Multiple white-pink to brown macules with an overlying fine scale	Vitiligo: non-scaly chalk-white lesions. Seborrheic dermatitis: yellow greasy scales involving the chest as well as the scalp.
Cutaneous candidiasis	Moist areas, skin folds, particularly the groin	A "beefy red" edematous area with irregular edges with many small papules (satellite lesions) outside of the borders.	Tinea corporis or cruris: well-defined borders, no satellite lesions and the scrotum is not involved. Contact dermatitis: will not have satellite lesions. Psoriasis: symmetrical with well-defined borders and no satellite lesions.

Table 6: **Nonprescription Topical Antifungal Agents**[37,38]

Drug	Dosage	Duration of therapy	Adverse effects
Azoles			
Clotrimazole 1%	Twice daily	Tinea cruris × 2 wks Tinea corporis × 4 wks Cutaneous candidiasis × 2-3 wks Pityriasis versicolor × 2 wks	Irritation, erythema, pruritus, stinging. Rare: Hypersensitivity reactions.
Miconazole 2%	Twice daily	Tinea cruris × 2 wks Tinea corporis × 4 wks Cutaneous candidiasis × 2-3 wks Pityriasis versicolor × 2 wks	Itching, burning, stinging
Tioconazole 1%	Twice daily	Tinea cruris × 2 wks Tinea corporis × 4 wks Cutaneous candidiasis × 2-4 wk Pityriasis versicolor × 2 wks	Itching, burning, stinging
Ketoconazole 2% shampoo (used as a lotion)	Single application or once daily × 3 days	Pityriasis versicolor × 1 or 3 days	Itching, burning, stinging
Other			
Tolnaftate 1%	Twice daily	2-4 wks	Local skin irritation
Undecylenic acid	Twice daily	Tinea cruris × 2 wks Tinea corporis × 4 wks	Itching, burning, stinging
Nystatin 100,000 units/g	Two or three times daily	Cutaneous candidiasis × 2-3 wks	Rarely: Irritation
Salicylic Acid 6%/ Benzoic Acid 6%	Twice daily	4-6 wks	Irritation, salicylate toxicity if used on extensive skin areas

Because they are rubbed into the skin, creams and lotions are generally considered to be more effective than sprays or powders, which are often used adjunctively. Lotions are preferred in intertriginous areas. Creams may be more occlusive than lotions possibly causing maceration.

Before the advent of effective antifungal agents, keratolytics such as Whitfield's ointment containing benzoic acid 12% and salicylic acid 6% were used to produce desquamation of the fungal-containing epidermis. The preparation can be irritating and if used over a large surface area, can lead to salicylate

toxicity.[36] Safer and more effective antifungal agents are generally preferred.

Topical antifungal creams or lotions should be applied to the affected area including 2 to 3 cm beyond its border twice daily for a minimum of two weeks (or until the lesion is cleared), plus one to two weeks after the lesion has cleared.

Prescription Therapy

Terbinafine, a topical prescription allylamine, can be applied once daily[11,39] and produces similar cure rates within one week of treatment.[40] Patients with widespread disease, persistent recurrence or who are immunocompromised may require systemic antifungal therapy (e.g., terbinafine, fluconazole).

Monitoring of Therapy

Table 7 provides a monitoring plan for patients with fungal skin infections.

Yeast Infections

Pityriasis Versicolor (Tinea Versicolor)
Pathophysiology

Pityriasis versicolor is an infection of the stratum corneum of the skin where sebaceous glands are present, especially the upper trunk. Since the term tinea refers to diseases caused by dermatophytes, the preferred term is pityriasis (meaning scaling) for this yeast infection. *M. furfur* (also called *Pityrosporum orbiculare or Pityrosporum ovale*) normally colonizes the skin but causes an opportunistic infection in association with immunosuppression, pregnancy, malnutrition, oily skin, or use of corticosteroids or oral contraceptives. It affects about 1% of the general population and occurs most commonly in postpubertal adults and in warm, humid climates.[9,11]

The most common presentation is multiple white to reddish-brown macules that may coalesce to form large patches of various colors ranging from white to tan. A fine scale is apparent when scratched. The lesions tend to be darker than the surrounding skin in fair-skinned patients and lighter in dark-skinned patients. This is primarily a cosmetic problem where the lesions do not tan along with the surrounding normal skin. Recurrences rates are as high as 60% to 80%.[41] (See photo on page PS-5.)

Goals of Therapy

- Reduce or eliminate yeast elements
- Reduce or eliminate skin lesions and symptoms
- Prevent recurrences of infection

Patient Assessment[9,11]

Characteristics and differential diagnosis of pityriasis versicolor can be found in Table 5. Patients with pityriasis versicolor usually only have cosmetic manifestations; pruritus is unusual. Self-care measures are appropriate for those with pityriasis versicolor. If the etiology of the infection is unclear, patients should see a physician.

Nonpharmacologic Therapy

Because yeasts thrive in moist environments, controlling excess heat and humidity may be helpful. Avoid application of oil to the skin as *M. furfur* can overgrow in these areas.

Pharmacologic Therapy

Topical treatment with a variety of different agents can produce equivalent mycological cure rates in excess of 80%.[42] Traditional treatment involves **selenium sulfide** 2.5% shampoo applied to the affected area then washed off 10 to 15 minutes later. This is repeated once daily for 7 to 14 days then used once to twice monthly to prevent recurrences.[29,42] Two-week applications of topical azole creams (e.g., **miconazole**) appear to be as effective as selenium sulfide but are more costly alternatives when the condition is widespread.[9,42] **Ketoconazole** 2% shampoo used as either a single application or once daily for three days produced clinical cure rates of about 70%.[43] Other nonspecific topical agents such as sulfur 2%, salicylic acid, zinc pyrithione 1%, benzoyl peroxide or propylene glycol 50% have demonstrated limited efficacy in older trials.[36]

Prescription Therapy

Topical, not oral terbinafine, is also effective, as are ciclopirox and ketoconazole cream.[42] Oral therapy for patients with extensive infection, or who are intolerant of or unable to use topical therapy includes ketoconazole (400 mg single dose), fluconazole (400 mg single dose) or itraconazole (200 mg daily for seven days).[16,44,45]

Monitoring of Therapy

A monitoring plan for patients with pityriasis versicolor is provided in Table 7. Resolution of scaling occurs promptly but the pigmentary changes may take weeks to months to resolve. Preventive treatment with once-monthly applications of selenium sulfide shampoo can reduce the recurrence rate to less than 15%.[11]

Cutaneous Candidiasis
Pathophysiology

Candida yeasts are part of the normal flora of the skin, oropharynx, intestinal tract and vagina. Infections arise when skin pH is increased, competing bacteria are removed by antibiotic treatments, glucose content in sweat increases as in diabetes and/or the surrounding environment is warm and moist.[9] With impaired host defenses, infections may affect not only skin, nails or mucous membranes but also rarely lead to systemic infections. Risk factors for cutaneous candidiasis include diabetes mellitus, obesity, tropical environment, neutropenia, HIV infection, psoriasis, contact dermatitis and use of corticosteroids or antibiotics.[46] (See photo on page PS-3.)

The most common form of *C. albicans* infection is intertrigo. Any skin fold area such as the gluteal fold, axillae (armpit), interdigital spaces, under breasts, or abdominal folds can be affected. These occlusive areas create moist, warm environments ideal for *C. albicans* to flourish.

Candidal paronychia occurs in individuals who have their hands in water excessively. This condition consists of painful, reddened and swollen nail folds. Chronic infection can lead to nail involvement with yellowish discoloration and separation of the nail plate from the nail bed (onycholysis).[1]

Goals of Therapy

- Eradicate or reduce the yeast elements
- Eliminate or reduce lesions and symptoms
- Prevent spread of infection
- Prevent recurrences

Table 7: **Monitoring Therapy for Fungal Skin Infections**

Symptoms	Monitoring	Endpoint of Treatment	Actions
Lesions specific for each fungal infection	**Patient:** daily for lesions decreasing in size and no more new lesions developing **Pharmacist:** Next visit	Clearing of all lesions within 4 wks	If no improvement or spreading of lesions by 1 wk, refer patient to a physician.
Pain, swelling, redness, or drainage	**Patient:** daily for any evidence of new onset of these symptoms **Pharmacist:** Next visit	No development of these symptoms	Refer patient to a physician if these symptoms develop as it may indicate a bacterial superinfection.
Recurrent lesions	**Patient:** watch for recurrence of any new lesions for weeks or months following initial infection	No new lesions	Refer patient to physician to rule out any underlying predisposing conditions. Emphasize preventative measures.
Inflammation being treated with corticosteroids	**Patient:** daily	Resolution of inflamed areas	If no improvement or lesion is worsening by 1 wk, refer patient to a physician. Emphasize correct use of cool compresses.
Allergy	**Patient:** daily while on therapy. **Pharmacist/Physician:** after 1 wk or next pharmacy visit	No allergy	Stop therapy. See physician.
Irritation caused by topical agents		Little to no irritation that subsides with continued use	Stop therapy if no improvement after several doses.

Patient Assessment

A description and differential diagnosis of cutaneous candidiasis is provided in Table 5. The lesions are red, macerated patches with irregular scalloped borders. Papules and pustules called satellite lesions form outside of the borders. Symptoms of pruritus and soreness are common.[11]

Patients with widespread, systemic or persistent, recurrent infection or those who are immunocompromised should be referred to a physician for management.

Nonpharmacologic Therapy

Good hygiene measures such as daily bathing and avoiding tight-fitting clothing aid in skin dryness, making a less desirable environment for yeasts. Measures to keep the area dry by using cool water or astringent soaks (aluminum acetate) for 15 to 20 minutes three times daily are useful. The affected area should be air dried afterwards. Applying nonmedicated powders several times daily helps to reduce the moisture in the skin folds and may help prevent the infection. The use of cornstarch should be avoided as this may promote the growth of candida organisms.[9,10]

Pharmacologic Therapy

Nystatin and **azoles** (miconazole, clotrimazole) are effective nonprescription topical agents when applied for two to three weeks. Tolnaftate and undecylenic acid are ineffective. To reduce inflammation, topical corticosteroids (e.g., **hydrocortisone** 0.5%) may be used sparingly twice daily for short periods (of one to two weeks) in conjunction with antifungals.[10,46] Nonmedicated powders can also be applied a few times daily to decrease moisture in intertriginous areas (Table 6).

Prescription Therapy

In widespread cutaneous disease and immunocompromised patients, oral anti-yeast medications (e.g., fluconazole, ketoconazole, itraconazole) may be indicated. A physician referral is necessary.

Alternative Therapy

Table 8 lists herbal therapies that have been used for a variety of fungal and bacterial skin infections. There is no adequate clinical evidence of efficacy available for any of these herbs.

Table 8: **Herbals Used for Skin Infections**[47]

Herb	Proposed action/ Effect(s)	Dose/Form	Adverse effect(s)	Comments
Goldenseal (*Hydrastis canadensis*)	Antiseptic, antimicrobial, astringent	External use for boils and fungal infections	Mucocutaneous irritation	Oral ingestion can cause CNS stimulation, increased cardiac and uterine contractility.
Purple cornflower (*Echinacea angustifolia* or *Echinacea purpurea*)	Antiseptic, antimicrobial, antiinflammatory, immune modulator	External use for boils, ulcerations, yeast infections	Dermatitis	Oral use: Trials as an immune modulator to prevent colds and flu show mixed results.
Slippery elm bark (*Ulmus fulva*)	Emollient, antiviral	External use for minor skin irritations, boils	Dermatitis	Oral ingestion has been used to induce abortions.
St. John's wort	Astringent, antimicrobial, antiinflammatory, immunomodulator	External use for wounds, contusions	Photosensitivity is rare	Oral use: More trials available in mild-moderate depression.

Monitoring of Therapy

Substantial improvement should be evident within one week of topical treatment.

Persistent candidal infection may be a sign of immunosuppression and should be referred to a physician for investigation. Table 7 suggests a monitoring plan for patients with fungal infections.

Viral Infections

Warts (Verrucae)
Pathophysiology

Warts are common viral infections of the skin caused by any of 70 distinct DNA (deoxyribonucleic acid) viruses in the human papillomavirus (HPV) family. The Latin term "verruca," which means "a steep place," was given because warts resemble small hills on the skin. Children and young adults are most commonly affected. Handlers of meat, poultry and fish have a high incidence of warts. It has been estimated that 25% of the population have a wart at some time. Warts are usually spread by direct skin-to-skin inoculation of the virus from an infected person, although transmission by fomites such as in swimming pools may also occur. There is a variable time between inoculation and the appearance of a lesion, ranging from two to six months for common warts. Cell-mediated immune responses to the virus are important in host resistance. Predisposing conditions for more extensive or recalcitrant warts may include atopic dermatitis and immunosuppressive states.[10] Based on their location, there are several different forms of warts including common warts (hands), flat warts (face), and plantar warts (foot).[48] See Chapter 40 for plantar warts.

Common Warts

Common warts are hyperkeratotic papulonodules most often seen on the fingers, hands and around the nails. They can occur anywhere on the skin. The lesions typically are small, hard, raised growths with a rough surface that looks like cauliflower. Spontaneous remission occurs in about two-thirds of affected patients within two years. Recurrence is common.[49] (See photo on page PS-4.)

Flat Warts

Flat warts frequently present as several small and subtle papules with a smooth surface affecting the face or neck. Pigmentary changes may be the most disturbing feature for the patient.[48]

Goals of Therapy

- Remove the virus-containing wart with minimal destruction of normal tissue
- Prevent spread of the wart

Patient Assessment[9-11]

A description and differential diagnosis of warts can be found in Table 9. Warts may cause pain and bleed if irritated, otherwise they produce no symptoms and are harmless.

Patients presenting with warts on the face or genitals should be referred to a physician, as should patients with flat warts and those with resistant or widespread lesions. Patients with neuropathies such as diabetes or circulatory disorders should not self-medicate with caustic substances, because they are unable to judge the extent of the therapy and are more likely to have poor healing.[10]

Nonpharmacologic Therapy

Patients should avoid scratching or biting the wart. This will prevent the development of pain or bleeding and will reduce the spread of the virus. Patients should not share personal items such as towels that have been in contact with the wart. Watchful waiting in children is appropriate since 60% of untreated warts will disappear within two years.[9,10] However, warts can enlarge and multiply if untreated.[10]

A benign treatment for periungual (around the nails) warts that avoids damage to the nail bed from chemicals or cryosurgery, is adhesive tape ("wart tape") therapy.[50] This is accomplished by wrapping several layers of waterproof adhesive tape around the

Table 9: **Characteristics and Differential Diagnosis of Warts**[9-11]

Condition	Distribution	Lesion	Differential diagnosis
Common warts	Hands, surrounding or beneath the nails, or sites of trauma	Flesh-toned or gray-brown papule, studded with black dots occurring singly or in groups	Callus: has skin lines. Seborrheic keratosis: greasy, pigmented (dirty yellow to black color) appearance, affects middle-aged and elderly persons. Molluscum contagiosum: a small flesh colored, firm, domed papule with a central pore indentation. A cheesy white material can be expressed. It affects primarily children and sexually active young adults. Comedone (whitehead): contents can be expressed. Occurs in the presence of other acne lesions e.g., pustules (pimples). Skin tags: flesh-colored papules that lack the roughness of warts. Squamous cell carcinoma: an asymptomatic skin-colored to reddish-brown firm tumor on damaged skin. Usually there is a central ulceration. It occurs in sun-exposed areas and appears later in life.
Flat warts	Face; backs of hands	Flat warts: reddish, smooth, flat or slightly elevated papules occurring in multiples	

affected finger and leaving it on for 6.5 days. The tape is removed for 12 hours to air dry the area then reapplied for another 6.5 days. This cycle is repeated for four to six weeks or until the virus can no longer survive in the occlusive environment and the wart disappears.[50,51]

Pharmacologic Therapy

Topical therapy is used to remove the virus-containing wart with minimal destruction of normal tissue. The type of therapy depends on the location, degree of symptoms, and the patient's immune status and cooperation. Scarring can occur with more destructive therapies. Therapy may take several weeks or months.

There is considerable lack of evidence to make a rational selection of local treatments for common warts.[52] Common warts can be self-treated topically with **salicylic acid** which has produced a cure rate of 75% compared to 48% in control groups.[52]

Salicylic acid is commercially available in a variety of strengths and dosage forms that may be combined with **lactic acid**. Generally strengths of about 17% in liquid (collodion) form are useful for common warts and multiple warts, whereas strengths of 40% as plasters are preferred for thicker skin areas such as in

plantar warts[10] (Table 10). Instructions for use can be found in the Patient Information section. A dimethyl-ether/propane mixture is available for cryotherapy. It does not appear to be effective in achieving the low temperatures necessary for cellular necrosis.[53]

Prescription Therapy

Physician-directed topical treatments include bichloracetic acid, cantharidin or liquid nitrogen. Other prescription therapies include liquid nitrogen, topical 5-fluorouracil or tretinoin. Resistant warts require cryotherapy every 10 to 14 days combined with salicylic acid or curettage and electrodessication.[49]

In extensive recalcitrant warts, a variety of other physician-directed treatment modalities have been used with limited evidence of benefits and risks. Oral cimetidine 30 to 50 mg/kg per day (usually four times daily) for up to three months may have immunomodulatory activity and some trials have suggested benefit.[54,55] Dermatologists may offer immunotherapy (induction of an allergic reaction with dinitrochlorobenzene),[52] intralesional bleomycin or laser.[48,49]

Monitoring of Therapy

Table 11 presents a monitoring framework for patients with warts.

Table 10: **Nonprescription Wart Treatment**[49]

Treatment	Common warts	Flat warts	Useful in young children	Cure rate	Pain with application	Comments
Salicylic acid liquid/ Patches	Yes	Yes	Yes	75%	No	Best supportive evidence for efficacy. Use 40% for thick areas and 17% for thin warts. Lactic acid 17% combination is useful. Assess response after 2-3 wks. Apply for up to several months. Continue treatment for 1-2 wks after clinical removal of wart to ensure complete elimination of virus. Stop treatment for a few days if treated area becomes painful and excessively irritated.

Table 11: **Monitoring Therapy for Warts**

Symptoms	Monitoring	Endpoint of therapy	Actions[50]
Wart size (treatment with salicylic acid)	**Patient:** daily, watching for dead skin and reduction in the size of the wart **Pharmacist:** review response in 2-3 wks	Reduction in the size of the wart within 2-3 wks Disappearance of the wart within 4 or more wks. Return of normal healthy skin	Pharmacist should review technique of application and evaluate dosage form if no improvement in 2-3 wks. Refer to physician if there is no improvement in the wart after 12 wks of treatment.
Wart color or shape suggesting it may not be a wart	**Patient:** daily, watching for any unexpected dramatic change in color or shape **Pharmacist:** Next visit	Disappearance of the wart/lesion	Refer patient to physician if there is any unusual change in color or shape of the lesion. Need to rule out cancers.
Bleeding after minimal trauma	**Patient:** daily **Pharmacist:** Next visit	Absence of bleeding	Refer patient to a physician if there is any unexplained bleeding. Need to rule out cancers.
Signs of infection such as redness, pain and pus	**Patient:** daily **Pharmacist:** Next visit	Absence of infection	Refer patient to a physician if signs are suggestive of a secondarily infected lesion.
Warts that are growing quickly	**Patient:** daily	Absence of enlarging or new warts	Refer patient to a physician.
Allergy	**Patient:** daily while on therapy	No allergy	Stop therapy. Refer to physician.
Irritation caused by topical agents	**Pharmacist/Physician:** next visit.	Little to no irritation that subsides with continued use	Stop therapy if no improvement after reinforcing method of application. Refer to physician.

Parasitic Infections

Lice (Pediculosis)
Pathophysiology

Lice are tiny blood-sucking insects that are specific parasites of humans. Worldwide, there are hundreds of millions of cases of pediculosis annually. Outbreaks in institutions such as schools and long-term care facilities are common. Three species of lice exist: head lice (*pediculus humanus capitis*), body lice (*pediculus humanus corporis*) and pubic lice (*phthirus pubis* or "crabs").

Lice are 1 to 3 mm long with three pairs of legs that end with claws. Head and pubic lice live on the skin, whereas body lice live in the seams of clothing. The adult female life cycle is up to 30 days and she lays 7 to 10 eggs daily. The body louse lays her eggs in clothing, while head and pubic lice lay their eggs at the base of hair shafts. These eggs are cemented to the hair in egg casings called nits. The eggs hatch 8 to 10 days later and mature into adult forms within 8 to 15 days for head and body lice, but 14 to 22 days for pubic lice. Since lice are obligate human parasites, survival time off the human host varies from 3 days for head lice, 10 days for body lice, and 24 hours for pubic lice. Nits can survive away from the human host for up to 10 days. In contrast to head and pubic lice, the body louse is a vector of a variety of human diseases such as typhus, relapsing fever and trench fever.

Transmission for head lice is by hair-to-hair contact and by fomites such as clothing or hair accessories; for pubic lice, sexual or close body contact and fomites such as bed linens and towels; for body lice, clothing and linens. Poor hygiene has a major role only in the epidemiology of body lice.[56,57]

Head Lice
Pruritus particularly around the back and sides of the scalp is the main symptom of louse infestation. Physical examination of the scalp should detect nits (eggs) attached to the base of hair shafts in the warmer parts of the scalp (back and sides). The height of the nits above the scalp indicates how long the infestation has been present on the growing hair.

Itchy papules can develop as a hypersensitivity reaction to the bites.[56,57] Secondary bacterial infection may occur as a result of scratching.

Body Lice
The body louse lives and lays eggs in the seams of clothing and usually emerges at night to take a blood meal from the host. Consequently, nocturnal pruritus is a common symptom. Erythematous papules with a central puncture point (bite sites) are evident often around the waist and axillae where seams of clothing contact the skin. Hypersensitivity reactions to the bites can develop and the resultant pruritus is accompanied by excoriations that may become secondarily infected. Lice and eggs are found in clothing seams.[57,58]

Pubic Lice
Nits attached at the base of the hair follicles are more difficult to find than with head lice. The lice may appear as small, yellow-brown to gray dots. Small brown specks on undergarments result from lice excreta. With heavy infestations, bite sites may reveal a blue-gray skin discoloration known as *maculae ceruleae*, the result of injected louse anticoagulant saliva during feeding.[9,57,58] Pruritus in the genital area is the main symptom, with hypersensitivity reaction and secondary infection also possible.

Eyelashes, eyebrows, beards and other hairy areas can also be infested. Itching, burning and eye irritation can occur when the eyelashes are involved.[58]

Goals of Therapy
- Exterminate head, body or pubic lice
- Relieve pruritus
- Prevent secondary bacterial infections
- Prevent spread of the infestation

Patient Assessment
Refer patients with recurrent or unresponsive head lice and pubic lice to a physician. Patient assessment of lice is found in Table 12.

Table 12: **Assessment of Pediculosis**[9,10,58]

	Head lice	Body lice	Pubic lice
Type of primary lesions	Papules	Papules	Papules
Type of secondary lesions	Excoriations, crusts; pustules with secondary infections	Excoriations, crusts; pustules with secondary infections	Excoriations, crusts; blue-gray pigmentation; pustules with secondary infections
Distribution of lesions and pruritus	Scalp	Waist and axillae (trunk)	Pubic area
Presence of lice or nits	Scalp hair	Seams of clothing	Pubic hair, eyelashes, eyebrows
Transmission	Head-to-head contact; sharing hats or combs	Clothing or bedding; conditions of poor hygiene	Sexual exposure to an infected person
Differential diagnosis	Dandruff Seborrheic dermatitis Accumulation of hair cosmetics	Seborrheic dermatitis Flea bites or other insect bites Eczema Impetigo Folliculitis	Seborrheic dermatitis Folliculitis Dermatophytosis
Host	Children	Persons with poor hygiene	Sexually active adults

Nonpharmacologic Therapy

Contact with infected persons promotes the spread of the infestation. Avoid sharing personal items such as clothing, combs, hats and bedding of an infected person.

Clothes, linens, scarves and hats should be dry-cleaned, washed in hot water and dried in the hot cycle, or stored in plastic bags for at least 10 days. Furniture should be vacuumed. Combs and brushes should be soaked in hot water for 5 to 10 minutes or washed with a pediculicide shampoo.[58,59]

Pharmacologic Therapy

Application of a pediculicide such as permethrin 1%, pyrethrins or lindane 1% is highly effective.[58] There is no evidence that one agent is more effective than another. The best choice depends on local resistance patterns[60,61] and safety considerations. Table 13 discusses nonprescription products available for the treatment of pediculosis.

Head Lice

For scalp and hair infestations, the pediculicide, **permethrin** 1% cream rinse applied to towel-dried hair and left on for 10 minutes is considered the drug of choice due to its low toxicity and high ovicidal activity. Although activity persists for about two weeks after the application, a second treatment 7 to 10 days later is advised.[59]

Pyrethrins with piperonyl butoxide shampoos have low ovicidal activity and no residual activity so retreatment 7 to 10 days later is necessary to kill recently hatched lice. Persons allergic to ragweed or chrysanthemum must avoid both pyrethrins and permethrin. **Lindane** 1% shampoo is applied for four minutes and repeated 7 to 10 days later. It has the highest potential for neurotoxicity upon systemic absorption and is contraindicated in persons with seizure disorders. Caution must be exercised in pregnant and lactating women, children younger than two years, and inflamed skin conditions.

Family members and close contacts should be examined and treated if infested.[59] Bedmates should be treated prophylactically.[63]

Table 13: **Nonprescription Products Used to Treat Lice and Scabies**[62]

	Pyrethrins with piperonyl butoxide	Permethrin	Lindane
Description	Pyrethrin is a fast acting insecticide extracted from chrysanthemum genus flowers.	Synthetic pyrethroid	Gamma benzene hexachloride
Treatment	Pediculosis and scabies	Pediculosis and scabies	Pediculosis and scabies
Precautions		Caution in children less than 2 mos old	Caution: children < 10 yrs old, elderly, pregnancy or lactation, seizure disorders
Efficacy	45% after first application; 94% after second application. Killing time 10-20 minutes. No residual effect so repeat treatment 7-10 days later. Sprays: uncertain efficacy for inanimate objects.	96%-100% Good ovicidal activity (70% to 80%)	67-92% Killing time 6 h. Poor ovicidal activity and has no residual effect on the hair so repeat treatment 7-10 days later in pediculosis
Kinetics	Minimal absorption Rapidly metabolized	2% systemic absorption Rapidly inactivated No active metabolites Renally excreted in 72 h	10% systemic absorption and accumulates with repeated exposures
Contraindications	Allergies to ragweed, Chrysanthemum, or petroleum products which may lead to cross-sensitivity.	Allergies to ragweed and chrysanthemum which may lead to cross-sensitivity	Patients with extensively excoriated skin, elderly and children may have enhanced percutaneous absorption and increased potential for toxicity.
Side effects	Contact dermatitis due to the petroleum distillates used for solvent purposes in the formulation	Mild, transient itching, redness and swelling. Uncommon adverse effects include burning, stinging, rash, tingling, and numbness	Slight local irritation. Neurotoxic (dizziness, nausea, vomiting, hallucinations, abnormal movements, seizures)

After treatment, nits will remain attached to the hair. This is primarily a cosmetic concern since dead nits cannot spread the infestation. Several methods of removing nits have been suggested. The glue by which nits are attached can be loosened by either soaking the hair with **white vinegar** (3% to 5% acetic acid) then wrapping the hair in a towel (soaked in the vinegar) for 30 to 60 minutes, or by applying a commercial **formic acid 8%** rinse (e.g., Step-2®). Although the clinical benefit has not been documented[64], the nits may then be more easily removed with a fine-tooth nit comb.[59]

A combing method known as "BugBusting" requires combing of wet hair for 30 minutes every third or fourth day using a fine-toothed comb. This method is considered unfeasible to implement and there is no evidence to support its effectiveness.[60,65]

Control measures for outbreaks of head lice in schools that included the "no-nit" policy requiring children be free of nits before returning to school have not been effective in preventing spread of the infestation. Consequently, it is recommended that parents of the affected child be notified, that the child not be sent home early but merely treated with an effective pediculicide that evening and return to school the next morning.[57,59]

Treatment Failures of Head Lice
Several cases of *pediculosis capitis* resistant to permethrin 1% and to lindane have been reported. When a

properly applied treatment fails, try switching to a product of a different pharmacologic class.[57] A number of alternative therapies have been investigated for difficult cases unresponsive to the usual agents. Permethrin 5% cream left on the hair overnight covered with a plastic shower cap[66] or prescribed oral ivermectin 200 µg per kilogram (available through the Special Access Program in Canada)[67] or the combination of oral co-trimoxosole 10 mg/kg per day (usually twice daily for 10 days) plus permethrin 1% applied for 10 minutes on day 1 and day 7 may be effective for cases resistant to all topical pediculicides.[68] Itching caused by an inflammatory response to the pediculicide may persist for several days after treatment. An oral antihistamine or topical corticosteroid (e.g., hydrocortisone 0.5% cream) may be required for relief.[59]

An acetomicellar complex of acetic acid, citronella oil and camphor is available for the treatment of lice; its efficacy may require further study.

Pubic Lice

The pediculicides used to treat head lice are effective for pubic lice with retreatment in seven to ten days.

If eyelashes are infested, nits and lice can be removed with tweezers, followed by an application of white petrolatum two to four times daily for 10 days to asphyxiate the remaining lice.[56] More data are needed to determine the efficacy of occlusive agents such as petroleum jelly, olive oil or mayonnaise.[59] Sexual contacts should be treated if infested. Again, itching caused by the pediculicide can be treated with an oral antihistamine or topical corticosteroid.[59]

Body Lice

Pediculicides are unnecessary. Simple hygienic measures, including bathing and laundering of infested clothing and linens in hot water, are effective management. Alternative strategies for items that cannot be washed are drycleaning or storing them in a sealed plastic bag for at least 10 days.[58,59]

Alternative Therapy

Several alternative therapies used as pediculicides can be found in Table 14. There is no adequate clinical evidence of efficacy for any of these herbs.[65,70]

Monitoring of Therapy

After treatment of head and pubic lice, the dead nits will still be attached to the hair. They can be removed with fingertips, tweezers or a fine-toothed (nit) comb. Observe for any recurrence of lice and nits. Refer patients with recurrent or unresponsive head lice and pubic lice to a physician.

For body lice infestations, inspect clothing and other personal items for the presence of lice.

A secondary bacterial skin infection with redness and pus may develop and may require topical antibacterial treatment. A monitoring plan for patients with pediculosis can be found in Table 15.

Scabies
Pathophysiology

Scabies is a highly contagious infestation of the skin with the human mite, *Sarcoptes scabiei var hominis*. Women have a higher number of infestations than men but the highest prevalence is seen in children under two years of age. Epidemics occur in poor living conditions and in institutions.

Scabies infestations are most commonly transmitted by close personal contact, particularly sexual contact. Spread by fomites such as furniture and towels is rare. The impregnated female mite, which has a rounded body and four pairs of legs, burrows (i.e., creates a tunnel) into the epidermis and lays two or three eggs daily. Three or four days later, the eggs hatch into larvae that travel from the burrow to the skin surface where they mature into adult mites within 14 to 17 days. The smaller male mite lives predominantly on the skin surface and dies shortly after mating with the female mite. The adult female has a life span of about 30 days.[56,57,73]

With a first infection, pruritus, which is worst at night, occurs after several weeks as a result of sensitization to the mites, eggs or feces. After a reinfestation, pruritus may occur within 24 hours. Burrows (silvery lines) may be apparent and an immune response to the scabies mite results in erythematous papules on the trunk. The face and scalp are spared in adults but unfortunately not in infants and young children. Scratching leads to excoriations that may become

Table 14: **Herbal Treatments Listed as Scabicides and Pediculicides**[69]

Herb	Proposed action/ Effect(s)	Dosage/Form	Adverse reaction(s)	Comments
Anacyclus pyrethrum (root)	Stimulates skin nerve endings resulting in redness and irritation	No precise information is available	Skin irritation	
Anamirta cocculus (*Cocculus indicus*) (ripe, dried fruit)	Stimulates the parasympathetic nervous system if absorbed	Was used as a powder for scabies. 1-5 mg orally is used in dizziness	Vomiting, headaches, central nervous system depression, spastic twitching	Very poisonous. 2-3 cocculus kernels can be fatal.
Chrysanthemum cinerariifolium (Pyrethrum) (flowers)	Neurotoxic effect on the sodium canal of insects	External application of a liquid extract. Rinse after use.	Limited toxicity when up to 2 g of the drug are ingested	Overdose results in headache, tinnitus, nausea, paresthesias, respiratory disturbances.
Delphinium staphisagria (Stavesocre) (ripe dried seeds)	Actions similar to aconitine	Ointments and washes for lice are available	Redness, contact dermatitis	Oral ingestion (especially extracts made from seeds) is poisonous – cardio-pulmonary collapse
Knautia arvensis (Field scabious) (stem and flower)	Astringent, antiseptic properties	30 g in 1 L of water – applied externally for scabies	No health hazards are known	
Lawsonia inermis (Henna) (pulverized leaves, fruit and bark)	Astringent and antibacterial effects	External preparations are used for scabies (strength not available)	Health risks not recorded	Stomach complaints if ingested orally
Melaleuca alternifolia (Tea tree oil)	Antimicrobial, anti-septic properties	External preparations for lice and scabies	Local irritation, allergic contact dermatitis	Not to be taken orally
Piper nigrum (Black pepper) (berries and dried fruit)	Antimicrobial and insecticidal effects	External preparations for scabies (strength not available)	External irritant. No health hazards are known.	
Ranunculus sceleratus (Poisonous buttercup)	Skin and mucous membrane irritant	Available as a tincture for topical use in scabies	Extended skin contact can cause blisters and is irritating	Overdose with internal use has resulted in death from asphyxiation.

secondarily infected leading to pustules.[54,66,73] (See photo on page PS-4.)

Immunocompromised hosts such as patients with HIV infection, institutionalized persons or pregnant women may develop an atypical, hyperkeratotic and more contagious form of scabies called crusted scabies (also referred to as Norwegian scabies). Patients present with pronounced scaling of the hands and feet or may be generalized. Pruritus is minimal where burrows and erythematous papules are less common. Infested persons have huge numbers of mites (e.g., 2 million) compared with 20 mites with the classic type of scabies.[74,75]

Goals of Therapy

- Exterminate the scabies mite
- Relieve the pruritus

Table 15: **Monitoring Therapy for Pediculosis**[71,72]

Symptoms	Monitoring	Endpoint of treatment	Actions
Detection of live lice	**Patient:** daily for 2 wks	Absence of live lice after 10 min of applying pediculicide	Treat again with pediculicide
Presence of nits	**Patient:** daily for 2 wks	Absence of nits	Vinegar, formic acid, nit comb to physically remove dead nits
Pruritus	**Patient:** daily for 2 wks	Relief of pruritus	Oral antihistamines, topical corticosteroids
Inflammatory pustules	**Patient:** daily for 2 wks	Clearing of any lesions and return to normal appearance of the skin within one week of treatment	If mild, topical antibiotics (e.g., mupirocin). If unresponsive or extensive, refer patient to a physician as systemic antibiotics may be necessary.

- Prevent secondary bacterial infections
- Prevent the spread of the infestation

Patient Assessment[9,10,76]

Intense pruritus that worsens at night is the most common presenting symptom. Affected patients exhibit silvery lines known as burrows on the hands (especially the web spaces), flexor surfaces of the wrists and genitalia, but occasionally other sites such as the axillae, buttocks and nipples may be involved. Papules may be present on the trunk. Children may have atypical lesions but they are often concentrated on hands, feet, scalp and body folds.[77] Table 16 provides characteristics and differential diagnosis of scabies.

Suspect scabies in all patients with a pruritic rash, especially if it worsens at night. Papules appearing on the genitalia and breasts when other household members have similar signs and symptoms strengthen the diagnosis. However, a definitive diagnosis should be made by a physician prior to treatment.[78]

Nonpharmacologic Therapy

Clothes and linens should be washed in soap and hot water (60°C), drycleaned or stored in plastic bags for five to seven days. All surfaces, rugs, furniture and unwashable items should be vacuumed. The mite does not survive off the skin for more than two days. Avoid body contact with others until completion of treatment and follow-up.

Pharmacologic Therapy

Infested persons and their close physical contacts from the previous two months should be treated at the same time, whether or not symptoms are present.

Table 16: **Characteristics and Differential Diagnosis of Scabies**[9,10,76]

Condition	Lesions	Distribution	Differential diagnosis
Scabies	Primary lesions are linear or wavy burrows (2-5 mm long) with papules and vesicles near burrows. Secondary lesions as a result of excessive scratching are excoriations or eczema. Secondary infections with impetigo or pustules are possible.	Fingerwebs, wrists, sides of hands and feet, axilla, groin, breasts, belt line	Flea or insect bites: lesions are usually single or multiple papules. Atopic dermatitis: distribution is behind knees or in fold of elbows. Seborrheic dermatitis: scales in a distribution involving the scalp and face. Impetigo: exhibits honey-colored exudates and crusting. This may appear as a secondary infection.

A topical scabicide should be applied to the entire body including face and scalp after a tepid bath or shower and drying. Clean clothing is then put on. The scabicide must be washed off after 12 hours.[79]

Permethrin 5% may be more effective than other scabicides[80] and has reduced systemic absorption.[81] Currently it is the preferred treatment for adults and children older than two months of age. **Lindane** 1% has caused convulsions when used on patients with extensive skin disease and in children. Permethrin and lindane are more effective than crotamiton and probably sulfur.[80]

The preferred treatment in pregnancy, lactation and children less than two months old is **precipitated sulfur 6% in petrolatum**.[16] For three days, the preparation is applied daily after a bath and left on for 24 hours. It has the disadvantages of unpleasant odor and local irritation.[82]

Prescription Therapy
Crusted scabies is more difficult to treat and the failure rate is significant with the usual treatments. Oral ivermectin 200 μg/kg as a single dose combined with topical permethrin 5% cream may be effective for crusted scabies (Norwegian scabies).[83] Early reports of deaths in elderly people using this combination of medications[84] have not been confirmed. Currently ivermectin is reserved for special forms of scabies not eradicated with approved agents.

Monitoring of Therapy[9,10]
The appearance of new burrows at any stage after treatment is an indication for further treatment. Itch can persist for several weeks and may be relieved with topical corticosteroids, and/or oral antihistamines. Mites separated from the host die in 72 hours. Table 17 presents a monitoring plan for patients with scabies.

Suggested Readings

Anon. Drugs for head lice. *Med Lett* 1997;39:6-7.

Baddour LM. Impetigo, folliculitis, furunculosis, and carbuncles. *UpToDate* 2001. Available at: http://www.utdol.com.

Chosidow O. Scabies and pediculosis. *Lancet* 2000; 355:819-27.

Crissey JT. Dermatophyte (tinea) infections. *UpToDate* 2001. Available at http://www.utdol.com.

Crissey JT. Pediculosis. *UpToDate* 2001. Available at: http://www.utdol.com.

Crissey JT. Scabies. *UpToDate* 2001. Available at: http://www.utdol.com.

Goldstein BG, Goldstein AO. Cutaneous warts. *UpToDate* 2001. Available at: http://www.utdol.com.

Gupta AK, Einarson TR, Summerbell RC, Shear NH. An overview of topical antifungal therapy in dermatomycoses. *Drugs* 1998;55:645-74.

Table 17: **Monitoring Therapy for Scabies**[9,10]

Symptoms	Monitoring	Endpoint of treatment	Actions
Burrows	**Patient:** daily for the following 2 wks **Pharmacist:** Next visit	Clearing of burrows over the following 2 wks and return to normal skin appearance	If new burrows are detected, then retreatment with a scabicide is necessary. Ensure nonpharmacologic measures are utilized.
Papules	**Patient:** daily for the following 2 wks **Pharmacist:** Next visit	Clearing of papules and return to normal skin appearance	If new papules are detected, then retreatment with a scabicide is necessary. Ensure nonpharmacologic measures are utilized.
Pruritus	**Patient:** daily for several wks **Pharmacist:** Next visit	Itching should resolve within several (2-3) wks	If itching persists, refer patient to a physician.
Pustules, impetigo	**Patient:** daily for several wks **Pharmacist:** Next visit	This secondary infection should improve with 3 days of antibacterial (mupirocin) treatment.	If no improvement or getting worse within 3 days of treatment, refer patient to a physician.

Noble SL, Forbes RC, Stamm PL. Diagnosis and management of common tinea infections. *Am Fam Physician* 1998;58:163-74.

O'Dell ML. Skin and wound infections: an overview. *Am Fam Physician* 1995;57:2424-32.

References

1. Dale DC, ed. *Scientific American Medline* SAM-CD. Seattle: Scientific American; 1998.
2. Baddour LM. Primary skin infections in primary care: an update. *Infect Med* 1993;10:42.
3. Hayden GF. Skin diseases encountered in a pediatric clinic. *Am J Dis Child* 1985;139:36-8.
4. Lewis LS. Impetigo. *eMed J* May 25, 2001;2(5).
5. Park R. Impetigo. *eMed J* June 27, 2001;2(6).
6. Ratz J, Ward DB. Impetigo. *eMed J* Sept 9, 2001;2(9).
7. Baddour LM. Impetigo, folliculitis, furunculosis, and carbuncles. *UpToDate* 2001. http://utdol.com/application/topic.
8. Amagai M, Matsuyoshi N, Wang ZH et al. Toxin in bullous impetigo and staphylococcal scalded skin syndrome targets desmoglein 1. *Nat Med* 2000;6:1275.
9. Hooper BJ, Goldman MP. *Primary Dermatologic Care.* St. Louis: Mosby; 1999.
10. Goldstein BG, Goldstein AO. *Practical Dermatology.* 2nd ed. 1997;71-7.
11. Lookingbill DP, Marks JG. *Principles of Dermatology.* 3rd ed. Philadelphia, PA: Saunders; 2000.
12. Ontario Anti-infective Review Panel. *Anti-infective Guidelines for Community-acquired Infections.* 3rd ed. Toronto; 2001.
13. Ho VC. Bacterial skin infections In: Gray J, ed. *Therapeutic Choices.* 3rd ed. Ottawa: Canadian Pharmacists Association; 2000.
14. Britton JW, Fajardo JE, Krafte-Jacobs B. Comparison of mupirocin and erythromycin in the treatment of impetigo. *J Pediatr* 1990;117:827.
15. Sutton JB. Efficacy and acceptability of fusidic acid cream and mupirocin ointment in facial impetigo. *Curr Ther Res* 1992;51:673-8.
16. Gilbert DN, Moellering RC, Sande MA. *The Sanford Guide to Antimicrobial Therapy.* 31st ed. Hyde Park, VT: Antimicrobial Therapy: 2001.
17. Kumar A, Murray DL, Hann CB et al. Comparative study of cephalexin hydrochloride and cephalexin monohydrate in the treatment of skin and soft tissue infections. *Antimicrob Agents Chemother* 1998;32:882.
18. Demidovich CW, Wittler RR, Rugg ME, Bass JW, Browning WC. Impetigo: current etiology and comparison of penicillin, erythromycin and cephalexin therapies. *Am J Dis Child* 1990;144:1313-5.
19. Rhody C. Bacterial infections of the skin. *Primary Care; Clin Off Pract* 2000;27.
20. Sosin DM, Gunn RA, Ford WL, Skaggs JW. An outbreak of furunculosis among high school athletes. *Am J Sports Med* 1989;20:403.
21. *Furuncle; Carbuncle.* November 2001. Available at: http://www.dynamicmedical.com.
22. Wright RC. Traumatic folliculitis of the legs. A persistent case associated with use of a home epilating device. *J Am Acad Dermatol* 1992;27:771-4.
23. Raz R, Miron D, Colodner R, Staler Z, Samara Z, Keness Y. A 1-year trial of nasal mupirocin in the prevention of recurrent staphylococcal nasal colonization and skin infection. *Arch Intern Med* 1996;156(10):1109-12.
24. Levy R, Shriker O, Porath A et al. Vitamin C for the treatment of recurrent furunculosis in patients with impaired neutrophil functions. *J Infect Dis* 1996;173:1502.
25. Klempner MS, Syrt B. Prevention of recurrent staphylococcal skin infections with low-dose oral clindamycin therapy. *JAMA* 1988;260:2682.
26. Crissey JT. Dermatophyte (tinea) infections. *UpToDate* 2001. www.utdol.com. Accessed April 2001.
27. Noble SL, Forbes RC, Stamm PL. Diagnosis and management of common tinea infections. *Am Fam Physician* 1998;58: 163-74.
28. Zuber TJ, Baddam K. Superficial fungal infection of the skin. Where and how it appears help determine therapy. *Postgrad Med* 2001;109:117-32.
29. Rupke SJ. Fungal skin disorders. *Primary Care; Clin Off Pract* 2000;27.
30. Berg D, Erickson P. Fungal infections in children. New developments and treatments. *Postgrad Med* 2001;110:83-94.
31. American Academy of Dermatology. Guidelines of care for superficial mycotic infections of the skin: tinea corporis, tinea cruris, tinea faciei, tinea manuum, and tinea pedis. *J Am Acad Dermatol* 1996;34:282-7.
32. American Academy of Dermatology. Guidelines of care for superficial mycotic infections of the skin: tinea capitis and tinea barbae. *J Am Acad Dermatol* 1996;34:290-4.
33. Crawford F, Hart R, Bell-Syer S, Torgerson D, Young P, Russell I. Topical treatments for fungal infections of the skin and nails of the foot. (Cochrane Review). In: *The Cochrane Library.* 1. Oxford: UpdateSoftware; 2000.
34. Hart R, Bell-Syer S, Crawford F, Torgerson D, Young P, Russell I. Systematic review of topical treatments for fungal infections of the skin and nails of the feet. *BMJ* 1999;319: 79-82.
35. Shear NH, Einarson TR, Arikian SR et al. Pharmacoeconomic analysis of topical treatments for tinea infections. *Pharmacoeconomics* 1995;7:251-67.
36. Gupta AK, Einarson TR, Summerbell RC, Shear NH. An overview of topical antifungal therapy in dermatomycoses. A North American perspective. *Drugs* 1998;55:645-74.
37. Gupta AK, Sauder D, Shear N. Antifungal agents: an overview. Part I. *J Am Acad Dermatol* 1994;30:677-98.
38. Gupta AK, Sauder D, Shear N. Antifungal agents: an overview. Part II. *J Am Acad Dermatol* 1994;30:911-33.
39. Patel JM, Blankenship R. Ringworm, body. *EMed Consumer J,* April 12, 2001;2(4).
40. Evans EGV. A comparison of terbinafine 1% cream given for one week with clotrimazole 1% cream given for four weeks in the treatment of tinea pedis. *Br J Dermatol* 1994;130:2-4.
41. Faergemann J. Pityriasis versicolor. *Semin Dermatol* 1993; 12:276.
42. Savin R. Diagnosis and treatment of tinea versicolor. *J Fam Pract* 1996;43:127-32.
43. Lange DS, Richards HM, Guarnieri J et al. Ketoconazole 2% shampoo in the treatment of tinea versicolor: a multicenter, randomized, double-blind, placebo-controlled trial. *J Am Acad Dermatol* 1998;39:944-50.
44. Faergemann J. Treatment of pityriasis versicolor with a single dose of fluconazole. *Acta Derm Venereol* 1992;72:74-5.
45. Hickman J. A double-blind, randomized, placebo-controlled evaluation of short-term treatment with oral itraconazole in

patients with tinea versicolor. *J Am Acad Dermatol* 1996; 34:785.

46. American Academy of Dermatology. Guidelines of care for superficial mycotic infections of the skin: mucocutaneous candidiasis. *J Am Acad Dermatol* 1996;34:110-5.

47. Gardiner R, Kemper KJ. Herbs in pediatric and adolescent medicine. *Pediatric Rev* 2000;21:44-56.

48. *Cutaneous Manifestations of Human Papilloma Virus.* Available at: http://telemedicine.org/warts/cutmanhpv.htm. Accessed June 13, 2001.

49. Goldstein BG, Goldstein AO. Cutaneous warts. *UpToDate.* 2001. Available at: http://www.utdol.com/application/ topic/print.asp?file =pri_derm/8201.

50. Eidenberg ME, Sheridan BJ. Warts. *EMed Consumer J,* Feb 24, 2001;2(2).

51. *Verruca Vulgaris.* www.dynamicmedical.com. Updated Nov 23, 2001.

52. Gibbs S, Harvey I, Sterling JC, Stark R. Local treatments for cutaneous warts. In: *The Cochrane Library.* 4. 2001.

53. Sterling JC, Handfield-Jones S, Hudson PM. Guidelines for the management of cutaneous warts. *Br J Dermatol* 2001; 144:4-11.

54. Orlow SJ, Paller A. Cimetidine therapy for multiple viral warts in children. *J Am Acad Dermatol* 1993;28:794.

55. Glass AT, Solomon BA. Cimetidine therapy for recalcitrant warts in adults. *Arch Dermatol* 1996;132:680.

56. Angel TA, Nigro J, Levy ML. Infestations in the pediatric patient. *Pediatr Clin North Am* 2000;47(4):921-35.

57. Chowsidow O. Scabies and pediculosis. *Lancet* 2000;355: 819-27.

58. Crissey JT. Pediculosis. *UpToDate* Online. April 2001. Available at: http://www.uptodate.com.

59. Pickering LK, ed. *2000 Red Book: Report of the Committee of Infectious Diseases.* 25th ed. Elk Grove Village, IL: American Academy of Pediatrics; 2000

60. Dodd CS. Interventions for treating headlice. In: *The Cochrane Library.* 1. Available at: http://www.update-soft-ware.com/abstracts. Accessed May 27, 2001.

61. Burgess I. Head lice. What are the effects of treatment for head lice? Insecticide based pharmaceutical products. *Clinical Evidence. BMJ* [serial online]. Jan 2001; Issue 6.

62. McEvoy, GK ed. *AHFS Drug Information.* Bethesda, Md: American Society of Health System Pharmacists; 2001.

63. Infectious Diseases and Immunization Committee. Canadian Paediatric Society. Head lice infestations. A persistent itchy 'pest'. *Pediatr Child Health* 1996;1(3):237-40.

64. Burkhart CN, Burkhart CG, Pchalek I, Arbogast J. The adherent cylindrical nit structure and its chemical denaturation in vitro: an assessment with therapeutic implications for head lice. *Arch Pediatr Adolesc Med* 1998;152:711-2.

65. Burgess I. Headlice. What are the effects of treatment for head lice? Mechanical removal of lice or viable eggs by combing. *Clinical Evidence. BMJ* [serial online]. Jan 2001; Issue 6.

66. Schachner LA. Treatment resistant head lice: alternative therapeutic approaches. *Pediatr Dermatol* 1997;14:409-10.

67. Burkhart CN, Burkhart CG. Another look at ivermectin in the treatment of scabies and head lice. *Int J Dermatol* 1999; 38:235.

68. Hipolito RB, Mallorca FG, Zuniga-Macaraig ZO, Apolinaro PC, Wheeler-Sherman J. Head lice infestation: single drug versus combination therapy with one percent permethrin and trimethoprim/sulfamethoxazole. *Pediatrics* 2001;107:E30.

69. Gruenwald J, Brendler T, Juenicke C. *PDR Physicians Desk Reference for Herbal Medicines.* Montvale, NJ: Medical Economics; 1998.

70. Burgess I. Head lice. What are the effects of treatment for head lice? Herbal treatments and aromatherapy. *Clinical Evidence. BMJ.* [serial online]. Jan 2001; Issue 6.

71. Stichele RHV, Dezeure EM, Gogaert MG. Systematic review of clinical efficacy for topical treatments for head lice. *BMJ* 1995;311:604-8.

72. Meinking TL, Entzel P, Villar ME, Vicaria M, Lemard FA, Porcelain SL. Comparative efficacy of treatments for pediculosis capitis infestations. Update 2000. *Arch Dermatol* 2001;137:287-92.

73. Crissey JT. Scabies. *UpToDate* 2001. Oct 10, 2000. Available at: www.uptodate.com.

74. Walton FW, McBroom J, Mathews JD, Kemp DJ, Currie BJ. Crusted scabies: a molecular analysis of Sarcoptes Scabiei variety hominis populations from patients with repeated infestations. *Clin Infect Dis* 1999;29:1226-30.

75. Molinaro MJ, Schwartz RA, Janniger CK. Scabies. *Cutis.* 1995;56:317-21.

76. Malerba A, Kauffman CL. Scabies. *EMed J* Nov 20, 2001; 2(11).

77. Canadian Paediatric Society Statement. Scabies management. *Pediatr Child Health* 2001(6)10:775-8.

78. Potts J. Eradication of ectoparasites in children. How to treat infestations of lice, scabies and chiggers. *Postgrad Med* 2001;110:57-64.

79. Clinical Effectiveness Group. Association for Genitourinary Medicine and Medical Society for the Study of Venereal Diseases. National guideline for the management of scabies. *Sex Transm Infect* 1999;75(suppl 1):S76-7.

80. Walker G, Johnstone P. Scabies. What are the effects of topical treatments? Permethrin; gamma benzene hexachloride; crotamiton; Sulphur compounds. *Clinical Evidence. BMJ* [serial online]. May 2000.

81. Franz TJ, Lehman PA, Franz SF, Guin JD. Comparative percutaneous absorption of lindane and permethrin. *Arch Dermatol* 1996;132:901-5.

82. Goldstein BG, Goldstein AO, eds. *Practical Dermatology.* 2nd ed. St. Louis, MO: Mosby; 1997:58.

83. Chouela EN, Abeldano AM, Pellerano G. Equivalent therapeutic efficacy and safety of ivermectin and lindane in the treatment of human scabies. *Arch Dermatol* 1999;135:651-5.

84. Barkwell R, Shield S. Deaths associated with ivermectin treatment in scabies. *Lancet* 1997;349:1144-5.

Patient Information adapted from the following references:

85. Goldstein BG, Goldstein AO, eds. *Practical Dermatology.* 2nd ed. St. Louis, MO: Mosby; 1997.

86. Hooper BJ, Goldman MP, eds. *Primary Dermatologic Care.* St. Louis, MO: Mosby; 1999.

87. Edwards L, ed. *Dermatology in Emergency Care.* New York: Churchill Livingstone; 1997.

88. Epstein E. *Common Skin Disorders.* Philadelphia, PA: Saunders; 2001.

89. *Information on Kids Health.* Available at: http://www. kidshealth.org.

90. *Patient Education Handouts – MD Consult.* Available at: http://home.mdconsult.com.

91. *American Academy of Dermatology Patient Information.* Available at: http://www.aad.org/pamphlets.

92. *Information from Your Family Doctor.* Available at: http:// www.familydoctor.org.

Impetigo—Patient Information

What is impetigo?

- Impetigo is a contagious skin infection that commonly affects the nose and mouth area of children. It can also affect other parts of the body, usually where the skin has been damaged such as insect bites or scrapes. Adults can also get impetigo.
- It starts as little oozing round spots (blisters) that grow larger every day. The oozing fluid dries up to form a crust that looks like honey. Another less common form of impetigo is a very large blister.

How do we get impetigo?

- Impetigo is caused by one or two bacteria called *Staphylococcus aureus* ("staph") and *group A Streptococcus* ("strep"). It is spread by touching the infected skin or sharing towels or linens.

What are the symptoms?

- Impetigo infects the upper layer of the skin and may cause a little itching. It is generally not painful.

How is impetigo treated?

- If there are only a few small spots, impetigo can be treated with a topical antibiotic ointment called mupirocin. It should be applied three times daily until healed. This may take five to seven days. Other over-the-counter topical antibiotics are not effective.

- If there are thick crusts, remove them before applying the antibiotic ointment. Apply warm compresses (a clean facecloth soaked in warm soapy water or saline) to the area for 10 to 15 minutes then, gently scrub off the crust.
- Cover the draining sores with gauze and tape to avoid spreading the infection.
- See your doctor if the impetigo is more than just a few small spots; you may need oral antibiotic treatment.

How can we prevent the spread of impetigo?

- Avoid close contact with people who have impetigo.
- After two days of antibiotic treatment, the impetigo will no longer be contagious.
- Wash and change clothes, towels and bedding daily for the first two days of antibiotic treatment.
- Keep any scratches or cuts on other areas of the body very clean and covered with bandages.
- Tell children not to touch or pick the sores or the infection may spread.

When should I see my doctor?

- If the skin does not begin to heal after three days of treatment.
- If a fever develops.
- If the infected area worsens with redness, warmth or pain.

Boils (Furuncles and Carbuncles)—Patient Information

What are boils?

- Boils or furuncles are skin infections that cause painful, red, pus-filled swellings surrounding the base of hair strands. Carbuncles are very large boils or groups of boils that are the result of a spread of the infection.

How do we get boils?

- Boils are caused by a bacteria called *Staphylococcus aureus* ("staph") that can live harmlessly on the skin in the rectum, genitals and lining of the nose. If the skin is damaged, the bacteria can invade the hair follicle (the skin pocket where the hair strands grow) to cause an infection.
- Some people with weakened resistance to infection, such as kidney or liver disease or diabetes, are more likely to get boils.

What are the symptoms?

- The first sign of infection is a tiny white or yellow headed pimple at the base of the hair strand. This condition is called folliculitis. The infection can spread wider and deeper into the skin to cause a painful, red swelling (lump) that is about 1 or 2 cm wide. This is a boil or furuncle. After several days, the center of the boil becomes soft and filled with pus. Eventually, this pus will drain and relieve the pain.
- Carbuncles cause similar but more severe symptoms than furuncles.
- Boils most commonly occur in hairy, moist areas of the body such as the back of the neck, face, armpits and buttocks.

How are boils treated?

- A furuncle can often be managed with self-treatment. Carbuncles need to be treated by a doctor.

- Apply warm compresses (a clean washcloth soaked in warm water) three times daily for 20 to 30 minutes. This will help the boil to come to a "head."
- Clean the boil with antiseptic soap and cover it with a loose gauze dressing.
- The boil will usually burst and drain on its own over several days.
- Do not squeeze the boil as this may cause the bacteria to spread into the blood and cause a more serious infection.
- Until the boil drains, it is very painful. Sometimes the boil may need opening. This is best done by your doctor.
- Carbuncles often require antibiotic treatment prescribed by your doctor.

How can we prevent the spread of boils?

- The pus is contagious and can spread to other parts of the skin or infect other people.
- Daily showering and hair washing with antibacterial soap will decrease the bacteria on the skin and lessen the chance of boils spreading.
- Wash clothes touching the boils in hot soapy water and dry in the hot cycle of the dryer.
- Wash hands after touching the boils.
- Do not share facecloths and towels.
- Topical antibiotics do not help heal boils but they may help prevent the spread.

When should I see my doctor?

- If the boil has come to a head and needs to be opened for it to drain.
- If you develop recurrent boils or other family members also develop boils.
- If the condition worsens and a fever is present.

Fungal (Tinea) Infections—Patient Information

Tinea Infections

What is a tinea infection?

- Tinea or "ringworm" are common names used to describe a variety of fungal skin infections. Different terms are used to describe the infection depending on the location of the infection. Tinea corporis is "ringworm" of the body, tinea capitis is "ringworm" of the scalp, tinea pedis is "athlete's foot," tinea cruris is "jock itch" or a groin infection.

How do we get tinea infections?

- Tinea infections are caused by a group of fungi called dermatophytes. They are normally present in soil, animals (cats and dogs) and on people. Fungi like to live where it is warm, dark and moist. Dermatophytes live harmlessly on the surface of the skin until there is a cut or scrape in the skin.

What are the symptoms?

- Tinea infections may cause mild itching. The affected skin may be light red and scaly.
- The term "ringworm" is used because the fungus infection causes ring-shaped spots that can be 1 to 2 cm in size. At the edge of these rings is a raised border that looks like a worm is under the skin. The skin in the middle of the ring looks normal. The infection spreads as the ring slowly gets bigger.
- Dermatophyte infections of the scalp (tinea capitis) may appear like dandruff with patchy scaling spots and broken stubbles of hair.
- Dermatophyte infections of the groin (tinea cruris) may cause burning and itching. The skin is often excessively moist.

How is tinea treated?

- Tinea can be treated with antifungal creams, lotions or shampoos. Examples are products containing miconazole and clotrimazole which are very effective. Tolnaftate is another example. After washing and drying the affected area, apply these creams to the rash as well as 2 to 3 cm outside its borders twice daily. Treat jock itch (tinea cruris) for two weeks and ringworm of the body (tinea corporis) for four weeks.
- If the infection involves large areas, or does not get better with topical treatment, oral antifungal medicine will be prescribed by your doctor. Infections of the nails and scalp should be treated with oral antifungals.

How can we prevent the spread of tinea?

- Keep the skin clean, cool and dry. This will discourage the fungal growth.
- Wear clean cotton clothing that allows fresh air to circulate.
- Apply powders to absorb sweat and prevent rubbing.

When should I see my doctor?

- If the ringworm continues to spread after one week of topical treatment.
- If the rash has not cleared after two weeks of topical treatment for jock itch, after four weeks for ringworm of the body.
- If the rash recurs.
- If the nails or scalp are infected, since prescription antifungals are necessary.

Warts—Patient Information

What are warts?

- Warts are small, round, hard bumps on the skin with a rough cauliflower-like surface. They may be white, pink or brown in color and may have little black specks inside. They commonly grow on fingers, hands, and soles of the feet. Warts can grow on any part of the body. They are usually painless except when they are on the bottom of the feet.

What causes warts?

- Warts are caused by a virus called the Human papilloma virus. This virus can be spread from person to person by touching the wart. Some people will get warts easily while others never do. It is not known why this happens.

How are warts treated?

- Warts are harmless and disappear in months or sometimes in two to three years without treatment. If they cause pain and bleed when bumped or cause embarrassment, treatment is available. Removal of the wart may also prevent spread to other areas of the body or to other people. Wart treatments kill the skin that contains the virus while not harming the normal skin. There are many different ways to get rid of warts.

Home Treatment

Follow these steps for treating your warts.

- Soak the wart in water for about 10 minutes. Then dry the skin lightly.
- Apply petroleum jelly to the normal skin surrounding the wart to protect it.
- Carefully apply salicylic acid to the wart. You may need to use a toothpick to apply some solutions. Let the liquid dry for five minutes.
- Cover the wart with adhesive tape. This keeps the skin moist so that the medicine will penetrate and work better.

- After 24 hours, remove the tape. The surface of the wart will have turned gray which means the chemical has started to destroy the wart. You need to remove this dead skin by filing it away with a pumice stone or emery board. Always wash your hands after touching the wart.
- Repeat this process daily until the wart is gone. This may take several weeks or even months.
- If the wart becomes sore, stop the treatment for a few days.

When should I visit my doctor?

- Warts on the face, genitals or surrounding the fingernails should be treated by your doctor.
- See your doctor if your warts are still present after eight weeks of home treatment.

What different treatments will the doctor suggest?

- There are several different chemicals that a doctor may use, such as cantharidin or trichloroacetic acid.
- Other ways of destroying warts include applying liquid nitrogen to freeze the wart, burning off the wart with electricity, cutting out the wart or removing it with a laser. Some of these treatments may be painful and leave a scar.
- Dermatologists may use methods such as interferon or bleomycin injections into the wart, to stimulate your own immune system to fight off the infecting virus.
- Several treatments may be required, but the wart will usually fall off within a few days.

Will the warts come back?

- Even though the wart looks like it is gone, the virus may still be in nearby skin. No treatment works 100% of the time. If you get more warts, treat them as before, being very careful to follow the directions. To reduce the spread of the virus, avoid scratching, biting or chewing warts.

Lice—Patient Information

What are lice?
- Lice are tiny wingless insects that live mainly on hairy parts of humans.
- There are three different kinds of lice: head lice, body lice and pubic lice. They feed on human blood. The female louse lays eggs (called nits) that attach to the base of hairs in the scalp, eyelashes, underarms and pubic area. The body louse actually lives in the seams of clothing and lays its eggs there. Eggs hatch in 8 to 10 days and eventually mature to produce more lice. Each louse lives for about a month. They can survive away from humans for several days.
- It is very common for children to get head lice. Body lice affects persons with very poor hygiene. Pubic lice occurs with infected sexual partners.

How do we get lice?
- Lice is spread by coming into close contact with someone who has lice or by sharing personal items such as combs, brushes, hats, towels and bedding of an infected person.

What are the symptoms?
- Itching in the areas where the louse bites is a common complaint. Frequent scratching may cause redness and infection with pus. You may see nits, which are tiny white dots attached to the hair. They cannot be brushed off easily.
- Pubic lice may cause the affected skin area to turn bluish gray.
- Body lice can spread serious diseases such as typhus, trench fever and relapsing fever.

Treatment of Head Lice or Pubic Lice
- A safe product is a hair rinse containing permethrin 1%. After shampooing, apply the cream rinse, leave it on for 10 minutes, then rinse thoroughly with water.
- Another useful product is a shampoo containing pyrethrins with piperonyl butoxide. Apply the medication to dry hair, leave on for 10 minutes, then add a small amount of water to lather. Rinse thoroughly with water.
- An alternate shampoo containing lindane must be used with caution as it can be absorbed and cause convulsions if used incorrectly. When it is recommended in special situations, apply lindane shampoo to dry hair, leave on for four minutes then add a small amount of water to form a lather. Rinse thoroughly with water.
- A second treatment with any of these products is recommended 7 to 10 days later to ensure the lice and any hatched eggs are gone.
- After the treatment, the dead nits will still be attached to your hair. They must be removed with your fingertips, tweezers or a fine-toothed (nit) comb. Start at the scalp and comb to the end of the hair. Clean the comb with soap and hot water after use. Wetting the hair with vinegar and water or applying a product that contains formic acid 8% may help loosen the nits for easier removal.
- Treat all family members and close contacts at the same time to prevent re-infection.
- Dryclean clothes, linens, scarves and hats, or wash them in hot water and dry in a hot cycle, or store them in plastic bags for at least 10 days. Vaccuum rugs and furniture.

Treatment of Body Lice
- Since these lice live in clothing that is in contact with the skin and are found on the skin only when they are feeding, topical treatments are not usually necessary.
- Clean clothing and other personal items thoroughly as instructed above.

When should I visit my doctor?
- If treatment fails, you should see your doctor. One of the other medications will work.
- See your doctor if you continue to have an excessive itch. It is normal to be itchy for several weeks after the treatment but you may require a steroid (hydrocortisone) cream or antihistamine for relief.
- If you develop a skin infection with redness and pus, you may need antibiotic treatment.

Scabies—Patient Information

What is scabies?

- Scabies is a skin infection caused by a small mite called *Sarcoptes scabiei*. After mating, female mites burrow into the top surface of the skin to live and lay two or three eggs daily. The eggs hatch three to four days later and mature in about 14 days to repeat the cycle. They can live for two or three days in clothing, bedding or dust.

How do we get scabies?

- Scabies is spread by coming in close contact with someone who has scabies mites, by sharing the same bed or clothing, or from sexual partners.

What are the symptoms?

- You may notice the mite's burrows as short, wavy, threadlike lines on the skin surface of the webs of the fingers, inner side of the wrists and underarms. Other areas that may be involved can be the elbows, breasts, genitals and buttocks. In infants, the face and head may be affected.
- The most disturbing symptom is itchiness that is more persistent at night or when the body is warm. You may actually be infected for several weeks before you begin to get itchy and you may continue to itch several weeks after you have been treated. This itching is caused by a sensitivity response your body has to the mite, eggs or feces in the burrow.
- Scratching the affected areas can cause skin injury leading to a bacterial infection with redness, swelling and pus.

How is scabies treated?

- There are several different lotions and creams to get rid of scabies. They are called pesticides or scabicides.
- Apply these creams or lotions to the entire skin surface from the neck down, including under the nails, and leave it on for a specified time period then wash it off. In children under two, apply the scabicide to the head as well. One treatment is usually effective. Repeating treatments may irritate the skin further.
- Permethrin 5% lotion is left on for 8 to 14 hours before washing it off.
- Lindane cream or lotion should be washed off after six hours. Avoid this product in young children, pregnant or lactating women, as it can be absorbed in dangerous amounts and cause harm.
- Crotamiton cream is applied for two nights in a row and washed off 48 hours later.
- Sulfur ointment is applied for three nights in a row then washed off on day four.

How can we prevent the spread of scabies?

- Treat all family members and close contacts at the same time even if they have no symptoms of scabies.
- Since the scabies mite can live in clothing and bedding for two or three days, be sure to wash all clothing and linens that have been in contact with the infected person during the past week.
- Items that cannot be washed should be drycleaned, dried in a hot dryer cycle or stored in plastic bags for 14 days. Vacuum rugs and furniture .

When should I visit my doctor?

- If the condition worsens you should see the doctor. Occasionally a second treatment with a scabicide is required, or you may be reinfected.
- See your doctor if the itching continues beyond a few weeks and is not being relieved with hydrocortisone 0.5% cream or oral antihistamines. The itch normally lasts for several weeks after the scabicide treatment.
- If you develop a skin infection with redness and pus, you may need antibiotic treatment.

First Aid Treatment of Skin Conditions

Dale Wright, BSP, MSc, MDE

Arthropod Bites and Stings

Pathophysiology

Arthropods include spiders, scorpions, ticks, fleas, caterpillars, centipedes, ants and flying insects such as bees, wasps, mosquitoes and flies. They may sting (e.g., bees, wasps, fire ants, scorpions), bite (e.g., spiders, ticks, centipedes, mosquitoes, ants, black flies, horse flies), emit a toxic secretion (e.g., caterpillars), or have irritant hairs (e.g., some caterpillars or spiders).[1] The most common injury is a localized, self-limiting skin reaction. Occasionally serious sequelae can result from systemic effects of envenomation or significant allergic reactions. Deaths from arthropod exposures are rare in North America and usually result from anaphylaxis.[1]

Spiders

Most spiders are venomous but few deliver sufficient venom in a human bite to cause systemic symptoms. Most spider bites cause an initial stinging sensation followed by localized swelling, tenderness, redness and sometimes itching that lasts for about two days.[1] Spiders in the widow family (*Lactrodectus* species) have a neurotoxic venom. Local piloerection and sweating at the bite site within minutes may progress to spasms of the abdomen and lower limbs, generalized sweating, headache, dizziness, nausea and vomiting.[2,3] Symptoms gradually decline over two to three days. Spiders such as the brown recluse, wolf spider and hobo spider sometimes cause localized skin necrosis at the bite site. Within eight hours, the initial red, itchy lesion may become painful, blistered and purplish in color. It may progress to a central necrosis accompanied by fever, malaise, cramps and

hematuria.[2,3] These types of spiders are usually found only in the southern-most regions of Canada.

Ticks

Ticks attach to their victims with specialized mouth parts and feed for about a week until they are engorged with blood. The most common reaction is a red papule at the bite site, but swelling, blistering, bruising, itching or secondary skin infection may develop.[4] Occasionally a neurotoxin injected by the tick can cause a serious motor neuron paralysis in children.[4] Ticks can carry diseases such as Rocky Mountain spotted fever,[3] and Lyme disease in some areas of southwestern BC and southwestern Ontario.[5] However, there are few areas in Canada that are considered even "moderate risk areas" for Lyme disease.[5] Lyme disease typically presents with a rash that expands outward from the bite site in a ring pattern. (See photo on page PS-4.) It is usually accompanied by flu-like symptoms: fever, lethargy, fatigue, headache. The most common sequela of untreated Lyme disease is arthritis. Neurologic or cardiac complications are less common.[5] Prompt removal of ticks minimizes systemic reactions and risk of tick-borne diseases.

Hymenoptera Insects

The venom of stinging insects of the order *Hymenoptera*, which includes bees, wasps, hornets and ants, contains biogenic amines (e.g., histamine, dopamine, serotonin) as well as enzymes that can cause local tissue damage.[6] While most ants cause only a minor bite wound, fire ants, found in the southern United States, are venomous.[4] The most common reaction to a sting from a hymenoptera insect is localized pain, redness and swelling that is intense for a few minutes then subsides over a few hours. Occasionally there may be an extensive local reaction with swelling over a large area (e.g., the whole limb) peaking at 48 hours and subsiding over the next week. With a subsequent sting, 10% of people with this reaction will have a more severe reaction, although only 5% will experience anaphylaxis.[7] The most serious reaction to insect stings is anaphylaxis, which has an incidence of 0.3 to 3% in the general population.[7] Within minutes, patients experience generalized warmth, flushing and itching that can progress to hives, airway edema with throat tightness and difficulty breathing, bronchospasm, and in severe cases shock with hypotension.[3,6] Multiple stings are more likely to result in serious systemic reactions because of the dose of histamine delivered.[3]

Mosquitoes

Biting insects such as mosquitoes deposit salivary secretions into the skin that commonly cause local histamine reactions with redness, swelling, and intense itchiness. Reddened, itchy papules develop within hours then subside slowly over a few days. Some people may develop antibodies that contribute to formation of large welts. Anaphylaxis is rare.[7] Systemic disease from biting insects is uncommon in Canada, but in other countries mosquitoes can carry encephalitis, malaria or yellow fever.[3]

Goals of Therapy

- Prevent bites and stings
- Provide symptomatic relief for localized reactions

Patient Assessment

Self-management is appropriate for most arthropod exposures in Canada because localized skin reactions are the most common consequence. Refer patients to a doctor for treatment of more extensive local reactions, or systemic symptoms that suggest significant envenomation. Suspect significant envenomation when a patient has suffered multiple stings from a venomous insect. Suspected anaphylaxis is a medical emergency. Note that patients on beta-blockers may have a delayed onset of anaphylaxis and respond poorly to treatment.[6] An assessment plan for patients

with arthropod bites and stings is presented in Figure 1.

Prevention

To prevent stings and bites from flying insects, people should avoid use of scented cosmetics, perfumes and hairsprays that can attract insects. Light-colored clothing is preferable to bright or dark colors.[8] Good personal hygiene may also deter mosquitoes, which are attracted to volatile compounds in sweat.[8] Electronic bug "zappers," and ultrasonic devices or plants purported to repel mosquitoes are ineffective.[8] Burning plain or citronella candles may reduce but not eliminate mosquito bites.[8] Eliminating sources of standing water, such as rain barrels, clogged gutters and bird baths is the best way to reduce the local mosquito population.[8]

People with a history of anaphylaxis to insect stings should consider physical protection with long pants, long sleeves, shoes and socks when they are in fields or grassy areas where wasps like to nest. They should wear gloves when gardening, and take care while cooking and eating outdoors.[6,7] Physical protection against insect bites with clothing or netting is also recommended for infants less than six months of age and travelers to areas where mosquito-borne illness is endemic.[9]

To protect against ticks, pants and shirts should be tight at the ankles and wrists, or tucked into socks and gloves. Light-colored clothing makes ticks more visible. A hat should be worn in areas with tall grass or brush. Prompt removal of ticks will prevent most sequelae, so daily inspection of skin in ankle, wrist and neck areas is important.[4,5]

Nonpharmacologic Therapy

The bite site should be cleaned with warm water and soap to help prevent secondary infection. Ice or cool compresses applied to the site provide symptomatic relief.[5] In addition, cold from an ice pack can reduce absorption of venom and slow tissue release of histamine. Apply ice intermittently for no more than 15 minutes at a time, to prevent frostbite. Home remedies such as baking soda poultices or toothpaste applied to the site may also help relieve symptoms, and are not toxic, although they have never been tested in clinical trials.[3,8]

Figure 1: **Assessment of Patients with Insect Stings/Bites**

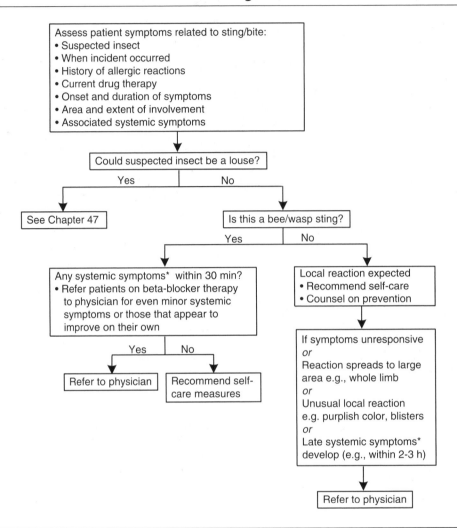

Systemic symptoms: Generalized itching, flushing, sneezing, watery eyes, hives, nausea, vomiting, muscle cramps, dizziness, fainting, hoarseness, lump in throat, difficulty breathing, changes in heart rate (faster or slower).

The bee's stinger has multiple barbs that often cause it to detach and remain in the wound.[3,6] Remove the stinger by gently scraping with a fingernail or knife blade to avoid squeezing more venom into the wound.[3] Ticks are best removed by using tweezers to pull gently on the tick until it releases. This can take 30 to 60 seconds. Methods of tick removal such as applying caustic substances, heat from a match, or occlusive substances such as petrolatum or nail polish do not work and may be harmful.[5]

Pharmacologic Therapy
Insect Repellents
Insect repellents (Table 1) can deter biting insects such as mosquitoes, black flies and ticks, but not

Table 1: Insect Repellents*[8,10-13]

Ingredient	Action	Dose/Dosage Forms	Side Effects	Comments
DEET (N,N-diethyl-m-toluamide)[8,11,12]	Vapor thought to have offensive smell or taste to insects. Effective against mosquitoes, black flies, ticks, chiggers, fleas. Duration of effect variable. 15% DEET protects about 5 h against black flies or mosquitoes. 5% DEET protects for about 2 h. Long-acting formulation lasts for about 8 h.	Concentration 5–95%. Products with lower concentrations of DEET are just as effective as higher concentrations but remain effective for shorter periods. Apply sparingly to exposed skin as needed. May apply to clothing. Cream, lotion, liquid, spray, towelette forms. Long-acting formulations now available.	Irritating to mucous membranes and open wounds. Contact dermatitis (rash, redness, itching) reported. Absorbed through intact skin. Rare reports of neurologic toxicity (lethargy, confusion, ataxia, tremors, seizures). Lower dermal absorption and toxicity with long-acting formulation.	Can damage plastics, acetate, rayon, spandex, pigmented leather, painted surfaces. Reduces effectiveness of sunscreens. Avoid excessive or prolonged use. This is the only personal repellent effective against ticks.
Soybean oil[10]	Thought to mask attractants given off by host and/or by cooling skin surface temperature. At least as effective as DEET against mosquitoes and black flies. Longer duration of effect against black flies than mosquitoes.	Concentration 2%. Apply to exposed skin as needed. Oil, lotion, spray forms. Oil form has longer lasting effect than lotion or spray.	Very low toxicity. Skin irritation reported rarely. Low potential for hypersensitivity reactions. No systemic absorption through skin.	For use against mosquitoes and black flies only. Do not use to protect against ticks.
Oil of citronella[8,11,12]	Thought to have offensive smell or taste to insects. Tested against mosquitoes only. Products registered in Canada have duration of less than 1 h.	Concentration 0.05–15%. Apply to exposed skin as needed. Oil, lotion, spray, towelette forms.	Low toxicity. Skin irritation (redness, rash, itchiness) may occur. Hypersensitivity reactions possible.	For use against mosquitoes only. Frequent reapplication needed. Currently use not recommended in children less than 2 yrs old.
Other essential plant oils (e.g., lavender, cedar, verbena, pennyroyal, pine, geranium, cajeput, cinnamon, rosemary, basil, thyme, allspice, garlic, peppermint)[8,12] Skin-So-Soft®[8]	Thought to have offensive smell or taste to insects. Tested against mosquitoes only. Limited effectiveness — oil of lavender products registered in Canada have duration of less than 30 min.	Concentrations variable. Typically found in combination. Apply sparingly as needed. Oil, lotion, spray forms. Note: Repellents under the Skin-So-Soft® brand now contain a recognized repellent, usually DEET.	Presumed to be of low toxicity but information lacking. Watch for skin irritation or local hypersensitivity reactions.	For use against mosquitoes only. Frequent application required for prolonged effect. Currently not recommended in children less than 2 yrs old due to lack of toxicity information.
Permethrin, pyrethrum[8,11]	Contact insecticide that is neurotoxic to insects causing knock-down or death. Effective against many insects, including mosquitoes and ticks. Permethrin is a synthetic pyrethroid related to the plant alkaloid pyrethrum.	Permethrin concentration 0.5%. Not for use on skin. Spray on clothing, tents, netting as needed. Spray form, mosquito coils.	Low mammalian toxicity, poor absorption through skin. May cause skin irritation (redness, burning, itchiness).	Spray on protective items for 30–45 sec until moist. Allow clothing to dry for 2–4 h before wearing. Effect maintained for at least 2 wks, even with washing.

*Repellents no longer registered in Canada for use as personal insect repellents include citronyl, dimethylphthalate, ethyl hexanediol, di-n-propyl-isocinchomeronate (MGK 326), and n-octylbicycloheptane dicarboxamide (MGK 264). Products containing these chemicals will be removed from Canadian retail outlets during 2002.[13]

stinging insects.[8,11] They must be applied to all exposed skin, since unprotected skin even close to a treated area is vulnerable to bites.[8] Repellent activity and duration of effect is highly variable, depending on the chemical and its concentration, the individual and how active they are, the environment and the insect.[11]

The most effective compound against the broadest spectrum of insects is **diethyltoluamide (DEET)**. Despite scattered case reports of neurotoxicity with DEET, when used appropriately it is considered safe in adults, including pregnant and lactating women, and children over the age of six months (See Insect Bites and Stings—Patient Information).[8,11,12] Concentrations less than 10% are preferred for children under 12 years of age. DEET should be applied no more than once a day in children less than two years of age, and up to three times a day in older children.[12] Although DEET is considered safe in pregnant and lactating women, it is prudent to use nonchemical bite prevention methods whenever possible. When DEET is required, recommend a low concentration (e.g., < 10%) applied sparingly. Microencapsulated forms of DEET are now available that provide a longer-lasting effect with lower toxicity.[8] Combination products containing DEET and sunscreens are not recommended. The application rates for the two products are different (DEET must be applied sparingly and sunscreens should be applied liberally) and DEET appears to reduce the effectiveness of sunscreens.[8]

Soybean oil is a new insect repellent approved for use against mosquitoes and black flies, but not ticks. It is as effective as DEET with very low toxicity.[10] It is safe for use on children. This is a promising product but more experience is required to determine its place in therapy.

Repellents containing **essential plant oils** such as citronella oil or lavender oil are less effective, and have a shorter duration of effect than DEET.[8] **Permethrin** is a contact insecticide that can be applied to clothing or other fabrics (e.g., netting, tents) but not skin. It is very effective against ticks and in conditions with a high density of mosquitoes and other biting insects.[8] Burning mosquito coils containing permethrin can reduce mosquito concentrations in enclosed areas. Mosquito coils are recommended as a supplement to netting at night for travelers to areas with endemic mosquito-borne illness.[9]

Symptomatic Relief

A variety of nonprescription treatments can be used to relieve symptoms from local reactions to bites and stings. For pain, consider usual doses of oral **analgesics** such as acetaminophen, ASA or ibuprofen. **Oral antihistamines** relieve acute itchiness and swelling, and can be used prophylactically to reduce the reaction to mosquito bites in sensitized individuals.[8] Effectiveness of antihistamines in relieving local symptoms of bee and wasp stings is unproven, although systemic antihistamines are an important adjunctive measure in managing systemic reactions.[3]

Topical products for symptomatic relief of bites and stings (Tables 2, 3) often contain local anesthetics, antihistamines, astringents (e.g., calamine, zinc oxide) and/or irritants (e.g., menthol, camphor, ammonia) alone or in combination.[14] It is difficult to recommend one product over another since evidence on the degree of effectiveness or comparative efficacy of topical antipruritics is lacking. Laboratory evidence is available confirming the effectiveness of pramoxine 1% lotion,[17] menthol 1% solution,[18] and hydrocortisone 2.5% cream[19] in controlling histamine-induced itch, but clinical evidence is lacking. Products are usually applied in the recommended dosage (Tables 2, 3) for two or three days until the symptoms subside.

Avoid the use of **benzocaine**, which is widely available in many first aid products, because it is a well-known sensitizer with cross-allergenicity to other ester class local anesthetics and PABA derivatives, including sulfonamides.[15] **Tetracaine** is found in a few products, but should not be used because it carries a high risk of sensitization and systemic toxicity.[14] **Lidocaine** and **dibucaine** are less likely to cause sensitization and systemic toxicity, but should be used infrequently and only for short periods to avoid development of an allergy to important parenterally administered local anesthetics.[15] **Pramoxine** is a good alternative to "caine" anesthetics for topical use because it is effective with low toxicity and sensitization potential. Topical **diphenhydramine** also should be used sparingly because it occasionally causes allergic contact dermatitis and sensitization to antihistamines of the ethanolamine class (e.g., dimenhydrinate, doxylamine).[15] Judicious use of

Table 2: **Topical Local Anesthetics**[14-16]

Anesthetic	Action	Dose/Dosage forms	Side effects	Comments
Dibucaine	Reduces conduction of sensory nerve impulses in skin resulting in reversible loss of sensation. Class: amide	Concentration 0.5-1%. Apply as needed 3-4 times daily. Ointment, cream forms	Skin irritation and sensitization possible but uncommon. High potency for systemic effects with absorption through open skin: restlessness-nervousness, tremors, twitching, nausea, vomiting.	Avoid frequent application or application to large open wounds or large areas of broken skin. Keep out of reach of children.
Lidocaine	Reduces conduction of sensory nerve impulses in skin resulting in reversible loss of sensation. Class: amide	Concentration 0.5-9.6%. Apply as needed up to 5 times a day; sprays no more than twice an hour. Ointment, cream, lotion, liquid, gel, spray forms	Skin irritation and sensitization possible but uncommon. Poor absorption through intact skin. Systemic effects possible with absorption through open skin.	Lower concentrations preferred for self-care. Avoid frequent application or application to large open wounds or large areas of broken skin. Keep all local anesthetics of amide or ester type out of reach of small children since methemoglobinemia can occur with accidental ingestion.
Pramoxine	Reduces conduction of sensory nerve impulses in skin resulting in reversible loss of sensation. Class: structurally unique	Concentration 1%. Apply as needed up to 4 times a day. Cream, lotion, gel forms	Local irritation with burning, stinging possible, especially of mucous membranes. Low sensitization potential, no cross-allergenicity.	Avoid application near eyes or nose. Preferred choice of topical anesthetic because of low potential for sensitization and low toxicity.

Table 3: **Topical Antipruritics**[14]

Ingredient	Action	Dose/Dosage forms	Side effects	Comments
Ammonia Ammonium hydroxide	Local cooling sensation from rubefacient effect (see menthol). Irritant effect contributes to local analgesia.	Concentration 3.5%. Apply sparingly as needed. Liquid form only	Skin irritation with burning, redness. Burns have occurred when topped with a dressing. Very irritating to mucous membranes and open skin. Inhalation causes sneezing, coughing.	Keep away from eyes, nose, mouth. Avoid inhaling vapors. Do not apply to abraded skin or open wounds. Do not apply under dressings.
Calamine (zinc carbonate or zinc oxide colored with ferric oxide) **Zinc oxide**	Mild astringents (protein precipitation at cell surface reduces edema, inflammation) and protectants. Soothing effect on irritated skin	Concentration 1-16%. Apply liberally as needed. Ointment, cream, lotion, pad-impregnated forms	Well-tolerated, no hypersensitivity reactions, no systemic absorption	
Camphor	Cooling sensation from rubefacient effect. Mild local analgesia and anti-itch effects from local irritant effect. Irritants stimulate local sensory nerves reducing transmission of pain signals.	Concentration 0.13-10.5% (most are < 1%). Apply sparingly as needed. Ointment, gel, liquid, lotion, pad forms	Skin irritation (burning, redness) at higher concentrations. Readily absorbed through intact and broken skin. Systemic toxicity includes nausea, vomiting, headache, dizziness, tremors.	Lower concentration products preferred. Do not apply to large areas of skin or open wounds. Keep high concentration products out of reach of small children.
Diphenhydramine	Blocks histamine H_1 receptors. Effect at sensory nerve endings reduces itching. In allergic reactions also reduces local redness, swelling.	Concentration 2%. Apply as needed up to four times daily. Cream, lotion, gel, spray forms	Hypersensitivity reactions (rash, itching, inflammation) and photoallergic dermatitis reported occasionally with topical use. Systemic absorption from skin possible, but side effects rare.	Avoid prolonged topical use to prevent sensitization. Oral administration preferred and more effective for itching.
Menthol Peppermint oil	Dilate blood vessels in skin causing cooling sensation (rubefacient). Also have local irritant effects (see camphor).	Concentration 0.2-1.3%. Apply sparingly as needed. Ointment, cream, liquid, lotion, gel, spray forms	Hypersensitivity, contact dermatitis (rash, itching) reported. Skin irritation (burning, redness) possible.	
Papain	Proteolytic enzyme that hydrolyses polypeptides. No information on action or effectiveness as an antipruritic	Concentration 3.5%. Apply as needed. Lotion form only	Skin irritation with burning, redness possible. Local hypersensitivity reactions (rash, redness, itching) have been reported.	
Phenol	Mild local analgesia and anti-itch effects from local irritant effect (see Camphor). Antiseptic at concentrations > 1%	Concentration 0.18-1.5%. Apply sparingly as needed. Ointment, liquid forms	Skin irritation with burning, itching, redness. Readily absorbed through intact and broken skin. Systemic toxicity may include CNS/CVS excitation followed by depression.	Lower concentration products preferred. Do not apply to large areas of skin. Suitable for very small minor wounds only.

combination topical first aid products is advised because these are common ingredients.

Topical **corticosteroids** (e.g., hydrocortisone 0.5%) are sometimes recommended to relieve itchiness, swelling and redness associated with mosquito bites.[7] However, a concentration of at least 2.5% hydrocortisone may be needed to effectively reduce intensity and duration of histamine-induced itch.[19] Hydrocortisone products are applied sparingly up to four times a day until itching subsides. They should be used for no longer than seven days. Avoid application to large areas of the body.

If a secondary infection appears to develop at the bite site (increasing redness, swelling, and tenderness beyond that expected for the insect), **topical antibiotics** may be applied after cleansing the area with soap and water.[3]

Prescription Treatment

Suspected anaphylaxis requires immediate referral to an emergency room for treatment with subcutaneous epinephrine, parenteral diphenhydramine, corticosteroids and supportive care as necessary.[6,7] All patients who have had an anaphylactic reaction should carry an emergency epinephrine kit.[6] Beta-blocker therapy should be avoided in these patients.[6]

Extensive local reactions to bee and wasp stings that do not respond to oral diphenhydramine may require treatment with a short course of oral prednisone.[6,7]

Although a Lyme disease vaccine is available, there are very few, if any, locations in Canada where its routine use is warranted.[5]

Table 4 provides a monitoring framework for therapy of arthropod stings and bites.

Table 4: **Monitoring Therapy for Arthropod Stings and Bites**

Symptom	Monitoring	Endpoint	Actions
Pain	**Patient:** Degree and duration of pain relief with each analgesic dose. Pain should subside within 24 h. **Health care provider:** Next visit	Pain reduced to a tolerable level	Contact a health professional if inadequate response or significant symptoms continue past 24 h.
Itching	**Patient:** Degree and duration of relief with each application. **Health care provider:** Next visit. If topical agents are inadequate, consider oral antihistamines.	Itching reduced to a tolerable level	Oral diphenhydramine considered the "gold standard". Contact a health professional if no relief with oral diphenhydramine after 48 h.
Swelling, redness	**Patient:** Inspect daily. **Health care provider:** Next visit. Swelling and redness should subside over 24-48 h.	Minimal swelling, redness	Contact a health professional if extensive swelling occurs (e.g., if whole limb is involved).
Local infection e.g., unusual swelling, redness, or tenderness at bite site, pus or fever.	**Patient:** Inspect daily. **Health care provider:** Next visit. If symptoms develop, try topical antibiotics for 48 h.	No signs or symptoms of infection	Refer to a physician if signs and symptoms of local infection do not respond to topical antibiotics within 48 h.
Suspected anaphylaxis – Mild: generalized itching, flushing, hives, sneezing Moderate: dizziness, nausea, cramps, incontinence Severe: Fainting, seizures, hoarseness, lump in throat, chest tightness, difficulty breathing, fast or slow heart beat	**Patient:** Watch for symptoms within 30 min of exposure. **Health care provider:** Ask if any symptoms within 30 min of exposure. Observe for 6 h if symptoms noted. May give oral diphenhydramine 1 mg/kg to 75 mg/dose for mild symptoms, but still refer patient.	Symptoms subside and do not recur or worsen during 6 h of observation	Refer all cases of suspected anaphylaxis to a physician for observation and management.

Minor Cuts and Wounds

Pathophysiology

A wound occurs when the skin barrier is broken from mechanical trauma. There are six main types of wounds: *abrasions* where scraping causes loss of superficial skin layers, *lacerations* where the tissue is cut or torn, *crush* injuries from the impact of an object, *punctures* with small openings of unknown depth, *avulsion* where a portion of tissue is completely removed or left hanging, and *combination* wounds.[20] Partial-thickness wounds affect the epidermis and outer dermal layers, while deeper full-thickness wounds penetrate to subcutaneous tissues such as fat, muscle or bone.[21] Blunt trauma can produce a superficial bruise or deeper hematoma from leakage of blood from small venules and arterioles.[22] Minor wounds are extremely common and have a multitude of causes including abrasions from scratching, minor household or workplace accidents, falls, sports injuries (see Chapter 37) and animal encounters.

All wounds are contaminated with bacteria to some extent, and infection is possible if the wound is not dealt with promptly. Both gram-negative and gram-positive bacteria are involved in burn wound infections.[21] Factors affecting the risk of infection include: time lapse before the wound is treated, presence and type of foreign matter in the wound, location of the wound, injury to underlying structures such as bone or muscle, and presence of devitalized tissue. Patient factors related to infection risk include age, underlying medical conditions (e.g., diabetes, peripheral vascular disease), malnutrition, smoking, obesity and drug therapy affecting the immune system.[20]

Infection and poor wound management practices can interfere with wound healing. The normal healing process begins with an immediate inflammatory reaction that brings cells and mediators to stop bleeding, remove bacteria and debris, and stimulate tissue repair. Within 24 to 48 hours, tissue repair begins with production of collagen and new blood vessels.[21] Epithelial cells start to form from the edge of the wound, and skin along the edges of the wound contracts toward the centre to try to close the wound. Epithelialization is complete by 9 to 21 days, depending on the size and depth of the wound. In four to five days, collagen forms early scar tissue that holds the

wound edges together and gives it strength. Collagen continues to remodel and strengthen the wound for up to a year or more.[20,21] Minor wounds usually heal without scarring. Large or deep wounds may leave a visible ridge or puckering of excess collagen at the healed wound site.

Goals of Therapy

- Optimize conditions for normal wound healing
- Prevent infection
- Minimize patient discomfort

Patient Assessment

Generally, superficial wounds that are fairly small and accompanied by limited bleeding are suitable for self-management. Refer patients to a physician for treatment if they have underlying medical conditions or drug therapy that put them at risk for infection or delayed healing. In addition, refer those with large or complicated wounds, such as wounds that continue to bleed, potentially deep puncture wounds, gaping wounds or those that expose fat, muscle or bone, mammalian bites, wounds with visible foreign material or dirt, and any wound causing severe pain.[20] Finally, many patients should be referred for a tetanus booster, even if they can manage the wound care themselves (see Pharmacologic Therapy). Patient assessment of minor wounds is presented in Figure 2.

Nonpharmacologic Therapy

Discomfort from bruising in closed wounds can be relieved by applying ice packs wrapped in a towel for 20-minute periods every two hours for the first day. Subsequently, application of local heat and elevation of the site are recommended for symptom relief while blood is spontaneously resorbed from tissues.[22]

For open wounds, cleaning the wound is an essential first step. It removes bacteria, foreign debris and devitalized tissue that can interfere with wound healing and lead to infection. Before cleaning a wound, patients or caregivers should always wash their hands with soap and water, avoiding soap contact with wounds on the hand.[20] The most

Figure 2: **Assessment of Patients with Minor Acute Wounds**

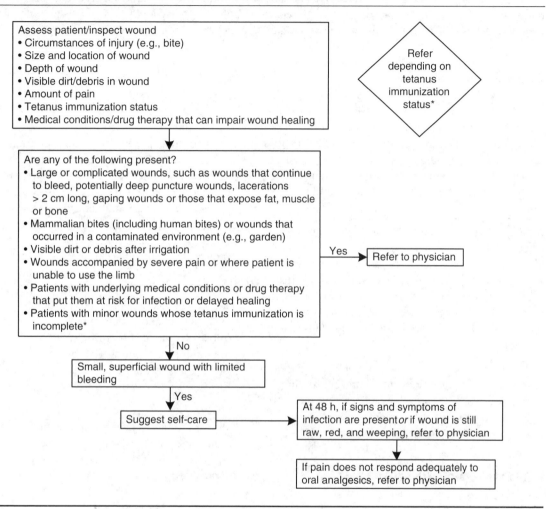

Patients with minor wounds whose tetanus immunization is incomplete (i.e., less than 3 doses), those uncertain when last tetanus shot was, or if it was known to be more than 10 years ago.

effective wound cleaning agent is tap water or normal saline applied under pressure.[20,23] Advise patients to squirt water onto the wound from a water bottle or a large syringe with no needle, hold the wound under a moderately running tap, or pour water from a cup onto the area. Visible pieces of dirt or other foreign material that remain after irrigation can be gently picked out of the wound with tweezers cleaned in rubbing alcohol or by brushing gently with clean gauze.

After cleaning, a dressing should be applied for at least 24 to 48 hours to protect the wound from contamination and prevent infection, keep the wound moist to promote healing, absorb excess wound secretions, immobilize the area and improve patient comfort.[20,21,23,24] Wounds open to air can be painful and prone to dehydration that can delay healing.[20] Most dressings have three layers: a nonadherent contact layer to prevent the wound surface from sticking and to protect the regenerating epithelium, an absorbent layer (e.g., gauze) to absorb wound secretions and provide further protection, and an outer layer to hold the dressing in place.[20] A wide variety of dressing products are available. Some contain all three layers, such as self-adhesive strips used for small wounds. Others serve one or more of these purposes and are selected based on the size and characteristics of the wound. See Dermatologic Appendix: Dressings for a discussion of dressings. Self-adhesive strips or gauze dressings held in place with tape or stretch gauze are usually sufficient for self-management of minor wounds. Applying a small amount of petrolatum or antibiotic ointment to the wound before covering it with a dressing helps prevent sticking.[20,21]

Although some specialty dressings may be left in place for days, most dressings should be changed at least daily, or more often if they appear to be dirty or wet with wound secretions. Remove blood or crusty exudates by washing gently with mild soap and water before applying a clean dressing. After 48 hours, the dressing should be removed and the wound inspected for signs of infection.

After cleaning, the edges of small cuts can be held together with skin tapes to promote healing.[23] Larger cuts where the edges won't stay together, the edges are jagged, or the wound is deep may need referral for stitches. Stitches reduce scarring.

Pharmacologic Therapy

Cleaning Agents
Antiseptics should not be used for routine wound cleaning or care. They can damage exposed tissues and interfere with the healing process, and they do not reduce the risk of infection.[20,23] Hydrogen peroxide is sometimes recommended to aid in removing dirt from wounds by its effervescent action, however, it is irritating and destroys regenerating epithelium. It may have a place in removing encrusted blood from skin around a wound or helping remove blood-soaked dressings.[20]

Antibacterials
Topical antibacterials (Table 5) have not been conclusively shown to reduce infection rates in managing minor wounds.[23] They are probably most helpful in

reducing crust formation that can interfere with wound healing, and to prevent dressings from adhering to wounds.[20] A small amount of topical antibiotic applied to the wound before the dressing prevents it from sticking.[20]

Pain Relief
Topical anesthetics (Table 2) are common ingredients in first aid products that reduce the pain of minor scrapes and cuts. As previously noted (Arthropod Bites and Stings), benzocaine and tetracaine should not be used because of the potential for sensitization (benzocaine) and systemic toxicity (tetracaine). Lidocaine and dibucaine should be used sparingly and only for a short duration of time to avoid sensitization. They should not be applied to large open wounds, which can increase their systemic absorption.[14] **Pramoxine** is an effective alternative that has low toxicity and does not cause sensitization. **Ethyl chloride** spray is available for sports-related injuries, but is of limited benefit because the duration of action is very short, about one minute, and it can cause frostbite if used inappropriately. It should never be used on open wounds or abraded skin because systemic absorption can cause liver and kidney toxicity.

Avoid oral or topical antiinflammatory drugs such as ibuprofen for acute pain relief of open wounds. They can interfere with the normal wound healing process.[20] Acetaminophen or narcotic analgesics (e.g., codeine) are preferred.

Prescription Management
Tetanus is a potential complication of any wound in those whose tetanus immunization is incomplete or has lapsed.[26] Even patients with apparently minor, clean wounds should be referred for a tetanus booster if their immunization was incomplete (i.e., less than three doses), they are uncertain when their last tetanus shot was, or if it is known to be more than 10 years ago. Patients with dirty or complicated wounds require tetanus prophylaxis if more than five years has lapsed since their last tetanus booster.[26] Rabies is usually only a consideration in bites from unprovoked animal attacks, especially where wild animals such as raccoons, skunks, foxes or bats are involved.[23]

Table 5: **Topical Antibacterials**[14,16,25]

Antibacterial	Action/Spectrum	Dose/Dosage forms	Side effects	Comments
Bacitracin	Blocks bacterial cell wall formation. Mainly gram-positive spectrum. Resistance uncommon, no cross-resistance. Activity not impaired by blood, pus, devitalized tissue.	Apply sparingly 1-3 times daily. Available in ointment, cream, or pad-impregnated forms. Available alone or in combination with polymyxin and/or neomycin to extend spectrum.	Minimal systemic absorption. Well-tolerated. Contact allergy with local pruritus, burning, redness possible. Anaphylactoid reactions with generalized itching, facial swelling, sweating, chest tightness reported but rare.	Cross-sensitivity with neomycin allergy reported.
Gramicidin	No information available on action. Mainly gram-positive spectrum.	Apply sparingly 1-3 times daily. Available in ointment or cream in combination with polymyxin.	No information available on kinetics or local side effects. Significant systemic toxicity. Damages sensory epithelium of nose.	Avoid use on broken skin. Do not apply to nasal membranes.
Mupirocin (Prescription in most provinces)	Inhibits bacterial protein and RNA synthesis. Mainly gram-positive, especially staphylococci and streptococci. Resistance uncommon, cross-resistance unlikely.	Apply sparingly 1-3 times daily. Available in ointment or cream form as a single-ingredient product only.	Minimal systemic absorption. Well-tolerated but local itching, burning, stinging, redness, dryness reported. Minimal contact allergy. Polyethylene glycol (PEG) vehicle absorbed through large open wounds and renal toxicity possible.	Avoid use in patients with renal failure or use on extensive open wounds or burns.
Polymyxin	Disrupts bacterial membranes by a surfactant-like effect. Mainly gram-negative including E.coli and species of Pseudomonas, Enterobacter, and Klebsiella. Resistance uncommon, cross-resistance not reported.	Apply sparingly 1-3 times daily. Available in ointment, cream or pad-impregnated forms. Available only in combination with bacitracin, neomycin, and/or gramicidin.	Minimal systemic absorption. Well-tolerated. Contact allergy uncommon but may cross-react in patients sensitive to bacitracin.	

Prophylactic oral antibiotics are not routinely used because they have not been shown to reduce the rate of infection from most wounds, including bite wounds.[20,23]

Monitoring of Therapy

Table 6 sets out a plan for monitoring therapy of minor cuts and wounds.

Table 6: **Monitoring Therapy for Minor Cuts and Wounds**

Sign/Symptom	Monitoring	Endpoint	Actions
Bleeding	**Patient** – Assess response after 5 min of direct pressure applied over the wound.	Bleeding significantly slows or stops within 5 min of direct pressure	Refer to a physician if blood is spurting or significant bleeding persists after 5 min of direct pressure.
Infection e.g., swelling, surrounding redness that is tender to touch, red streaks from the wound, pus or fever.	**Patient** – Inspect daily at dressing change. **Health care provider** – Follow-up at 48 h.	No signs or symptoms of infection present at 48 h.	Refer to a physician if signs and symptoms of infection are present at 48 h.
Wound healing	**Patient** – Inspect daily at dressing change **Health care provider** – Follow-up at 48 h.	Normally healing wounds appear pink or red with tiny opalescent islands of epithelium throughout and no secretions. Scab formation is a normal protective mechanism for minor wounds.	Refer to a physician if wound continues to weep, remains raw and red, or does not appear to be closing.

Burns

Pathophysiology

Burns encompass a spectrum of tissue injury with cell death and protein denaturation caused by heat (e.g., flame, scalding liquids, hot objects, gases), radiation (e.g., sunburn), electricity or chemical exposures (e.g., caustic cleaners, solvents, laboratory reagents).[27,28] The potential seriousness of the burn is related to the body location and skin thickness, type and duration of exposure, and extent of the burn.[27,28] In particular, depth of the burn impacts healing time and potential sequelae of scarring and contractures. Patient factors that increase the risk of burn wound infections or delayed burn healing include age (very young or elderly), underlying medical conditions such as diabetes or vascular disease, malnutrition, smoking and drug therapy affecting the immune system.[27,28]

Superficial burns affecting only the epidermis (e.g., sunburn) heal quickly and cause little scarring. Slightly deeper burns penetrating the upper layer of the dermis take longer to heal, but scarring is unusual. Burns involving deeper layers of the dermis and embedded appendages such as sweat glands, hair follicles, nerve endings and blood vessels have prolonged healing times and a high likelihood of scarring. Full-thickness burns in which the epidermis and dermis are both destroyed will not heal and require surgery and skin grafting to reduce scarring and contractures. Burn wound characteristics are summarized in Table 7.[27-29] Note that electrical and chemical burns can be difficult to assess because tissue damage may be deeper or more extensive than is apparent from the burn's appearance.[27] Some chemicals, such as hydrofluoric acid, can continue to cause tissue injury if not managed properly.[27]

The extent and seriousness of partial-thickness to full-thickness burns, and thus their appropriate treatment, is determined in part by estimating the total body surface area (TBSA) affected by the burn. Superficial burns are *not* included in TBSA calculations of burn wounds. Ninety-five per cent of burns treated in a clinic or emergency room fall into the minor category: < 10% TBSA burn in an adult or < 5% TBSA burn in a child, and < 2% full-thickness burn. Most of these burns can be successfully managed by a physician on an outpatient basis.

Goals of Therapy

- Minimize further damage from the suspected agent
- Promote healing that will prevent or minimize disfiguring sequelae
- Prevent infection
- Control pain

Patient Assessment

Self-management is appropriate for most superficial burns or small burns with minimal blistering (few, small blisters of limited distribution on the body). A TBSA estimation is not appropriate to guide assessment of burns for self-management, since this calculation pertains only to partial- or full-thickness burns. Refer patients with burns of any size that are more serious than the mildest partial-thickness burn (i.e., minimal blistering) to a physician. Appropriate referral minimizes the risk of infection and scarring.

Even patients who have burns with minimal blistering should be referred if they involve thin skin areas (e.g., inner surface of arm, perineum, around eyes), individuals presumed to have thin skin (e.g., children less than 5 years or adults older than 55 years), or patients with underlying conditions that put them at risk of infection or delayed healing (e.g., diabetes, chronic alcohol abuse, immunocompromised).[27,28] Electrical burns and chemical burns involving concentrated products or hydrofluoric acid should also be referred even if they appear to be minor, since the injury may be deeper than the appearance of the burn suggests.[28] Hydrofluoric acid burns may initially look innocuous but can progress to deep tissue necrosis within 24 hours. Patient assessment of burns is summarized in Figure 3.

Nonpharmacologic Therapy

To minimize further damage from the burning agent, remove clothing that is burnt, hot or contaminated by chemicals. In addition, remove jewelry from the affected area. Cooling can limit the extent of injury

Table 7: **Burn Wound Characteristics**

Category	Example	Appearance	Healing
Superficial (epidermis only)	Sunburn, very brief thermal contact or flash	Dry, red, blanches with pressure, painful	3-7 days, no scarring
Superficial partial thickness (epidermis, upper dermis)	Scald (spill, splash), brief flame, thermal contact or exposure to dilute chemicals	Moist, weeping, red, small blisters, blanches with pressure, painful	7-21 days, scarring unusual, potential pigment changes
Deep partial thickness (epidermis, deep dermis with some hair follicle, sweat gland damage)	Scald, oil or grease, flame, prolonged exposure to dilute chemicals	Wet or waxy, dry, color variable (red, patchy, white), blisters, no blanching with pressure, pain only with pressure	> 21 days, risk of scarring and contracture
Full thickness (epidermis, dermis to subcutaneous layer)	Scald (immersion), steam, flame, concentrated chemical, hydrofluoric acid, high voltage electrical	Dry, waxy white to leathery gray to charred and black, no blanching with pressure, pain with deep pressure only	Never heals spontaneously, requires surgery/grafts, very severe risk of scarring and contractures

Adapted with permission from Clayton MC, Solem LD. No ice, no butter. Advice on management of burns for primary care physicians. *Postgrad Med* 1995;97(5):151-5, 159-60, 165, and Morgan ED, Bledsoe SC, Barker J. Ambulatory management of burns. *Am Fam Physician* 2000;62(9):2015-26.

Figure 3: **Assessment of Patients with Burns**

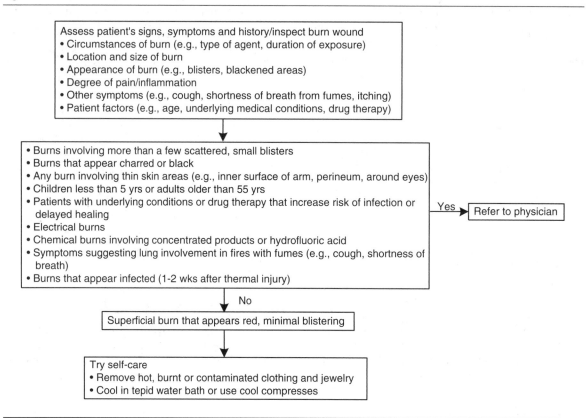

Assess patient's signs, symptoms and history/inspect burn wound
- Circumstances of burn (e.g., type of agent, duration of exposure)
- Location and size of burn
- Appearance of burn (e.g., blisters, blackened areas)
- Degree of pain/inflammation
- Other symptoms (e.g., cough, shortness of breath from fumes, itching)
- Patient factors (e.g., age, underlying medical conditions, drug therapy)

- Burns involving more than a few scattered, small blisters
- Burns that appear charred or black
- Any burn involving thin skin areas (e.g., inner surface of arm, perineum, around eyes)
- Children less than 5 yrs or adults older than 55 yrs
- Patients with underlying conditions or drug therapy that increase risk of infection or delayed healing
- Electrical burns
- Chemical burns involving concentrated products or hydrofluoric acid
- Symptoms suggesting lung involvement in fires with fumes (e.g., cough, shortness of breath)
- Burns that appear infected (1-2 wks after thermal injury)

Yes → Refer to physician

No

Superficial burn that appears red, minimal blistering

Try self-care
- Remove hot, burnt or contaminated clothing and jewelry
- Cool in tepid water bath or use cool compresses

and provide some pain relief, and should be started as soon as possible.[28] Cool the burn for 15 to 30 minutes with tepid tap water irrigations (cool to touch), immersion in tepid water, or application of cool tap water compresses (12°C). If the burn is serious enough to require medical attention, cooling can be continued with cool compresses during transport. Ice application is not recommended because it can cause vasoconstriction that may worsen the injury. Home remedies such as butter, grease or powder should never be used. Attempts to neutralize a chemical burn can make things worse. Instead, chemical burns should be irrigated with copious amounts of luke-warm water poured over the burn site. Burns from concentrated alkaline chemicals often require irrigation for several hours and therefore are best managed in an emergency department.

Dry, superficial burns where the skin is not broken do not require a dressing. All partial- and full-thickness burns should be covered with nonadherent dressings similar to those recommended for minor wound care. The dressing is usually changed daily or more often if it becomes soaked with wound secretions.[27,28] Small blisters should be left intact and never drained. Large blisters require medical attention for debridement to prevent infection.[27] Baking soda baths may provide relief of itching.

Pharmacologic Therapy

Discourage the use of disinfectants to clean burn wounds because they may impair healing.[28] Tap water and mild soap can be used to gently clean secretions and wound debris away at each dressing change.

Superficial burns with no blistering or open areas do not require topical antibiotics.[24] All other burns should be treated with topical antibiotics (Table 5) to prevent infection and keep dressings from adhering to the wound. **Bacitracin**, which is effective against gram-positive organisms,[25] is the nonprescription topical antibiotic most often recommended for outpatient burn management.[28] The antibacterial spectrum can be expanded by combining it with other antibiotics such as polymyxin or the prescription topical antibiotic neomycin.[25]

Usual doses of nonprescription **analgesics** (acetaminophen or ibuprofen) are often sufficient to control pain in minor burns. ASA should be avoided because platelet inhibition poses a risk of bleeding in the presence of open wounds.[28] Deeper burns with open areas often require narcotics for adequate pain management.[28,25] In sunburns, full antiinflammatory doses of **ibuprofen** (400 mg q6h in adults) for 48 hours may reduce redness and burn severity.[29] Local anesthetics (Table 2) are a common ingredient in products for treatment of minor burns. As previously noted (Arthropod Bites and Stings), benzocaine and tetracaine should not be used, and lidocaine and dibucaine should be used sparingly. **Pramoxine** is a suitable alternative. Local anesthetics should never be applied to blistered or open areas of skin because of the risk of systemic absorption.

Deeper burn wounds can take six months to two years to heal completely. Itching is common during the healing phase of burn wounds. Moisturizing lotions and colloidal oatmeal baths may provide symptomatic relief. Systemic antihistamines such as **diphenhydramine** are often used to relieve symptoms as well.[28] Avoid use of topical antihistamines and "caine" family local anesthetics in this situation since the risk of sensitization and allergic contact dermatitis increases with prolonged use. **Pramoxine** and **menthol** are safe antipruritic options. The area will also be more sensitive to sun and extremes of heat and cold. High SPF (25 or greater) sunscreens should be used until the wound has healed completely to prevent permanent hyperpigmentation from repeated injury.[27,28]

Topical **aloe vera gel** is a common herbal remedy recommended for sunburn and minor wounds. Animal studies show that it has antiinflammatory properties and can stimulate collagen synthesis. In animal models it increases tissue survival in frostbite injuries, accelerates burn healing, and promotes wound healing.[30] However, studies in humans are limited and of poor quality.[31] Results have been variable, ranging from impaired wound healing in a study of post-surgical wounds, to no effect on radiation-induced skin injury, to improved epithelialization in partial thickness burns.[30,31] Its major benefit is as a topical moisturizer or protectant in minor burns such as sunburn. The potential of aloe vera to impair wound healing suggests it should not be used on open wounds. Some patients experience mild side effects of burning sensation, contact dermatitis or mild itching with topical application.[31]

Prescription Treatment

Silver sulfadiazine is a prescription, broad spectrum topical antibiotic that is frequently used to prevent burn wound infections.[27,28,32] It should not be used on the face, in patients with sulfonamide hypersensitivity, in newborns, in women who are pregnant or breast-feeding, or in infants under two months of age.[28] Oral antibiotics are not effective in preventing burn wound infections.

Use of corticosteroids in the treatment of sunburn is disputed. Systemic and topical steroids may have little or no clinically important effect in the management of sunburn.[33] However, for serious sunburn, some recommend oral prednisone[32] or potent prescription topical corticosteroids to reduce redness, stinging and itching.[29] Steroids do not reduce sun-induced skin damage.[29]

Tetanus prophylaxis is recommended for deeper partial-thickness and full-thickness burns.

Monitoring of Therapy

Table 8 provides a monitoring plan for burn therapy.

Table 8: **Monitoring Therapy for Burns**

Symptom	Monitoring	Endpoint	Actions
Pain	**Patient:** Every 4-6 h and at dressing changes **Health care provider:** daily or at dressing changes. Assess pain on a scale of 0-10 where 0 is no pain and 10 is the worst possible pain. Assess if pain interferes with sleep or usual activities.	The patient's worst pain score should be less than 5. Higher pain scores interfere with sleep, activity, mood.	Refer to a physician patients whose pain is not responding adequately to regular (q6h) doses of nonprescription analgesics. Narcotic analgesics will be required.
Burn healing	**Patient:** daily **Health care provider:** daily for 2-3 days, then weekly until epithelialization is complete, then every 4-6 wks to assess scar formation. For most outpatient-managed burns, epithelialization should be complete by 2 wks.	Sunburn erythema should be markedly reduced by 48 h. Peeling is normal. In partial-thickness burns, when epithelialization is complete, wound appears pink or red with tiny opalescent islands of epithelium throughout and no secretions.	If epithelialization is not complete by 2 wks, there is a significant risk of scarring. Refer patients for possible grafting.
Itching	**Patient:** Every 4-6 h **Health care provider:** daily Consider oral antihistamines for itching not responding to supportive measures such as moisturizing lotions, cool compresses, or bathing.	Itching does not interfere with sleep or normal activities.	Itching not responding to oral diphenhydramine should be referred to a physician. Prescription antihistamines or potent topical steroids may be required.
Infection e.g., swelling, surrounding redness that is tender to touch, red streaks from the wound, pus, fever, swollen or tender lumps in the groin or armpit.	**Patient:** Inspect daily at dressing change. **Health care provider:** Follow-up at 48 h then weekly until epithelialization complete.	No signs or symptoms of infection noted before epithelialization is complete. Risk is low after this point.	Refer to a physician if signs and symptoms of infection are noted.

Frostbite

Pathophysiology

Frostbite refers to cold-induced injuries where ice crystals form in tissues.[34] Resulting tissue injury occurs through direct and indirect mechanisms. Formation of extracellular, and later intracellular, ice crystals results in cellular dehydration and physical damage to cell membranes and vascular structures. This leads to progressive microvascular collapse and initiates a series of events that in serious frostbite leads to progressive ischemia, thrombosis and tissue necrosis.[35,36] The severity of injury and degree of irreversible damage is related to the duration of exposure and length of time the tissue remains frozen, rather than solely to air temperature. Wind chill and high humidity can increase the risk of injury at a given air temperature.[34]

Risk factors for frostbite include alcohol consumption (combination of vasodilation and loss of judgment), psychiatric illness, vagrancy, inadequate clothing and previous history of cold injury.[34,35] Conditions that impair peripheral circulation, such as constrictive clothing, immobilization, vasoconstricting medication, smoking, diabetes, atherosclerosis, and vasospastic diseases (e.g., Raynaud's phenomenon) predispose individuals to frostbite.[36] Hands and feet account for 90% of cases, but the face, ears and penis are other common sites.[34]

Frostnip is a pre-freeze, superficial injury in which cooling of tissues to less than 10°C results in a blue-white discoloration of skin, and loss of sensation, transient numbness and tingling. Symptoms resolve quickly with rewarming and may be accompanied by erythema and mild edema, but there is no tissue damage.[35,36] In true frostbite the frozen area appears as a waxy white, yellowish or mottled blue-white plaque surrounded by erythema.[35,36] The area feels numb, hard and wooden. With deep freezing, tissue is not moveable over underlying bone. If the hands are involved, movements may be clumsy or lack fine motor control. With deep frostbite involving muscles and nerves, use of the extremity is lost.

Because most frostbite injuries appear similar during the frozen state, the risk of sequelae can be assessed only after rewarming.[34] Rewarming is typically accompanied by edema, flushing and intense throbbing or burning pain. Areas with minor frostbite will develop normal sensation, color and warmth, and the tissue will be soft and pliable. Large blisters filled with clear fluid may form in 6 to 24 hours. After rewarming, areas with significant damage appear blanched or cyanotic (blue-grey), feel hard, and develop dark fluid-filled blisters.[36] In the most serious injuries, skin necrosis occurs resulting in mummification and autoamputation at 22 to 45 days.[34,35] Long-term sequelae of frostbite can include tingling and burning sensations from ischemic neuritis lasting for weeks. Cold sensitivity, loss of sensation, pigmentation changes, nail deformities or hyperhidrosis may persist for years.[34-36]

Two other cold-related injuries that do not involve freezing are *chilblains* from repetitive exposure to mild, dry cold, and *trench foot* from prolonged exposure to wet cold.[36] In chilblains, persistent vasospasm and vasculitis results in pruritus, redness, and mild edema of the face, hands, feet and shins which can progress to development of plaques, bluish nodules, and ulceration. In trench foot, neurovascular damage occurs in the absence of ice crystal formation. Feet initially appear pale and cyanotic, and feel cold, numb

and tingly. After rewarming, the skin remains very painful to touch, blisters are common and may ulcerate. Pain, cold sensitivity and hyperhidrosis may last for years.[36]

Goals of Therapy
- Prevent further acute heat loss
- Minimize tissue damage during rewarming
- Control pain
- Prevent infection in damaged tissues

Patient Assessment

Because the severity of the injury is difficult to assess while tissue is still frozen, referral to a physician for proper rewarming and post-warming assessment is preferred for all patients with still-frozen areas of skin. If immediate referral is not possible, provide instructions for rewarming and observation. Patients presenting after rewarming should be referred if there are large, blistered areas, especially if the blisters are filled with a milky or blackish fluid, or if they have pain that is not controlled with usual doses of non-prescription analgesics. Assessment of patients with cold-related injuries is presented in Figure 4.

Nonpharmacologic Therapy

To prevent further acute heat loss, wet and/or constricting clothing should be removed from the affected area. The area should not be rubbed since friction can increase tissue damage. If rewarming in warm water cannot be started right away, the area should be insulated as much as possible and kept away from sources of heat to prevent partial thawing and refreezing that can worsen tissue damage.[34,36]

The area should be rewarmed by immersing in warm water (40 to 42°C – comfortably warm bath) for 10 to 30 minutes until it feels pliable and appears red.[36] After rewarming, the area is elevated to minimize edema, and a sterile dressing is applied for protection. If blisters develop, clear or white blisters are usually debrided by a health professional, while blackish blisters are left intact.[34,35]

Frostnip responds quickly to rewarming with no sequelae.[35,36] Chilblains are treated conservatively with warmth, elevation of the area, and application of soothing moisturizers.[35] Trench foot can be prevented by taking measures to keep feet dry when active outside for long periods, such as choosing synthetic fibres that wick moisture away from the skin, changing socks regularly, and inspecting feet often.[36]

Figure 4: **Assessment of Patients with Frostbite**

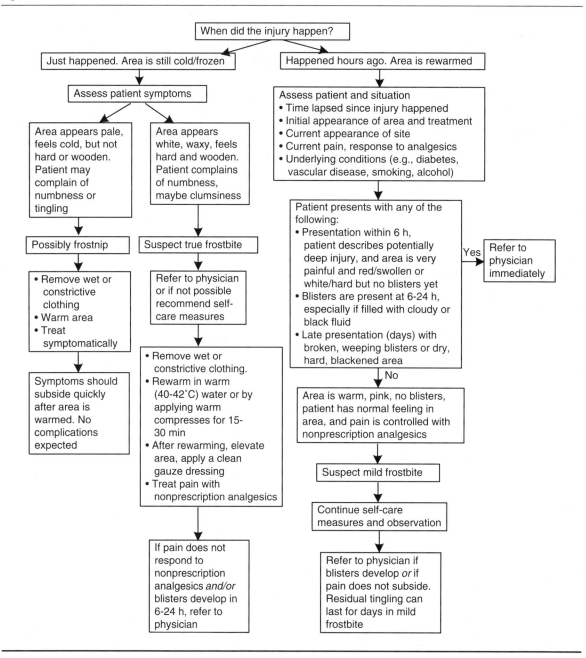

Table 9: **Monitoring Therapy for Frostbite**

Symptom	Monitoring	Endpoint	Actions
Hard, whitish, frozen-looking tissue	**Patient:** Continuously until area has rewarmed. **Health care provider:** After 15-30 min of immersion for initial rewarming. After 24 h for sequelae	Rewarmed tissue will be warm, red, and pliable. It may be swollen. Areas of minor frostbite will develop normal color and warmth with no blisters at 24 h.	After rewarming, areas that appear whitish and hard, or areas that develop large blisters at 6-24 h (filled with clear, cloudy or dark fluid) should be assessed by a physician.
Numbness, tingling, pain	**Patient:** Symptoms are normal during rewarming; every 6 h after rewarming before each analgesic dose **Health care provider:** Every 4-6 h for first day then daily. Pain not responding to nonprescription analgesics may require narcotics.	Symptoms of tingling and pain are tolerable by patient.	Patients with continued pain and tingling at 24 h should be assessed by a physician, even if they have apparently minor frostbite.

Pharmacologic Therapy

No specific treatment is required for minor frostbite. When blisters form in more serious frostbite, application of topical **aloe vera** to the lesions every six hours appears to improve tissue survival.[34] Aloe vera inhibits local production of thromboxane A2, thought to be involved in the pathogenesis of progressive dermal ischemia.[34] **Ibuprofen** is recommended as an analgesic because it may also suppress harmful prostaglandin activity.[34]

Prescription Treatment

In serious frostbite, narcotic analgesics may be required for pain not responding adequately to nonprescription analgesics. Frostbite injuries that develop blisters are prone to tetanus and therefore tetanus prophylaxis is indicated. Use of systemic antibiotics for infection prophylaxis is controversial; however, they are sometimes used in cases of significant tissue loss.[34]

Table 9 provides a monitoring plan for frostbite therapy.

Suggested Readings

Bites and Stings

Fradin MS. Mosquitoes and mosquito repellents: a clinician's guide. *Ann Intern Med* 1998;128(11): 931-40.

Kemp ED. Bites and stings of the arthropod kind. *Postgrad Med* 1998;103(6):88-90,93-6,102-4,106.

Minor Wounds

Eastman SR. Basics of wound care. *US Pharmacist* 1996;21(8):91-8.

Gouin S, Patel H. Office management of minor wounds. *Can Fam Physician* 2001;47:769-4.

Burns

Clayton MC, Solem LD. No ice, no butter. Advice on management of burns for primary care physicians. *Postgrad Med* 1995;97(5):151-5,159-60,165.

Morgan ED, Bledsoe SC, Barker J. Ambulatory management of burns. *Am Fam Physician* 2000;62(9): 2015-26.

Frostbite

Murphy JV, Banwell PE, Roberts AH et al. Frostbite: pathogenesis and treatment. *J Trauma* 2000;48(1): 171-8.

References

1. Russell FE. Venomous arthropods. *Vet Hum Toxicol* 1991;33 (5):505-8.
2. Allen C. Arachnid envenomations. *Emerg Med Clin North Am* 1992;19(2):269-98.
3. Kemp ED. Bites and stings of the arthropod kind. *Postgrad Med* 1998;103(6):88-90,93-6,102-4,106.
4. Metry DW, Hebert AA. Insect and arachnid stings, bites, infestations, and repellents. *Ped Ann* 2000;29(1):39-48.

5. National Advisory Committee on Immunization. Statement on immunization for Lyme disease. *Can Comm Dis Rep* 2000; 26(ACS-3).

6. Jerrard DA. ED management of insect stings. *Am J Emerg Med* 1996;14:429-33.

7. Reisman RE. Insect stings. *N Engl J Med* 1994;331(8):523-7.

8. Fradin MS. Mosquitoes and mosquito repellents: a clinician's guide. *Ann Intern Med* 1998;128(11):931-40.

9. Population and Public Health Branch, Health Canada. Vectors of diseases hazards and risks for travellers: Part III. *Can Comm Dis Rep* 2000;27(17):146-8. Available at: www.hc-sc.gc.ca/pphb-dgspsp/publicat/ccdr-rmtc/01pdf/cdr2717.pdf. Accessed Dec 14, 2001.

10. Pest Management Regulatory Agency, Health Canada. *Proposed Regulatory Decision Document: Soybean Oil.* Ottawa: Minister of Public Works and Government Services Canada, May 14, 1999. Available at: www.hc-sc.gc.ca/pmraarla/english/pdf/prdd/prdd9902-e.pdf. Accessed Dec 14, 2001.

11. Brown M, Hebert AA. Insect repellents: an overview. *J Am Acad Dermatol* 1997;36:243-9.

12. Population and Public Health Branch, Health Canada. *Safety Tips on Using Personal Insect Repellents.* Ottawa: Health Canada, May 2001. Available at: www.hc-sc.gc.ca/pphb-dgspsp/ publicat/info/repell_e.html. Accessed Dec 14, 2001.

13. *Pest Management Regulatory Agency, Health Canada. Re-evaluation Decision Document: n-octylbicycloheptane Dicarboxamide (MGK Repellent 264).* Ottawa: Minister of Public Works and Government Services Canada, Dec 12, 2001. Available at: www.hc-sc.gc.ca/pmra-arla/english/pdf/rrd/ RRD2001-02-e.pdf. Accessed Dec 14, 2001.

14. Parfitt K, ed. *Martindale – The Complete Drug Reference.* 32nd ed. London: Pharmaceutical Press; 1999.

15. Rietschel RL, Fowler JF. *Fisher's Contact Dermatitis.* Philadelphia: Lippincott Williams & Wilkins; 2001.

16. McEvoy GK, ed. *AHFS Drug Information.* Bethesda: American Society of Health-System Pharmacists; 2001.

17. Yosipovitch G, Maibach HI. Effect of topical pramoxine on experimentally induced pruritus in humans. *J Am Acad Dermatol* 1997;37(2pt1):278-80.

18. Bromm B, Scharein E, Darsow U, Ring J. Effects of menthol and cold on histamine-induced itch and skin reactions in man. *Neurosci Lett* 1995;187:157-60.

19. Zhai H, Frisch S, Pelosi A et al. Antipruritic and thermal sensation effects of hydrocortisone creams in human skin. *Skin Pharmacol Appl Skin Physiol* 2000;13(6):352-7.

20. Lammers RL. Principles of wound management. In: Roberts JR, Hedges JR, eds. *Clinical Procedures in Emergency Medicine.* 3rd ed. Philadelphia: Saunders; 1998:533-9.

21. Eastman SR. Basics of wound care. *US Pharmacist* 1996;21 (8):91-8.

22. Trued ST. Minor soft tissue injuries and infections. In: Dornbrand L, Hoole AJ, Fletcher RH. *Manual of Clinical Problems in Adult Ambulatory Care.* Philadelphia: Lippincott-Raven; 1997:714-20.

23. Gouin S, Patel H. Office management of minor wounds. *Can Fam Physician* 2001;47:769-74.

24. Pearson AS, Wolford RW. Management of skin trauma. *Primary Care* 2000;27(2):475-92.

25. Kaye ET. Topical antibacterial agents. *Infect Dis Clin North Am* 2000;14(2):321-39.

26. National Advisory Committee on Immunization. *Canadian Immunization Guide.* 5th ed. Ottawa: Canadian Medical Association; 1998:166.

27. Clayton MC, Solem LD. No ice, no butter. Advice on management of burns for primary care physicians. *Postgrad Med* 1995;97(5):151-5,159-60,165.

28. Morgan ED, Bledsoe SC, Barker J. Ambulatory management of burns. *Am Fam Physician* 2000;62(9):2015-26.

29. Guenther L. Sunburn. In: Gray J, ed. *Therapeutic Choices.* 3rd ed. Ottawa: Canadian Pharmacists Association; 2000: 507-18.

30. Combest WL. Aloe vera. *US Pharmacist* 2000;25(4):64-74.

31. Vogler BK, Ernst E. Aloe vera: a systematic review of its clinical effectiveness. *Br J Gen Pract* 1999;49:823-8.

32. Peate WF. Outpatient management of burns. *Am Fam Physician* 1992;1321-30.

33. Driscoll MS, Wagner RF. Clinical management of the acute sunburn reaction. *Cutis* 2000;66(1):53-8.

34. Murphy JV, Banwell PE, Roberts AH et al. Frostbite: pathogenesis and treatment. *J Trauma* 2000;48(1):171-8.

35. Kanzenback TL, Dexter WW. Cold injuries – protecting your patients from the dangers of hypothermia and frostbite. *Postgrad Med* 1999;105(1):72-6.

36. Danzl DF. Frostbite. In: Rosen P, Barkin R, eds. *Emergency Medicine – Concepts and Clinical Practice.* St. Louis: Mosby-Year Book; 1998:953-62.

Insect Bites and Stings—Patient Information

- Use insect repellents to prevent bites from insects such as mosquitoes, black flies and ticks. They do not work against stinging insects such as bees and wasps.
- DEET is the most effective insect repellent. Restrict use in children aged six months to two years, and in women who are pregnant or breastfeeding.
- Do not use repellents containing citronella or lavender oil on children under two years of age, because there is less information on these products.
- Physical protection (e.g., clothing, netting) is preferred for infants and small children.
- Products containing soybean oil appear to be as effective as DEET against mosquitoes and black flies and are very safe. They can be used by pregnant or breastfeeding women and small children. They do not protect against ticks.
- Tips for safe use of insect repellents include:
  —Apply sparingly and only to exposed skin. Do not apply to open wounds or irritated skin. Avoid applying to a child's hands or face. Wash off when protection is no longer needed.
  —Use a low concentration (< 10% DEET) on infants and children, and pregnant or breastfeeding women. Use only once a day in children less than two years, and up to three times a day in older children. A maximum concentration of 30% is usually adequate for adults.
  —Use aerosol products in a well-ventilated area. If you accidentally get the product in your eyes or mouth, rinse thoroughly with warm water.
  —Products containing permethrin are for use on clothing, tents or equipment only. Never use them on skin.
- Travelers to areas where mosquito-borne illness is common are advised to wear light-colored, tightly woven clothing that covers arms and legs. Apply DEET-containing repellents to all exposed skin areas, including neck, wrists and ankles. At night, burn a mosquito coil in your sleeping area, and protect yourself with a mosquito net. Spray clothing, tents and netting with an insecticide such as permethrin to improve their repellent ability.

- Travelers to tick-infested areas should wear light-colored clothing that is tight at the wrists and ankles or tucked into gloves and socks. Use a DEET-containing repellent on all exposed skin areas. Spray clothing and boots with an insecticide such as permethrin to improve their tick-repelling effect. Inspect skin daily for ticks and remove any ticks promptly. Use tweezers to grab the tick and pull gently until the tick detaches. This may take up to a minute of steady pulling. Applying poisons, heat or substances to cover the tick will not work and may be harmful.
- When you get a bite or sting, wash the site(s) with warm water and soap. Apply ice or cool compresses to relieve the irritation. Do not apply ice for longer than 15 minutes at a time to avoid frostbite. For pain, use a pain reliever such as acetaminophen, ASA or ibuprofen. For itching, try anti-itch lotions, creams or sprays, hydrocortisone creams, or oral antihistamines. Swelling sometimes responds to hydrocortisone creams or oral antihistamines.
- If the symptoms do not improve or get worse over 24 to 48 hours, see a health professional.
- Serious reactions to insect bites or stings are uncommon but can occur. See a doctor immediately if you develop any of the following symptoms within 30 minutes:
  —flushing or itching all over your body
  —sneezing or watery eyes
  —hives
  —nausea, vomiting
  —cramps
  —dizziness, fainting
  —hoarse voice or lump in throat
  —difficulty breathing
  —changes in heart rate (fast or slow)
  Also, contact a doctor if you develop a rash, the bite reaction spreads to a large area (e.g., involves your whole arm or leg), or if you develop an unusual reaction at the bite site such as a purplish color or blisters.
- If you develop an allergy to bee or wasp stings carry appropriate medical information like a Medic Alert bracelet. Your doctor may also suggest you carry an emergency medical kit.

Minor Cuts and Wounds—Patient Information

- Cleaning your wound properly is the most important thing you can do. Wash your hands with soap and water first, unless the wound is on your hand.
- Clean the wound using only warm tap water. Do not use soap, antiseptic solutions or hydrogen peroxide on your wound. These can be irritating and interfere with wound healing.
- If possible, apply water to the wound with some pressure — squirt water onto the wound from a water bottle or a large syringe with no needle, or hold the wound under a moderately running tap.
- If you can see any pieces of dirt or other material (e.g., glass, metal, gravel) in the wound, try to remove them using a pair of tweezers soaked in rubbing alcohol, or by rubbing gently with a clean gauze pad.
- After the wound is clean, apply a small amount of petrolatum or antibiotic ointment to the wound. Then cover with a clean adhesive strip bandage or a gauze pad and tape. Change the bandage every day or more often if it looks dirty or damp. Wash the area gently with water and mild soap before applying more ointment and a clean bandage.
- You can usually remove the bandage after 48 hours. Look for signs of infection such as reddened, puffy areas around the wound site that are tender to touch, red streaks coming from the wound, throbbing pain in the wound area, or pus (creamy yellowish-gray fluid) in the wound. Other signs of infection include fever, chills, or tender lumps or swelling in your armpit, groin or neck.
- See your doctor if you have any signs of infection, or if the wound is still bleeding or leaking fluid after 48 hours.

Burns—Patient Information

- Burns that are safe for self-care include sunburns and minor burns that look like sunburns – red, painful, minimal blistering (small blisters in only a few areas). See a doctor for all other burns. This includes:
  —Burns with small blisters in thin skin areas (e.g., inner surface of arm, groin area, around eyes), *or* in people with thin skin (children less than 5 years or adults older than 55 years), *or* in people with conditions that put them at risk of infection or delayed healing (e.g., diabetes, chronic alcohol abuse, suppressed immune systems);
  —Electrical burns and chemical burns involving concentrated products or hydrofluoric acid, even if they appear to be minor. These burns are often worse than they look;
  —Burns from smoky fires where you are coughing, short of breath, or it hurts to breathe;
  —Burns whose pain is not adequately controlled with cooling or nonprescription pain relievers.
- Remove clothing that is burnt, hot or contaminated by chemicals. Remove jewelry from the affected area.
- Cooling the burn is the most important first aid measure you can take. Hold the area under a moderately running tap with tepid water (cool to touch but not cold) or immerse the area in tepid tap water for at least 15 minutes. You can also apply cloths or gauze soaked in cold tap water for 15 to 30 minutes. If you need to seek medical attention, keep the cold wet cloths on the area until you get to a doctor.

- *Do not* use ice, or home remedies such as butter, grease or powder on a burn. *Do not* try to neutralize chemical burns by putting a different kind of chemical on the burn. These actions make things worse.
- Minor burns are often painful. Cooling helps relieve the pain. You can also try pain relievers such as acetaminophen or ibuprofen but ASA or Aspirin® should not be used in this situation. Ibuprofen is particularly helpful for sunburns.
- Minor burns are sometimes itchy. Avoid scratching. Apply moisturizing creams often. If this doesn't work, you can try a nonprescription hydrocortisone cream or an oral antihistamine such as diphenhydramine.
- Minor burns in which the skin is not broken do not need a bandage, dressing or antibiotic cream. They usually heal in three to six days. Peeling is normal. Burned areas will be more sensitive to sunlight for up to one year, so be sure to wear a sunscreen with an SPF of at least 25 during that time.
- Infection is a possibility in burns where the skin is broken (e.g., deeper burns, blisters that break, scratching itchy burns). Apply an antibiotic cream and cover loosely with a bandage or gauze dressing. Change the bandage or dressing every day until the area is dry. Clean the area with tap water and mild soap before putting on a clean dressing. Watch for signs of infection such as an increase in redness, swelling and tenderness at the site, yellowish discharge (pus), or fever and tender lumps in your armpit or groin. See a doctor if you have any signs of infection.

Frostbite—Patient Information

- Ears, nose, fingers and toes are the body parts most likely to suffer frostbite. People who drink alcohol, smoke, or have medical conditions that affect blood flow to their skin (e.g., diabetes, vascular disease) are more prone to develop frostbite.
- Prevent frostbite by wearing warm clothing that protects these areas when you have to be outdoors in very cold weather. Wind and high humidity increase the risk of frostbite.
- The first sign of frostbite is numbness and tingling in the area. Your skin may look pale. This is a sign to go indoors, or at least to warm the area and cover it. Feeling to the area should be restored quickly when you warm it (e.g., by holding your hand over it).
- When the skin is frozen in true frostbite, it feels hard, wooden and numb, and looks a waxy whitish, yellow, or blue-white color. If your hands or feet are affected, you may feel clumsy. If the frostbite is very deep and extends to your muscles, you may not be able to move that part of your body.

- If you think you have true frostbite, do not rub the area or apply heat to it (e.g., heating pad) or hold it in front of a heat source (e.g., fire, heater). Remove any wet or tight clothing around the area. Cover it with dry clothing and get indoors as soon as possible.
- Rewarm frozen areas by immersing them in warm water until the area looks reddened, and feels warm and soft. If this is not possible (e.g., ears, nose), use warm compresses. Rewarming usually takes about 15 to 30 minutes. Do not rub the area while it is under water. Once the area is rewarmed, keep it elevated and apply a clean, dry gauze dressing to protect it.
- It is normal to feel pain and tingling when the frozen area is rewarmed. If this is not relieved by nonprescription analgesics, or does not subside in 24 hours, see a doctor.
- In serious frostbite, blisters filled with clear, cloudy, or blackish fluid will form in the area in 6 to 24 hours. If this happens, see a doctor. The injury can progress to gangrene and infection if it is not treated properly.

Dressings

Marie Berry, BScPharm, BA, LLB

Dressings are intended to protect a wound from damage and contamination, and in some cases promote healing. The simplest dressing is gauze covering a wound, held in place by adhesive tape. Minor cuts and scrapes are often covered by self-adhesive strips that combine both gauze and adhesive tape in a pre-packaged format.

Wounds can be chronic in nature; for example ulcerations secondary to conditions such as diabetes, peripheral vascular ulcers, and pressure ulcers or "bed sores." Wounds may be extensive in nature, such as a deep wound or one that has had tissue torn from it. All wounds, even minor ones, require dressings that are specific for the type of wound, as do post-surgical wounds.

Dressings first and foremost assist in stopping bleeding and protect the wound from debris and micro-organisms as well as further damage.[1] However, dressings may serve other purposes. An ideal dressing maintains a moist environment while removing excess exudate to prevent maceration. Wounds that are painful benefit from dressings that are able to "soothe" nerve endings – hydrogels, hydrocolloids, sheet gels. Table 1 lists some of the common characteristics of dressings.

Bandages

Bandages are most commonly a combination of gauze and adhesive tape. They may be self-adhesive or require further adhesive material.[2]

Gauze acts as an absorbent and protectant. It is made by weaving bleached cotton into an open-mesh cloth. The natural waxes and impurities are removed from the cotton to increase its absorbing capacity. Gauze is classified either according to its mesh or to the number of threads per inch. Self-adherent gauze clings to itself; available as pads or rolls, it can be used to wrap a wound without adhesive tape e.g., head wound. Viscous rayon and regenerated cellulose are also used in bandages, sometimes in conjunction with gauze.

Nonadherent gauze is easily removable, yet still protective. It is preferred as the primary dressing, next to the wound, because of increased comfort. When removed, nonadherent gauze does not leave gauze threads on the wound surface nor does it disturb the wound surface by "pulling" or removing parts of the wound surface. It is prepared by impregnating viscous rayon with an oil-in-water emulsion or by covering the gauze with a perforated plastic film.

Table 1: **Characteristics of an Ideal Dressing**

Provides a moist environment – a moist environment will accelerate epidermal migration and dermal repair.

Provides thermal insulation – a drop in temperature below 37°C delays mitotic activity for up to four 4 h.

Is highly absorptive – excess exudate can macerate healthy tissue.

Is impermeable to bacteria – bacteria and other micro-organisms can colonize a wound.

Is free of contaminants – sterile technique is paramount in the application of sterile dressings.

Is nonadherent – dressings that adhere to wounds can cause further tissue damage.

Is non-toxic – some antiseptics and hypochlorites are toxic to tissue.

Adhesive tape is used to secure a gauze dressing to a wound. Several kinds are available, including waterproof, cloth, clear, and paper. The choice of tape depends upon the type of wound, potential skin sensitivities, and personal preference. In general, hypoallergenic and easy-to-remove adhesive tapes are preferred. For maximal adhesion, apply tape to dry skin. For wounds that require protection from water or even dirt, choose a waterproof tape. Paper or cloth tape reduces the risk of skin damage for wounds that require frequent dressing changes.

Adhesive tape is a fabric or film evenly coated with a pressure-sensitive adhesive mixture. Today, most adhesives are acrylate-based; historically they were rubber-based. Acrylate-based adhesives tend to produce fewer allergic reactions, and thus are generally termed hypoallergenic. True allergic reactions comprise a small fraction of reactions to adhesive tape. Rather, the irritation may be caused by the mechanics of tape removal, either repeated removal or skin stripping. Combined with an existing dermatitis or a fragile skin surface, adhesive tape reactions may be severe.

Self-adhesive bandages are convenient alternatives to gauze and tape; however, the correct size needs to be chosen for the wound. The bandage should be large enough to cover the wound completely, yet not too large. If the bandage is too small, the adhesive may adhere to the wound, making removal difficult, or alternatively a portion of the wound will be exposed. If the bandage is too large, the wound will not be covered securely, impairing healing, and the bandage itself may "bunch" and come loose from the wound. For wounds on body areas that are difficult to bandage such as fingertips and knuckles, specially shaped bandages are available. Butterfly closures are self-adhesive bandages that pull and hold the edges of small wounds together to encourage healing. Butterfly closures are not a substitute for stitches in larger wounds.

Medicated Dressings

Gauze bandages may be impregnated with pharmaceutical agents. Medicated gauze allows easy removal and provides a delivery system for antibiotics and antiseptics. Petrolatum gauze removes easily and acts as a protectant for the underlying skin.

Antiseptic-impregnated gauze contains chlorhexidine or povidone-iodine to prevent infection and to ease removal of the dressing. Antibiotics, such as framycetin sulfate, may be added to gauze to prevent and treat infections.[3]

Protective Dressings

Protective dressings are either mechanical or physical or a combination of both. Compared to physical dressings which simply provide a physical barrier, mechanical dressings actually perform other functions. Some act as tissue adhesives, absorbents for exudate, and wound debridement agents. Most require a secondary dressing of gauze and adhesive tape to secure them. Table 2 lists suitable dressings depending on the wound to be treated.

- *Collodion* is a viscous solution of pyroxylon in ether and alcohol. Flexible collodion is collodion containing camphor and castor oil. Traditionally, both have been used to seal small wounds. More recently, cyanoacrylate compounds have been developed as tissue adhesives to close small wounds.[4]
- *Alginates* are made from seaweed and create a moist environment while absorbing exudate as well as blood. Some are higher in galuronic acid, which means they retain their shape and can be lifted off the wound in one piece. Others are higher in mannuronic acid and less likely to retain their shape. They are easily washed out of the wound with sterile saline.
- *Film dressings* are semipermeable and can be used alone or in conjunction with other dressings. They prevent bacterial contamination but do not absorb exudate; however, they do allow fluid to evaporate while keeping the wound moist. For the patient, film dressings are comfortable and resistant to shear.
- *Foams* are the product of advanced polymer technology. They do not adhere to the wound, yet absorb exudate. Hydrophilic polyurethane dressings can absorb several times their weight in exudate.
- *Hydrocolloids* consist of a mixture of pectins, gelatins, and sodium carboxymethylcellulose. Ideal for sloughing or necrotic wounds, they provide an occlusive environment and remove exudate by mixing with it.
- *Hydrogels* are matrices containing a high percentage of water and are available as both sheets and gels.

The sheets are polysaccharides cross-linked with polyacrylamide and are ideal for shallow wounds like burns. Gels are more suitable for deeper wounds. A secondary dressing is usually needed to keep the hydrogel dressing in place and moist.

Potential Problems when Applying a Dressing
The most commonly used dressings are self-adhesive bandages. Their application is straightforward; however, care must be taken to ensure the gauze pad is not contaminated through handling. Proper use and

Table 2: **Dressing Selection According to Wound**

Wound description/Symptom	Types of suitable dressing
Black surface, hard eschar requiring rehydration and/or debridement	Enzymatic Hydrogel Hydrocolloid
Soft black surface requiring removal	Cadexamer iodine dressings
Green surface which may be malodorous, requiring infection control	Film dressings Antiseptic, such as povidone-iodine-impregnated dressings. Antiinfective, such as framycetin sulfate-impregnated dressings.
Yellow surface	Hydrogel Hydrocolloid
Clinical infection requiring treatment of infection and control of exudate and odor	Film dressings Antiseptic such as povidone-iodine-impregnated dressings Antiinfective such as framycetin sulfate-impregnated dressings
Granulating surface requiring creation of moist environment and management of exudate	Alginates Foam dressings Film dressings Hydrocolloid
Epithelialising surface requiring creation of moist environment	Film dressings Foam dressings Thin hydrocolloid
Pain requiring dressings that protect nerve endings	Hydrogels, hydrocolloids, and sheet gels are good choices. Hydrophilic dressings such as sugar paste or cadexamer exert an osmotic pull and may increase the pain.
Odor is most often caused by gram-negative bacteria such as pseudomonas	Silver sulfadiazine cream reduces colonization. Povidone-iodine has antiseptic activity, but is quickly deactivated in the presence of pus, thus an iodine cadexamer dressing may be preferred in that it allows for a slower release of antiseptic, extending the antiseptic activity.
Excessive exudate requiring a balance between the need for a moist environment and prevention of maceration	Foam and hydrocolloid dressings are good choices to absorb exudate. Some types of wounds, for example venous ulcers, and wounds in some types of medical conditions, for example hypertension coupled with venous disease, produce more exudate. In this situation compression dressings are useful.
Bleeding needs to be controlled	Alginates have hemostatic properties.
Infection may need to be controlled by systemic antibiotic treatment	Antiseptic- or antibiotic-impregnated gauze may be useful.

application of any dressing is essential for maximum effectiveness.[5]

- Use the correct size. A dressing should be large enough to cover the wound, yet not so large it bunches.
- Use sterile technique to apply the dressing with clean hands or gloves. The dressing surface and wound itself should not be touched. Table 3 describes the steps in applying a dressing.
- Whatever is applied to the wound will eventually have to be removed. Greasy substances are best avoided as they may be difficult to remove, causing more damage to the wound. Lint from loosely woven gauze can also be problematic.
- The wound must be cleaned prior to applying any dressing. Applying a dressing to a contaminated wound increases the risk of infection. Flushing the wound with water or sterile saline may be sufficient.
- If a wound requires debridement, it should be performed before a dressing is applied. Bleeding should be controlled before applying a dressing. The exception are dressings specifically designed for debridement or control of bleeding.
- Sutures may be needed; dressings, even butterfly closures, do not replace necessary sutures.
- Always consider potential complications. These include excessive bleeding and infection. SHARP is an acronym for the signs of infection – swelling, heat, ache, redness, pus. A malodorous wound is usually infected.

- Remember that some patients have a higher risk for complications. Individuals with diabetes have both impaired peripheral circulation and wound healing ability. Nutritional deficiencies may delay healing, and the use of some medications, for example anticoagulants or nonsteroidal antiinflammatory drugs, may predispose individuals to bleeding.
- Different dressings require changing at different intervals. It is a misconception that once a dressing is applied there is no need to change it.

Suggested Readings

Brown CD, Zitelli JA. A review of topical agents for wounds and methods of wounding: guidelines for wound management. *J Dermatol Surg Oncol* 1993; 19:732.

Ovington LG, Eastman SR. Moist wound healing. *US Pharmacist* 2001;March:99-108.

References

1. Jeter KF, Tittle TE. Wound dressings of the nineties: indications and contraindications. *Clin Podiatr Med Surg* 1991; 8:799.
2. Bolton L, van Rijswijk L. Wound dressings: meeting clinical and biological needs. *Dermatology* 1991;3:146.
3. Brown CD, Zitelli JA. A review of topical agents for wounds and methods of wounding: guidelines for wound management. *J Dermatol Surg Oncol* 1993;19:732.
4. Edlich RF, Vikram RR. 5th Annual David R. Boyd, MD Lecture: Revolutionary advances in wound repair in emergency medicine during the last three decades. A view toward the new millennium. *J Emerg Med* 2001;20(2):167.
5. Szycher M, Lee SJ. Modern wound dressings: a systemic approach to wounds. *J Biomater Appl* 1992;7:142.

Table 3: **Application of a Dressing**

Wash hands and work in a clean area. Wearing gloves is an option; table or countertop may need to be cleaned with a disinfectant.

Assess wound. If wound is deep or bleeding excessively, seek medical attention.

Control bleeding. The wound should be allowed to bleed slightly then apply gentle pressure to stop bleeding. A puncture wound should not be squeezed because the puncturing object may be pushed further into the wound.

Clean wound. Remove large foreign particles, debride if necessary by flushing with water, wash with soap and water.

Check for symptoms of infection — swelling, heat, ache, redness or pus, and if present, seek medical attention.

Apply dressing. Cover the wound with a dry, sterile gauze dressing using commercially available materials whenever possible. Ensure the dressing extends beyond the edges of the wound, use adhesive tape to secure the dressing and do not impede circulation by bandaging the wound too tightly.

Reproductive, Gynecologic and Genitourinary Health Section Highlights

Chapter 49: **Contraception**

Nonhormonal contraception
Sympto-thermal method (basal temperature, saliva monitoring, fertility monitors)
Spermicides (foams/gels/film/sponge)
Barrier methods (male and female condoms, diaphragm, cervical cap)
IUDs
Emergency contraception

Chapter 50: **Vaginal Symptoms**

Genital hygiene (douching, towlettes, sprays)
Toxic shock syndrome
Vaginal dryness
Vaginal candidiasis

Chapter 51: **Dysmenorrhea and Premenstrual Syndrome**

Dysmenorrhea
Premenstrual syndrome (PMS)
Sample monitoring chart for PMS symptoms
DSM-IV criteria for premenstrual dysphoric disorder

Chapter 52: **Menopause and Perimenopause**

Management of symptoms

Chapter 53: **Prenatal and Postpartum Care**

General principles of nonprescription drug use in pregnancy and lactation
Pregnancy-associated nausea and vomiting
Allergic rhinitis during pregnancy
Other common conditions in pregnancy (constipation, hemorrhoids, reflux esophagitis, backache, headache, common cold, nutrition)
Postpartum perineal care and postepisiotomy pain
Postpartum depression
Postpartum contraception
Nonprescription medications during lactation

Chapter 49

Contraception

Denis Bélanger, BScPhm

Introduction

Despite significant advances in contraceptive technology, unplanned pregnancies are a common occurrence in Canada. According to a Health Canada report in 1996, there were a total of 21,597 live births to mothers 15 to 19 years of age. Over the past two decades, the live birth rate has declined for teens aged 15 to 19 years, from 35.6 per 1000 in 1974 to 22.1 per 1000 in 1996.[1] During this same period, the number of induced abortions in this age group increased.

Healthy sexual practices are important; unsafe sexual behaviors may lead to infertility, unplanned pregnancy, human immunodeficiency virus (HIV) or other sexually transmitted diseases (STDs). However, among Canadians aged 15 to 59 in a relationship of less than 12 months' duration, 16% did not use a condom the last time they had sex, and 8% reported never using a condom.[1]

There are many options available for effective contraception, each with specific advantages and disadvantages. The health care professional is in an excellent position to help determine which is best for the individual. This chapter focuses on nonhormonal contraceptive methods, and includes a discussion of emergency contraception.

Nonhormonal Contraception
Pathophysiology

The female reproductive cycle is comprised of two main phases, the follicular or preovulatory phase and the luteal or postovulatory phase. The first day of menses marks the beginning of the follicular phase. During the follicular phase, follicle-stimulating hormone promotes the maturation of 6 to 12 ovarian follicles. After about seven days, one follicle predominates and development of the other follicles stops. Just prior to ovulation, there is a dramatic surge in luteinizing hormone, which causes final maturation of the follicle and release of the ovum into the fallopian tube. Release of the ovum from the follicle marks the beginning of the luteal phase. Once the follicle ruptures and releases the ovum, the remaining cells of the follicle become the corpus luteum, which secretes large amounts of estrogen and progesterone. If the ovum is not fertilized, the corpus luteum degenerates and levels of estrogen and progesterone drop quickly. This fall in hormones causes menses and the cycle starts over again.[2]

The luteal phase lasts 14 ± 2 days and is the more consistent of the two phases. The follicular phase however, can vary by several days, making it difficult to predict when ovulation will occur. The usual menstrual cycle lasts 28 days; however, it can vary from as short as 20 to as long as 40 days.[2]

A woman can become pregnant from puberty until menopause. If pregnancy is not desired, it is important that she use an effective method of birth control during this entire period, including perimenopause.

"Natural" Contraceptive Methods (Nonpharmacologic and Nonmechanical)
Sympto-thermal Method

The sympto-thermal method of contraception (also known as the "basal temperature" or "mucus" method), uses several indices to determine the fertile period including calendar calculations, changes in cervical mucus and changes in basal temperature (the temperature that occurs just before rising for the day).[3-5]

During the follicular phase, the *basal temperature* is stable. There is a slight drop in basal temperature about 12 to 24 hours before ovulation, followed by a sharp rise in temperature due to the progesterone secreted by the corpus luteum after ovulation. The basal temperature remains elevated until menses. Basal thermometers (similar to regular thermometers but with a wider calibration set) are required to easily distinguish the slight variations in temperature. The temperature is usually taken orally, rectally or vaginally before the woman rises for the day. It should be taken at the same time and by the same route each day. The woman should avoid speaking, eating, drinking or smoking before taking a reading. Factors that can affect basal temperature include fever or infection, travel, emotional changes and certain medications (e.g., hormones, corticosteroids). Electric basal thermometers are preferred over mercury thermometers. They are easier to use and read, and they store the readings in memory until the data are needed.[3-5]

Cervical mucus can be used as an indicator of fertility, as it changes over the course of the menstrual cycle. Cervical mucus is almost non-existent after menses. During the follicular phase, it is opaque, white or yellowish in color, viscous and sticky. The mucus increases in volume and takes on the appearance of uncooked egg whites (clear, thin and stretchable) as ovulation approaches. After ovulation the mucus becomes opaque and viscous until menses. The changes in mucus are the result of an increase in estrogen. Around the time of ovulation, the character of the mucus provides a favorable environment for sperm.[3,4]

Advantages
The sympto-thermal method offers the advantage of not requiring a device or pharmacologic agents and is supported by various religious organizations. It also increases a couple's knowledge of the menstrual cycle and can be used to determine the fertile period in a cycle if conception is desired.

Disadvantages
This method is not recommended for women with irregular menstrual cycles as the level of predictability decreases. It also requires that the woman be highly

motivated and disciplined, and precludes sexual intercourse for at least seven days of each cycle.

Failure Rate
The average failure rate is 3 to 22%.[5]

Fertility Monitors
Fertility monitors are used by women to help determine their fertile and infertile periods. Although marketed for patients with infertility, these monitors can be used by all women to obtain a better understanding of their menstrual cycles, and to help identify periods of infertility for the means of contraception. At the present time four fertility monitoring devices are licensed by Health Canada (Luna Fertility Indicator®, Ovu-Trac Natural Fertility Tester®, Clearplan Easy Fertility Monitor® and PSC Fertility Monitor®).[6-9] The Luna® and Ovu-Trac® devices use the principle of saliva ferning to help determine the fertile period.[6,7] These devices contain a magnifying lense to help the woman detect the presence or absence of a fern-like pattern in her saliva.

The Clearplan Easy Fertility Monitor® is an electronic device that requires the use of urine dip sticks to monitor surges in estrogen and luteinizing hormone.[8] The computer stores the data from the dip sticks to construct a woman's menstrual cycle and identify her period of maximum fertility.

The PSC (Pheromone Sciences Corp.) Fertility Monitor® is a small wristwatch-like device that contains an interactive microprocessor and a chemical sensor.[9] The chemical sensor rests on the skin surface and monitors variances in ion concentration on the surface of the skin. This is based on the theory that women produce a surge in sweat ions approximately five to six days prior to ovulation and again around the time of ovulation, which leads to a change in the pH of perspiration on the skin. The watch indicates whether the woman is in her fertile or infertile period. The watch can be placed onto a base and data can be transferred to a computer to print out a 30-day ovulation chart.

Other electric fertility monitors that are marketed by various contraception Internet sites include Bioself®, Persona® and Lady-Comp®. The Lady-Comp® and Bioself® use the calendar rhythm along with the woman's basal temperature to identify infertile days in the menstrual cycle.[10-12]

The Lady-Comp® does not give a readout of temperature but rather a green, red or yellow light. The green light means infertility, the red light fertility and a yellow light that indicates possible or probable fertility. The Bioself® displays the basal temperature along with the indication of "fertile" or "infertile". The Bioself® 2000 (an advancement on the Bioself®) monitor can interface with a personal computer and the stored data can be displayed as fertility charts.[10]

Researchers in Germany evaluated the efficacy of the Lady-Comp® by sending out questionnaires to 648 women who purchased the device.[13] Of the 648 women enrolled in the study, 597 used the device for contraceptive purposes (i.e., to avoid pregnancy) over a total of 10,275 months. Thirty-three women who did not want to conceive, became pregnant. Using life-table analysis, the researchers determined that there was a 5.3% unintended pregnancy rate after one year, 6.8% after two years of use and 8.3% after three years. The average length of the fertile period that the monitor identified was 14.3 days.

The Persona® device is a hand-held monitor that uses built-in data from thousands of women plus information that the user inserts with the use of a urine dipstick. The woman uses the urine dipstick eight times per month. The unit interprets the results and indicates to the woman if she is in a fertile or infertile period.[11]

These devices can be purchased from various Internet sites including www.babytech.com, www.birthcontrol.com, www.persona.org.uk.

Advantages

These devices are supported by various religious organizations and increase a woman's knowledge of her menstrual cycle, and can be used to determine the fertile period in a cycle if conception is desired. They do not generally require as much discipline or motivation to use as the sympto-thermal method.

Disadvantages

These devices are not recommended for women with irregular menstrual cycles as the level of predictability decreases, and they preclude sexual intercourse for at least seven days of each cycle. The electronic devices are also expensive (prices range from $200 to $560).

Failure Rate

The average failure rate of these devices is 5.3 to 8.3%.[13]

Pharmacologic Methods (Spermicides)

Spermicidal products usually contain **nonoxynol-9**, a surfactant that interferes with sperm motility, making the sperm unviable.[14] Spermicides can be used alone or in combination with condoms, cervical caps, diaphragms or intrauterine devices. Spermicides are available in various forms including jellies, foams, sponges and films. Sponges and films also act as physical barriers in preventing conception.

Spermicidal agents containing nonoxynol-9 have also been reported to reduce the transmission of human immunodeficiency virus (HIV) and other sexually transmitted diseases (STDs).[15] A meta-analysis concluded that nonoxynol-9 does reduce the risk of chlamydia and gonorrhea, but there were insufficient data to draw any conclusions about HIV transmission.[16] Later controlled trials, however, have shown that nonoxynol-9 does not reduce the transmission of HIV and in one study the use of nonoxynol-9 was associated with an increased incidence of gonorrhea. Therefore, the effect of nonoxynol-9 on STD transmission is controversial.[17, 18]

Foams and Jellies

Counsel women using contraceptive foams to mix the spermicide well by shaking the container about 20 times before use. Most products require the use of one applicatorful, but quantities vary among brands, and the directions on the package insert should be followed. The applicator should be placed on the container and pressure applied until the applicator is full. While lying down, the applicator is inserted into the vagina as deep as possible, then the plunger is pushed to release the dose. Intercourse should take place within 20 to 30 minutes after insertion. More foam/gel should be inserted if it has been more than 30 minutes since the first dose was inserted, and for every time the couple engages in intercourse.[14]

There is less leakage with foam than gel; hence, these agents are usually preferred for esthetic reasons. Contraceptive foams can be used alone or with condoms. The contraceptive jellies can be used alone, in combination with condoms or with a diaphragm or cervical cap.

Advantages

These products are widely available and are easy to use and to carry. They may reduce the risk of STDs including HIV and herpes, although this is controversial.

Disadvantages

They need to be applied before intercourse and may interfere with the mood. They are messy and sometimes pads have to be worn after intercourse to absorb the extra fluid. They may irritate the vagina or penis.

Failure Rate

When used alone spermicidal agents have a failure rate of 21%.[14] When used with a diaphragm or condom, the failure rate is around 2 to 8%.[14]

Contraceptive Sponges (Figure 1)

The sponge (e.g., Protectaid® by Axcan Pharma) is a piece of soft foam filled with three types of spermicide (nonoxynol-9, benzalkonium chloride and sodium cholate).[19,20] When inserted properly, it covers the cervix. It has two slots that help when inserting and removing the sponge. It functions by two mechanisms: firstly, the sponge acts as a physical barrier by blocking the entrance to the uterus; secondly, the chemicals inside the sponge act on sperm as well as bacteria and viruses that can cause STDs. The sponge can be inserted at any time before sexual intercourse and must be kept in place for at least six hours afterwards, for a maximum of 12 hours after being inserted.

Advantages

It is small, comfortable, easy to use and easy to carry. It may offer some protection against STDs.

Disadvantages

It has a relatively high failure rate if used alone and it is relatively expensive (approximately $3.60 per sponge).

Failure Rate

The failure rate of the sponge alone is 40% for parous women and 20% for nulliparous women.[21] When used in combination with a male condom the failure rate is decreased.[21]

Figure 1: **Contraceptive Sponge**

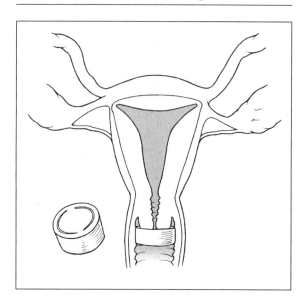

Contraceptive Vaginal Film

This product, VCF® by Apothecus Pharmaceutical Corp., contains nonoxynol-9 in a film base.[22,23] The VCF® dissolves completely and quickly into a gel after insertion high into the vagina against the cervix. It can be inserted from 15 to 60 minutes before intercourse. The gel acts as a barrier to block sperm from entering the cervix and the nonoxynol-9 is spermicidal. To insert the film, the VCF® is removed from the packaging, folded in half, placed on the tip of the second or third finger and then inserted into the vagina and applied against the cervix. A new film should be applied every time the couple engages in intercourse. Women should not douche after intercourse; the gel will disappear on its own.

Advantages

It is discreet, easy to use and carry and relatively inexpensive (approximately $1.50 per sheet).

Disadvantages

May cause irritation to the vagina or penis and requires application before intercourse.

Failure Rate

When combined with a condom, the contraceptive vaginal film has a failure rate of about 2%.[23]

Mechanical ("Barrier") Methods

Male Condoms (Figure 2)

The history of condoms goes back to medieval times when sheaths of linen or animal intestine were used. Today, the condom is a sheath of processed lamb cecum ("lambskin"), latex or polyurethane that fits over the erect penis. It provides a receptacle that prevents semen from reaching the vagina and cervix. The use of latex condoms as a component of "safer sex" is widely publicized and encouraged as a means of reducing the risk of transmission of STDs, including HIV.[24,25]

In 2001, the Department of Health and Human Services published a report that summarized the scientific evidence on latex condom effectiveness for STD prevention.[26] The report concluded that consistent use of condoms reduced the risk of HIV transmission by 85% for both males and females and reduced the risk of gonorrhea by 25 to 75% in males. The reports states that there was adequate evidence to conclude that condoms do not reduce the risk of human papillomavirus infection in females. For most STDs including gonorrhea in females, and chlamydia, trichomonas, genital herpes, chancroid and syphilis in both males and females, there was inadequate data upon which to reach any conclusions about protection offered by condom usage. This report has generated much debate in the field of infectious diseases and will most likely stimulate further well-controlled research on the effectiveness of condoms for the prevention of STD transmission.

Theoretically, condoms should be completely effective in preventing contraception. In the real world, however, they are not so effective. The broad range in reported efficacy may result from study design, patient demographics and socioeconomic status. Condom failure can be attributed to either breakage or slippage. The incidences of breakage and slippage have been reported to be between 0.5 and 2.5% and 0.6 and 2%, respectively.[27-30] Risk factors associated with breakage include low income and low education of the user, opening the package with sharp objects, unrolling condoms before donning, lack of sex education or experience in using condoms, and a larger penile circumference.[27-31] Risk factors for slippage include lengthy or intense intercourse and unrolling condoms before donning. In one study the use of lubricants was associated with increased slippage in vaginal intercourse and reduced slippage in anal intercourse.[27]

Alcohol and drug use have also been shown to be associated with an increased incidence of condom failure (both breakage and slippage).[27-31] The other leading cause of condom failure relates to user attitudes that lead to inconsistent use (e.g., reduction in physical sensations, uncomfortable feeling, interruption in sexual activity, perception that sexual activity must be less vigorous, fear of sending a message that either the user or partner is unclean).

Condoms should not be used after the expiry date. They should be kept in a cool, dry place and condoms with clear packaging should be kept out of the sunlight. Use condoms with water-based lubricants only. Oil-based lubricants (e.g., massage oil, Vaseline®) should never be used with latex condoms as they cause the latex to deteriorate. Condoms should not be disposed of in the toilet. After use, they should be wrapped in tissue and disposed of in the garbage.

Latex condoms are more elastic than lambskin and as a result, are more likely to remain in place on the penis during intercourse and on withdrawal. Electron microscopic examination of the surface of a latex condom reveals no breaks or pores, which is the reason latex condoms are considered impenetrable to organisms that cause STDs, including HIV. Latex condoms are available with a variety of features: reservoir end, lubricated (wet or dry), lubricated with spermicide (nonoxynol-9), thin latex, extra strength, tapered, contoured, ribbed, studded, textured internal surface, colored and flavored. Most are produced in a standard size; however smaller and larger sizes are also available.

It is estimated that up to 10% of the population is allergic to latex. Repeated exposure to certain proteins in the latex is thought to be the cause of allergies. The most common symptoms for both men and women is genital inflammation with redness, itching and burning. In more severe cases, intraepidermal edema leads to the formation of vesicles. Once the vesicles rupture, the skin weeps, oozes and crusts. The easiest approach to dealing with this problem is to switch to polyurethane or lamb cecum condoms or the female condom. Before polyurethane products were introduced, couples would use a lambskin condom along with a latex condom for STD protection (i.e., if the allergy is exhibited by the woman, a lambskin condom could be worn over a latex condom; if the man is allergic, a lambskin condom could be worn under the latex condom).

Polyurethane (non-latex) condoms are also available in Canada (e.g., Trojan Supra®, Avanti Superthin® by Durex). Polyurethane is stronger than latex; therefore, the condoms are thinner and allow for greater sensation. Polyurethane offers the same level of protection against pregnancy and STDs as latex condoms.

Lambskin condoms are not noted for elasticity and may slip off the penis during intercourse or withdrawal. It is claimed they provide better transmission of body heat and therefore greater sensitivity. Magnification of natural membrane condoms show a surface riddled with pores of differing diameters which can allow for the transmission of STDs and HIV. They are also more expensive.

Advantages

- Easy and convenient to obtain and to use
- They prolong intercourse (less stimulation)
- Arousing to put on
- Protect both men and women from STDs (latex and poylurethane only)
- Inexpensive
- Good option for people who engage in sexual acts infrequently
- Can be used without medical supervision

Disadvantages

- Interruption in lovemaking
- Reduced sensation
- Necessity of prompt withdrawal after intercourse
- Awareness of its presence
- Less vigorous intercourse because condom may slip
- Difficulty in putting it on correctly
- Embarrassment
- Sometimes does not stay in place
- Difficult to dispose of
- Messy to use

Failure Rate

When used alone, condoms have a failure rate of 14%,[21] but when used with a spermicidal agent, the failure rate is less than 2%.[14]

Female Condoms (Figure 3)

The female condom (Reality Condom®) is the first female barrier contraceptive that protects against STD

Figure 2: **Male Condom**

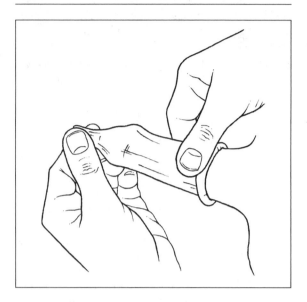

transmission and pregnancy.[32] It is a polyurethane pouch with rings at each end that help to keep the condom in place. The closed end is inserted into the vagina and covers the cervix. The ring on the closed end helps anchor it in place like a diaphragm. The open end hangs out of the vagina. The ring on this end is placed against the body and helps prevent the condom from entering the vagina. After intercourse the condom is removed and discarded. A new condom must be used for repeated intercourse.

Advantages

This product gives women more control over contraception. In contrast to the male condom, it can be inserted several hours in advance so it is less likely to spoil the mood. Any lubricant can be used with this product since it is not latex-based. It offers protection against STDs as well as unwanted pregnancy. It can be used in latex-allergic individuals.

Disadvantages

The condom is large and unattractive. More skill is required to use it correctly when compared to a male condom. It hangs outside the vagina and may make rustling noises prior to and during intercourse. Female condoms are not widely available and may be difficult to procure.

Figure 3: **Female Condom**

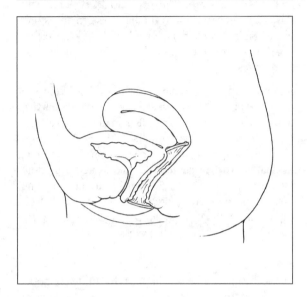

Failure Rate

Failure can range from as low as 5% when used correctly and consistently, to as high as 21% for occasional users.[33]

Diaphragm (Figure 4)

A diaphragm is a small, soft rubber dome with a covered flexible spring at the outer edge, that is used in conjunction with a spermicidal gel or cream.[34,35] The diaphragm holds the spermicide close to the cervix. Proper use of the diaphragm and contraceptive cream or gel prevents the sperm from entering the uterus, reducing the chance of pregnancy. The use of a diaphragm offers some protection against STDs but no protection against HIV. Although a diaphragm does not require a prescription, a woman must be properly fitted by a physician or trained nurse. Women also usually receive appropriate counseling about the use of their diaphragm by the same professional. If not, provide the following information to these women.

To apply the contraceptive gel or cream, the diaphragm should be held dome-side down and about one tablespoon of gel or cream squeezed into the dome. A little of the gel or cream is applied to the rim of the diaphragm with a finger. A diaphragm can be inserted up to six hours before intercourse and should stay in place for at least six hours after intercourse, but must be removed within 24 hours to reduce the risk of toxic shock syndrome. To insert the diaphragm, it must first be folded and then inserted into the vaginal canal. The diaphragm is pushed along the back of the vagina as far as it will go. The front rim is tucked up along the roof of the vagina behind the pubic bone and the back rim of the diaphragm is below and behind the cervix. This is usually done with the woman standing with one foot propped up, squatting or lying on her back. When the diaphragm is properly in place, the woman should not feel it, nor should the male partner be aware of its presence.

The diaphragm can be removed by hooking the index finger behind the front rim and pulling down and out. Alternatively, the woman can assume a squatting position and push downward with her abdominal muscles (bearing down as one would for a bowel movement). Once removed, it should be washed with mild soap and water, rinsed, dried with a towel and then stored in its plastic container. Applying talcum powder or perfumed powder can damage the diaphragm, so this practice should be strongly discouraged. Oil-based lubricants can decrease the integrity of a diaphragm. Only water-soluble lubricants should be used if required.

Advantages

Since the diaphragm can be inserted in advance, it need not interfere with the sexual encounter.

Disadvantages

Because the diaphragm is made from latex, it cannot be used in latex allergic patients. It can be difficult to insert and remove and can become dislodged during sexual intercourse. Diaphragms require refitting after childbirth or significant weight change (i.e., 5 to 10 kg).

Failure Rate

When used correctly and consistently, the diaphragm has a failure rate of 6%; however, typical failure rates of 18% have been quoted in the literature.[34,35]

Cervical Cap (Figure 5)

The cervical cap is a dome-shaped device made of latex or silicone that fits snugly over the cervix.[36] The groove on the inside of the cap creates a seal and

Figure 4: **Diaphragm in Place**

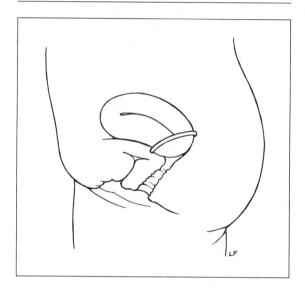

keeps the cap in place with support of the vaginal wall. Although they do not require a prescription, cervical caps should be fitted by a trained health care professional. Proper fit of the cervical cap is necessary for maximum efficacy. Like the diaphragm, the cervical cap is a barrier that blocks passage of sperm from the vagina through the cervix and is used in conjunction with a spermicide. If lubrication is required, oil-based products (e.g., Vaseline®) are not recommended as they can decrease the integrity of the cap. Only water-soluble lubricants should be used.

The following directions should be followed when using a cervical cap. The cap should be filled to about one-third full with spermicide. The rim of a cervical cap should *not* be covered with spermicide. The rim should be squeezed between the thumb and forefinger and inserted into the vagina. The cap is pushed as deep into the vagina as it will go. Suction is produced by pressing on the dome and twisting the cap like the lid on a jar. Proper fitting is verified by running a finger along the rim and firmly tugging down on the dome. The cap should remain in place and there should be a sensation of the cervix being pulled. To remove it, the cap is tilted to one side and a finger is hooked under the rim to pull it out. The cap should be left in place for at least eight hours after intercourse and for a total no longer than 48 hours.

Once removed, the cap is washed with mild soap and warm water. The groove of the inner rim is cleaned with a cotton swab. The cap should be dried and dusted with cornstarch to inhibit moisture and stored in its original container. For additional cleansing the cap can be soaked in bleach, alcohol or vinegar for 10 minutes.

A cervical cap by the name of "Oves®" is being sold on the Internet.[37] This cervical cap is a disposable cap that is worn for three days. It is made from silicone, and can be used in patients with latex allergies. According to the manufacturer this product is being evaluated in a large trial in the United Kingdom. Preliminary data in only 12 women are encouraging, but it is far too early to predict its efficacy. The Oves® cap comes in three sizes (26, 28, 30 mm) and requires proper fitting by a trained professional.

Advantages
Cervical caps can be left in place for up to 48 hours, allowing spontaneous protected sex. Less spermicide is required than with the diaphragm and the cap is smaller and even less noticeable to the partner. Caps can often be worn when a diaphragm doesn't fit well. They can be a good alternative for women who cannot use the diaphragm due to poor vaginal muscle tone and/or a history of chronic bladder infections.

Disadvantages
They may not be suitable for every woman (size, shape and position of the cervix are determining factors in a fit). They can be more difficult to insert than a diaphragm and can be dislodged from the cervix during intercourse. An unpleasant odor can occur when the cap is used for longer than the recommended maximum (48 hours).

Failure Rate
When used correctly and consistently, the cervical cap has a failure rate of 9%. Typical failure rates of 18% have been quoted in the literature.[36]

Intrauterine Devices (Figure 6)
An intrauterine device (IUD) is a small T-shaped device that is inserted into the uterus to prevent pregnancy.[38,39] There are currently two IUDs on the market: a copper IUD and a levonorgestrel IUD. Both require a prescription. Although the precise

Figure 5: **Diaphragm and Cervical Cap**

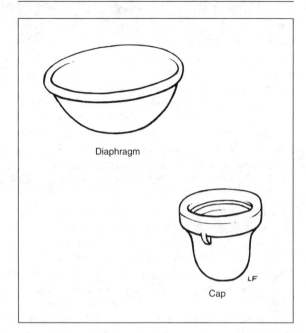

Diaphragm

Cap

LF

mechanism of action of IUDs is unknown, it is generally accepted that **copper IUDs** work by impeding ascent of sperm to the fallopian tubes or by reducing the ability of the sperm to fertilize an ovum. A foreign body reaction in the uterus causes both cellular and biochemical changes that may be toxic to sperm. The **levonorgestrel-containing IUD** offers the same "foreign body" mechanism plus the levonorgestrel causes thickening of the cervical mucus, an antiproliferative effect on the endometrium and possibly, suppression of ovulation in some women. The copper IUD should be replaced within 30 months and the levonorgestrel IUD should be replaced within five years. IUDs are inserted by a trained health care professional.

Advantages
IUDs are highly effective forms of contraception. They do not require application prior to sexual relations and can remain inserted for up to 30 months (copper IUD) or five years (levonorgestrel IUD). The IUD is relatively inexpensive over the long term and may be associated with a lower risk of endometrial and cervical cancer.[40]

Disadvantages
There is a possibility of perforation of the uterus. IUDs can be associated with bleeding and cramping which can result in removal in 10 to 15% of cases.

Failure Rate
In a comparative clinical trial copper IUDs had a failure rate of 5.9% and the levonorgestrel IUD had a failure rate of 0.5%.[39]

Figure 6: **Intrauterine Device (IUD)**

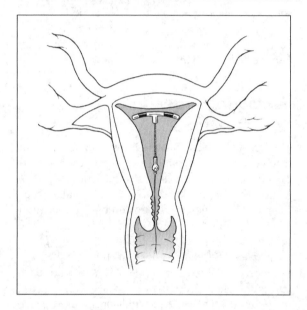

Emergency Contraception
Introduction

It is estimated that about half of all pregnancies are unplanned and a quarter of them end in abortions.[40] Emergency contraception (EC) is a means by which unplanned pregnancies can be avoided, thus reducing the need for abortions. ECs are methods used to protect against unplanned pregnancies after having unprotected sex. They offer no protection against sexually transmitted diseases (STDs). EC is meant to be used after an isolated act and should not be relied upon as a usual method of contraception because it is not as effective as regularly used contraceptives. Situations that warrant EC include completely unprotected intercourse, a broken condom, displacement of a diaphragm or cervical cap during intercourse, sexual assault, missed doses of regular birth control, unplanned sexual encounter where a condom was not available.

There are many methods of EC, the most common being oral estrogen/progestin combinations, progestin alone or insertion of an IUD.

Hormonal EC is normally used within 72 hours of unprotected intercourse and is more effective the earlier it is used. There is some evidence that combined hormonal EC (estrogen/progestin) may be somewhat effective beyond the 72-hour period, up to five days after intercourse. Insertion of an IUD can be used as a method of EC up to seven days after unprotected intercourse.

Estrogen/Progestin Combinations

The use of an estrogen/progestin combination for emergency contraception was first described by Yuzpe et al, in 1974 and has subsequently been named the "Yuzpe method."[41] The original study examined the efficacy of a single dose of 100 μg of ethinyl estradiol (EE) with 1.0 mg of norgestrel. The dosing was subsequently altered to the above regimen given twice, with the first dose taken within 72 hours of unprotected intercourse and the second dose 12 hours later. In Canada, Ovral® (EE 50 μg, norgestrel 0.5 mg) has been traditionally used in the Yuzpe method. Other oral contraceptives can also be used to obtain the same doses of hormones, but they require more tablets to make up the total doses

needed (Table 1). The Preven® kit was the first product to be officially indicated for EC in Canada. It was later withdrawn due to lack of sales.

Mechanism of Action

Several possible mechanisms of action have been proposed for the Yuzpe method. These mechanisms depend on the point in the menstrual cycle at which the hormones are consumed. EC will either delay ovulation, or result in anovulation if taken before ovulation occurs.[42] The progestin component will also cause thickening of the cervical mucus.[42] If EC is taken after ovulation, it may interfere with implantation.[42]

Efficacy

Failure rates reported in trials using the Yuzpe method have ranged from 0.2 to 7.4%.[43] A meta-analysis of pooled data from eight studies estimated that the Yuzpe method probably prevented 74% of pregnancies.[44] The efficacy of the Yuzpe method is higher when taken closer to the time of unprotected intercourse and decreases over time. A World Health Organization Task Force study showed that delaying the first dose of the Yuzpe method from 12 to 24 hours after intercourse increased the risk of pregnancy by up to 50%.[43]

Side Effects

Nausea (30 to 70%) and vomiting (15 to 25%) were the most commonly reported adverse effects of the Yuzpe method.[45] For this reason, the use of an antinauseant (i.e., dimenhydrinate) one hour before the hormone doses is recommended. Most references recommend repeating the dose if vomiting occurs up to three hours after the dose.[45] One study incorporating an

Table 1: **Estrogen/Progestin Combinations for Emergency Contraception**

Trade name	Estrogen	Progestin	1st Dose	2nd Dose
Ovral	ethinyl estradiol 50 μg	norgestrel 0.5 mg	2 tablets	2 tablets
MinOvral	ethinyl estradiol 30 μg	levonorgestrel 150 μg	4 tablets	4 tablets
Alesse	ethinyl estradiol 20 μg	levonorgestrel 100 μg	5 tablets	5 tablets
Triquilar	ethinyl estradiol 30 μg	levonorgestrel 125 μg	4 yellow tablets	4 yellow tablets
Triphasil	ethinyl estradiol 30 μg	levonorgestrel 125 μg	4 yellow tablets	4 yellow tablets

antinauseant showed the lowest nausea and vomiting incidence, 28 and 9.6% respectively.[42] Other possible side effects include headache, dizziness, fatigue, mood changes, menstrual irregularities, vaginal bleeding, and abdominal pain.[46] Regular menses should occur on the expected day, but the Yuzpe method can delay menses by a few days. Approximately 11.5% of women have a delay of greater than three days beyond expected menses.[47]

The only true contraindication to the Yuzpe method is pregnancy (because it is ineffective); however, past history of thromboembolism and migraine with aura are also considered contraindications by some authors.[43,48] Researchers believe that pregnancy itself poses a far greater risk of thromboembolism to women with a previous history of embolic events than the Yuzpe method.[46] The risk of thromboembolism due to pregnancy in this population has been estimated to be 60 per 100,000 women.[46] The risk of thromboembolism due to the Yuzpe method has not been systematically studied, but there have been three cases of venous thromboembolism reported in the United Kingdom after approximately four million users.[48]

Progestin-Only

The use of levonorgestrel alone (two doses of 0.75 mg given 12 hours apart) was first reported by Ho and Kwan in 1993.[47] It has been used for many years in Europe and China for EC.[46] This regimen was introduced to the Canadian market in the summer of 2000 under the trade name Plan B®.

Mechanism of Action

The precise mechanism of action of levonorgestrel in EC is not known. It is believed that levonorgestrel prevents ovulation by suppressing follicular growth and corpus luteum development.[46] It is also accepted that levonorgestrel may inhibit fertilization by altering the tubal transportation of the sperm or ova.[46] Levonorgestrel may also interfere with implantation by altering the endometrium.

Efficacy

In a comparative clinical trial of almost 2000 women, the levonorgestrel method produced a slightly better response than the Yuzpe method.[50] The pregnancy rates were 3.2 and 1.1% with the Yuzpe and

levonorgestrel methods, respectively. Efficacy was highly dependent on the timing of first dose relative to the time of unprotected intercourse. If the first dose was given within 24 hours, the pregnancy rate was 2 to 0.4% for Yuzpe and levonorgestrel, respectively. At 25 to 48 hours post-intercourse, the pregnancy rate rose to 4.1 and 1.2%. At 49 to 72 hours, the pregnancy rate was 4.7 and 2.2%.

Side Effects

The levonorgestrel regimen offers the advantage of fewer adverse effects than the Yuzpe method. In the comparative trial the incidences of adverse effects from the levonorgestrel and Yuzpe groups were nausea (23.1 vs. 50.5%), vomiting (5.6 vs. 18.8%), dizziness (11.2 vs. 16.7%), fatigue (16.9 vs. 28.5%), headache (16.8 vs. 20.2%), breast tenderness (10.8 vs. 12.1%), and lower abdominal pain (17.6 vs. 20.9%).[50] Clearly, the levonorgestrel regimen was better tolerated than the Yuzpe method.

Despite levonorgestrel not being recognized as a major teratogen, pregnancy is still considered a contraindication to its use for EC. Levonorgestrel has no known adverse effects on clotting factors, so its use in women with a history of thromboembolism and migraine with aura is safer than the Yuzpe method.[51]

Intrauterine Devices (IUDs)

The postcoital insertion of a copper IUD is a highly effective means of EC.[46] In Canada there is only one copper IUD on the market (Nova-T®). The added benefit of IUDs for EC is that they can be inserted up to 10 days after unprotected intercourse and retain their effectiveness,[46] although the Society of Obstetricians and Gynecologists of Canada recommends they be used for EC only up to seven days after unprotected intercourse.

Another benefit of the use of an IUD for EC is that it can be left in place and used as an effective contraceptive method for the life of the device. Obtaining an IUD for this indication is not as easy as the Yuzpe or levonorgestrel options. Insertion of an IUD requires a trained professional and a pelvic examination.

Mechanism of Action

The copper IUD has never been a popular choice for EC because some people believe IUDs function as an abortifacient.[52] This is based on the proposed mechanism of action of IUDs. Some argue that IUDs function by preventing implantation of a fertilized ovum. A scientific statement from the World Health Organization argued that it was unlikely that the efficacy of IUDs was based mainly or exclusively on their ability to interfere with implantation.[53] They added that IUDs most likely interfere with steps in the reproductive process that occur before fertilization of the ovum (e.g., direct toxic effect on the sperm). After reviewing the available evidence, the American College of Obstetricians and Gynecologists also concluded that IUDs do not function as an abortifacient.[54]

Efficacy

The copper IUD is a highly effective means of EC. A review of the studies concluded that the pregnancy rate was less than 0.1%.[55]

Side Effects

IUDs can cause vaginal bleeding and uterine cramping. Insertion of the IUD can be painful.

Other Methods of Emergency Contraception

Androgens

Danazol, a semisynthetic steroid androgen, was first reported to be an effective form of EC in 1983.[56] Mixed results from clinical trials, however, have limited its use for this indication.[43]

Mechanism of Action

Danazol blocks steroidogenesis in the ovary and after ovulation has an effect on endometrial receptors.[46]

Efficacy

In the first study, danazol, given as two doses of 400 mg 12 hours apart, produced a pregnancy rate of 6%.[56] In a larger study, single doses of danazol 800 mg or 1200 mg produced pregnancy rates of 1.7 and 0.8%, respectively.[57] In a trial that compared danazol 600 mg given as two doses 12 hours apart to the Yuzpe regimen, the pregnancy rates were 4.66 and 2.66%, respectively.[58] This difference was statistically significant.

Side Effects

Danazol causes less nausea than the Yuzpe method (approximate incidence of 10%).[57] Other reported adverse effects include headache, vomiting, breast pain or tenderness, pelvic pain, lethargy, fatigue, dizziness.[57]

Antiprogesterones

Mifepristone, also known as RU-486, is a controversial oral abortifacient agent. It has been used in Europe for many years as an abortifacient and is now available in the United States for this indication on a limited basis. Mifepristone is also an effective agent when used for EC. It is currently the leading form of EC in China.[49] Mifepristone is currently available through the Special Access Programme, Health Canada, and is undergoing clinical trials in Canada as an abortifacient, hence its access is limited to use within trial protocols.

Mechanism of Action

Mifepristone binds to progesterone receptors in a competitive manner.[46] When given before ovulation, mifepristone interrupts follicular maturation. It may also disrupt the midcycle surge and cause regression of the dominant follicle. Since progesterone plays such an important role in the maintenance of the endometrium, mifepristone has a marked effect on the endometrium.[59]

Efficacy

A single dose of mifepristone 600 mg given within 72 hours of unprotected intercourse was superior in efficacy to the Yuzpe method in two comparative trials.[60,61] A dose-finding study examined the efficacy of 10, 50, and 600 mg of mifepristone when given within five days of unprotected intercourse.[62] Pregnancy rates were 1.2, 1.1, and 1.3% in the 10, 50, and 600 mg dose groups, respectively. The authors estimated that mifepristone, used for EC would prevent 84 to 86% of pregnancies when using an estimate of expected recognizable pregnancies. There was no difference in efficacy of mifepristone with respect to administration of dose from time of unprotected intercourse.

Side Effects

Side effects reported with mifepristone for EC include nausea (17.4%), headache (12.6%), dizziness (12.6%), and vomiting (1.7%).[62] Delay in expected menses of three days or more was reported in 18, 23, and 26% of women with mifepristone 10, 50, and 600 mg doses, respectively. This can lead to much anxiety in the patient.

Access to EC

The prescription status of levonorgestrel EC regimens is currently being reviewed in Canada. At present, women can access all methods of EC through a physician in any province. However, some provinces have made hormonal EC available directly from pharmacists without the woman having to first visit a physician. For information on the current prescription status of hormonal EC in individual provinces, contact the provincial pharmacy licensing body.

Lack of knowledge is a major limiting factor to the use of EC. The general population is largely unaware of the concept, as are many health care professionals. National campaigns are needed to make women aware of these methods to prevent unplanned pregnancies.

Resource Tips

Sexualityand**u**.ca, developed by the Society of Obstetricians and Gynecologists of Canada: www.sexualityandu.ca.

Fertility devices: www.babytech.com; www.birthcontrol.com; www.persona.org.uk

Planned Parenthood Federation of Canada http://www.ppfc.ca/index.html.

Suggested Readings

American College of Obstetricians and Gynecologists. Emergency Oral Contraception. *ACOG Practice Bulletin*. Number 25. Washington, DC: The American College of Obstetrics and Gynecologists, March, 2001.

American Health Consultants. *Contraceptive Technology Update: A Monthly Newsletter for Health Professionals*. Available from: http://www.hc-sc.gc.ca/hppb/srh/e_links.html.

Canadian Consensus Conference on Contraception. *Journal SOGC* 1998;20(5,6,7,8). Available from:

http://sogc.medical.org/SOGCnet/sogc_docs/common/guide/pdfs/CSOeng.pdf.

Davis V, Dunn S. Emergency Postcoital Contraception: SOGC Clinical Practice Guidelines. *Journal SOGC* July 2000;92:1-5. Available from: http://sogc.medical.org/SOGCnet/sogc_docs/common/guide/pdfs/ps9.pdf.

Ho PC. Emergency contraception: methods and efficacy. *Curr Opin Obst Gynecol* 2000;12:175-9.

LaVelleur J. Emergency contraception. *Obstet Gynecol Clin North Am* 2000;27(4): 817-39.

Montreal Health Press. *Birth Control Handbook*. 1999. P.O. Box 1000, Station Place du Parc, Montreal, Quebec, H2W 2N1. Tel.: (514) 282-1171; Fax: (514) 282-0262.

Thomas MA. Postcoital contraception. *Clin Obstet Gynecol* 2001;44:101-5.

References

1. Health Canada: Health Promotion Online. Available from: http://www.hc-sc.gc.ca/hppb/srh/e_factsheet.html. Accessed June 17, 2000.
2. Carr BR, Wilson JD. Disorders of the ovary and female reproductive tract. Chapter 340. In: Isselbacher et al, eds. *Harrison's Principles of Internal Medicine*, 13th ed. Toronto, ON: McGraw-Hill Inc., 1994.
3. Parenteau-Carreau S. The sypto-thermal methods. *International Journal of Fertility* 1981;26(3):170-81.
4. Rice FJ, Lanctot CA, Garcia-Devesa C. Effectiveness of the sympto-thermal method of natural family planning: an international study. *International Journal of Fertility* 1981;26(3): 222-30.
5. de Leizaola MA. Prospective study of the efficacy of a recent sympto-thermal method of natural family planning. *Journal de Gynecologie, Ostetrique et Biologie de la Reproduction* 1998;27(2):174-80.
6. Ovu-Trac Natural Fertility Tester. Available from: http://www.birthcontrol.com/vu.html. Accessed November 2, 2001.
7. *Luna Fertility Indicator*. Available from: http://www.lunafert.com/howit.html. Accessed November 2, 2001.
8. ClearPlan Easy Fertility Monitor. *ClearPlan ClearResults*. Available from: http://clearplan.com/canada/. Accessed November 2, 2001.
9. Pheromone Sciences Corp. Fertility Monitor Project. Available from: http://pheromonesciences.com. Accessed November 2, 2001.
10. Babytech.com *Bioself Fertility Monitor*. Available from: http://www. babytech.com/bioself.html. Accessed June 28, 2001.
11. Persona. Available from: http://www.persona.org.uk/. Accessed June 28, 2001.
12. NaturalMethods Lady-Comp. Available from: http://www. naturalmethods.com/MainFrame.html. Accessed June 28, 2001.

13. Fruendl G, Frank-Hermann P, Godehardt E, et al. Retrospective clinical trial of contraceptive effectiveness of the electronic fertility indicator Ladycomp/Babycomp. *Adv Contracept* 1998; 14:97-108.

14. Contraception – Spermicidal Agents. Available from: http://www.well-net. com/womenshealth/contraception/contraceptionspermacidalagents-1.html. Accessed July 27, 2001.

15. Malow RM, Ziskind D, Jones DL. Use of female controlled microbicidal products for HIV risk reduction. *AIDS Care* 2000;12(5):581-8.

16. Cook RL, Rosenberg MJ. Do spermicides containing nonoxynol-9 prevent sexually transmitted infections? A meta-analysis. *Sex Trans Dis* 1998;25(3):144-50.

17. Richardson BA, Lavreys L, Martin HL, et al. Evaluation of a low-dose nonoxynol-9 gel for the prevention of sexually transmitted diseases: a randomized clinical trial. *Sex Trans Dis* 2001;28(7):394-400.

18. Roddy RE, Zekeng L, Ryan KA et al. A controlled trial of nonoxynol-9 film to reduce male-to-female transmission of sexually transmitted diseases. *N Engl J Med* 1998;339(8):504-10.

19. Courtot AM, Nikas G, Gravanis A, et al. Effects of cholic acid and "Protectaid" formulations on human sperm motility and ultrastructure. *Hum Reprod* 1994;9(11):1999-2005.

20. Psychoyos A, Creatsas G, Hassan E et al. Spermicidal and antiviral properties of cholic acid: contraceptive efficacy of a new vaginal sponge (Protectaid) containing sodium cholate. *Hum Reprod* 1993;8(6):866-9.

21. Hatcher RA, Trussel J, Stewart F, et al. *Contraceptive Technology.* 17th revised ed. New York, NY: Irvington Publishers, 1998.

22. Mauck CK, Baker JM, Barr SP et al. A phase I comparative study of three contraceptive vaginal films containing nonoxynol-9. Postcoital testing and colpsocopy. *Contraception* 1997;56(2):97-102.

23. Mauck CK, Allen S, Baker JM et al. An evaluation of the amount of nonoxynol-9 remaining in the vagina up to 4 hours after insertion of a vaginal contraceptive film (VCF) containing 70 mg nonoxynol-9. *Contraception* 1997;56(2):103-10.

24. Wellesley College Health Service. *A word about condoms.* Available from: http://www.wellesley.edu/Health/education/contracepts/condoms.html. Accessed July 27, 2001.

25. Health Education Associates. *Condoms – contraception & safe sex.* Available from: http://www.well-net.com/womenshealth/contraception/ condomscontraceptionsafesex.html. Accessed July 27, 2001.

26. National Institute of Allegy and Infectious Diseases, National Institutes of Health, Department of Health and Human Services. *Workshop Summary: Scientific evidence on condom effectiveness for sexually transmitted disease prevention.* July 20, 2001. Available from: http://www.niaid.nih. gov/dmid/stds/condomreport.pdf. Accessed November 2, 2001.

27. Smith AM, Jolley D, Hocking J et al. Does additional lubrication affect condom slippage and breakage. *Int J STD AIDS* 1998;9(6):330-5.

28. Spruyt A, Steiner MJ, Joanis C et al. Identifying condom users at risk for breakage and slippage: findings from three international studies. *Am J Pub Health* 1998;88 (2):239-44.

29. Rosenberg MJ, Waugh MS. Latex condom breakage and slippage in a controlled clinical trial. *Contraception* 1997;56(1): 17-21.

30. Lindberg LD, Sonenstein FL, Ku L et al. Young men's experience with condom breakage. *Fam Plann Perspect* 1997;29(3):128-31.

31. Smith AD, Jolley D, Hocking J et al. Does penis size influence condom slippage and breackage. *Int J STD AIDS* 1998;9(8):444-7.

32. Emory Department of Gynecology & Obstetrics. *Condoms for Women: The Reality Female Condom.* Available from: http://www.emory.edu/WHSC/MED/FAMPLAN/reality.html: Accessed July 27, 2001.

33. Anne Rose's Ulimate Birth Control Links Page. Available from: http://www.ultimatebirthcontrol.org/. Accessed July 27, 2001.

34. Indiana University Health Centre. *Diaphragm.* Available from: http://www.indiana.edu/~health/diaph.html. Accessed July 27, 2001.

35. University of Toronto Sexual Education and Peer Counselling Centre. *Diaphragm and Spermicidal Jelly.* Available from: http://www.campuslife.utoronto.ca/services/sec/dia. html. Accessed July 27, 2001.

36. Indiana University Health Centre. *Cervical cap.* Available from: http://www.indiana.edu/~health/cervcap.html. Accessed July 27, 2001.

37. Veos UK. *Ovès: the new contraceptive cap.* Available from: http://www.oves.com/english/index.htm. Accessed July 27, 2001.

38. Roberto R, Yacobson I, Grimes D. The mechanism of action of hormonal contraception and intrauterine contraceptive devices. *Am J Obs Gyn* 1999;181(5, part 1):1263-9.

39. Andersson K, Odlind V, Rybo G. Levonorgestrel-releasing and copper-releasing (Nova T) IUDs during five years of use: A randomized comparative trial. *Contraception* 1994; 49(1):56-72.

40. Endometrial and cervical cancer risk may be lower with IUD use. *Contraception Rpt* 1998;9(5):9-10.

41. Yuzpe AA, Thurlow HJ, Pamzy I et al. Post coital contraception: A pilot study. *J Reprod Med* 1974;13:53-7.

42. Chiou VM, Shrier LY, Emans SJ. Emergency postcoital contraception. *J Pediatr Adolesc Gynecol* 1998;11:61-72.

43. Ho PC. Emergency contraception: methods and efficacy. *Curr Opin Obstet Gynecol* 2000;12:175-9.

44. Trussell J, Rodriguez G, Ellertson C. Updated estimates of the effectiveness of the Yuzpe regimen of emergency contraception. *Contraception* 1999;59:147-51.

45. Van Look PFA, Stewart F. Emergency contraception. In: Hatcher RA, Trussell J, Stewart F, et al., eds. *Contraceptive Technology,* 17th ed. New York, NY: Ardent Media, 1998.

46. LaVelleur J. Emergency contraception. *Obstet Gynecol Clin North Am* 2000;27(4):817-39.

47. Ho PC, Kwan MSW. A prospective randomized comparison of levonorgestrel with the Yuzpe regimen in post-coital contraception. *Hum Reprod* 1993;8:389-92.

48. Trussell J, Rodriguez G, Ellertson C. New estimates of the effectiveness of the Yuzpe method of emergency contraception. *Contraception* 1998;57:363-9.

49. Glasier A. Emergency postcoital contraception. *N Engl J Med* 1997;337:1058-64.

50. World Health Organization Task Force on Postovulatory Methods of Fertility Regulation, Randomized controlled trial of levonorgestrel versus the Yuzpe regimen of combined oral contraceptives for emergency contraception. *Lancet* 1998;352:428-33.

51. Glasier A. Safety of emergency contraception. *JAMA* 1998; 53:219-21.

52. Sivin I. IUDs are contraceptives, not abortifacients: a comment on research and belief. *Stud Fam Plann* 1989;20:355-9.

53. World Health Organization Scientific Group. *Mechanism of action, safety and effiacy of intrauterine devices.* Geneva: World Health Organization; 1987. Technical Report Series 753.

54. American College of Obstetricians and Gynecologists. *The intrauterine device.* Washington: The College, 1987. Technical Bulletin 104.

55. Trussell J, Ellertson C. Efficacy of emergency contraception. *Fertil Cont Rev* 1995;4:8-11.

56. Rowlands S, Guillebaud J, Bounds W et al. Side effects of danazol compared with an ethinylestradiol/norgestrel combination when used for postcoital contraception. *Contraception* 1983;27:39-49.

57. Zuliani G, Colombo UF, Molla R. Hormonal postcoital contraception with an ethinylestradiol-norgestrel combination and two danazol regimens. *Eur J Obstet Gynecol Reprod Biol* 1990;37:253-60.

58. Webb AMC, Russell J, Elstein M. Comparison of Yuzpe regimen, danazol, and mifepristone (RU486) in oral postcoital contraception. *BMJ* 1992;305:927-31.

59. Swahn ML, Danielsson MG, Bygdeman M. Contraception with anti-progesterone. *Bailliere's Clin Obstet Gynecol* 1996; 10:43-53.

60. Glasier A, Thong KJ, Dewar M et al. Mifepristone (RU-486) compared with high-dose estrogen and progestogen for emergency contraception. *N Engl J Med* 1992;327:1041-4.

61. Webb AMC, Russell J, Elstein M. Comparison of Yuzpe regimen, danazol, and mifepristone (RU486) in oral postcoital contraception. *BMJ* 1992;305:927-31.

62. Task Force on Postovulatory Methods of Fertility Regulation. Comparison of three single doses of mifepristone as emergency contraception: A randomized trial. *Lancet* 1999;353: 697-702.

Nonhormonal Birth Control—Patient Information

Nonhormonal birth control choices include sponges, diaphragms, cervical caps, spermicides, male and female condoms, and intrauterine devices (IUDs). Male and female condoms, diaphragms and cervical caps are much more effective when used with spermicides. Talk to your pharmacist or doctor about which method might be best for you and how to use it properly to get the most protection from pregnancy and sexually transmitted diseases (STDs). Here are some tips on using these birth control methods:

Male Condoms
- Latex condoms are much more effective when used in combination with vaginal spermicides. When used correctly, they protect against pregnancy and STDs such as AIDs.
- If you are allergic to latex, talk to your pharmacist about other choices.
- Check the expiry date before using condoms and store them in a cool dry place. Wallets and cars are not ideal places to store condoms for a long time.
- Fingernails and jewelry can tear condoms so be careful.
- For lubrication, use only water-based products such as K-Y® jelly. Oil-based products can decrease the effectiveness of latex condoms by degrading the latex.
- If the condom doesn't come with a reservoir at the end, make sure to leave some room between the tip of the penis and the tip of the condom, to collect the sperm when you ejaculate.
- After having sex, withdraw the penis right away. Hold the rim of the condom so that it doesn't slip off when you withdraw.
- If a condom breaks, the female partner should insert some spermicide into the vagina. She might want to talk to the doctor or pharmacist about emergency contraception as well.
- Used condoms should be wrapped in tissue and thrown in the garbage, not the toilet.

Female Condoms
- Safe for people with allergy to latex.
- The closed end goes inside the vagina, up near the cervix. The open end fits around the outside of the vagina.
- They are more effective when used with spermicide.

Diaphragm
- Rubber dome that fits over the cervix to stop the sperm from reaching the uterus.
- You have to be fitted by a trained health professional before ordering a diaphragm.
- Before inserting a diaphragm, put about a tablespoonful of spermicide inside the dome and a bit on the rim.
- You can insert a diaphragm up to six hours before having sex and should leave it in place for at least six hours after.
- If you have sex more than once while wearing your diaphragm, insert spermicide into the vagina before each time.
- To reduce the risk of toxic shock syndrome, a diaphragm should *never* be left in place for more than 24 hours, and don't use it if you have vaginal bleeding (during your period or after having a baby, for example).
- After having a baby, you will have to be refitted for a diaphragm about six to eight weeks after delivery, because you may need a different size.

Cervical Cap
- Looks like a diaphragm only smaller.
- The cervical cap fits snugly over the cervix and has to be in the right position to work best. Talk to your doctor or pharmacist about this.
- Fill the inside of the cap to about one-third full with spermicide, but *don't* put any on the rim.
- The cervical cap must be left in place for eight hours after having sex. It can be left in place for a total of up to 48 hours and you don't have to insert more spermicide if you have sex more than once during that time.
- Don't use the cervical cap if you have menstrual bleeding or had a baby within the last six weeks.
- After having a baby, you will need to be refitted for a cervical cap about six to eight weeks after delivery, because you may need a different size.

Contraceptive Sponge
- The sponge has three types of spermicide in it. When it is inserted properly, it covers the cervix.

- The sponge can be inserted up to six hours before having sex and should be left in place for six hours after, for a total of no more than 12 hours at a time.
- You can have sex more than once while the sponge is in place, as long as it is left in place for six hours after the last time, and *not* more than 12 hours in total.

Contraceptive Film
- Insert the film into the vagina 10 to 60 minutes before you have sex. It contains spermicide and dissolves into a gel once inside the vagina.

- A new one has to be inserted every time you have sex.
- The gel disappears on its own after sex. Douching is not necessary and not recommended.

Intrauterine Devices (IUDs)
- IUDs have to be inserted by your doctor. They protect against pregnancy, but not STDs.
- They can last for several years, depending on the type.
- Some people have heavy bleeding and cramps after their IUD is inserted.

Emergency Contraception (Birth Control)— Patient Information

Emergency contraception (EC) means using a birth control method after having unprotected sex, or when another method of birth control fails. There are two main types of EC: the "morning after pill" and intrauterine devices (IUDs).

The "morning after pill" can actually be used for up to 72 hours after unprotected sex, so the name is misleading. You have to take two doses of hormone pills, similar to regular birth control pills, 12 hours apart. Taking EC pills can decrease your chances of getting pregnant by 75%. The sooner they are taken, the better they work. Taking EC pills is not a good way to prevent pregnancy all the time. There are other more effective ways to do that.

The other main type of emergency birth control is having an IUD inserted. This can be done up to seven days after unprotected sex. One of the advantages is that it is a reliable form of birth control for several years after being inserted. Neither EC pills nor IUDs protect you from sexually transmitted diseases like AIDS.

Some things to know about using EC:
- The timing of the second dose is very important. It has to be 12 hours after the first, so you might want to time the first dose so that you are awake to take the second.
- The pills can make you sick to your stomach. You should take a medication to prevent nausea (e.g., dimenhydrinate or Gravol®) 30 to 60 minutes before each dose.
- If you vomit within three hours after taking a dose, you have to repeat the dose.
- If you can't take hormones or if it has been longer than 72 hours and less than 7 days since unprotected sex, ask your doctor about having an IUD inserted. You will have to have an examination first.
- After taking EC pills, your period should arrive on time, or it might be a few days early or late. If it is more than a week late, or if it arrives more than three weeks after you take the pills, you need to have a pregnancy test, either at home or through your doctor.
- Check with your pharmacist to see if EC pills are available without a prescription in the province you live in. You can do this by telephone, to save time.
- Talk to your pharmacist or doctor about a regular method of birth control. They can answer questions about the effectiveness, risks and prevention of STDs associated with different methods.

Chapter 50

Vaginal Symptoms

Laura-Lynn Pollock, BSc(Pharm), RPh, NARTC, Dip AC

Vaginal Physiology[1-4]

The vagina is a fibromuscular structure that connects the external genitalia, or vulva, with the internal cervix and uterus. It provides a channel for the removal of menstrual discharge, and the transverse folds or rugae of the vaginal wall allow the flexibility of size and shape that are required for sexual intercourse and childbirth.

Normal vaginal length is variable but is usually between 8 and 10 cm. The vagina is positioned at a 45° angle, upwards and posteriorly. It is in close proximity to the bladder, urethra, perineum and rectum (Figure 1).

A healthy vaginal environment is maintained through a balance among many host factors including the local bacterial flora, hormonal influences and the epithelial cells lining the vaginal wall. Estrogen induces the maturation of the epithelial cells and stimulates the proliferation of epithelial basal cells. It also increases the cells' ability to store glycogen, which is subsequently metabolized to lactic acid by the vaginal bacterium, *L. vaginalis*, making the vagina acidic with a pH of 3.5 to 5.5. The nonpathogenic Lactobacilli thrive in the acidic environment while the proliferation of more troublesome microflora is controlled.

There is normally a vaginal discharge that varies in quantity, consistency and appearance throughout the menstrual cycle. This discharge can be due to mucus production of the cervical glands, a transudate from the capillaries of the vaginal walls, and/or from various other sources such as the uterus. Monthly hormone fluctuations are responsible for the changing characteristics of the discharge. Sometimes the discharge is pasty, white and scanty. Other times it is

Figure 1: **Female Reproductive System**

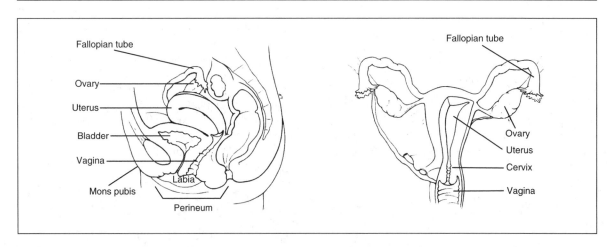

wet, slippery and has the consistency of uncooked egg white (around the time of ovulation). There is often no apparent discharge on the days immediately after menses has stopped. Vaginal discharge contributes to the health of the vagina and helps to maintain the pH and normal microflora. It should not cause irritation, burning or itching.

A mild odor may occur when vaginal discharge combines with secretions from glands in the vulvar area. This odor should not be unpleasant or cause concern. Causes of unusual or unpleasant odor, genital irritation or itching may include poor hygiene, allergic or sensitivity reactions to products used, vaginal infections or a forgotten tampon.

Genital Hygiene[1,2]

Proper genital hygiene can be achieved very simply. The perineal area should be washed daily using warm water and mild soap. The outer labia should be gently separated and the clitoral area cleaned and rinsed. This area can be sensitive to perfumes and harsh ingredients in some soaps, so only mild products should be used. After cleansing, the perineal area should be rinsed well with warm water to remove soap residue.

The vagina cleanses itself naturally through its secretions and does not require further cleansing.

Although normal genital hygiene does not require the use of nonprescription products, there are a number of products marketed for just that purpose. Some women choose to use vaginal douches, genital towlettes and feminine deodorant sprays even though they are rarely necessary and may carry risks for the users.

Vaginal Douching

Douching is a process of instilling fluid into the vagina and flushing the cavity. It has been used for hygienic reasons, and although not effective for these purposes, it has been used by some women to decrease vaginal irritation and itching, to treat a suspected vaginal infection, or postcoitally as attempted birth control.[5,6]

There are no substantiated benefits to routine douching and it can be associated with significant adverse outcomes:

- Douching may disrupt the normal vaginal environment, increasing the risk of irritation or infection.
- Douching may play a role in the development of ascending infections of the genital tract (e.g., salpingitis and pelvic inflammatory disease), ectopic pregnancy and possibly cancer of the cervix.[7,8]

- Douching postcoitally is not an effective contraceptive method. It should be avoided until at least six hours after intercourse if a vaginal spermicide has been used, because douching can decrease the effectiveness of the spermicide.
- It should also be avoided within 24 hours prior to a vaginal examination as this may hinder detection of a vaginal infection.

Despite this, douching is still used by women for a variety of reasons. To decrease potential risks, it is important to provide sound advice to these women to help prevent adverse effects. The use of suitable solutions and appropriate technique are important safety factors. Douching should be avoided during pregnancy unless it is on a physician's advice. Douching is never recommended as a contraceptive method or as a treatment for suspected vaginal infections.

Examples of douching solutions include:

- Plain warm water (simple and least likely to be harmful)
- Vinegar and water (available commercially or can be made at home by adding 15 to 30 mL vinegar to a litre of warm water; produces transient decrease in vaginal microflora, similar to flushing with saline[9])
- Commercially available products containing perfumes, astringents, antiinfectives or proteolytics (these ingredients do not increase effectiveness and can be irritating)

Instillation of the solution is by means of a vaginal syringe. There are two basic kinds of syringes – the fountain syringe and the bulb syringe. The fountain syringe consists of a piece of tubing attached to a bag (like a hot water bottle). A rounded plastic nozzle is on the end of the tubing for insertion into the vagina. Gravity creates the flow of the solution. The bulb syringe has no tubing. The vaginal tip is attached directly to a small bag or bottle. The fluid is forced out of the bulb by squeezing the device or by the inward pressure exerted by the distended walls of the bulb.

Proper technique is essential for safe douching. The pressure used to instill the solution should be gentle, not forceful. Too much pressure may cause reflux of the solution (and possibly bacteria) into the uterus, and increase the risk of pelvic infection. Correct technique is outlined in Vaginal Douching – Patient Information.

Genital Towlettes

Genital towlettes (e.g., Tucks®, Massengill® towlettes) are premoistened disposable wipes that are generally safe for occasional use. They contain ingredients such as perfumes, astringents, emmollients and antiinfectives and can be irritating or cause allergic reactions. Mild soap and warm water is preferred for daily cleansing.

Genital Deodorant Sprays

Genital deodorant sprays (e.g., FDS®) contain ingredients such as perfumes and propellants and are marketed to reduce genital odor. Their use is not recommended. They can mask odors of infections and cause treatment delays. They have a high incidence of irritation and allergic reactions. If they are used, they must not be applied to the inside of the vagina. For more information, see Genital Deodorant Sprays – Patient Information.

Toxic Shock Syndrome

Pathophysiology

Toxic shock syndrome (TSS) is a severe, life-threatening condition resulting from toxin-producing strains of *S. aureus*. Menstrual TSS became a significant concern with the introduction of hyperabsorbable tampons in the late 1970s. These products had the ability to act as a reservoir for *S. aureus*. Since the removal of these products from the market, the rate of TSS has decreased. The prevalence of menstrual TSS is 1 to 5 per 100 000 women of menstrual age per year. It primarily affects young women (15 to 25 years of age) who use tampons during menses.[10] Tampon use is a major risk factor for the development of menstrual TSS. Other risk factors include the use of diaphragms, cervical caps and contraceptive sponges.[11]

TSS can evolve clinically in rapid fashion, with a healthy woman becoming very ill in less than 12 hours. Criteria for diagnosis include:
- Temperature > 38.9°C;
- Hypotension;
- Rash with subsequent desquamation, particularly on the hands and feet;
- Involvement of at least three of the following systems: GI (vomiting, profuse diarrhea); muscular (severe myalgia); mucus membranes (hyperemia); kidney (renal insufficiency); liver (increased enzymes); blood (thrombocytopenia); and CNS (disorientation, confusion).[10]

If left untreated, TSS can be fatal.

Goals of Therapy

- Educate patients about signs and symptoms of TSS and how to avoid it
- Reduce the risk of TSS as much as possible
- Know how to ask key questions to identify possible TSS and to refer for immediate medical attention when indicated

Patient Assessment

If a young woman presents with symptoms including fever, rash, vomiting, profuse diarrhea, dizziness and/or faintness, TSS should be among the diagnoses considered. Asking the patient how the onset of illness relates temporally to her menstrual period, whether she uses tampons and what contraceptive method she uses can help determine the likelihood of TSS. If symptoms are consistent with those of TSS and can be temporally associated with the use of tampons, a diaphragm, cervical cap or contraceptive sponge, the intravaginal product should be removed immediately and she should be referred for immediate medical attention. Treatment of TSS includes aggressive fluid replacement and intravenous antibiotic therapy.[10,11]

Prevention

Risk reduction is the key to minimizing the occurrence of TSS that is associated with menstruation and/or contraceptive devices. Advise women on proper use of tampons and barrier contraceptives that are associated with an increased risk of TSS (see Toxic Shock Syndrome — Patient Information).

Vaginal Dryness

Pathophysiology

It is common to have periods of time when vaginal lubrication is decreased. Low estrogen levels during perimenopause or menopause, in the postpartum period, during lactation and immediately following menses, may result in vaginal dryness. Sometimes tampons can decrease vaginal lubrication, and occasionally women find that oral contraceptives or other medications can also contribute (Table 1). This decreased lubrication may be transient, or it may be long-term, as is often the case for peri- or postmenopausal women.[12-15] For more information on menopause and perimenopause, see Chapter 52.

Reduced levels of estrogen cause thinning of the vaginal tissue, loss of collagen support and reduced production of vaginal lubrication even when sexual arousal has occurred. These changes are associated with a number of vaginal symptoms, including vaginal dryness (Table 2).[12-15]

Goals of Therapy

- Provide lubrication to vaginal tissue
- Decrease symptoms associated with vaginal dryness
- Increase level of comfort during sexual intercourse.

Patient Assessment

The majority of women seeking advice and relief from vaginal dryness are in peri- or postmenopause. Refer women with moderate to severe or chronic vaginal dryness to their physician for assessment. It is reasonable to recommend a trial of nonprescription lubricants to women with occasional, mild to moderate symptoms.

Table 1: **Medications Associated with Decreased Vaginal Lubrication**[6,12-15]

Oral contraceptives	Antihypertensives
Antihistamines	Chemotherapy
Antidepressants	Antiarrhythmics

Table 2: **Vaginal Symptoms of Low Estrogen**[6,12-15]

Vaginal dryness
Slow production of lubrication with sexual arousal
Pruritus
Dyspareunia (pain during sexual intercourse)
Abnormal bleeding
Discharge

Nonpharmacologic Therapy

Some relief from vaginal dryness may result from increasing blood flow to the pelvic region through sexual stimulation. Intercourse is not necessary to achieve this effect and should be avoided if it is painful. Any form of sexual activity may help restore vaginal moisture.

Pharmacologic Therapy

Nonprescription Therapy

Nonprescription options consist mainly of lubricants,[12-15,17,18] which can provide rapid, short-term relief. Water-based products are generally safe for external and internal application. For dyspareunia they can be applied to the penis and the opening of the vagina to decrease discomfort. Gels (e.g., K-Y

Jelly®) are short-acting and require frequent reapplication. Bioadhesive polymers (e.g., Replens®), attach to the vaginal epithelium and provide water and electrolytes to the cells. They have a longer duration of action (two to three days) and are used on a continuous basis, not immediately prior to intercourse.

Oil-based products should be avoided because they can be irritating, difficult to remove, and can damage condoms, diaphragms and cervical caps.

Prescription Therapy

Hormonal supplementation with **estrogens** and **progestins** is a prescription option.

They can be in the form of systemic hormone replacement therapy or by vaginal application of estrogen. Topical formulations include cream or ring-shaped devices that are inserted into the vagina and deliver estrogen over a 90-day period (e.g., Estring®).

Estrogen replacement reverses the vaginal changes seen with menopause and provides relief of symptoms. Systemic hormone supplementation is particularly useful if there are a number of menopausal symptoms to control, or for possible long-term benefits such as decreased risk of osteoporosis (see Chapters 34 and 52).[10,14,16]

Herbal Remedies

Black cohosh has been used in the management of menopausal symptoms including vaginal dryness, although the evidence for its efficacy is not strong. It can cause nausea and headache and is contraindicated in pregnancy and lactation. The usual dose is 3 to 6 mL of a 1:5 tincture in 60% ethanol per day, or 500 to 1000 mg dried root or rhizome two to three times daily. It should be used with caution in women already taking estrogen and there is concern about its ability to potentiate hypotensive drugs.[17,18]

Vaginal Candidiasis

Pathophysiology[16,19]

The healthy vagina is host to a number of microorganisms including Lactobacilli, Streptococci, Staphylococci, G. vaginalis, C. albicans (and other Candida species), anaerobes and U. urealyticum. The types and numbers of these organisms vary from woman to woman due to such factors as age, sexual history, contraceptive method, pregnancy, menstruation, antibiotic use, vaginal trauma (e.g., surgery) and even tampon use.[4,16,19]

Normally, the organisms live in balance in the vaginal environment without adverse effects. When this harmony is disrupted it can allow for overproduction of host organisms or colonization by acquired pathogens. These changes set the stage for the development of vaginitis.[20,21]

Vaginitis (or vaginosis) describes a group of conditions that have similar symptoms but a variety of causes (Table 3). Treatment for vaginitis is specific to the cause, so the correct diagnosis is important. Only candidiasis is recommended for self-treatment.

Table 3: **Common Causes of Vaginitis**[20-22]

Cause	Common symptoms	Vaginal pH
Bacterial vaginosis*	"Fishy" odor Creamy discharge (yellow/grey)	5-6
Candidiasis	Severe pruritus of vulva and vaginal areas Stinging/burning "Cottage cheese" discharge	< 4.5
Trichomoniasis	Frothy, wet discharge Pruritus possible	≥ 6
Atrophy	Vaginal discharge Spotting Soreness, burning	7

The most common cause of vaginitis. Polymicrobial infection involving deficiency of lactobacilli and overgrowth of anaerobes, often (but not always) including G. vaginalis.[22]

Goals of Therapy

- Relieve symptoms
- Cure the infection

- Prevent recurrence
- Prevent misdiagnosis and delayed treatment of another condition

Patient Assessment[19-21,23]

The decision to recommend self-treatment for vaginal candidiasis must be made with care. Other forms of vaginitis or sexually transmitted diseases (which can have similar symptoms[24]) and allergic or adverse reactions must be ruled out. Refer patients to a physician if:

- They are pre-pubertal – vaginal candidiasis is not common in this group and should be assessed;
- They are presenting with vaginal symptoms for the first time;
- They have an underlying illness such as diabetes, or are pregnant;
- They have a recurrence of vaginal candidiasis within two months of the last episode (complicated

cases may require prescription or other therapy);
- They are at risk of a sexually transmitted disease (STD) (e.g., history of unprotected intercourse, multiple partners, casual sexual encounters).

Women who have symptoms of vaginal candidiasis and have had a previous diagnosis of candidiasis may be eligible for self-treatment. An assessment approach is outlined in Figure 2.

Prevention of Resistance

Reports of azole-resistant candidiasis are of concern. Among speculated, yet unproven, causes is the self-treatment of vaginal infections. Misdiagnosis and inappropriate or incomplete courses of therapy are among possible causes of this resistance. Although not substantiated, it is a reminder that correct diagnosis and appropriate product use is important for proper self-treatment with vaginal antifungals. *C. glabrata* is one of the organisms found in resistant cases. *C. glabrata* tends to be found in older women who

---

Figure 2: **Assessment of Patients with Vaginal Candidiasis**

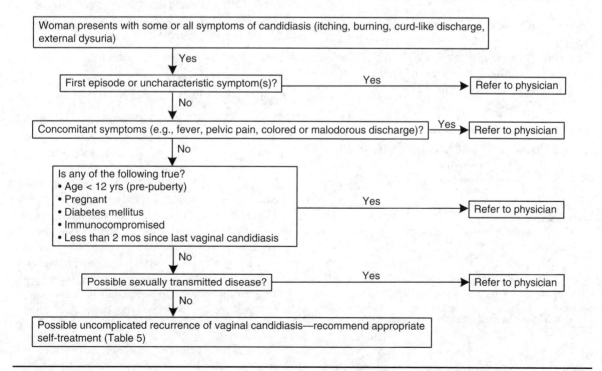

have used azole therapy and who have a complicating underlying illness such as diabetes mellitus.[25] Women with recurrent symptoms of vaginitis should be referred to a physician for diagnosis to ensure appropriate treatment.

Nonpharmacologic Therapy[19-21,23]

Although there is no specific nonpharmacologic therapy for vaginal candidiasis, there are suggested preventive measures for women wishing to avoid recurrences.

Prevention[25]

Next to bacterial vaginosis, *Candida* is the second most common cause of vaginitis. Many women are prone to recurrent or resistant infections. They, in particular, may wish to try to control their symptoms by trying preventive measures. These generally include modifying potential predisposing factors, where possible (Table 4). There is a lack of evidence to support the use of preventive measures such as clothing and dietary modifications but they may be worth trying in recurrent, resistant cases and generally do not cause adverse outcomes.

Good genital hygiene measures are important to keep the tissue healthy and free from irritation. Vaginal deodorants, douching, harsh soaps and perfumed products for genital use should be avoided as irritation or allergic reactions may occur.

Table 4: **Possible Predisposing Factors for Vaginal Candidiasis**[19-21,23]

Menses	
Pregnancy	
Medications:	Antibiotics
	Corticosteroids
	Oral contraceptives, HRT
	Chemotherapy
	Tamoxifen
Poorly controlled diabetes mellitus	
Immunocompromised conditions (e.g., HIV/AIDS)	
Stress	
Chemical irritants – deodorants, soaps, antiseptics	
Diet	
Tight-fitting clothing	
Synthetic undergarments	

Tight clothing and synthetic underwear should be avoided to minimize the development of warm, moist, irritated skin where *Candida* can proliferate. Cotton underwear and loose fitting undergarments and pants are recommended.

Dietary modifications have been tried with varying success. Some women feel that it may be helpful to avoid high sugar foods and increase the consumption of yogurt (containing active *Lactobacillus* species cultures). It was once believed that loss of Lactobacillus species in the gut would predispose a woman to candidal infections. Studies have not supported this. Bacterial vaginosis, on the other hand, often occurs in the presence of low levels of vaginal Lactobacilli.

Severe dietary restrictions such as yeast-free diets can be tried but are difficult to follow and are generally not effective.

Probiotics, such as *L. acidophilus* capsules, have been used orally and sometimes vaginally, during courses of oral antibiotic therapy, in an attempt to normalize the vaginal flora and prevent vaginal candidiasis. This measure has not been shown to be effective in decreasing vaginal candidiasis.[19] If a woman wants to use such a bacterial replacement while taking antibiotics it will not interfere with therapy but the effectiveness may not be satisfactory.

Pharmacologic Therapy[16,19,21,22,24-26]

After the woman has been assessed to verify that vaginal candidasis is the likely cause of symptoms, self-treatment can be considered. Simple, uncomplicated cases (i.e., women with previous history of diagnosed vaginal candidiasis and no complicating medical conditions who experience infrequent, mild to moderate symptoms)[19,21] can be treated with non-prescription vaginal antifungals. Short-course therapy (one to three days) is effective, convenient and may increase compliance due to its simplicity; however, it does not achieve results more quickly than longer course treatment (six to seven days). If successful, symptoms resolve within seven days of beginning treatment.

Women with persistent symptoms that have not responded to self-treatment and women with severe symptoms or complications (e.g., diabetes mellitus, pregnancy, immunosuppression, HIV infection and risk of other STDs) should be referred for physician assessment prior to treatment. Persistent cases may respond better to the longer course of therapy (6, 7 or 14 days) or a change in the antifungal product. Complicated cases must be treated individually according to physician recommendation.[16,19,21,26]

Nonprescription Therapy

Several nonprescription vaginal antifungal products are available (Table 5). Effectiveness rates are similar among the various antifungal agents and products (70 to 90%).[22,24,25,27] Selection is generally determined by length of therapy desired, dosage form preferred and the woman's previous experience.

It is important to provide directions to the user to ensure correct use and compliance with the chosen regimen. The product is usually administered vaginally at bedtime to increase contact time with vaginal tissue and should be continued through menses if it commences during therapy. The complete course of treatment should be used even if symptoms resolve before completion of the doses. If vulvar symptoms are significant, a topical antifungal can be used adjunctively (Table 5).

If the therapy is ineffective, the woman should be referred to a physician before retrying self-treatment. Prescription therapy may be required.

Boric acid 600 mg capsules, intravaginally, once or twice daily for 14 days has also shown some success in the treatment of resistant vaginal candidiasis.[28,29]

Generally, the woman's sexual partner is not treated for candidal infection; however, in resistant or recurrent vaginal infection it may be appropriate to recommend that the male partner use antifungal cream on his penis daily for seven days while the woman is receiving treatment.[23] Refraining from sexual intercourse is also recommended during treatment.

For a listing of available nonprescription vaginal antifungals, see the *Compendium of Self-Care Products*, published annually by the Canadian Pharmacists Association.

Prescription Therapy[16,21,23,25,27,30]

Prescription medication is used for persistent or recurrent cases of vaginal candidiasis, for women with a greater tendency to develop candidiasis (e.g., immunocompromised patients) or for the convenience of short-course oral therapy. Prescription topical antifungals are available, but the oral antifungals offer the most successful alternatives to nonprescription products. Single dose oral therapy with such agents as fluconazole (150 mg) is an effective option with high patient acceptability and compliance.

Prophylaxis[19,21,26,27,30]

Prophylactic therapy is sometimes prescribed for women with recurrent candidiasis. Single dose daily, weekly or biweekly treatments of oral or topical therapy can be used to help reduce recurrence of candidiasis. Resistance is a concern with prophylactic treatment, so it should only be used in women with a persistent problem and under a physician's supervision.

Monitoring of Therapy

Monitoring may be difficult for the pharmacist, as women with vaginal candidiasis are often otherwise healthy individuals who may not be regular clients. It is important that the woman understand that symptoms should resolve within seven days of the start of treatment, no matter which regimen is used. She should also know what to do in case of adverse effects or if treatment is not successful (Table 6).

Resource Tips

Office of Communications and Public Liaison
National Institute of Allergy and Infectious Diseases
National Institutes of Health
Bethesda, MD 20892
http://www.niaid.nih.gov/factsheets/stdvag.htm

Calgary Health Region – Education Services
http://www.crha-health.ab.ca/hlthconn/items/vag-dc.htm

Suggested Readings

Bengtson JM. The Vagina. In: Ryan KJ, ed. *Kistner's Gynecology & Women's Health*. 7th ed. St. Louis, MI: Mosby, Inc., 1999:81-92.

Table 5: **Nonprescription Therapy for Vaginal Candidiasis**[28,29,31]

Drug	Formulation		Dosage	Adverse effects	Comments
Clotrimazole (e.g., Canesten®)	Vaginal cream	1%	One applicatorful vaginally at bedtime for 6 nights.	Uncommon; irritation, headache, abdominal cramps, allergy	Irritation can be dose-related; choosing longer course with lower strength formulation may help.
		2%	One applicatorful vaginally at bedtime for 3 nights.		
		10%	One applicatorful vaginally at bedtime for 1 night.		
	Vaginal tablet	100 mg	One tablet vaginally at bedtime for 6 nights.		
		200 mg	One tablet vaginally at bedtime for 3 nights.		
		500 mg	One tablet vaginally at bedtime for 1 night.		
	Topical cream*	1%	Apply small amount to vulva up to twice daily as needed for up to 7 days.		
Miconazole (e.g., Monistat®)	Vaginal cream	2%	One applicatorful at bedtime for 7 nights.	As above	As above. *Drug interaction:* Topical miconazole may cause increased INRs and bleeding in women taking warfarin. If necessary to use the two together, discuss increased INR monitoring with physician (e.g., every 2 days). Caution patient to watch for signs of bleeding.
	Vaginal suppository	100 mg	One suppository vaginally at bedtime for 7 nights.		
	Vaginal ovule	400 mg	One ovule vaginally at bedtime for 3 nights.		
		1200 mg	One ovule vaginally at bedtime for 1 night.		
	Topical cream*	2%	Apply small amount to vulva up to twice daily as needed for up to 7 days.		
Tioconazole (e.g., Gynecure®)	Vaginal ointment	6.5%	One applicatorful vaginally at bedtime for one night.	As above	Irritation can be dose-related; choosing longer course with lower strength formulation may help.
	Vaginal ovule	300 mg	One ovule vaginally at bedtime for 1 night.		
	Topical cream*	1%	Apply small amount to vulva up to twice daily as needed for up to 7 days.		
Boric acid	600 mg gelatin capsules (extemporaneously prepared)		One capsule vaginally once or twice daily for 14 to 28 days	Irritation more common than with azoles	NOT to be taken by mouth. Not first-line, although reported to be > 90% effective. Option if first-line agents are unsuccessful or irritating or if infection is resistant. Prepare capsules by filling #1 gelatin capsule shell with 600 mg boric acid powder USP.

Often included as part of combination packaging.

Table 6: **Monitoring Therapy for Vaginal Candidiasis**

Symptoms	Monitoring	Endpoint of therapy	Actions
Vulvovaginal itching and burning, dyspareunia discharge	Patient: daily for 7-10 days Pharmacist: after 7 days or next pharmacy visit	Eradication of symptoms	If symptoms still present after 1 wk from start of therapy, refer to physician.
Increased irritation that may indicate adverse reaction to product or inappropriate therapy	As above	As above	Increased severity of symptom(s) should be assessed promptly; discontinue therapy and refer to physician.

General Reference on Women's Health: Boston Women's Health Book Collective. *The New Our Bodies, Ourselves*. 25th anniversary ed. New York, NY: Touchstone; 1992.

Reife CM. Office Gynecology for the Primary Care Physician, Part 1. *Med Clin North Am* 1996;80(2): 299-319.

Sobel JD, Faro S, Force RW et al. Clinical opinion – vulvovaginal candidiasis: Epidemiologic, diagnostic, and therapeutic considerations? *Am J Obstet Gynecol* 1998;178(2):203-11.

References

1. Bengtson JM. The Vagina. In: Ryan KJ, ed. *Kistner's Gynecology & Women's Health*. 7th ed. St. Louis, MI: Mosby Inc. 1999: 81-92. Available from: http://Home.mdconsult.com/das/book/body/38464112/866/11.html.

2. Rome E. Anatomy and physiology of sexuality and reproduction. In: The Boston Women's Health Book Collective. *The New Our Bodies, Ourselves*. 25th anniversary ed. New York, NY: Touchstone, 1992:241-58.

3. Newton ER, Piper JM, Shain R et al. Predictors of the vaginal microflora. *Am J Obstet Gynecol* 2001;184(5):845-55.

4. Donders GGG, Bosmans E, Dekeersmaecker et al. Pathogenesis of abnormal bacterial vaginal flora. *Am J Obstet Gynecol* 2000;182(4):872-8.

5. Rosenberg MJ, Phillips RS, Holmes MD. Vaginal douching—who and why? *J Reprod Med* 1991; 36(10):753-8.

6. Sanford W, Hawley NP, McGee E. Sexuality. In: The Boston Women's Health Book Collective. *The New Our Bodies, Ourselves*. 25th anniversary ed. New York, NY: Touchstone; 1992.

7. Thomas Zhang J, Leybovich E. Vaginal douching and adverse health effects: a meta-analysis. *Am J Public Health* 1997;87(7):1207-11.

8. Ness RB, Soper DE, Holley RL et al. Douching and endometritis: results from the PID evaluation and clinical health (PEACH) study. *Sex Transm Dis* 2001;28(4):240-5.

9. Onderdonk AB, Delaney ML, Hinkson PL. Quantitative and qualitative effects of douche preparations on vaginal microflora. *Obstet Gynecol* 1993;80(3):333-8.

10. Waldvogel F. Staphylococcus aureus (including toxic shock syndrome). In: Mandell GL, Bennett JE, Dolin R, eds. *Mandell, Douglas and Bennett's Principles and Practice of Infectious Diseases*. 4th ed. New York, NY: Churchill Livingstone,1995;1765-7.

11. Lebherz TB. Infectious and benign diseases of the vagina, cervix and vulva. In: Hacker NF, Moore JG, eds. *Essentials of Obstetrics and Gynecology*. 3rd ed: Philadelphia, PA: WB Saunders, 1998;393-411.

12. Kelly S. Coping with vaginal dryness. *Clin Prac Sexual* 1992;8(8/9):1-4.

13. Bachmann GA, Notelovitz M, Kelly SJ et al. Long term non-hormonal treatment of vaginal dryness. *Clin Prac Sexual* 1992,8(8/9):3-8.

14. Product Information Replens® moisturizer and lubricant. Roberts Pharmaceutical Canada Inc., Missisauga,1996.

15. Hendrix SL. Nonestrogen management of menopausal symptoms. *Endocrinol Metab Clin North Am* 1997;26(2):379-90.

16. Reife CM. Office gynecology for the primary care physician, part 1. Vaginitis, the Papanicolaou smear and postmenopausal estrogen replacement. *Med Clin North Am* 1996; 80(2):299-319.

17. McKenna DJ. Black cohosh: efficacy, safety, and use in clinical and preclinical applications. *Altern Ther Health Med* 2001;7(3):93-100.

18. Hardy ML. Herbs of special interest to women. *J Am Pharm Assoc* 200;40(2):234-42.

19. Sobel JD, Faro S, Force RW. Vulvovaginal candidiasis: epidemiologic, diagnostic, and therapeutic considerations? *Am J Obstet Gynecol* 1998;178(2):203-11.

20. Weisenfeld HC, Macio I. The infrequent use of office-based diagnostic tests for vaginitis. *Am J Obstet Gynecol* 1999; 181(1):39-41.

21. Sobel JD. Vulvovaginitis, when *Candida* becomes a problem. *Derm Clin* 1998;16(4):763-8.

22. Nyiresy P. Chronic vulvovaginal candidiasis. *Am Fam Physician* 2001;63(4):697-702.

23. Hay RJ. The management of superficial candidiasis. *J Am Acad Dermatol* 1999;40(6Pt2):s35-42.

24. Ferris DG, Dekle C, Litaker MS. Women's use of over-the-counter antifungal medications for gynaecological symptoms. *J Fam Pract* 1996;42:595-600.

25. Kemper DW. Women's Health. In: *BC HealthGuide*. 14th ed. British Columbia: Healthwise Publications, 2000.

26. Abramowicz M, ed. Drugs for sexually transmitted infections. *Med Let* 1999;41(1062):1-6.

27. Abramowicz M, ed. Drugs for vulvovaginal candidiasis. *Med Let* 2001;43(1095):3-4.

28. Jovanovic R, Congema E, Nguyen HT. Antifungal agents vs. boric acid for treating chronic mycotic vulvovaginitis *J Repro Med* 1991;36(8):593-7.

29. Sobel JD, Chaim W. Treatment of Candida glabrata vaginitis: A retrospective review of boric acid therapy *Clin Infect Dis* 1997;24:649-652.

30. Korn AP, Abercrombie PD. Gynecology and family planning for the woman infected with HIV. *Obstet Gynecol Clin* 1997;24(4):855-72.

31. Tatro DS, ed. *Drug Interaction Facts* St. Louis, MI: Facts and Comparisons, 2001:72.

Genital Hygiene—Patient Information

- Wash the area around the outside of the vagina daily with warm water and mild soap. Rinse well.
- The inside of the vagina cleanses itself naturally. Douching is not necessary and not recommended.
- A mild genital odor is normal. Simple cleaning (as above) each day can keep the normal odor to a minimum.

- Poor hygiene, infection or a forgotten tampon can cause an unusual or unpleasant odor, itching or irritation. If washing with soap and water does not help, see your doctor.

Vaginal Douching—Patient Information

Douching is not a necessary part of genital cleanliness and it can be harmful. It does not work as birth control. If you choose to douche, be sure to do it properly and that it's safe for you to do:

- Use only occasionally, and never because you think you have a vaginal infection.
- Do not douche if you are pregnant, unless your doctor advises you to.
- Do not douche within six hours after sexual intercourse if you have used a vaginal spermicide. It can lessen the effectiveness of the spermicide.
- Genital irritation or unusual odor might mean that you have a vaginal infection. Even though douching might relieve the symptoms, only proper diagnosis and treatment will cure the infection. See your doctor if you think you have a vaginal infection.
- Do not douche for at least 24 hours before having a vaginal examination.
- Wash reusable douching equipment with hot water and soap every time you use it.

Technique
Proper technique is important for safe douching.
- For a *fountain syringe*, fill the bag with solution, clamp off the tubing and hang the bag about 30 cm

(1 foot) above your hips. Don't hang it higher than recommended. It could cause the pressure to be too high.
- If you're using a *bulb* syringe, fill the bag or bottle with solution.
- Lie on your back in the tub with your knees bent.
- Gently insert the plastic tip into the vagina and slip it in as far as it will go comfortably.
- Release the clamp on the fountain syringe or gently squeeze the bulb syringe to start the flow of fluid into the vagina.
- When enough fluid is inside, you will have a mild feeling of fullness in the pelvic area. Putting in too much fluid or putting it in too forcefully can push fluid into the uterus, and this could lead to irritation and infection.
- Gently remove the tip from the vagina and use one hand to hold the labia (on either side of the opening to the vagina) together to keep the fluid from flowing out of the vagina.
- Release after one minute and let the fluid come out.
- Dispose of the douching equipment. If it is reusable, wash it with soap and hot water.

Genital Deodorant Sprays—Patient Information

Important: Apply to external genital area only. *Do not* apply to the inside of vagina.

Proper Use
- Shake the canister.
- Hold the canister at least 20 cm (8 inches) from your genital area. Irritation can occur if too much spray is applied or from the propellants in the spray.
- Press down on the nozzle to release the spray.
- Do not use the spray before sexual intercourse. Irritation can occur if the spray comes in contact with sensitive areas like the penis or vagina.

- Do not insert tampons right after you use the spray.
- Don't use the spray on irritated or broken skin.
- Don't use the spray when you're wearing menstrual pads. It may cause irritation.
- If the spray causes any burning, irritation or itching, stop using it and wash the area with warm water and mild soap. If the symptoms don't improve, see your doctor.

Toxic Shock Syndrome—Patient Information

Toxic shock syndrome (TSS) is a life-threatening infection caused by bacteria that produce deadly toxins. In the 1980s it was learned that women using tampons, contraceptive sponges, diaphragms or cervical caps were at higher risk of developing TSS.

The treatment of TSS requires immediate medical attention. People with TSS can suddenly become very sick, with symptoms such as:
- High fever
- Sunburn-like rash
- Low blood pressure (shock)
- Dizziness
- Fainting
- Vomiting
- Diarrhea
- Confusion

Here are some things you can do to lower your risk of TSS:
- Use sanitary pads instead of tampons during your period, especially overnight.

- If you use tampons, use the lowest absorbency that meets your needs. Change tampons four to six times a day and never wear one longer than eight hours at once.
- Do not use contraceptive sponges, diaphragms or cervical caps during your period.
- If you recently gave birth, do not use tampons for postpartum bleeding. Do not use contraceptive sponges, diaphragms or cervical caps while your are still bleeding. In addition, diaphragms and cervical caps have to be refitted six to eight weeks after you have a baby.
- If you have the symptoms described above and think you might be at risk for TSS, see your doctor right away. If left untreated, TSS can be very dangerous and even fatal.

Vaginal Candidiasis (Yeast Infection)—Patient Information

To get the most out of your treatment:
- Maintain good genital hygiene.
- Use the medicine exactly as recommended by your pharmacist or health care provider.
- Use the product at bedtime to decrease leakage of the medication from the vagina.
- Continue treatment even if your period starts.
- Use menstrual pads or panty liners if you want to use something to absorb leakage, or if your period starts. Don't use tampons because they can absorb the medication and decrease its effectiveness.
- Finish all the treatment even if your symptoms go away before it is finished.
- Wash all reusable applicators with water and soap after each use. Throw out disposable applicators after one use.
- Do not share applicators with anyone else.

Other things that might help:
- Wear loose fitting, natural fibre (cotton) panties and pants and avoid synthetic fabrics.
- Wear pantyhose with a cotton crotch piece.
- Eat less sugar and more yogurt.

Things to remember:
- Nonprescription treatments for vaginal yeast infections are meant to be used only if you have had a previous yeast infection that was diagnosed by a doctor. If this is your first yeast infection, if you have diabetes or are pregnant, or if you are not sure if this is a yeast infection, see your doctor before using nonprescription medicine for it.
- Nonprescription medicines for vaginal yeast infections are used in the vagina, but the cream can be applied on the external area to help reduce itching, burning or irritation outside the vagina, only if it's caused by the same infection.
- Your symptoms should clear within seven days of starting treatment. See your doctor if they don't go away in seven days or if they get worse during treatment.
- This treatment will only work if you have a vaginal *Candida* ("yeast") infection. It is not effective for any other type of vaginitis.
- Do not have intercourse during your treatment, to avoid infecting your partner. Also, be aware that vaginal treatments for yeast infections could decrease the effectiveness of spermicides, condoms, diaphragms and cervical caps – during treatment and for up to three days after.

Chapter 51

Dysmenorrhea and Premenstrual Syndrome

Thomas E.R. Brown, PharmD and Christinne Campbell, BScPhm

Reproductive Physiology[1]

Female reproductive physiology revolves around the menstrual cycle. The average length of a menstrual cycle is 28 days, but it can range from 23 to 35 days. On average, a woman will menstruate 400 times from the onset of menarche to menopause.

Female reproduction is regulated by the hypothalamic-pituitary-ovarian (HPO) axis. A normal menstrual cycle begins with the pulsatile release of gonadotropin-releasing hormone (GnRH) from the hypothalamus. The release of GnRH stimulates the pituitary to release follicle stimulating hormone (FSH) and luteinizing hormone (LH). The rate and amplitude of GnRH pulses from the hypothalamus determine which hormone (FSH or LH) is released by the pituitary. The first day of the menstrual cycle is identified as the first day of menstruation, when recruitment of follicles in the ovary begins. At the start of each new menstrual cycle, FSH stimulates a group of follicles in the ovary. These follicles produce and secrete estradiol. This is known as the *follicular* phase of the menstrual cycle. By around the seventh day, one follicle becomes dominant, continues to grow, secretes estradiol and at the time of ovulation, releases an egg. The other follicles undergo atresia (i.e., they cease to grow and eventually die). Estradiol concentrations rise throughout the follicular phase and peak just prior to ovulation.

The follicular phase of the menstrual cycle in the ovary corresponds to the proliferative phase in the endometrium. Estradiol released through stimulation of the follicles in the ovaries causes the endometrial lining to proliferate.

Ovulation occurs around day 14 of the menstrual cycle. At this time the pituitary decreases the amount of FSH that is secreted and increases the secretion of LH. A surge in LH signals the dominant follicle to rupture and release the egg into the fallopian tube. This is known as ovulation. The ruptured follicle undergoes luteinization and becomes the corpus luteum. Progesterone and some estradiol are produced and secreted by the corpus luteum.[1] This second half of the menstrual cycle is referred to as the luteal phase. Progesterone and estradiol concentrations rise during the luteal phase. The corpus luteum has a 14-day life span; therefore, if fertilization does not occur, the corpus luteum undergoes atresia and progesterone and estradiol concentrations fall.

The *luteal phase* of the menstrual cycle corresponds to the secretory phase in the endometrium. Progesterone stimulates glandular cells in the endometrium to produce glycogen, mucus and prostaglandins. These changes in the endometrial tissue are known as secretory changes.

If fertilization and implantation do not occur by around day 23 of the menstrual cycle, the corpus luteum regresses, progesterone and estradiol concentrations decline, the endometrium undergoes involution and menstruation begins.

Dysmenorrhea

Pathophysiology

Definition

Dysmenorrhea is defined as painful menstruation, and can be primary or secondary. Primary dysmenorrhea is attributed to uterine contractions, whereas secondary dysmenorrhea is due to pelvic disease such as endometriosis, inflammatory disease uterine polyps.[2] The main focus of this section is primary dysmenorrhea.

Prevalence

The reported prevalence of dysmenorrhea ranges from 6 to 80%, with the most common being 50%. The peak incidence is in women between 20 and 24 years of age, and it decreases with age. It is the most common cause of missed school or workdays in young women. Approximately 10% of women will suffer from severe symptoms.[2]

Etiology

Dysmenorrhea occurs in ovulatory cycles. During anovulatory cycles, the endometrial tissue contains smaller amounts of prostaglandins; therefore, these cycles are usually painless.[2] Prostaglandins are released during endometrial cell lysis, which occurs just prior to menstruation,[2] and have a direct effect on the endometrium and surrounding tissues, resulting in the signs and symptoms of dysmenorrhea.[2]

The role of prostaglandins in the pathogenesis of dysmenorrhea is well-established. Women with dysmenorrhea have higher concentrations of $PGF_2\alpha$ and PGE_2 in their menstrual fluid than women who do not complain of pain on menstruation.[2] Moreover, administering these prostaglandins by infusion induces the same discomfort and symptoms experienced by women with dysmenorrhea.

Women with dysmenorrhea have increased uterine activity, resulting in increased resting tone, increased strength and frequency of contractions and/or dysrhythmic contractions.[2]

Dysmenorrhea usually begins 6 to 12 months after menarche and only occurs with ovulatory cycles. It tends to decrease with age, when the woman begins engaging in sexual intercourse and after childbirth.[3]

Clinical Presentation

The diagnosis of dysmenorrhea is based on the presence of symptoms, normal pelvic exam and the patient's response to therapy.[3] Individuals who do not respond to a proven therapy should be investigated for causes of secondary dysmenorrhea.[2] Menstrual pain occurs a few hours before or just after menstruation begins. It usually lasts for 48 to 72 hours. The pain is described as cramps and is most intense over the lower abdomen, but it may radiate to the back and legs. Associated symptoms include nausea and vomiting, fatigue, diarrhea and headache.[2]

Goals of Therapy

- Relieve symptoms
- Minimize time lost from work, school and other activities
- Identify patients who may have secondary dysmenorrhea and refer them to their physician for assessment

Patient Assessment

Assess patients with dysmenorrhea to confirm that their complaints are consistent with the etiology, signs and symptoms of dysmenorrhea (Figure 1). Response to a proven therapy for dysmenorrhea is usually a confirmation of the diagnosis.

Nonpharmacologic Therapy

Regular aerobic exercise has been shown to reduce symptoms of dysmenorrhea. It can also decrease stress, which may be a contributing factor.[3] Warm baths or applying heating pads or a hot water bottle to the abdomen may reduce discomfort. In a randomized, controlled study, heating pads were found to provide pain relief equivalent to the use of ibuprofen. When both heating pads and ibuprofen were used together there was no more pain relief than with either agent used alone; however, pain relief occurred faster when both therapies were combined.[4] Association with diet is unclear; however, decreasing fat intake may be of some benefit.[3] For most women, drug therapy is required, and nonpharmacologic measures are used adjunctively.[3]

Figure 1: **Assessment of Dysmenorrhea**

Patient presents with pelvic pain, possibly radiating to back and/or legs, that begins with onset of menses and lasts 2-3 days, and initial onset was within 2 yrs of menarche

↓

If birth control also required, refer to physician for possible oral contraceptive therapy for dysmenorrhea

↓

If birth control not required (or patient does not wish to explore that option), recommend nonpharmacologic measures and if no contraindication, ibuprofen for a 3- to 6-cycle trial

↓

If ibuprofen contraindicated or ineffective, refer to physician for possible prescription therapy

Pharmacologic Therapy

Pharmacologic agents that decrease the amount of prostaglandins in endometrial tissue or inhibit prostaglandin synthesis are considered first-line therapies for the treatment of dysmenorrhea.

Nonprescription Therapy
Ibuprofen
Like other NSAIDs, ibuprofen decreases endometrial and menstrual fluid prostaglandin concentrations[5] and is highly effective in the treatment of dysmenorrhea. Symptom relief with ibuprofen ranges from 60 to greater than 85%.[6]

If there are no contraindications to use of a NSAID (see Chapter 36), ibuprofen should be administered at the onset of pain or menses and continued for 72 hours, as the peak concentration of prostaglandins occurs in the first 48 hours.[7] A loading dose is usually unnecessary.[8] Women who do not get adequate relief of symptoms may start ibuprofen when their basal body temperature declines prior to menses.[3] The recommended dose of ibuprofen is 400 mg every four to six hours. Ibuprofen should be tried for three to six cycles before being declared a treatment failure.[3] Refer women to their physician if symptoms are not relieved, or if pain becomes worse.[3]

Potential adverse effects of ibuprofen in the management of dysmenorrhea are similar to those seen generally with NSAID use and include GI disturbances, CNS effects and hypersensitivity reactions (see Chapter 36).

Acetylsalicylic Acid (ASA) and Acetaminophen
Studies have shown that ASA and acetaminophen do not decrease concentrations of prostaglandins in menstrual fluid.[9] In many studies, neither of these agents was better in providing pain relief than placebo.[10,11]

In addition, caution is advised regarding the use of ASA in adolescents or young adults because of the possible association with Reye's syndrome when ASA is used for certain conditions such as influenza or varicella.

Prescription Therapy
Prescription therapy for dysmenorrhea may include an NSAID, an oral contraceptive agent or a combination of the two.

Many NSAIDs have been used in the management of dysmenorrhea. Type I prostaglandin (PG) synthetase inhibitors such as acetic acids (e.g., indomethacin), propionic acids (e.g., ibuprofen, naproxen) and fenamates (e.g., mefenamic acid) are considered the agents of choice, relieving dysmenorrhea by reducing prostaglandin concentrations in endometrial and menstrual fluid.[3] Because of where they work on the prostaglandin synthesis cascade, type II PG inhibitors like oxicams (e.g., piroxicam, meloxicam, tenoxicam) and phenylbutazone may not prevent the production of uterotoxic endoperoxides, and may be less effective for dysmenorrhea.[3] Mefenamic acid may have an advantage, as it not only inhibits the formation of prostaglandins but can also block prostaglandins at the receptor site, although the clinical significance of this has been questioned.[3]

If NSAID therapy is contraindicated, fails or if birth control is also required, an oral contraceptive agent is often used to treat dysmenorrhea. Oral contraceptives relieve dysmenorrhea symptoms by reducing the amount of prostaglandins in menstrual fluid (because they reduce the actual amount of fluid), and by inhibiting ovulation (dysmenorrhea occurs only in ovulatory cycles).[3] Oral contraceptives are up to 90% effective in relieving dysmenorrhea symptoms.[12]

The combination of an oral contraceptive and an NSAID may also be beneficial. About 10% of women do not respond to treatment with NSAIDs, oral contraceptives or both.[12] If prescription drug therapy fails, the woman should be assessed for possible causes of secondary dysmenorrhea.[3]

Alternative Therapies

Alternative approaches for managing refractory dysmenorrhea have been investigated, including transcutaneous electric nerve stimulation (TENS), acupuncture, omega-3 fatty acids, transdermal nitroglycerin and magnesium supplementation.[12] These therapies require further study to determine their role in treating dysmenorrhea. Women who do not respond to standard therapy should discuss these options with their physician.

Monitoring of Therapy

Refer patients who fail to respond to a three- to six-cycle trial of nonprescription ibuprofen in conjunction with nonpharmacologic measures to their physician.

Instruct patients taking ibuprofen or other NSAIDs to report any signs of serious adverse effects to their physician (see Chapter 36).

Premenstrual Syndrome (PMS)

Pathophysiology

Definition

The term PMS refers to the cyclic recurrence of physical, behavioral and psychological symptoms during the luteal phase of the menstrual cycle (after ovulation), that ameliorate at the start of menses.[13] A severe subtype of PMS that includes significant mood changes and impairment of functioning, formerly known as late luteal phase dysphoric disorder, is now referred to as premenstrual dysphoric disorder (PMDD).[14]

PMS affects up to 40% of women of reproductive age,[13,15] whereas PMDD affects approximately 5% of women.[16]

Etiology

The etiology of PMS has not been fully elucidated.[17] Several theories have been proposed involving fluctuations in hormonal control of the menstrual cycle, dysregulation of neurotransmitter systems and nutritional deficiencies.

Increased sensitivity to normal fluctuations in sex steroid hormones (estradiol and progesterone) during the menstrual cycle has been proposed as a possible etiologic factor in PMS.[13] A study of premenstrual women demonstrated that the occurrence of symptoms was due to an abnormal response to normal hormonal fluctuations.[18] Because ovarian sex hormones can affect the synthesis, release, reuptake and inactivation of neurotransmitters,[15] fluctuations in

these hormones may lead to PMS or PMDD in susceptible women.[13]

Serotonin is a neurotransmitter that plays a role in modulating mood and behavior.[19] Studies have shown that women with PMS have lower whole blood serotonin concentrations and decreased platelet uptake of serotonin during the late luteal phase of the menstrual cycle, compared to control subjects.[19] Decreased serotonergic neurotransmission may be associated with depressed mood, irritability, anger, aggression, poor impulse control and appetite disturbances.[19]

Although evidence for serotonin abnormalities in PMS is the most convincing, abnormalities in the catcholaminergic, gamma-aminobutyric acid (GABAergic) and opioid neurotransmitter systems have been observed in women with PMS.[13,20]

Risk Factors

Deficiencies in certain nutrients such as calcium, magnesium, manganese, vitamin B_6, vitamin E and linoleic acid have been reported in PMS.[13] However, consistent excess or deficiency in dietary factors has not been clearly documented in women with PMS as compared to control subjects.[21]

PMS is twice as prevalent in identical twins as in fraternal twins, suggesting the likelihood of a genetic predisposition for PMS.[13]

Other factors such as low parity, oral contraceptive use, menstrual cycle characteristics and socioeconomic or lifestyle variables are not consistently associated with the development of PMS.[13]

Clinical Presentation

PMS is frequently a diagnosis of exclusion, as there is no currently accepted diagnostic test for this condition.[13,14] The differential diagnosis may include anemia, diabetes, thyroid disorders, chronic fatigue syndrome, endometriosis, fibrocystic breast disease and various psychiatric disorders.[13,16] These conditions should be ruled out before a firm diagnosis of PMS is made.

There is general agreement that the diagnosis of PMS requires that:
- Symptoms be present during the luteal phase of the menstrual cycle.
- Symptoms reach their peak shortly before the beginning of menstruation and remit at the onset of menses or shortly thereafter.[13]
- Symptoms must be severe enough to interfere with daily functioning and interpersonal relationships.[13,17]
- There is a symptom-free period during the follicular phase of the menstrual cycle.[13,16]

The diagnosis of PMS is confirmed through prospective monitoring of a woman's symptoms during at least two menstrual cycles.[13,16,22] A daily symptom calendar can be used to determine whether the woman's symptoms are cyclic in nature and are confined to the luteal phase (Figure 2).

Over the last several decades, research into PMS has identified over 100 premenstrual symptoms.[23] Symptoms of PMS can be divided into two broad categories: cognitive or affective, and physical[17] (Figure 2). The onset of PMS and related symptoms can occur at any time after puberty.[16] Typically, the onset of symptoms occurs in the mid-twenties[13] and women usually seek treatment in their thirties.[13,16] Perimenopausal women can suffer from PMS, but it subsides after menopause.

The number of symptoms required for a diagnosis of PMS is not consistent among different authorities.[16] The criteria developed by American College of Obstetricians and Gynecologists require the presence of at least one symptom from a list of specific affective and somatic symptoms, during the 5 days prior to menses and occurring over several cycles.[24] To prevent over-diagnosis of this condition, some suggest that the presence of five or more symptoms, that change in severity throughout the menstrual cycle is appropriate for a diagnosis of PMS.[16]

Goals of Therapy[14]

- Relieve symptoms
- Minimize functional impairment
- Optimize overall health
- Rule out or identify other possible conditions that can have similar symptoms, and refer for proper assessment and treatment

Patient Assessment (Figure 3)

For a diagnosis of PMS, patients should have symptoms in the latter half of their menstrual cycle. These complaints should be cyclic in nature; therefore, they should resolve at the start of menses and not be present during the entire menstrual cycle (Pathophysiology, Clinical Presentation). Patients with severe, debilitating symptoms with a strong affective or psychological component should be referred to a physician for assessment of possible PMDD (Table 1).

Nonpharmacologic Therapy

Lifestyle Modifications

Relaxation and stress reduction techniques, although not rigorously studied in PMS trials, can be recommended to women suffering from PMS as a means of promoting a healthy lifestyle.[25] Because symptoms of PMS can include both insomnia and hypersomnia, appropriate sleep hygiene techniques should also be encouraged[13] (see Chapter 6).

Data suggest that regular moderate exercise has a beneficial effect on the symptoms of PMS[13,16] including breast tenderness, fluid retention, stress and depression.[13] Therefore, encourage women to engage in moderate aerobic activity three to four times weekly as a method of alleviating their symptoms.[13]

Dietary Modifications

Caffeine

Improvement in breast symptoms was noted in a large proportion of women who refrained from consuming methylxanthine-containing foods and beverages.[21] Although the data are limited, it is appropriate to recommend that women who suffer from PMS limit their intake of coffee, tea, chocolate and caffeine-containing soft drinks.[21]

Figure 2: **Sample Monitoring Chart for Premenstrual Symptoms***

Day of menstrual cycle	1**	2	3	4	5	6	7	8	9	10	11	12	13	14	15	16	17	18	19	20	21	22	23	24	25	26	27	28	(29)	(30)	(31)	(32)	(33)
Affective or cognitive symptoms																																	
Aggression																																	
Anger																																	
Anxiety																																	
Depression																																	
Fatigue																																	
Forgetfulness																																	
Hostility																																	
Irritability																																	
Lethargy (lack of energy)																																	
Mood lability (sudden mood changes)																																	
Panic attacks																																	
Poor concentration																																	
Reduced coping skills																																	
Physical Symptoms																																	
Acne																																	
Appetite change																																	
Bloating, fluid retention, oliguria (less urine than usual)																																	

(cont'd)

Figure 2: **Sample Monitoring Chart for Premenstrual Symptoms*** (cont'd)

Day of menstrual cycle	1**	2	3	4	5	6	7	8	9	10	11	12	13	14	15	16	17	18	19	20	21	22	23	24	25	26	27	28	(29)	(30)	(31)	(32)	(33)
Physical symptoms (cont'd)																																	
Breast pain or swelling																																	
Constipation																																	
Dizziness or vertigo																																	
Fatigue																																	
Headaches																																	
Hot flashes																																	
Muscle aches																																	
Nausea and vomiting																																	
Pelvic heaviness or pressure																																	
Weight gain																																	

*Rate symptoms according to severity (e.g., 3 = severe, 2 = moderate, 1 = mild, 0 = absent).
**First day of menstrual period.

Figure 3: **Assessment of Patients with Premenstrual Syndrome (PMS)**

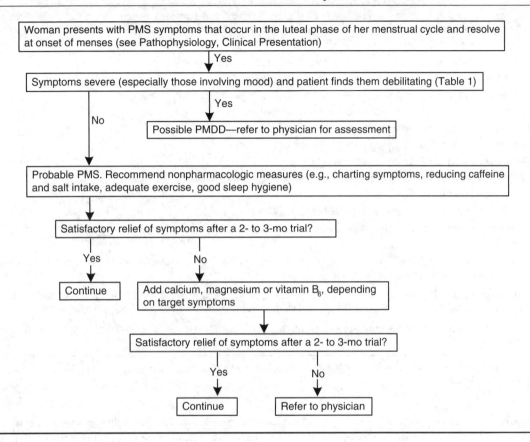

Salt

Restricting salt intake in the premenstrual phase has been suggested as a method of alleviating PMS symptoms of fluid retention, weight gain, bloating and breast swelling and tenderness.[16] Although clinical trials have not examined this intervention, it is a reasonable recommendation both as an attempt to decrease PMS symptoms and to promote general good health.[16]

Pharmacologic Therapy

Nonprescription Therapy

Ibuprofen

The use of prostaglandin inhibitors is based on a theory that PMS results from an excess of prosta-

glandins.[16] Nonprescription NSAID choices include ibuprofen. Based on studies with other prostaglandin inhibitors, ibuprofen would be expected to provide pain relief in PMS.[13,16] Recommend ibuprofen in the lowest effective dose for short-term therapy.[14]

Calcium

A randomized, controlled trial showed that 1200 mg elemental calcium daily (in the form of calcium carbonate) is more effective than placebo for reducing symptoms of negative affect, water retention, food cravings and pain in women with PMS. The authors speculated that calcium supplementation might act to replace a calcium deficit, leading to decreased parathyroid hormone secretion and reduced neuromuscular irritability and vascular reactivity.[26]

Table 1: **DSM-IV Criteria for Premenstrual Dysphoric Disorder (PMDD)**

A. In most menstrual cycles during the past year, five or more of the following symptoms were present for most of the time during the last week of the luteal phase, began to remit within a few days after onset of the follicular phase, and were absent in the week postmenses, with at least one of the symptoms being number 1, 2, 3 or 4:

 1. Markedly depressed mood, feelings of hopelessness or self-deprecating thoughts
 2. Marked anxiety, tension, feelings of being "keyed up" or "on edge."
 3. Marked affective lability (e.g., feeling suddenly sad or tearful or increased sensitivity to rejection)
 4. Persistent and marked anger or irritability or increased interpersonal conflicts
 5. Decreased interest in usual activities (e.g., work, school, friends, hobbies)
 6. Subjective sense of difficulty in concentrating
 7. Lethargy, easy fatigability or marked lack of energy
 8. Marked change in appetite, overeating or specific food cravings
 9. Hypersomnia or insomnia
 10. A subjective sense of being overwhelmed or out of control
 11. Other physical symptoms such as breast tenderness or swelling, headaches, joint or muscle pain a sensation of "bloating," weight gain

B. The disturbance *markedly* interferes with work or school or with usual social activities and relationships with others (e.g., avoidance of social activities, decreased productivity and efficiency at work or school).

C. The disturbance is *not* merely an exacerbation of the symptoms of another disorder, such as Major Depressive Disorder, Panic Disorder, Dysthymic Disorder, or a Personality Disorder (although it may be superimposed on any of these disorders).

Criteria A, B and C must be confirmed by prospective daily ratings during at least two consecutive symptomatic cycles. (The diagnosis may be made provisionally prior to this confirmation.)

Reprinted with permission from the *Diagnostic and Statistical Manual of Mental Disorders*, Fourth Edition, Text Revision. Copyright 2000 American Psychiatric Association.

Magnesium

Several small, randomized, placebo-controlled trials have shown magnesium to be a promising treatment alternative for premenstrual symptoms such as fluid retention.[13,16] Although the evidence is not definitive for magnesium,[24] if a woman chooses to try this supplement, a dose of 200 to 400 mg daily can be recommended.[13] A mild laxative effect with magnesium has been observed at higher doses.[13]

Vitamin B$_6$

The rationale for using vitamin B$_6$ in the treatment of PMS stems from the fact that it is a cofactor in the synthesis of dopamine and the metabolism of tryptophan (a serotonin precursor).[21] Vitamin B$_6$ increases the inhibitory to excitatory amine ratio, which could theoretically alleviate PMS, as several symptoms are thought to represent an excitatory state of the CNS.[21] Some evidence supports the use of vitamin B$_6$ in the treatment of premenstrual symptoms.[27] A meta-analysis of nine trials studying the use of vitamin B$_6$ in PMS

concluded that it is likely beneficial in treating premenstrual symptoms and premenstrual depression.[27] Vitamin B$_6$ can be recommended in doses of 50 to 100 mg daily.[27] Doses exceeding 200 mg daily have been associated with peripheral neuropathy.[27]

Vitamin E

Although vitamin E has been proposed as a potential treatment of PMS, there is no definitive evidence that supports its efficacy.[16]

Combination Products

Several nonprescription preparations include an analgesic as well as parabom (a diuretic) and/or pyrilamine (an antihistamine). Evidence that the addition of these two agents offers superior efficacy over an analgesic alone comes from very old data that has not been reproduced in the last 30 to 40 years. Most experts believe that if these two agents have added benefit, their effects are mild at best.

Prescription Therapy

Prescription alternatives are available that target specific symptoms of PMS (e.g., fluoxetine for cognitive symptoms, spironolactone for fluid retention and bromocriptine for mastalgia). Prescription medication that blocks ovulation is also available (GnRH analogs, danazol and oral contraceptives). A woman should consult her physician to discuss the appropriateness of these more complex strategies in the treatment of her symptoms.

Herbal Remedies

Several herbal products have been promoted to relieve the symptoms of PMS, although none have been proven to be effective.[17] Oil of evening primrose has been shown to be no better than placebo in relief of PMS-related symptoms. Chaste berry has been recommended; however, the studies that suggest it is effective have been small and poorly designed. At this time, there is insufficient evidence to recommend these strategies as appropriate methods of treating premenstrual symptoms.

Monitoring of Therapy

Encourage women to self-monitor their response to various treatment measures by charting their symptoms regularly (Figure 2). Women with unrelenting or progressive symptoms, especially if they might indicate the presence of PMDD (Table 1), should be referred to their physician.

Resource Tips

National Association for PMS:
www.pms.org.uk

Readers Digest Canada:
readersdigest.ca/mag/1998/10/living_0l.html

University of Pennsylvania Health System:
www.obgyn.upenn.edu.mudd/PMSarticle.html

Suggested Readings

Coco A. Primary Dysmenorrhea. *Am Fam Physician* 1999;60(2):489-96.

Eden JA. Dysmenorrhea and premenstrual syndrome. In: Hacker NF, Moore JG, eds. *Essentials of Obstetrics and Gynecology* 3rd ed. Philadelphia, PA: WB Saunders, 1998:386-392.

Frackiewicz EJ, Shiovitz TM. Evaluation and management of premenstrual syndrome and premenstrual dysphoric disorder. *J Am Pharm Assoc.* 2001;41(3): 437-47.

Johnson SR. Clinician's approach to the diagnosis and management of premenstrual syndrome. *Clin Obstet Gynecol* 1992;35(3):637-657.

Moline ML, Zendell SM. Evaluating and managing premenstrual syndrome. *Medscape Women's Health* 5(2), 2000. Available from http://www.medscape. com/Medscape/WomensHealth/journal/2000/v05.n 02/wh3025.moli/wh3025.moli-01.html.

Pearlstein T, Stone AB. Premenstrual syndrome. *Psychiatr Clin North Am* 1998;21(3):577-590.

Sagraves R, Parent-Stevens L, Hardman J. Gynecologic disorders. In: Koda-Kimble MA, Young LY, eds. *Applied Therapeutics: The Clinical Use of Drugs.* 7th ed. Philadelphia, PA: Lippincott Williams & Wilkins, 2001;46-11 to 46-16.

References

1. Surrey ES, Lu JKH, Toot PJ. The menstrual cycle, ovulation, fertilization, implantation and the placenta. In: Hacker NF, Moore JG, eds. *Essentials of Obstetrics and Gynecology.* 3rd ed. Philadelphia, PA: WB Saunders; 1998:59-75.

2. Eden JA: Dysmenorrhea and premenstrual syndrome. In: Hacker NF, Moore JG, eds. *Essentials of Obstetrics and Gynecology.* 3rd ed. Philadelphia, PA: WB Saunders; 1998: 386-392.

3. Sagraves R, Parent-Stevens L, Hardman J. Gynecologic disorders. In: Koda-Kimble MA, Young LY, eds. *Applied Therapeutics: The Clinical Use of Drugs.* 7th ed. Philadelphia, PA: Lippincott Williams & Wilkins; 2001;46-11 to 46-16.

4. Akin MD, Weingand KW, Hengehold DA, Goodale MB, Hinkle RT, Smith RP. Continuous low-level topical heat in the treatment of dysmenorrhea. *Obstet Gynecol* 2001;97:343-9.

5. Zhang WY, Li WPA. Efficacy of minor analgesics in primary dysmennorhoea: a systematic review. *Br J Obstet Gynaecol* 1998;105:780-9.

6. Chan WY, Darwood MY, Fuchs F. Relief of dysmenorrhea with the prostaglandin synthetase inhibitor ibuprofen: effect on prostaglandin levels in menstrual fluid. *Am J Obstet Gynecol* 1979;135:102-8.

7. Chan WY Dawood MY, Fuchs F. Prostaglandin in primary dysmenorrhea: comparison of prophylactic and non-prophylactic treatment with ibuprofen and use of oral contraceptive. *Am J Med* 1981;70:535-41.

8. Shapiro SS. Treatment of dysmenorrhea and premenstrual syndrome with non-steroidal anti-inflammatory drugs. *Drugs* 1988;36:475-90.

9. Pebdergrass PB, Ream LJ, Scott JN, Agna MA. Do aspirin and acetaminophen affect total menstrual loss? *Gynecol Obstet Invest* 1984;18:129-33.

10. Janbu T, Lokken P, Nesheim BI. Effect of acetylsalicylic acid, paracetamol and placebo on pain and blood loss in dysmenorrheic women. *Acta Obstet Gynecol* (Scand suppl) 1979;87:81-5.

11. Zhang WY, Po ALW. Efficacy of minor analgesics in dysmenorrhea: a systematic review. *Br J Obstet Gynaecol* 1998; 105;780-9.

12. Coco A. Primary dysmenorrhea. *Am Fam Physician* 1999; 60(2):489-96.

13. Frackiewicz EJ, Shiovitz TM. Evaluation and management of premenstrual syndrome and premenstrual dysphoric disorder. *J Am Pharm Ass* 2001;41(3):437-47.

14. Daugherty JE. Treatment strategies for premenstrual syndrome. *Am Fam Physician* 1998;183-92,197-8.

15. Pearlstein TB. Hormones and depression: what are the facts about premenstrual syndrome, menopause, and hormone replacement therapy? *Am J Obstet Gynecol* 1995;173:646-53.

16. Moline ML, Zendell SM. Evaluating and managing premenstrual syndrome. *Medscape Women's Health* 5(2), 2000. Available from: http://www.medscape.com/Medscape/ Womens Health/journal/2000/v05.n02/wh3025.moli/wh3025. moli-01.html.

17. Frye GM, Silverman SD. Is it premenstrual syndrome? Keys to focused diagnosis, therapies for multiple symptoms. *Post Grad Med* 2000;107(5):151-9.

18. Schmidt PJ et al. Differential behavioural effects of gonadal steroids in women with and in those without premenstrual syndrome. *N Engl J Med* 1998;338(4):209-16.

19. Rapkin AJ. The role of serotonin in premenstrual syndrome. *Clin Obstet Gynecol* 1992;35(3):629-36.

20. Pearlstein T, Steiner M. Non-antidepressant treatment of premenstrual syndrome. *J Clin Psych* 2000;61(suppl 12):22-7.

21. Chuong CJ, Dawson EB. Critical evaluation of nutritional factors in the pathophysiology and treatment of premenstrual syndrome. *Clin Obstet Gynecol* 1992;35(3):679-92.

22. Johnson SR. Clinician's approach to the diagnosis and management of premenstrual syndrome. *Clin Obstet Gynecol* 1992;35(3):637-57.

23. Pearlstein T, Stone AB. Premenstrual syndrome. *Psychiatr Clin North Am* 1998;21(3):577-90.

24. American College of Obstetricians and Gynecologists. Premenstrual Syndrome: *Clinical Management Guidelines for Obstetrician-Gynecologists.* ACOG Practice Bulletin. 2000;15:1-9.

25. Stevinson C, Ernst E. Complementary/alternative therapies for premenstrual syndrome: a systematic review of randomized controlled trials. *Am J Obstet Gynecol* 2001;185:227-35.

26. Thys-Jacobs S et al. Calcium carbonate and the premenstrual syndrome: effects on premenstrual and menstrual symptoms. *Am J Obstet Gynecol* 1998;179:444-52.

27. Wyatt KM et al. Efficacy of vitamin B-6 in the treatment of premenstrual syndrome: systematic review. *BMJ* 1999;318: 1375-81.

Dysmenorrhea—Patient Information

Abdominal cramps and pain in the back and legs are very common symptoms during a woman's menstrual period. Some women also have nausea, vomiting, diarrhea, headache or feel very tired. It usually starts a few hours before, or right at the beginning of your period and lasts about two to three days.

Things you can do to feel better include:
- Comfort measures like a warm bath, or a heating pad or hot water bottle on your belly.
- Get regular aerobic exercise – this may prevent symptoms on an on-going basis.

- Take ibuprofen during your period for three to six months. Your pharmacist can help you decide if ibuprofen is appropriate for you, and tell you exactly how to take it and what to watch for. (Some people should not take ibuprofen).
- If these measures do not relieve your symptoms, or if the medication makes you feel worse, see your doctor.
- If you also require a method of birth control, ask your doctor about going on the pill to relieve your painful menstrual periods.

Premenstrual Syndrome (PMS)—Patient Information

PMS is a group of physical and psychological symptoms that bother some women in the last half of their menstrual cycle (leading up to their period).

These symptoms can include:

Psychological	**Physical**
• Aggression	• Acne
• Anger	• Changes in appetite (food cravings)
• Nervousness	
• Depression	• Bloating, fluid retention
• Forgetfulness	• Pain or swelling in breasts
• Sudden mood changes	
• Panic attacks	• Constipation
• Lack of concentration	• Dizziness
• Fewer coping skills	• Fatigue
	• Headaches
	• Hot flashes
	• Muscle aches
	• Nausea and vomiting
	• Pressure in the pelvic area

Here are some things you can do to relieve your symptoms:
- Try relaxation techniques and reduce the stress in your life.
- Reduce your caffeine intake. This might relieve breast soreness. Caffeine is found in coffee, tea, chocolate and many soft drinks.
- Reduce your salt intake. It might help reduce bloating.

- Get regular exercise (three to four times a week). This can help reduce many symptoms of PMS.
- Nonprescription anti-inflammatory medicines such as ibuprofen (e.g., Advil®, Motrin®) might help relieve pain or headache. Some people should not take these medicines. Your pharmacist can help you decide if these medicines are right for you, help you select a product and tell you exactly how to take it.
- Calcium supplements have helped many women relieve symptoms of abdominal pain, mood changes, bloating and food cravings. Ask your pharmacist if you should take calcium carbonate 1200 mg daily. If you do decide to try calcium, don't take it within three hours of any other medications, and take it with a meal.
- Some women have found that taking magnesium supplements (200 to 400 mg daily) has helped relieved some PMS symptoms.
- Taking vitamin B_6 (50 to 100 mg daily) might help. Another name for vitamin B_6 is pyridoxine. Do not take more than the recommended dose.
- Some herbal remedies have been promoted for the relief of PMS, but so far studies have not shown that they work.

If you have psychological symptoms that are severe and you feel you are not functioning well when you have PMS, or if you have tried self-treatment for your physical or psychological symptoms and it hasn't worked, see your doctor. There are prescription options available to help manage PMS.

Patient Self-Care (PSC), 2002

Menopause and Perimenopause

Thomas E.R. Brown, PharmD

Pathophysiology

Definition

Menopause is the cessation of menses for at least 12 consecutive months.[1] This may be a naturally occurring event or it can be related to the removal or destruction of the ovaries. On average, natural menopause occurs at 51 years of age.[1] A menopause that occurs before the age of 40 is defined as a premature menopause, and menopause occurring after 55 years of age is considered a late menopause.[1] Perimenopause refers to the time leading up to menopause, typically characterized by missed menstrual periods with or without symptoms of hypoestrogenism.[1] Perimenopause has an average duration of four years with a range of two to eight years. The climacteric is an older term that refers to perimenopause, menopause and postmenopause.

Physiology

At the time of menopause, the ovary has no follicles left that respond to the stimulation of follicle stimulating hormone (FSH).[2] The lack of follicular stimulation and development signals the end of the regular menstrual cycle and the monthly fluctuations in both estradiol and progesterone concentrations.[2] Without follicular development and the designation of a Graafian (dominant) follicle, estradiol concentrations remain low and ovulation does not occur; therefore, progesterone concentrations remain low as well.[2] As a result, endometrial proliferation occurs rarely and there are no secretory changes. The pituitary gland increases the production and release of both FSH and leuteinizing hormone (LH) in an attempt to entice the ovary to initiate follicular development.[2] The ovary cannot respond; therefore, FSH and LH concentrations remain elevated while estradiol and progesterone concentrations remain low.[2]

The postmenopausal female continues to produce estrogen in the adipose tissue as a result of the conversion of androstenedione (from the adrenal gland) to estrone.[2] The amount of estrone produced depends on the amount of adipose tissue present. Estrone has a weaker effect on the endometrium than estradiol; therefore, proliferation of endometrial tissue is rare, except in women who are obese.

During perimenopause, cessation of menses, along with the increase in FSH and LH and decrease in estradiol and progesterone, occurs gradually over several months to years.[2] The ovary becomes slow to respond to FSH and LH. Therefore, it can take longer for follicular development and endometrial proliferation to occur; however, unlike in menopause, the follicles in the ovary are still able to respond and ovulation does still occur.[2]

Perimenopausal women may suffer from vasomotor symptoms as well as vaginal dryness. The approach to therapy in these individuals is similar to menopausal women. However, it is important to note that many of the nonprescription therapies have been studied only in postmenopausal women. Perimenopausal women can also suffer from premenstrual symptoms (see Chapter 51) and must still consider the possibility of becoming pregnant.

Clinical Presentation

For the most part, menopause can be diagnosed based on the absence of menses for 12 consecutive months and the symptoms an individual is experiencing. Blood tests are seldom of value in diagnosing menopause.

The most common symptoms are vasomotor symptoms and signs of urogenital aging. Vasomotor symptoms are often referred to as either hot flashes or hot flushes. If they occur during sleep they are referred to as night sweats. Approximately 85% of women experience some form of vasomotor symptom and in 25% the symptoms can be severe. Night sweats can lead to insomnia, fatigue and irritability. Vasomotor symptoms last an average of five years in 75% of women; the remainder may have the symptoms for the rest of their lives.[3] Urogenital aging occurs after menopause and consists of vaginal dryness, pain with intercourse and urinary incontinence.[3] Other symptoms of menopause can include changes in the skin (e.g., increased wrinkling), decreased libido and loss of memory. It is uncertain whether these symptoms are a result of decreased hormone concentrations or secondary to vasomotor and urogenital symptoms.

Long-term Implications

There are several different signs and symptoms of hypoestrogenism and their onset can vary widely among women. They can start in the perimenopausal period or present several years after menopause.[1] Initially, a woman may experience changes in menstrual function such as irregular and/or heavy periods, and she may also experience hot flashes. These symptoms may begin in the perimenopause. The menstrual irregularities end at the time of menopause; however, the peak incidence of hot flashes occurs at the time of menopause and for the majority of women these symptoms last up to five years. Mood disturbances may also accompany menopause but most appear to resolve by the age of 60.

The most rapid bone loss occurs in the first 15 years following menopause, after which bone loss continues at a much slower rate. For information on osteoporosis, see Chapter 34.

Urogenital atrophy begins around the time of menopause and tends to progress as a woman ages. Other disease states including Alzheimer's, colon cancer and cardiovascular disease also increase in incidence as a woman ages. Several trials are being conducted to determine the relationship between these conditions and hormone replacement therapy.

Goals of Therapy

- Relieve undesirable vasomotor or urogenital symptoms of perimenopause and menopause

- Help the woman maintain the highest possible quality of life
- Educate the woman on all aspects of menopause, including long-term health implications and options for their treatment or prevention

Patient Assessment

Encourage women presenting for the first time with questions about menopause or bothersome menopausal symptoms to make an appointment with their physician to discuss all the implications of menopause and the various options for treatment and prevention of its possible sequelae. In the meantime, provide them with information about menopause and the nonpharmacologic measures and nonprescription drug therapies that may relieve symptoms.

It is important to determine which symptoms a woman is experiencing and the degree to which they are bothersome. The general approach for women with mild symptoms is to institute as many nonpharmacologic approaches as possible and then to try a pharmacologic therapy that has been shown to be superior to placebo (e.g., soya supplements, vitamin E, black cohosh or Replens®). Women who do not respond to these therapies, or who have moderate to severe symptoms, should be referred to a physician for possible prescription therapy (Figure 1).

Nonpharmacologic Therapy

Exercise

A study of women in Norway showed that aerobic exercise reduced the number of hot flashes by 40%.[4] Therefore, by increasing aerobic exercise, a woman may experience fewer vasomotor symptoms and also benefit from its effects on the bones and heart.

Sexual Activity

Increasing blood flow to the pelvic region may relieve vaginal dryness and pain on intercourse. This is usually done through sexual stimulation. Therefore, in women who are experiencing vaginal dryness, increasing sexual activity, rather than avoiding it due to discomfort, may be beneficial.[5] To increase lubrication, sexual intercourse itself is not necessary if it is uncomfortable; any form of sexual activity will help restore vaginal moisture.

Figure 1: **Assessment of Patients with Menopausal Symptoms**

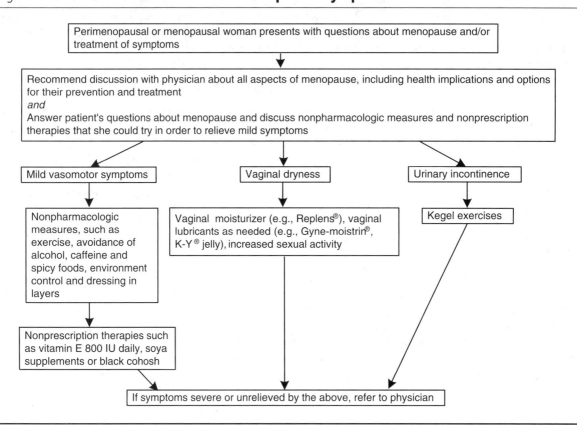

Pelvic Floor Exercises

Kegel exercises may be of value in women who are experiencing incontinence.[6] Kegel exercises involve alternating contraction and relaxation of the pelvic muscles. The contraction is similar to trying to stop urinating. When done correctly, the abdominal and leg muscles are not recruited. The contraction should be held for 4 to 8 seconds. These can be done several times a day.

Dietary Measures

Vasomotor symptoms can be exacerbated by the ingestion of spicy foods, alcohol or caffeine. Therefore, the simplest strategy to reduce the number of hot flashes and night sweats is to avoid spicy foods and to limit alcohol and caffeine intake.

There has been considerable discussion about the potential benefit of ingesting *phytoestrogens* to relieve menopausal symptoms. These are plant-based substances that may have weak estrogenic and/or antiestrogenic activity. They are found in a variety of food substances. There are two main types of phytoestrogens, lignans and isoflavones. The richest source of lignans is flax seed and the richest source of isoflavones is soya products, including tofu and tempeh.[7] Observational studies between Western and Asian women have shown that Asian women have less vasomotor symptoms.[8] This may be attributed to differences in the amounts of dietary phytoestrogens ingested between these two populations.[9] However, it is difficult to confirm this through prospective studies. The results of studies looking at increasing the amount of phytoestrogens through diet have been variable, with the positive studies showing only mild improvement in vasomotor symptoms. The amount of phytoestrogens that need to be consumed remains unknown and their effects seem to be mild at best.[10]

Temperature Control

Vasomotor symptoms can be exacerbated by a warm environment. To minimize this possibility, the indoor temperature should be kept comfortably cool, and it is recommended that a woman dress in layers so that clothes may be removed as needed to maintain comfort.

Nonprescription Therapy

Vitamin E

A randomized, placebo-controlled study in women with breast cancer showed a statistically significant reduction in hot flashes with the use of vitamin E compared to placebo. The dose of vitamin E in the trial was 800 IU per day.[11]

There is no evidence to support the use of intravaginal administration of vitamin E capsules for the relief of vaginal dryness.

Bioadhesive Vaginal Moisturizer

There are two types of vaginal products that are used to reduce the discomfort of vaginal dryness. First are the vaginal lubricants (e.g., Gyne-moistrin®, K-Y® jelly), which are used prior to intercourse to provide lubrication. Second is a bioadhesive vaginal moisturizer (i.e., Replens®), which increases vaginal moisture. A randomized, controlled trial comparing Replens® to conjugated equine estrogen vaginal cream showed that both products increase vaginal moisture and help restore the vaginal epithelium.[12] Replens® should be instilled into the vagina every three days on a continuous basis. It should not be used prior to intercourse as a substitute for a vaginal lubricant.

Soya Protein Supplements

Many formulations of soya protein are available for menopausal women to supplement their dietary intake. Some studies have shown mild positive effects of these on vasomotor symptoms, bone density and lipid profiles.[10,13] The results are variable and can only be applied to the standardized formulation used in the specific studies. Supplements contain varying amounts of isoflavones and soya protein, many of which might not be standardized. The daily dose suggested to achieve beneficial effects is 150 mg of isoflavones or 50 g of soya protein.[13] Additionally, those who recommend the use of soya supplements suggest that it may take up to six months or longer before an effect is seen on vasomotor symptoms. The dose and duration of therapy have not been determined through research trials but come from anecdotal suggestions.

Herbal Remedies

Flax Seed Oil

Women may try to increase the amount of lignans through supplementation with flax seed oil. This may be difficult as the active substance in lignans, enterolactone, is not present in flax seed oil.[8] Enterolactone must be added to the oil. Therefore, flax seed oil without the addition of enterolactone is probably of little value for vasomotor symptoms. Whether or not flax seed oil that contains enterolactone has any effect on vasomotor symptoms has yet to be determined and the dose remains unknown.

Black Cohosh

Black cohosh is the most commonly used herbal preparation for the treatment of vasomotor symptoms in Germany. A small, randomized trial comparing black cohosh to conjugated equine estrogens demonstrated that the two therapies were equivalent in their reduction of vasomotor symptoms.[14] However, a subsequent study comparing black cohosh to placebo in women with breast cancer showed no difference between therapies.[15] Side effects reported with black cohosh include GI upset and decreased blood pressure. The safety of black cohosh use in women with breast cancer is not known.

Oil of Evening Primrose

A randomized, placebo-controlled trial assessing the effect on vasomotor symptoms demonstrated that oil of evening primrose was comparable to, but not better than, placebo.[16] Both groups in this trial reported a 20 to 30% reduction in the number of hot flashes.

Dong Quai

Dong quai is a commonly used Chinese herbal menopause remedy. It has been shown to be equivalent to, but no better than, placebo in a randomized, controlled trial assessing vasomotor symptoms.[17] It has also been shown that dong quai has no estrogenic effects on the endometrium or vagina.

Ginseng

In a clinical trial, ginseng extract had no effect on vasomotor symptoms or FSH concentrations in 400 postmenopausal women, when compared to placebo.[18] However, the extract was able to enhance the patient's sense of well-being, compared to placebo. Another placebo-controlled trial showed no difference between ginseng and placebo on work performance and energy metabolism in women.[19]

Red Clover

Two studies of preparations containing red clover in postmenopausal women showed that it was no better than placebo in reducing the number of hot flashes or other menopausal symptoms.[20]

Prescription Therapy

The gold standard prescription alternative for treating symptoms of menopause is estrogen. *Estrogen* may be administered by the oral or transdermal route.

There are several differences between oral and transdermal estrogens. Oral estrogens cause an increase in HDL-cholesterol, a decrease in LDL-cholesterol and an increase in triglycerides. Transdermal estrogens primarily lower LDL-cholesterol with little change in HDL-cholesterol and no effect on triglycerides. Transdermal estrogen also has less impact on the coagulation cascade and gall bladder compared to oral estrogen. Smoking induces liver enzyme activity; therefore, smokers may achieve higher concentrations of estrogens from a transdermal system compared to oral therapy. Vaginal therapy may be used for the treatment of urogenital aging.

Progestins are combined with estrogen to reduce the risk of endometrial cancer. Therefore, in a woman who has had a hysterectomy, estrogens are often used alone. Estrogen is usually given in a continuous manner whereas progestins can be administered either cyclically (12 to 14 days each month) or continuously. Estrogens with cyclic progestins will often produce a regular menstrual period, whereas estrogen with continuous progestin should induce amenorrhea after six to eight months of therapy.

There are different types of progestins available.[21] Oral micronized progesterone (i.e., Prometrium®) does not blunt the positive effects that estrogen has on HDL-cholesterol; whereas, both medroxyprogesterone acetate and norethindrone acetate can blunt estrogen's positive effect. Oral micronized progesterone may also cause sedation; therefore, it should be taken at bedtime.

Alternatives to estrogen for the treatment of vasomotor symptoms include progestin therapy alone, clonidine, venlafaxine and gabapentin.[13,22] The data proving efficacy with these agents varies from well-controlled trials to case reports.

Monitoring of Therapy

Nonpharmacologic and nonprescription therapies usually require several weeks to months of use before efficacy can be established. The length of therapy is variable. The treatment of vasomotor symptoms may continue for up to 5 years after which the majority of women do not suffer from hot flashes, or it may continue indefinitely for the treatment of urogenital atrophy.

Every woman must make a subjective decision about the intrusiveness or tolerability of a given symptom and participate fully in the decision-making process *vis-à-vis* therapy. Armed with accurate, current information, she can make both short- and long-term decisions about symptom control and prevention of heart disease, osteoporosis and other menopause or age-related health issues. Monitoring can include asking the patient at each visit about the efficacy and side effects of her therapy, checking for interactions if she begins (or has already started) a new nonprescription therapy and answering any questions she may have.

Resource Tips

Society of Obstetricians and Gynecologists of Canada
http://sogc.medical.org/SOGCnet/index.html

The North American Menopause Society
http://www.menopause.org/otherwebresources/edu.html

Suggested Readings

Fluker M, Montemuro S. Canadian Consensus Conference. Menopause: Complimentary Approaches. *J Obstet Gynaecol Can* 2001;1204-1213.

Smith T, Contestabile E. Executive summary, Canadian Consensus on Menopause and Osteoporosis. *J Obstet Gynaecol Can* 2001;23:829-35

Wren B. Menopause. In: Hacker NF, Moore JG, eds. *Essentials of Obstetrics and Gynecology* 3rd ed. Philadelphia, PA: WB Saunders, 1998:602-9.

References

1. Smith T, Contestabile E, Executive summary, Canadian Consensus on Menopause and Osteoporosis. *J Obstet Gynaecol Can* 2001;23:829-35.
2. Wren B, Menopause. In: Hacker NF, Moore JG, eds. *Essentials of Obstetrics and Gynecology* 3rd ed. Philadelphia, PA: WB Saunders, 1998:602-9.
3. Canadian Consensus Conference. Urogenital health. *J Soc Obstet Gynaecol Can* 1998;20:13-21.
4. Hammar M, Berg G, Lindgren R. Does physical exercise influence the frequency of postmenopausal hot flushes? *Acta Obstet Gynecol Scand* 1990;69:409-12.
5. Canadian Consensus Conference. Psychosexual aspects. *J Soc Obstet Gynaecol Can* 1998;20:9-12.
6. Bo K, Hagen RH, Kvarstein B, Jorgensen J, Larsen S. Pelvic floor muscle exercise for the treatment of female stress incontinence: III. Effects of two different degrees of pelvic floor muscle exercies. *Neurol Urodyn* 1990:489-502.
7. Murkies AL, Wilcox G, Davis S. Phytoestrogens, *J Clin Endocrinol Metab* 1998;83:297-303.
8. Tham DM, Gardner CD, Haskell WL. Potential health benefits of dietary phytoestrogens: a review of the clinical epidemiological and mechanistic evidence. *L Clin Endocrinol Metab* 1998;83:2223-35.
9. Lock M. Ambiguities of aging: Japanese experience and perceptions of menopause. *Cult Med Psychiatry* 1986;10:23-46.
10. Davis SR. Phytoestrogen therapy for menopause\al symptoms? *BMJ* 2001;323:354-5.
11. Barton DL, Loprinzi CL, Quella SK et al. Prospective evaluation of vitamin E for hot flashes in breast cancer survivors. *J Clin Oncol* 1998;16:495-500.
12. Nachtigall LE. Comparative study: Replens versus local estrogen therapy in menopausal women. *Fert Steril* 1994;61:178-80.
13. Fluker M, Montemuro S. Canadian Consensus Conference. Menopause: Complimentary Approaches. *J Obstet Gynaecol Can* 2001;1204-1213.
14. Liske E. Therpaeutic efficacy and safety of Cimicifuga racemosa for gynecological disorders. *Adv Therapy* 1998;15:43-51.
15. Jacobson JS, Troxel AB, Evans J, et al. Randomized trial of black cohosh for the treatment of hot flashes among women with a history of breast cancer. *J Clin Oncol* 2001;19:2739-45.
16. Chenoy R, Hussain S, Taylor Y, O'Brien PMS, Moss MY, Morse PF. Effect of gamolenic acid from primrose oil on menopausal flushing. *BMJ* 1994;308:501-3.
17. Hirata JD, Sweirsz LM, Zell B, Small R, Ettinger B. Does dong quai have estrogenic effects in postmenopausal women? A double-blind, placebo controlled trial. *Fert Steril* 1997;68:981-6.
18. Wiklund IK, Mattsson LA, Lindgren R, Limoni C. Effects of a standardized ginseng extract on quality of life and physiological parameters in symptomatic postmenopausal women: a double-blind, placebo controlled trial. *Int J Clin Pharmacol Res* 1999;19:89-99.
19. Engles HJ, Said J. Failure of chronic ginseng supplementation to affect work performance and energy metabolism in healthy adult females. *Nut Res* 1996;16:1295-1305.
20. Fugh-Berman A, Kronenberg F. Red clover (trifolium pratense) for menopausal women:current state of knowledge. *Menopause* 2001;8:333-7.
21. Ferreira E, Brown TER. Canadian Consensus Conference. Menopause: Pharmacotherapy. *J Obstet Gynaecol Can* 2001;1104-1114.
22. Gottoso TJ. Gabapentin's effects on hot flashes and hypothermia. *Neurology* 2000;54:2161-3.

Menopause and Perimenopause—Patient Information

Menopause is a normal part of life for every woman, signifying the end of the childbearing years. Although some physical changes will occur, menopause does not have to mean the end of your sex life or good health.

Symptoms of menopause and perimenopause can include:
- Hot flashes (sometimes called hot flushes, or night sweats if they happen at night)
- Vaginal dryness
- Painful sexual intercourse
- Loss of bladder control
- Skin changes (increased wrinkling)
- Lower sex drive
- Memory loss

Some things you could try to help minimize your symptoms include:
- Avoiding spicy foods, alcohol and caffeine.
- Keeping your environment comfortably cool.
- Dressing in layers in case you get too warm.
- Staying tobacco-free.
- Getting regular aerobic exercise.
- For vaginal dryness, lubricants can be used prior to intercourse if it is painful. A vaginal moisturizer can be used on a regular basis to relieve dryness. Any sexual activity will help restore vaginal moisture, even without intercourse.
- Kegel exercises can help improve bladder control. Kegel exercises are squeezing movements of the pelvic muscles, similar to trying to stop urinating. You shouldn't tense any other muscles like your stomach, back or leg muscles. Try holding the contraction for a count of four to eight, then relaxing. Repeat the contracting and relaxing for about five minutes, several times daily.

Therapies you could try:
- Vitamin E supplements may help relieve hot flashes.
- Herbal remedies such as soya supplements, black cohosh, oil of evening primrose, dong quai, ginseng and red clover have been promoted for the relief of menopausal symptoms. Of these, the ones that have been shown to work at least a little are soya supplements and black cohosh.
- Vaginal lubricants such as K-Y® jelly or Gyne-Moistrin® prior to intercourse or moisturizers such as Replens® on a continuous basis, to relieve vaginal dryness.

Hormone Therapy

There are pros and cons to everything, including hormone replacement therapy. Whether to take HRT is a very personal decision. Every woman is different in terms of the benefit she might get from HRT, and the potential risks involved.

If you're experiencing menopause, talk to your doctor about whether HRT is right for you, and for how long. Ask about all of the options for preventing osteoporosis or heart disease after menopause. You and your doctor can decide what screening tests you may need or want to have, and what to do to stay as healthy as possible as you get older.

Prenatal and Postpartum Care

Shelita Dattani, BSc(Pharm), PharmD

The management of common medical conditions during pregnancy and lactation often includes self-medication. It can be a therapeutic challenge to appropriately identify the efficacy and safety of management strategies in this patient population. This chapter provides an overview of some of the common self-care situations encountered in pregnancy and the postpartum period.

General Principles of Nonprescription Drug Use in Pregnancy and Lactation[1-3]

Although little information is available about drug effects on the fetus, many women take both prescription and nonprescription medications during

Table 1: Myths and Facts Regarding Drug Therapy in Pregnancy and Lactation[2-6]

Myths	Facts
Women who are pregnant should not take any medications.	Although only a few medications are specifically indicated for use during pregnancy, many medications are safe for use in pregnancy.
The fetus is only susceptible to teratogenic effects from drug therapy administered in the first three months of pregnancy.	The first three months of gestation may be the most critical in terms of fetal structural malformations, but functional and behavioral defects are also associated with later exposure when the brain is still developing. Teratogenic agents are defined as those that are capable of producing structural or functional abnormalities in the fetus.
This drug causes malformations in animals, so it should not be used in pregnancy.	Animal data cannot always be extrapolated to human situations (e.g., erythromycin is considered a safe antibiotic to use in pregnancy, but it has been reported to cause malformations in rats).
Due to ease of availability, it can be assumed that nonprescription drug therapies are safe to use in pregnancy and lactation.	There are many nonprescription drugs that are not safe for use in pregnancy/lactation or that lack human safety data (e.g., ASA, NSAIDs, loratadine, dextromethorphan).
Due to ease of availability, herbal products can be considered safe in pregnancy and lactation.	In many cases, there is little reliable human data about the safety of herbal products during pregnancy or lactation. Certain herbs such as St. John's wort are specifically contraindicated due to empirical evidence that they can act as abortifacients. As with any other medicine, one must weigh the risks and possible benefits of using herbal products during pregnancy.
If a drug is excreted in breast milk, it is contraindicated in a lactating mother.	In many cases, very low concentrations of drugs are present in breast milk but they are still considered safe to use in lactation. In general, taking drugs during breastfeeding poses much less risk to the infant than drug therapy during pregnancy. Health care professionals should consult specific references to determine drug safety in lactation.

Table 2: **Principles of Recommending Nonprescription Drug Therapy to Pregnant and Lactating Women**[2,4]

Recommend nonpharmacologic therapy first.
Evaluate whether the drug is really necessary.
Consider whether the benefits of drug therapy outweigh the risks.
Choose the most effective agent with the least amount of risk in the lowest possible dose for the shortest possible duration.
Consider local application of drugs whenever possible to minimize systemic absorption.
Any prolonged use of drug therapy (greater than 3 days) should be approved by a physician.
Refer to physician if nonprescription therapy fails to provide relief after 3 days.
Schedule doses so that the least amount of drug gets into the breast milk (e.g., right after breastfeeding or before the baby is expected to have a long sleep period). The rationale for this is that drug diffuses from the milk back to the vascular compartment as plasma drug concentration falls, so that the lowest levels in milk occur just prior to the next dose. Avoid sustained-release products or drugs with long half-lives. If several drugs are equally useful, select the drug that is excreted in breast milk in the lowest concentration with the least effect on the infant.

pregnancy. When treating common medical conditions in a pregnant or lactating woman, the risks and benefits to the patient, fetus and nursing infant must be weighed carefully to help the patient make an informed decision about medication use. Take care to provide accurate, current and relevant information in a calm, nonalarming manner, putting into perspective that even if a woman does not take any medication during pregnancy, there is always a baseline risk of 1 to 5% for major fetal malformations. Tables 1 and 2 provide some guiding principles for medication use during pregnancy and lactation.

Pregnancy-associated Nausea and Vomiting

Pathophysiology

Pregnancy-associated nausea and vomiting (PANV), commonly referred to as "morning sickness," occurs in about 70% of pregnant women.[7] Approximately half of these women have mild nausea and vomiting and half experience moderate symptoms requiring treatment. Morning sickness usually appears by 4 to 8 weeks gestation and disappears by 14 to 16 weeks gestation.[3,7] The nausea and/or vomiting is usually self-limiting and not associated with any adverse fetal outcome.[3] Severe vomiting may be associated with low birth weight babies.[8]

The etiology of PANV is unknown, although increased concentrations of HCG have been implicated.[7,8] Progesterone-induced relaxation of gastric smooth muscle and a delay in gastric emptying may also play a role. Although it occurs rarely, severe morning sickness, or hyperemesis gravidarum, may lead to dehydration, malnutrition and weight loss, and hospitalization may be required.[8] Hyperemesis gravidarum affects 0.05 to 0.1% of pregnancies and is usually a diagnosis of exclusion. Onset is always in the first trimester, usually between weeks six and eight. Hyperemesis gravidarum may last the duration of the pregnancy, but usually becomes less extreme as the pregnancy progresses. It tends to recur in subsequent pregnancies, so a previous history makes the diagnosis more likely.[3,8]

Goals of Therapy

- Improve patient's quality of life
- Maintain adequate nutrition
- Prevent dehydration and significant weight loss

Patient Assessment

Patients with adequate hydration and nutrition despite PANV can be counseled on nonpharmacologic measures to relieve symptoms. For more severe nausea and vomiting with signs of dehydration or weight loss, refer patients to a physician immediately. More information on PANV can be found in Chapter 20.

Nonpharmacologic Therapy[3,8]

There are many measures pregnant women can take to alleviate PANV. Avoiding aggravating factors such as certain smells, fried or spicy food, an empty stomach, stress and fatigue is key. Taking prenatal vitamins and/or iron supplements after meals, rather than on an empty stomach, is also suggested. Information for patients on management of morning sickness is found at the end of the chapter.

Although there are no data to support their efficacy, acupressure wrist bands (e.g., Seabands®) have been used in the management of nausea and vomiting and appear to be safe in pregnancy.

Pharmacologic Therapy

Nonprescription Therapy

Antiemetics are indicated for the treatment of moderate PANV that fails to respond to nonpharmacologic interventions. Table 3 lists nonprescription therapies used in the management of PANV. Patients should not take the medications outlined in Table 3 without approval from their physician, due to the lack of evidence supporting these therapies.

Ginger may be helpful in reducing nausea. It has been used in many forms such as ginger tea, gingerale, gingersnaps or powdered gingerroot. Although data on safety of ginger are lacking, the usual dose is up to 1000 mg per day, based on a calculation that up to 1000 mg of ginger is taken through normal diet in some cultures. The effects of large amounts of ginger on the fetus are still not known,[8] and it should be used only on the advice of a physician.

Prescription Therapy

The therapy of choice in the management of PANV that is unresponsive to nonpharmacologic measures is

Table 3: **Nonprescription Drug Therapy for Pregnancy-associated Nausea and Vomiting**[*7-10]

Drug	Effective dose	Mechanism of effect	Onset	Side effects	Monitoring of therapy
Dimenhydrinate	50 to100 mg orally or rectally every 4 h as necessary (maximum 200 mg per day); can also be given parenterally. Minimal data on efficacy	Binds to H_1 receptors and blocks effects of histamine; blocks chemoreceptor trigger zone	15-30 min	Sedation; anti-cholinergic effects. No known teratogenic effects	Monitor patient for signs and symptoms of sedation and anticholinergic effects (e.g., dry mouth, constipation). Refer to physician if nausea and vomiting not improved or side effects intolerable, after 3 days.
Pyridoxine (vitamin B_6)	Unknown; 10 mg or 25 mg TID have been studied. One study showed that 25 mg every 8 h was significantly better than placebo in decreasing vomiting in all patients and decreasing nausea in patients with severe symptoms.	Unknown	Unknown	No known teratogenic or adverse effects in doses used for nausea and vomiting	Refer to physician if nausea and vomiting not improved in 3 days.

*To be used only on the advice of a physician.

Diclectin®, a combination delayed-release product containing doxylamine 10 mg and pyridoxine 10 mg. It is the only product that has Health Canada approval for PANV.[3,8] It has been studied in over 200 000 pregnant women to date and has not been found to increase the risk of teratogenesis.[10] It is first-line therapy if conservative nonpharmacologic methods fail.[10] Two tablets are taken at bedtime for early morning symptoms. One additional tablet can be taken in the morning and midafternoon if needed for nausea. Diclectin™ can cause drowsiness, headache, dizziness or irritability.

Other prescription agents that have been used in nausea and vomiting during pregnancy include meclizine, metoclopramide, ondansetron and phenothiazines (e.g., chlorpromazine and prochloperazine). Although these agents have not been associated with increased teratogenicity, they have not been as well studied as Diclectin®. Newborns may experience extrapyramidal effects if phenothiazines are given near term. Corticosteroids have been used safely in severe cases of morning sickness.[3,10]

Allergic Rhinitis During Pregnancy

Pathophysiology

Allergic rhinitis affects approximately one-third of women of childbearing age. Common symptoms include nasal itchiness, rhinorrhea and sneezing.[1] More information on this condition can be found in Chapter 12.

Goals of Therapy[1,3]

- Relieve symptoms
- Minimize risk of complications, such as sinusitis

Nonpharmacologic Therapy[1,3]

The mainstay of nonpharmacologic management of allergic rhinitis during pregnancy is minimizing exposure to allergens such as pollen, animal dander, dust mites or mold growth, and remaining indoors when necessary.

Pharmacologic Therapy[1,10,11]

Nonprescription Therapy

The nonprescription therapies in Table 4 should be used only under the supervision of a physician. Antihistamines should be used as first-line agents in the treatment of allergic rhinitis and of the therapies listed in Table 4, first-generation antihistamines (e.g., **chlorpheniramine, diphenhydramine**) should be tried initially. Due to limited safety data, second-line antihistamines such as **cetirizine** can be used if first-generation agents are not tolerated by the patient. Although **brompheniramine** is contraindicated during pregnancy, it is the antihistamine of choice in lactation.[1]

Decongestant medication can be utilized supplementally for additional symptom relief; topical decongestants should be tried first (**normal saline** should be tried as a first-line agent – **systemic decongestants** should not be used unless **topical decongestants** have failed and the benefit outweighs any potential risk (see Table 4). Antitussives should only be used supplementally for relief of dry cough if expected benefit is great. **Dextromethorphan** should be considered first-line due to its established safety in pregnancy. **Codeine** can be used in the short-term for symptoms unresponsive to dextromethorphan (see Table 4).

Prescription Therapy

Intranasal **sodium cromoglycate** is recommended for patients with daily symptoms that are unresponsive to antihistamine use alone. It is well tolerated with very few adverse effects and is considered safe in pregnancy and lactation, as it is minimally absorbed across nasal membranes.[1]

Intranasal **beclomethasone** is reserved for symptoms unresponsive to antihistamines and/or cromolyn. Systemic absorption is minimal and its use in pregnancy has not been associated with an increased risk of congenital abnormalities. Some beclomethasone may be excreted into breast milk but it is unlikely to be clinically significant. Currently, there are limited data on the safety of intranasal corticosteroids other than beclomethasone during pregnancy and lactation.[1]

The antileukotrienes, **zafirlukast** and **montelukast**, have been used in the treatment of allergic rhinitis

Table 4: **Nonprescription Drug Therapy for Allergic Rhinitis in Pregnancy and Lactation**[1,10,11]

Drug	Effective dose	Expected clinical benefit	Onset	Side effects	Monitoring of therapy	Comments Pregnancy	Comments Lactation
Antihistamines							
Brompheniramine	4 mg every 4-6 h	Relief of nasal congestion through inhibition of histamine release	15-30 min	Drowsiness, irritability	Monitor infants of lactating mothers for signs of irritability, excessive crying and altered sleep. If infant experiences these effects or if mother's symptoms do not improve after 1 wk, refer to physician.	Inconclusive data; avoid use	Considered first-line antihistamine during lactation, based on available information.
Cetirizine	5-10 mg daily	Relief of nasal congestion through inhibition of histamine release	20-60 min	Preferred by patients due to ease of administration and because it is nonsedating	Monitor patient for sedation, headache or anticholinergic effects (e.g., dry mouth). Refer to physician if side effects intolerable or if symptoms not improved after 1 wk.	Because of limited safety data, should be considered a second-line antihistamine if first-generation agents (e.g., chlorpheniramine, diphenhydramine) not tolerated.	Excreted in breast milk, although adverse effects on nursing infants have not been reported. Avoid use
Chlorpheniramine	4 mg every 4-6 h (maximum 24 mg per day)	Relief of nasal congestion through inhibition of histamine release	15-30 min	Sedation (less than with diphenhydramine); anticholinergic effects, including mucosal drying, which may inhibit lactation. Use smallest possible dose to minimize adverse effects.	Monitor patient for sedation or anticholinergic effects (e.g., dry mouth). Refer to physician if side effects intolerable or symptoms not improved after 1 wk.	Most data support no increased risk of congenital effects in pregnant women.	No information on use in lactation. Avoid use

(cont'd)

Table 4: Nonprescription Drug Therapy for Allergic Rhinitis in Pregnancy and Lactation[1,10,11] (cont'd)

Drug	Effective dose	Expected clinical benefit	Onset	Side effects	Monitoring of therapy	Comments — Pregnancy	Comments — Lactation
Antihistamines (cont'd)							
Diphenhydramine	25 to 50 mg every 6-8 h	Relief of nasal congestion through inhibition of histamine release	15-30 min	Sedation; anticholinergic effects including mucosal drying which may inhibit lactation. Use smallest possible dose to minimize adverse effects.	Monitor for sedation, palpitations, dizziness or anticholinergic effects (e.g., dry mouth). Refer to physician if side effects intolerable or symptoms not improved after 1 wk.	Most data support no increased risk of congenital effects in pregnant women.	Manufacturer cautions against use in lactation due to increased sensitivity of newborns to antihistamines.
Loratadine	10 mg daily	Relief of nasal congestion through inhibition of histamine release	1-3 h	Headache, drowsiness, anticholinergic effects including dry mouth	Monitor for sedation, headache or anticholinergic effects (e.g., dry mouth). Refer to physician if side effects intolerable or symptoms not improved in 1 wk.	Inconclusive data; avoid use	Considered first-line antihistamine during lactation, based on available information.
Decongestants							
Systemic: Pseudoephedrine	30 to 60 mg every 4-6 h (maximum 120 mg per day)	Relief of congestion through vasoconstriction of respiratory mucosa	15-30 min	Signs and symptoms of adrenergic stimulation, palpitations, nervousness, insomnia, dizziness	If side effects intolerable or symptoms do not improve after 1 wk (with concurrent antihistamine use) refer to physician.	Avoid during first trimester due to recent association between use of pseudoephedrine and rare birth defect known as gastrochisis. Use cautiously, and only if topical decongestants have failed and expected benefit is great.	Excreted in breast milk but considered compatible with breastfeeding. Infants should be monitored for signs and symptoms of α-adrenergic stimulation (e.g., irritability, excessive crying, altered sleep patterns).

Drug	Dose	Action	Onset	Side effects	Comments	Pregnancy	Lactation
Topical (intranasal): normal saline, oxymetazoline, xylometazoline	Use lowest effective dose, according to manufacturer's instructions.	Relief of congestion through vasoconstriction of respiratory mucosa (oxymetazoline, xylometazoline). Osmotic effect (normal saline)	5-10 min	Use topical decongestants (oxymetazoline, xylometazoline) sparingly (maximum 3-5 days), to minimize tolerance or rebound congestion.	If symptoms not improved after 1 wk (with concurrent antihistamine use) refer to physician.	Normal saline spray should be used as a first-line intranasal decongestant, due to its established safety profile. Topical decongestants (oxymetazoline, xylometazoline) have not been associated with birth defects but limited data available.	Normal saline spray can be used in pregnancy. Safety of topical decongestants (oxymetazoline, xylometazoline) in lactation not established; avoid use.

Antitussives

Drug	Dose	Action	Onset	Side effects	Comments	Pregnancy	Lactation
Dextromethorphan	10-20 mg every 4 h or 30 mg every 6-8 h.	Relief of cough through centrally mediated cough suppression	15-30 min	Minimal	If symptoms do not improve after 1 wk (with concurrent antihistamine use), refer to physician.	Safe in pregnancy. Use only if expected benefit is great, on an as-needed basis. Avoid products that contain ethanol.	No data available on use in lactation; do not encourage routine use.
Codeine	10-20 mg every 4-6 h as needed.	Relief of cough through centrally mediated cough suppression	30-60 min	Drowsiness, constipation, palpitations, dizziness	If side effects are intolerable or symptoms do not improve (with concurrent antihistamine use) after 1 wk, refer to physician.	Short-term use of low doses acceptable in pregnancy. Avoid high doses close to term (risk of neonatal opiate withdrawal). Use only if expected benefit is great, on an as-needed basis.	Codeine not excreted in breast milk to a significant degree; short-term use of low doses acceptable.

after conventional treatments have failed. Harmful effects have not been seen in animal studies with either of these agents but there are very limited data in human pregnancy and use should be avoided unless benefit clearly outweighs risk. Safety of these agents in lactating mothers has not been established and use should be avoided.[1,11]

Other Common Conditions

Table 5 describes the management of some conditions commonly encountered in pregnancy. Each condition is covered in detail in specific chapters of this book, as outlined in the footnotes.

Postpartum Perineal Care and Postepisiotomy Pain
Pathophysiology

Perineal pain affects approximately 25% of women in the first eight weeks of the postpartum period.[12] Postpartum perineal pain is usually due to episiotomy or extensive tearing during delivery. The perineum is an extremely tender site for a cut or stitches and women report a wide range of pain, from mild to excruciating. Typically, the pain is felt for 7 to 10 days, which is the time usually required for the wound to heal.

Goals of Therapy

- Relief of perineal pain
- Prevention of complications such as infection

Patient Assessment

When perineal pain is severe or associated with foul-smelling discharge, burning, bleeding or high fever, refer patients to a physician immediately.

Nonpharmacologic Therapy[12,13,14]

A list of nonpharmacologic measures can be found in the patient information section on perineal care/episiotomy pain.

Pharmacologic Therapy
Nonprescription Therapy

Short-term relief of perineal pain can be obtained with one of the local agents listed in Table 6. Medicated anesthetic creams containing lidocaine are also available but should only be used under the direction of a physician due to the risk of systemic absorption from the area of trauma. Analgesics such as acetaminophen and ibuprofen can also be used effectively and safely in this situation. Opioid analgesics such as codeine can be used safely in the postpartum period but are not ideal due to limiting side effects such as constipation and nausea.[15]

Postpartum Depression
Pathophysiology

Emotional disturbances after childbirth are generally classified as the more common postpartum blues ("baby blues") or the more serious postpartum depression. Postpartum blues is a common disorder that is estimated to occur in 26 to 85% of new mothers.[16] The disorder generally begins sometime in the first week after delivery and symptoms may include insomnia, tearfulness, depression, fatigue, anxiety and poor appetite. Postpartum blues has only a minimal effect on the mother's ability to function and the disorder usually resolves spontaneously within a few weeks.[16]

Postpartum depression occurs in approximately 10% of new mothers. The condition is more disabling and persistent and the mother often finds it difficult to take care of her infant. The incidence is highest in the first three months postpartum with a peak onset in the first four to six weeks, but may occur anytime in the first six months after delivery. The symptoms are very similar to regular depression and can include lowered energy, disturbed sleep and changes in appetite. Depressive symptoms can lead to disorders of mother-to-infant bonding such as feelings of detachment, lack of love, or resentment or hostility towards the baby.[16,17] Thoughts of self-harm or suicide can also be present.[3,17]

Most women will recover naturally over a three to six month period without any treatment. Supportive counseling is recommended if symptoms persist for

Table 5: **Management of Other Common Conditions in Pregnancy**[1,3,7,13,18]

Condition	Cause	Nonpharmacologic therapy	Pharmacologic therapy	Monitoring	Comments
Constipation*	Compression of intestines by enlarging uterus; reduced GI motility due to increased progesterone levels; increased water resorption by colon; iron and calcium supplementation; bedrest.	Eat foods high in fibre (whole grains, vegetables, fruits, high fibre cereals). Increase fluid intake (6–8 glasses of water daily in addition to mealtime beverages); discuss reduction of iron supplementation with physician (if taking more than 30 mg per day); exercise.	Bulk laxatives safest (e.g., psyllium) on an as-needed basis (not absorbed and pose least threat to fetus); stool softeners (e.g., docusate) have also been used.	Refer to physician if symptoms do not improve after 5–7 days.	Avoid repeat administration of osmotic (e.g., lactulose) and stimulant (e.g., bisacodyl) laxatives, including castor oil, due to excess fluid and electrolyte loss; mineral oil and castor oil may interfere with absorption of nutrients such as Vitamin K (could decrease availability to fetus) and other fat-soluble vitamins.
Hemorrhoids†	Increased venous pressure below the uterus; constipation; vessel walls relaxed by progesterone (can lead to swelling)	Maintain normal bowel function; prevent constipation and straining; ice pack or cold compress to help relieve itching; keep anal area clean to avoid irritation; clean anal area with soap and water after each bowel movement; warm water sitz baths for 15 minutes as needed for comfort.	Stool softeners (e.g., docusate) may relieve some discomfort. External products preferred because those inserted into rectum may be readily absorbed from rectal mucosa. Astringents (e.g., witch hazel pads) or rectally applied petroleum jelly can be used to clean and soothe the hemorrhoid area.	Refer to physician if symptoms do not improve after 5 days.	Ointments or suppositories containing topical anesthetics (e.g., benzocaine, pramoxine) or hydrocortisone should not be used (except under supervision of a physician) due to possible systemic absorption with consequent effects on the fetus.
Reflux esophagitis‡	Occurs in approximately 30% of women — usually in third trimester; upward displacement of stomach by uterus and decreased GI motility can lead to gastric reflux; esophageal sphincter relaxed by progesterone.	Avoid large meals; eat slowly; avoid foods that cause heartburn; eat in an upright position; drink warm milk; avoid eating just before going to bed; elevate the head of the bed using blocks, or use two extra pillows to raise the head; avoid stooping, bending or assuming other positions that tend to worsen reflux.	Aluminum and/or magnesium containing antacids as well as products containing alginic acid or simethicone. Calcium products may provide additional benefits in pregnancy and lactation. Data evaluating safety of H_2 receptor antagonists in pregnancy are lacking; refer to physician — risk vs. benefit must be carefully weighed.	Monitor for signs and symptoms of reflux. Refer to physician if symptoms do not improve after 7 days.	ASA (e.g., Alka Seltzer®) is a particular risk in third trimester but probably should be avoided throughout pregnancy except under direction of physician. Sodium bicarbonate not recommended due to short duration of effect, possible rebound symptoms and metabolic alkalosis with chronic use.

(cont'd)

Table 5: **Management of Other Common Conditions in Pregnancy**[1,3,7,13,18] *(cont'd)*

Condition	Cause	Nonpharmacologic therapy	Pharmacologic therapy	Monitoring	Comments
Backache[π], headache[#]	Back muscles under strain due to growing abdomen; weight of uterus can contribute; headache commonly resulting from muscle tension.	Relaxation exercises; massage; rest in recumbent position; good posture and lifting techniques; moderate exercise; pelvic tilts; elevation of one leg while standing; cool wet cloth to forehead for headaches.	Acetaminophen alone or with codeine if necessary; codeine should only be used in smallest dose for shortest treatment possible.	Refer to physician if symptoms do not improve after 5 days. With codeine, monitor patient for side effects such as constipation or drowsiness and refer to physician if side effects are not tolerable.	Avoid ASA or other NSAIDs if possible — especially in third trimester, due to increased risk of prolonged gestation and labor and premature closure of ductus arteriosus. Refer to physician immediately if headache associated with blurred vision or nausea.
Common cold[**]	Viral	Bedrest; maintain fluid intake; humidify air	Use only under supervision of physician; many products contain more than one ingredient including analgesic, decongestant, cough suppressant or expectorant and/or antihistamine. Use of topical decongestants is preferred over systemic products. Cough and throat lozenges are unlikely to have systemic effects. If drugs are needed, they should be used sparingly and for the shortest treatment period possible (Table 4).	Refer to physician if symptoms are associated with fever, nausea or vomiting. With codeine, monitor patient for side effects such as constipation or drowsiness and refer to physician if side effects are not tolerable.	Avoid high doses of codeine close to term (risk of neonatal opiate withdrawal).

| **Nutrition**[††] | Some nutrient requirements are increased due to needs of growing fetus. | Eat a well-balanced diet with special attention to adequate protein, calcium (total of 1200-1500 mg elemental calcium per day), iron (extra 30 mg elemental iron per day), and folic acid (400 µg daily). | Prenatal vitamin supplementation should be done under supervision of a physician. Folic acid supplementation is recommended (400 µg), starting before conception and continuing through pregnancy. Most acceptable prenatal multivitamin preparations contain the appropriate amount of folic acid. Calcium may have to be supplemented depending on dietary intake. Iron may have to supplemented in addition to prenatal vitamin, depending on lab findings. | If patient is not getting adequate nutrition from diet, refer to physician for dietary counseling. | Women with a family history of neural tube defects should take 5 mg of folic acid daily under physician supervision. High doses of vitamin A may cause birth defects. The maximum dose of supplementary vitamin A before and during pregnancy is 5000 IU per day. |

*For more information, see Chapter 21.
[†]For more information, see Chapter 27.
[‡]For more information, see Chapter 23.
[¤]For more information, see Chapter 35.
[#]For more information, see Chapter 8.
[**]For more information, see Chapter 13.
[††]For more information, see Chapter 31.

Table 6: **Nonprescription Drug Therapy for Perineal Care and Postepisiotomy Pain**[15]

Drug	Dose	Side effects	Monitoring of therapy	Comments
Local agents Witch hazel liquid or pads (e.g., Tucks® medicated pads).	Use as needed for comfort	Not applicable	If pain not relieved after 2 days, recommend a trial of oral analgesics.	May reduce itching and pain. If pain not relieved, a trial of an oral analgesic may be warranted (see below).
Analgesics Acetaminophen	325-1000 mg every 4-6 h as necessary	Minimal	If pain not relieved after 2 days, refer to physician.	Considered safe in breast-feeding mothers
Ibuprofen	400 mg every 4-6 h as necessary	GI effects, dizziness, rash		Considered safe in breast-feeding mothers

longer than two weeks, to help reduce the severity or prevent progression of the depression. Up to 10% of women diagnosed with postpartum depression will still display some symptoms of depression one year after delivery.[17]

Goals of Therapy

- Relieve depressive symptoms
- Identify patients at risk of serious depression
- Educate patients on recognizing danger signs

Patient Assessment

Postpartum women should be monitored carefully by their health care providers. The checklist provided at the end of the chapter can be used as a tool for recognition of signs of postpartum depression. If any of the signs on the checklist apply to a postpartum patient, the pharmacist should actively advise her to get help by immediately referring her to her physician for counseling and/or specialized mental health treatment.

Nonpharmacologic Therapy

Milder symptoms can usually be treated with supportive counseling.

Pharmacologic Therapy

Nonprescription Therapy

St. John's wort has been used in the treatment of mild to moderate depression; however, there is no reliable information regarding its use in lactation. It should be avoided in lactating mothers with postpartum depressive symptoms.[6] Although depression can also affect women during pregnancy, St. John's wort should not be used in pregnant women because of evidence suggesting it may increase uterine muscle tone.[6]

Prescription Therapy

More severe or prolonged depression requires medication, and rarely, hospitalization to prevent suicide or infanticide.[14] Antidepressant medications considered compatible with breastfeeding include sertraline, paroxetine, amitriptyline and desipramine.[12,17]

Postpartum Contraception
General Principles

Most health care providers suggest waiting about four to six weeks before resuming intercourse, to allow the woman's body to heal. The uterus and vagina must return to their prepregnancy size, a process that usually occurs more quickly in breastfeeding women.

Many variables can influence this time frame, such as fatigue, postpartum depression and decreased sex drive. Furthermore, many women take much longer before they feel like resuming intercourse. Couples need to make individual decisions based on comfort level.

Ovulation usually resumes within five weeks after delivery in nonlactating mothers and within 8 to 10 weeks in mothers who breastfeed their infants without supplementation. Hence, breastfeeding should not be considered a form of contraception.

Oral Contraceptives

The risk of thromboembolic disease is increased in women taking oral contraceptives (OCs) less than three weeks after delivery. A recent review recommends waiting to start OCs until at least two weeks after delivery in women without other risk factors for venous thrombosis, and until four to six weeks after delivery in women with risk factors such as history of DVT, surgery, immobilization, chronic disease, smoking, or age > 35 years.[19]

Combination OCs may be used for nursing mothers but may cause a decrease in the quantity of milk produced if they are introduced prior to established lactation.[14] Nursing mothers should wait until at least six weeks after delivery to begin OCs to allow establishment of milk supply.[20] For mothers with low milk supply, progestin-only contraceptives may be used as they do not appear to affect milk volume.[19,20]

Refer patients to their physician for a discussion of oral contraceptive options.

Barrier Methods[13,21]

Barrier methods include male and female condoms, sponges, diaphragms and cervical caps, all supplemented by spermicides. Male condoms can be used almost immediately postpartum. To decrease the risk of toxic shock syndrome, contraceptive sponges, cervical caps and diaphragms should not be used while there is continued postpartum bleeding.

Diaphragm and cervical cap fitting or refitting should be performed six to eight weeks after delivery, to allow for completion of uterine involution.

For more information on barrier contraceptive devices, see Chapter 49.

Other

Levonorgestrel (silastic capsules implanted subdermally in the upper arm during onset of menses), medroxyprogesterone (intra-muscular injection) and intrauterine devices are also effective contraceptive alternatives.[20] Fewer side effects are encountered with these methods when they are started after uterine involution is complete, which typically occurs four to six weeks after delivery.[15,20]

Nonprescription Therapy During Lactation

Nearly all drugs will be present in breast milk to some degree following maternal ingestion.[2] Many lists of drugs that are acceptable to ingest during lactation have been developed, but they differ and are based on subjective interpretation of data. Most of the published data come from single case reports, and reports of drug concentration in breast milk are often based on single dose measurements, not accounting for effects of drug accumulation. Therefore, it is difficult to interpret the clinical significance of this information.[2]

Table 7 compiles some of the information pertaining to nonprescription medication use during lactation.

Resource Tips

Motherisk (conducting studies on the health of expectant mothers and their unborn children):
(416) 813-6780 www.motherisk.org

Motherisk nausea and vomiting in pregnancy (NVP) hotline: Toll free: 1-800-436-8477

Society of Obstetricians and Gynecologists of Canada: www.sogc.org

Planned Parenthood Federation of Canada: www. ppfc.ca

Women's Health (general): www.stjosephs.london. on.ca/SJHC/programs/women/women.htm

Information and support for postpartum depression: http://www.sickkids.on.ca/fetalcentre/Bereavement PostPartum.asp

Table 7: **Nonprescription Medications Usually Considered Compatible with Breast-feeding**[1,2,9]

Drug class	Comments
Analgesics	Analgesics such as acetaminophen, ASA, ibuprofen and codeine are compatible with breast-feeding when take occasionally at therapeutic doses. Chronically administered ASA, especially at higher doses, is associated with bleeding and metabolic acidosis (one case) and has the potential to have adverse effects on platelet function in the nursing infant.
Laxatives	Bulk-forming agents are the safest agents to the nursing infant as they are not absorbed. Senna and cascara have been used with little or no adverse effects (few reports of infant diarrhea but causality questionable); docusate has been associated with one known report of infant diarrhea but causality unknown.
Antidiarrheals	May be safest to prescribe least absorbable compounds for occasional use such as kaolin/pectin. Loperamide has been used safely. Bismuth subsalicylate should be avoided during lactation because of systemic salicylate absorption.
Nasal decongestants	Pseudoephedrine considered safe in breastfeeding mothers. No data available for nasal sprays; normal saline spray preferred.
Antihistamines	Generally thought to pose no hazard to nursing infant; diphenhydramine and brompheniramine may be associated with symptoms of irritability and lethargy. Anticholinergic effects may inhibit lactation.
Antacids	Problems related to acid-base balance are minimal with nonsystemic antacids since they are relatively nonabsorbable; however, cations such as magnesium and aluminum are absorbed from the gastrointestinal tract and, in theory, may pass into breast milk in significant amounts.
Vitamins	Appropriate when used in normal doses. Maternal ingestion of pharmacologic doses of vitamin D may cause hypercalcemia in the nursing infant; monitor infant's serum calcium levels.

Suggested Readings

Briggs GG, Freeman RK, Yaffe SJ. *Drugs in pregnancy and lactation.* 5th ed. Baltimore, MD: Williams and Wilkins; 1998.

Koren G. *Maternal-fetal toxicology.* 2nd ed. New York, NY: Marcel Dekker; 1994.

Micholaus A, McIness DK, Ensom MH. Allergies: A motherhood issue. *Pharm Pract* 2000;16(2):49-58.

Taddio A. Treatment of chronic conditions during pregnancy. *Pharm Pract* 1996;12(8): Continuing education insert.

Vicars M, ed. *Healthy Beginnings: Your handbook for pregnancy and birth.* 2nd ed. Ottawa, ON: The Society of Obstetricians and Gynecologists of Canada; 2000.

References

1. Michoulas A, McIness DK, Ensom MH. Allergies: A motherhood issue. *Pharm Pract* 2000;16(2):49-58.
2. Yoshida E. Pregnancy and lactation. In: Carruthers-Czyzewski P, ed. *Nonprescription Drug Reference for Health Professionals.* Premier edition. Ottawa, ON: Canadian Pharmaceutical Association; 1996:289-90.
3. Taddio A. Treatment of chronic conditions during pregnancy. *Pharm Pract* 1996;12(8): Continuing education insert.
4. Einarrson A. Patient advice on drug use in pregnancy and lactation. *Pharmacy Connection* Jan/Feb 1995.
5. Moretti ME, Lee A, Ito S. Which drugs are contraindicated during breastfeeding? Practice guidelines. *Can Fam Physician* 2000;46:1753-7.
6. Jellin JM, Batz F, Hitchens K. *Pharmacist's Letter Natural Medicines Comprehensive Database.* Stockton, CA: Therapeutic Research Faculty; 1999;864-6.
7. Steinlauf AF, Traube M. Gastrointestinal complications. In: Burrow GB, Duffy TP, eds. *Medical complications during*

pregnancy. 5th ed. Philadelphia, PA: WB Saunders Company; 1999: 255-8.

8. Perrier H. Morning sickness. *Can Pharm J* 1998;131(2):24.

9. Briggs GG, Freeman RK, Yaffe SJ. *Drugs in pregnancy and lactation.* 5th ed. Baltimore, MD: Williams and Wilkins; 1998.

10. Mazotta P, Gupta A, Maltepe C, Koren G, Magee L. Pharmacologic treatment of nausea and vomiting during pregnancy. *Can Fam Physician* 1998;44:1455-7.

11. Dombrowski MP, Huff R, Lipkowitz M, Schatz M. The use of newer asthma and allergy medications during pregnancy. *Ann Allergy Asthma Immunol* 2000;84:475-80.

12. Montgomery AM. Breastfeeding and postpartum maternal care. *Prim Care* 2000;27(1):237-49.

13. Vicars M, ed. *Healthy Beginnings: Your handbook for - pregnancy and birth,* 2nd ed. Ottawa, ON: The Society of Obstetricians and Gynecologists of Canada; 2000.

14. Acheson LS, Danner SC. Postpartum care and breastfeeding. *Prim Care* 1993;20(3):729-46.

15. Peter, EA, Janssen PA, Grange CS, et al. Ibuprofen versus acetaminophen with codeine for the relief of perineal pain after childbirth: a randomized, controlled trial. *CMAJ* 2001; 154(9):1203-9.

16. Bright DA. Postpartum mental disorders. *Am Fam Physician* 1994;50(3):595-8.

17. Belanger D. Postpartum Depression *Can Pharm J* 2000;133 (8):20.

18. Scarr EM, Simmons LN. Constipation. In: Shopkow S, ed. *Ambulatory Obstetrics.* 3rd ed. San Francisco, CA: UCSF Nursing Press; 1999: 237-242.

19. Kennedy KI. Baillieres. *Clin Obstet Gynaecol* 1996;10:25-41.

20. Stover AM, Marnejon JG. Postpartum care. *Am Fam Physician* 1995;52(7):1465-72.

21. Canadian Consensus Conference on Contraception. *Journal SOGC* 1998;20(7):43-6.

Nonprescription Drug Use During Pregnancy and Lactation—Patient Information

If you are considering taking a nonprescription or herbal medication and you are pregnant or breastfeeding:

- Discuss nondrug therapy options first with your pharmacist and/or physician.
- Consult your physician or pharmacist before taking any nonprescription or herbal medication. Not every medication poses a risk to your unborn baby, but some do. Weigh the benefits against the risks to make an informed decision.

- Ask your pharmacist or physician if you can take a locally acting product (e.g., nose spray, ointment) instead of a pill to minimize the amount of medication you might pass on to your baby.
- Do not assume that because herbal medication is "natural" and accessible, that it is safe in pregnant and breastfeeding mothers.
- If you are taking medication while breastfeeding, try scheduling your doses right after a feed or when the baby goes down for a long nap.

Morning Sickness—Patient Information

If you are suffering from morning sickness during pregnancy:

- Avoid smells that make you feel nauseated.
- Eat crackers or dry toast before you get out of bed.
- Eat whatever food you want that looks and smells appealing and that relieves your nausea.
- Eat small amounts of dry food every one to two hours. An empty stomach can make you feel sick.
- Avoid warm places because feeling hot can add to nausea.

- Try to avoid stress and fatigue as both may aggravate morning sickness.
- Take your prenatal vitamins or iron supplements after meals, rather than on an empty stomach.
- Try sipping ginger ale or eating some gingersnaps.

If none of these methods help, talk to your doctor about taking medication to relieve your morning sickness.

Perineal Care and Episiotomy Pain—Patient Information

After delivering a baby, many women feel soreness or pain in the external vagina and surrounding area (perineum), due to an episiotomy or tearing during delivery. Here are some things you can do to relieve symptoms and help with healing:

- Avoid touching the area.
- Change sanitary pads at least every four to six hours. Do not use tampons for postpartum bleeding.
- Use medicated wipes (e.g., Tucks®) to cleanse and soothe the area.
- Use a perineal squirt bottle to pour warm water over the perineal area after going to the bathroom.
- Use a sitz bath (warm water, either in the bathtub or a special sitz bath that fits over the toilet seat) after bowel movements.
- Always pat the area dry from front to back to avoid bringing germs from the rectum into the vaginal area.

- Apply ice packs (wrapped in a towel) off and on for the first 12 to 24 hours (10 to 15 minutes at a time), to reduce swelling. A comfortable position for this might be to rest on your side with the ice pack between your legs.
- Avoid constipation by eating fibre-rich foods and drinking lots of water.
- Use a small pillow when sitting.
- Avoid standing or sitting for long periods, as this can further strain the perineum.
- Do Kegel exercises to increase circulation and help promote healing. Kegel exercises are small squeezing movements of the vaginal muscles, similar to when you try to stop urinating. Try holding the contraction for up to 8 seconds, then relax. Repeat the contracting and relaxing several times a day.
- Ask your pharmacist or physician about using oral acetaminophen or ibuprofen for pain.
- If you have severe pain, a foul-smelling discharge or high fever, see your doctor.

Postpartum Depression—Patient Information

Recognizing Signs of Postpartum Depression

If any of these signs apply to you, get help from your doctor:

- ❏ My mood hasn't gone away after two weeks.
- ❏ I have strong feelings of sadness or guilt.
- ❏ I have strong feelings of hopelessness or helplessness.
- ❏ I can't sleep, even when tired.
- ❏ I sleep all the time, even when my baby is awake.
- ❏ I am not able to eat, even when hungry.
- ❏ I am not able to eat because I am never hungry or because I feel sick.
- ❏ I worry about the baby a lot; I'm obsessed with the baby.
- ❏ I don't worry about the baby at all; it's almost like I don't care.
- ❏ I am having panic attacks.
- ❏ I have feelings of anger toward the baby.
- ❏ I think about harming myself or the baby.

If you have any of these signs, get help right away. If you know a new mother who has these signs of depression, get help for her. Counseling and treatment can help mothers manage these feelings. Don't wait, call your doctor.

Reprinted with permission from Vicars, M, ed. *Healthy Beginnings: Your handbook for pregnancy and birth* 2nd ed. Ottawa The Society of Obstetricians and Gynecologists of Canada, 2000. The book is available for sale from the Society.

Erectile Dysfunction

Denis Bélanger, BScPhm

Pathophysiology

The term "impotence" has traditionally been used to describe the inability of the male to attain and maintain erection of the penis sufficient to permit satisfactory sexual intercourse. A more precise term, "erectile dysfunction," signifies an inability of the male to achieve an erect penis as part of the overall process of male sexual function.[1]

Erectile dysfunction affects at least two million men in Canada. It is often, incorrectly, assumed to be a natural part of the aging process. For many men, erectile dysfunction creates mental stress that affects their interactions with family and associates. The prevalence of erectile dysfunction has been found to be associated with age. A prevalence of about 5% is observed at age 40, increasing to 15 to 25% at age 65 and older.[1]

Causes contributing to erectile dysfunction can be classified into two categories: organic and psychological.[2] Even though many patients' erectile dysfunction is thought to be organic in nature, psychological aspects of self-confidence, anxiety, partner communication and conflict are often important factors.[3,4]

The male erection is a vascular event that is initiated by neuronal action and maintained by a complex interplay between vascular and neurologic events.[4] Parasympathetic input causes relaxation of trabecular smooth muscle and dilation of the helicine arteries of the penis. This leads to expansion of the lacunar spaces and entrapment of blood in the cavernous spaces. Increasing pressure within these spaces causes the penis to become erect, resulting in compression of the venules against the tunica albuginea. The tunica albuginea must have sufficient stiffness to compress the venules penetrating it, blocking venous outflow and maintaining tumescence and rigidity.[4]

Most commonly, a combination of both organic and psychogenic factors is involved in erectile dysfunction. Psychological conditions, such as depression, anxiety and relationship problems, can impair erectile functioning by reducing erotic focus. This may lead to inability to initiate or maintain an erection. The organic causes can be further broken down into endocrine, local, neurologic, vascular and drug causes. The first four are presented in Table 1 and drug causes are presented in Table 2.[1-7]

Goals of Therapy

- Educate the patient about erectile dysfunction and correct any misunderstandings or misinformation the patient may have
- Reinstate normal sexual functioning of the patient

The pharmacist can support these goals by:
- Reviewing the medication history to identify any drugs that may increase the incidence of erectile dysfunction.
- Discussing alternative medications (that have a lower risk of causing erectile dysfunction), with the patient (nonprescription medications) and/or physician.
- Counseling the patient on the appropriate use of the therapy prescribed by the physician.
- Helping the patient locate a support group/referral centre (see Resource Tips).

Patient Assessment

Refer patients with erectile dysfunction to their physician. The central issue in the evaluation of erectile dysfunction is to separate the cases due to psychological factors from those due to organic causes. A thorough history is imperative for a proper diagnosis.

Table 1: **Organic Causes of Erectile Dysfunction**[1,2]

Category	Potential causes
Endocrine causes	Decreased testosterone due to testicular failure (primary or secondary) Hyperprolactinemia (pituitary tumors) Diabetes Hypo-/hyperthyroidism
Local/Penile causes	Peyronie's disease Previous priapism Penile trauma
Medical or surgical procedures	Lumbar sympathectomy Renal transplant Spinal cord resection
Neurologic diseases	Anterior temporal lobe lesions Diseases of the spinal cord Loss of sensory input Cerebral vascular disease Disease of peripheral nerves Diabetic neuropathy and various polyneuropathies
Vascular diseases	Aortic occlusion Atherosclerotic occlusion/stenosis of the pudendal and/or cavernosa arteries Arterial damage from pelvic radiation Venous leak Disease of the sinusoidal spaces

Men with psychogenic erectile dysfunction (except when caused by severe depression) usually have normal nocturnal and early morning erections. If the patient indicates the presence of rigid erections (often when awakening), the efferent neurologic and circulatory systems that mediate erections are intact, and the dysfunction is probably psychogenic in nature.[7]

If the patient is uncertain whether he experiences nocturnal erections, measurements of nocturnal penile tumescence (NPT) can be made by using a snap gauge or home monitor.[2] Examples of such devices are presented in Table 3.

Patients with vasculogenic erectile dysfunction may have some degree of NPT without the development of adequate rigidity, which may lead to a false positive NPT test. If psychogenic causes can be eliminated, the differential diagnosis of the organic etiology must then be considered.[8] The physician should perform a complete history and physical examination, to identify potential contributing causes such as diabetes, peripheral neuropathy, prior pelvic surgery or pelvic trauma.

Appropriate arteriographic, neurologic, hormonal and vasculogenic tests can be performed to help identify the exact organic etiology.[2]

A detailed medication history should always be performed, as an estimated 25% of cases of erectile dysfunction may be attributable to medications for other conditions.[1] The pharmacist can play an integral role by performing a medication history, identifying potential causative agents and recommending alternative medications (that have little or no risk of inducing erectile dysfunction) directly to the treating physician. Normally this medication history is pursuant to an initial evaluation by the patient's physician. In some instances, either waiting to see if tolerance to the sexual side effect develops or reducing the dose of the offending agent is attempted before switching to another medication. If a decision is made to remove an offending agent, the pharmacist should advise the physician and patient if there are any potential risks associated with an abrupt discontinuation, and recommend an appropriate withdrawal schedule.

Table 2: **Drugs Causing Erectile Dysfunction**[*1-7]

Drug	Infrequent side effect	Frequent side effect	Very frequent side effect
Antihypertensives			
Beta-blockers		Atenolol	Labetolol Propranolol
Diuretics	Amiloride Indapamide	Chlorthalidone Spironolactone	Hydrochlorothiazide
Sympatholytics		Methyldopa Reserpine	Clonidine Guanethidine
Alpha-blockers	Prazosin		
Antidepressants			
Cyclic antidepressants		Amitriptyline Amoxapine Imipramine	Clomipramine
Serotonin-norepinephrine reuptake inhibitors	Venlafaxine		
Other	Bupropion		
Antipsychotics		Chlorpromazine Lithium Pimozide	Fluphenazine Thioridazine
Barbiturates		All	
Miscellaneous	Famotidine	Acetazolamide Alcohol Carbamazepine Cimetidine Clofibrate Digoxin Methazolamide Norethindrone Phenytoin Primidone Smoking	Finasteride Ketoconazole Methadone

*Many drugs, such as SSRIs, commonly cause other types of sexual dysfunction. This table deals specifically with drugs that cause erectile dysfunction.

Therapy

Management of erectile dysfunction consists of psychotherapy/behavioral therapy, medical treatment or (most commonly) a combination of the two.

Nonpharmacologic Therapy

Psychotherapy/Behavioral Therapy

Careful attention to psychological factors and attempts to alleviate sexual anxieties should be a part of the therapeutic intervention in all patients with erectile dysfunction. Psychotherapy/behavioral therapy alone may be beneficial for patients in whom no organic causes are detected, or in cases where patients refuse medical/surgical interventions. Focus should be on treating coexistent problems such as issues related to the loss of a partner, dysfunctional relationships, psychotic disorders or substance abuse.[1,2,8] This approach has been reported to relieve depression and anxiety and improve sexual function; however, outcome data have not been quantified and success of specific techniques is poorly documented.

Table 3: **Devices for the Diagnosis of Erectile Dysfunction**

Name of product	Description	Manufacturer
Snap-Gauge®	Nonstretchable fabric band that joins together by a "hook-and-loop" closure. Three plastic elements attached to the device break sequentially at three specific levels of force. Worn around the penis during sleep. Normal erection will break all 3 elements.	Timm Medical Technologies, 6585 City West Parkway, Eden Prairie, MN 55344 USA 1-800-438-8592 or (612) 947-9410
RigiScan®	Ambulatory rigidity and tumescence monitor that measures the rigidity, duration and frequency of erections during the night. Frequency of nocturnal erections in a normal male is 3-6 events/8-h night with an average duration of 10-15 min per event.	Timm Medical Technologies, 6585 City West Parkway, Eden Prairie, MN 55344 USA 1-800-438-8592 or (612) 947-9410

Vacuum Constrictive Devices

Vacuum constriction devices are effective in all cases of erectile dysfunction, irrespective of the pathogenesis (Table 4). Erection is induced by creating a vacuum around the penis, and it is maintained by using a constriction band. The devices are difficult for some patients to use. These agents may impair ejaculation, which can cause some discomfort. Some men may experience petechiae and ecchymosis.[9,10] Petechiae (reddish pinpoint-sized dots) are caused by placing the penis under negative pressure too rapidly, and ecchymosis (bruising) is due to the penis being held under vacuum pressure too long. The major drawback of these devices is the necessity for precoital application, making acceptance by the sexual partner of major importance. Refer patients to their urologist for proper selection of a vacuum constriction device.[9,10]

Vascular Surgery

Surgery of the penile venous system, generally involving venous ligation, has been reported to be effective in patients with demonstrated venous leakage.[1] Decreased effectiveness of this procedure has been reported as data from longer-term follow-up periods have been obtained. Arterial revascularization procedures have a limited role and should be restricted to the clinical investigation setting in medical centres with experienced personnel.[1] Difficulties persist with the techniques used to assess the success of surgical therapy. Further investigation to clarify their value and role in this regard is indicated.

Penile Prostheses

Three forms of penile prostheses are available for patients who fail or refuse other forms of therapy: semi-rigid malleable rods; multicomponent, inflatable devices and self-contained implants (inflatable or mechanical).[1] The effectiveness, complications and acceptability vary among the three types of prostheses, with the main problems being mechanical failure, infection and erosions. The surgery permanently alters the corpora, ending most hope of return to natural erections. There is also a risk of the need for repeat surgery with all of the devices.[1] Descriptions of the different types of prostheses and their advantages and disadvantages are presented in Table 5.

Pharmacologic Therapy

Prescription Therapy

Various prescription medications are available for the treatment of erectile dysfunction.[4,11-34] Agents that treat erectile dysfunction systemically include **testosterone** supplementation (oral, injectable or transdermal patches), **bromocriptine, sildenafil, yohimbine** and **trazodone**. Local therapy involves intracavernous injections (i.e., **alprostadil** alone or in combination with **papaverine** and **phentolamine**) or intraurethral administration of alprostadil pellets.

Testosterone

Androgen supplementation has historically been the drug of choice for the treatment of erectile dysfunction,

Table 4: **Vacuum Constriction Systems for Erectile Dysfunction**

Product name/Description	Manufacturer/Distributor
ErecAid® – Hand grip pump system (manual)	Timm Medical Technologies, 6585 City West Parkway, Eden Prairie, MN 55344 USA 1-800-438-8592 or (612) 947-9410
Pos-T-Vac®: AVP-1000 – Battery operated system MVP-700 – Manual pump system	Pos-T-Vac, Inc. 1701 N 14th – P.O. Box 1436 Dodge City, KS 67801 USA 1-800-279-7434
Encore® – Manual pump system Eru-1® – Ring constriction system (used with pump)	Encore Medical Products Inc. 4820 U.S. 42 Ste. 7 Louisville, Kentucky, USA 40222-6355 1-800 221-6603
Vacuum Therapy System®	Wilkinson Technologies www.treat-impotence-safely.com

but now it should be reserved for patients with laboratory-confirmed hypogonadism.[12-14]

Bromocriptine

For men suffering from hyperprolactinemia (approximately 2 to 5% of patients with erectile dysfunction), bromocriptine therapy is often effective in normalizing the prolactin level and improving sexual function.[15,16] It is usually initiated in small divided doses and progressively increased until a total daily dose of 5 to 7.5 mg is achieved.

Sildenafil

Sildenafil was marketed in March, 1999, and is responsible for generating much of the recent publicity on erectile dysfunction. It has an overall efficacy of 70% and can be used for erectile dysfunction of various etiologies.[17-21] Common side effects include flushing, headache and dyspepsia. It should not be used in patients who are advised to avoid sexual activity because of their cardiovascular status, or in anyone taking nitrates.

Yohimbine

Yohimbine is an alkaloid with α-2 adrenergic blocking properties. Yohimbine appears to be most effective in treating erectile dysfunction of a psychogenic cause, or in patients with diabetes or hypertension.[22,23] Doses range from 5 mg three times daily to 30 mg per day.

Trazodone

Trazodone is a nontricyclic andidepressant that was found to cause priapism as an adverse effect in clinical trials. Doses range from 50 to 100 mg daily.[24,25] It is usually used synergistically with yohimbine and rarely used as monotherapy.[26]

Intracavernous Injections

These injections contain alprostadil (synthetic prostaglandin E_1), either alone, or in combination with papaverine and phentolamine ("triple p" therapy). They are effective in treating erectile dysfunction of vascular, neurogenic or psychogenic causes. Good results are attained in 70 to 80% of patients.[27-30] The drugs are self-injected into the corpus cavernosum through the lateral aspect of the shaft of the penis, after cleansing the area with alcohol.

Transurethral Alprostadil

Alprostadil pellets are inserted into the urethra with a special device. It is effective in approximately 43% of

Table 5: **Types of Penile Prostheses**[1]

Type	Description/Operation	Advantages	Disadvantages
Semi-rigid malleable rods	Two identical rods made of parallel silver or stainless steel wires, normally covered in silicone. There are no moving parts. The penis is always in an erect state. To prepare for sexual activity, the penis is simply bent into ready position for intercourse.	The penis is always erect and ready for sexual activity. Lowest complication rate of all implants. Lowest cost due to design. Inserted on an outpatient basis under local anesthetic.	Penis is always erect (hence difficult to conceal underneath certain clothing). Time between surgery and first sexual intercourse is 4-6 weeks.
Multi-component inflatable devices	Components are two plastic balloon-type cylinders, one reservoir of fluid and one pump. One cylinder is inserted into each corpus cavernosum, the pump is placed in the scrotum, and the fluid reservoir is placed in the lower abdomen. The erection is activated by squeezing the pump, causing the fluid to transfer from the reservoir to the cylinders inside the penis, which provides rigidity and adds girth to the penis. To return the penis to the flaccid state, the deflation part of the scrotal pump is activated.	Patient gets to control the erection. The penis has a natural appearance whether erect or flaccid. The girth of the penis grows when the device is used and shrinks when it is deflated.	Permanent failure occurs in about 5% of these implants during the first 5 yrs, increasing the risk of infection. These are the most expensive implants and involve the most complicated surgery.
Self-contained implants (inflatable)	Sealed cylinder placed in each corpus cavernosum. Each cylinder contains: fluid, pumping mechanism, release valve. When the head of the penis is squeezed, the twin pumps move fluid from a reservoir into the main area, creating rigidity. To stop the erection, the penis is bent near the glans, releasing fluid back to storage area.	Patient controls when he wants an erection. The penis appears natural in either the erect state or when flaccid. Cost is less than the multi-component implant. Lower failure rate than multi-component implant.	Implant failure does occur, necessitating surgery and removal. Infection is possible. Penis does not increase in girth when erect.
Self-contained implants (mechanical)	An intricate series of interlocking plastic blocks, with a spring-loaded stainless steel cable passing through them. With the cable slack, the blocks are not tightly positioned (flaccid). With the cable taut, each block fits snugly against the next (erect). If the penis is bent a certain way, a spring inside tightens the cable, producing an erection. When the penis is bent a second time, cable tension goes slack, ending the erection.	Patient controls when he wants an erection. The penis appears natural in either the erect state or when flaccid. Cost is less than the multi-component implant. No fluid is used.	Malfunctions can occur. This device is difficult to operate. Penis does not increase in girth when erect.

patients. The most common adverse effects include penile pain (32%) and urethral pain or burning (12%).[32-34]

Monitoring of Therapy

- Ensure patients know how to properly administer their therapy (this is especially important with intra-cavernous injections).
- Inquire during regular visits about the success or failures associated with the therapy.
- Offer patients a list of referral/support groups where they can find more information about their condition and its treatments (see Resource Tips).
- If the patient is taking sildenafil, enquire about any side effects at refill times and ensure that the patient is not experiencing any cardiovascular symptoms.

Resource Tips

Impotence Causes, Treatment of Male Sexual Dysfunction, http://www.impotence-causes-treatment-male-sexual-dysfunction.com/drug-for-impotence.htm

Impotence Information Center, P.O. Box 9, Minneapolis, MN, 55440

Impotence Information and Support Clinic, North York, Ontario. Run out of Sunnybrook/Women's College Health Science Centre, (416) 480-4024.

Impotence Institute of America, 8201 Corporate Drive, Suite 320, Landover MD 20785 USA, (301) 577-0650.

Impotence World Association, 119 S. Ruth St., Maryville, TN 37803, http://www.impotenceworld.org.

Suggested Readings

American Association of Clinical Endocrinologists and American College of Endocrinology. *AACE Clinical Practice Guidelines For The Evaluation and Treatment of Male Sexual Dysfunction*. Available from: http://www.aace.com/ clin/guides/sexualdysfunction.html.

Chun SS. Overview on current treatment options for managing erectile dysfunction. *Drugs and Therapeutics for Maritime Practitioners* 2001;24(1):1-6.

Lue TF. Erectile dysfunction. *N Engl J Med* 2000;342;24: 1802-13.

Montague DK, Barada JH, Belker AM et al. Clinical guidelines panel on erectile dysfunction: summary report on the treatment of organic erectile dysfunction. American Urological Association. *J Urol* 1996 Dec;156(6):2007-11.

National Institute of Health. *Consensus statement on impotence* 1992;10(4). Available from: http://odp. od.nih.gov/consensus/cons/ 091/091_intro.htm.

References

1. National Institute of Health, Consensus Development Panel on Impotence. Impotence. *JAMA* 1993;270(1):83-90.
2. Wilson JD, McConnell JD. Alterations in reproductive and sexual function. In: *Harrison's Principles of Internal Medicine*. 13th ed. Toronto, ON: McGraw-Hill Inc., 1994:262-5.
3. Montorsi F, Guazzoni G, Rigatti P, Pozza G. Pharmacological management of erectile dysfunction. *Drugs* 1995;50(3): 465-79.
4. Lue TF. Erectile dysfunction. *N Eng J Med* 2000;342:1802-13.
5. American Association of Clinical Endocrinologists and American College of Endocrinology. *AACE Clinical Practice Guidelines For The Evaluation and Treatment of Male Sexual Dysfunction*. Available from: http://www.aace.com/ clin/guidelines/sexdysguid.pdf.
6. Leung M. Drug induced sexual dysfunction. *Pharm Pract* 1998;14(9):44-50.
7. Finger WW, Lund M, Slagle MA et al. Medications that contribute to sexual disorders. A guide to assessment and treatment in family practice. *J Fam Pract* 1997;44:33-43.
8. Montague DK, Barada JH, Belker AM et al. Clinical guidelines panel on erectile dysfunction: summary report on the treatment of organic erectile dysfunction. American Urological Association. *J Urol* 1996;156(6):2007-11.
9. Obson JB. *A Patient's Guide for the Treatment of Impotence*. Augusta, GA: Obson Medical System, Charter Publishing Company, 1992.
10. Salvatore FT, Sharman GM, Hellstrom WJG. Vacuum constriction devices and the clinical urologist: an informed selection. *Urology* 1991;38(4):323-7.
11. Chun SS. Overview on current treatment options for managing erectile dysfunction. *Drugs and Therapeutics for Maritime Practitioners* 2001;24(1):1-6.
12. Chiavi RC, White D, Mandeli J, Levine AC. Effect of testosterone administration on sexual behavior and mood in men with erectile dysfunction. *Arch Sex Behav* 1997;26:231-41.
13. Morales A, Johnston B, Heaton JW, Clark A. Oral androgens in the treatment of hypogonadal impotent men. *J Urol* 1994;152:1115-8.
14. Arver S, Dods AS, Meikle AW et al. Improvement in sexual function in testosterone deficient men treated for 1 year with a permeation enhanced testosterone transdermal system. *J Urol* 1996;155:1604-8.
15. March CM. Bromocriptine in the treatment of hypogonadism and male impotence. *Drugs* 1979;17:349-58.
16. Cooper AJ. Bromocriptine in impotence. *Lancet* 1977;2:567.
17. Boolell M , Allen MJ, Ballard SA et al. Sildenafil: an orally active type 5 cyclic GMP-specific phosphodiesterase inhibitor for the treatment of penile erectile dysfunction. *Int J Impot Res* 1996;8:47-52.

18. Goldstein I, Lue T, Padma-Nathan H et al. Oral sildenafil in the treatment of erectile dysfunction. *N Engl J Med* 1998;338: 1397-1404.

19. Morales A, Gingell C, Collins M et al. Clinical safety of oral sildenafil citrate in the treatment of erectile dysfunction. *Int J Impot Res* 1998;10:69-73.

20. Kloner RA, Zusman RM. Cardiovascular effects of sildenafil citrate and recommendations for its use. *Am J Cardiol* 1999;84:11N-17N.

21. Webb DJ, Freestone S, Allen MJ et al. Sildenafil citrate and blood pressure lowering drugs: results of drug interaction studies with an organic nitrate and calcium antagonist. *Am J Cardiol* 1999;83:21C-28C.

22. Reid K, Surridge DR, Morales A et al. Is yohimbine effective in the treatment of organic impotence? Results of a controlled trial. *J Urol* 1987;137:1168-72.

23. Ernst E, Pittler MH. Yohimbine for erectile dysfunction: a systematic review and meta-analysis of randomized clinical trials. *J Urol* 1998;159(2):433-6.

24. Kurt U, Ozkardes H, Altug U et al. The efficacy of antiserotoninergic agents in the treatment of erectile dysfunction. *J Urol* 1994;152:407-9.

25. Albo M, Steers WD. Oral trazodone as initial therapy for management of impotence. *J Urol* 1993;149:344A.

26. Montorsi F, Ferini Stambi L, Guazzoni G, et al. Effect of yohimbine-trazodone on psychogenic impotence: a randomized, bouble-blind, placebo-controlled study. *Urology* 1994; 44:732-6.

27. Schramek R, Plas EG, Hubner WA et al. Intracavernous injection of prostaglandin E1 plus procaine in the treatment of erectile dysfunction. *J Urol* 1994;152:1108-10.

28. Viraq R, Shoukry K, Floresco J et al. Intracavernous self-injection of vasoactive drugs in the treatment of impotence: 8-year experience with 615 cases. *J Urol* 1991;145:287-91.

29. Edwards S, ed. Intracavernous injections for impotence. *New Drugs/Drug News* 1995;13(3):3-4.

30. Govier FE, et al. Experience with triple-drug therapy in a pharmacological erection program. *J Urol* 1993;150:1822.

31. Montorsi F, Guazzoni G, Bergamaschi F et al. Clinical reliability of multi-drug intracavernous vasoactive pharmacotherapy for diabetic impotence. *Acta Diabetol* 1994;31:1-5.

32. Padma-Nathan H, Keller T, Proppiti R et al. Hemodynamic effects of intraurethral alprostadil: the medicated urethral system for erection (MUSE). *Int J Impot Res* 1994;6(suppl 1): A42.

33. Porst H. Transurethral alprostadil with MUSE (medicated urethral system for erection) vs intracavernous alprostadil - a comparative study in 103 patients with erectile dysfunction. *Int J Impot Res* 1997;9:187-92.

34. Williams G, Abbou CC, Armar ET et al. Efficacy and safety of alprostadil therapy in men with erectile dysfunction. MUSE Study Group. *Br J Urol* 1998;81:889-94.

Impotence (Erectile Dysfunction)—Patient Information

Erectile dysfunction (ED) is the inability to get or maintain an erection sufficient for intercourse. About two to three million men in Canada have ED. Unfortunately, very few seek medical attention and up to two-thirds don't talk to their doctor *or* partner about it. It is more common as men get older. About 1 in 20 men at the age of 40 and about 1 in 5 at the age of 65 experience ED. Yet, it is *not* a normal part of aging.

There are several possible causes of ED. They can generally be broken down into two types, physical and psychological, but in some cases it can be a combination of both types.

The majority of cases are due to physical causes such as:
- Problems with nerve impulses in the brain, spinal cord or area of the penis
- Fibrous tissues in the penis
- Damage to the veins or arteries of the penis
- Medications
- Diseases such as diabetes, kidney disease, chronic alcoholism, multiple sclerosis, atherosclerosis and blood vessel diseases
- Smoking
- Hormone imbalances

Psychological causes are involved in up to one in five cases and include:
- Stress
- Anxiety
- Feelings of guilt
- Low self-esteem
- Fear of sexual failure (performance anxiety)

Treatment of ED depends on the cause. Options that your doctor might suggest include:
- Adjustment of your medications
- Therapy to help you deal with psychological causes
- If another disease is causing your ED, the doctor may make changes to your treatment for that condition
- Mechanical devices that help cause erections
- Pumps that are surgically implanted in the penis
- Drugs that are taken orally
- Drugs that are placed inside the penis directly

If you have ED, talk to your doctor and partner about the problem. A thorough medical examination is essential for a successful outcome. Because of important advances in recent years, there are several options available today to help men with ED.

Chapter 55

Premature Ejaculation

Denis Bélanger, BScPhm

Pathophysiology

Premature ejaculation is the most prevalent male sexual dysfunction.[1] Studies that attempt to establish incidence and prevalence are difficult to compare because of varying definitions for the dysfunction. However, the disorder is common, with prevalence estimates ranging between 22 and 38%.[1,2] Historically, sexual dysfunctions of all kinds were regarded as a byproduct of severe psychopathology. In the recent past, however, sexual dysfunctions have been viewed as problems amenable to treatment, and effective interventions have begun to emerge.

Premature ejaculation has been defined in terms of varying duration of intravaginal contact, number of thrusts prior to ejaculation, number of partner-achieved orgasms, or the ratio of intercourse frequency to partner satisfaction.[3] Masters and Johnson defined premature ejaculation as the man's inability to inhibit ejaculation long enough for his partner to reach orgasm 50% of the time.[4] The revised fourth edition of the *Diagnostic and Statistical Manual of Mental Disorders* (DSM-IV) defines premature ejaculation with the following three criteria:

- Persistent or recurrent ejaculation with minimal sexual stimulation before, upon, or shortly after penetration and before the person wishes it;
- Marked distress or interpersonal difficulty;
- Symptoms not due exclusively to the direct effects of a substance (e.g., opiate withdrawal).[5]

There is no reliable documentation identifying the cause or causes of premature ejaculation, although theories abound, spanning from physiological to psychological viewpoints. One theory views premature ejaculation as the consequence of hypersensitivity in the glans penis, resulting in excessive stimulation of the spinal cord section that elicits ejaculation.[6]

A review of 1130 cases, however, concluded that physiologic explanations accounted for fewer than 4%.[7] Psychoanalytic theories attribute premature ejaculation to generalized anxiety, passive-aggressive disorder, castration anxiety or unconscious negative feelings towards women.[8]

A few biological approaches have been presented. One behavioral approach links the role of anxiety with decreased ejaculatory latency. Since anxiety and ejaculation are sympathetically mediated responses, it was speculated that sympathetic arousal related to anxiety could accelerate ejaculation.[4] More recent knowledge, however, indicates that ejaculation appears to be mediated by both sympathetic and parasympathetic innervation, with the sympathetic nervous system controlling emission of semen into the posterior urethra and the parasympathetic nervous system responsible for the delivery of ejaculate.[9]

Another behavioral explanation for premature ejaculation identifies the role of learning and conditioning in the etiology of the disorder.[4] Situations such as sex with a prostitute or sex in situations where discovery might be imminent (e.g., in a car, or at home when parents may return) condition the male to pair rapid ejaculation with sexual intercourse. Masturbation practices have also been suggested in the etiology of premature ejaculation. When masturbation is hurried out of anxiety, fear of discovery or guilt, a speedy response may follow.

Causes of premature ejaculation may be divided into two general subtypes (i.e., physiological and psychological).[9] These two general classes may be further divided into four subclasses. The subclasses of physiological premature ejaculation include:

- Neurologic (biological predisposition to ejaculate quickly);

- Physical illness (e.g., prostatitis, urinary tract infection);
- Physical injury (e.g., spinal cord injury);
- Pharmacologic side effects (e.g., opiate or antipsychotic withdrawal).

The subclasses of psychological premature ejaculation include:
- Chronic psychological disorders [e.g., obsessive compulsive disorder, bipolar disorder, anxiety, personality disorder, psychological distress (e.g., adjustment disorder, reactive depression, sexual shame)];
- Relationship stress (e.g., unresolved emotional relationship conflicts);
- Psychosexual skills deficit (e.g., lack of sexual experience, difficulty focusing on one's own sensations).

Goals of Therapy

- Help control symptoms and improve sexual functioning of the patient
- Improve quality of relationship between patient and sexual partner

Patient Assessment

The assessment of premature ejaculation should be multidimensional to reach a sound treatment decision. These include self-reporting, behavioral, physiological and medical evaluations. Refer patients to their physician for the proper diagnosis of premature ejaculation.

Organic factors are implicated in a relatively small proportion of cases of premature ejaculation. These include trauma to the sympathetic nervous system, prostatic hypertrophy, prostatitis, urethritis, alcoholism, diabetes, arteriosclerosis, cardiovascular disease, venous leakage and polyneuritis. Premature ejaculation has been described following withdrawal from antipsychotics and opiates.[10-12] It is associated with the use of desipramine, nonprescription sympathomimetics (e.g., pseudoephedrine), and with alcohol-related peripheral neuropathy.[13] Medical evaluation of premature ejaculation should include inquiry into genitourinary symptoms, symptoms of generalized or localized neurological disease, previous abdominal or pelvic trauma, and use of prescription and nonprescription drugs.

Nonpharmacologic Therapy

Various nonpharmacologic treatments (i.e., cognitive-behavioral strategies) exist for men suffering from premature ejaculation. Rarely will one technique suffice in managing the problem. Frequently men will have to use a combination of four to five techniques to obtain the desired results. Cognitive-behavioral techniques can be taught to the individual or to the couple. Examples of individual procedures include physiologic relaxation training (e.g., focusing on breathing, body awareness and muscle relaxation exercises), sensual awareness training (e.g., teaching the man to become aroused by his own sensations instead of partner interaction), pubococcygeal muscle control training, pelvic floor rehabilitation training, pacing techniques (e.g., stop-start technique, pause-squeeze technique), and testicular restraint technique. Examples of techniques taught to couples include sensate focus pleasuring exercises, partner genital exploration/relaxation exercises, pacing techniques and intercourse acclimatization.[9]

The "pause-squeeze" technique by Masters and Johnson is considered by some specialists to offer the best results. In this technique the partner puts one thumb on the frenulum of the penis, with the first and second fingers of the same hand just above and before the coronal ridge. A firm grasping pressure is applied for four seconds and then released. The pressure is applied front-to-back with the specific pressure proportional to the degree of erection present: a firm squeeze with an erect penis; a moderate squeeze when the penis is more flaccid. The squeeze may lead to a temporary 10 to 25% decrease in the erection. Masters and Johnson initially reported an overall failure rate of only 2.7%.[4] Others, however, have not been able to replicate these results with overall improvement rates in the range of 43% to 65%.[7] Most of the data are based on uncontrolled case reports or program description, hence success rates may be confounded by other treatment modalities which make them difficult to compare. This technique is less effective when it is self-applied.[4] The pause-squeeze technique is part of an elaborate treatment regimen that the couple must follow. Initially this technique is used during mutual masturbation. After several days of practice the couple is instructed to transfer this process to coitus. Later, a basilar squeeze technique may be taught, where the partner applies the squeeze technique to the base of the penis, to minimize interruptions to lovemaking.

The testicular restraint technique is a physiological aid to help delay orgasm by preventing the testicles from ascending into the perineum. Some men can benefit from cuffing the testicles and gently pulling down. Alternatively, Velcro®-type devices and leather straps can be used to achieve the same effects. These items are available at most stores that sell erotic material.[9]

Pharmacologic Therapy

A variety of pharmacologic agents have been reported to delay or block an ejaculatory response. These include topical anesthetics, neuroleptics, antidepressants, alpha-blockers, beta-blockers, anxiolytics and intracavernous injections of smooth muscle relaxants.[6,14-28] Of these, only topical anesthetics are available to patients without a prescription.

Nonprescription Therapy

In one study, **dibucaine** 1% ointment showed improvement in ejaculatory latency.[14] The authors stated that if sexual intercourse was undertaken at the height of anesthesia (i.e., two to three hours after application) the males were able to prolong the act for whatever period of time, usually 10 to 30 minutes, necessary for their partners to reach climax. The dibucaine neither prevented orgasm nor diminished its intensity. Before intercourse, the penis was washed free of all remaining ointment and dried, and there was no anesthetic affect on the vaginal mucosa of the partner. Limitations identified were reduced sexual sensation and the need to plan sexual relations in advance in order to apply the ointment two to three hours prior to the act.

The effect of **benzocaine** 3% cream in delaying climax was studied in 13 men who complained of premature ejaculation.[6] Prior to treatment, 11 men reported that orgasm occurred before the penis was inserted into the vagina; in one case it took place immediately on intromission, and in another case about one minute later. Approximately 2 g of the cream was massaged over the glans of the penis. After five minutes the excess cream was wiped off and the volunteer proceeded to engage in coitus. The degree of anesthesia produced by the application was complete in 10 cases and partial in three with an average duration of 25.2 minutes. The average interval between intromission of the penis into the vagina and orgasm was lengthened to 1.6 minutes (range 0.5 to 5). There were no untoward effects in any case. The local anesthetic did not affect the female partner's sensation in any way.

Researchers in Toronto examined the effects of **lidocaine/prilocaine** cream (25mg/g each) in 11 healthy, married men with premature ejaculation in an open pilot, unblinded study.[28] Men were instructed to apply 2.5 g of the cream to the penis 30 minutes before intercourse and to cover the penis with a condom. Five patients reported excellent results (i.e., ejaculation occurred 15 to 20 minutes after penetration) and four patients reported satisfactory results (i.e., ejaculation occurred 5 to 10 minutes after penetration). Two patients were not satisfied with the cream; however, one of these patients reported a delayed ejaculation of over 20 minutes after penetration.

In patients who choose to try the topical anesthetics after seeing their physician, encourage application of a condom to reduce transfer of the anesthetic to the vagina during intercourse.[29]

Prescription Therapy

Various prescription medications including antipsychotics, antidepressants, alpha-blockers, beta-blockers, anxiolytics (e.g., alprazolam, lorazepam), and intracavernous injections of smooth muscle relaxants have been reported to offer benefits to patients with premature ejaculation.[15-27] Most of the latest work in this area tends to focus on antidepressants. The selective serotonin reuptake inhibitor (SSRI) class of antidepressants appears to neurologically slow down ejaculation by 2 to 10 minutes. Benefits with fluoxetine, paroxetine and sertraline have been shown in case reports and small trials.[27] Tricyclic antidepressants, specifically amitriptyline, clomipramine, and desipramine, have also been shown to offer some benefit to patients suffering from premature ejaculation.[27]

Monitoring of Therapy

Pharmacists can support the goals of therapy for premature ejaculation by:

- Ensuring that patients know how to properly administer their therapy;

- Inquiring during regular visits about the success or failures associated with the therapy;
- Offering patients a source of referral/support groups where they can find more information about their condition and its treatments (see Resource Tips).

Resource Tips

Impotence Causes, Treatment of Male Sexual Dysfunction (series of links, including premature ejaculation): http://www.impotence-causes-treatment-male-sexual-dysfunction.com/drug-for-impotence.htm

Suggested Readings

Balon R. Antidepressants in the treatment of premature ejaculation. *J Sex Marital Ther* 1996;22:85-96.

Epperly TD, Moore KE. Health issues in men: part I: common genitourinary disorders. *Am Fam Physician* 2000;61:3657-64.

McMahon CG, Samali R. Pharmacological treatment of premature ejaculation. *Curr Opin Urol* 1999;9: 553-61.

Metz ME, Pryor JL. Premature ejaculation: a psycho-physiologic approach for assessment and management. *J Sex Marital Ther* 2000;26: 293-320.

J Sex Martial Ther Metz ME, Pryor JL, Nesvaxil LJ et al. Premature ejaculation – a psychophysiologic review. 1997;23:3-23.

Rowland DL. A psychophysiological approach to assessing premature ejaculation. *Int J Impot Res* 1998;10 (suppl 2): S44-8.

References

1. Frank E, Anderson C, Rubinstein D. Frequency of sexual dysfunction in "normal" couples. *N Engl J Med* 1978;299: 111-5.
2. Nettelbladt P, Uddenberg N. Sexual dysfunction and sexual satisfaction in 58 unmarried Swedish male. *J Urol* 1979;23: 141-7.
3. Kaplan HS. *The New Sex Therapy.* Brunner/Mazel, New York, 1974.
4. Masters WH and Johnson VE. *Human Sexual Inadequacy*, Boston, Mass: Little, Brown and Company, 1970.
5. American Psychiatric Association, *Diagnostic and Statistical Manual of Mental Disorders* 4th ed. American Psychiatric Association, Washington, D.C., 1994.
6. Damrav F. Premature ejaculation: Use of ethyl amino benzoate to prolong coitus. *J Urol* 1963;89:936-9.
7. Shapiro B. Premature ejaculation: a review of 1130 cases. *J Urol* 1943;50:374-9.
8. Stanley E. Premature ejaculation. *BMJ* 1981;282:1521.
9. Metz ME, Pryor JL. Premature ejaculation: a psychophysiological approach for assessment and management. *J Sex Marital Ther* 2000;26:293-320.
10. Keitner GI, Selub S. Spontaneous ejaculation and neuroleptics. *J Clin Psychopharmacol* 1983;3:34-6.
11. Blachly PM. Management of the opiate abstinence syndrome. *Am J Psych* 1966;122:742-4.
12. Buffum J. Pharmacosexology: the effects of drugs on sexual function: A review. *Journal of Psychoactive Drugs* 1982;14: 5-44.
13. Williams W. Secondary premature ejaculation. *Aust N Z J Psychiatry* 1984;18:333-40.
14. Aycock L. The medical management of premature ejaculation. *J Urol* 1949;63:432.
15. Mellgren A. Treatment of ejaculation praecox with thioridazine. *Psychosomatique* 1987;15:454.
16. Bennet D. Treatment of ejaculation praecox with monoamine oxidase inhibitors. *Lancet.* 1961;2:1309.
17. Rapp MS. Two cases of ejaculatory impairment related to phenelzine. *Am J Psych* 1979;136:1200-1.
18. Nininger JE. Inhibition of ejaculation by amitriptylline. *Am J Psych* 1978;135:750-1.
19. Goodman RE. An assessment of clomipramine in the treatment of premature ejaculation. *J Int Med Res* 1980;8 (suppl3): 53-9.
20. Girgis SM, El-Hagger S, El-Hermouzy S. A double blind trial of clomipramine in premature ejaculation. *Andrologia* 1992; 14:364-8.
21. Homonnai ZT, Shilon M, Paz GF. Phenoxybenzamine – Am effective male contraceptive pill. *Contraception* 1984;29: 479-91.
22. Beretta G, Chelo E, Zanolla F. Effect of alpha-blocking agent in the management of premature ejaculation. *Acta Europa Fertilatis* 1986;17:442-5.
23. Cooper AG. A clinical trial of the beta blocker propranolol in premature ejaculation. *J Psychosom Res* 1984;28:331-4.
24. Hughes JM. Failure to ejaculate with chlordiazepoxide. *Am J Psych* 1964;121:610-1.
25. Segraves RT. Treatment of premature ejaculation with lorazepam. *Am J Psych* 1987;144:1240.
26. Fein RL. Intracavernous medication for treatment of premature ejaculation. *Urology* 1990;35:301-3.
27. Balon R. Antidepressants in the treatment of premature ejaculation. *J Sex Marital Ther* 1996;22:85-96.
28. Berkovitch M, Keresteci AG, Koren G. Efficacy of prilocaine-lidocaine cream in the treatment of premature ejaculation. *J Urol* 1995;154:1360-1.
29. Sahin H, Bircan MK. Re: efficacy of prilocaine-lidocaine cream in the treatment of premature ejaculation. *J Urol* 1996; 156:1783-4.

Premature Ejaculation—Patient Information

Premature ejaculation is the unintentional and unsatisfying speed of male ejaculation. It is the most common form of male sexual problems, affecting approximately 29% of all men. It can cause stress in men affected by it and can put strain on a relationship.

There are many possible causes of premature ejaculation. These can be physical or psychological or both. Psychological causes can include early sexual experiences (e.g., masturbating quickly to avoid being caught by parents), performance anxiety, and psychiatric conditions (e.g., obsessive compulsive disorder, depression). Physical causes can include medical conditions (e.g., prostatitis, spinal cord injury) or the use of certain medications.

Premature ejaculation can only be diagnosed by a physician. Your doctor will examine you and ask you many questions in order to make a proper diagnosis. You may be referred to a specialist such as a neurologist, urologist, psychiatrist or sex therapist for treatment. There are different options for treating premature ejaculation. Special techniques can be used to control ejaculation. These techniques can only be taught by someone specializing in this area. Various medications can also help with premature ejaculation. You can obtain local anesthetics (i.e., benzocaine, lidocaine/prilocaine combination) from your pharmacist, that help reduce sensation and delay ejaculation. Other drugs (e.g., antidepressants, antianxiety medications) might be prescribed by your doctor to help lengthen the duration of intercourse and delay ejaculation.

In the past, there were few options open to men suffering from this condition. Now, however, more research is being conducted in this field to help physicians better diagnose and help patients affected by premature ejaculation. Ask your doctor what treatment is best for you.

Chapter 56

Benign Prostatic Hyperplasia

Denis Bélanger, BScPhm

Pathophysiology

Benign prostatic hyperplasia (BPH), formerly known as benign prostatic hypertrophy, is a condition where a male's prostate becomes enlarged to the point that it causes discomfort.[1,2] It is the most common benign neoplasm in the aging human male. The prostate is a walnut-sized gland at the base of the bladder that completely surrounds the male urethra (Figure 1). Its functions include constriction of the prostatic urethra during ejaculation (to prevent contamination of the ejaculate with urine) and contributing fluid to the ejaculate. The prostate goes through two main periods of growth during a normal male's life.[3] The first is puberty, where the prostate doubles in size. The gland begins to grow again at age 25. This second stage of growth is what may cause BPH much later in life.[3] Symptoms of BPH rarely become apparent before age 40. The incidence, however, increases to about 50% for men in their 60s and about 90% for men in their 70s and 80s.[3]

The pathogenesis of BPH is not clearly understood; however, it is related to androgens and aging. Increases in circulating androgens appear to be responsible for the increases in both glandular and

---

Figure 1: **Male Reproductive Anatomy**

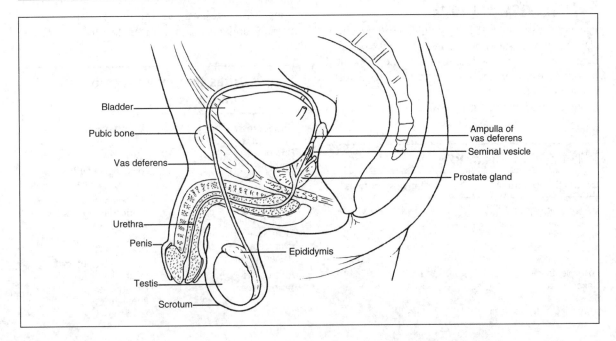

Bladder

Pubic bone

Vas deferens

Urethra

Penis

Testis

Scrotum

Epididymis

Ampulla of vas deferens

Seminal vesicle

Prostate gland

fibromuscular tissues that comprise the prostate gland.[4] Dihydrotestosterone (DHT), a metabolite of testosterone, is believed to be the main androgen responsible for both normal and hyperplastic prostate growth.[4] Testosterone is metabolized to DHT by the enzyme 5-alpha-reductase. At the beginning, BPH is manifested as microscopic nodules in the periurethral and transition zones, followed by progressive nodular proliferation that leads to bladder outlet obstruction and subsequent symptoms of BPH.[4]

Symptoms of BPH can be divided into two groups, obstructive and irritative (Table 1).[1,2] For most men, the symptoms appear gradually. In some men, however, symptoms appear acutely. Various factors can contribute to acute onset, including medications (e.g., decongestants), cold temperatures, alcohol consumption and prolonged immobility. If left untreated, BPH can lead to hypernephrosis, bladder infections, stone formation and recurrent urinary tract infections.[1,4]

Goals of Therapy

- Alleviate symptoms of BPH
- Improve patient's quality of life
- Prevent serious outcomes associated with poorly controlled BPH

Patient Assessment

Patients with suspected BPH should see their physician. Various tests and procedures are used to make a diagnosis of BPH, including a complete medical history focusing on the urinary tract, a digital rectal exam and urinalysis.[1] Additional diagnostic tests, including ultrasound, urine flow study, intravenous pyelogram and cystoscopy, are available to assess patients with BPH. The value of using these tests for the routine diagnosis of BPH has been questioned.[1] They may be useful, nonetheless, in selected patients if the diagnosis of BPH is uncertain after the initial evaluation.[1]

Several medications may exacerbate symptoms of BPH (Table 2).[5] Some of these drugs possess anticholinergic properties and inhibit bladder contraction; others possess alpha-adrenergic properties and increase urethral resistance. Anabolic steroids, which are commonly abused by men who want to improve their physical appearance, can also affect the prostate size.[6] A case report describes a 49-year-old bodybuilder who was consuming a "cocktail" of various anabolic steroids and agreed to have his prostate function measured over a seven-week period.[6] His prostate volume increased from 24.9 to 47.3 cm² (i.e., a 90% increase in volume) and his urine flow decreased from 18.8 to 15.7 mL/s (i.e., a 16.5% decrease). The patient also complained of nocturnal urinary frequency.

Symptom assessment can be performed using the American Urological Association (AUA) symptom index scale (Table 3).[1,2,4] This is a simple scale that can be administered by the patient or their health-care provider, for quantifying the severity of BPH symptoms. This index can be performed at the onset of therapy and periodically thereafter, to monitor the

Table 1: **Symptoms of BPH**[1,2,4]

Obstructive symptoms	Irritative symptoms
Weak urinary stream	Urinary frequency
Difficulty initiating stream	Nocturia
Stream starts and stops	Pain during micturition
Inability to terminate micturition	Urinary urgency
Post-void dripping	
Urinary retention	
Sensation of incomplete emptying of the bladder	

Table 2: **Drugs that may Exacerbate Symptoms of BPH**[5,6]

Antidepressants	**Antipsychotics**
Amitriptyline	Fluphenazine
Doxepin	Loxapine
Nortriptyline	**Muscle relaxants**
Trimipramine	Cyclobenzaprine
Antihistamines	**Miscellaneous**
Brompheniramine	**(anticholinergic properties)**
Chlorpheniramine	Atropine
Clemastine	Bethanechol
Cyproheptadine	Glycopyrrolate
Diphenhydramine	Hyoscine butylbromide
Androgens	Ipratropium
Testosterone	Procyclidine
	Pizotifen
	Selegiline

Table 3: American Urological Association Symptom Index for BPH Assessment

Circle one number on each line

Questions to be answered	Not at all	Less than 1 time in 5	Less than half the time	About half the time	More than half the time	Almost always
1. Over the past month, how often have you had a sensation of not emptying your bladder completely after you finished urinating?	0	1	2	3	4	5
2. Over the past month, how often have you had to urinate again less than 2 h after you finished urinating?	0	1	2	3	4	5
3. Over the past month, how often have you found you stopped and started again several times when you urinated?	0	1	2	3	4	5
4. Over the past month, how often have you found it difficult to postpone urination?	0	1	2	3	4	5
5. Over the past month, how often have you had a weak urinary stream?	0	1	2	3	4	5
6. Over the past month, how often have you had to push or strain to begin urination?	0	1	2	3	4	5
7. Over the past month, how many times, most typically, did you get up to urinate from the time you went to bed at night until the time you got up in the morning?	0	1	2	3	4	5

Sum of 7 circled numbers (AUA Symptom Score): _____

Symptoms are classified as: Score 0-7 = Mild
Score 8-19 = Moderate
Score 20-35 = Severe

Reproduced with permission from Lippincott Williams & Wilkins. Barry NJ, Fowler FJ, O'Leary MP et al. The American Urological Association Symptom Index for BPH. *J Urol* 1992;148:1549-1557.

success of treatment. It should not be used as the sole method of diagnosing BPH, because the symptoms are not specific to BPH.

Therapy

Treatment is recommended only when BPH poses a health risk for the patient or when it becomes very bothersome.[7] Mild BPH does not require treatment and in up to one third of cases, symptoms will disappear without treatment.[1,7] Treatment of BPH can include surgical or nonsurgical procedures, or drug therapy.

Nonpharmacologic Therapy

Watchful Waiting

Watchful waiting is an appropriate approach for the majority of men with BPH, since in most cases symptoms will disappear spontaneously.[1] Watchful waiting may be offered to patients who present to their physician with mild symptoms. These patients should be reassessed at regular intervals (e.g., yearly).

Surgical Procedures

Of all the treatment options available, prostate surgery offers the best chance for improvement in symptoms.[1] These procedures, however, also present the highest risk of complications among treatment options for BPH. The surgical procedures available to patients with BPH are presented in Table 4.

Pharmacologic Therapy

Nonprescription Therapy

The only nonprescription products that have been evaluated for BPH are the herbal remedies, saw palmetto, pygeum, stinging nettle and pumpkin seeds.

Herbal Remedies

Saw palmetto, pygeum, stinging nettle and pumpkin seeds are widely promoted for the treatment of mild symptoms of BPH. Although they have been shown to be beneficial in a limited number of studies, their role in treating BPH remains unclear. Studies evaluating these agents used specific commercial products that may not be available in Canada. Determining the

Table 4: **Surgical Procedures for Managing BPH**[1]

Procedure	Indication	Advantages
Transurethral incision of the prostate (TUIP)	For smaller prostates	Lower incidence of complications and retrograde ejaculation and fewer days in hospital than with open surgery or TURP. Takes only minutes to perform procedure
Transurethral resection of the prostate (TURP)	For moderately enlarged prostates	Fewer work days lost and fewer days in hospital than with open surgery. Highest degree of symptom improvement of all procedures
Open prostatectomy	For large prostates or patients with specific concomitant conditions	Most thorough excision of adenoma of all the procedures
Balloon dilatation	Temporary procedure for patients with definite contraindications to surgery	Produces immediate benefit, although effect only lasts about a year. Fewest days of work lost and fewest days in hospital
Electrosurgical ablation of the prostate	For prostates of any size	Can be done as outpatient procedure, less blood loss than with most other procedures
Visual laser ablation of the prostate	For patients taking anticoagulants or with coagulopathies	Can be done as outpatient procedure, least blood loss of all procedures
Urethral stent	Temporary or permanent procedure for poor surgical candidates	Can be done as outpatient procedure

comparative potency of different products is difficult. In many cases, the products evaluated contained a combination of two or more of these herbs at specific concentrations. Until herbals are fully regulated by Health Canada, the quality of products is difficult to assess and it is impossible to compare the efficacy of different herbs. For these reasons, recommending herbal remedies for patients with BPH should only be undertaken in concert with the treating physician and the patient, and they should only be used in men with mild symptoms such as those taking the watchful waiting approach.

Information on herbal remedies used in the management of mild symptoms of BPH is presented in Table 5.[8-14] Pharmacists can educate patients on how to use these products properly and on their potential benefits and side effects. Encourage patients to discuss the use of these remedies with their physician first. The pharmacist may want to discuss a patient's use of herbal remedies for BPH with their physician (with the patient's permission), to ensure that their use will not interfere with any decisions the physician has made concerning the patient's care.

Prescription Therapy

Prescription medications used for treating BPH belong to two classes, the 5-alpha-reductase inhibitors (e.g., **finasteride**) and the alpha-adrenergic antagonists (e.g., **alfuzosin, doxazosin, prazosin, tamsulosin** and **terazosin**).[15,16]

Between 20 and 30% of BPH tissue is composed of glandular tissue and 70 to 80% is composed of stromal or fibromuscular tissue.[17] Growth of glandular tissue is stimulated by DHT. Finasteride selectively inhibits 5-alpha-reductase (type 2) in the prostate, hence reducing the concentrations of DHT locally.

Stromal and fibromuscular tissues are under alpha-adrenergic control. The alpha-adrenergic antagonists reduce sympathetic stimulation to BPH tissue, which results in relaxation of smooth muscle around the bladder neck and the prostatic urethra.[16] Generally, the lag time to attain full therapeutic effect with alpha-adrenergic antagonists is between four and six weeks.[16] This delay is mostly due to the time it takes to attain full therapeutic doses. To minimize adverse effects such as dizziness or postural hypotension, these agents are started at low doses and titrated upward.[16] Alpha-adrenergic antagonists will improve

symptoms associated with voiding in approximately 60 to 80% of patients.[16] The peak onset of effect with finasteride occurs after 6 to 12 months of therapy,[15] at which point about 30 to 40% of patients will show symptomatic improvement. It is not uncommon to combine finasteride with an alpha-adrenergic antagonist.[15]

Monitoring of Therapy

Patients with BPH should be monitored on a regular basis by their physician. Pharmacists can also play a role in monitoring patients by applying the AUA Symptom Index (Table 3). This is especially important for patients who have chosen the natural products route and/or are not being followed closely by a physician.

Patients taking an alpha-adrenergic antagonist or finasteride should be questioned about the success of their therapy at every refill. Counsel patients being started on an alpha-adrenergic antagonist on how to slowly titrate their dosing regimen to avoid adverse effects (e.g., dizziness, postural hypotension).

Resource Tips

Enlarged prostate guide, new information about herbal remedies:
www.prostatehealing.com/bph.html

Health A to Z, search word: BPH
www.healthatoz.com/atoz/default.asp

MEDLINEplus Nedical encyclopedia: Support Group – BPH
www.nlm.nih.gov/medlineplus/ency/article/003977.htm

Suggested Readings

Cuellar DC, Kyprianou N. Future concepts in the medical therapy of benign prostatic hyperplasia. *Curr Opin Urol* 2001;11(1):27-33.

Kirby RS. The natural history of benign prostatic hyperplasia: what have we learned in the last decade? *Urology* 2000;56(5 suppl 1):3-6.

Lee M, Sharifi R. Benign prostatic hyperplasia: diagnosis and treatment guideline. *Ann Pharmacother* 1997;31:481-6.

Table 5: **Herbal Remedies Used in BPH**[8-14]

Herb	Dose	Proposed mechanism of action	Onset of action	Side effects
Pumpkin seed (*Cucurbita pepo*)	10 g of seeds per day or equivalent	Inhibition of conversion of testosterone to DHT	3 mos	None known
African plum (*Pygeum*)	50-100 mg (extract) twice daily or 5-20 g (dried bark) twice daily*	Inhibition of 5-alpha reductase, antiandrogenic effects	2 mos	GI upset ranging from nausea to severe pain
Saw palmetto (*Serenoa repens, Sabal fructus*)	160 mg (lipophilic extract) twice daily or 1-2 g (berries) daily†	Inhibition of 5-alpha reductase, antiandrogenic effects	1-6 mos	Headache, GI upset, hypertension, impotence, decreased libido
Stinging nettle (*Urtica dioica*)	150-300 mg (root extract) daily	Inhibits the binding of sex hormone-binding globulin to its receptors	2 mos	GI upset

*50-100 mg twice daily is the dose for an extract standardized to a 14% content of sterols (recommended for BPH) and 5-20 g twice daily is the dose for the dried pygeum bark. Studies with pygeum for BPH were with the extract formulation.
†160 mg twice daily is the dose for the lipophilic extract product (recommended for BPH) and 1-2 g daily is the dose for the saw palmetto berry. Studies with saw palmetto for BPH were with the extract formulation.

McGuirt Franklin R, Barron D. Use of natural products in benign prostatic hyperplasia. *US Pharmacist* 1999; 24(5):63-8.

Shapiro E, Lepor H. Pathophysiology of clinical benign prostatic hyperplasia. *Urol Clin North Am* 1995;22:285-90.

References

1. Benign prostatic hyperplasia guidelines. *Benign prostatic hyperplasia: diagnosis and treatment.* Rockville, MD: US Department of Health and Human Services Public Health Service, Agency for Health Care Policy and Research, 1994.
2. Turner CL. Treatment options in benign prostatic hyperplasia. *Pharm Pract* 1993;9(8):1-8 (CE lesson).
3. Kirby RS. The natural history of benign prostatic hyperplasia: what have we learned in the last decade? *Urology* 2000;56(5 suppl 1):3-6.
4. Shapiro E, Lepor H. Pathophysiology of clinical benign prostatic hyperplasia. *Urol Clin North Am* 1995;22:285-90.
5. Repchinsky C, ed. *Compendium of Pharmaceuticals and Specialties* 36th ed. Ottawa, ON: Canadian Pharmacists Association, 2001.
6. Pray WS. Prostate health and OTC medications. *US Pharmacist* 1999;24(11):16-28.
7. Cuellar DC, Kyprianou N. Future concepts in the medical therapy of benign prostatic hyperplasia. *Curr Opin Urol* 2001;11(1):27-33.
8. McGuirt FR, Barron D. BPH: Use of natural products in benign prostatic hyperplasia. *US Pharmacist* 1999;24(5):63-8.
9. Wilt TJ, Ishani A, Stark G et al. Saw palmetto extracts for treatment of benign prostatic hyperplasia: a systematic review. *JAMA* 1998;280:1604-9.
10. Anon. Saw palmetto for benign prostatic hyperplasia. *Med Let* 1999;41(1046):18.
11. Awang DVC. Saw palmetto, african prune and stinging nettle for benign prostatic hyperplasia (BPH). *Can Pharm J* 1997;130(9): 37-44.
12. McQueen CE, Bryant PJ. Pygeum. *Am J Health-Syst Pharm* 2001;58:120-3.
13. Blumenthal M, ed. *The Complete German Commission E Monographs: Therapeutic Guide to Herbal Medicine.* Austin, TX: American Botanical Council, 1998.
14. Burnham TH, ed. *The Review of Natural Products.* St. Louis, MI: Facts and Comparisons, 2001.
15. Wilde M, Goa JL. Finasteride: An update of its use in the management of symptomatic benign prostatic hyperplasia. *Drugs* 1999;57(4):557-81.
16. Cooper KL, McKiernan JM, Kaplan SA. Alpha-adrenoceptor antagoists in the treatment of benign prostatic hyperplasia. *Drugs* 1999;57(1):9-17.
17. Lee M, Sharifi R. Benign prostatic hyperplasia: diagnosis and treatment guideline. *Ann Pharmacother* 1997;31:481-6.

Benign Prostatic Hyperplasia—Patient Information

Benign prostatic hyperplasia (BPH) is a condition where a male's prostate gland enlarges to the point that it causes discomfort. The prostate is a walnut-sized gland that is part of the male reproductive system. The prostate surrounds the urethra, the canal through which urine passes out of the body.

Symptoms of BPH are rare before age 40. It is more common as men age, affecting half of men in their 60s and 9 out of 10 men in their 70s and 80s. Symptoms only occur when the enlarged prostate starts to push against the urethra, much like clamping a garden hose. This causes the lining of the bladder wall to thicken and become irritable. The bladder starts to contract even when it only contains small amounts of urine. Over time, the bladder weakens and loses its ability to empty itself completely, leaving behind urine.

Common symptoms of BPH include:
- A hesitant, interrupted, weak urine stream;
- Leaking or dribbling of urine between trips to the bathroom;
- More frequent urination (especially at night).

Although BPH and prostate cancer have similar symptoms, having BPH does not increase the chances of getting prostate cancer. For most men, the symptoms come on slowly. For some men, however, symptoms appear all of a sudden. Causes of sudden onset of symptoms can include: certain medications (for example, decongestants), cold temperatures, alcohol and being immobile for a long time.

Your doctor might do tests to diagnose your symptoms, such as a rectal exam or ultrasound. Men with possible BPH are often referred to a urologist for diagnosis and treatment.

Treatment is only necessary when BPH puts your health at risk or when it becomes very bothersome. Mild BPH does not require treatment and in up to one third of cases, symptoms will disappear without treatment. Treatment of BPH can include surgery, other procedures, or medications such as finasteride, terazosin, prazosin, tamsulosin, alfuzosin or doxazosin.

Herbal products containing saw palmetto, stinging nettle, pygeum (African plum tree) and pumpkin seeds have also been used to treat mild cases of BPH with varying degrees of success.

If you have symptoms of BPH, see your doctor. If the doctor recommends drug therapy or a herbal remedy, your pharmacist can help you get the most out of your medicine.

Pregnancy and Fertility Testing

Marie Berry, BScPharm, BA, LLB

Pregnancy Testing

If an ovum is fertilized and implanted in the endometrial wall, human chorionic gonadotropin (HCG) is detectable in the blood and urine about nine days later. In healthy women, HCG is a specific marker for pregnancy, because it is only produced by the placenta.

HCG, a glycoprotein produced by the trophoblastic cells of the placenta, maintains the corpus luteum. It replaces luteinizing hormone (LH). HCG can be detected as soon as six to eight days after conception, and is highest in concentration between 9 am and 12 pm. Its concentration in the blood doubles about every two days, reaching a peak in 60 to 70 days. It then decreases to a lower level for the rest of the pregnancy. The half-life of HCG is about 5.6 hours. Following parturition it returns to a baseline within 10 days. The detection of HCG is the basis of pregnancy testing kits.

Prior to the advent of a biological assay for HCG, pregnancy tests were performed by injecting a woman's urine into a female rabbit. After five days, the rabbit was sacrificed. HCG causes swelling of the corpus luteum and of the uterus; the rabbit's uterus was examined and a heavy uterus meant that the woman was most likely pregnant.

In the 1960s, immunoassay technology allowed synthesis of an antibody which would combine with HCG to produce a precipitant or change a colored substrate. The pregnancy testing kits in use today represent the third generation in terms of pregnancy testing technology.

First-generation Tests

These tests used polyclonal antibodies, which recognized multiple binding sites on HCG. Unfortunately, these antibodies also reacted with other substances such as LH and follicle-stimulating hormone (FSH), resulting in false positive results. This generation of tests has been replaced by second and third generation tests which do not require sample collection and preparation, an incubation period, or technical skill.

Second-generation Tests

Modern pregnancy tests employ monoclonal technology, and so are more specific. In second-generation testing kits, the anti-HCG antibody is bound to a solid surface such as a stick, bead, or filter paper. If HCG is present, it complexes with the antibody to produce a change in color of a chromogen-reactive enzyme. The HCG actually becomes sandwiched between the two antibodies, one attached to the test surface and the other attached to the color-producing enzyme.

Second-generation tests can detect HCG as early as the first day of a missed menstrual period and take a shorter time (1 to 30 minutes) to perform.

Third-generation Tests

The tests available today for home use are third-generation tests (e.g., Clear Blue®, Answer Now®). The technology is even more refined in third-generation testing kits. One anti-beta-subunit HCG monoclonal antibody is linked to a colored substrate. If present, HCG binds to this antibody and the resulting complex binds to a second monoclonal antibody bound to a solid surface. The second monoclonal antibody is the alpha-subunit and elicits the color change. Ease of use and accuracy are significant advantages of third-generation tests.

Proper Use

False positive and false negative results are possible regardless of which generation of test is used. Human error (e.g., holding wrong end of wand or stick in urine stream, exposing the wand or stick to the urine for less than the required length of time) is usually the cause of erroneous results. The easier a test is to use, the less likely errors will occur. Most third-generation tests have controls built into them, to combat this problem.

Other errors leading to false results include:
- Testing too early after conception;
- Testing too late (after 60 to 70 days, when HCG levels decline);
- Soap residue, blood or protein in the urine sample;
- Cloudy, pink or red urine;
- Strong urine odor;
- Warm or hot water rinses of the test surface;
- Use of fertility drugs, hormones, corticosteroids;
- Ectopic production of HCG by nontrophoblastic tumours;
- Conducting the test after missed or incomplete abortion.

Pregnancy testing kits afford early detection of pregnancy in privacy, and earlier detection can permit earlier prenatal care.[1] They also enable earlier avoidance of harmful chemicals, X-rays, drugs (e.g., retinoic acid analogs, misoprostol), and elective surgery, all of which could potentially harm a developing fetus. The tests are easy to use, readily available and about 96 to 99% accurate. They offer speed, convenience and confidentiality, along with an economical cost.

For a listing of available pregnancy tests, see the *Compendium of Self-Care Products*, published annually by the Canadian Pharmacists Association.

Fertility Testing
Basal Thermometers
Basal body temperature is the temperature that occurs prior to rising in the morning. It can be taken orally, rectally or vaginally but must be done in the same way and at the same time each day, consistently. The daily temperatures are recorded on a graph.

The range of temperatures recorded by a basal thermometer is smaller (e.g., 96 to 99° F or 36 to 38°C), and they are easier to read than fever thermometers. However, digital thermometers that measure to two decimal points may be used, and may be even easier to read. Some patients learn to use sympto-thermal charting, which combines symptoms (e.g., mucus, pain, breast tenderness, spotting) and basal body temperatures, allowing the fertile period to be more accurately pinpointed.

Progesterone is thermogenic; elevated levels cause a rise in body temperature. About 12 to 24 hours prior to ovulation, a drop in temperature occurs; however, it is not always possible to detect the drop. With ovulation, the corpus luteum releases progesterone causing a significant rise in temperature that is detectable and lasts for several days. The temperature increase is about 0.5°F or 0.28°C and is measurable by a basal thermometer.[2] This temperature rise occurs over a period of up to three days and is usually maintained until the first day of menses – day one of the next cycle. It is not the temperature itself that is significant, but the maintained high temperature. With several cycles of data, a pattern may emerge (e.g., the usual day of ovulation in a woman's cycle).[3]

Being able to identify a rise in temperature enables a woman to determine when she is most fertile and likely to conceive. Sexual intercourse (ideally every two days) during this time will increase the chance of conception. Conversely, a woman will also know when to avoid sexual intercourse if she does not want to conceive. For more information on contraception, see Chapter 49.

Ovulation Prediction Kits
While basal thermometers identify the rise in temperature that accompanies progesterone release, ovulation prediction tests identify the LH surge that precedes ovulation by measuring its concentration in the urine. A woman will know when she is most likely to ovulate and can plan her sexual activity to increase the chances of conception.[4]

These tests employ polyclonal and monoclonal antibody technology. One antibody is bound to a test surface and another to an enzyme. If LH is present, it becomes sandwiched between the two antibodies and produces a color change on the test surface. With no LH in the urine, the second antibody bound to the enzyme is washed away and no color change occurs. The color intensity depends upon the amount of LH present.

Most ovulation tests are mixtures of polyclonal and monoclonal antibodies. The polyclonal antibodies may bind with either the alpha- or beta-subunit of LH or even the entire molecule. The monoclonal antibodies are usually specific for the beta-subunit, which is a more accurate identifier of LH.[5]

More recently, tests are beta-subunit specific antibodies bound to colored latex particles. The second monoclonal antibody is bound to the test surface. Without LH, the antibody bound to the colored latex is washed away.

Usually kits contain five daily tests that require 3 to 60 minutes to perform. Using the average length of her cycle, a woman uses a chart to determine the day of her cycle she should begin testing. Some test results are compared to baseline color charts, some to the previous test, and others to a control window. These tests are up to 98.3% accurate if performed properly.

Fertility testing technology has advanced to include software programs that more specifically pinpoint fertility. In these test kits, the use of monitors containing the software is combined with urine testing. The software programming tracks the cycle day, indicates when a urine test should be performed, and reports the degree of fertility as low, high or peak.

These advanced tests use monoclonal technology, and not only test for LH, but also for estrone-3-glucuronide (E3G), which is a urinary metabolite of estradiol. Estradiol stimulates the secretion of cervical mucus that is favorable for the survival and transport of sperm. The rise in estradiol levels corresponds to the appearance of sperm-supportive cervical mucus. Estradiol levels gradually rise in the early stage of the cycle, reaching a threshold that triggers the LH surge. With these tests, the stick is not read visually, but rather inserted into the monitor, which optically reads the test and displays the result.

For all of these kits, urine should be collected at the same time each day, and while some tests are to be done on the first urine in the morning, others can be performed anytime during the day as long as there is a sufficient volume to ensure an effective concentration of LH. Human error accounts for the majority of false readings. The inclusion of test controls and comparison of the results to the previous days' results reduce the chance of errors.

Table 1 compares various methods of predicting the time of ovulation.

Proper Use
Home diagnostic kits give an approximate time of ovulation and an indication of when a woman may be more fertile. Each kit has a chart or graph that can be used to determine, based on the woman's cycle, when testing should begin. These instructions should be followed for best results.

Couples using home ovulation predictor kits and/or basal body temperature charts should be instructed in

Table 1: **Predicting Ovulation**

Test	Indicators of ovulation
Basal body temperature	Elevation of basal temperature (0.5°F, 0.28°C) over up to 3 days, lasting at least 11 days, usually to day 1 of menses
Cervical mucus	Abundant watery discharge; fern-like pattern on glass slide; stretchability of mucus
Endometrial biopsy (late luteal phase)	Histology within 2 days of chronological cycle day based on LH surge
Menstrual cycle history	Most cycles 26-30 days (range 23-35 days) with ovulation mid-cycle, (e.g., around day 14 for a 28-day cycle). The postovulatory phase is usually more likely to be around 14 days consistently (e.g., in a 35-day cycle, ovulation might occur around day 21)
Midluteal serum progesterone	Values greater than 10 ng/mL
Urinary LH kits (ovulation prediction kits)	Color change 12-24 h before ovulation

their interpretation for detecting ovulation. Intercourse should begin before the expected day of ovulation and should occur at approximately two-day intervals. This timing takes advantage of the fact that sperm survive for at least two days in the female reproductive tract, even longer in good cervical mucus. Because sperm reserves of the male require at least two days for replenishment, more frequent intercourse may result in small volumes and a slightly lower sperm count. The use of artificial lubricants (e.g., K-Y® jelly) during intercourse may interfere with fertility because they decrease sperm motility. For a listing of available ovulation prediction kits, see the *Compendium of Self-Care Products*, published annually by the Canadian Pharmacists Association.

References

1. Gannon K. Who is most apt to turn to a home pregnancy test? *Drug Topics* 1992;136:46.
2. Downs KA, Gibson M. Basal body temperature graph and the luteal phase defect. *Fertil Steril* 1983;40:466.
3. Moghissi KS. Accuracy of basal body temperature for ovulation detection. *Fertil Steril* 1976;27:1415.
4. Corsan GH, et al., Home urinary luteinizing hormone immunoassays: clinical applications. *Fertil Steril* 1990;53:591.
5. Engle JP. Ovulation predictors. *Am Druggist* 1993;207:55.

Dental Care Section Highlights

Chapter 57: **Teething**

>   Dental anatomy
>   Normal tooth eruption times
>   Delayed tooth eruption
>   Eruption cysts
>   Teething pain
>   Pericoronitis or pericoronal abscess

Chapter 58: **Oral Hygiene**

>   Pathophysiology of plaque, calculus and caries
>   Plaque control
>   Tooth brushing
>   Flossing
>   Toothpastes
>   Mouth rinses
>   Caries prevention
>   Fluoride

Chapter 59: **Periodontal Conditions**

>   Pathophysiology of gingivitis and periodontitis
>   Risk factors
>   Prevalence
>   Management of gingivitis and periodontitis
>   Oral hygiene
>   Dental office procedures
>   Mouth rinses
>   Local and systemic antiinfectives

Chapter 60: **Dental Conditions**

>   Dentin hypersensitivity
>   Cracked tooth syndrome
>   Postendodontic discomfort
>   Dry socket
>   Pulpal diseases
>   Pulpitis
>   Necrotic pulp
>   Periapical diseases
>   Acute apical periodontitis
>   Chronic apical periodontitis
>   Suppurative apical periodontitis

Chapter 57

Teething

Michelle Bourassa, BPharm, MSc, DMD

Pathophysiology

The normal primary dentition (also called deciduous or milk teeth) is composed of a total of 20 teeth, divided as follows: four incisors, two canines (cuspids) and four molars on each arch. The complete permanent (adult) dentition includes a total of 32 teeth: four incisors, two canines, four premolars and six molars in each arch.[1-3] Figure 1 represents the normal anatomy of an adult molar and its related structures.

Table 1 presents the usual age range for tooth eruption.[1,2] Figure 2 depicts the normal primary and permanent dentition.

Primary Teeth

The eruption of the primary teeth is accompanied by signs and symptoms in about two-thirds of infants.[4,5] Usually the symptoms are transient.[1-7] They may appear up to four days prior to the emergence of the tooth. The peak in incidence and severity is usually on the day of eruption or one or two days before. These symptoms generally resolve within three days after eruption.[4]

For a few days prior to eruption, the gum overlying the tooth may show signs of inflammation such as redness, irritation, swelling and tenderness. The child may have a greater tendency to rub the gum by biting

Figure 1: **Anatomy of a Molar**

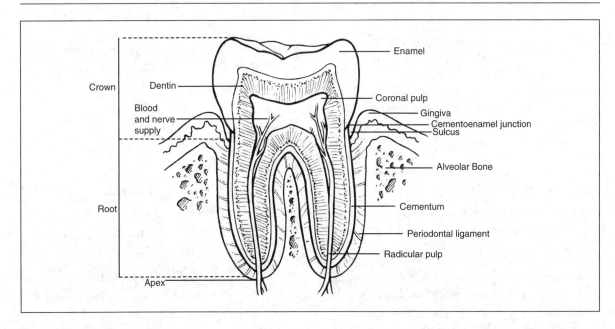

Table 1: **Usual Tooth Eruption Times**

	Upper (maxillary)	Lower (mandibular)
Primary teeth		
Central incisors	7-13 mos	6-10 mos
Lateral incisors	8-13 mos	10-16 mos
Canines (cuspids)	16-23 mos	16-23 mos
First molars	13-19 mos	12-19 mos
Second molars	25-33 mos	23-31 mos
Permanent teeth		
Central incisors	7-8 yrs	6-7 yrs
Lateral incisors	8-9 yrs	7-8 yrs
Canines (cuspids)	11-12 yrs	9-10 yrs
First premolars	10-11 yrs	10-12 yrs
Second premolars	10-12 yrs	11-12 yrs
First molars	6-7 yrs	6-7 yrs
Second molars	12-13 yrs	11-13 yrs
Third molars ("wisdom teeth")	17-21 yrs	17-21 yrs

Figure 2: **Occlusal Surface of Primary Teeth (upper and lower), and Permanent Teeth (upper and lower)**

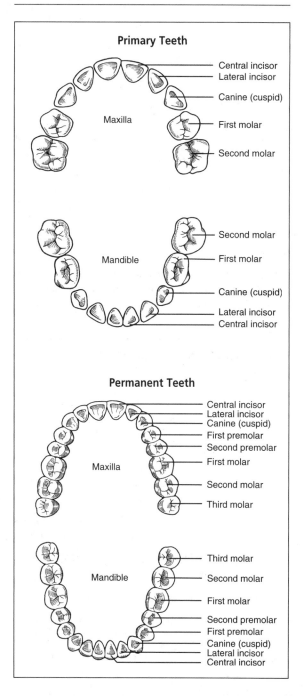

their fingers, lip, toys or some other object. This action induces more salivation and drooling, which can cause some facial irritation or skin rash. The local inflammation may be sufficient to explain the irritability of the child, which may manifest as agitation, restlessness, crying and insomnia. Other reported symptoms include a decrease in appetite for solid food, increased thirst, mild increase in body temperature (up to 37.7°C)[8], loose stools, ear rubbing and nasal congestion.[1,2,4-7,9,10]

Symptoms associated with an erupting tooth may coincide with an infectious process and the latter should not be overlooked when more severe symptoms are present. Fever, diarrhea, vomiting or symptoms of upper respiratory tract infection should be evaluated and not presumed to be caused by teething.[2,4,5]

Permanent Teeth

The eruption of a permanent tooth may be associated with the same gingival manifestations as with primary teeth, but the symptoms are usually much less pronounced. There may be local inflammation on the gum over and around the erupting tooth, from a few days prior to emergence of the tooth, to a few days after eruption.[2] Part of the gingiva may overlie the distal portion of the surface of the tooth for a relatively long period of time before completely receding. This part of the mucosa is called the operculum. Usually no symptoms result from its presence, but it can be problematic, particularly around the third molars, in the presence of mechanical trauma or plaque. Severe inflammation and marked swelling might then be seen at the operculum. This condition is called *pericoronitis* and is most often seen in teenagers and young adults. The patient may present with localized or diffuse pain, swelling and/or trauma at the operculum, bad breath and a foul taste in the mouth. When pus is present, the condition is called *pericoronal abscess*, and immediate dental or medical attention is recommended because the infection may spread into the oropharyngeal area and medially to the base of the tongue.[11] The swelling may extend to the adjacent tissue, and the patient may experience limitation in opening the mouth, lymphadenopathy and low-grade fever.[2,12-14]

Delayed Tooth Eruption[1]

There is a wide range in eruption times of primary and permanent teeth, due to individual variation (see Table 1). Developmental age is more important than chronological age in assessing delays in eruption. In an otherwise healthy child, a delay of up to 12 months is usually of no clinical significance. Delays can be caused by local factors such as the presence of a tooth in the erupting path, insufficient space in the arch or a dental infection. Rarely, systemic conditions or iatrogenic factors such as chemotherapy or radiotherapy of the head and neck can delay tooth eruption. Table 2 summarizes the possible causes of delayed tooth eruption. A dentist should be consulted when delays of more than 12 months are encountered.

Eruption Cysts

Occasionally, a localized, dome-shaped, fluctuant, bluish, swollen area, sometimes surrounded by

Table 2: **Causes of Delayed Tooth Eruption**[1,5]

Local causes	Systemic causes (infrequent)
Lack of arch space	Down syndrome
Anchylosis of the predecessor	Cleidocranial dysplasia
Premature loss of the predecessor	Congenital hypopituitarism
Cysts	Congenital hypothyroidism
Supernumerary teeth	Gaucher's disease
(extra teeth)	Osteoporosis
	Ectodermal dysplasia
Iatrogenic causes	Hypovitaminosis D
Chemotherapy	
Radiotherapy of the head and neck	

inflammation, appears on the gum overlying the crown of an erupting tooth. The space is filled with tissue, fluid and blood. This condition is called an eruption cyst and is more often seen over erupting molars. Eruption cysts may be encountered in the first and second decades and there is no gender predilection.[5,6,15]

Goals of Therapy

- Minimize pain, irritability and sleep disruption associated with teething pain
- Prevent complications through involvement of medical or dental professionals when indicated for systemic illness, eruption cysts, delayed tooth eruption, pericoronitis or pericoronal abscess

Patient Assessment

Table 3 lists circumstances in which referral to a dentist or physician is indicated.

Nonpharmacologic Therapy[2,3,5,6]

Teething Pain

Local measures can help minimize a child's discomfort during tooth eruption. Something hard, smooth and clean may be given to the child to bite and chew on, such as a frozen facecloth. Safe teethers, cooled in the refrigerator before use, can be very effective in reducing the local symptoms. They should not have any

Table 3: **When to Refer Patients with Teething Problems**

Condition	Recommendation
Pericoronitis	Dental consultation as soon as possible
Pericoronal abscess	Urgent dental or medical consultation
Delays of over 12 mos in tooth eruption	Dental consultation as soon as possible
Suspected systemic illness in a young child (e.g., fever, vomiting, diarrhea, symptoms of upper respiratory infection)	Medical consultation when appropriate (these symptoms are not normally associated with teething)
Eruption cysts that do not spontaneously drain, or that cause discomfort and/or interfere with feeding	Dental consultation as soon as possible

small parts that could break off and cause the child to choke. The Canadian Dental Association recommends rubbing the back of a small, cold spoon on the gum (See Resource Tips).

Pharmacologic Therapy[3,5,6]

Teething Pain

Nonprescription Therapy

For teething pain in infants that is not relieved by nonpharmacologic measures, oral analgesics, such as acetaminophen or ibuprofen, can be used at the usual dose (see Chapter 8). Systemic analgesics should never be rubbed on the gum.

Although their use is controversial, topical anesthetic agents (benzocaine 7.5 to 10% in a gel formulation) may be applied in a thin layer to the affected gum using a cotton swab or finger, up to four times daily.[2,5,6] The duration of action is 30-45 minutes. Because of concern about disabling the gag reflex if the child swallows the anesthetic, it is recommended that the caregiver wait for an hour before feeding the child, if a local anesthetic has been applied to the gum.

Treatment of Pericoronitis or Pericoronal Abscess

These conditions require a dental consultation for appropriate treatment. They can be treated by the dentist with careful debridement of the area with curettage, followed by an irrigation with physiologic saline solution, chlorhexidine 0.12% solution or hydrogen peroxide 3%. Some cases require surgical removal of the operculum, extraction or selective grinding of the opposing tooth, or extraction of the involved tooth.[13]

When systemic manifestations or extensive swelling are present, an antibacterial agent targeting gram-negative anaerobes (e.g., penicillin V, clindamycin or metronidazole)[11,12] is usually prescribed along with irrigation and extraction.

Mild analgesics (e.g., acetaminophen or ibuprofen) in the usual analgesic dose may be used to control the pain and decrease the fever when present. The patient may be instructed to rinse at home with lukewarm salt water (about 15 mL table salt in a litre of water) every two to three hours for two to three days.[2,12,14]

Treatment of Eruption Cysts

Eruption cysts usually rupture spontaneously. In rare cases, marsupialization (surgical excision of a small amount of gum tissue from the roof of the cyst) under local anaesthesia may be indicated if significant discomfort or interference with feeding occurs.[15]

Resource Tips

Canadian Dental Association: www.cda-adc.ca

Suggested Readings

Holt R, Roberts G, Scully C. Oral health and disease. In: Scully C, ed. *ABC of Oral Health*. London, UK: BMJ Books, 2001:1-4.

Twetman S, Garcia-Godoy F, Goepferd SJ. Infant Oral Health. *Dent Clin North Am* 2000;44(3): 487-505.

References

1. Holt R, Roberts G, Scully C. Oral health and disease. In: Scully C, ed. *ABC of Oral Health*. London: BMJ Books; 2001:1-4.
2. Nowak A, Crall J. Prevention of dental disease. In: Pinkham JR, ed. *Pediatric Dentistry Infancy through Adolescence*. 2nd ed. Philadelphia, PA: WB Saunders Co.; 1994:192-208.
3. Mitchell L, Mitchell DA. Preventive and community dentistry. In: Mitchell L, Mitchell DA, eds. *Oxford Handbook of Clinical Dentistry*. 3rd ed. Oxford, UK: Oxford University Press; 1999: 58-127
4. Macknin ML, Piedmonte M, Jacobs J, Skibinski C. Symptoms associated with infant teething: a prospective study. *Pediatrics* 2000;105:747-52.
5. Norén J, Koch G, Rasmussen P. Disturbances in tooth development and eruption. In: Koch G, Modéer T, Poulsen S, Rasmussen P, eds. *Pedodontics, A clinical Approach*. 1st ed. Copenhagen: Munksgaad; 1991:250-74.
6. Parkin SF. Some oral and dental diseases of childhood. In: Parkin S ed. *Notes on paediatric dentistry*. Oxford: Wright; 1991:170-82.
7. Denbensten P. Is teething associated with diarrhea? *West J Med* 2000;173:137.
8. Jaber L, Cohen IJ, Mor A. Fever associated with teething. *Arch Dis Child* 1992;67:233-4.
9. Wake M, Hesketh K, Lucas J. Teething and tooth eruption in infants: a cohort study. *Pediatrics* 2000;106:1374-9.
10. Hulland SA, Lucas JO, Wake MA, Hesketh KD. Eruption of the primary dentition in human infants: a prospective descriptive study. *Pediatr Dent* 2000;22(5):415-21.
11. Meng HX. Periodontal Abscess. *Ann Periodontol* 1999;4: 79-82.
12. Peterson LJ. Principles of management of impacted teeth. In: Peterson LJ, Ellis III E, Hupp JR, Tucker MR, eds. *Contemporary Oral and Maxillofacial Surgery*. St. Louis, MI: Mosby, 1993:225-60.
13. Holland GR. Management of Dental Pain. In: Lund JP, Lavigne GJ, Dubner R, Sessle BJ, eds. *Orafacial Pain From Basic Science to Clinical Management*. Chicago, IL: Quintessence Publishing Co, Inc.; 2001:211-20.
14. Abrams H, Jasper SJ. Diagnosis and management of Acute Periodontal Problems. In: Falace DA, ed. *Emergency Dental Care Diagnosis and Management of Urgent Dental Problems*. Baltimore, MD: Williams and Wilkins; 1995:132-50.
15. Flaitz CM. Oral Pathologic conditions and soft tissue anomalies. In: Pinkham JR, ed. *Pediatric Dentistry Infancy through Adolescence*. 2nd ed. Philadelphia, PA: WB Saunders; 1994:29-56.

Teething Pain—Patient Information

Primary teeth ("baby" teeth) begin to poke through the gums at about six months of age and continue arriving until there is a total of 20. About two-thirds of infants will experience some discomfort when teeth come in.

Symptoms of teething can include:
- Redness, swelling or tenderness in the gum over the arriving tooth;
- Irritability, restlessness, crying, not sleeping well;
- Less hungry for solid food, more thirsty than usual;
- Drooling, rubbing the gum.

Symptoms of teething do *not* include:
- Fever (above 37.7°C or 100°F)
- Diarrhea;
- Common cold symptoms;
- Vomiting.

If these are present, do *not* assume they are caused by teething, and see your doctor if necessary.

What you can *do* to relieve the pain:
- Give the child a cool, safe object to chew on, such as a safe teether or frozen facecloth. Make sure it can't break into small pieces that could cause choking. If the child already has one or more teeth, avoid liquid-filled teethers. The teeth could puncture the teether and break off a small piece that could choke the child.
- Rub the gums gently with the back of a cool, small spoon or with a clean finger.

- Give a pain-relieving medicine like acetaminophen or ibuprofen in the appropriate dose for the child. Your pharmacist can help select a product and tell you how to use it. ASA (aspirin, acetylsalicylic acid) should *not* be given to a child unless recommended by your doctor.
- Although local anesthetics such as benzocaine gel can be rubbed on the gum with a cotton swab, they only numb the area for about 30 to 45 minutes and might interfere with swallowing if the child swallows the anesthetic. If you choose to use these products, wait for an hour before feeding the child and use a very small amount, no more than four times a day. Your pharmacist can help you select the appropriate product for your child.

What you should *not do* for teething pain:
- Do not give the child teething biscuits. They may contain sugar or have hidden sugars – prolonged contact with sugar is bad for the teeth and gums.
- Do not rub oral pain relievers like acetaminophen or ibuprofen (especially not aspirin or ASA) directly on the gums.
- If a blister develops on top of the arriving tooth, do not try to break it. These little cysts are not usually dangerous and they almost always open and drain on their own. If the blister does not go away or if it seems to be causing pain or interfering with feeding, see your dentist.

Chapter 58

Oral Hygiene

Michelle Bourassa, BPharm, MSc, DMD

Pathophysiology

Dental Plaque

Dental plaque is defined as a gelatinous deposit adherent to the tooth surfaces, fillings or dental prostheses. Plaque is composed of aerobic and anaerobic bacteria in a matrix of bacterial or salivary glycoproteins and dextrans. Dental plaque is also referred to as "biofilm".[1,2]

When freshly-cleaned teeth are exposed to saliva, a layer of salivary glycoproteins adheres to the surface of the teeth. For an illustration of dental anatomy, see Figure 1, Chapter 57. Oral microorganisms can attach to the glycoproteins or to the tooth enamel itself. The sticky dextrans and levans produced by the bacteria constitute the matrix that permits colonization and aggregation of more bacteria. Initially, the plaque is made of gram-positive cocci and rods; with time, gram-negative rods and spirochetes join the previous microorganisms and the volume of plaque increases.[3,5]

Dental plaque can be divided into two types based on its location relative to the gum (i.e., supragingival or subgingival). Supragingival plaque is usually white to yellow in color and can be detected around the collar of the teeth with a probe or a disclosing solution when present in small amounts. When the volume is large the eye can easily identify it.[5,6]

Subgingival plaque is responsible for periodontopathies. On the tooth surface of the subgingival plaque, the stages of plaque formation and its initial constituents may be the same as for supragingival plaque. The plaque surface adjacent to the gingiva, however, is somewhat different. The structure appears less dense, the matrix is reduced and the bacteria are more free. With time and with progression of the periodontal disease, the types of microorganisms change and anaerobic gram-bacilli become dominant.[5,6]

Microbiology of Plaque[3-5,7,8]

The microbiology of dental plaque varies greatly on an individual basis and from one area to another in the same mouth. Gram-positive bacteria predominate and are mainly from the Streptococcus and Actinomyces species. In most dental plaque, Veillonella, Neisseria and some gram-positive organisms and filaments are also found, to a lesser extent. Facultative anaerobic Streptococci represent a significant proportion of bacteria encountered in plaque. The type and the relative amounts of microorganisms evolve with time, eventually producing an ecologic environment favoring anaerobes.

Consequences of Plaque

The presence of plaque plays an important role in two pathologic processes in the mouth, the development of caries (cavities) and periodontal diseases.[4,6]

Cariogenic Effect

Dietary sucrose increases plaque formation and the resulting plaque is more cariogenic. Studies have shown that ingestion of sucrose favors the colonization and aggregation of microorganisms on teeth and prosthetic devices. *S. mutans* seems to play the primary role in cariogenic plaque. One of its actions is to metabolize the sucrose into an acid that causes demineralization of the enamel and with time, tooth decay.[3,4,9]

Periopathogenic Effect

In order to initiate and maintain periodontal disease, plaque has to be present at the tooth surface. The pathogenic role of dental plaque is described in Chapter 59.

Calculus[3,5,10]

Dental calculus (tartar) is defined as the calcification of existing deposits on the teeth or any other hard surface in the mouth (fillings, fixed or removable prostheses). It can be located supragingivally or subgingivally. When visible, it has a yellowish color that may be darkened by dietary or exogenous pigmentation (e.g., coffee, tea, red wine, nicotine). Its formation starts in areas close to the salivary gland openings, i.e., lingual (tongue) side of the inferior incisors, and the buccal (cheek) side of the upper molars. When located under the margin of the gingiva, the calculus often takes on a dark color and is very adherent to the cementum of the tooth.

The surface of the calculus is usually rough and favors plaque retention, which can subsequently lead to irritation and periodontal inflammation.

The presence of dental plaque is a prerequisite for calculus formation. In most patients, calcification occurs within 48 hours in newly formed plaque. The amount of calculus being formed varies greatly from one individual to another, and depends on many factors such as the composition of saliva and the concentration of certain enzymes. Therefore, control of calculus formation begins with controlling plaque formation. Calculus requires removal by a professional, with ultrasonic, sonic or sharp instruments. In contrast, plaque can be controlled with good oral hygiene.

Plaque Control

Mechanical Methods

Mechanical removal of plaque may be achieved by brushing the teeth after every meal and at bedtime, and flossing once a day, preferably at bedtime. Using toothpaste is recommended; studies show that plaque removal is more effective when toothpaste is used.[11] In some patients, tools such as interproximal brushes, dental woodsticks and interspace brushes may be useful to help remove plaque from areas difficult to access with a toothbrush and floss.

Irrigating devices (e.g., Water-pik®) may also be useful in patients with bridges, orthodontic appliances or after oral surgery. They can remove food debris but do not remove plaque. Therefore, they can be recommended as adjunctive devices only. Some studies suggest that a greater reduction of gingival inflammation may result from subgingival irrigation by the dentist with chlorhexidine.[3,12,13]

Table 1 presents a nonexhaustive list of devices and their role in removing plaque:[3,11,14]

Tooth Brushing

Many techniques are described in the literature. The most recommended one is the sulcular method, which focuses on removal of the plaque adjacent to and within the sulcus (see Figure 1, Chapter 57).[3,11,13] It has been shown to be a very effective method for the removal of plaque, particularly from the gingival area of the tooth and gingival crevice (sulcus). Three to four minutes is probably the minimum time required to perform an effective plaque removal.[14,15] The detailed technique is described in the Patient Information Section.

Toothbrushes

A suitable toothbrush is one with soft or extra-soft, flexible, rounded bristles that can penetrate into the gingival crevice to effectively remove plaque without

Table 1: **Dental Cleaning Devices**

Device	Role
Toothbrush	Removes plaque from buccal (cheek) and lingual (tongue) sides and occlusal (biting) surfaces of the teeth
Dental floss	Removes plaque from interproximal surfaces (between the teeth)
Interdental brush, interproximal brush Toothpick Rubber tip	Removes plaque from concave root surfaces when attachment loss (detachment of the gingiva due to bone loss) is present, and from other difficult-to-reach areas
Stimulator (rod curved at one end with a sharp rubber tip)	Removes plaque by applying contouring pressure to hyperplastic gingival papillae (noninflammatory enlargement of the gingivae)[13]

causing trauma to soft and hard tissues. It should also be small enough to easily reach all areas of the mouth.[12,13] Replacement of a toothbrush is recommended every three months, or as soon as the bristles start to splay.[11] Studies have found no consistent superiority of one design over another for either plaque removal or gingival inflammation reduction.[14]

Many mechanical toothbrushes are now available. Studies have shown that when a patient has a good understanding of proper tooth brushing technique and has the ability to manipulate a manual toothbrush, little or no benefit is derived from using a mechanical toothbrush instead. In long-term studies, the electric brush shows little superiority in plaque removal.[13] The use of a mechanical brush may be beneficial when the manual technique has failed after a number of attempts, for patients with limited dexterity or for patients with orthodontic appliances.[12,14]

Toothpaste

The main roles of toothpaste are:[15]

- Minimizing the accumulation of plaque and tartar
- Strengthening the enamel against caries
- Cleaning the teeth by removing food debris and some stains
- Freshening the mouth

Toothpastes contain various combinations of the ingredients found in Table 2.[16]

Table 2: **Ingredients of Toothpastes**[16]

Ingredient	Role	Comments
Detergents (e.g., sodium lauryl sulfate, sodium-N-lauryl sarcosinate)	Foaming action may increase the solubility of plaque during brushing	Adverse effects (e.g., development of aphthous ulcers) in small percentage of patients may necessitate switching to a toothpaste without these agents.
Flavoring agents (e.g., sweetening agents)	Improve palatablility	
Humectants (e.g., glycerol, propylene glycol, sorbitol)	Prevent toothpaste from drying out	
Thickening agents (e.g., mineral colloids, natural gums, seaweed colloids, synthetic celluloses)	Stabilize the formulation	
Abrasive agents (e.g., calcium carbonate, dehydrated silica gels, hydrated aluminum oxides, magnesium carbonate, phosphate salts)	Remove debris and residual stains; whiten teeth	May cause burning sensation, drying of mucous membranes, taste alteration, gingival abrasion or enamel erosion. Some stains cannot be removed by toothpastes containing these whiteners (e.g., tetracycline staining, mottling).
Peroxides, sodium triphosphate	Whiteners	May work by breaking down pigments that accumulate on or in the tooth enamel
Pyrophosphates, triclosan, zinc citrate	Prevent calculus (tartar) formation	Mechanism not established. One hypothesis is the reduction of crystal growth on the tooth surface through chelation of cations.
Stannous fluoride, triclosan, zinc citrate	Prevent gingival inflammation	Reduce plaque accumulation through antibacterial activity. Stannous fluoride (and other toothpaste ingredients) may interact with chlorhexidine mouth rinse, rendering both agents less effective. Use them 30 min apart.
Fluoride	Reduces caries formation	Makes enamel more resistant to demineralization. Excess amounts can cause fluorosis (see Dental Caries, fluoride).

Studies have show that toothpaste with an attractive appearance and flavor encourages prolonged and regular use.[15] The market is overwhelmed with toothbrushes and toothpastes. Products that have obtained the Canadian Dental Association (CDA) seal respond to the needs of most patients. Particular needs should be discussed with the patient's dentist or dental hygienist.

Flossing

Dental floss and tape, waxed or unwaxed, are equally effective for cleaning proximal surfaces. Individual factors such as contacts (where two adjacent teeth come together), restorations, tooth alignment and manual dexterity determine the type of floss used. The floss should slip easily between the teeth and pass the margin of the fillings without tearing and becoming lodged in the interproximal spaces. Unwaxed floss is suitable for most people; if it does not slide easily between the teeth, a waxed floss can be used. For persistent problems with tearing or fraying, brands such as Glide®, Colgate Total® or EEZ-thru® can be tried.

Floss-holding devices have proven effective for some patients who have difficulty guiding the floss with their fingers.[13]

Chemical Methods
Mouth Rinses

A number of commercially available mouth rinses may be good adjuncts in helping control the development of supragingival plaque and in reducing subsequent gingivitis (Table 3). Oxygenating agents (e.g., hydrogen peroxide, carbamide peroxide) are not recommended because of lack of efficacy and potential adverse effects such as chemical burns of oral mucosa, decalcification of teeth and black hairy tongue.

Dental Caries

Dental caries is a localized and progressive dissolution and destruction of the calcified tissues of the teeth resulting from an infectious process.[9]

Bacteria from dental plaque are capable of producing organic acids from the metabolism of dietary carbohydrates as well as from proteolytic enzymes. S. mutans has a major role in this process. In response to the decrease in pH at the tooth surface, calcium and phosphate ions diffuse out of the enamel, and demineralization takes place. With an increase in pH, the process may be reversed. With time, disintegration of the mineral component of enamel and dentin occurs with subsequent formation of a cavity.

Table 3: **Mouth Rinses**[16-19]

Active ingredient(s)	Plaque and gingivitis reduction	Comments
Cetylpyridinium Chloride (e.g., Cepacol®	Moderate	Less effective than chlorhexidine. May cause staining of teeth
Chlorhexidine (e.g., Peridex▣)	High	Gold standard. Requires prescription. Limit use to once or twice daily; prolonged use may cause tooth staining, taste disturbances discoloration of tongue. Other adverse effects include taste disturbances, discoloration of tongue, local irritation or allergic reactions.
Essential oils (thymol, menthol, eucalyptol and methysalicylate (e.g., Listerine®)	High	Use for 30 seconds 4-6 times daily; high alcohol content in some products; may cause burning sensation, bitter taste or mucosal drying; not recommended for children because of alcohol content.
Sanguinaria canadensis (e.g., Viadent®)	Moderate	May cause allergic reactions, burning sensation in oral mucosa, bitter taste
Triclosan (e.g., Oral Plan Antimicrobial Mouthrinse®)	Moderate	Available only in combination with cetylpyridinium chloride and fluoride

Patients with xerostomia (dry mouth) have a higher risk for and incidence of caries (see Chapter 65).

Enamel Caries[20]

Initially, the lesion appears as a white spot due to demineralization of the enamel. With repeated exposure to acid, the surface changes from smooth to rough and may become stained. If left untreated, pitting and then cavitation occurs.

Dentin Caries[20]

In the dentin, demineralization is followed by bacterial invasion. Dentin shows the ability to produce secondary dentin in an attempt to protect the pulp, but its proximity to the pulp also represents a risk of bacterial invasion into the tooth structure.

Arrested Caries[20]

Under favorable conditions, the lesional process may stop, become inactive and may even regress. Most of the time, arrested enamel caries have a brown coloration and arrested dentin caries have a hard or leathery consistency and a darker color than dentin decay.

Susceptible Sites[9,20]

The sites on the tooth where plaque can accumulate are more prone to decay: proximal surfaces, cervical margins, pits and fissures (occlusal surface for the posteriors and palatal surface for the anteriors). Susceptibility is also dependent upon the volume and composition of the saliva, which represent the host factors.

Caries Prevention[9,20-22]

Caries prevention may be achieved by:
- Protecting the teeth or strengthening the tooth structures;
- Reducing the amount of substrate available to the bacteria;
- Removing plaque and calculus through mechanical or chemical procedures.

Those goals may be achieved by combining the following interventions:[21,23,24]
- Topical and/or systemic fluorides.
- Good, regular oral hygiene methods;
- Diet low in sugar and dietary acids;
- Regular professional dental care.

Role of Saliva[9,20]

Saliva plays various protective roles against tooth decay:
- Acts as a reservoir of calcium, phosphate and fluoride ions, and therefore favors remineralization;
- Contains IgA, lysozyme and peroxidase, which provide some antibacterial action;
- Decreases plaque accumulation and helps eliminate food debris;
- At high flow rates, it has an alkaline pH which helps buffer against organic acids.

Fluoride

The use of fluoride to prevent and control dental caries is well documented, safe and effective.[25-27] Systemic fluoride improves the crsytallinity and decreases the acid solubility of enamel formed in the pre-eruptive phase of tooth development. In addition, it may affect tooth anatomy and reduce the risk of caries associated with pits and fissures in the teeth. Locally administered fluoride benefits the enamel by reducing demineralization and promoting remineralization of early caries. The resulting remineralized enamel has improved resistance to acid attack. In the presence of fluoride, acid production by bacteria in plaque is decreased, as is the synthesis of extracellular polysaccharides.[9,19,23]

The addition of fluoride to drinking water is recognized as a cost-effective public health measure.[25,26] In areas where the water is not fluoridated, supplemental oral fluoride is recommended.[25,26]

For caries prevention in children, the monitored use of fluoridated dentifrice (pea-sized amount on the toothbrush) is recommended until the child is able to expectorate the dentifrice, which is around the age of six.[25-27] It is important for the caregiver to ensure the child does not swallow the toothpaste, to minimize the risk of fluorosis. A nonfluoridated dentifrice may be considered until the age of three.[27] In some cases, based on the individual child's risk of caries, professionally applied fluoride may be indicated. For children considered at high risk for caries, home protocols may be recommended by the dentist on an individual basis.[25,26]

Excessive amounts of fluoride may result in dental fluorosis, which is manifested by white specks on the child's teeth. It is a permanent cosmetic alteration of the enamel; there is no evidence that it affects the health of the child. It affects mainly younger children.[25,27] To minimize the risk of fluorosis, the total daily dose of fluoride should not exceed 0.05 to 0.07 mg F/kg of body weight.[25]

According to the Canadian Dental Association, the optimal level of fluoride in drinking water is between 0.8 and 1.0 ppm, as fluoride may come from other sources.[25]

Fluoride supplements should be considered for children living in areas where the drinking water is deficient in fluoride (the American Dental Association considers a concentration less than 0.6 ppm to be deficient in fluoride[26]). Before prescribing fluoride supplements, a careful evaluation of all daily sources of fluoride (drinking water at home, day care, school, other dietary sources) should be done by a dentist. Table 4 lists a daily dosing schedule for supplemental fluoride in children.[26,27]

Children who may be at higher risk for caries due to orthodontic or prosthodontic appliances or reduced salivary function, or children with high caries activity, should be considered for fluoride suppplements.[26,27]

Fluoride supplements are available as lozenges, chewable tablets or drops. A lozenge or chewable tablet containing 1 mg of fluoride delivers the same amount of fluoride as 1 g (average amount used) of a 1000 ppm fluoride toothpaste.[25]

Gastric distress, headache and weakness have been reported in cases of excessive ingestion. Allergic reactions such as rash and other idiosyncratic reactions have been rarely reported.[27] When taken as directed, no adverse effects have been reported.[27]

In order to prevent overdoses, no more than 120 mg of fluoride should be dispensed per household at one time.[27]

Fluoride tablets should be taken with a glass of water or juice. Calcium from milk or other dairy products may bind with fluoride causing both to be poorly absorbed.[27]

Care of Prostheses[28-30]
Any removable prosthesis should be cleaned after eating and before going to bed. Plaque and tartar can accumulate on artificial teeth as on natural ones. A soft toothbrush may be used to clean the prosthesis using a regular toothpaste. The gums and the remaining teeth should be cleaned carefully as well, with a soft tooth brush. The toothbrush is not sufficient to remove debris; therefore, immersing the device in a commercial denture cleaning solution is helpful. The patient should soak the dentures for 15 minutes once daily in the cleaning solution, then brush them with a dentifrice. Sodium hypochlorite solutions are effective denture cleaners; however, they should be avoided for dentures with metal parts since they have a tendency to cause corrosion of the metal. Household products should be avoided because they are too abrasive for use on acrylic resin surfaces. Dentures should be cleaned over a basin filled with water so that if they are accidentally dropped, the water will prevent breakage.

In spite of proper cleaning techniques, calculus may build up on some protheses. Calculus should be removed in the dental office with an ultrasonic cleaner.

Dentures should not be worn at night unless recommended by the dentist. They should be placed in a container and soaked (completely covered) in lukewarm water to prevent dehydration and subsequent dimensional change.

Table 4: **Fluoride Supplementation in Children**

Age	Recommended daily dose of fluoride based on concentration of fluoride in drinking water:		
	< 0.3 ppm	0.3 to 0.6 ppm	> 0.6 ppm
Birth to < 6 mos	0	0	0
6 mos to < 3 yrs	0.25 mg	0	0
3 to < 6 yrs	0.5 mg	0.25 mg	0
6 yrs to at least 16 yrs	1.0 mg	0.5mg	0

If the patient is not able to brush the dentures after the midday meal, they should at least thoroughly rinse the dentures and mouth.

Implants should be brushed and flossed carefully every day. All sides of the implant should be brushed, and floss used with caution where the implant meets the gum line.

Resource Tips

Canadian Dental Association: www.cda-adc.ca

Suggested Readings

Lundeen TF, Toberson TM. Cariology: The Lesion, Etiology, Prevention, and Control. In: Sturdevant CM, Roberson TM, Heymann HO, Sturdevant JR, eds. *The Art and Science of Operative Dentistry* 3rd ed. St. Louis, MI: Mosby, 1995:60-129.

References

1. Flemmig TF. Periodontitis. *Ann Periodontol* 1999;4:32-7.
2. Slots J, Jorgensen MG. Efficient antimicrobial treatment in periodontal maintenance care. *JADA* 2000 Sept;131:1293-1304.
3. Flamand Y, Bercy P. Prophylaxie du patient. In: Bercy, Tenenbaum eds. *Parodontologie, Du Diagnostic à la pratique.* Paris: De Boek & Larcier, 1996:91-104.
4. Rölla G, Waaler SM, Kjaerheim V. Concepts in Dental Plaque Formation. In: Busscher HJ, Evans LV, eds. *Oralbiofilms and plaque control.* Amsterdam: OPA, 1998:1-17.
5. Manson JD, Eley BM. The oral environment in health and disease. In: Manson JD, Eley BM, eds. *Outline of periodontics* 4th ed. Oxford, UK: Wright, 2000:26-33.
6. McHugh WD. Dental Plaque: Thirty Years On. In: Newman HN, Wilson M, eds. *Dental Plaque Revisited.* Cardiff: Bioline, 1999:1-4.
7. Marsh PD, Bradshaw DJ. Microbial Community Aspects in Dental Plaque. In: Busscher HJ, Evans LV, eds. *Oralbiofilms and plaque control.* Amsterdam: OPA, 1998:43-55.
8. Jones CG. Chlorhexidine: is it still the gold standard? *Periodont 2000* 1997;15:55-62.
9. Lundeen TF, Toberson TM. Cariology: the lesion, etiology, prevention, and control. In: Sturdevant CM, Roberson TM, Heymann HO, Sturdevant JR, eds. *The Art and Science of Operative Dentistry* 3rd ed. St. Louis, MI: Mosby, 1995: 60-129.
10. Davies RM, Ellwood RP, Volpe AR, Petrone ME. Supragingival calculus and periodontal disease. *Periodontol 2000* 1997;15:74-83.
11. Manson JD, Eley BM. Prevention of periodontal disease. In: Manson JD, Eley BM, eds. *Outline of periodontics* 4th ed. Oxford, UK: Wright, 2000:132-144.
12. Forgas L. Plaque Control. In: Fedi PF, Vernino AR, Gray JL, eds. *The Periodontic Syllabus* 4th ed. Baltimore, MD: Lippincott Williams & Wilkins, 2000:75-85.
13. Wilson TG, Kornman KS. Treating Plaque-Associated Gingivitis. In: Wilson TG, Kornman KS, eds. *Fundamentals of periodontics.* Chicago, IL: Quintessence Publishing Co. Inc, 1996:319-347.
14. Handcock EB, Newell DH. Preventive strategies and supportive treatment. *Periodontol 2000* 2001;25:59-76.
15. Forward GC, James AH, Barnett P, Jackson RJ. Gum health product formulations what is in them and why? *Periodontol 2000* 1997;15:32-9.
16. Mariotti AJ, Burrell KH. Mouthrinses and dentifrices. In: Cianclo SG, ed. *ADA guide to dental therapeutics* 2nd ed. Chicago, IL: ADA Publishing Co., 2000:211-29.
17. Cummings D. Vehicles: how to deliver the goods. *Periodontol 2000* 1997;15:55-62.
18. Drisko CH. Nonsurgical periodontal therapy. *Periodontol 2000* 2001;25:77-88.
19. Jackson RJ. Metal salts, essential oils and phenols – old or new? *Periodontol 2000* 1997;(15):52-4.
20. Mitchell L, Mitchell DA. Preventive and community dentistry. In: Mitchell L, Mitchell DA, eds. *Oxford Handbook of Clinical Dentistry.* 3rd ed. Oxford University Press, 1999:26-56.
21. Parkin SF. Preventive dentistry. In: Parkin SF, ed. *Notes on Paediatric Dentistry.* Oxford, UK: Wright, 1991:36-49.
22. Stookey GK. Current status of caries prevention. *Compendium 2000,* 21(10A):862-7.
23. Nowak A, Crall J. Prevention of dental disease. In: Pinkham JR, ed. *Pediatric Dentistry Infancy Through Adolescence.* 2nd ed. Philadelphia, PA: WB Saunders 1994:192-208.
24. Twetman S, Garcia-Godoy F, Goepferd SJ. Infant Oral Health. *Dent Clin North Am* 2000 44(3):487-505.
25. Candadian Dental Association Statement on fluoridation. Available from: www.cda-adc.ca. Accessed January 15, 2002.
26. Pediatric Dentistry, Guidelines for Fluoride Therapy, special issue, Reference Manual 2000-2001:22(7):45.
27. Burrel KH, Chan JT, Systemic and Topical Fluorides, *ADA guide to Dental Therapeutics,* 2nd ed. Chicago, IL: ADA Publishing, 2000:230-41.
28. McGivney GP. In: McGivney GP, Castlebeery DJ, eds. *McCracken's Removable Partial Prosthodontics.* 9th ed. St. Louis, MI: Mosby, 1995:442-3.
29. American Dental Association web site: www.ada.org. Accessed January 16, 2002.
30. Canadian Dental Association web site: www.cda-adc.ca. Accessed January 16 2002.

Oral Hygiene—Patient Information

Dental Check-ups
- See your dentist and hygienist as often as they recommend, but no less than once a year.

Brushing your Teeth
- Brush your teeth after each meal and before going to bed.
- Use a toothpaste that you like and that has the seal of the Canadian Dental Association (CDA), or one recommended by your dentist or hygienist.
- Replace your toothbrush with a new one every three months.
- Make sure you use a toothbrush with soft or ultra-soft bristles.

How to Brush Properly
- Place your brush at a 45° angle to your teeth. The bristles should reach the place where the gum and the teeth meet.
- Move your brush in a gentle circles, starting at the gum and moving towards the top of the tooth. Do not scrub your gums hard. You could damage them and get gum disease.
- Use this gentle circle technique to clean the cheek side and tongue side of each tooth. For the tongue side of the front teeth, use the tip of your toothbrush. Finish by cleaning the chewing surface of each tooth.
- To do a thorough job, brush for about three to four minutes.

Flossing
- Flossing is very important because it removes plaque that you can't reach with your toothbrush.
- Flossing every day helps your gums remain healthy and prevents tartar from forming. Tartar is like hardened plaque. You can't remove it yourself. Only your dentist or hygienist can do it.

How to Floss Properly
- Take about 40 to 50 cm (16 to 20 inches) of floss (about the length between your hand and your shoulder).

- Wrap each end around your middle fingers, leaving about 8 to 10 cm (3 to 4 inches) between your hands.
- Hold the floss between your thumb and index finger of each hand, leaving about 2.5 to 5 cm (1 to 2 inches) in between.
- To clean the teeth of the lower jaw, the index fingers of both hands guide the floss between the teeth.
- For the upper jaw, the index finger of one hand and the thumb of the other will guide the floss. *Never* snap the floss into the gums.
- Slide the floss between your teeth and when the floss reaches the gum line, wrap it into a "C" shape around the tooth and move it *gently* under the gum line.
- Holding the floss tightly against the tooth, glide it up and down two or three times.
- Floss both sides of each tooth. Don't forget the back of your last upper and lower molars.
- Change to a new section of the floss as it wears.
- For a better result, brush your teeth *after* flossing.

Mouth Rinses
If your dentist prescribes a mouth rinse for you called Chlorhexidine (Peridex®), this is how you should use it:
- Brush your teeth carefully.
- Rinse your mouth well with water to remove any toothpaste that is still in your mouth.
- Measure the amount of mouth rinse prescribed.
- Swish it in your mouth for 30 seconds, then spit it out.
- Repeat these steps as often as your dentist recommends.
- Do not use it for more than the number of days your dentist recommended. It can cause dark stains on your teeth and fillings if you use it too long.

Chapter 59

Periodontal Conditions

Michelle Bourassa, BPharm, MSc, DMD

Pathophysiology

Periodontal disease includes any pathologic process involving the periodontium (tissues supporting the teeth, including the cementum, periodontal ligament, alveolar bone and gingiva – see Figure 1, Chapter 57). Bacterial irritation is now recognized as the primary cause of periodontal disease. Dental plaque is a prerequisite, and many local or systemic factors[1-7] influence the inflammatory response of the peridontium to plaque. Examples of local factors include:

- Anatomic factors (e.g., root morphology, position of tooth in arch, root proximity)
- Iatrogenic factors (e.g., dental procedures, restorative material, dentures)
- Traumatic injury (e.g., toothbrush abrasion, food impaction, fingernail scratch, orthodontics)
- Chemical injury (e.g., ASA tablets applied to the gum)[2]
- Smoking

Systemic factors can include:
- Aging
- Endocrine imbalance
- Hematologic disorder
- Emotional or psychological stress
- Medications
- Nutritional deficiencies
- Genetic disorders
- Neoplasms, leukemia, multiple myeloma

Pathogenesis of Periodontal Disease[4,8]

Plaque accumulates at the gingival or supragingival level. If not disrupted, it matures microbiologically, and an inflammatory reaction can be initiated. The tissue reaction produces intermediate products that serve as nutrients for gram-negative anaerobic bacteria. Concomitantly, the inflammation and bacterial enzymes increase tissue permeability, allowing high molecular weight products from the bacteria to penetrate the superficial tissues. Eventually, a balance between the bacterial challenge and the host responses is achieved, resulting in a chronic inflammatory process known as gingivitis.

Little is known about what causes the shift from stable, chronic gingivitis to periodontitis. The induction and progression of periodontitis most likely involves disruption in the balance between the bacteria and the host defences. The bacterial population may change, or host defences could be transiently or permanently altered by such things as psychological stress, viral infection or smoking.

In the chronic state, microorganisms such as *P. gingivalis, P. intermedia, B. forsythus,* and *F. nucleatum* are found, as well as many others. These bacteria produce factors that may be responsible for tissue destruction and alteration of host defences. Clinical signs of the disease may be partially explained by the normal inflammatory and immune processes detected in the periodontal tissues. The accumulation of bacteria induces the entry of chemotactic products into the tissue, which stimulates the migration of inflammatory and immune cells (e.g., polymorphonuclear cells, macrophages and lymphocytes).

There appears to be local control of the response based on the antibody patterns. After prolonged exposure to endotoxins, the protective effect of the antibodies tends to decline. Dental interventions such as scaling and root planing have been shown to reactivate the antibodies and provide better protection. Enzymes such as collagenases from the polymorphonuclear cells and fibroblasts, along with inflammatory mediators (e.g., interleukin-1-β and prostaglandin E_2) may be potentially destructive to the connective tissues and bone. When inflammation is allowed to become chronic, the epithelial cells in the junctional epithelium tend to migrate toward the apex.

Prevalence

Gingivitis

The prevalence and severity of gingivitis vary significantly with age.[5] In young children, the gingiva around the deciduous teeth seems to be resistant to plaque-induced inflammation. The results of an Australian study in children showed a high prevalence of mild inflammation and a poor correlation between oral hygiene and the severity of inflammation. Those findings may be explained by a difference in the intensity of the immunologic response or in the microbial flora of the gingival fluid.[9]

From the age of five or six years to puberty, gingivitis is reported very frequently. In fact, chronic gingivitis has been found in 80% of children under the age of 12 and in almost 100% at the age of 14. The incidence of inflammation peaks at around age 12 for girls and age 14 for boys. At puberty it seems that the gingival tissue reacts more severely to plaque deposition than after puberty.[9]

In a group of teens (15 to 19 years of age), 79% of subjects showed some gingival inflammation. The prevalence of gingivitis was 54% in the group aged 19 to 44 and declined to 44% at age 45 to 64 and to 36% in subjects of 65 years of age. In most cases the gingivitis was limited to a few teeth.[9,10]

In western countries, acute necrotizing ulcerative gingivitis is usually seen in the 16 to 30 age group. It has a low prevalence in rich countries and a higher one in poorer countries, often affecting malnourished children.[9]

Periodontitis

In children, periodontal disease is often associated with systemic conditions such as juvenile diabetes mellitus, Down's syndrome and many others. Juvenile periodontitis, a form of aggressive periodontitis, was found in 1.5% of Black and 0.3% of Caucasian children under the age 15. Amongst the Caucasian children the ratio of males to females was 1:4 and in the other group it was 1:1.[9]

In the 15- to 19-year-old group, the more prevalent condition was the presence of calculus with or without gingival bleeding. It was encountered much more often in the non-industrialized countries.[9]

The WHO global Oral Dental Bank, based on data from over 50 countries, looked at the prevalence of periodontitis in the age groups 35 to 44 and 45 to 74 years. It was found that the most frequent condition observed (5 to 20%) was calculus and shallow pocketing. The mean number of deep pockets per person was small and had a tendency to increase with age.[10]

In a study conducted in 1989 in the American population, Brown reported that 29% of people aged 19 to 44 years and almost 50% of people of 45 years and older had at least one site affected. Periodontitis was diagnosed in about 50% of the elderly.[10] Moderate periodontits was found in 28% of the general population and 8% had advanced disease. As age increased, the prevalence of both conditions increased. Moderate periodontitis was diagnosed in 28% of people between 19 and 44 years of age and in 44% of people 45 years or older. Advanced disease occurred in 3% of the < 45 years group and in 15% in the group 45 years or older.[10]

Risk Factors

Both prevalence and severity of periodontal disease increase with age and it seems to become clinically significant in the fourth decade of life.[5,9] For all age groups, the disease seems to be 1.5 times more prevalent in men than in women. The Black population had twice the risk of having pockets, compared to the Caucasian population.[10] Socioeconomic status is also a contributing factor, since pockets and loss of attachment are seen in a higher percentage of people with less than a Grade 12 education and in people with a lower income.[4,10,11] Genetic variation may explain why in equal age groups, the transition from gingivitis to periodontitis appears to be earlier and more severe in the Asian population than in the European population.[5,9] Studies estimate the risk for periodontitis in a smoker to be 2.5 to 7.0 times greater than in nonsmokers.[4]

It is difficult to reliably predict who will progress from gingivitis to periodontitis. Considerable variations have been found in the clinical presentation and the rates of disease progression of chronic periodontitis.[9]

Goals of Therapy

- Prevent progression of periodontal disease

- Restore and maintain optimal gingival and periodontal health
- Motivate the patient to maintain a rigorous oral hygiene routine

Patient Assessment

Periodontal disease is assessed and managed by dentists and dental hygienists. Other health care professionals can support their role in preventing periodontal disease by encouraging patients to maintain good oral hygiene and to see their dentist regularly. The recommended frequency varies according to the needs of each patient, but is never less than once yearly.

Gingivitis[12-15]

Gingivitis is defined as inflammation of the gingiva. There are many subtypes of gingivitis (Figure 1), but they share the following characteristics:

Figure 1: **Classification of Periodontal Diseases**[14]

---

1. Gingival Diseases
   - a. Dental plaque-induced gingival diseases
     - i.   Gingivitis associated with dental plaque only
     - ii. Gingival diseases modified by systemic factors
       - 1- Associated with the endocrine system
       - 2- Associated with blood dyscrasias
     - iii. Gingival diseases modified by medications
       - 1- Gingival hyperplasia (cyclosporine, phenytoin, calcium channel blockers)
       - 2- Oral contraceptive-associated gingivitis
     - iv. Gingival diseases modified by malnutrition
   - b. Non-plaque-induced gingival lesions
     - i.   Gingival diseases of specific bacterial origin
     - ii.   Gingival diseases of viral origin
     - iii. Gingival diseases of fungal origin
     - iv.   Gingival lesions of genetic origin
     - v.   Gingival manifestations of systemic conditions
       - 1- Mucocutaneous disorders
       - 2- Allergic reactions
     - vi.   Traumatic lesions
     - vii. Foreign body reactions
     - viii. Not otherwise specified

2. Chronic periodontitis*

3. Aggressive periodontitis*

4. Periodontitis as a manifestation of systemic disease
   - a. Associated with hematological disorders
   - b. Associated with genetic disorders
   - c. Not otherwise specified

5. Necrotizing periodontal diseases
   - a. Necrotizing ulcerative gingivitis
   - b. Necrotizing ulcerative periodontitis

6. Abscesses of the periodontium
   - a. Gingival abscess
   - b. Periodontal abscess
   - c. Pericoronal abscess (see Chapter 57)

7. Periodontitis associated with endodontic lesions

8. Developmental or acquired deformities and conditions
   - a. Localized tooth-related factors that modify or predispose to plaque-induced gingival diseases/periodontitis
   - b. Mucogingival deformities and conditions around teeth
   - b. Mucogingival deformities and conditions on edentulous ridges
   - d. Occlusal trauma

---

*May be generalized or localized.

- Discoloration of gingival tissue (red or red-blue);
- Signs of inflammation such as:
  —bleeding on brushing or gentle probing
  —swelling, puffiness
  —loss of stippling of the gingival (surface becomes smoother)
  —loss of gingival tone
  —firm and leathery texture of the gingival tissue
- The gingival margin is located at or coronal to the cementoenamel junction. Pseudo-pockets may be encountered if swelling or hyperplasia is present;
- Probing depths are between 1 and 3 mm or more if swelling is present (Figure 2);
- Pain is uncommon.

Periodontitis[11,13,16]

Periodontitis involves progression of gingivitis to include apical migration of the junctional epithelium, attachment loss, loss of bone and pocketing. The usual clinical findings are:

- Discoloration of gingival tissue (red or red-blue), or it may appear normal;
- Signs of inflammation such as:
  —bleeding on brushing or probing
  —smooth, shiny gingival surface
  —loss of stippling of the gingiva
  —suppuration on occasion
  —exposed root surface(s)
- The gingival margin may be located anywhere relative to the cementoenamel junction;
- Probing depths are in the range of 4 mm or more (Figure 2);
- Occasional pain.

Nonpharmacologic Therapy

Gingivitis[11,17-19]

By far, the most common form of gingivitis is plaque-induced gingivitis. The other forms of gingivitis are very rare and specialized references could be consulted for more information.

Plaque control is the gold standard of treatment for gingivitis induced by dental plaque.

Periodontitis[11,12,17,20]

Periodontitis is treated by dental professionals. Most periodontal diseases can be successfully arrested if the treatment plan can achieve the following objectives:

- Removal of the causative factors;
- Reduction or elimination of all pockets and establishment of a normal sulcus depth;
- Restoration of physiologic gingival and bone architecture;
- Establishment of a functional occlusion by occlusal adjustment and restorative procedure;
- Maintenance of periodontal health through adequate plaque control by the patient, and regular visits to the dentist for close follow-up and early intervention, in case of recurrence.

The following interventions may be required to achieve the previous objectives:

Phase I

- Scaling and root planing
- Removal of overhanging restorations and other plaque retentive areas
- Extraction of tooth or teeth
- Preliminary occlusal adjustment (selective grinding of teeth to establish a stable bite) and odontoplasty (modification of tooth contours)
- Patient motivation and instruction in proper oral hygiene procedures
- Evaluation of the results

Phase II

- Surgical treatment. This phase includes all procedures designed to reduce or eliminate pockets by resecting or relocating the gingival margin. It may also include the correction of mucogingival defects and the placement of dental implants.

Phase III

- Restorative treatment. When indicated, this step involves completion of occlusal adjustment, operative dentistry, replacement of missing tooth or teeth by fixed and/or removable prostheses and permanent splinting.

Phase IV

- Maintenance treatment. Patients must continue maintenance therapy for their lifetime. Patients who have been diagnosed with moderate to advanced periodontitis may require maintenance recalls as often as every three months. The interval between recall appointments is dictated by the level of disease control achieved by the patient at home.

Figure 2: **Progressive Changes in Periodontal Conditions**

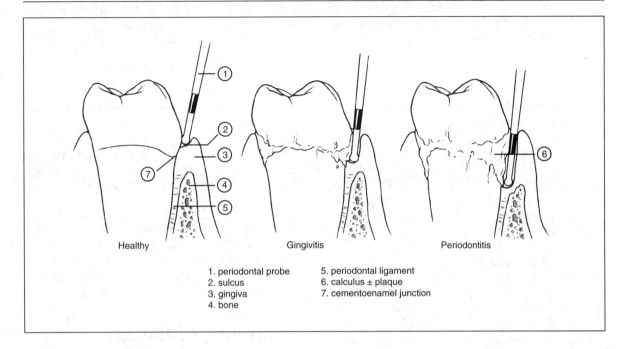

Healthy   Gingivitis   Periodontitis

1. periodontal probe   5. periodontal ligament
2. sulcus   6. calculus ± plaque
3. gingiva   7. cementoenamel junction
4. bone

Pharmacologic Therapy

Gingivitis

If plaque control cannot be achieved manually (due to lack of dexterity, for example) or in systemically compromised or post-op patients, topical antimicrobial products may be used as an adjunct to regular plaque control measures. The Canadian Dental Association has approved several mouth rinses to help in plaque control and gingivitis reduction. More information about these products, as well as information for patients on proper brushing, flossing and use of chlorhexidine mouth rinse, can be found in Chapter 58.

Periodontitis

Dental Office Procedures

The effectiveness of scaling and root planing may be slightly increased when combined with irrigation of the crevice with a antimicrobial agent such as chlorhexidine. Povidone-iodine (Betadine®) has also been used as irrigation solution.[21,22] Staining of the tooth may result from its use. Iodine derivatives are contraindicated in pregnant or nursing women, in patients with sensitivity to iodine and those with susceptibility to hypothyroidism.[23]

Chlorine-releasing agents (e.g., sodium hypochlorite, chlorine dioxide, chloramines-T) have also been employed in periodontal therapy. Their effectiveness remains to be determined. For irrigation at home, patients may have to use a diluted chlorine solution (0.1% or less) depending upon taste tolerance.[23]

Topical Antibacterials

As an adjunct to tooth brushing and flossing, some authors recommend the use of chlorhexidine mouth rinse to reduce the salivary levels of periodontal pathogens. Chlorhexidine has shown broad-spectrum efficacy, good adherence to tooth surfaces and oral mucosa, and a low irritation potential. This mouth rinse should be used under the supervision of a dentist and for a limited period of time, due to the potential for reversible staining of the teeth and irreversible staining of fillings associated with prolonged use.[19,21,22,24,25] Information for the patient on proper use of chlorhexidine mouth rinse can be found in Chapter 58.

Triclosan has shown moderate in vivo efficacy and is available as a toothpaste and as a pre-brushing rinse. *Sanguinaria canadensis*, available as a toothpaste, has demonstrated moderate efficacy in plaque and gingivitis reduction in short- and long-term studies. The best results were obtained when the two were combined.[19,26]

Anti-infective agents may also be placed subgingivally in vehicles that will allow slow release of the agent into the periodontal pocket. Agents studied include chlorhexidine chips[27], tetracycline fibres, doxycycline gel[28], minocycline gel and metronidazole gel. Of these, only doxycycline gel is currently available in Canada (Atridox®). Studies have shown little benefit when these products were used as adjuncts to mechanical therapy. They are not recommended as single therapy.[11,19,26]

Systemic Antibacterials

Patients with plaque-induced gingivitis or chronic periodontitis usually respond well to mechanical periodontal therapy and little or no additional benefit is expected from the use of any antiinfective agent. However, some patients may benefit from the use of systemic antibacterial therapy.[21,29] The addition of an antimicrobial agent should be used as a complement to mechanical periodontal treatment. Its goal is to support host defences in overcoming the infection by destroying subgingival microorganisms remaining after local treatment. The best candidates are patients with continuing loss of periodontal attachment despite appropriate local therapy, refractory periodontitis, early onset periodontitis, medical conditions predisposing to periodontitis, or acute or severe periodontal infections (e.g., periodontal abscess, acute necrotizing gingivitis/periodontitis).[21,29]

Unfortunately, only a few studies have examined selection of an agent, and the dosage regimens have been established empirically rather than through systematic research. Therefore, the optimal agent and dosage regimen, especially for refractory periodontitis, remain unclear.

The adult oral dosages of antibacterials commonly prescribed for treatment of periodontitis are presented in Table 1.[6,29]

Antibacterial regimens recommended for acute periodontal abscesses are:
Amoxicillin: Oral loading dose of 1.0 g followed by a maintenance dose of 500 mg three times daily for three days, followed by a patient evaluation to determine whether further antibiotic therapy or dosage adjustment is required.

For patients with allergy to beta-lactam antibacterials: Azithromycin: Oral loading dose 1.0 g on day 1, followed by 500 mg once daily on days 2 and 3; *or* Clindamycin: Oral loading dose of 600 mg, followed by 300 mg four times daily for three days.

Monitoring of Therapy

Encourage patients with gingivitis who are attempting to prevent progression to periodontitis and even eliminate their gingivitis to adhere to their dentist's recommended oral hygiene regimen. Encourage patients who are undergoing treatment for periodontitis to keep their scheduled dental appointments and to adhere to prescribed therapy. Pharmacists can monitor the patient's use of chlorhexidine mouth rinse to help avoid staining due to prolonged usage.

Information for the Patient

See Chapter 58.

Table 1: **Antibacterial Regimens for Periodontitis**[6,29]

Drug	Dose
Ciprofloxacin	500 mg twice daily for 8 days
Metronidazole	500 mg three times daily for 8 days
Metronidazole plus amoxicillin	250 mg of each three times daily for 8 days
Metronidazole plus ciprofloxacin	500 mg of each twice daily for 8 days
Tetracycline	500 mg three times daily for 21 days

Resource Tips

Canadian Dental Association:
http://www.cda-adc.ca

Suggested Readings

Cummings D. Vehicles: how to deliver the goods. *Periodontol 2000* 1997;15:55-62.

Flemmig TF. Periodontitis. *Ann Periodontol* 1999;4: 32-7.

Jones CG. Chlorhexidine: is it still the gold standard? *Periodontol 2000* 1997;15:55-62.

Jorgensen MG, Slots J. Practical Antimicrobial Periodontal Therapy. *Compendium* 2000;21(2):111-22.

Kinane DF. Causation and pathogenesis of periodontal disease. *Periodontol 2000* 2001;25:8-20.

References

1. Vernino AR. Etiology of Periodontal Disease. In: Fedi PF, Vernino AR, Gray JL, eds. *The Periodontic Syllabus* 4th ed. Baltimore, MD: Lippincott Williams & Wilkins, 2000:14-21.
2. Rees T. Systemic Contributing Factors. In: Fedi PF, Vernino AR, Gray JL, eds. *The Periodontic Syllabus* 4th ed. Baltimore, MD: Lippincott Williams & Wilkins, 2000:22-31.
3. Manson JD, Eley BM. The effect of systemic factors on the periodontal tissues. In: Manson JD, Eley BM, eds. *Outline of Periodontics* 4th ed. Oxford, UK: Wright, 2000:187-202.
4. Kinane DF. Causation and pathogenesis of periodontal disease. *Periodontology 2000* 2001;25:8-20.
5. Tessier JF, Baehni PC. Epidémiologie et étiologie des maladies parodontales. In: Bercy P, Tenenbaum H, eds. *Parodontologie, Du Diagnostic à la pratique.* Paris: De Boek & Larcier;1996:25-35.
6. Oringer RJ, Williams RC. Assessment and management of periodontal infections: a medical-surgical approach. *Compendium* 2000 Oct:21(10A):906-18.
7. McLeod DE. A practical approach to the diagnosis and treatment of periodontal disease. *JADA* 2000 April;131:483-91.
8. Kornman KS. The pathogenesis of periodontal diseases: An Overview. Wilson TG, Kornman KS, eds. *Fundamentals of periodontics.* Chicago, IL: Quintessence Publishing Co, Inc. 1996:1-45.
9. Manson JD, Eley BM. Epidemiology of pariodontal disease (the size of the problem). In: Manson JD, Eley BM, eds. *Outline of Periodontics* 4th ed. Oxford, UK: Wright, 2000:119-31.
10. Brown LJ, Löe H, Prevalence, extent, severity and progression of periodontal disease. *Periodontology 2000* 1993;2, 57-71.
11. Research, Science and Therapy Committee of The American Academy of Periodontology. Position Paper. Treatment of Gingivitis and Periodontitis. *J Periodontol* 1997;68:1246-53.
12. Wilson TG, Kornman KS. The Periodontium in Health and Disease. In:. Wilson TG, Kornman KS, eds. *Fundamentals of periodontics.* Chicago, IL: Quintessence Publishing Co, Inc., 1996:281-3.
13. Gray J. Plaque-Related Periodontal Diseases: Pathogenesis. In: Fedi PF, Vernino AR, Gray JL, eds. *The Periodontic Syllabus* 4th ed. Baltimore, MD: Lippincott Williams & Wilkins, 2000:31-40.
14. Mariotti A, Dental Plaque-Induced Gingival Diseases. *Ann Periodontol* 1999;4:7-17.
15. Tenenbaum H. Classification des maladies parodontales. In: Bercy P, Tenenbaum H, eds. *Parodontologie, Du Diagnostic à la pratique.* Paris: De Boek & Larcier;1996:49-64.
16. Fleming TF. Periodontitis. *Ann Periodontol* 1999;4:32-7.
17. Pihlstrom BL. Periodontal risk assessment, diagnosis and treatment planning. *Periodontology 2000* 2001;25:37-58.
18. Jackson RJ. Metal salts, essential oils and phenols – old or new? *Periodontology 2000* 1997;(15):52-4.
19. Wilson TG. Kornman KS. Treating Plaque-Associated Gingivitis. In: Wilson TG, Kornman KS, eds. *Fundamentals of periodontics.* Chicago, IL: Quintessence Publishing Co, Inc., 1996:319-47.
20. Gray J. Host Defenses and Periodontal Disease. In: Fedi PF, Vernino AR, Gray JL. *The Periodontic Syllabus* 4th ed. Baltimore, MD: Lippincott Williams & Wilkins, 2000:51-69.
21. Slots J, Jorgensen MG. Efficient antimicrobial treatment in periodontal maintenance care. *JADA* 2000 Sept;131: 1293-1304.
22. Jorgensen MG, Slots J. Practical antimicrobial periodontal therapy. *Compendium* 2000;21(2):111-22.
23. Slots J. Primer for antimicrobial periodontal therapy. *J Periodontal Res* 2000;35(2):108-14.
24. Jones CG. Chlorhexidine: is it still the gold standard? *Periodontology 2000* 1997;15:55-62.
25. Addy M, Moran JM. Clinical indications for the use of chemical adjuncts to plaque control: chlorhexidine formulations. *Periodontology 2000* 1997;15:52-4.
26. Cummings D. Vehicles: how to deliver the goods. *Periodontology 2000* 1997;15:55-62.
27. Ciancio SG. Local delivery of chlorhexidine. *Compendium* 1999;20(5):427-32.
28. Garrett S. Local delivery of doxycycline for the treatment of periodontitis. *Compendium* 1999;20(5):437-46.
29. Research, Science and Therapy Committee of The American Academy of Periodontology. Position Paper. Systemic Antibiotics in Periodontitis. *J Periodontol* 1996;67:831-8.

Chapter 60

Dental Conditions

Michelle Bourassa, BPharm, MSc, DMD

Patient Assessment (Figure 1)
Dentin Hypersensitivity[1-3]
Pathophysiology

The dentin is composed of tubules containing fluid that is in contact with the pulp (see Figure 1, Chapter 57). External stimuli disturb the fluid content or cause movement, which stimulates the nociceptive receptors in the pulp and leads to the perception of pain.

Dentin hypersensitivity is characterized by a transient pain in response to different types of stimuli such as chemical (e.g., acid), thermal (e.g., cold or hot drinks or food, exposure to air), mechanical (e.g., toothbrush, probe, fingernails) or osmotic (e.g., sugar, gel) when applied to exposed dentin. This condition may be the result of root denudation (exposure) due to gingival recession from toothbrush abrasion, periodontal disease or surgery, erosion or abfraction (a noncarious lesion occurring at the cementoenamel junction on the lingual or buccal side of the tooth).

Dentin hypersensitivity is associated with no pathological lesion. Rather, it is an exaggerated response to stimuli that would provoke no symptoms in a healthy tooth. The pain may be characterized as sharp, of rapid onset and short duration.

Between 8.7 and 30% of adults experience dentin hypersensitivity. The sites most often affected are the buccal surfaces of the canines and premolars (see Figure 2, Chapter 57). Significant gingival recession is seen in 68% of cases of hypersensitive teeth, and most of the remaining cases are associated with gingival abrasion or erosion. This condition is encountered more often in young individuals with root exposure due to rapid gingival recession.

Therapy[1,4,5]

Treatment of dentin hypersensitivity is aimed at chemical or physical blockade of the patent dentinal tubules to prevent movement of the fluid inside. Physical techniques may involve application of fluoride varnishes, sealants, resins, glass ionomer cements or soft tissue grafts. Chemical desensitization involves blocking pulpal nociceptor activity or occluding the tubules with a protein precipitate, a crystallized oxalate deposit or potassium formulations.

Desensitizing toothpastes exert their effect by the latter mechanism (i.e., chemically). They are the mainstay of treatment of this condition.

The patient may be prescribed desensitizing toothpaste to use along with a soft or ultra-soft toothbrush. The toothpaste may contain as active ingredients: potassium salt(s), strontium salts or stannous fluoride. Among the commercially available products, several have received the Canadian Dental Association (CDA) seal of approval (e.g., Sensodyne F®, Gel Kam®, Crest Sensitivity Protection®). The dentist may also apply highly concentrated fluoride preparations (varnishes or solutions) or oxalate salt preparations. In resistant or recurrent cases, the dentist may employ physical techniques to achieve a fast and more sustained resolution of the pain.

If pain persists for longer than four weeks, a dentist should be consulted.[6]

Cracked Tooth Syndrome[1,2,5]

For illustration of tooth anatomy, see Figure 1, Chapter 57.

Figure 1: **Assessment of Patients with Dental Conditions**

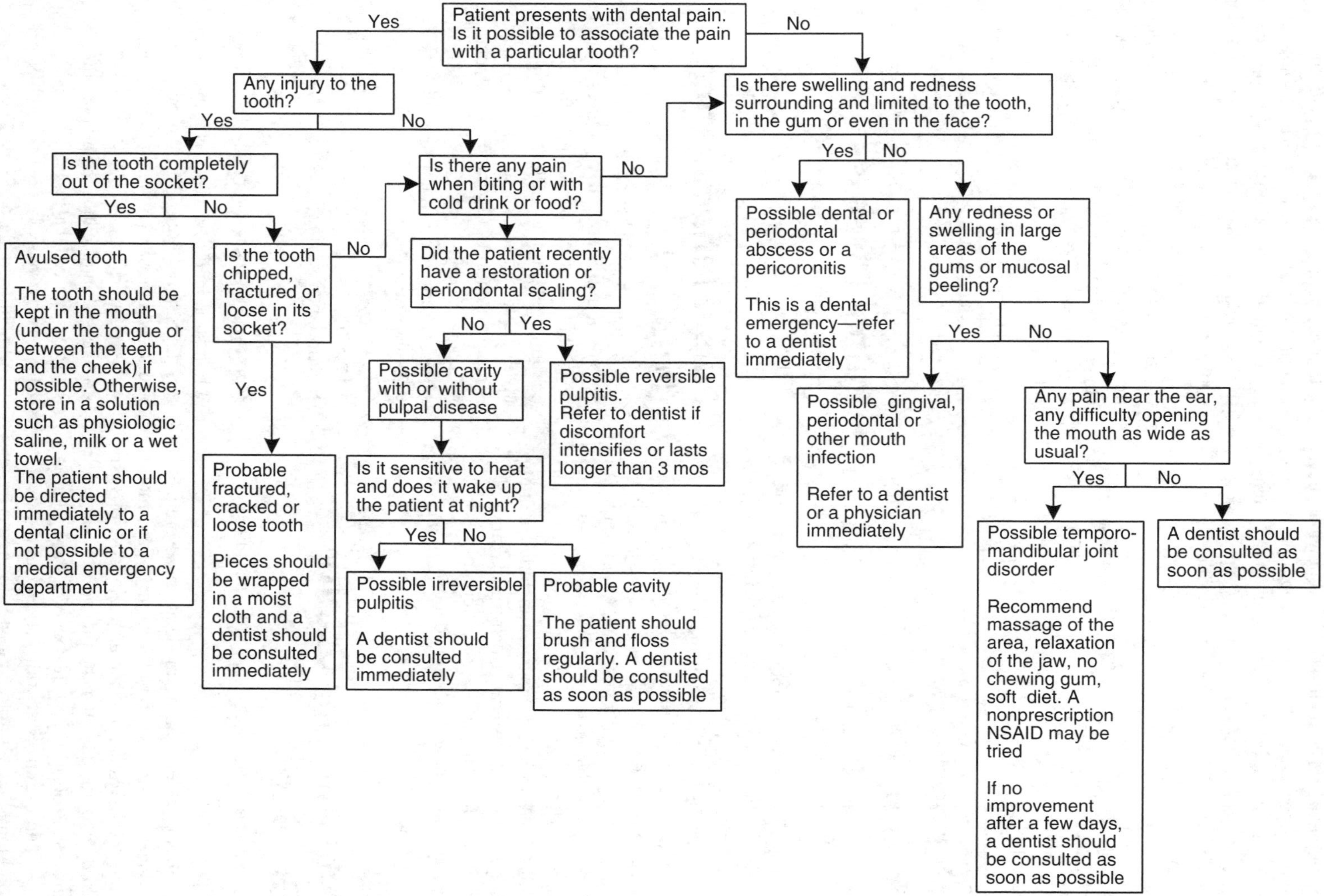

Patient presents with dental pain. Is it possible to associate the pain with a particular tooth?

Any injury to the tooth?

No → Is there swelling and redness surrounding and limited to the tooth, in the gum or even in the face?

Yes → Any injury?

Is the tooth completely out of the socket?

Yes → Avulsed tooth

The tooth should be kept in the mouth (under the tongue or between the teeth and the cheek) if possible. Otherwise, store in a solution such as physiologic saline, milk or a wet towel.
The patient should be directed immediately to a dental clinic or if not possible to a medical emergency department

No → Is the tooth chipped, fractured or loose in its socket?

Yes → Probable fractured, cracked or loose tooth

Pieces should be wrapped in a moist cloth and a dentist should be consulted immediately

No → Is there any pain when biting or with cold drink or food?

Did the patient recently have a restoration or periondontal scaling?

Yes → Possible reversible pulpitis.
Refer to dentist if discomfort intensifies or lasts longer than 3 mos

No → Possible cavity with or without pulpal disease

Is it sensitive to heat and does it wake up the patient at night?

Yes → Possible irreversible pulpitis

A dentist should be consulted immediately

No → Probable cavity

The patient should brush and floss regularly. A dentist should be consulted as soon as possible

Is there swelling and redness surrounding and limited to the tooth, in the gum or even in the face?

Yes → Possible dental or periodontal abscess or a pericoronitis

This is a dental emergency—refer to a dentist immediately

No → Any redness or swelling in large areas of the gums or mucosal peeling?

Yes → Possible gingival, periodontal or other mouth infection

Refer to a dentist or a physician immediately

No → Any pain near the ear, any difficulty opening the mouth as wide as usual?

Yes → Possible temporo-mandibular joint disorder

Recommend massage of the area, relaxation of the jaw, no chewing gum, soft diet. A nonprescription NSAID may be tried

If no improvement after a few days, a dentist should be consulted as soon as possible

No → A dentist should be consulted as soon as possible

Sharp, momentary pain on mastication (chewing) may be felt by the patient with a cracked tooth. A cracked tooth can occur as a result of trauma, extensive filling, or in an intact tooth with an opposing cusp occluding against a marginal ridge. The pain may originate from the pulp or the periodontum. The usual stimulus is biting.

Cracked teeth may be treated by various restorative techniques. Vertically fractured teeth usually require extraction. The prognosis depends on the type and the extent of the crack.

Postendodontic Discomfort[1,7]

For illustration of tooth anatomy, see Figure 1, Chapter 57.

Discomfort following endodontic treatment (root canal) is frequent. The apical extrusion of debris produced during the procedure leads to apical periodontitis. Usually the pain is mild and requires no medication, or can be relieved by mild analgesics (e.g., acetaminophen, ibuprofen). The discomfort generally subsides within a few days. On occasion, an acute periapical abscess may occur, causing swelling and pain. The patient should consult a dentist immediately. Appropriate treatment includes draining the abscess through the canal or by incision, and a prescription for an NSAID or a combination of analgesics. An antibacterial should be considered if systemic signs of infection are present.

Acute Alveolar Osteitis ("Dry Socket")[1,8]

For illustration of tooth anatomy, see Figure 1, Chapter 57.

Acute alveolar osteitis causes moderate to severe pain, occurring as a complication of a surgical third molar (wisdom tooth) extraction. Pain generally develops on the third or fourth day after the procedure. The healing process is delayed and the bone of the socket is exposed and extremely sensitive. The pain is usually dull and throbbing and often radiates to the ear. The extraction site may have a foul odor and impart a bad taste in the patient's mouth. The etiology is not completely understood but increased fibrinolytic activity at the surgical site is suspected. The patient should consult a dentist as soon as possible if this presentation arises. Treatment generally consists of gentle irrigation of the site with normal saline followed by the insertion of iodoform gauze soaked with either eugenol or benzocaine, for pain relief. The dressing is changed every day for three to six days until the pain subsides.

Even without intervention, the patient would not have any sequelae other than pain throughout the healing period.[8]

Pulpal Diseases

For illustration of tooth anatomy, see Figure 1, Chapter 57.

Pulpal Inflammation (Pulpitis)

This condition usually manifests initially as reversible pulpitis; if untreated it may progress to an irreversible pulpitis. The reversible form is the most commonly encountered and a variety of etiologies may be involved. Reversibility may be preserved if the cause is rapidly removed. Common causes include:[2,5]

- Caries
- Recent restoration (filling)
- Faulty restorations
- Trauma
- Exposed tubules
- Periodontal scaling

Pathophysiology[1,4]

When submitted to a noxious stimulus, an inflammatory reaction is induced in the pulp with the classic manifestations of:

- Vasodilation
- Increased intracellular tissue pressure
- Increase in cellular infiltrates
- Increased levels of mediators such as prostaglandins and neuropeptides

Although initially reversible (enough reparative cells remain in the pulp to allow recovery), the condition could continue to degenerate and endodontic therapy may be necessary to stop the process.[2]

The main symptom of *reversible pulpitis* is sensitivity or mild pain of brief duration after stimulation with cold, sweets and sometimes heat. The pain subsides upon removal of the stimulus. There is no spontaneous pain nor pain on biting. Usually a cause can be identified on dental examination.

With *irreversible pulpitis*, the pain may be more prolonged after the initial stimulus and it can occur spontaneously. Irreversible pulpitis results from significant pulpal injury (e.g., from caries, trauma or cumulative effect of multiple restorations) and does not respond to removal of the causative factor.[2,5] The type of insult and the patient's age are important factors that affect whether the pulp can recover. With aging, the ability of the pulp to repair itself diminishes.

Therapy[1,2,5]

The treatment of reversible pulpitis is based on correcting the cause. If the symptoms result from a recent restoration or periodontal scaling, reassure the patient that the discomfort should diminish and disappear over a period of up to three months. Symptomatic treatment may be offered (e.g., a desensitizing toothpaste) and symptoms should be monitored. If the discomfort intensifies or lasts longer than 3 months, refer the patient to a dentist.

Caries should be treated by removing the decay and placing a filling to occlude the dentinal tubules (see Figure 1, Chapter 57). If the cavity is extensive, the pulp may be exposed when removing the decay and if it is carious, the pulpitis is classified as irreversible and a root canal is the treatment of choice.

A root canal involves mechanical and biochemical debridement and treatment of the canal system of a tooth, to eliminate pulpal and periapical diseases. In some cases, extraction may be necessary. Pain is usually controlled with nonprescription analgesics (e.g., acetaminophen or ibuprofen) or prescription NSAIDs.[1,2]

Necrotic Pulp
Pathophysiology

For illustration of tooth anatomy, see Figure 1, Chapter 57.

This condition may result from degeneration of an inflamed pulp, with the same causes as those identified for irreversible pulpitis. In this case, the reparative potential of the pulp is totally absent and the pulp lacks viable tissue. Inflammation of the periapical tissue may be associated with necrotic pulp.[2,5]

Often, the history includes a previous episode of symptoms related to irreversible pulpitis. When it is necrotic, the pulp does not respond to stimuli such as cold or heat. The patient may feel some spontaneous dull and throbbing pain that worsens when the patient is lying down or that is stimulated by biting. The latter suggests an inflammation of the periapical tissues.[2,4]

Therapy

The appropriate treatment options are extraction or endodontic therapy (root canal). An NSAID or mild analgesic may be prescribed by the dentist for a few days for possible postoperative pain or discomfort.[2]

Periapical Diseases
Acute Apical Periodontitis
Pathophysiology

This condition defines a moderate to severe inflammatory process of the periodontal tissues located near the apex of a tooth (see Figure 1, Chapter 57). Although it is most frequently associated with a pulpal condition (reversibly or irreversibly inflamed or necrotic pulp), other nonpulpal causes have been identified such as trauma or bruxism (grinding or clenching the upper and lower teeth together, often while sleeping). The periapical tissues show a marked inflammatory response with vasodilation and polymorphonuclear lymphocyte infiltration.[2,7]

Therapy

The appropriate treatment options are extraction or endodontic therapy. If endodontic treatment is chosen, canal debridement and drainage should be performed by a dentist on an emergency basis. Generally, the drainage provides partial to complete relief of the pain. Some discomfort may persist for a few days and a mild analgesic or an NSAID may suffice. In some cases opioids may be required, but they should be used for a short period of time. If swelling increases, incision and drainage may be required. If extraoral swelling occurs, the patient should consult a dentist immediately. If a dentist is not available, refer to a physician. An antibiotic (e.g., penicillin V, clindamycin or a combination of metronidazole and amoxicillin, erythromycin or clarithromycin) should be prescribed.[2,7] The infection may spread through the surrounding tissues and structures or disseminate, and serious complications may arise. Severe cases have required extraoral drainage of pus.[9]

Chronic Apical Periodontitis
Pathophysiology

Also called granuloma, this condition results from an apical inflammation with a low-grade, long-standing response to canal bacteria and irritants. It is usually asymptomatic and is evidenced by an apical radiolucency on X-ray. The cause is generally necrotic pulp, but it may be associated with other conditions including central giant cell granuloma or cemental dysplasia.[7]

The patient may be completely asymptomatic and unaware of the problem or may experience some mild sensitivity on biting or percussion (the dentist may test by tapping on the tooth).[7]

Therapy

The same treatment modalities as for necrotic pulp are indicated (i.e., extraction or root canal). Analgesics may be indicated to relieve some potential postprocedural discomfort, but antibiotics are usually not indicated.[7]

Suppurative Apical Periodontitis

This condition refers to an apical lesion that has established drainage through a sinus tract.[7,10] The patient may report a "gumboil" or a foul taste in the mouth. Gentle pressure on the gum may expel pus from the fistula.[7,10] Suppurative apical periodontitis shares the same causes and treatment modalities (e.g., extraction or root canal) as for chronic apical periodontitis.

Suggested Readings

Bender IB. Pulpal pain diagnosis – a review. *Journal of Endodontics* 2000;26(3):175-9.

Cailleteau JC. Diagnosis and Management of Toothaches of Dental Origin. In: Falace DA, ed. *Emergency Dental Care, Diagnosis and Management of Urgent Dental Problems.* Malvern, PA: Williams and Wilkins, 1995:25-66.

Simon JHS. Periapical Pathology. In: Cohen S, Burns RC, eds. *Pathways of the Pulp.* 7th ed. St. Louis, MI: Mosby Inc, 199:425-62.

References

1. Holland GR. Management of Dental Pain. In: Lund JP, Lavigne GJ, Dubner R, Sessle BJ, eds. *Orafacial Pain From Basic Science to Clinical Management.* Chicago, IL: Quintessence Publishing Co, Inc; 2001:211-20.
2. Cailleteau JC. Diagnosis and Management of Toothaches of Dental Origin. In: Falace DA, ed. *Emergency Dental Care, Diagnosis and Management of Urgent Dental Problems.* Malvern, PA: Williams and Wilkins; 1995:25-66.
3. Vreven J, Van Nieuwenhuysen JP. Relations pulpo-parodontales. In: Bercy, Tenenbaum, eds. *Parodontologie, Du Diagnostic à la pratique.* Paris: De Boek & Larcier, 1996:223-36.
4. Bender IB, Pulpal pain diagnosis – a review. *Journal of Endodontics* 2000;26(3):175-9.
5. Gluskin AH, Cohen AS, Brown DC. Orofacial Dental Pain Emergencies: Endodontic Diagnosis and Management. In: Cohen S, Burns RC, eds. *Pathways of the Pulp.* 7th ed. St. Louis, MI: Mosby Inc, 1998:20-49.
6. Somerman M, Chan JT. Desensitizing agents. In: *ADA Guide to Dental Therapeutics,* 2nd ed. Chicago, IL: ADA Publishing, 2000:242-9.
7. Simon JHS. Periapical Pathology. In: Cohen S, Burns RC, eds. *Pathways of the Pulp.* 7th ed. St. Louis, MI: Mosby Inc, 1998:425-62.
8. Peterson LJ. Prevention and Management of Surgical Complications. In: Peterson LJ, Ellis III E, Hupp JR, Tucker MR, eds. *Contemporary Oral and Maxillofacial Surgery.* St. Louis, MI: Mosby, 1993:269-88.
9. Furst IM, Ersil P, Caminiti M. A rare complication of tooth abscess-Ludwig's angina and mediastinitis. *J Can Dent Asssoc* 2001;67:324-7.
10. Roberts G, Scully C, Shotts R. Dental emergencies. In: Scully C, ed. *ABC of Oral Health.* London, UK: BMJ Books, 2001:35-8.

Dental Conditions—Patient Information

Urgent Problems

See your dentist immediately if you have any of the following:

- A tooth that is sensitive to cold or heat or biting, and wakes you up at night with pain.
- Swelling and redness around one tooth, in the gums or even in the face.
- Peeling gums.

Cracked or Chipped Tooth

- If you crack or chip a tooth, keep the pieces in a moist cloth and take them with you to see a dentist, immediately.

Loose Tooth

- If the whole tooth is loose or out of its socket, keep it in your mouth, under your tongue or between your teeth and cheek, and see a dentist immediately.
- If you can't see a dentist, go to a medical emergency department.
- If you don't keep the tooth in your mouth, store it in normal saline solution, milk or a wet towel. You can make normal saline solution by adding 1.25 mL (one-quarter teaspoon) of table salt to 250 mL (one cup) of water.

Mouth Conditions Section Highlights

       Potential complications
       Drugs causes

Chapter 61

Aphthous Ulcers
(Canker Sores)

Mary E. MacCara, PharmD

Pathophysiology

Aphthous ulcers (aphthous stomatitis, canker sores) and recurrent aphthous ulcers (recurrent aphthous stomatitis) represent a noninfectious oral problem of unknown etiology.[1-3] They are the most prevalent oral lesions in the general population with a frequency of 5 to 25% and a three-month recurrence rate of 50%.[1,3] The first occurrence is usually between the ages of 10 and 20[4] with more than one-third of school-age children experiencing these oral lesions.[5] Individuals in middle and upper-middle class socioeconomic groups have a higher frequency of aphthous ulcers than the general population.[6] Local trauma and stress are thought to be the most likely precipitating factors, with allergies, genetic predisposition, nutritional deficiencies, systemic disease and medication use also playing a role.[1-3] Patients with aphthae may have considerable pain which leads to difficulty eating, speaking and swallowing.[1-3] Persistent and recurring ulcers can result in weight loss and a decrease in quality of life.[1]

There are three types of aphthous ulcers: minor, major and herpetiform. The most common are minor aphthae, occurring in 70 to 87% of cases.[1,3] *Minor* aphthae appear as recurrent, small, round or oval, clearly defined, painful ulcers with shallow necrotic centres, raised margins and erythematous halos.[3] They are usually smaller than 1 cm in diameter and have a whitish gray pseudomembrane. Lesions may appear as single or multiple ulcers (1 to 5 ulcers) usually on movable oral mucosa including the mucosa of the lips and cheeks, the floor of the mouth, the underside of the tongue and the soft palate.[1,3,6] Minor aphthae heal spontaneously without scarring within 7 to 10 days. A vague localized feeling of discomfort may precede the actual appearance of the lesion by a couple of days.[6]

Major aphthae are less common, occurring in 7 to 20% of affected patients and are more severe than minor aphthae. Although they are similar in appearance to minor aphthae, they are larger, exceeding 1 cm in diameter, deeper and appear in larger numbers (1 to 10).[1] They often scar and can persist for weeks to months causing significant difficulty swallowing.[1,3] They are frequently found in patients infected with human immunodeficiency virus (HIV).[3]

Herpetiform aphthous ulcers are the least common, affecting 5 to 10% of cases. They appear as multiple small clusters of pinpoint ulcers, 2 to 3 mm in diameter, 10 to 100 in number but they may coalesce into wide-spread, irregular lesions.[3] These ulcers may last 7 to 30 days and have the potential to scar. As their name indicates, they are herpetiform in nature, but herpes simplex virus cannot be cultured from these lesions.

Goals of Therapy[1]

Infrequent, minor aphthous ulcers:
- Control local pain

Major, herpetiform, or frequent, recurrent, minor aphthous ulcers:
- Control local pain
- Reduce duration of ulcers
- Restore normal oral function
- Ensure adequate food and fluid intake
- Decrease frequency and severity of recurrences

Patient Assessment (Figures 1,2)

When evaluating a patient with symptoms suggestive of aphthous ulcers, consider other conditions with oral ulcerative manifestations. These include infections (viral, treponemal, fungal), autoimmune diseases (e.g., Behcet's syndrome, inflammatory bowel disease, lupus erythematosus), hematologic diseases (cyclic neutropenia) and neoplasms (squamous cell carcinoma). Patients with white thickened patches on the mucosa of the cheeks, gums or tongue may have leukoplakia, a precancerous lesion associated with the use of tobacco products. (See photos on page PS-4.)

Aphthous ulcers normally are not preceded by fever or vesicles and occur almost exclusively on movable oral mucosa (inside of the cheeks and lips, tongue, floor of mouth and soft palate). When patients present with a mouth lesion that is not easily distinguished as an aphthous ulcer or have additional symptoms, such as fever, skin lesions, uveitis, genital ulceration, recurrent bloody or mucous diarrhea, head/neck adenopathy, or malar rash, they may be suffering from some other type of lesion or a systemic disorder and should be referred to a physician.[2]

Figure 1: **Assessment of Patients with Aphthous Ulcers**

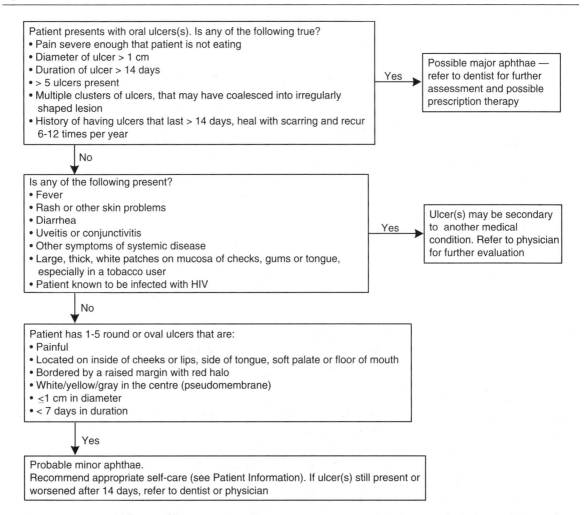

Figure 2: **Anatomy of the Mouth**

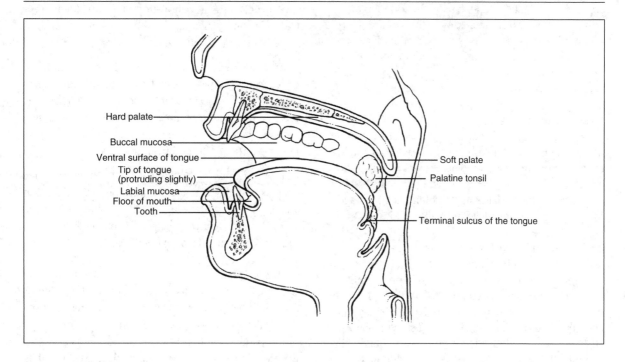

Hard palate
Buccal mucosa
Ventral surface of tongue
Tip of tongue (protruding slightly)
Labial mucosa
Floor of mouth
Tooth

Soft palate
Palatine tonsil

Terminal sulcus of the tongue

Prevention

Several well-recognized causes may contribute to the development of aphthous ulcers.

Local Trauma

If accidental self-biting leads to the development of aphthous ulcers, advise the patient to chew carefully and slowly, using extra caution or avoiding sharp-edged foods such as hard candy, crackers or potato chips. Teeth, dental procedures and devices can also cause trauma, which leads to aphthous ulcers. Patients should consult with their dentist if their teeth or dental appliances have sharp points. Taking care while brushing and the early replacement of toothbrushes to prevent injury from "splayed" bristles can also help prevent trauma to the oral mucosa.

Emotional and Environmental Stress

Stress may precede 60% of initial ulcers and may be involved in 21% of recurrent cases.[1] Frequency of aphthous ulcers is three times greater in medical and dental students than in the general population[1]

Relaxation and imagery training have significantly reduced aphthous ulcers.[1]

Nutritional Deficiencies

Deficiencies involving iron, folic acid, zinc and vitamins B_1, B_2, B_6 and B_{12} are more common in patients with aphthous ulcers than in people without aphthous ulcers.[1,3] Calcium and vitamin C may also be deficient in patients with aphthous ulcers.[7] Referral to a physician for hematologic screening in children and in patients with a history of ulcers exceeding six months may detect these deficiencies.[3] Patients with nutritional deficiencies respond well to replacement therapy.[1]

Allergies

Oral hypersensitivity reactions to various food additives, essential oils, mints and dental materials[3] and antibodies to cow's milk and wheat protein have been seen in patients with recurrent aphthous ulcers (RAU).[1] Strict elimination diets involving cow's milk or glutens have provided resolution or improvement in

RAU.[1] If an allergic or hypersensitivity reaction is suspected, referral to an allergist is warranted.[3] Sodium lauryl sulfate (SLS), commonly found in toothpastes, can cause an increase in the occurrence of aphthous ulcers. Patients with SLS-related adverse reactions should use toothpastes that do not contain this detergent.[3] Biotene® toothpaste does not contain sodium lauryl sulfate.

Drug-induced Causes

It has been suggested that patients with RAU have a higher medication intake than those without.[8] Medications associated with RAU include opioid analgesics, NSAIDs and beta-blockers.[8] Smoking appears to offer a protective effect,[2,8] although smoking is a risk factor for other oral lesions including leukoplakia.

Treatment of Underlying Systemic Disease

Identification and treatment of certain systemic diseases has been associated with improvement of RAU. These systemic conditions include: Crohn's disease, Behcet's disease, various types of neutropenia, pernicious anemia, systemic lupus erythematosus, HIV infection, periodic fever, aphthosis, pharyngitis and adenitis (PFAPA) syndrome, and mouth and genital ulcers with inflamed cartilage (MAGIC) syndrome.[3]

Nonpharmacologic Therapy

All patients with aphthous ulcers can benefit from avoiding foods that cause pain. These include foods that are hard, crusty, sharp, spicy, salty, acidic or difficult to chew, such as crackers, potato chips, pickles, tomatoes, citrus fruits and juices. Alcoholic beverages and chocolate may also cause pain and should be avoided when ulcers are present.

Pharmacologic Therapy

Nonprescription Therapy

Infrequent minor aphthous ulcers resolve on their own and may require only short-term pain management. Patients seeking temporary pain relief can apply a product containing a topical anesthetic such as benzocaine or lidocaine. Their duration of action is relatively short (20 to 45 minutes) and they should be used with oral analgesics and protectants to provide longer pain relief.

Local Anesthetics

Gels, ointments and pastes can be applied directly on the ulcer using a cotton-tipped swab, such as a Q-Tip®, four times a day, before meals and at bedtime, for up to one week.[5,9]

Local anesthetics should be used with caution in children under two years of age.[9] Increased absorption of benzocaine in infants and young children has led to methemoglobemia. The use of excessive amounts can lead to choking from difficulty swallowing and to being burned from hot food.

Gel formulations have a high alcohol content and may cause an initial stinging or burning on application which can be distressing to children. Applying ice before using a gel may help prevent this side effect[5] or another dosage form may be selected.

Oral Analgesics

Oral analgesics, such as acetaminophen, ibuprofen or acetylsalicylic acid (ASA), may be recommended for pain relief using dosages based on the age or weight of the patient. Caution is advised with the use of ASA in children, adolescents or young adults because of its possible association with Reye's syndrome when used in this population for conditions such as influenza or varicella.

Protectants

Placing a mucosal adherent agent (e.g., Orabase®, Zilactin®) over the ulcer may provide temporary pain relief and protection. The hydroxycellulose base found in Zilactin® adheres to mucosa significantly longer than Orabase®.[3]

Oral Hygiene

Encourage patients to maintain regular daily oral hygiene, which includes brushing and flossing the teeth (see Chapter 58). Aphthae can be cleansed by rinsing the mouth with salt and water (2.5 to 5 mL table salt per 250 mL warm water) several times a day, especially after meals. There is no evidence to suggest that other cleansing rinses (e.g., sodium perborate, found in Amosan®) or half-strength hydrogen peroxide (i.e., diluted to 1.5%) provide an advantage over saline rinses.

Other Treatments

Chlorhexidine mouthwash has no significant effect on the pain or duration of RAU.[1] Silver nitrate sticks have been used to cauterize aphthae. Their application is quite painful and should not be recommended for self-treatment due to the possibility of causing local necrosis and delaying healing.[2]

Prescription Therapy

Refer patients with major or herpetiform aphthous ulcers or frequent minor aphthous ulcers who experience multiple episodes each month and/or who have severe pain, difficulty eating, drinking, chewing and swallowing to a dentist or physician for further evaluation and more extensive drug therapy. Topical agents are first-line therapy and the corticosteroids, **fluocinonide**, **clobetasol** and **triamcinolone**, have demonstrated efficacy in pain relief of RAU.[1,3] The efficacy of corticosteroids can be increased if they are started during the early phase of ulceration, when lymphocyte activity is at its maximum.[3]

Establishing effective topical delivery of these agents is a problem because they are readily rubbed or washed away within the mouth. Using the more potent **corticosteroids** and compounding them with a mucosal adherent provides for more effective delivery. Triamcinolone in Orabase® is available commercially and Flaitz and Baker[5] reported that corticosteroid ointment formulations mix well with equal parts of Orabase®, providing for better adherence to the oral mucosa. In addition, advise the patient not to eat or drink for 30 minutes following application.[5]

Oropharyngeal candidiasis is a potential side effect with the administration of topical corticosteroids and patients should be monitored for this (see Chapter 64).

Amlexanox 5% paste (Apthera®) increases healing rate and pain relief in RAU.[1] It has antiinflammatory and antiallergic properties. In addition, **tetracycline** mouthrinse has been shown to significantly reduced the pain and duration of RAU as compared to placebo.[1] The dosage studied was tetracycline 250 mg four times a day, administered as a solution that was retained in the mouth for one to two minutes then spit out. Use of this oral rinse for more than five days may predispose patients to oral fungal infections.[1]

In severe cases of major RAU that are unresponsive to topical prescription therapy, systemic medications (e.g., **prednisone, levamisole and thalidomide**) may be indicated.[1,3]

Anecdotal Therapies

Therapies that have been suggested for aphthous ulcers but have received little or no study are listed in Table 1.

Table 1: **Anecdotal Therapies for Aphthous Ulcers**[2,3,10-12]

Acidophilus
Calendula
Deglycyrrhizinated licorice
l-Lysine
Mixtures *
Nicotine patches
2-octyl cyanoacrylate (tissue adhesive)
Sucralfate suspension as mouth rinse
Thiamine
Vitamin B complex
Vitamin C
Zinc lozenges

---

*1. *Various combinations of tetracycline, lidocaine, diphenhydramine, dyclonine or dexamethasone mixed 1:1 with sucralfate suspension, attapulgite suspension or aluminum hydroxide/ magnesium hydroxide suspension.[3]*

2. *One part prednisolone syrup 15 mg/5 mL or dexamethasone elixir 0.5 mg/5 mL, 2 parts diphenhydramine elixir 12.5 mg/5 mL, 3 parts doxycycline 25 mg/5 mL or minocycline 50 mg/5 mL, 6 parts lidocaine 2% viscous; used as rinse or applied to ulcer.[13]*

Monitoring of Therapy

If the ulcer is still present or has worsened after 14 days of self-care, advise the patient to see a physician or dentist.

Resource Tips

MayoClinic.Com. Diseases & Conditions A-Z. Canker sores. http://www.mayoclinic.com/home?id=5.1.1.3.18

Suggested Readings

Barrons RW. Treatment strategies for recurrent oral aphthous ulcers. *Am J Health Syst Pharm* 2001; 58(1):41-50; quiz 51-3.

Boulinguez S, Reix S, Bedane C, et al. Role of drug exposure in aphthous ulcers: a case-control study. *Br J Dermatol* 2000;143(6):1261-5.

Flaitz CM, Baker KA. Treatment approaches to common symptomatic oral lesions in children. *Dent Clin North Am* 2000;44(3):671-96.

McBride DR. Management of aphthous ulcers. *Am Fam Physician* 2000;62(1):149-54,160.

Pray WS. Advising patients about oral ulcers. *US Pharm* 2000;25:15-16, 21, 25-26.

Ship JA, Chavez EM, Doerr PA, Henson BS, Sarmadi M. Recurrent aphthous stomatitis. *Quintessence Int* 2000;31(2):95-112.

References

1. Barrons RW. Treatment strategies for recurrent oral aphthous ulcers. *Am J Health Syst Pharm* 2001;58(1):41-50; quiz 51-3.
2. McBride DR. Management of aphthous ulcers. *Am Fam Physician* 2000;62(1):149-54,160.
3. Ship JA, Chavez EM, Doerr PA, Henson BS, Sarmadi M. Recurrent aphthous stomatitis. *Quintessence Int.* 2000;31(2): 95-112.
4. MayoClinic.Com. Diseases & Conditions A-Z. Canker sores. Available from: http://www.mayoclinic.com/home?id= 5.1.1.3.18. Accessed July 25, 2001.
5. Flaitz CM, Baker KA. Treatment approaches to common symptomatic oral lesions in children. *Dent Clin North Am* 2000;44(3):671-96.
6. Sonis A, Zaragoza S. Dental health for the pediatrician. *Curr Opin Pediatr* 2001;13(3):289-95.
7. Ogura M, Yamamoto T, Morita M, Watanabe T. A case-control study on food intake of patients with recurrent aphthous stomatitis. *Oral Surg Oral Med Oral Pathol Oral Radiol Endod* 2001;91(1):45-9.
8. Boulinguez S, Reix S, Bedane C, Debrock C, Bouyssou-Gauthier ML, Sparsa A, et al. Role of drug exposure in aphthous ulcers: a case-control study. *Br J Dermatol* 2000; 143(6):1261-5.
9. Pray WS. Advising patients about oral ulcers. *US Pharm* 2000;25:15-6, 21, 25-6.
10. The Natural Pharmacist. TNP.com. Conditions. Canker sores. Available from: http://www.tnp.com/encyclopedia/condition/22/. Accessed July 25, 2001.
11. Scheid P, Bohadana A, Martinet Y. Nicotine patches for aphthous ulcers due to Behcet's syndrome. *N Engl J Med* 2000;343(24):1816-7.
12. Kutcher MJ, Ludlow JB, Samuelson AD, Campbell T, Pusek SN. Evaluation of a bioadhesive device for the management of aphthous ulcers. *J Am Dent Assoc* 2001;132(3):368-76.
13. Landow K. Help for canker sores? *Postgrad Med* 2000; 107(1):255-6.

Canker Sores (Aphthous Ulcers)—Patient Information

To help your canker sore feel better:

- Avoid foods that hurt – foods that are hard, crusty, sharp, spicy, salty, acidic or hard to chew. Examples are: crackers, potato chips, pickles, oranges, lemons, tomatoes and fruit juices.
- Take care to keep your teeth and gums clean but be careful not to hurt the canker sore. Brush your teeth using a *soft* toothbrush twice a day and use dental floss once a day. Use a new *soft* toothbrush if your old one has splayed or broken bristles that can hurt your mouth or the canker sore.
- Rinse your mouth with one-half to one teaspoonful (2.5 to 5 mL) of table salt dissolved in one cup of warm water several times a day to help soothe the canker sore. Use this rinse after meals to remove bits of food that may bother the canker sore. Be sure to spit out the salt water after rinsing.
- Most mouthwashes for bad breath have a high alcohol content and using them will make the canker sore sting. Don't use these mouthwashes when you have a canker sore.
- A canker sore should get better on its own in 10 to 14 days. Your pharmacist may suggest you use an ointment with an anesthetic in it to help the pain for a short time. You may use this four times a day for no longer than 14 days. Put a small amount of anesthetic ointment on the canker sore, using a cotton tipped swab (Q-Tip®), before eating meals and before going to bed.
- Your pharmacist may suggest that you cover the canker sore with a small amount of Orabase® or Zilactin® to help lessen the pain.

- You may use a nonprescription pain medicine such as acetaminophen, ibuprofen or ASA to help reduce the pain. Your pharmacist can help you choose a pain medicine that is right for you and tell you how to take it.

To help prevent canker sores:

- If you sometimes bite the inside of your cheek and a canker sore appears at that spot, take extra care while chewing. Chew your food slowly and try not to talk while you are chewing.
- If you have any teeth or dental work with sharp points, see your dentist so that the sharp points can be made less irritating.
- Most toothpastes have an ingredient called sodium lauryl sulphate. Some people have fewer canker sores when they use a toothpaste that does not have this ingredient in it. Your pharmacist can suggest a toothpaste, if you want to try this approach.

You should see a doctor or dentist if:

- The canker sore is still there after 14 days.
- If the canker sore has gotten larger or if more canker sores have developed.
- The pain is not controlled when using the medication recommended, and you have difficulty chewing or swallowing.
- If you also feel sick, have a fever, pain in the joints, irritated eyes or many, watery bowel movements.

Chapter 62

Cold Sores
(Herpes Labialis)

Mary E. MacCara, PharmD

Pathophysiology

There are two main herpes simplex viruses (HSV): herpes simplex-1 (HSV-1) and herpes simplex-2 (HSV-2). HSV-1, which is most commonly transmitted via saliva, causes the majority of oral herpes infections; HSV-2, which is present in genital secretions, causes the majority of genital herpes infections. However, oral-genital contact may cause a primary infection of either type in either the oral or genital region. Both HSV-1 and HSV-2 can cause a primary and recurrent infection. Primary herpes infections are frequently subclinical, or cause symptoms difficult to differentiate from other upper respiratory tract infections. When it is symptomatic, and its symptoms involve the oral region, it is known as primary herpes gingivostomatitis. Although not inevitable, about 20 to 40% of patients who experience a primary herpes infection develop subsequent recurrent herpes infections caused by reactivation of HSV that remains latent in neural ganglion cells. Recurrences in the oral region most commonly affect the lips, and are known as herpes labialis, cold sores or fever blisters.[1]

Babies generally acquire anti-HSV antibodies from their mothers, which protects them from infection until around six months of age.[1] The incidence of primary herpetic infection with HSV-1 increases between the ages of two and three years, with new cases generally occurring in preschool children. Primary infection can occur at any age, however, in both children and adults. The incidence of infection with HSV-2 increases after sexual activity begins, with risk factors including being female, a history of sexually transmitted disease and multiple sexual partners.[1,2]

Goals of Therapy[3]

- Reduce pain and itching
- Reduce viral shedding
- Decrease duration of lesions
- Prevent secondary bacterial infection
- Prevent recurrences

Patient Assessment (Figure 1)

A primary herpetic gingivostomatitis infection may be so mild it goes unnoticed, or it may be characterized by malaise, fever, lymphadenopathy and multiple crops of painful vesicles and ulcerative erosions on the tongue, palate, gingiva, buccal mucosa and lips. The ulcers rupture readily, leaving small ulcers covered with a pseudomembrane and surrounded by erythema.[4] This primary infection lasts one to three weeks without scarring.[2] Oral shedding of the virus continues for up to 23 days.[2]

Cold sores (herpes labialis, fever blisters), are the manifestation of recurrent HSV around the mouth. They are a common problem affecting 20 to 40% of the general population[4] and approximately 33% of school-aged children.[5] The virus may reactivate two or three times a year, but this varies.[2] The typical manifestation is a painful, unilateral vesicular lesion surrounded by erythema, appearing on the vermilion border of the lip and around the nostrils.[2,4,6] The vesicles break, leaking a clear, sticky fluid, then crust over and heal without scarring within 7 to 10 days.[2,4,7] A prodromal tingling and burning sensation in the location of the eruption may occur 2 to 24 hours before the appearance of the vesicles,[2,4,6] but this does not occur in all cases. The lesion appears over one to two days and viral shedding occurs over three to five days, which is the time it takes for the lesion to crust over.[2] Generally there are no systemic symptoms and the patient complains only of the unsightly appearance, pain and sometimes, itching.[7]

Sun exposure, especially that which results in sunburn and frequently occurs on beaches or mountain ski areas, is the most common factor associated with the development of recurrences of herpes labialis.[7,8] A variety of other known triggers include stress, surgical trauma, dental extraction, menses and other hormonal changes, infectious febrile conditions and hyperthermia.[4,9]

Patients who are immunosuppressed by disease or drug therapy are at a high risk of recurrences of HSV. This includes persons receiving cancer chemotherapy or drugs to suppress rejection of organ transplantation and patients with acquired immunodeficiency syndrome (AIDS). Atopic individuals may develop a rapidly progressing HSV cutaneous infection.

Nonpharmacologic Therapy

Caution patients to keep the lesion clean with gentle washing using a mild soap and water. This can also be accomplished by soaking the area with cool compresses of tap water.[10] Patients should avoid excessive touching of the lesion and should wash their hands frequently to prevent autoinnoculation and spread of HSV.

Pharmacologic Therapy

Nonprescription Therapy

Primary and recurrent oral HSV infections in immunocompetent patients are self-limited and generally

---

Figure 1: **Assessment of Patients with Cold Sores**

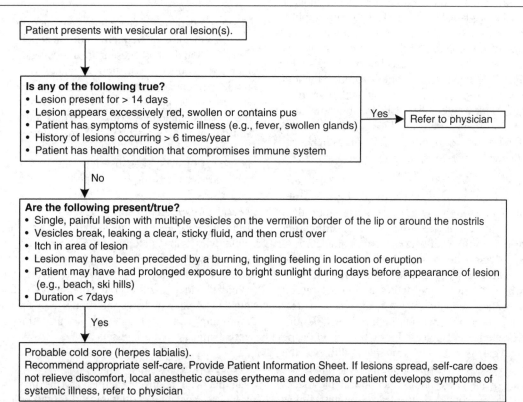

require only symptomatic treatment.[11] Pharmacists can recommend the use of topical products that contain protectants (e.g., **petrolatum, zinc oxide, cocoa butter, allantoin** or **calamine**) to prevent cracking and excessive drying of the lesion.[12] Should a secondary bacterial infection occur, topical application of a nonprescription antibiotic ointment three or four times daily is appropriate.[10] The use of systemic analgesics (e.g., acetaminophen, ibuprofen or acetylsalicylic acid) is also reasonable if the cold sore is very painful.[10]

Local Anesthetics

Products containing local anesthetics offer temporary relief from pain and itching of cold sores. Preliminary evidence suggests that they may be of benefit in preventing eruptions or in shortening the duration of lesions.[13,14] It has been suggested that local anesthetics have inhibitory effects on HSV, inhibiting its activation or membrane penetration and preventing its spread through lymph capillaries.[13] **Tetracaine** 1.8 % cream has been studied in immunocompetent patients and found to significantly reduce the healing time of recurrent herpes labialis lesions. The patients applied tetracaine cream or placebo cream six times a day from time of prodrome, and the time to healing was reduced from 7.2 days with placebo to 5.1 days with tetracaine.[14] Patients also reported significantly less itching with the tetracaine product, although pain relief was similar with the placebo and tetracaine groups.[14] Further research is needed to determine the role of tetracaine and other local anaesthetics in preventing cold sores or shortening their duration.

Topical local anesthetics can be contact sensitizers. Those with the ester structure (e.g., **benzocaine**, tetracaine) are more likely to cause sensitization than are those with an amide structure (e.g., **lidocaine**, **dibucaine**). Those with a nonester/nonamide structure (e.g., **dyclonine**, **pramoxine**) are thought to be the least sensitizing. Purcell and Dickson reported two cases where 1% dyclonine hydrochloride gel caused allergic contact dermatitis while being used to treat herpes labialis.[15] The patients believed their lesions were worsening and increased the application of the dyclonine gel, thereby delaying recognition of the contact dermatitis.[15] Pharmacists must be aware of the possibility of allergic reactions due to local anesthetics and that allergic contact dermatitis can be mistaken as widespread herpes simplex infection.

External Analgesics

The Food and Drug Administration in the United States has reviewed nonprescription products for the treatment of herpes labialis and has classified external analgesics, alcohols, ketones and certain local anesthetics as safe and effective.[16] Examples of these ingredients include: **camphor**, **menthol**, **benzyl alcohol**, benzocaine, dibucaine and dyclonine HCl. Camphor at a concentration greater than 3% and menthol greater than 1% have counterirritant effects and are contraindicated in the treatment of cold sores due to the irritation and inflammation they can cause.[17]

Astringents

Highly astringent ingredients such as tannic acid and zinc sulphate are not recommended for treatment of cold sores. They have the potential to cause excessive drying of the area with resultant fissuring, discomfort and potential bacterial superinfection.[10,12] In addition, the herpes virus may be fractionated by astringents causing resistant strains to emerge.[12,17]

Others

There is no published literature regarding the safety and effectiveness of **heparin** in the treatment of cold sores, although it is present in a frequently recommended product.[18] Caustic substances (e.g., silver nitrate, phenol) may create further damage and should not be applied to cold sores. Corticosteroids are not recommended for use in oral inflammation caused by viruses, as they may mask the spread of infection and suppress the normal immune responce.[19] However, their use topically in conjunction with antivirals is being investigated.[20]

Acetylsalicylic Acid (ASA)

Herpetic episodes were noted to disappear in an adult male who was treated with ASA post myocardial infarction. Preliminary testing suggests that ASA, administered orally at 125 mg per day, at the first clinical evidence of a cold sore, may reduce the number of days of active infection.[21] ASA may act by inhibiting viral protein synthesis and through its antiinflammatory mechanisms.[21]

Prescription Therapy

Patients with recurrent herpes labialis may benefit from systemic antiviral therapy and should be referred to a physician or dentist for evaluation.

Several antiviral agents (e.g., **acyclovir, famciclovir, penciclovir, valacyclovir**) have been studied clinically for either the treatment or prophylaxis of herpes labialis. Acyclovir, famciclovir and valacyclovir are all marketed as prescription agents in Canada, although none of these drugs has an official indication for herpes labialis in the general population. One of famciclovir's official indications is for recurrent episodes of mucocutaneous herpes simplex infections in HIV-infected patients. Penciclovir is not currently marketed in Canada.

Evidence supports the use of oral **acyclovir** in the treatment of herpes labialis and the prevention of recurrent herpes labialis. Acyclovir, at a dosage of 400 mg orally five times daily for five days, started within one hour of the first symptoms of recurrence of herpes labialis, reduced the duration of pain by 36% and the time to loss of crust by 27%.[22] When given to healthy adults with at least six recurrences of lesions per year, acyclovir at a dosage of 400 mg twice daily for four months resulted in a 53% reduction in the number of recurrences of herpes labialis and a 71% reduction in the amount of viral shedding.[23] Reduction of viral shedding should lead to a reduction in HSV transmission.[24] Oral acyclovir has also been shown to alter the severity of sun-reactivated herpes labialis during high risk situations such as sun exposure on ski hills.[24,25]

Although commonly used in the treatment and prophylaxis of recurrent episodes of herpes labialis, topical acyclovir has not been shown to be effective.[24,25] Possibly this is because there is poor penetration of topically applied acyclovir to the neural ganglion, the site of viral replication.[25]

Famciclovir was successful in decreasing lesion size and healing time in ultraviolet radiation-induced herpes labialis.[26] This was a dose-ranging trial and doses of 500 mg three times daily increased healing time significantly more than did a dose of 125 or 250 mg three times a day. **Fluocinonide** 0.5% gel was used with famciclovir 500 mg orally, both three times a day for five days in ultraviolet radiation-induced herpes labialis.[20] This combination resulted in significantly reduced lesion size and a significant reduction in the number of patients experiencing lesion pain as compared to patients treated with famciclovir alone.

The authors claim this to be the first published clinical trial where a topical corticosteroid was used in the treatment of recurrent herpes labialis.[20]

Alternative Therapy

There is some evidence that a cream of **lemon balm** (*Melissa officinalis*) containing 1% of a 70:1 leaf extract, applied to the site of a cold sore during the prodromal stage, reduces the number and size of lesions, although the overall severity of the outbreak is not lessened.[27,28] When used for treatment it is applied thickly four times a day; a twice-daily application is used for prevention.[27]

Lysine, one of the 10 essential amino acids, is marketed for prevention and treatment of herpes labialis. Evidence regarding the effectiveness of lysine for this indication varies. Its efficacy in prevention of herpes labialis appears to be dose-dependent. Older studies using lower dosages (e.g., 624 mg daily) did not show benefit whereas newer studies using dosages ranging from 750 to 4000 mg daily support the claim of decreasing the frequency of outbreaks.[29,30] Studies do not support the use of lysine for decreasing the severity or duration of outbreaks.[30] Large amounts of nitrogen are produced with the metabolism of lysine. Persons with renal or hepatic disease may have difficulty eliminating this nitrogen and therefore its use as a supplement is contraindicated in these patients. Lysine can increase the absorption and decrease the elimination of calcium.[29,30]

Prevention

Protecting affected areas from sun exposure, especially on the beach and at ski hills, might reduce the frequency of cold sore recurrences.[2,3] A sunscreen with an SPF of 30 or higher should be applied to the lips and face 30 minutes prior to exposure.

Reducing stress (e.g., eating well, getting enough sleep and exercise, relaxation) can also help prevent recurrences in individuals for whom stress is a known trigger.[3,4]

Avoid spread of cold sores to other parts of the body and to other people by frequent hand washing and avoiding skin-to-skin contact with others until after the blister has dried up and crusted over.

Monitoring of Therapy

Cold sores are expected to resolve within two weeks. If self-treatment does not relieve the discomfort, the lesions spread, or the patient develops symptoms of systemic illness (e.g., fever, malaise, swollen glands), the patient should see a physician. If application of a product containing a local anesthetic causes increased erythema and edema in the area of the lesion, contact dermatitis should be suspected and the product discontinued.

Resource Tips

MayoClinic.Com. Diseases & Conditions A-Z.Cold Sore. http://www.mayoclinic.com/home?id=5.1.1.3.29

MedicineNet.com. Herpes Simplex Infections (non-genital) http://www.medicinenet.com/Script/Main/Art.asp?li=MNI&ArticleKey=9632&page

Centers for Disease Control and Prevention. Issues in Child Care Settings. What you should know about.... cold sores in the child care setting. http://www.cdc.gov/ncidod/hip/abc/facts06.htm

Suggested Readings

Birek C. Herpesvirus-induced diseases: oral manifestations and current treatment options. *J Calif Dent Assoc.* 2000;28(12):911-21.

Flaitz CM, Baker KA. Treatment approaches to common symptomatic oral lesions in children. *Dent Clin North Am.* 2000;44(3):671-96.

Greenberg MS. Herpesvirus infections. *Dent Clin North Am.* 1996;40(2):359-68.

Leflore S, Anderson PL, Fletcher CV. A risk-benefit evaluation of aciclovir for the treatment and prophylaxis of herpes simplex virus infections. *Drug Saf.* 2000;23(2):131-42.

MayoClinic.com. What are cold sores? Available from: http://www.mayoclinic.com/home?id=5.1.1.3.29. Accessed July 25, 2001.

Whitley RJ, Roizman B. Herpes simplex virus infections. *Lancet.* 2001;357(9267):1513-8.

References

1. Greenberg MS. Herpesvirus infections. *Dent Clin North Am.* 1996;40(2):359-68.

2. Emmert DH. Treatment of common cutaneous herpes simplex virus infections. *Am Fam Physician.* 2000;61(6):1697-706, 1708.

3. Nadelman CM, Newcomer VD. Herpes simplex virus infections. New treatment approaches make early diagnosis even more important. *Postgrad Med.* 2000;107(3):189-95, 199-200.

4. Birek C. Herpesvirus-induced diseases: oral manifestations and current treatment options. *J Calif Dent Assoc.* 2000;28(12):911-21.

5. Flaitz CM, Baker KA. Treatment approaches to common symptomatic oral lesions in children. *Dent Clin North Am.* 2000;44(3):671-96.

6. Australian Herpes Management Forum. Managing oral herpes. Guidelines for clinicians on the treatment of oral herpes simplex. Available from: http://www.herpes.on.net/cold_sores/Default.htm. Accessed July 25, 2001.

7. Sonis A, Zaragoza S. Dental health for the pediatrician. *Curr Opin Pediatr.* 2001;13(3):289-95.

8. Raborn GW, Martel AY, Grace MG, McGaw WT. Herpes labialis in skiers: randomized clinical trial of acyclovir cream versus placebo. *Oral Surg Oral Med Oral Pathol Oral Radiol Endod.* 1997;84(6):641-5.

9. Guerriere-Kovach PM, Brodell RT. Recurrent herpes simplex virus infection. Suppressive, reactive, and preventive antiviral regimens. *Postgrad Med.* 2000;107(6):139-40, 143, 147.

10. Covington TR, ed. *Nonprescription Drug Therapy. Guiding Patient Self-care.* St. Louis, MI: Facts and Comparisons; 2001.

11. MayoClinic.com. What are cold sores? Available from: http://www.mayoclinic.com/home?id=5.1.1.3.29. Accessed July 25, 2001.

12. Pray SW. *Nonprescription Products Therapeutics.* Philadephia, PA: Lippincott Williams & Wilkins; 1999.

13. Cassuto J. Topical local anaesthetics and herpes simplex. *Lancet.* 1989;1(8629):100-1.

14. Kaminester LH, Pariser RJ, Pariser DM, et al. A double-blind, placebo-controlled study of topical tetracaine in the treatment of herpes labialis. *J Am Acad Dermatol.* 1999;41(6):996-1001.

15. Purcell SM, Dixon SL. Allergic contact dermatitis to dyclonine hydrochloride simulating extensive herpes simplex labialis. *J Am Acad Dermatol.* 1985;12(2 pt 1):231-4.

16. Federal Register, 1990;55:3362, 3370.

17. Federal Register, 1993;58:27636.

18. Pharmacy Post's 6th survey on OTC counselling and recommendations. *Pharmacy Post.* 2000;8(3):27-44.

19. American Dental Association. *ADA Guide to Dental Therapeutics.* 1st ed. Chicago: ADA Publishing Co, Inc.; 1998.

20. Spruance SL, McKeough MB. Combination treatment with famciclovir and a topical corticosteroid gel versus famciclovir alone for experimental ultraviolet radiation-induced herpes simplex labialis: a pilot study. *J Infect Dis.* 2000;181(6):1906-10.

21. Karadi I, Karpati S, Romics L. Aspirin in the management of recurrent herpes simplex virus infection. *Ann Intern Med.* 1998;128(8):696-7.

22. Rooney JF, Straus SE, Mannix ML, et al. Oral acyclovir to suppress frequently recurrent herpes labialis. A double-blind, placebo-controlled trial. *Ann Intern Med.* 1993;118(4):268-72.

23. Spruance SL, Stewart JC, Rowe NH, McKeough MB, Wenerstrom G, Freeman DJ. Treatment of recurrent herpes simplex labialis with oral acyclovir. *J Infect Dis.* 1990;161(2):185-90.

24. Leflore S, Anderson PL, Fletcher CV. A risk-benefit evaluation of aciclovir for the treatment and prophylaxis of herpes simplex virus infections. *Drug Saf.* 2000;23(2):131-42.

25. Vander Straten M, Carrasco D, Lee P, Tyring SK. A review of antiviral therapy for herpes labialis. *Arch Dermatol.* 2001; 137(9):1232-5.

26. Spruance SL, Rowe NH, Raborn GW, Thibodeau EA, D'Ambrosio JA, Bernstein DI. Peroral famciclovir in the treatment of experimental ultraviolet radiation-induced herpes simplex labialis: A double-blind, dose-ranging, placebo-controlled, multicenter trial. *J Infect Dis.* 1999;179(2):303-10.

27. The natural pharmacist. TNP.com. Herbs & supplements. Lemon balm. Available from: http://www.tnp.com/encyclopedia/substance/71. Accessed July 25, 2001.

28. Koytchev R, Alken RG, Dundarov S. Balm mint extract (Lo-701) for topical treatment of recurring herpes labialis. *Phytomedicine.* 1999;6(4):225-30.

29. The natural pharmacist. TNP.com. Herbs & supplements. Lysine. Avaible from: http://www.tnp.com/encyclopedia/substance/159/ Accessed July 25, 2001.

30. Tomblin FA Jr, Lucas KH. Lysine for management of herpes labialis. *Am J Health Syst Pharm.* 2001;58(4):298-300, 304.

Cold Sores (Herpes Labialis)—Patient Information

Cold sores are caused by the herpes simplex virus. A person with a cold sore can pass the virus on to another person and they could get a cold sore. Cold sores are most contagious from the time they appear until they dry and crust over. To keep from spreading the virus:

- Do not have skin-to-skin contact with young children, people with eczema, cancer, AIDs or an organ transplant while you have a cold sore.
- Do not share forks, spoons, drinking containers, razors or towels while you have a cold sore.
- Do not kiss others while you have a cold sore.

Take care of a cold sore by:

- Gently washing with mild soap and water to keep the cold sore clean.
- Avoid touching the cold sore with your fingers.
- Wash your hands often with soap and water to avoid getting a bacterial infection in the cold sore. Washing your hands also helps stop the spread of the virus.
- Always use your own towel and do not let others use yours.
- Putting an ointment on the cold sore helps to keep the cold sore from cracking and drying. This helps prevent a bacterial infection in the cold sore. Your pharmacist may suggest that you use a plain ointment, such as Vaseline®, to keep the cold sore from cracking. Your pharmacist may also suggest that you use an ointment that contains a local anesthetic. The anesthetic may help lessen the pain and itching. Once the scab falls off, you no longer need to use the ointment. Before putting ointment on with your finger, wash your hands.

- If the cold sore is very painful you may use a non-prescription pain medicine such as acetaminophen, ibuprofen or ASA. Ask your pharmacist which medicine is appropriate for you to take.

Contact your pharmacist if:

- The cold sore becomes more red and you think it may have developed another infection.
- You are putting a local anesthetic ointment on the cold sore and the area around the cold sore becomes red and swollen. Stop using the ointment.

You should see a doctor if:

- The cold sore does not go away after 14 days of care.
- The cold sore spreads or you feel sick with a fever or swollen glands.

Preventing cold sores:

- Bright sunlight at the beach or on ski hills causes some people to have cold sores. If you think that being in bright sunlight causes you to have cold sores, apply sunscreen (minimum SPF 30) on lips and face 30 minutes before going out into the sunlight. Wearing a wide-brimmed hat can also help.
- If you think that stress causes you to have cold sores, try to learn how to minimize the stress in your life or learn effective ways to deal with it. Getting regular exercise, enough sleep and eating well can help.

If you have six or more cold sores per year, ask your doctor about prescription medicines that can help decrease the number of cold sores you get.

Chapter 63

Halitosis

Mary E. MacCara, PharmD

Pathophysiology

Halitosis, bad breath, *fetor ex ore* and malodor are all terms used to describe unpleasant or offensive odors emitted in exhaled breath. In its simplest form, bad breath is related to substances ingested (e.g., herbs, spices, garlic, tobacco or alcohol) or is associated with dryness in the mouth upon awakening (morning breath). It can be of great concern to patients.

There is growing interest in the diagnosis and treatment of bad breath. Five international conferences on this topic were held between 1993 and 2001. Diagnosis and treatment of halitosis is being incorporated into routine dental care, and specialized dental and multidisciplinary clinics are being set-up solely for the treatment of patients with halitosis.[1]

Halitosis can be broadly classified into situations when odor is present (*genuine halitosis*) and situations when odour is of concern to the patient, but is not perceived by others (*pseudo-halitosis* and *halitophobia*).[2] Genuine halitosis is further classified as physiologic and pathologic.

Physiologic halitosis arises from the putrefactive process within the mouth, especially at the back of the tongue. Pathological halitosis is caused by disease or malfunction of the oral tissues (e.g., gingivitis, dental abscesses) and includes halitosis due to periodontal disease and xerostomia. The major elements in the production of oral malodor are volatile sulphur compounds (VSCs), primarily hydrogen sulfide, methyl mercaptan and dimethyl sulfide. These VSCs are produced on the dorsum of the tongue through microflora putrefaction. This generally occurs when there is a shift from gram-positive to gram-negative bacteria contributed to by a decreased salivary flow, a reduction in carbohydrate substrate and a rise in pH.[3] The oral cavity is generally considered to be the main source of halitosis in most healthy individuals.[3]

Extraoral pathologic halitosis arises when malodor comes from sources other than the mouth. These include the nasal, paranasal and laryngeal regions, the upper digestive tract, the lungs, or from disorders in any other body system (e.g., diabetes mellitus, hepatic cirrhosis, uremia or internal bleeding). Pseudo-halitosis and halitophobia have a psychological component and can be difficult to treat.

There is no reliable way for people to properly assess their breath odor. There also are extremes in whether or not people recognize bad breath in themselves. Some have a life-long concern about having bad breath, while others don't seem to notice that their breath is offensive. Dentists are being called upon more frequently to deal with malodor problems, and pharmacists can provide a service to their clients by referring them to an appropriate dental clinic if bad breath is an on-going concern.[4]

Goals of Therapy

- Encourage patients to seek regular dental care
- Encourage good oral hygiene
- Help the patient minimize symptoms and refer when necessary
- Discourage prolonged use of mouth rinses that have a high alcohol content or contain an antibacterial agent

Patient Assessment (Figure 1)

Evaluate patients seeking help for bad breath based on their personal, dental and medical history. Information collected should include foods ingested, tobacco and alcohol use, and whether there are any specific times when bad breath is most noticeable. Certain foods (e.g., garlic) are known to cause bad breath, and tobacco and alcohol use can also cause halitosis. Most people have bad breath upon awakening. Irregular eating can lead to hunger ketosis and bad breath.

Assess oral hygiene. Poor dental hygiene and/or dental pathology is a major cause of bad breath (see Chapter 58). Pain or discomfort in the mouth and oral cavity may signify pathology that requires treatment. Patients who wear dentures must be assessed to determine proper denture hygiene.

Consider xerostomia due to medication use or radiation therapy as a possible cause of bad breath. Ingestion of systemic antibiotics or regular use of an antibacterial mouth rinse can put the patient at risk for

Figure 1: **Assessment of Patients with Halitosis**

Patient presents with halitosis. Is any of the following true?
- Patient has painful, red swollen areas around the gums or tongue or any pus-filled area within the mouth (These can be signs of candidiasis, bacterial infection or gingivitis.)
- Patient has recently had a dental extraction or other dental surgery

Yes → Refer to dentist

No ↓

Is any of the following true?
- Patient has symptoms of respiratory disease, sinusitis, tonsillitis or rhinitis
- Patient is concerned about bad breath but friends and family do not share this concern

Yes → Refer to physician

No ↓

Does the patient:
- Wake up in the morning with a dry mouth and bad breath?
- Eat garlic or spicy foods?
- Eat irregular meals (hunger ketosis)?
- Smoke tobacco or use smokeless tobacco?
- Go to sleep at night without removing dentures?
- Have poor denture hygiene?
- Have poor oral hygiene habits?
- Use a mouthwash with a high alcohol content or which contains an antibacterial agent (for period longer than one week)?
- Use medications which can cause dry mouth (see Chapter 65)?
- Require a dental check-up and cleaning (has not seen dentist in past 12 mos)?

Yes to 1 or more questions ↓

Pharmacist can, as appropriate:
- Recommend avoiding potential causes (specific foods , tobacco, delaying meals, leaving dentures in the mouth at night)
- Recommend practicing good oral hygiene (which includes good denture hygiene, if appropriate) and having regular dental check-ups (see Chapter 58)
- Recommend cleaning the tongue gently
- If medication is the likely cause of dry mouth and resulting bad breath (see Chapter 65), follow up with physician for possible adjustment of medication (with patient's permission)
- If patient wishes to try a mouth rinse, recommend a product containing essential oils and/or zinc chloride, with the lowest alcohol content available, for use at bedtime for 1 wk
- Discourage long-term use of products with high alcohol content.
- Provide Patient Information sheet

overgrowth of anaerobic, odoriferous bacteria or fungi that can be a source of bad breath.[5] Regular use of a mouth rinse with a high alcohol content can cause drying of the mucosa and bad breath. Respiratory disease (e.g., chronic sinusitis) or chronic illness (e.g., diabetes mellitus or alcoholic cirrhosis) can be extraoral causes of bad breath. Bad breath perceived by the patient but not by others usually has a psychological component and requires management by a mental health specialist.

Nonpharmacologic Therapy

The oral cavity is the source of bad breath in the majority of patients, and good oral hygiene along with treatment of any periodontal or other oral diseases is necessary to relieve the problem. Encourage patients to visit a dentist and dental hygienist for removal of dental plaque and accumulated bacteria on the dorsum of the tongue and in periodontal pockets, and for assessment of oral diseases. Encourage good oral hygiene, which includes brushing with a soft-bristled toothbrush at least twice a day, and flossing daily.[6]

A clean tongue is a healthy, pink color. A whitish haze on the tongue can indicate bacterial buildup.[7] Cleaning the tongue, along with other oral hygiene measures, is a very effective means of decreasing physiologic halitosis. Tongue cleaning can be accomplished through use of a small-headed child's toothbrush, or by using a specially designed tongue cleaner or a tongue scraper[8] The tongue is stroked from the back to the tip with the brush or cleaner, then the mouth is rinsed with water. The posterior portion of the tongue is most important to clean. Show patients the terminal sulcus of the tongue so that they are aware of the anatomical limits for cleaning (Figure 2, Chapter 61).[2] Extending these limits can lead to gagging.

It is important that patients understand that they should not be overzealous in their cleaning, to avoid causing damage to and bleeding of the tongue surface. Tongue scrapers must be used cautiously and adult toothbrushes are not recommended for tongue cleaning.[2] A clinical trial has shown that cleaning the tongue with either a cleaner or a scraper reduced VSC levels more than by cleaning with a toothbrush. However, 30 minutes after the procedure, there was no significant difference in the levels of VSC in the subjects regardless of method of cleaning.[8] It has been suggested that regular use of a tongue cleaning procedure may reduce bacterial flora from the tongue and that use of toothpaste in the cleaning process may extend the effect of tongue cleaning.[8]

Cleaning the mouth after eating or drinking dairy products or eating meat or fish, and drinking plenty of fluids[9] are adjunctive measures for treating bad breath. Saliva has many functions in keeping the mouth healthy, including lubrication, oxygenation, buffering and antimicrobial action. Increasing saliva flow and tongue action helps decrease bad breath. Chewing sugarless gum and munching on fibrous vegetables such as raw carrots and celery can help accomplish this.[7,10]

Pharmacologic Therapy

Nonprescription Therapy

Oral rinses (mouthwashes) may supplement oral hygiene. Most commercial mouth rinses mask odors and provide antiseptic properties for a relatively short time period (less than 30 minutes).[5] Rinsing with water is of little help because water offers no antiseptic properties and can wash away saliva which does have these properties.[7] The duration of action of mouth rinses is probably optimized if they are used prior to going to bed. Residues of the mouth rinse may remain in the mouth longer because the individual is not eating or drinking; this is also the time when bacterial activity is at its highest due to decreased saliva flow.[11]

Although mouth rinses are often recommended for treatment of bad breath, few have been evaluated for efficacy in the treatment of bad breath.[12] Loesche reviewed double-blind clinical trials wherein mouthwashes were tested to determine their effect on malodor. Rinses containing essential oils or zinc chloride were successful in reducing moderate malodor.[12] Long-term use of mouth rinses that contain alcohol may cause drying of the oral tissues[7] and this in itself can cause bad breath.

Prescription Therapy

Chlorhexidene appears to be successful in reducing malodor, but has many side effects including tooth staining, taste disturbances and sloughing of oral tissues.[12] There are no other prescription medications indicated for the treatment of bad breath, unless it is caused by lack of saliva (see Chapter 65).

Herbal Remedies

Chlorophyll and parsley have been known as breath fresheners for many years. There are no scientific studies to either promote or refute their use for this purpose.

Monitoring of Therapy

After one week of practising good oral hygiene, including gentle cleaning of the tongue, the patient should see an improvement in their bad breath, and this routine should be continued. If the patient's tongue hurts or bleeds following cleaning, or the patient complains that tongue cleaning causes excessive gagging, it is likely they require further instruction on tongue cleaning. Dentists and dental hygienists may be better situated to give these instructions.

Mouth rinses containing essential oils and/or zinc chloride, used at bedtime, may be helpful in reducing bad breath. Products with high alcohol content are not recommended for long-term use as they may cause dryness which can exacerbate bad breath. Monitor the duration of use of these products where possible and discourage long-term use of products with high alcohol content.

Resource Tips

American Dental Association (ADA.org). Frequently Asked Questions, bad breath (halitosis): http://www.ada.org/public/faq/breath.html

Mayo Clinic (MayoClinic.com). Diseases & Conditions A-Z: Halitosis: http://www.mayoclinic.com/home?id=5.1.1.8.1

Harvard Health Letter. Oral health. Bad breath. 2001 Jun;26(8):5. http://www.health.harvard.edu/medline/Health/L601d.html

Suggested Readings

Loesche WJ. The effects of antimicrobial mouthrinses on oral malodor and their status relative to US Food and Drug Administration regulations. *Quintessence Int.* 1999;30(5):311-8.

Messadi DV. Oral and nonoral sources of halitosis. *J Calif Dent Assoc.* 1997;25(2):127-31.

Nachnani S. The effects of oral rinses on halitosis. *J Calif Dent Assoc.* 1997;25(2):145-50.

Rosenberg M. Clinical assessment of bad breath: current concepts. *J Am Dent Assoc.* 1996;127(4):475-82.

Weinberg. MA. Halitosis: the "bad breath" syndrome. *US Pharmacist* 2001;26(3):46,48,51-52,57.

Yaegaki K, Coil JM. Examination, classification, and treatment of halitosis; clinical perspectives. *J Can Dent Assoc.* 2000;66(5):257-61.

References

1. Neiders M, Ramos B. Operation of bad breath clinics. *Quintessence Int.* 1999;30(5):295-301.
2. Yaegaki K, Coil JM. Examination, classification, and treatment of halitosis; clinical perspectives. *J Can Dent Assoc.* 2000;66(5):257-61.
3. Messadi DV. Oral and nonoral sources of halitosis. *J Calif Dent Assoc.* 1997;25(2):127-31.
4. Eli I, Baht R, Koriat H, Rosenberg M. Self-perception of breath odor. *J Am Dent Assoc.* 2001;132(5):621-6.
5. Clark GT, Nachnani S, Messadi DV. Detecting and treating oral and nonoral malodors. *J Calif Dent Assoc.* 1997;25(2): 133-44.
6. Weinberg. MA. Halitosis: the "bad breath" syndrome. *US Pharmacist* 2001;26(3):46,48,51-52,57.
7. Nachnani S. The effects of oral rinses on halitosis. *J Calif Dent Assoc.* 1997;25(2):145-50.
8. Seeman R, Kison A, Bizhang M, Zimmer S. Effectiveness of mechanical tongue cleaning on oral levels of volatile sulfur compounds. *J Am Dent Assoc.* 2001;132(9):1263-7.
9. Carlson-Mann L. The use of tongue cleaners in the treatment of halitosis. *Probe.* 1998;32(3):114-5.
10. Reingewirtz Y, Girault O, Reingewirtz N, Senger B, Tenenbaum H. Mechanical effects and volatile sulfur compound-reducing effects of chewing gums: comparison between test and base gums and a control group. *Quintessence Int.* 1999; 30(5):319-23.
11. Rosenberg M. Clinical assessment of bad breath: current concepts. *J Am Dent Assoc.* 1996;127(4):475-82.
12. Loesche WJ. The effects of antimicrobial mouthrinses on oral malodor and their status relative to US Food and Drug Administration regulations. *Quintessence Int.* 1999;30(5): 311-8.

Bad Breath (Halitosis)—Patient Information

The reason for bad breath is usually found within your mouth. If you have not been to see your dentist or dental hygienist recently, make an appointment to see them. They can find out if there is a problem with your teeth or gums that is causing the bad breath.

Things you can do to help stop bad breath:

- Take good care of your teeth and gums. Brush your teeth twice a day using a soft toothbrush (that does not have splayed bristles) and floss between your teeth once a day.
- A child's soft toothbrush can be used to gently brush the tongue to remove bacterial build-up. Brushing the back of the tongue is important. Do not brush too hard.
- Visit the dentist and dental hygienist regularly (at least once a year, preferably every six months).
- Avoid the use of tobacco and alcohol. They can cause bad breath.
- Snack on foods that require lots of chewing, such as raw celery and carrot sticks. Chewing these vegetables will cause saliva to flow and this helps keep the breath fresh.
- Chew sugarless gum (gum sweetened with xylitol). This will also cause saliva to flow.

- You may want to use a mouthwash at bedtime. Mouthwashes tend to cover up bad breath for a short time (less than 30 minutes). They do not remove the cause of bad breath. Mouthwashes tend to work a bit longer if you do not eat or drink right after using them.
- Many mouthwashes have a lot of alcohol in them. These can make the problem worse by making your mouth dry if they are used regularly for a long time. Some mouthwashes contain an ingredient that can stain your teeth. Check with your pharmacist before choosing a mouthwash.
- If you wear dentures, take them out at bedtime and practise good denture hygiene (e.g., clean dentures and gums with a soft toothbrush two to three times a day and soak dentures for 15 minutes every day in denture cleaning solution).
- A dry mouth can cause bad breath; it can also cause problems with your teeth and with eating. Many medications can cause a dry mouth. If you have a dry mouth, talk to your pharmacist and/or dentist about this problem.
- Nose and throat problems and some diseases can cause bad breath. If you think you may be sick, talk to your doctor.

Chapter 64

Oral Candidiasis

Mary E. MacCara, PharmD

Pathophysiology

Candida organisms are fungi that normally live in the mouth, the GI tract, mucous membranes and the skin. When changes occur in the host environment to cause an imbalance of flora or a decrease in resistance, *Candida* becomes an opportunistic pathogen.[1] Clinical problems can range from mild candidiasis to chronic, recurrent and life-threatening disseminated disease.[1]

C. albicans, the most common cause of oral candidiasis, is also known as moniliasis, thrush or candidosis.[2] It can occur following recent use of antibiotics, corticosteroids, immunosuppressive drugs, cytotoxic chemotherapy or irradiation.[2,3] Patients with immunodeficiencies such as leukemia or AIDS, or hypoendocrine states such as hypothyroidism, Addison's disease or diabetes mellitus, are at risk of developing candidiasis.[2-4] Xerostomia (dry mouth) that is due to drug use, irradiation and disease, or wearing of dentures, also predisposes a patient to developing oral candidiasis.[3,4] *C. albicans* can be transferred to an infant's mouth during passage through the birth canal.[5] Newborn babies, especially if premature, are susceptible to this infection.[5] Healthy infants who suck on pacifiers have a higher colonization rate of *Candida* in the mouth.[6,7] Candidiasis may also occur in pregnant women and individuals who are malnourished.[2]

Goals of Therapy

- Resolve infection
- Prevent recurrences
- Ensure accurate diagnosis of candidiasis and proper assessment and management of potential causes (e.g., inhaled corticosteroid use, denture wear) through appropriate referral

Patient Assessment (Figure 1)

Because candidal infections are opportunistic and often associated with predisposing factors, identification and correction of the underlying factors is essential. Hence, the pharmacist needs to take a referring role, confirming with the patient that there may be an oral problem that needs appropriate identification by a physician or dentist. Oral candidiasis can be classified as:

- Acute pseudomembranous candidiasis (thrush)
- Atrophic candidiasis
- Chronic atrophic candidiasis (denture stomatitis)

It is possible for candidiasis to appear with more than one group of symptoms simultaneously.[3,4]

Acute pseudomembranous candidiasis, or thrush, appears as soft, creamy yellow, slightly elevated plaques (pseudomembranes) on any mucosal surface of the mouth, but most frequently on the inside of the cheeks and on the upper surface of the tongue.[4] The plaques can easily be rubbed off, exposing a red area of underlying epithelium. The surrounding mucosa is not inflamed. This form of the disease is found most commonly in infants, the elderly and the terminally ill.[3]

Loss of the pseudomembrane by the *Candida* organism causes small to generalized large red lesions with inflammation of the surrounding tissues. This condition is known as *atrophic candidiasis*. These lesions are most commonly seen on the palate and on the tongue, which shows depapillation and dekeratinization.[4] Atrophic lesions follow the use of broad-spectrum antibiotics or the use of inhaled corticosteroids[4] and may be associated with HIV infection.[3]

Chronic atrophic candidiasis (denture stomatitis) presents as erythematous, edematous lesions with a

Figure 1: **Assessment of Patients with Oral Candidiasis**

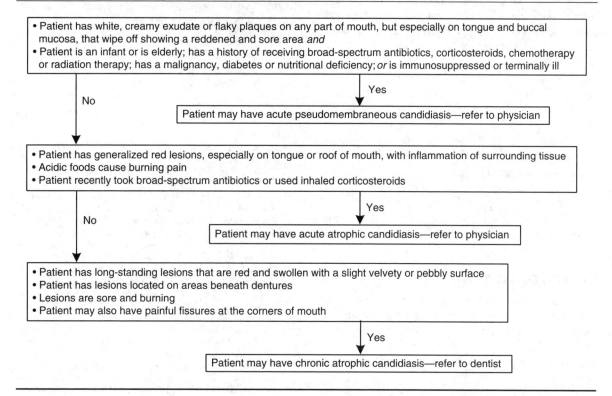

- Patient has white, creamy exudate or flaky plaques on any part of mouth, but especially on tongue and buccal mucosa, that wipe off showing a reddened and sore area *and*
- Patient is an infant or is elderly; has a history of receiving broad-spectrum antibiotics, corticosteroids, chemotherapy or radiation therapy; has a malignancy, diabetes or nutritional deficiency; *or* is immunosuppressed or terminally ill

No

Yes

Patient may have acute pseudomembraneous candidiasis—refer to physician

- Patient has generalized red lesions, especially on tongue or roof of mouth, with inflammation of surrounding tissue
- Acidic foods cause burning pain
- Patient recently took broad-spectrum antibiotics or used inhaled corticosteroids

No

Yes

Patient may have acute atrophic candidiasis—refer to physician

- Patient has long-standing lesions that are red and swollen with a slight velvety or pebbly surface
- Patient has lesions located on areas beneath dentures
- Lesions are sore and burning
- Patient may also have painful fissures at the corners of mouth

Yes

Patient may have chronic atrophic candidiasis—refer to dentist

slight velvety/pebbly surface located on the palate and upper and lower edentulous ridges, typically below the entire denture-bearing area. The area may be sore and there may be a burning sensation. It is present in approximately 50% of complete denture wearers.[3] Angular cheilitis (sore, erythematous fissured lesions affecting the angles of the mouth) is commonly associated with chronic atrophic candidiasis.[3,4]

Oral psoriasis, discoid lupus erythematosus, pernicious anemia, white keratoic lesions (leukoplakia) and early erythema multiforme can all present with oral symptoms similar to oral candidiasis.[1,2,8]

Pharmacologic Therapy

Refer patients with suspected oral candidiasis to their physician or dentist. Elimination of the underlying factors responsible for the opportunistic infection may be sufficient to allow the microflora to return to normal and thus resolve the condition; however, prescription therapy with an antifungal agent may also be necessary.[1] Previously, gentian violet was used for the management of oral candidiasis but more effective, nonst'aining pharmacologic agents are now preferred.

Prescription Therapy
Pharmacologic therapy falls into three categories: the polyenes (**nystatin** and **amphotericin B**), the azoles (e.g., **ketoconazole**, **clotrimazole, fluconazole** and **itraconazole**) and **5-flucytosine**.[9] A systematic review examined the evidence concerning treatment and prevention of oropharyngeal candidiasis in people with HIV infection, denture stomatitis, diabetes mellitus, in those receiving chemotherapy and in infants and children.[10] Antifungal resistance, especially in AIDS-associated infections, is a concern.[9]

Monitoring of Therapy

People who wear dentures, especially for longer than 24 hours at a time, have poor oral hygiene or mucosal trauma from poorly fitting dentures are at risk of developing oral candidiasis. People with complaints of dry mouth, which can be drug-induced, are also at risk (see chapter 65.) Patients taking broad-spectrum antibiotics, undergoing chemotherapy or radiation therapy or who take corticosteroids systemically or by inhalation should be monitored for signs and symptoms of oral candidiasis. Preventive measures for oral candidiasis during steroid inhalation include the use of a spacer device and rinsing the mouth with water following inhalation. If signs or symptoms of oral candidiasis are identified in a person with oral complaints, refer them to a physician or dentist for evaluation and possible treatment.

Resource Tips

Centers for Disease Control and Prevention. Issues in the Child Care Setting. What you should know about...Yeast infections (thrush) in the child care setting:

http://www.cdc.gov/ncidod/hip/abc/facts43.htm

Suggested Readings

Appleton SS. Candidiasis: pathogenesis, clinical characteristics, and treatment. *J Calif Dent Assoc.* 2000; 28(12):942-8.

Clinical Evidence Online. *Oral health. Oropharyngeal candidiasis.* 2000 BMJ Publishing Group. Available from: http://www.clinicalevidenceonline.org/.

Farah CS, Ashman RB, Challacombe SJ. Oral candidosis. *Clin Dermatol.* 2000;18(5):553-62.

Scully C, Porter S. ABC of oral health. Swellings and red, white, and pigmented lesions. *BMJ.* 2000;321 (7255):225-8.

References

1. Farah CS, Ashman RB, Challacombe SJ. Oral candidosis. *Clin Dermatol.* 2000;18(5):553-62.
2. Scully C, Porter S. ABC of oral health. Swellings and red, white, and pigmented lesions. *BMJ.* 2000;321(7255):225-8.
3. Fotos PG, Lilly JP. Clinical management of oral and perioral candidosis. *Dermatol Clin.* 1996;14(2):273-80.
4. Appleton SS. Candidiasis: pathogenesis, clinical characteristics, and treatment. *J Calif Dent Assoc.* 2000;28(12):942-8.
5. Habif TP. *Clinical dermatology. A color guide to diagnosis and therapy.* 3rd ed. St. Louis, MI: Mosby; 1996:394.
6. Mattos-Graner RO, de Moraes AB, Rontani RM, Birman EG. Relation of oral yeast infection in Brazilian infants and use of a pacifier. *ASDC J Dent Child.* 2001;68(1):33-6, 10.
7. Darwazeh AM, al-Bashir A. Oral candidal flora in healthy infants. *J Oral Pathol Med.* 1995;24(8):361-4.
8. Brice DM, Danesh-Meyer MJ. Oral lesions in patients with psoriasis: clinical presentation and management. *J Periodontol.* 2000;71(12):1896-903.
9. Ellepola AN, Samaranayake LP. Antimycotic agents in oral candidosis: an overview: 2. Treatment of oral candidosis. *Dent Update.* 2000;27(4):165-70, 172-4.
10. Clinical Evidence Online. *Oral health. Oropharyngeal candidiasis.* 2000 BMJ Publishing Group. Available from: http://www.clinicalevidenceonline.org/

Thrush (Oral Candidiasis)—Patient Information

Thrush or oral candidiasis is caused by a yeast infection in your mouth. This can happen more often when you have certain diseases (for example, diabetes mellitus, leukemia and hypothyroidism). It can also happen after you have taken certain medications (for example, antibiotics, steroids, chemotherapy) or have had radiation therapy. People who wear dentures are at risk of getting this infection. Healthy newborn babies and infants who suck on pacifiers may also get thrush. As people get older they tend to get a dry mouth. Having a dry mouth can lead to thrush.

You can help prevent oral candidiasis:

- Tell your pharmacist, dentist or doctor if you have problems with a dry mouth. They can help decrease this problem and make you more comfortable.
- Don't use a mouthwash that has a high alcohol content for a long time. These mouthwashes can cause your mouth to become dry.
- If you wear dentures, take them out at night. Be sure to clean them properly.
- If you use an inhaled corticosteroid, rinse your mouth with water after using it. Ask your pharmacist about using a spacer with your inhaled corticosteroid. A spacer can help decrease the chance of oral candidiasis.

When you have oral candidiasis:

- See your doctor or dentist so you can receive medication to treat this infection.
- Once the infection has cleared you should throw out your old toothbrush and start using a new one.
- If you wear dentures, ask your pharmacist or dentist about a special solution for soaking your dentures at night while you have the infection (hypochlorite 0.1% solution).

Chapter 65

Dry Mouth

Mary E. MacCara, PharmD

Pathophysiology

Dry mouth (xerostomia) describes a patient's perception of insufficient moisture within the mouth. It is more than a problem of inconvenience and its presence should not be considered trivial.

Xerostomia is usually associated with salivary hypofunction in which there are both decreased saliva production and qualitative changes in saliva. Saliva has various protective functions including maintaining the neutral pH of the mouth, promoting remineralization of teeth, coating the teeth and lubricating the oral mucosa, providing local antimicrobial activity and assisting in the taste mechanism.[1] The loss of saliva's protective functions can affect all of the mouth's functions as well as a person's general well-being and quality of life (Table 1).[2,3]

Table 1: **Potential Complications of Dry Mouth**[2,3]

Impaired ability or willingness to talk
Increased dental caries
Tooth loss
Oral infections, e.g., candidiasis, gingivitis
Decreased ability to chew and swallow
Decreased nutritional status
Inhibition of taste sensation
Avoidance of some foods that are difficult to chew/swallow
Wearing dentures becomes uncomfortable or impossible

Xerostomia can occur at any age but is more common in older people, affecting 25% of women and 16% of men in that age group.[3] It is also associated with chronic diseases including depression, uncontrolled hypertension, Alzheimer's disease, Addison's disease, alcoholic cirrhosis, hyperlipidemia, Sjögren's syndrome, uncontrolled diabetes mellitus, HIV infection and absent or malformed salivary glands.[1,2]

Dry mouth is one of the more common adverse effects of medications. Many classes of drugs can cause dry mouth including antidepressants, antipsychotics, antihistamines, decongestants, antiparkinson agents, anticholinergics, urinary antispasmodics, benzodiazepines, antiemetics, opioids and adrenergic agonists.[4-6] Drugs that cause significant dry mouth in more than 10% of patients are identified in Table 2.[6]

The risk of dry mouth is also increased by smoking and the intake of caffeine-containing beverages.[2]

Xerostomia is common in cancer patients. It can occur in patients who have had therapeutic radiation to the head and neck and can be a component of graft-versus-host disease following bone marrow transplantation.[1,3] Mouth breathing due to dyspnea, nasal obstruction or delivery of oxygen via nasal prongs can be a major cause of dry mouth in the terminally ill.[7]

Xerostomia can also be of a short-term nature. Anxiety, dehydration, viral infections (e.g., mumps) and short-term drug use can all cause temporary salivary hypofunction leading to dry mouth.[1]

Goals of Therapy

- Identify patients with dry mouth and advise appropriate self-care
- Advise patients with suspected underlying pathology to see a physician
- Advise patients with long-term xerostomia to see a dentist, to minimize damage to teeth

---

Table 2: **Drugs Causing Significant Dry Mouth in More Than 10% of Patients**[6]

Adrenergic agonists; bronchodilators
Isoproterenol

Alpha-adrenergic receptor agonists
Clonidine

Alpha-adrenergic receptor blockers
Reserpine

Antiarrhythmics
Propafenone

Anticholinergics
Atropine sulfate
Belladonna and opium
Benztropine mesylate
Diphenoxylate and atropine
Glycopyrrolate
Hyoscyamine sulfate
Ipratropium bromide

Anticonvulsants
Clonazepam

Antidepressants
Amitriptyline HCl
Amoxapine
Bupropion
Clomipramine HCl
Desipramine HCl
Doxepin HCl
Maprotiline HCl
Nefazodone
Paroxetine
Phenelzine
Protriptyline HCl
Trimipramine
Venlafaxine

Antiemetics
Nabilone
Prochlorperazine

Antihistamines
Loratadine

Antiparkinson Agents
Selegiline
Trihexyphenidyl

Antispasmodics
Dicyclomine
Flavoxate
Oxybutynin

Antipsychotics
Loxapine

Benzodiazepines
Alprazolam
Chlordiazepoxide
Clorazepate dipotassium
Diazepam
Flurazepam
Lorazepam
Oxazepam
Temazepam

Biologic response modulators
Interferon alpha-2a
Interferon alpha-2b

Ergot alkaloids
Ergotamine

Retinoic acid derivatives
Isotretinoin

Skeletal muscle relaxants
Cyclobenzaprine

Patient Assessment (Figure 1)

Patients have differing perceptions of whether or not their mouths are dry. Some have sufficient saliva flow, but complain of dry mouth. In contrast, some patients have true xerostomia yet do not recognize that their mouths are dry. Advise patients who complain of dry mouth to see their physician or dentist so the underlying reason can be identified. Difficulty eating (e.g., mouth feels dry while eating, patient has difficulty swallowing food and needs to sip water to swallow dry food), is suggestive of salivary hypofunction as the cause of dry mouth.[1] The continuous presence of dry mouth symptoms during the day is associated with more significant salivary hypofunction than if there is gradual onset of symptoms over the course of the day. Symptoms of dry mouth that occur only at night are usually not associated with salivary hypofunction because salivary function normally approaches zero during sleep.[1]

Patients may experience regional or generalized mucosal pain, often described as "burning," or they may describe the inability to eat acidic or spicy foods such that they have had to make changes in their diet.[1] This can be suggestive of chronic atrophic candidiasis, secondary to dry mouth. Patients with chronic atrophic candidiasis frequently also have angular cheilitis, seen as "cracks in the corners of the mouth." Refer patients suspected of having chronic atrophic candidiasis to a physician or dentist for proper diagnosis and treatment (see Chapter 64).

Pharmacists should be aware of the prescription medications that cause dry mouth and counsel patients taking these medications to report dry mouth symptoms to their physician. In addition, pharmacists can ask about the occurrence of this side effect when the patient returns for a refill. Instruct patients with dry mouth due to a prescription medication to not reduce the dosage of the medication or stop taking it without first consulting their physician.[2]

Pharmacists can assess whether a nonprescription medication may be causing a patient's dry mouth, and advise the patient regarding possible adjustment of therapy.

Figure 1: **Assessment of Patients with Dry Mouth**

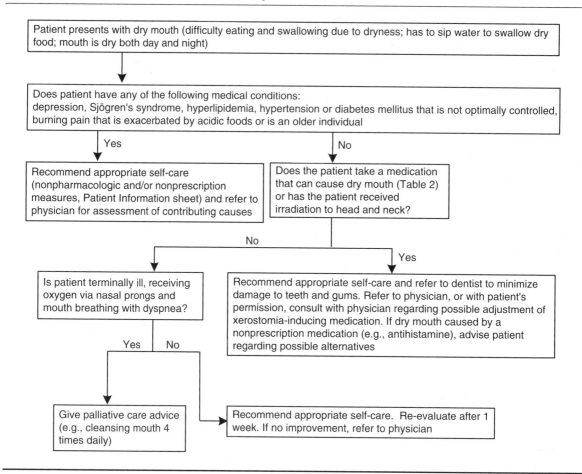

Pharmacists should also assess the ability of patients with dry mouth to swallow solid dosage forms and assist in exploring alternative options.

Nonpharmacologic Therapy

Treatment is directed towards easing patient discomfort and preventing dental caries.

Dental Care[1]

Inform patients they are at increased risk of dental caries because of their decreased saliva. They should visit their dentist and dental hygienist and practise regular brushing and flossing of the teeth. The use of fluoride is very important in preventing dental caries. It is applied professionally by the dentist or hygienist and maintained by the patient through daily use of high fluoride-containing toothpastes (e.g., Prevident®) or mouth rinses (e.g., Oral B® Fluoride 0.05%, alcohol-free). Remind patients that reduction of sugar in the diet will help prevent dental caries. They should try to restrict sugar intake to mealtime, avoiding between-meal sugary snacks (see Chapter 58).

Salivary Flow Stimulation[1,2]

If the patient's salivary glands are still functioning, physiologic stimulation of saliva flow can be accomplished through masticatory or gustatory stimuli. Encourage patients to chew sugarless gum or suck sugarless hard candies as needed throughout the day. These substances are sweetened using an alcohol sugar such as xylitol, mannitol, maltitol, lactitol or erythritol, which do not promote dental caries.[8] Labels should be carefully read to ensure the product does not contain simple sugars such as glucose, fructose, sucrose, lactose and maltose, which are cariogenic.[9]

Water Consumption
For general good health it is important that people have sufficient fluid intake. However, unless xerostomia is due to dehydration, patients should not assume that drinking large volumes of water will overcome oral dryness. Frequent small sips of water during the day will help relieve oral symptoms. The use of saliva substitutes may be more convenient for patients awakened at night with dry mouth symptoms. Frequent intake of water at night can lead to nocturia and interrupted sleep.

Pharmacologic Therapy
Nonprescription Therapy
Saliva Substitutes
Artificial saliva products can help moisten the mouth. None replaces all the functions of saliva and their action is short-lived due to swallowing.[1,10] Their use has not been shown to prevent caries or oral candidiasis.[1] These products are most convenient for patients to use while traveling, while talking and at night, to prevent nocturia from increased fluid intake during the night.

Moi-Stir®, available as a spray or swabs, contains electrolytes normally present in saliva, including the chloride salts of calcium, magnesium, potassium and sodium, as well as sodium phosphate dibasic. Mouth Kote® is a herbal remedy mouth moisturizer composed of yerba santa, water, xylitol, sorbitol and citric acid. Yerba santa (*Eriodictyon californicum*) is said to have expectorant properties and is used as a flavoring agent.[11,12]

Oralbalance® gel is an oral moisturizer containing a synthetic polymer, polyglycerylmethacrylate, and the salivary enzymes, lactoperoxidase and glucose oxidase. In patients with dry mouth secondary to radiation of the salivary glands, it offered more relief to patients with severe xerostomia than to those with moderate xerostomia.[13] The duration of its moistening

effect averaged one hour during the daytime and more than four hours during the night.[13]

Other Products for Dry Mouth
The Biotene® line of dry mouth products, including toothpaste, mouthwash and gum, contain salivary enzymes, lactoperoxidase, glucose oxidase and lysozyme, the goal being to replace the missing salivary enzyme activity in patients with salivary hypofunction. Patients with dry mouth due to radiation therapy for head and neck cancer have anecdotally reported improvement in their oral symptoms with the use of these products.[14,15] Patients with xerostomia following radiation therapy preferred the taste and consistency of Biotene® toothpaste and Oralbalance® gel over commercial toothpastes and carboxymethylcellulose gel; however, symptom improvement with these products, in the same study, did not reach statistical significance.[15]

Lozenges containing 200 mg of anhydrous crystalline maltose were found to increase unstimulated whole saliva flow in patients with primary Sjögren's syndrome and to significantly reduce dry mouth symptoms. The lozenges were administered three times a day for 24 weeks. Improvement in dry mouth symptoms were seen within 12 weeks and reached statistical significance after 12 weeks of use. Side effects were mild and included sinusitis, headache, cheilitis, salivary gland enlargement and fatigue.[16] Anhydrous crystalline maltose is classified as a nutritional supplement. It has the potential to cause dental caries.

Prescription Therapy
Pharmacologic stimulation of the salivary glands can be accomplished through the use of the cholinergic agonist, pilocarpine.[1] It is administered orally at a dosage of 5 mg three or four times daily. Its most frequent adverse effect is increased perspiration with other unwanted effects being nausea, increased urination, lacrimation, headache and dizziness. Pilocarpine is indicated for the treatment of dry mouth symptoms including hypofunction of salivary glands due to radiotherapy for head or neck cancer and in Sjögren's syndrome. Its use to treat xerostomia due to chronic medication ingestion is not a Health Canada approved indication. Always consider the potential for drug interactions.

Monitoring of Therapy

Patients advised to practise appropriate self-care for dry mouth should be reassessed after one week. If they are achieving improved mouth comfort through increased intake of fluids, use of sugarless candy and are practising good dental hygiene, they should be encouraged to continue these measures. They should also be encouraged to seek the advice of a dentist for evaluation of the cause of their dry mouth and for advice on the care of their teeth. Patient acceptance of a saliva substitute (taste, dosage form, degree of comfort attained) will dictate whether or not it will be used. Encourage patients who are not achieving mouth comfort with one product to try another.[10] If mouth complications arise (e.g., candidiasis) or the dryness worsens, the patient should be evaluated by a dentist or physician.

If pilocarpine has been prescribed, the patient should be monitored for excessive cholinergic side effects. If no improvement in mouth discomfort is noted after one week, consultation with a physician may be necessary for dosage adjustment.

Resource Tips

Mayo Clinic Condition Centers: What is dry mouth? http://www.mayoclinic.com/findinformation/conditioncenters/invoke.cfm?objectid=50B3D1EF-C44D-46A3-A5E06F9AC4F2A836

National Institute of Dental and Craniofacial Research. Dry Mouth http://www.nohic.nidcr.nih.gov/pubs/drymouth/dmouth.htm

The Sjögren's Syndrome Foundation Inc http://www.sjogrens.com/ offers useful resources for people with Sjögren's syndrome, including management of dry mouth. Contact them for information concerning *The Moisture Seekers Newsletter*.

The University of Ottawa Institute of Palliative Care offers in its Online Education Centre useful information for health professionals and caregivers on palliative mouth care for patients with a dry mouth. http://www.pallcare.org/educate/index.html

Suggested Readings

Daniels TE, Wu AJ. Xerostomia – clinical evaluation and treatment in general practice. *J Calif Dent Assoc* 2000;28(12):933-41.

Holmes S, Xerostomia: aetiology and management in cancer patients. *Support Care Cancer* 1998;6(4):348-55.

Pray SW. Help for patients with dry mouth. *US Pharmacist* 2000;25:16,19-22.

Sreebny LM, Schwartz SS. A reference guide to drugs and dry mouth. 2nd ed. *Gerodontology* 1997;14(1):33-47.

Wynn RL, Meiller TF. Drugs and dry mouth. *Gen Dent* 2001;49(1):10-4.

References

1. Daniels TE, Wu AJ. Xerostomia – clinical evaluation and treatment in general practice. *J Calif Dent Assoc* 2000; 28(12):933-41.
2. Pray SW. Help for patients with dry mouth. *US Pharmacist* 2000;25:16,19-22.
3. Holmes S, Xerostomia: aetiology and management in cancer patients. *Support Care Cancer* 1998;6:348-55.
4. American Dental Association. *ADA Guide to Dental Therapeutics.* 1st ed. Chicago, IL: ADA Publishing Co, Inc., 1998.
5. Sreebny LM, Schwartz SS. A reference guide to drugs and dry mouth. 2nd ed. *Gerodontology* 1997;14(1):33-47.
6. Wynn RL, Meiller TF. Drugs and dry mouth. *Gen Dent* 2001; 49(1):10-4.
7. University of Ottawa Institute of Palliative Care. Online education centre. Palliative mouth care. Risk factors. Available from: http://www.pallcare.org/educate/index.html. Accessed July 26, 2001.
8. Kurtzweil P. Staking a claim to good health. FDA Consumer 1998;32(6). Available from: http://www.fda.gov/fdac/features/1998/698_labl.html. Accessed July 26, 2001.
9. Mount G, Hume R. Dental caries. A learning program on the nature and management of dental caries. UCLA Dentistry Continuing Education. Available from: http://www.dent.ucla.edu/ce/caries/. Accessed July 26, 2001.
10. Wynn RL, Meiller TF. Artificial saliva products and drugs used to treat xerostomia. *Gen Dent* 2000;48(6):630-6.
11. Review of Natural Products. Yerba santa monograph. St. Louis, MI: Facts and Comparisons; 1991.
12. The Natural Pharmacist. TNP.com. Herbs & Supplements. Yerba santa. Available from: http//www.tnp.com/encyclopedia/substance/99/388. Accessed July 26, 2001.
13. Regelink G, Vissink A, Reintsema H, Nauta JM. Efficacy of a synthetic polymer saliva substitute in reducing oral complaints of patients suffering from irradiation-induced xerostomia. *Quintessence Int.* 1998;29(6):383-8.
14. Warde P, Kroll B, O'Sullivan B, et al. A phase II study of Biotene in the treatment of postradiation xerostomia in patients with head and neck cancer. *Support Care Cancer.* 2000;8(3):203-8.
15. Epstein JB, Emerton S, Le ND, Stevenson-Moore P. A double-blind crossover trial of Oral Balance gel and Biotene toothpaste versus placebo in patients with xerostomia following radiation therapy. *Oral Oncol* 1999;35(2):132-7.
16. Fox PC, Cummins MJ, Cummins JM. Use of orally administered anhydrous crystalline maltose for relief of dry mouth. *J Altern Complement Med* 2001;7(1):33-43.

Dry Mouth (Xerostomia)—Patient Information

A dry mouth is not pleasant and can cause problems. It can cause teeth to decay more easily and it can make eating hard to do. If you have a dry mouth, visit your dentist and your doctor. They can help find out why your mouth is dry and your dentist can help you protect your teeth from cavities while your mouth is dry.

Things you can do to relieve dry mouth:
- Sip water often during the day.
- Avoid or cut down on caffeine-containing drinks such as coffee, tea and cola. Caffeine causes your mouth to become more dry.
- Do not use tobacco or alcohol. They both cause your mouth to be dry.
- Chew sugar-free gum or suck on sugar-free candy during the day. This will help keep the mouth moist and won't cause cavities.
- Keep your teeth and gums clean. Brush your teeth twice a day with a soft toothbrush and floss between the teeth once a day.
- Use a fluoride-containing toothpaste daily or rinse with a fluoride-containing mouthwash. This will help prevent cavities.
- An artificial saliva product may help make your mouth feel more moist. Your pharmacist may suggest a product to use at night or when you are bothered by dryness, such as when you are talking. Artificial saliva does not protect your teeth like real saliva. Tell your dentist if you are using one of these products.
- If you have a hard time swallowing your medicine in tablet or capsule form, ask your pharmacist if the same medicine can be taken as a liquid. Some people find it easier to swallow capsules and tablets if they sip some water first, then swallow the capsule or tablet using a full glass of water.
- Use a humidifier or vaporizer to help keep the air moist in your house and make you more comfortable.
- If you have a hard time eating food, try sipping water throughout your meal, and choose soft or puréed foods when you can.

General Appendices

A. **Medical Devices and Aids to Daily Living**

B. **Home Testing**

C. **Complementary and Alternative Therapies**

D. **Information for the Traveler**

E. **Microorganism Abbreviations**

Medical Devices and Aids to Daily Living

Marie Berry, BScPharm, BA, LLB

Medical devices and aids to daily living (ADLs) are an integral part of contemporary home health care market. It is estimated that in Canada over $30 million annually is spent on both. The market itself is broad and includes not only such traditional items as medical equipment, but first aid and wound care products, sports medicine items, incontinence aids, palliative care products, and diagnostic equipment.

Several factors have combined to create this expanded market – longer life expectancies, technological advances and economies involved in modern health care.

The Canadian population is living longer because of advances in medical knowledge and technology. Over time, more older people will be living in their homes, requiring medical devices to carry on their day-to-day living.

Improved technology enables individuals to stay at home or to go home earlier from hospital, and also permits earlier diagnosis and self care.

In general, treatment in hospitals is expensive, and both medical devices and ADLs allow less costly home-based treatment. Patients are discharged earlier from hospital with home recovery, and not-for-admission or "day" surgery is more common.

Use of medical devices and ADLs not only has economic advantages, but it provides an improved quality of life, reducing or even eliminating a person's disability. Orthopedic patients (e.g., those with hip replacements or fractures) can be more mobile. Individuals with brain damage (e.g., stroke patients or accident victims who have suffered hemiplegia) can be better equipped to cope with every day life. Rheumatoid arthritis, amyotrophic lateral sclerosis

(ALS), and multiple sclerosis (MS) patients are able to cope better with their diseases. Amputees do not have to be institutionalized. Caregivers, as well, find their tasks much less onerous.

Medical Devices

Medical devices include a wide range of items. The legal definition is any article, instrument, apparatus, or contrivance, including any component, part or accessory thereof, manufactured, sold or represented for use in the diagnosis, treatment, mitigation or prevention of a disease, disorder, or abnormal physical state or its symptoms.[1] The definition also includes devices that could be used to restore, correct or modify a body function or body structure; to diagnose pregnancy; and to care for pregnant individuals and their offspring. It is a broad definition and includes both human beings and animals.

While a broad range of medical devices are listed in Table 1, this appendix focuses specifically on durable medical equipment, patient comfort aids, respiratory aids and home intravenous equipment. Diagnostic tests intended for home use, wound care products, incontinence aids, surgical sundries and sports and orthopedic products are discussed elsewhere in this book (see Index).

Durable Medical Equipment

Durable medical equipment can withstand day-to-day wear. At one time, high quality equipment was available only in hospital or institutional settings. Today, such equipment is intended for in-home use, either by the individual alone or with the assistance of a caregiver. Durable medical equipment can be

Table 1: **Medical Devices**

Category	Examples
Durable medical equipment	Commodes Shower chairs Walkers Wheelchairs
Home diagnostic tools	Blood glucose monitors, cholesterol testing kits, pregnancy testing kits, blood pressure monitors
Patient comfort aids	Pressure therapy Pillows Cushions Elastic compression stockings; back, neck and limb braces
Respiratory aids	Asthma nebulizers Peak flow meters Allergy sprays Vaporizers, humidifiers
Wound care products	First aid products Surgical bandages Specialized dressings
Incontinence aids	Undergarments Protectors Sheaths Drainage bags Bedwetting alarm systems
Surgical sundries	Personal hygiene products Ear plugs Gloves Medicine measuring devices Manicure accessories
Sports and orthopedic products	Belts Braces Supports Massagers Hot/cold therapy
Home intravenous products	Accessories such as tubing, infusion pumps, needles, syringes

divided into two groups that represent the majority of these types of devices: equipment for bathroom safety and equipment for mobility.

Equipment for Bathroom Safety
Approximately one-half of falls in the home occur in the bathroom, and of those, two-thirds involve getting into or out of the bathtub.[2] Bath oils and bubble bath make bathtubs slippery. Showers are an alternative, but some individuals have difficulty standing in a shower. Chairs designed to be used in the shower are an option. Something as simple as a bath mat with suction cups reduces the risk for falls. Bathtub and shower grab bars, along with tub rails, make a bathroom safer. Hand-held or portable showers are another alternative.

Shampoo Trays
For people confined to bed or in a wheelchair, shampoo trays make washing hair possible.

Inflatable Bathtubs

Inflatable vinyl tubs fit over a bed and come with a hand-held shower and hose, making bathing in bed a possibility.

Bath Boards

Bath boards sit across the tub and usually have hand-grips. They are ideal for storing soap and sponges within easy reach and for helping to maintain stability when stepping out of the bathtub.

Bath/Shower Seats

Bath seats are set right into the tub, or across the tub, allowing an individual to sit down while bathing. Some have backrests, and all have suction cups to prevent them from slipping. Shower seats are similar to bathtub seats. Suction cup legs, adjustable seat heights, back support, non-slip coverings and easy to clean surfaces are desirable features.

Bathtub Transfer Benches

Bathtub transfers are the greatest cause of anxiety in debilitated individuals, as this is when most falls occur. Requiring someone to assist in a bathtub transfer is also a sign of lost independence and privacy.

Transfer benches straddle the bathtub with two seating areas – one inside the tub and one outside. The individual sits on the seat outside the bathtub, much like they would in a chair. While seated they can move their legs one at a time over the bathtub edge and into the bathtub, finally pulling themselves over to the portion of the seat positioned above the bath water.

Transfer benches have adjustable heights. A couple of trial runs while fully clothed and without bath water are recommended, to adjust the bench to the correct height. The sitting surfaces must be slippery enough so that the transfer is easy, but not so slippery that someone may slide off the surface, especially when it is wet.

Transfer benches should be easy to clean and if not permanent, they should be light and easy to position. Suction cups are used to anchor the bench both to the bathtub and to the floor. Most have side grab bars and backrests. They should be adjustable so that a person can enter the tub from either the right or the left.

Raised Toilet Seats

Raised toilet seats ease sitting down and getting up from the toilet and facilitate transfers from a wheelchair to the toilet seat. Most raised toilet seats add 4 inches to the toilet height, although some are adjustable up to 6.5 inches. All raised toilet seats attach directly to the toilet bowl and some can be attached permanently by means of clips. Portable raised toilet seats are available for traveling.

Some raised toilet seats have cut-out areas that accommodate various lower extremity disabilities where limited range of movement or other conditions prevent a normal flexed sitting position.

Raised toilet seats might have armrests and safety rails. A safety bar can be attached to the wall next to the toilet. A trial run will help with the appropriate placement.

Miscellaneous

Wash mitts, wash sponges (some have a pocket for a bar of soap), long-handled scrubbing brushes/sponges and tap turners make bathing easier, and help prevent falls. The toilet tissue dispenser should be within easy reach. Toilet tissue aids enable individuals without manual dexterity to use toilet tissue. Splashguards can be attached to any toilet, raised seat or not.

Equipment for Mobility

Historically, decreased mobility for an individual meant being housebound, bedridden, or even institutionalized. Also, decreased mobility has associated health risks such as thromboembolism. Equipment for mobility includes canes, walkers and wheelchairs.

Canes and Walkers

Canes and walkers reduce instability and afford confidence and increased mobility. Wooden canes and walkers are less expensive, but are heavier. Aluminum canes and walkers are lightweight, thus more easily manoeuvred and ideal for individuals who, because of age or disease, do not have great muscle strength.

Canes and walkers should be measured to ensure a correct fit.[3] The distance from the top of a cane's handle to its tip should equal the distance from the wrist crease to the ground, when the arm is straight down at the side. The measurement should be performed with the individual standing erect and wearing everyday shoes.

If the cane is too short, the user will lean forward. If it is too long they will lean backward. Adjustable and telescopic canes enable an individual to find the correct fit. Walkers are measured in a similar manner, and most walkers are adjustable.

A cane handle should afford an easy, yet firm grip. A swan's neck handle is easier for balancing, and many handles have moulded grips. Metal and wood cane tips or walker feet tend to slip. Soft rubber tips are required, and are replaceable. A flip-back ice-gripping tip can be attached to the tip for extra stability in winter. Quad bases (four legs) add balance to canes. Although canes are most comfortably held in the dominant hand, holding the cane in the contralateral hand will provide greater balance.

Walkers may have wheels on two or four of the legs, and the wheels may be permanent or removable. Some walkers have wheels that can be attached to the two front legs, the two back legs, or all four legs; others have wheels that can be locked in place. Walker accessories include tote bags and attached seats. A folding walker eases transportation.

Wheelchairs

Wheelchairs should provide comfortable and functional mobility.[4] The everyday routine of the individual must be taken into consideration before choosing a wheelchair, because the choice can vary depending upon the individual's activities (e.g., going to work, participating in sports).

The method of propulsion of the wheelchair may be independent or assisted by another person. Independent propulsion refers not only to propelling wheels or hand rims manually, but also to the use of electrical controls with the hand, mouth, legs or feet.

Positioning of an individual in a wheelchair should provide adequate balance and support. The buttocks should bear equal loads, with adequate back support. Ideally, the shoulder should align vertically with the elbows, with the arms resting at right angles. The knees and ankles should be at right angles as well. More severely disabled people may not be able to

achieve the ideal position and adaptation of the chair is needed.

The wheelchair seat dimensions should fit with the body dimensions. A chair that is too large or too small does not function well for the user. The seat and back should not sag. The dimensions of an empty wheelchair are not the same as the dimensions of the chair with the user sitting in it. And, if a seat cushion is used, the dimensions also change.

The environment in which the chair will be used is a key factor.[5] If the chair is to be used indoors, its size and ability to manoeuvre must be considered as well as the architectural features of the building or room in question. Measuring doorways and checking the turning axis of the chair are required to ensure the wheelchair fits through doorways, both at home and at work.

Wheelchairs used outdoors should be able to negotiate uneven ground, slopes and curbs. This is a major limitation of wheelchairs in that they were designed to function on man-made surfaces, and they perform poorly outdoors (e.g., in the park, on the beach).

Wheelchairs used for leisure activities may require high performance features and should be easy to transport. Appearance and styling may be important. Certain sports (e.g., basketball, track) require specialized wheelchairs that are light and strong.

When traveling by car, close access to the car seat eases transferring between chair and car. Lightweight chairs with detachable or pivoting armrests and footrests make transfers and transportation easier.

Wheelchair accessories can increase comfort and mobility, and can sometimes reduce health risks. Wheelchair cushions can accommodate urinals, reduce pressure sores and support the head. Harnesses provide support and increase safety. Trays, bags, stump boards, umbrellas and rain hoods, pushing gloves and cuffs, portable ramps and transfer boards are other examples of wheelchair accessories.

Wheelchair manufacturers use different terms to describe the same features. Checking with the manufacturer will help to clarify the terms and descriptions.

Table 2 summarizes considerations involved in selecting a wheelchair.

Table 2: **Selecting a Wheelchair**

Features	Options/Considerations
Frame	Style Indoor or outdoor use Amputee Regular or lightweight construction
Seat height	Standard Hemiplegic
Arm rests	Fixed Removable Pivoting Full length Desk length Wrap-around
Backrest	Height Reclining Sectional
Footrests	Fixed Pivoting or swing-away Removable Elevated
Propulsion	Regular drive One-handed drive Electrical
Wheels	Spokes Composite Quick-release axle Caster width Pneumatic, semi-pneumatic or solid tires
Esthetics	Upholstery and frame colour Individual's self-image, personality, and preferences
Capabilities of chair	Home Work Leisure/Sports School Community Outdoor vs. indoor Terrain (An individual may need more than one wheelchair in order to perform different activities.)
Fit	Seating and postural needs Range of motion Size, weight, endurance, cognitive and perceptual status of user
Cost	Availability of funding Anticipated life expectancy of the wheelchair In the case of children, changes in size

Patient Comfort Aids

Patient comfort aids include pressure therapy, pillows, cushions, elastic compression stockings and back, neck and limb braces. Some of these devices are used therapeutically as well as to provide comfort.

Elastic Compression Stockings

Elastic compression stockings are also known as surgical or support stockings or hose. In the simplest form, support stockings are intended to relieve tired, aching legs and prevent swelling of feet, ankles and legs. Individuals who stand or sit for long periods of time or older individuals with compromised venous return are ideal candidates for these stockings. Prescribed compression stockings may be indicated for medical conditions such as varicose veins.

Elastic compression stockings decrease superficial venous pressure, increase the upward flow in unoccluded deep and superficial veins and raise local interstitial pressure. Compression of the leg also prevents some edema. They are designed to give gradual support with the most pressure exerted at the ankle, less at the calf and the least at the thigh.[6] Stockings vary in their compression and range from 12 to 60 mg Hg compression at the ankle.

A correct fit requires accurate measurements of the unedematous leg, first thing in the morning. To ensure effective compression, the stocking should be washed and dried according to the manufacturer's directions and replaced every two to three months. They are intended to be removed at night and put on in the morning before beginning daily activities. Manual dexterity is needed to put on or remove the stockings, and devices are available to assist with this.

Compression stockings are available as pantyhose, socks (above or below the knee), with open or closed toes and in various colors. The required compression and affected leg area should be the starting point in selection.

Antiembolism stockings are worn by the nonambulatory individual, to prevent venous emboli caused by inactivity. They provide less support and are not suitable for ambulatory individuals.

Respiratory Aids

Peak Flow Meters

Peak flow meters help predict and prevent exacerbations in a chronic obstructive pulmonary condition such as asthma. They allow home monitoring of a patient's lung function and titration of their medication in response to their lung function. The Canadian Asthma Consensus Conference recommends home monitoring by adult patients who are poor perceivers of airway obstruction and by patients with severe asthma.[7]

Peak flow meters measure the peak expiratory flow (PEF) rate, or the amount of air that can be forced out after the lungs are fully inflated. It is a mouthpiece with a gauge, an indicator and a scale. There are usually two sizes of mouthpieces to accommodate either children or adults.

After a complete exhalation, the individual inhales as deeply as possible, places the meter in their mouth, and blows out as hard and fast as possible. The final position of the indicator on the scale is the PEF measured in litres per minute. Three consecutive readings are taken, with the highest of the three being the result that is recorded. Children as young as four are able to perform this test.

It is recommended that daily measurements at 12-hour intervals are taken, for example 7 am and 7 pm, and recorded in a log or graph. Many meters come with a graph. If inhaled steroids or beta-agonists are used either before or after the test, a note is made. These values are compared to "predicted normal" values depending on age, race, gender, height and weight. A better approach is comparison to the individual's personal best.

A zoning system is usually used to make the test reading relevant for the patient. One zoning system frequently used is based on traffic lights. A result in the green zone correlates to 80 to 100% of the individual's personal best; yellow zone, 60 to 80%; and red zone, below 60%. In the yellow zone, medication may have to be re-evaluated, and in the red zone a bronchodilator is immediately required. If a reading appears in the red zone twice within a 48-hour period, medical attention should be sought.

Problems that can cause false readings include: the wrong size of mouth piece, the indicator not being at the bottom of the scale before the test is begun, fingers blocking some part of the mouthpiece opening, and atmospheric pressure effects.

Vaporizers/Humidifiers

Vaporizers use heat to disperse moisture in the air and, because they are hot, increase the temperature of the space in which they are used and can cause burns. Humidifiers require no heat. They increase humidity by physically dispersing water droplets in the air.

The use of distilled water prevents some mineral built-up in humidifiers; however, vaporizers require some minerals in the water in order for it to vaporize. Regular cleaning of both humidifiers and vaporizers is essential to remove debris and prevent growth of microorganisms, thus preventing infection and allergic reactions. Medication should not be added to humidifiers and if used with vaporizers, should only be placed in the medication cup (not the water reservoir).

Oxygen Therapy

Ambulatory respiratory and hospice patients may require oxygen therapy and with the available technology (e.g., face masks, nasal cannulae, oxygen concentrators, tracheal or endotracheal tubes), such therapy is more portable.

Oxygenated water and ozone therapy are touted as beneficial. Both, however, are expensive and lack evidence supporting their effectiveness.

Home Intravenous Products

Patients with chronic illness and serious infections may require long hospitalizations away from family, friends and work; however, they might be well enough to reside at home if they were able to obtain the required medication. Home intravenous programs have been developed to meet this need.

Home intravenous programs comprise one of the fastest growing segments of the home health care market. Several factors are responsible:

- More reliable equipment (e.g., better catheters, home infusion pumps);
- Increased patient awareness and involvement;
- Cost savings;
- Home health support from health care professionals.

Sixty per cent of home intravenous programs involve antibiotics, nutrition, or chemotherapy.[8] Other drugs (e.g., morphine in analgesic pumps) and fluid therapy account for the balance.

Examples of therapies that can be administered through home intravenous programs include:
- Antibiotic therapy for diseases such as infective endocarditis, septic arthritis, cystic fibrosis and osteomyelitis;
- Chemotherapy for breast cancer, Hodgkin's disease, leukemia or testicular cancer;
- Parenteral nutrition for patients with short bowel syndrome, inflammatory bowel disease, chronic intractable diarrhea or chronic idiopathic intestinal obstruction syndrome.

To succeed with a home intravenous program, a patient and their family must feel comfortable with the technology and skill required. The patient must have adequate cognitive function and no psychosis or drug addiction problems (Table 3).

Table 3: **Criteria for Candidates of Home Intravenous Programs**

Positive criteria	Negative criteria
Medical stability	Substance abuse
Manageable infection/ disease	Impaired vision
Adherence to program	Home without running water, electricity, refrigeration.
Sufficient cognitive function	
Venous access	

Most home intravenous patients have a venous catheter to which tubing and a prepared intravenous drug are attached. The drug infusion takes place over a specified period of time. The catheter is usually a long-term indwelling intravenous catheter (e.g., Broviac, Hickman or Groshong). These catheters require a heparin lock and the catheter site is usually rotated, to retain venous patency.

Subcutaneous infusion pumps are implanted devices used to infuse medication, blood products, fluids or nutrition. The pump appears as a raised area under the skin surface. There is a port with a self-sealing silicone rubber septum through which a Huber needle is inserted. The medication enters the body through tubing attached to the Huber needle.

Analgesic pumps are portable external devices that pump analgesic medications, typically morphine, through tubing and into a small needle placed in the subcutaneous tissue. The pump controls the flow of medication and is usually programmed to provide a set dose per time period. The pump can also be used manually with the patient having some control over dosage, but the pump is programmed to provide no more than a maximum quantity per time period. The pump is hung outside the tub when showering or bathing and placed under the pillow or hung on a hook when sleeping. Exposure of the pump to humidity, heat and freezing should be avoided.

Parenteral nutrition bypasses the GI tract completely and is infused into the circulation. With total parenteral nutrition (TPN) there may be a loss of GI function.

Complications

Phlebitis, infiltration and infection at the catheter site are the most common problems. Air emboli, dislodged catheters, migrating ports, catheter leaks and occlusion can also occur. The prepared intravenous solutions must be stored carefully, most often in the refrigerator and sometimes in the freezer.

Aids to Daily Living (ADLs)

The term "aids to daily living" refers to items that make day-to-day life easier for both an individual and their caregivers (e.g., clothing with Velcro® closures, handle grips for cutlery, wheelchairs and canes). ADLs can enable an individual to avoid institutionalization.[9]

ADLs are often recommended by occupational therapists who evaluate and recommend adaptations that enable an individual's daily living activities to continue. Mastering the correct technique for using an ADL can enable individuals to relearn an old skill, perform an old task in a new manner, or use equipment to perform a task.[10] The emphasis is on simplifying tasks, planning ahead, organizing the task, sitting and resting regularly when possible, and using correct body mechanics. Table 4 lists some common ADLs.

Tips for Using Medical Devices and ADLs

To gain the most benefit from medical devices and ADLs, they should to be used correctly:

- Measurements must be accurate in order to ensure a correct fit. Read the directions carefully and be sure the correct units are used (e.g., if the manufacturer lists sizes in inches, do the measurement in inches).
- With any medical device or ADL that requires assembly, read the instructions for assembly carefully. One option is to have it pre-assembled.
- All directions for use should be thoroughly understood prior to use of any medical device or ADL. If ambiguities exist, they should be clarified.
- Most medical devices and ADLs provide the manufacturer's contact information, such as a toll free number. Keeping this information handy makes it easier to investigate problems or ask questions.

Resource Tips

Provincial departments of health.

Health professionals in the related field (e.g., respiratory technologists for inhalation devices, occupational therapists for ADLs and mobility aids).

Organizations such as the Victoria Order of Nurses (VON) – in-home support for some types of medical devices and ADLs.

Retailers – including mail order and sports accessory retailers – may specialize in medical devices and ADLs.

Support groups:
The Arthritis Society
www.arthritis.ca
393 University Ave., Suite 1700, Toronto, ON
M5G 1E6   (416) 979-7228   1-800-321-1433

The Amyotrophic Lateral Sclerosis Society
www.als.ca
265 Yorkland Blvd. Suite 300, Toronto, ON   M2J 1S5
1-800-267-4ALS (4257)

The Canadian Head Injury Coalition
29 Pearce Ave., Winnipeg, MB   R2V 2K3

Table 4: **Examples of Aids to Daily Living**

Dishes	Partitioned; lip or raised edge; suction cup fixed on base; heated; food guards.
Cups	Easy-to-hold handles; detachable handles; attached straws and/or spouts; nose cut outs; weighted bases; insulated; holders to stabilize.
Utensils	Plastic coated spoons; weighted handles; easy to hold grips; swivel utensils; extension handles; specialized handles for odd angles; foam tubing to increase grip; putty to create a customized grip.
Kitchen	Electric and manual knives and peelers with easy-to-hold handles; cutting boards with nails to hold food for cutting; cutting boards with corner guards; easy-to-use and hold can and jar openers.
Home accessories	Doorknob and tap turners and grippers; easy-grip scissors; long reach sponge mops, dusters and vacuums; reading lights and magnifiers; book holders; reachers.
Personal care	Extension combs and brushes; handle grippers for tooth brushes; zipper pulls; elastic shoelaces; sock and panty hose aids; button hooks.
Communications	Games, stickers and communication boards; pen grips; computer accessories.
Recreation	Playing card holders and shufflers; knitting needle holders; hand cuffs and mobile bridges for pool cues.

The Lung Association
www.lung.ca
3 Raymond St., Suite 300 Ottawa, ON K1R 1A3
(613) 569-6411   1-800-972-2636

The Multiple Sclerosis Society of Canada
www.mssociety.ca
250 Bloor St. E., Toronto, ON M4W 3P9
(416) 922-6065   1-800-268-7582

Canadian Paraplegic Association Inc.
www.canparaplegic.org
1101 Prince of Wales Drive, Suite 230, Ottawa ON
K2C 3W7   1-800-720-4933

Canadian Rehabilitation Council for the Disabled
www.ccrw.org
302-500 University Ave, Toronto, ON M5G 1V7
1-800-664-0925

References

1. *Food and Drugs Act* R.S. 1985, C.F.-27, section 2.
2. Vassallo M, et al. Falls on integrated medical wards. *Gerontology* 2000;46:158.
3. Anonymous. Canes, walkers, and crutches. Don't let choosing one throw you off balance. *Mayo Clin Health Lett* 1999;17(1):4.
4. Minkel JL. Seating and mobility considerations for people with spinal cord injury. *Phys Ther* 2000;80:701.
5. Tomlinson JP. Managing maneuverability and rear stability of adjustable manual wheelchairs: an update. *Phys Ther* 2000; 80:904.
6. Agu O, et al. Graduated compression stockings in the prevention of venous thromboembolism. *Br J Surg* 1999;86:992.
7. Boulet L-P, et al. Canadian asthma consensus report, 1999. *CMAJ* 1999;161(11 suppl).
8. Anonymous. Five therapies account for 60% of home infusion. *US Pharmacist* 1993;18(4):16.
9. Finlayson M, Havixbeck K. A post-discharge study on the use of assistive devices. *Can J Occup Ther* 1992;59(4):201.
10. Pedretti MS, Zoltan B. *Occupational therapy practice skills for physical dysfunction.* 3rd ed. Toronto, ON: CV Mosby Company, 1990.

Home Testing

Marie Berry, BScPharm, BA, LLB

Home diagnostic devices are used for early diagnosis, to determine whether a certain therapy is effective, to monitor a medical condition, and for screening. Confidentiality and the ability to monitor or diagnose a condition at home make these devices popular. Advances in technology have also increased their accuracy. Two of the most commonly used home diagnostic devices are those for blood glucose levels and those for pregnancy or ovulation. These are discussed in the Diabetes Appendix: Diabetes Care Devices and the Reproductive Health Appendix: Pregnancy and Fertility Testing.

All home testing is meant to augment appropriate medical care. Home testing has been shown to increase compliance with treatment programs in some populations and gives individuals more understanding about their health.

Blood Pressure

Hypertension is termed a silent killer because it is asymptomatic. It is estimated that four million Canadians have hypertension, yet only half are treated and only 16% have adequate blood pressure control.[1,2]

Home blood pressure monitoring enables an individual to evaluate whether a new drug or treatment is working; to chart their course, which may act as motivation for compliance; and to avoid "white coat" hypertension. Both the 2000 Canadian hypertension guidelines and the American Association of Clinical Endocrinologists suggest that the use of home blood pressure monitoring be considered in people with diabetes.[2,3]

Home blood pressure monitoring should never be considered for self-diagnosis of hypertension. If the blood pressure is elevated with home blood pressure reading, medical advice should be sought for a definitive diagnosis of hypertension.[4]

Blood pressure is traditionally taken with a mercury sphygmomanometer, consisting of a cuff, a stethoscope, and a meter connected to a column of mercury. Sometimes the stethoscope is attached to the cuff itself. An aneroid blood pressure cuff is similar to a mercury sphygmomanometer but uses the air pressure from the cuff to move a needle on a circular gauge instead of forcing mercury up a column.

When inflated, the cuff becomes a tourniquet cutting off blood flow; the cuff is then loosened by releasing air. To measure blood pressure, an individual listens with the stethoscope for sounds (*Korotkoff sounds*) in the main artery of the arm, the brachial artery, as the cuff is slowly deflated. Korotkoff sounds are rhythmic beatings as the blood flows through the artery to the lower arm. While the cuff is inflated there is no flow and therefore no sounds, but once flow resumes the sounds resume. The pressure in the mercury column is read when the first Korotkoff sound (Figure 1) is heard and this represents the systolic pressure. As the cuff continues to deflate, the Korotkoff sounds become fainter, until they disappear. The pressure is measured again at the point where the sounds disappear, and this is the diastolic pressure.

Although sphygmomanometers, both mercury and aneroid models, are available for home use, they require coordination and experience for optimal use. Usually if the individual is right-handed the gauge is held in the left hand with the cuff on the left arm. Problems arise when the cuff is not positioned properly or there is inexperience in recognizing Korotkoff sounds. Many people mistake the third Korotkoff sound for the first, or the fourth for the fifth.

Figure 1: **Korotkoff Phases for Blood Pressure Measurement**

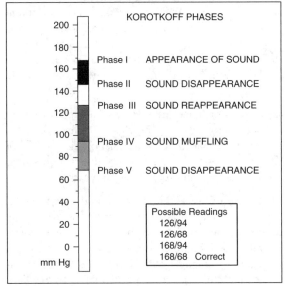

KOROTKOFF PHASES

Phase I	APPEARANCE OF SOUND
Phase II	SOUND DISAPPEARANCE
Phase III	SOUND REAPPEARANCE
Phase IV	SOUND MUFFLING
Phase V	SOUND DISAPPEARANCE

Possible Readings
126/94
126/68
168/94
168/68   Correct

Reproduced with permission from Evans, CE. *The Canadian Consensus on Hypertension Management—A Summary of Recommendations 1984-89.* Montreal: Canadian Hypertension Society; 1990:2.

Electronic Models

Electronic models are ideal for home use because they require less coordination than sphygmomanometers and there is no listening for Korotkoff sounds. There are two types of electronic blood pressure monitors available: *oscillometric* and *auscultatory*. Oscillometric models measure blood pressure by analyzing small changes in cuff pressure. The pressure in the inflated cuff changes as blood moves through expanding and contracting blood vessels. Auscultatory models detect Korotkoff sounds.

Some auscultatory models use a single microphone or sensor that must be positioned accurately over the brachial artery. Most electronic monitors have a liquid crystal diode display which makes reading the blood pressure numbers easy. Pulse readings are often provided along with blood pressure readings.

Accuracy can be a problem with electronic models. If the reading is consistently too high or too low, it may still be used to evaluate trends, but if the monitor reads too high one time and too low the next, the readings have no value. Once purchased, electronic models should be compared in accuracy to blood pressure readings done by a health care professional. This comparison should be repeated periodically. Both the British Hypertension Society and the US Association for the Advancement of Medical Instrumentation have formulated validation standards that indicate whether or not a particular model is accurate. The Canadian Coalition for the Prevention and Treatment of High Blood Pressure endorses electronic models that meet the validation standards of these organizations.

The proper technique for using blood pressure monitors is important, and should be checked from time to time to ensure no bad habits have developed. The blood pressure reading should be taken under the same circumstances and at approximately the same time of day. Blood pressure changes with daily cycles, and is typically the lowest during sleep. Public speaking can produce a 10 mm Hg rise in blood pressure; strenuous exercise 60 to 70 mm Hg rise; sex up to 100 mm Hg rise for men and 80 mm Hg rise for women; and a competitive video game 20 mm Hg rise. Some manufacturers recommend that cigarettes, caffeine and strenuous exercise be avoided for about an hour before the blood pressure measurement is taken.

It is recommended that two or three readings be taken at one time, resting several minutes between each reading. The readings can be compared and averaged. Keeping a log of the blood pressure readings will reflect what is normal for an individual and what effect various activities or medications have on the blood pressure reading.[5]

Electronic models that work on the wrist or finger have been developed. However, they are not as accurate as devices that work on the upper arm.[6,7]

Cholesterol

Elevated cholesterol levels increase the risk of coronary heart disease and stroke. Screening of high risk individuals, and lowering cholesterol levels with diet or medication reduce mortality and morbidity.[8]

Cholesterol home tests are appropriate for screening for hypercholesterolemia. They are not helpful in monitoring the effect of diet or drug therapy. These tests use an optical reader to determine total cholesterol in a blood sample. A drop of blood is drawn using a lancet and placed on a test strip. Most test strips do not require wiping, but rather use capillary action to move the blood sample to the optical reader.

The test strip is impregnated with a reagent that reacts with cholesterol in the blood sample to produce a color change. The optical reader uses light absorption to determine the degree of color change, and thus the cholesterol content of the sample. The results are expressed digitally on a liquid crystal diode display.

Test results take 3 to 15 minutes, and represent total cholesterol. Home tests do not distinguish between low density lipoproteins (LDL), high density lipoproteins (HDL) and triglycerides. To obtain a breakdown of the cholesterol fractions a laboratory procedure is required.

A record of results may be useful for observing trends in an individual's cholesterol levels over time and under various conditions.

Fecal Occult Blood

Colorectal cancer is the fourth most common cancer in Canada[9] and has a mortality rate as high as 60%. Cancerous lesions within the colon may bleed before they are well-developed.[10] A blood loss of 0.5 to 0.75 mL causes stools to appear dark red or black and tarry. However, with lower amounts of blood loss the stool appears normal. Detection of occult (hidden) blood in the stool is a useful screening tool in the early detection of bowel disease and bowel cancer.

People who have risk factors for colorectal cancer – over age 50, personal history of inflammatory bowel disease, polyps or colorectal cancer, family history of colorectal cancer – are candidates for screening via testing for fecal occult blood.[9]

Occult blood testing will also differentiate between blood and other substances causing stool discoloration (e.g., drugs such as phenazopyridine).

Two types of technology exist – *guaiac* tests and tests using monoclonal antibodies. In the guaiac test a positive reaction is the result of *pseudoperoxidase* activity. In the presence of hemoglobin in the stool

and hydrogen peroxide in the test reagent, guaiac undergoes oxidation turning the sample blue. The guaiac test is used both in the laboratory and at home.

Newer fecal occult blood tests use monoclonal antibody technology. An enzyme-linked immunosorbent assay (ELISA) for human hemoglobin is used and is more specific than the guaiac test for human hemoglobin. This type of test has fewer potential false positive results and is thus considered more accurate than the guaiac test.

Both types of home test consist of test pads that are dropped into the toilet bowl after defecation. This avoids the collection and transportation of stool samples necessary for a laboratory test, a process that individuals may find esthetically unpleasant.

A negative test for fecal occult blood does not necessarily rule out colorectal cancer. Some cancerous lesions do not bleed, and others may bleed infrequently. Dietary fibre encourages cancerous lesions to bleed, improving the accuracy of the test, and increasing dietary fibre prior to testing is recommended. Since cancerous lesions may bleed intermittently, three consecutive stool samples should be tested to minimize the possibility of a false negative.

Foods with peroxidase activity can cause false positive results with the guaiac test (Table 1). These should be avoided for 48 hours prior to performing the test and until after the third sample has been tested. This is not a problem with tests using monoclonal antibody technology.

Table 1: **Foods with Peroxidase Activity**

Artichoke	Meat (red or rare)
Broccoli	Mushrooms
Canteloupe	Parsnip
Horseradish	Turnip

A positive result does not necessarily mean the subject has bowel cancer. Many drugs and other physical conditions associated with GI bleeding or that result in blood being swallowed may also cause a positive result for occult blood in the stool (Table 2). Menstruation may also result in cross-contamination of the test pad and a false positive result. In the case of

Table 2: **Drugs and Physical Conditions**[10,11] **Associated with Fecal Occult Blood**

Drugs	Physical conditions
Colchicine	Anal fissures
Corticosteroids	Bleeding gums
Iron	Diverticulitis
NSAIDs	Dysentery
Reserpine	Hemorrhoids
Warfarin	Nosebleed
	Peptic ulcer disease
	Proctitis
	Ulcerative colitis

drugs, occult blood loss is considered an adverse effect and early detection enables a change in therapy and/or dosage.

For accurate results, the toilet bowl must be free of chemicals such as toilet bowel cleaners, disinfectants and deodorizers. Newer tests contain control tests that check for such contaminants.

A person with a positive fecal occult blood test should contact a physician immediately.

Menopause

Home diagnostic tests for menopause look for a constantly high level of follicle-stimulating hormone (FSH). During a normal menstrual cycle FSH levels vary, rising as an ovum matures in the ovaries and falling after the release of the ovum at midcycle. Closer to menopause, with decreasing ovarian function, the body produces less estrogen and as a result, FSH levels tend to remain constantly high.

The test is an immunochromatographic one-step test that uses an ELISA to detect FSH in urine. A positive result is indicated by a color change, and two positive tests taken a week apart indicate a constantly high level of FSH consistent with menopause. Therefore, if the first test is positive, it should be repeated one week later.

A control is built into the test to ensure the test itself is working; however, damaged or expired test material should not be used. The test should be performed using the first urine of the morning because it has the highest concentration of FSH. This also ensures the

two tests are performed at about the same time each day, minimizing the effect of diurnal variation.

Oral contraceptives can cause a false negative result by decreasing levels of FSH, and the manufacturer recommends that these be discontinued for at least six months prior to testing. During pregnancy FSH levels are elevated, and an undetected pregnancy will result in a false positive result. Most incorrect results are due to human error – damaging the absorbent end of the test wand, using too small or too large a urine sample, turning the wand upside down after sampling, reading the results too early or too late.

Menopause home tests do not indicate fertility, and should never be the basis of a contraceptive decision. Menopause occurs over months and years, thus menopause home test kits are limited in that they only capture FSH levels in a general quantitative way at a specific time.[12]

Helicobacter Pylori

H. pylori is a gram-negative bacteria that has been linked to peptic ulcer disease. Antibiotics are readily able to eradicate the bacteria and, in combination with acid suppressive therapy, treat the ulceration, effectively curing the ulcer disease.[13] *H. pylori* infection can be diagnosed by several methods: histologic testing of stomach tissue samples obtained during endoscopy, serologic testing for antibodies to *H. pylori,* and urea breath-testing.[14]

The home test is an immunochromatographic assay for antibodies to *H. pylori* in a blood sample using an ELISA of the antibodies. The test allows both the pretreatment of the whole blood sample and immunochromatographic detection to be done in one step.

H. pylori tests include a control, and the result of any test where the control test fails is invalid. There are limitations of such tests. It does not identify whether the infection is current or in remission. Because elevated antibody levels may persist for 6 or more months after successful eradication,[14] a false positive may result if testing is performed soon after the infection is cured with antibiotics. A false negative may result when antibody levels are below detection limits.

A positive test result should prompt a physician consultation.

Prostate Specific Antigen (PSA)

Once a man reaches 40 or 50 years of age, the prostate gland may begin to create new cells and become enlarged. About 80% of all men will have enlarged prostates by the time they reach the age of 80. This condition, *benign prostatic hyperplasia* (BPH), while not life threatening, can cause urinary and ejaculatory problems (see Chapter 56).

BPH symptoms include weak or interrupted urinary stream; a feeling that the bladder doesn't empty completely after urination; delay or hesitation at the start of voiding; the need to void often, especially at night; and urinary urgency. The symptoms of prostate cancer can overlap with those of BPH and include difficulty or pain when urinating or ejaculating, a weaker than usual stream of urine, dribbling after voiding, blood or pus in the urine or ejaculatory fluid, and pain in the hip or back.[15]

PSA levels are elevated in prostate cancer, and testing for elevated levels may mean early detection and treatment. The benefit of early detection and treatment is controversial.[16] The value of PSA screening is therefore unknown. However some authorities do recommend periodic monitoring of PSA levels to screen for prostate cancer.

Home tests use monoclonal antibody ELISA to detect PSA antibodies in a whole blood sample. A positive result is indicated by a color change. A control test is included and if the control does not work, the results are invalid.

Autoimmune disease and sexual activity within 48 hours of the test can elevate the PSA level and yield a false positive result. The minimum detectable concentration of PSA in standard solution is 3 to 4 ng/mL. False negative results occur in the presence of prostate cancer with PSA levels below this limit.

A positive result warrants medical consultation.

Multiple Drug Detection

Some drugs are abused, are potentially addictive and can impair cognitive functioning. As well, these drugs can result in health complications and individuals harming themselves while under the drug's influence.[17] Of special concern are marijuana, phencyclidine (PCP), methamphetamine, cocaine and opiates such as heroin.[18]

Home drug detection kits are urine tests that use ELISA technology. Drugs can be detected for 3 to 10 days after use, depending upon the drug.

False positive results can result from the use of legitimate medication (e.g., analgesics containing codeine), ingestion of foods containing poppy seeds or cocoa, or prolonged exposure to second-hand marijuana smoke. Adding bleach, alum or oxidizing agents to the urine sample will result in a negative test.

Blood Coagulation

Home blood coagulation monitors measure prothrombin time (PT) and calculate the International Normalized Ratio (INR).[19] With home monitoring, an individual would either contact their physician or anticoagulant clinic with the results and receive directions on adjusting their anticoagulant dosage, or alternatively use the results themselves to adjust anticoagulant dosages. Education regarding the effect of factors such as diet, illness, and disease on blood coagulation as well as a high degree of motivation is needed if a patient is to perform home monitoring of their blood coagulation.

These monitors use a whole blood sample applied to a cartridge, where it is drawn by capillary action into a channel coated with dried thromboplastin. When the thromboplastin has been rehydrated by the blood sample, coagulation begins. The mixture will continue to move along the channel until a blood clot forms. A laser photometer detects cessation of flow as a change in light scattering, resulting in a PT measurement that is then used to calculate the INR. Results take about two minutes.

Infections

Home tests for infections focus on streptococcal infections, influenza, and urinary tract infections.

With streptococcal throat infection test kits the throat is swabbed and the swab inserted into the chamber of a test cassette. The test is based on an ELISA for streptococcal antigens. Results are available in five minutes.

Throat and ear examination kits with fully illustrated guide books are also available. Both can be difficult to use with uncooperative children and as a result are not widely used or available.

Home diagnostic kits are available for detection of influenza. A nasal swab is used in a three-step procedure to produce results in 10 minutes. Both influenza A and B antigens are detectable. Again, appropriate medical consultation may be preferred.

Home test kits for urinary tract infections are urine dip tests that detect nitrites produced by gram-negative bacteria from nitrates. Some tests also detect leukocyte esterase, an enzyme that indicates the presence of leukocytes in the urine. False negative results may be caused by vegetarian diets, high intake of ascorbic acid and tetracycline.

Home testing for infections should be performed in conjunction with appropriate medical attention, based upon the patient's symptoms and medical history.

Human Immunodeficiency Virus

Human immunodeficiency virus (HIV) is the virus that causes acquired immunodeficiency syndrome (AIDS). With early detection precautions can be taken to prevent transmission to other individuals. Early detection also affords early treatment with an improved quality of life.

For home HIV tests, the blood sample is taken at home and sent to a central laboratory for processing.

The tests use ELISA technology to detect antibodies to the virus. False negative results may occur when the test is used too early or too late in the course of the disease. Antibodies to HIV do not develop until two to eight weeks after contracting the virus.[20] In late stage disease, antibody production can be too low to detect.

False positive results can occur in multiparous women, in individuals who have recently been vaccinated against influenza or hepatitis B, as the result of multiple blood transfusions, and in autoimmune disease. Any positive result must be confirmed by a physician.

Potential Home Diagnostic Testing Problems

Human error is the primary reason for failure or erroneous results when home testing. Care in preparing, administering, and interpreting the results is needed.

- Note the accuracy of the test as well as the substance for which the test is designed (e.g., cholesterol tests measure only total cholesterol and do not provide a lipid profile).
- Read all directions and identify all test components prior to testing.
- Check the kit expiry date. Do not use an expired test kit.
- A clean, undisturbed area is ideal for testing. Test surfaces should not be touched and hands should be washed prior to testing to reduce potential contamination.
- If the test equipment or monitor uses batteries, make sure they are charged.
- Directions for sample collection, including the best time of day for collection, should be followed carefully and any timing should be done accurately with a timer, watch, or clock with a minute hand.
- If the test uses a control and it fails, results are invalid and should not be used.
- Interpretation of the results is essential; for example, the meaning of a positive or negative result, and when to seek medical attention.
- The calibration of monitors should be checked on a routine basis.
- If testing is ongoing (e.g., blood pressure), keep a log or diary.
- If the subject resists the test procedure (e.g., taking a blood or urine sample, or throat swab) the sample may not be adequate and the result inaccurate. The required manual dexterity and eyesight is also essential.
- At each step of a test human error can occur, thus tests with fewer steps have less potential for human error.
- Many manufacturers have toll-free telephone numbers and web sites that are good resources.

References:

1. Joffres MR, Ghadirian P, Fodor JG, Petrasovits A, Chockalingham A, Hamet P. Awareness, treatment and control

of hypertension in Canada. *Amer J Hypertens* 1997;10: 1097-102.

2. Canadian Hypertension Society. *2000 Canadian Recommendations for the Management of Hypertension*. Available at: http://www.chs.md. Accessed March 7, 2002.

3. American Association of Clinical Endocrinologists. Medical guidelines for the management of diabetes mellitus: the AACE system of intensive diabetes self-management—2000 update. *Endocr Pract* 2000;6(1):43-84.

4. van Egmond J, Lenders JW, Weernink E, Thien T. Accuracy and reproducibility of 30 devices for self measurement of arterial blood pressure. *Am J Hypertension* 1993;6:873.

5. King DS, et al. Educating patients on hypertension and blood pressure monitoring. *Drug Topics* 1998;142(Nov suppl):1.

6. Bultemeier NC, White JR, Campbell RK. Home monitoring of blood pressure. *US Pharm* 2001;26(9):81-90.

7. Rotch AL, Dean JO, Kendrach MG, Wright SG, Wooley TW. Blood pressure monitoring with home monitors versus mercury sphygmomanometer. *Ann Pharmacother* 2001;35: 817-22.

8. Anonymous. Executive summary of the third report of the National Cholesterol Education Program (NCEP) Expert Panel on Detection, Evaluation, and Treatment of High Blood Cholesterol in Adults: Adult Treatment Panel III. *JAMA* 2001;285(19):2486-97.

9. Canadian Cancer Society. *What should I know about colorectal cancer?* Available at: http://www.cancer.ca/english/CI_S_CRC_allscreeningfaqs.asp. Accessed March 5, 2002.

10. Mandel JS, Bond JH, Church TR, et al. Reducing mortality from colorectal cancer by screening for fecal occult blood. *N Engl J Med* 1993;328:1365.

11. Finley RS, Lindley CM, LaCivita CL, Henry DW. Solid tumors. In: Young LY, Koda-Kimble MA, eds. *Applied Therapeutics: The Clinical Use of Drugs.* 6th ed. Vancouver, WA: Applied Therapeutics Inc; 1995:93-1 to 93-30.

12. Rousseau ME. Women's midlife health. Reframing menopause. *J Nurse Midwifery* 1998;43(3):208.

13. Tytgot GN. Treatment of peptic ulcer. *Digestion* 1998;59 (5):446.

14. van Zanten SJOV, Flook N, Chiba N, et al. An evidence-based approach to the management of uninvestigated dyspepsia in the era of *Helicobacter pylori. CMAJ* 2000;162 (12 Suppl):S3-S23.

15. Pienta KJ, Esper PS. Risk factors for prostate cancer. *Ann Intern Med* 1993;118:793.

16. Feightner JW. Screening for prostate cancer. In: *The Canadian Guide to Clinical Preventive Health Care.* Canadian Task Force on the Periodic Health Examination, 1994 (reviewed 1999). Available at: http://www.hc-sc.gc.ca/hppb/healthcare/pubs/clinical_preventive/pdf/s10c67e.pdf. Accessed March 5, 2002.

17. Floren AE. Urine drug testing and the family physician. *Am Fam Physician* 1994;49:1441-7.

18. Macdonald DI. Diagnosis and treatment of adolescent substance abuse. *Curr Probl Pediatr* 1989;19:389-94.

19. Riley RS, Rowe D, Fisher LM. Clinical utilization of the international normalized ratio (INR). *J Clin Lab Anal* 2000; 14(3):101-14.

20. Demeter LM, Reichman RC. Detection of human immunodeficiency virus infection. In: Mandell GL, Bennett JE, Dolin R, eds. *Mandell, Douglas and Bennett's Principles and Practice of Infectious Diseases.* 5th ed. Philadelphia, Penn: Churchill Livingstone; 2000:1369-1374.

Appendix C

Complementary and Alternative Therapies

Janet Webb, BSc(Pharm), MSc

Eighty per cent of the world's population relies upon traditional health care treatments that by North American standards would be considered "unconventional."[1,2] Increased human mobility and improved global communication leads to a greater awareness of and exposure to unfamiliar therapies; frustrations with or distrust of the conventional health care system prompts many to seek alternatives. A recent review of complementary and alternative medicine indicates that among nine western countries, Canada, at nearly 60%, was second only to Germany in prevalence of alternative medicine use.[3]

These therapeutic approaches bring with them terminologies and philosophies which can be confusing to those trained in the conventional medical sciences of North America. Even the widely used term "complementary and alternative medicine" (CAM) lacks clear definition, and is itself subject to interpretation.[4] The definition of complementary medicine adopted by the Cochrane Collaboration is as follows:

> Complementary and alternative medicine (CAM) is a broad domain of healing resources that encompasses all health systems, modalities, and practices and their accompanying theories and beliefs, other than those intrinsic to the politically dominant health system of a particular society or culture in a given historical period. CAM includes all such practices and ideas self-defined by their users as preventing or treating illness or promoting health and well-being. Boundaries within CAM and between the CAM domain and that of the dominant system are not always sharp or fixed.[5]

With the increasing use of these therapies, some of which are likely to become integrated into mainstream medical practice,[6] health care professionals must become familiar with terminologies used in CAM. The following provides definitions and brief descriptions of some terms which health care providers may encounter in this evolving area.

Scientific evidence to either disprove or support the perceived efficacy and hazards of CAM lags far behind that of conventional medicine. As well, although some of these approaches have been used for thousands of years, when used outside of their traditional cultural context and without the supervision of experienced practitioners, both their historical value and safety may be altered.[7] These limitations also apply when attempts are made to examine these therapies in a conventional setting where circumstance may not reflect the actual conditions of use.

Categories of CAM

The National Center for Complementary and Alternative Medicine in the United States groups CAM therapies into five major categories:[8]

- *Alternative Medical Systems*[8]

  These are complex and comprehensive systems of treatment, encompassing both theory and practice, which have developed outside the sphere of conventional medicine. Some have been in use for thousands of years (e.g., traditional oriental medicine) while others have been developed more recently (e.g., homeopathy).

- *Mind-body Interventions*[3,8-10]

  This type of therapy uses techniques meant to utilize the brain or mind to influence body function.

Theories suggest the connection between the nervous system and other body systems (e.g., the immune and endocrine systems) can be employed to promote self-healing and well-being. The connection between the mind and body has been explored in the use of support groups for cancer patients, and in the effect of exercise on altered mood (e.g., depression).

- *Biological-based Therapies*[8]

This describes the use of natural/biologic products, which can be derived from plants (e.g., herbs) or animals (e.g., shark cartilage), and also includes vitamins, minerals and diet therapies. Orthomolecular and megavitamin therapies are in this category.

- *Manipulative and Body-based Methods*[8,11,12]

These manual therapies involve manipulation or movement of the body, and include chiropractic, massage therapy, osteopathy and reflexology as examples. Some methods propose that bodily function depends on proper body alignment, and that misalignment or asymmetry results in illness, possibly at a site distant from the distortion. Correction of body symmetry optimizes the balance between the sensory and motor nervous systems.[11] Restoration of structural imbalance improves supply and draining of blood and lymph, promotes improved nutrition to tissues, and facilitates the body's ability to heal itself.[11]

- *Energy Therapies*[8]

These methods seek to manipulate energy fields within the body or those fields external to it. The theory of energy work maintains that the universe is permeated with a "life force" or "vital energy" which also surrounds and pervades the human body.[13] Imbalance or blockages of the energy may result in disease, and therapy is aimed at correcting these problems. When treating the malady, a close, cooperative participation between the practitioner and the patient is required. Therapeutic touch, reiki and Qigong are examples of energy therapies.

Definitions

Acupressure[11,14]

A manual therapy in which deep pressure is applied to certain acupuncture points. It is theorized that different noxious stimuli, including emotional trauma, cause energy to accumulate in particular pressure points situated along the channels or meridians through which qi (pronounced "chee," a vital force or energy, which circulates through the body in 12 major channels termed "meridians") flows. Application of pressure by the practitioner improves flow of qi, causing a release and dissipation of tension, alleviation of disease and relief of pain.[11] It has been studied for the treatment of nausea of pregnancy, headache, backache, stroke and traumatic brain injury.[14,15] Application of pressure to a particular point on the inside of the wrist has been promoted to alleviate motion sickness.[16]

Acupuncture

Can describe either a therapeutic discipline or a technique, which can vary with different traditional approaches.[17] Needles of various sizes, but commonly having a shaft of 25 mm and a diameter of 0.25 mm, are inserted at specific points on the body to regulate the flow of qi along chosen meridians (see Chinese Medicine).[18,19] In a more conventional approach, these acupuncture points are termed "trigger points" which correspond to areas of increased sensitivity that can produce referred pain in a characteristic manner.[20] Anatomically, these points correspond to peripheral nerve junctions, and are involved in pain transmission. The technique itself involves the insertion of several needles (usually 4 to 10), and may vary with respect to angle and depth of insertion, length of time retained (often 10 to 30 minutes), manipulation methods (e.g., twirling, electrical current), and frequency of treatment.[20] Areas of interest in acupuncture treatment include pain management including post-operative dental pain, headache, substance abuse, nausea, asthma, urticaria and stroke rehabilitation.[15,20-23]

Aromatherapy[24]

A treatment method using volatile (essential) oils whose fragrance or odor is deemed an integral part of therapy. The oils are extracted from plants, diluted with vegetable oil then often applied to the skin by massage, or they can be delivered in steam for inhalation of the scent.[14] When applied externally, the fragrance, the massage itself, and the dermal absorption of the constituents are all deemed beneficial,[25] although a psychological component cannot be ruled out.[3] In the United Kingdom, aromatherapy has been used in conventional settings such as hospices, palliative care units, cancer units and pediatric units.[24]

Ayurveda[8,14,26,27]

This is a major medical system, originating in India, and possibly dating back 5000 years. It is a sophisticated, complex system of theory and practice, which considers the body, mind and spirit, and attempts to achieve harmony and balance between them. It is believed that the body is a miniature representation of the universe. The same elements that form the universe form the human body; when the elements are out of balance, ill health results. Patient assessment includes physical examination as well as consideration of mental and social factors. Treatment choices include manipulation, diet, purification to rid the body of toxins (possibly involving vomiting, purgation, or enemas), and rejuvenation therapies to build the body's strength. Herbal therapies are employed, as well as minerals and metals, which might include heavy metals.[28] Yoga and meditation are also utilized.

Biofeedback[14]

A system which permits a patient to regulate body function (e.g., heart rate, blood pressure, degree of muscle contraction) by receiving feedback signals from instruments monitoring the function, and to adjust the physiologic process accordingly.

Chinese Medicine[1,12,14,17,18,29]

(Also known as Traditional Chinese Medicine or Traditional Oriental Medicine.)

A comprehensive and major medical system, dating back to 3000 BC, which comprises many traditions, philosophies and approaches to treatment. It is based on fundamental concepts which can be difficult for the uninitiated to grasp. These include a balance between yin and yang (opposing yet complementary phenomena that exist simultaneously throughout the universe, including the body), and unimpeded flow of qi. Health problems may reflect a lack of harmony within an individual, or between an individual and their environment. Diagnosis of the patient involves a multitude of techniques in addition to taking a medical history, which include assessing temperament, examining the tongue and properties of the pulse, and noting qualities of speech and breath. The practitioner evaluates how illness manifests itself in the patient, then treats the person, not the disease. Treatments are highly individualized, targeting the deep cause of the disease rather than only symptoms. Chosen methods

of therapy include diet, herbal therapy, acupuncture, moxibustion, cupping and bleeding, tui na and qigong.

Chinese Herbal Medicine

An integral part of Chinese medicine, which encompasses use of animal parts and minerals in addition to plant material.[18] *The Encyclopedia of Traditional Chinese Medicinal Substance*, published in 1977, lists over 5000 entries. Substances are categorized according to their properties, for example heat-clearing, wind-dispelling, or blood rectifying. The use of medicinal substances can be complex, with specific combinations selected considering their compatibility and complementary/synergistic effects.[30] They are usually consumed as a decoction (simmered tea) but also may be dispensed in solid dosage forms, or used externally.

Chiropractic

A manipulative therapy aimed at correcting misalignment within the musculoskeletal system.[11] Chiropractors apply a variety of manoeuvres, such as sharp thrusts, to the spine, pelvis and limbs in order to adjust alignment and correct disorders.[31] Although formerly advocated for treating a wide variety of complaints, today it is limited primarily to treating musculoskeletal disorders. It is used mainly for back and neck pain, but research is examining its use in other disorders such as headache.[31]

Craniosacral Therapy[32,33]

A manual technique in which gentle pressure is applied to the skull to adjust and normalize rhythmic pulsations of the cerebrospinal fluid. It has been purported to relieve pain (e.g., headache) and vertigo.

Cupping and Bleeding

A component of Chinese medicine in which a warm glass or bamboo cup is placed on the skin. As it cools, the suction created draws blood and lymph to the skin surface. It is used to assist circulation, and to remove cold and damp, which are considered external causes of disease.[18,32] Arabs believed that cupping would relieve a variety of ailments, from toothache to elephantiasis.[19]

Dietary Supplements

This term is defined in the United States by the *Dietary Supplement Health and Education Act* (1994) as products intended to supplement the diet which may contain vitamins, minerals, amino acids, herbs or other botanicals, or a "dietary substance for use to supplement the diet by increasing the total dietary intake."[34] The Act does not require either proof of efficacy or proof of safety.[2] In Canada, supplements are defined quite differently by Health Canada. Dietary vitamin supplements in Canada are not permitted to contain herbs, amino acids, digestive aids, enzymes or animal tissue.[35] The preferred regulatory term in Canada is Natural Health Product, but its definition is still under development.

Herbalism

An approach which uses plant materials not only as substitutes for pharmaceuticals, but to optimize health and wellness. The World Health Organization has taken the position that, in the absence of opposing scientific evidence, the traditional and historical use of herbal remedies provides evidence of their efficacy and safety.[7,36] The entire plant kingdom, including moss, algae and fungi may be utilized (although some herbal traditions also use animal parts, insects, metals, rocks, shells, etc.).[37] Concepts include the belief that the therapeutic response to a plant will be different than the response to an individual chemical component of the plant.[37] Growing conditions, collection and storage methods will also affect response, as will the expectations of the patient and the cultural significance of the plant (which may include a placebo component). Recognition is given to patients' involvement and responsibilities in their own self-care.

Holistic Medicine

An approach that takes into account the body, mind and spirit of an individual, as well as the interaction of the three to maintain health and well-being.[32,38] Critics may argue that competent physicians have always done this, and that this is not the exclusive domain of alternative practitioners.[39] What might be termed holistic approaches, involving multidisciplinary teams (physicians, spiritual healers, and psychological counselors) have been successfully incorporated into conventional medical practices.[40,41]

Homeopathy[12,17,42,43]

An alternative medical system, dating back to the early 19th century which is based on the philosophy that the body has an innate ability to heal itself, and that "like cures like." It teaches that symptoms are manifested when the body attempts to heal itself or to correct an imbalance. The constellation of symptoms guides therapy. A substance that produces a specific pattern of symptoms in a healthy person will, when given in minute doses, help fight an illness with identical symptomatology. By increasing symptoms, the body is thus encouraged further to overcome the affliction. When choosing a therapy, the homeopath considers the mental and emotional state of the patient, in addition to the physical. The closest match between the symptoms of the individual and the remedy are attempted, recognizing that different people will exhibit different symptom patterns. The homeopathic arsenal contains more than 2000 substances, derived from plants, minerals, metals, animal products and even diseased tissues. The substances are prepared in serial dilutions, which are vigorously shaken with each dilution, which is believed to increase potency. Potencies are typically noted as X or C, indicating 1:10 dilutions, or 1:100 dilutions, respectively (e.g., 6X will denote 6 dilutions of 1:10). Dilutions may be such that no molecules of the original substance exist in the final preparation. Paradoxically, the greater the dilution, the higher the potency. Preparations of highest potency are reserved for use under the direction of a homeopath. In North America, asthma, headache, depression, allergies, psychosocial problems and skin conditions are among the most frequent conditions treated by homeopaths.

Hydrotherapy[19,44]

The use of water as therapy, which encompasses a multitude of diverse applications including baths, saunas, douches, immersion, wraps and colonic irrigation.

Iridology[3,14]

A discredited method of diagnosis which examines changes in the iris to determine state of health.

Magnet Therapy[33,45]

The application of magnets to treat disorders by influencing ionic currents in the body causing stimulation of cells and enhanced blood flow. Unipolar or bipolar magnets are fastened into clothing, worn like jewelry (e.g., bracelets), held in place against the skin by adhesive, or used in bedding. They have been promoted to treat musculoskeletal complaints such as chronic low back pain, muscle pain in post-polio syndrome, and neuropathic pain in diabetes. It is not to be confused with magnetic healing, which was a form of hypnosis.

Massage Therapy[11]

A manipulative method that uses a variety of manual techniques (stroking, kneading, friction, vibration) applied to soft tissues. Human touch itself is considered to be a beneficial part of massage. It is used in traditional medical systems including Ayurveda and Chinese medicine. Massage is used to promote relaxation, relieve muscle tightness, alleviate pain, reduce anxiety and promote sleep.

Moxibustion[18]

A component of Chinese medicine that involves the burning of dried and powdered leaves of *artemesia vulgaris*. It can be burned in very small amounts directly on the skin, on a mediating substance placed between the burning material and the skin surface, or on the handle of an acupuncture needle. It is believed that the burning substance has the ability to warm and enter the meridians, and affect the flow of qi. Moxibustion is used in combination with acupuncture for a wide variety of conditions.

Naturopathic Medicine[44,46]

A system of treatment which emphasizes the healing power of nature, and which draws from a wide variety of therapeutic approaches. The use of nutrition, herbs and natural products is fundamental, with treatments borrowed from Chinese medicine, homeopathy, herbalism, Ayurveda, and manual therapies. As it does not identify with one particular mode of therapy, it is generally defined by its approach. This includes core principles of preventive medicine, treatment of the whole person, and determination of the cause of the disease. Its goal is to aid the body's efforts to heal itself and restore normal body function, rather than attempt to focus on the treatment of symptoms.

Orthomolecular Therapy[14,39]

A term derived from the Greek word "orthos," meaning straight or correct, it was first used by Linus Pauling in 1968 to describe the treatment of disease with large quantities of nutrients, especially vitamins. It is similar to megavitamin therapy but minerals, amino acids, hormones, and metabolic intermediates can also be administered. The amounts of nutrients administered may be 20 to 600 times the recommended daily intake.

Osteopathic Medicine[11,31,47]

A system which originated as a manipulative method, but which has evolved into mainstream medicine in the United States where practitioners receive a Doctor of Osteopathy (DO) degree and restrict themselves to conventional medicine. Depending on the practitioner, manual techniques may include thrusting (similar to chiropractic methods), lymphatic drainage and craniosacral therapy. Osteopathic methods attempt to correct symmetry, motion restriction, tissue texture changes and tenderness. Musculoskeletal problems such as soft tissue trauma, temporomandibular joint dysfunction, and lumbar and cervical pain are treated. In countries other than the United States, such as Great Britain, osteopaths earn Bachelor of Science degrees and have practices similar to that of chiropractors.

Qigong[18]

An energy therapy that is a major branch of Chinese medicine and is aimed at manipulating qi. It involves a wide variety of activities to balance, regulate, and harness qi in order to promote health, longevity, healing, and spiritual development. An internal form has the patient acting alone using exercise, breathing or relaxation methods. In the external form, a practitioner projects his or her qi into the patient via their hands, the use of needles, or visualization.

Reflexology (Zone Therapy)[11,25]

A manual technique involving application of deep pressure to the feet. Different zones on the feet are thought to correspond to areas on the body (equated with meridians). Pressure is applied using the fingers and thumbs to enhance the flow of energy through the body. It has been tried to relieve symptoms of chronic conditions such as asthma, headache, bladder and bowel problems. It has been studied in stroke, brain injury, and spinal cord injury patients.[15]

Reiki[11,13]

An energy therapy developed in mid-19th century Japan, whereby a practitioner channels reiki (universal life energy), attained through meditation and prayer, through their body to promote healing in another individual. Among other uses, it has been utilized to accelerate healing, relieve headache, and treat depression.

Rolfing[11,13]

A manipulation method which uses deep muscle massage to correct distortions in the body. It teaches that distortions in posture reflect a withdrawal response to past emotional and physical trauma, and restoring correct posture with manipulation will release the traumas, resulting in a feeling of lightness and well-being.

Shiatsu[11,14,48]

A Japanese massage technique in which pressure is applied to specific points on the body likened to acupuncture points. It may be combined with passive stretching to optimize the effect. It has been likened to acupressure in technique, but is used more for prevention of illness than treatment.

Therapeutic Touch[11,14,49]

An energy therapy developed in the late 1960s in which an operator moves their hands above the surface of a patient's body in an attempt to correct imbalance in the patient's energy field and facilitate healing. It is promoted for relaxation, relief of tension or migraine headaches, nausea and acute pain, including pain from burns.

Tui Na[11,18]

A manipulative practice within Chinese medicine, which involves trained practitioners manipulating soft tissues and joints. Attention is given to the flow of qi along meridians, and acupuncture points are stimulated. It is commonly used in orthopedic and neurological applications, and can be used in situations where acupuncture is considered inappropriate (e.g., pediatrics).

Suggested Readings

Astin JA. Why patients use alternative medicine: results of a national study. *JAMA* 1998;279:1548-53.

Ernst E. The role of complementary and alternative medicine. *BMJ* 2000;321:1133-5.

Oumeish OY. The philosophical, cultural, and historical aspects of complementary, alternative, unconventional, and integrative medicine in the old world. *Arch Dermatol* 1998;134:1373-86.

Tausk FA. Alternative medicine: Is it all in your mind? *Arch Dermatol* 1998;134:1422-5.

Zollman C, Vickers A. ABC of complementary medicine. Complementary medicine in conventional practice. *BMJ* 1999;319:901-4.

Zollman C, Vickers A. ABC of complementary medicine. What is complementary medicine? *BMJ* 1999; 319:693-6.

References

1. American Botanical Council. *Terminology*. Available at: http://www.herbalgram.org/browse.php/ed_terminology. Accessed June 29, 2001.
2. Winslow LC, Kroll DJ. Herbs as medicines. In: Fontanarosa PB, ed. *Alternative Medicine: an Objective Assessment*. Chicago: American Medical Association; 2000:254-64.
3. Ernst E. The role of complementary and alternative medicine. *BMJ* 2000;321:1133-5.
4. Berkenwald AD. In the name of medicine. *Ann Intern Med* 1998;128:246-50.
5. Zollman C, Vickers A. ABC of complementary medicine. What is complementary medicine? *BMJ* 1999;319:693-6.
6. *WHO information fact sheet N 134. Traditional medicine*. Available at: http://www.who.int/inf-fs/en/fact134.html. Accessed July 10, 2001.
7. McGuffin M, Hobbs C, Upton R, Goldberg A. *American Herbal Products Association's Botanical Safety Handbook: Guidelines for the Safe Use and Labeling for Herbs in Commerce*. Boca Raton, FL: CRC Press; 1997.
8. National Center for Complementary and Alternative Medicine, National Institutes of Health. *Major Domains of Complementary and Alternative Medicine*. Available at: http://nccam.nih.gov/fcp/classify/index.html. Accessed June 29, 2001.
9. Dacher E. The development of an integrated medical model: toward a postmodern medicine. In: Micozzi MS, ed. *Fundamentals of Complementary and Alternative Medicine*. 2nd ed. New York: Churchill Livingstone; 2001:57-71.
10. Gordon JS. Mind-body medicine: overview. In: Fontanarosa PB, ed. *Alternative Medicine: an Objective Assessment*. Chicago: American Medical Association; 2000:154-6.
11. Coughlin P. Manual therapies. In: Micozzi MS, ed. *Fundamentals of Complementary and Alternative Medicine*. 2nd ed. New York: Churchill Livingstone; 2001:100-27.
12. Micozzi MS. Translational issues in conventional and complementary medicine. In: Micozzi MS, ed. *Fundamentals of Complementary and Alternative Medicine*. 2nd ed. New York: Churchill Livingstone; 2001:9-17.
13. Hurwitz WL. Energy medicine. In: Micozzi MS, ed. *Fundamentals of Complementary and Alternative Medicine*. 2nd ed. New York: Churchill Livingstone; 2001:238-56.
14. Cassileth BR. *The Alternative Medicine Handbook: the Complete Reference Guide to Alternative and Complementary Therapies*. New York: Norton; 1998.
15. Diamond BJ, Shiflett SC, Schoenberger NE, Nayak S, Cotter AC, Zeitlin D. Complementary/alternative therapies in the

treatment of neurologic disorders. In: Spencer JW, Jacobs JJ, eds. *Complementary/alternative Medicine: an Evidence-based Approach.* Toronto: Mosby, 1999:170-207.

16. Kronenberg F, Murphy PA, Wade C. Complementary/alternative therapies in select populations: women. In: Spencer JW, Jacobs JJ, eds. *Complementary/alternative Medicine: an Evidence-based Approach.* Toronto: Mosby; 1999:341-62.

17. Cassidy CM. Social and cultural context of complementary and alternative medicine systems. In: Micozzi MS, ed. *Fundamentals of Complementary and Alternative Medicine.* 2nd ed. New York: Churchill Livingstone; 2001:18-42.

18. Ergil KV. Chinese medicine. In: Micozzi MS, ed. *Fundamentals of Complementary and Alternative Medicine.* 2nd ed. New York: Churchill Livingstone; 2001:303-44.

19. Oumeish OY. The philosophical, cultural, and historical aspects of complementary, alternative, unconventional, and integrative medicine in the old world. *Arch Dermatol* 1998; 134:1373-86.

20. Vickers A, Zollman C. ABC of complementary medicine. Acupuncture. *BMJ* 1999;319:973-6.

21. NIH Consensus Development Panel on Acupuncture. *JAMA* 1998;280:1518-24.

22. LaRiccia PL. Acupuncture: overview. In: Fontanarosa PB, ed. *Alternative Medicine: an Objective Assessment.* Chicago: American Medical Association; 2000:448-50.

23. Chen C-J, Yu H-S. Acupuncture treatment of urticaria. *Arch Dermatol* 1998;134:1397-9.

24. Stevensen CJ. Aromatherapy. In: Micozzi MS, ed. *Fundamentals of Complementary and Alternative Medicine.* 2nd ed. New York: Churchill Livingstone; 2001:146-58.

25. Vickers A, Zollman C. ABC of complementary medicine. Massage therapies. *BMJ* 1999;319:1254-7.

26. Zysk KG, Tetlow G. Traditional ayurveda. In: Micozzi MS, ed. *Fundamentals of Complementary and Alternative Medicine.* 2nd ed. New York: Churchill Livingstone; 2001: 345-65.

27. Lad DV. Ayurvedic medicine. In: Jonas WB, Levin JS, eds. *Essentials of Complementary and Alternative Medicine.* Philadelphia: Lippincott Williams & Wilkins; 1999:200-15.

28. Prpic-Majic D, Pizent A, Jurasovic J, Pongracic J, Restek-Samarzija N. Lead poisoning associated with the use of Ayurvedic metal-mineral tonics. *Clin Toxicol* 1996;34:417-23.

29. Lao L. Traditional Chinese medicine. In: Jonas WB, Levin JS, eds. *Essentials of Complementary and Alternative Medicine.* Philadelphia: Lippincott Williams & Wilkins; 1999: 216-32.

30. Koo J, Arain S. Traditional Chinese medicine for the treatment of dermatologic disorders. *Arch Dermatol* 1998;134: 1388-93.

31. Vickers A, Zollman C. ABC of complementary medicine. The manipulative therapies: osteopathy and chiropractic. *BMJ* 1999;319:1176-9.

32. Jonas WB, Levin JS, eds. *Essentials of Complementary and Alternative Medicine.* Philadelphia: Lippincott Williams & Wilkins; 1999.

33. Spencer JW, Jacobs JJ, eds. *Complementary/alternative Medicine: an Evidence-based Approach.* Toronto: Mosby; 1999.

34. NIH Office of Dietary Supplements. *What are Dietary Supplements?* National Institutes of Health Office of Dietary Supplements web site. Available at: http://ods.od.nih.gov/whatare/whatare.html. Accessed June 29, 2001.

35. *Dietary Vitamin Supplements: Category IV Monograph.* Health Canada website. Available at: http://www.hc-sc.gc.ca/hpb-dgps/therapeut/zfiles/english/guides/cat4/vitamin_e.html. Accessed June 29, 2001.

36. World Health Organization. *Research Guidelines for Evaluating the Safety and Efficacy of Herbal Medicines.* Geneva: World Health Organization; 1993.

37. Meserole L. Western herbalism. In: Micozzi MS, ed. *Fundamentals of Complementary and Alternative Medicine.* 2nd ed. New York: Churchill Livingstone; 2001:128-45.

38. Astin JA. Why patients use alternative medicine: results of a national study. *JAMA* 1998;279:1548-53

39. British Columbia Cancer Agency. *Information for Health Professionals: Alternative Therapies.* Available at: http://bccancer.bc.ca/pg_g_05.asp?PageID=1715&ParentID=4. Accessed June 29, 2001.

40. Watkins AD. Psychoneuroimmunology. In: Micozzi MS, ed. *Fundamentals of Complementary and Alternative Medicine.* 2nd ed. New York: Churchill Livingstone; 2001:200-14.

41. Zollman C, Vickers A. ABC of complementary medicine. Complementary medicine in conventional practice. *BMJ* 1999;319:901-4.

42. Jacobs J, Moskowitz R. Homeopathy. In: Micozzi MS, ed. *Fundamentals of Complementary and Alternative Medicine.* 2nd ed. New York: Churchill Livingstone; 2001:87-99.

43. Vickers A, Zollman C. ABC of complementary medicine. Homoeopathy. *BMJ* 1999;319:1115-8.

44. Pizzorno JE, Snider P. Naturopathic medicine. In: Micozzi MS, ed. *Fundamentals of Complementary and Alternative Medicine.* 2nd ed. New York: Churchill Livingstone; 2001: 159-92.

45. Collacott EA, Zimmerman JT, White DW, Rindone JP. Bipolar permanent magnets for the treatment of chronic low back pain. A pilot study. *JAMA* 2000;283:1322-5.

46. Murray MT, Pizzorno JE. Naturopathic medicine. In: Jonas WB, Levin JS, eds. *Essentials of Complementary and Alternative Medicine.* Philadelphia: Lippincott Williams & Wilkins; 1999:304-21.

47. Goodman H. Osteopathy. In: Jonas WB, Levin JS, eds. *Essentials of Complementary and Alternative Medicine.* Philadelphia: Lippincott Williams & Wilkins; 1999:289-303.

48. Field T. Massage therapy. In: Jonas WB, Levin JS, eds. *Essentials of Complementary and Alternative Medicine.* Philadelphia: Lippincott Williams & Wilkins; 1999:383-91.

49. Rosa L, Rosa E, Sarner L, Barrett S. A close look at therapeutic touch. In: Fontanarosa PB, ed. *Alternative Medicine: an Objective Assessment.* Chicago: American Medical Association; 2000:202-11.

Information for the Traveler

Helen Ng, BScPhm and Deanne Wong, BScPhm

Travelers may find themselves more prone to illness while away from home.[1,2] This may be due to exposure to new strains of organisms not common at home, insect bites, and adjustments to different climate and culture.[1,2] There is often a sense of reluctance by travelers to seek medical help for minor illnesses due to possible language barrier, high cost, poor accessibility and concerns of lower medical standards, especially in developing countries.[1,2] Advise travelers to plan ahead by taking a travel first aid kit for self-treatment of minor ailments.[1,2]

Travel insurance is recommended for travel outside Canada. In addition, advise travelers to practise safe sex while abroad. Many countries have high rates of HIV and STDs. Condoms should be purchased prior to travel.[3]

Travel First Aid Kit

Commercial first aid kits are available for purchase at St. John Ambulance offices or online at www.sja.ca. Alternatively, people can prepare their own travel first aid kit. Items for the first aid kit should be organized in a self-sealing plastic bag or a plastic box for easy portability. In general, a first aid kit for travelers can be divided into two sections: medications and first aid supplies (Table 1).

Medications

Analgesic: Acetaminophen or ibuprofen are effective for the relief of mild to moderate pain and the reduction of fever.[1,4]

Antihistamine: Antihistamines are used to treat minor allergic conditions. Sedating antihistamines (e.g., diphenhydramine) are effective as mild tranquilizers while the traveler adjusts to jet lag. Certain antihistamines (e.g., dimenhydrinate) are useful to control symptoms associated with motion sickness.[1,4,5]

Decongestant: Oral pseudoephedrine is useful for relieving congested eustachian tubes in adults during descent of an aircraft.[6,7] Topical decongestants are not useful.[6] See Barotrauma in General Ear Conditions, Chapter 16.

Hydrocortisone 0.5% cream: Hydrocortisone cream is useful in various skin conditions such as mild dermatitis and pruritus.[8]

Antiseptic: Either chlorhexidine or povidone-iodine can be used to disinfect minor cuts or abrasions to prevent skin infections.[9]

Topical antibiotic cream/ointment: Antibiotic cream/ointment (e.g., polymyxin B-gramicidin-bacitracin) can be used on superficial wounds to treat minor irritation/infection.[8]

Sunscreen: Broad-spectrum sunscreen with SPF 15 or greater helps prevent sunburn.[1,2,4]

Insect repellent: Insect repellents containing DEET (N, N-diethyl-m-toluamide) are effective against a variety of mosquitoes, ticks, fleas, chiggers and flies.[1,2,10] See Personal Protection Against Vectors.

Oil of cloves: Oil of cloves is useful for the temporary relief of dental pain until dental care is available.[1,2,5]

Antacid: An antacid (e.g., aluminum and magnesium hydroxide) is effective in the relief of indigestion and heartburn.[4]

Antidiarrheal: Both loperamide and bismuth subsalicylate are effective in the management of travelers' diarrhea (see Chapter 22).[11]

Oral rehydration solution sachets: Oral rehydration solution is effective in preventing dehydration due to travelers' diarrhea in high-risk travelers (see Chapter 22).[11]

Laxative: A laxative may be helpful in treating constipation arising from factors associated with travel (e.g., dietary changes).

First Aid Supplies
Recommend the following first aid supplies:[1,2,4,5,8]
- Adhesive bandages
- Sterile gauze
- Adhesive tape
- Safety pins
- Thermometer
- Scissors
- Fine tweezers (for the removal of splinters or ticks)
- Ice pack (to reduce swelling)

Jet Lag

Jet lag is defined as the disruption or desynchronization of circadian rhythms, usually as a result of rapid crossing of multiple time zones with air travel.[10,12,13] The effect of jet lag is individualized, with some people adjusting to time zone differences more rapidly than others.[12,14] Age may also play a factor on symptom severity and speed of recovery.[12] Jet lag is also more severe when traveling eastward than westward.[12,14] This is because it is easier for one to adjust by extending the day rather than shortening it.[14] Symptoms of jet lag are common with time changes of ≥ 5 hours and are typically manifested as fatigue, daytime sleepiness, insomnia, irritability and gastric discomfort.[12-14]

The key to the management of jet lag is avoidance. Recommendations on nonpharmacologic methods of avoiding or minimizing jet lag are listed below:[10,12, 14-16]
- Plan ahead and decide whether to stay on "home time" or new location time. Home time may be best if spending less than three days at the new destination.[15]
- Arrive at new destination in the early evening (local time).
- Anticipate the new time zone. Sleep on the plane if the arrival is in the morning and stay awake if arrival time is in the evening.
- Be well-rested prior to travel.
- Stay well-hydrated during the flight by drinking plenty of fluid; avoid in-flight alcohol and caffeine.
- Exercise during the flight by stretching and walking; this is particularly helpful when the traveler wants to remain awake.
- Exposure to outdoor daylight at the destination may help in resetting the circadian rhythm.
- Remain active during daylight hours on arrival at the destination and adopt local mealtimes.
- Plan on sleeping the same amount in a 24-hour period as when at home.

Melatonin
Endogenous melatonin is produced in the pineal gland.[12,14] Its production is regulated by circadian rhythms.[12,14] Light exposure inhibits melatonin secretion while darkness stimulates its secretion.[12,14] It is therefore widely believed that the use of melatonin at

Table 1: **Travel First Aid Kit**

Medications

Analgesic	Decongestant	Oil of cloves
Antacid	Hydrocortisone cream	Sunscreen
Antihistamine	Insect repellent	Topical antibiotic cream/ointment
Antiseptic agent		

First aid supplies

Adhesive bandages	Ice pack	Sterile gauze
Adhesive tape	Safety pins	Thermometer
Fine tweezers	Scissors	

the appropriate time can help reset the body's internal clock and minimize jet lag.[14] Although melatonin is considered an investigational drug in Canada, it may be readily available at the traveler's destination. A recent systematic review has concluded that melatonin is effective for jet lag and appears safe for occasional use.[17] Travelers should be aware that melatonin can cause headache, transient depressive symptoms, drowsiness, dizziness, abdominal cramps and irritability.[14] The use of melatonin in the prevention or management of jet lag cannot be recommended at this time due to lack of quality control.[17]

High Altitude Illness[18,19]

Travelers to destinations at altitudes above 2500 m are at risk of altitude-induced illness. This term encompasses acute mountain sickness (AMS), high-altitude cerebral edema (HACE) and high-altitude pulmonary edema (HAPE).[19] The clinical presentation of each is described in Table 2. HACE is the end-stage of AMS and can be fatal. The progression to HACE from mild AMS ranges from 12 hours to, more commonly, one to three days. HAPE can occur without pre-existing AMS and accounts for most deaths from high-altitude illness.[19]

The risk of illness increases directly with the rate of ascent, the altitude at which one sleeps (sleeping altitude) and the altitude reached.[18] Travelers to high attitudes should be aware of the possibility of high-altitude illness and its signs and symptoms so it can be treated early and its progression halted.

Gradual, step-wise ascent is the best method of prevention. Travelers should:
- Ascend slowly and avoid direct transport to altitudes above 3000 m;

- Spend two or three nights at 2500 to 3000 m before going higher;
- Above 3000 m, sleeping altitude should not be increased by more than 300 m per night, with a rest day (i.e., two nights at the same altitude) every two or three days.[18] Day trips to higher elevation accelerate acclimatization.[18]

Travelers should avoid alcohol, sedative hypnotics and heavy exertion.[18] In addition, prophylaxis with acetazolamide is indicated for rapid ascents (24 hours or less) to > 3000 m, rapid gains in sleeping altitude, and a past history of AMS or HAPE. Dexamethasone may be used as an alternative.[18]

A detailed description of management of high-altitude illness is beyond the scope of this text. However, treatment of AMS includes rest and acclimatization at the same altitude. This may take between 12 hours and four days. Descent of at least 500 m is indicated if AMS is severe, if symptoms progress during acclimatization, or if symptoms of HACE or HAPE occur.[18]

Heat-induced Illness

Those traveling from temperate areas to warmer climates are at risk of heat-induced illness, ranging from pedal edema to heat stroke. Travelers should be aware that the thermoregulatory system may take up to three weeks to fully adapt to increased demands placed on it by high temperatures and humidity.[20] Table 3 summarizes factors associated with heat-induced illness and preventive measures that travelers can employ. See Chapter 10 for a discussion of the signs and symptoms of various heat-related illnesses and their management.

Table 2: **Clinical Presentation of Variants of High-altitude Illness**

Mild acute mountain sickness	Moderate acute mountain sickness	High-altitude cerebral edema	High-altitude pulmonary edema
Headache with nausea, dizziness and fatigue during first 12 h after rapid ascent to high altitude (> 2500 m).	Moderate-to-severe headache with marked nausea, dizziness, lassitude, insomnia, fluid retention at high altitude for 12 h or more.	Acute mountain sickness for 24 h or more, severe lassitude, mental confusion, ataxia.	Dyspnea at rest, cough (dry at first, then moist), severe weakness, drowsiness, cyanosis, tachycardia, tachypnea, rales.

Adapted with permission from Hackett PH, Roach RC. High-altitude illness. *N Engl J Med* 2001; 345(2):107-14.

Table 3: **Factors Associated with Heat-induced Illness and Preventive Measures**

Factor	Preventive measures
Recent arrival	Graded physical activity in the first few weeks of arrival. Avoid long periods of continuous exertion
Lack of fitness and obesity	If strenuous activity is to be undertaken, build up fitness before travel
Inappropriate clothing	Advance planning of clothing and equipment
Certain drugs (diuretics, sympathomimetics) and alcohol	Avoid
Salt loss	Replace in food and/or beverages
Any skin condition that reduces sweating	Extra vigilance recommended
Insufficient fluid intake	Good supply of clean water consumed even if not thirsty

Reproduced with permission from Goodyer L. Environmental hazards. *Pharm J* 2001;266:577-80.

Personal Protection Against Vectors[21-24]

A vector is an organism that plays a role in the transmission of a pathogen between humans or from animal to human.[21] The best known vector is probably the *Anopheles* mosquito, responsible for transmission of malaria. Others include culicine mosquitoes (*Culex* and *Aedes* species), tsetse flies, blackflies, ticks and certain freshwater snails.

A traveler's risk of exposure to a vector depends on the type and location of accommodations, the duration of the visit and a number of behavioral aspects. For example, for business travelers who stay in a capital city and spend most of their time in air-conditioned facilities the risk of contracting a vector-borne disease is usually very small. However, the traveler who visits out-of-the-way destinations, stays in accommodations of lower standards, or stays for longer periods of time may have an increased risk.

Risk reduction measures include remaining in well-screened or air-conditioned areas, sleeping under mosquito nets (preferably insecticide-treated), wearing clothing (ideally insecticide-treated) that provides good coverage (e.g., long sleeves, trousers, socks), and using insect repellents containing **diethlytoluamide** (DEET).[24] In areas where schistosomiasis is endemic, contact with freshwater (e.g., lakes, slow running streams) should be avoided.[23] When hiking in tick endemic areas, trousers should be tucked into socks and boots worn instead of sandals.[25,26]

Screens and mosquito nets should have a mesh size of 1.5 mm or less and should be checked regularly for holes. Mosquito nets impregnated with insecticides are available and are significantly more effective in preventing malaria than nets without insecticide. Impregnated nets also deter entry by vectors smaller than the mesh size of the net (e.g., sandflies) and are safe for use by children and pregnant women. All mosquito nets should either reach the floor all around the bed or be tucked under the mattress.

A knockdown insecticide (i.e., spraycan) can be used prior to sleep to clear a room of insects that have gained entry during the day. Health Canada recommends the use of a spraycan in combination with a mosquito coil or net. Clothing can also be treated with the insecticide **permethrin** to increase protection against vectors.

Insect Repellents

The duration of effect of insect repellents varies according to a number of factors, including the concentration of repellent and amount applied, temperature and, possibly, wind conditions.[25] It is decreased by sweating, washing and abrasion. Health Canada recommends using a repellent containing DEET.[24] Various concentrations of DEET are available and these vary in their duration of effect. Using a formulation containing more than 50% DEET is not recommended, since the duration of effect is not lengthened above this concentration but the risk of toxicity may be increased.[24] In children, a product containing DEET 10% or less should be applied sparingly (not to hands or face) and washed off after the child comes indoors.[24] In Canada, DEET products are not recommended for use in children under two years of age. However, in areas where malaria is endemic, the risk of severe malarial disease outweighs any risk of properly applied products.[24]

Correct Application of Insect Repellent[24,25]

- Test for allergy before using a repellent for the first time by applying to a small patch of skin.
- Apply to exposed skin, including the face, wrists, ankles and neck. To apply to the face, dispense repellent into the hands, rub the hands together, then apply to face, taking care to avoid the mouth, eyes and nose.
- Wash hands after application to avoid inadvertent transfer of repellent to eyes, mouth and nose.
- Do not apply to broken or inflamed skin.
- Do not apply to children's hands or face.

Malaria[24]

Up to 30,000 travelers from industrialized countries contract malaria each year[27] and fatalities have been reported in North America. Areas where malaria is transmitted include most of sub-Saharan Africa and New Guinea; large areas of Southern Asia; parts of Southeast Asia, Oceania, Haiti, Central and South America; and limited areas of Mexico, the Dominican Republic, North Africa and the Middle East.[24] Any traveler to an area where malaria is endemic should understand the seriousness of the disease; their personal risk of becoming infected; measures to prevent infection, including personal protection against vectors and chemoprophylaxis, where appropriate; and the importance of *seeking medical attention immediately if they develop a fever during travel or within one year of their return home.*

Risk of infection varies widely. Factors that influence risk include geographic destination, time of year, travel destination within a geographic location (e.g., urban versus rural), type of accommodation, duration of travel, elevation of destination (transmission is rare above 2000 m), and efficacy and compliance with prophylactic measures.[27] Each traveler should have their individual risk of infection and the necessity of chemoprophylaxis assessed prior to travel.

Effective chemoprophylactic agents are available, though resistance is widespread in some parts of the world. Compliance with prophylaxis is important, but noncompliance rates are high. Even when used

appropriately, chemoprophylaxis is not 100% effective; therefore, compliance with bite-avoidance measures is important.

Children, pregnant women and immunocompromised hosts are predisposed to developing severe malarial infection. These groups should avoid travel to areas with significant transmission of malaria. If this is not possible, children, including breastfed infants, pregnant women and immunocompromised hosts should be well-protected against mosquito bites and receive appropriate chemoprophylaxis.[24]

Anyone who visits an area where malaria is a consideration should contact a physician *immediately* if they experience fever during travel or within one year of their return home. If necessary, they should remind the physician that they have visited an area where malaria is transmitted, that chemoprophylaxis is not always effective, and that blood smears are necessary to rule out malaria.[28]

Traveling with Medication

Any medication used on a regular basis should be brought along, as well as any emergency or intermittent use items (e.g., asthma inhalers, EpiPens®). Travelers are advised to take extra amounts of medications as well as a written prescription with the chemical name of the drug (universally recognized) in case of emergency.

All medication should be stored in the original labeled container to avoid problems at borders as well as to facilitate drug identification in case of emergency.[29] Medications should also be kept in carry-on luggage in case of flight delays or lost luggage, and to protect it from extreme temperatures.[30] Diabetics who are required to bring hypodermic syringes and needles should carry a letter from their physician authorizing such possession to avoid delays at customs. Syringes should be declared at Customs. Insulin that will not be used within one month, or any medication that requires refrigeration, can be kept cool in a wide-mouth thermos; the thermos should be cooled by filling it with cold or iced water and then pouring out the water before storage of medication.[30,31] The medication should then be refrigerated once the destination is reached.

If pills or capsules might experience rough handling (e.g., during backpacking), blisterpacking may prevent breakage. Alternatively, placing cotton wool in the prescription vial may be helpful.[32]

Before traveling, people who use controlled drugs or nonprescription codeine preparations should check with embassies or consulates of the destination country and any country through which the person will travel en route. Regulations vary from country to country, and what is legal in Canada may not be permitted in another country.

Travelers requiring oxygen therapy during air travel should contact the airline in advance.[13,16]

Most airlines will accommodate travelers with special diets if informed at least 24 hours in advance.[13]

Travel Clinics

In general, immunizations can be divided into two broad categories: routine and non-routine.[33] Routine immunizations include those that are normally given during childhood such as measles, mumps and rubella. Non-routine immunizations become important when traveling outside Canada or the United States. Examples of non-routine vaccinations include hepatitis A, typhoid and yellow fever.[33] It is recommended that when traveling outside Canada or the United States, travelers should plan a pre-trip visit to their health care provider or a travel clinic at least four to six weeks before their trip. This is important, as there are specific vaccination requirements that may vary depending on the planned destination. Travel clinics also provide other services such as assessment of malaria risk, of need for expanded medical kits and advice on personal protection against vectors.

There are travel clinics available across Canada. For a full listing, visit the Internet web site at http://www.hc-sc.gc.ca/hpb/lcdc/osh/trave/clinic or contact local public health authorities.

Travel Health Information Resources

Travelers seeking English-speaking physicians can inquire with hotel receptions, tour companies or Canadian embassies.[2] The International Association for Medical Assistance to Travelers (IAMAT) will supply a directory of English speaking physicians in 125 countries and territories (Table 4).[13,34] IAMAT physicians have agreed to provide services with set fee schedules.[34] Membership to IAMAT is free of charge although a small donation is requested to help support its work.

Table 4: **SUMMARY of IAMAT* Services**

- Membership card—entitles bearer to services and fixed IAMAT rates
- World directory—a directory of English-speaking physicians in 125 countries and territories who have agreed to a set payment schedule
- Traveler clinical record—a passport-size record completed by one's doctor prior to departure
- World immunization chart—provides information on preventive measures
- World malaria risk chart and protection guide—a guide to malaria prophylaxis
- World schistosomiasis risk chart and information brochure—provides information on preventive measures against schistosomiasis
- World climate chart—summary of climate in any part of the world

IAMAT* CANADA: 40 Regal Road, Guelph, Ontario N1K 1B5
Tel.: (519) 836-0102
Fax: (519) 836-3412
www.iamat.org

1287 St. Clair Avenue West, Toronto, Ontario M6E 1B8
Tel.: (416) 652-0137

*International Association for Medical Assistance to Travelers

There is a variety of commercial databases and Internet sources available for travel information. Even among reputable web sites, conflicting information can be found and careful consideration by the user is needed.[35] A listing of some useful web sites for travel information is listed in Tables 5 and 6. As well, there are services available that may provide helpful travel information (Table 7).

In addition, travelers may contact the Department of Foreign Affairs and International Trade for information on safety and security considerations (1-800-267-6788).

Table 5: **Web Sites for Travel Medicine Recommendations for the Health Care Provider**[35,36]

Web site	URL	Description
Centres for Disease Control and Prevention (CDC)	www.cdc.gov/travel	US recommendations; Yellow Book: Health Information for International Travel
World Health Organization (WHO)	www.who.int	General travel advice; country–specific malaria risk and antimalarial recommendations
Committee to Advise on Tropical Medicine and Travel (CATMAT)	www.hc-sc.gc.ca/hpb/ lcdc/osh/reccom_e.html #catmat	International travel health information for health professionals
Population and Public Health Branch, Health Canada	www.hc-sc.gc.ca/pphb-dgspsp/tmp-pmv/	Regularly updated including information on outbreaks and a list of clinics providing travel health services in Canada

Table 6: **Web Sites on Travel Medicine for the Consumer**[35]

Website	URL	Description
Travelhealth Online	www.tripprep.com	Comprehensive
Fit for Travel	www.fit-for-travel.de/en/index.html	Sophisticated user interface
Lonely Planet Health	www.lonelyplanet.com/health	Good quality, wide audience
Medicine Planet	www.medicineplanet.com/home	In development, sophisticated user interface

Table 7: **Other Health Information Resources**[36]

Population and Public Health Branch, Health Canada
Fax link: (613) 941-3900
(24-h service providing travel information for travelers and travel health professionals)

International Society of Travel Medicine
PO Box 15060
Atlanta, GA
30333-0060
USA

CDC Fax Information Service
Fax link: 1-888-232-3299
(To request fax information on travelers' health)

Water Treatment Methods for Travelers

Safe drinking water is essential for travelers to foreign countries, as well as for backpackers within Canada, who rely on water from streams, ponds, rivers and lakes.

Fluid Requirements

In general, the human body requires an average intake of 2 L of water a day to function optimally. A more accurate calculation is based on body surface area using the formula 1500 to 2000 mL/m^2 per day.[37] Fluid is replenished by consuming water, other beverages and solid foods. Because it is difficult to measure the total amount of fluid obtained by eating food, it is recommended that only drinking fluids be counted toward meeting the requirement of 2 L a day. Physical exertion by athletes or travelers in hot, humid or cold weather and at high altitudes increases fluid loss and more fluids should be consumed. Knowing the daily fluid requirements of each traveler will allow travelers to plan the quantity of fuel needed to boil water and the size of container needed to store the water. Enough fluid should be consumed to keep the urine clear and light in color.

Risks of Unsafe Water

Drinking unsafe water may result in acute infections within hours or days, marked by vomiting, diarrhea, fever, malaise and/or abdominal pain. Diseases contracted by drinking contaminated water may be of viral, bacterial or protozoal origin and include amebiasis (*E. histolytica*), cholera, cryptosporidiosis, *E. coli* enteritis, giardiasis (*G. lamblia*), hepatitis A, *Shigella* enteritis and typhoid fever.[37] Vaccines are not available to protect travelers against most of these diseases, except for typhoid and hepatitis A. Simple precautions should be taken to minimize the risk of infection. These are described in Chapter 22. This appendix describes treatment of water from streams, ponds, rivers and lakes. When necessary, these methods may also be used to treat well water.

Unsafe Water

Water treatment methods outlined in this text are directed at preventing infectious illnesses from bacteria, viruses and protozoa. However, other contaminants including radionucleides, inorganic materials such as copper, mercury or lead and organic contaminants such as solvents, pesticides and herbicides may exist in water that has not been processed for human consumption.[38] Testing for individual contaminants is not practical for travelers as it may involve sending samples to a licensed testing facility or carrying individual test kits for each contaminant (e.g., lead). It is best to verify with a local guide whether the drinking water source is suitable for humans. While physical appearance is not a reliable indicator of safety, there are some signs of unsafe water. Contaminated water may appear turbid (cloudy) and have a smell (rotten egg, gasoline, chemical smell other than chlorine/ iodine).[38]

Turbidity may not only indicate contamination, but may also interfere with disinfection.[39] Cloudy water should be strained through a clean cloth or filter.[26,39-43] It can then be boiled or chemically treated with iodine. Once purified, water should be stored in clean, covered containers to reduce the chance of recontamination. Purified water that has been stored in a clean container should be replaced after six months.[44]

Recommended Water Treatment Methods
Heat
Boiling water is the most reliable, and therefore the preferred, method of purifying water for drinking.[39] Boiling eliminates bacteria, viruses and protozoa. Water should be boiled vigorously for one minute then allowed to cool to room temperature.[26] At altitudes greater than 2000 m above sea level, water should be boiled for three minutes, or boiled for one minute then chemically treated with iodine.[26] Boiled water may taste flat; adding a pinch of salt or oxygenating the water by pouring the water back and forth between two clean containers can improve this.[26]

Iodination
Iodination is recommended only for short-term (i.e., a few weeks) use if boiling is not feasible.[26,39-43] Contact time of the iodine in water should be extended if the water is very cold or cloudy. In order to kill *Cryptosporidium*, iodinated water should be allowed to sit for 15 hours before consumption.[26] Ideally, in order to remove protozoal cysts such as *G. lamblia*, water should be first filtered through a filter with an

absolute pore size of one micrometer or less, then iodinated to kill viruses and bacteria.[26,39-41] Iodination should be used with caution in pregnant women, infants, children, and travelers with thyroid disease.[26,39-41] Prolonged ingestion of iodine may lead to hypothyroidism or hyperthyroidism, goitre, hypersensitivity, iodism or poisoning which is manifested by corrosion of the GI tract, metallic taste, vomiting and abdominal pain.[45] Iodine also crosses the placenta and is excreted into breastmilk.[45] The iodine may stain and it imparts an unpleasant taste to the water; palatability can be improved by adding a vitamin C tablet or powdered drink crystals prior to consumption.[40] Table 8 lists iodine products appropriate for water purification and describes their use. Other iodine-based products such as Lugol's solution or stainless iodine have different iodine concentrations and should not be recommended.

Other Water Treatment Methods[26,42,43]

Chlorine treatment is not as reliable as iodine.[39] Chlorine treatment alone may not kill some enteric viruses, *G. lamblia* and *E. histolytica* cysts and *Cryptosporidium* species.[26] If chlorine is used, add two drops (0.1 mL) chlorine household bleach to 1 L water (four drops if water is cloudy), mix and let stand 30 minutes (longer if water is very cold).[43]

Water treatment devices such as filters, micro filters or portable iodine-impregnated resin devices are available from camping equipment stores. Filters or micro filters are available with small pore sizes (0.1 to 0.3 micrometer). They may remove protozoa, *G. lamblia* cysts and large bacteria, but will not remove viruses.[26] Filtration alone is therefore inadequate to purify water. Although filtration is not mandatory, it complements heating or iodine treatment, if it is used first to remove large particles.

Filters with iodine-impregnated resins are more effective against bacteria than protozoa and viruses. The contact time with the iodine in the filter is too short to kill *Giardia* in cold water, *Cryptosporidium* and some viruses.[5] Depending on the brand, devices are available as a cup for single person use or as pumps for treating larger volumes of water. Some may have prefilters to remove large particles. Prefilters can be cleaned by back flushing or can be replaced at an additional cost. Units vary in price, size, and weight and in the maximum volume of water that can be treated. Proper selection, operation and maintenance of water treatment devices are essential in producing safe drinking water. There are insufficient published scientific reports to determine which devices are most effective at removing bacteria and viruses.

Suggested Readings

Backer H. Water disinfection for international and wilderness travelers. *Clin Infect Dis* 2002;34(3): 355-64.

Committee to Advise on Tropical Medicine and Travel (Canada). Statement on high-altitude illness. *Can Comm Dis Rep* 1998 Nov 15;24(ACS-4). Available at: http://www.hc-sc.gc.ca/hpb/lcdc/publicat/ccdr/98 vol24/24sup/acs4.html.

Table 8: **Iodine Products for Water Purification**[26,42,43]

Iodination	Procedure
Tincture of Iodine 2% solution*	Add 5 drops (0.25 mL) per litre of clear water or 10 drops (0.5 mL) per litre of cold (< 5°C) or cloudy water. Mix thoroughly and let stand for at least 30 min before drinking. Very cold or cloudy water should be allowed to stand several hours before use, if possible.
Saturated iodine solution†	Add 12.5 mL per litre of water and let stand for 15-20 min and 20 mL per litre for at least 20 min if cold or cloudy water.
Tetraglycine hydroperiodide†	Add one tablet/L of room temperature water and wait 15 min before use. Use 2 tablets per litre of cold or turbid water and wait 20 min.

Note: If *Cryptosporidum* is a risk, water should stand 15 h. Treated water should have a slight taste of iodine; if not, repeat procedure.

*Available in first aid kits and from pharmacies.
†Available at camping equipment stores and drug wholesalers.

Committee to Advise on Tropical Medicine and Travel (Canada). 2000 Canadian recommendations for the prevention and treatment of malaria among international travelers. *Can Comm Dis Rep* 2000 Mar;26S2. Available at: http://www.hc-sc.gc.ca/hpb/lcdc/publicat/ccdr/00vol26/26S2/26S2e_3.html

Thomas RE. Preparing patients to travel abroad safely – Part 1: Taking a travel history and identifying special risks. *Can Fam Physician* 2000;46:132-8.

References

1. First aid kits for travelers (editorial). *Pharmacy Today* 1993 (Oct).
2. Waler E, Williams G. ABC of health travel – first aid while abroad. *BMJ* 1983;286:1039-42.
3. Thomas RE. Preparing patients to travel abroad safely. Part 4: Reducing risk of accidents, diarrhea and sexually transmitted diseases. *Can Fam Physician* 2000;46:1634-8.
4. Seiden H, Cantarutti P, Thayer S. A customized first aid kit for home and vacation. *Can Fam Physician* 1985;31:2316-8.
5. Grant E, Grant P. Miscellaneous injuries and first aid equipment. *Pharm J* 1997;258:476-8.
6. Jones JJ, Sheffield W, Ehite LJ, Bloom MA. A double-blind comparison between oral pseudoephedrine and topical oxymetazoline in the prevention of barotrauma during air travel. *Am J Emerg Med* 1998;16:262-4.
7. Csortan E, Jones J, Haan M et al. Efficacy of pseudoephedrine for the prevention of barotrauma during air travel. *Ann Emerg Med* 1994;23:1324-7.
8. Facts & Comparisons. Home Medicine Cabinet – Basic Inventory. *Drug Newsletter* 1989;8(10):77.
9. Gouin S, Patel H. Office management of minor wounds. *Can Fam Physician* 2001;47:769-74.
10. Dyment SZ. The pharmacist and the traveler. *Pharmacy Practice* 1990;6(4):31-4.
11. Committee to Advise on Tropical Medicine and Travel (Canada). Statement on Travellers' Diarrhea. *Can Comm Dis Rep* 2001;27(ACS-3):1-12. Available at: http://www.hc-sc.gc.ca/hpb/lcdc/publicat/ccdr. Accessed October 31, 2001.
12. Committee to Advise on Tropical Medicine and Travel (Canada). Travel statement on jet lag. *Can Comm Dis Rep* 1995;21-16:148-51.
13. Skjenna OW, Evans JF, Moore M et al. Helping patients travel by air. *Can Med Assoc J* 1991;144(3):287-93.
14. Palacioz K. NADH for jet lag. Pharmacist's Letter/Prescriber's Letter Jan 2001. Online version (Document #170115).
15. Waterhouse J, Reilly T, Atkinson G. Jet-lag. *Lancet* 1997;350:1611-6.
16. Bettes TN, McKenas DK. Medical advice for commercial air travelers. *Am Fam Physician* 1999;60(3):801-9.
17. Herxheimer A, Petrie KJ. Melatonin for the prevention and treatment of jet lag (Cochrane Review). In: *The Cochrane Library*, Issue 1, 2002. Oxford: Update Software.
18. Committee to Advise on Tropical Medicine and Travel (Canada). Statement on high-altitude illness. *Can Comm Dis Rep* 1998, Nov 15; 24(ACS-4). Available at: http://www.hc-sc.gc.ca/hpb/lcdc/publicat/ccdr/98vol24/24sup/acs4.html. Accessed November 27, 2001.
19. Hackett PH, Roach RC. High-altitude illness. *N Engl J Med* 2001;345(2):107-14.
20. Goodyer L. Environmental hazards. *Pharm J* 2001;266:577-80.
21. Anonymous. Vectors and diseases. Hazards and risks for travellers: Part 1. *Can Comm Dis Rep* 2001;27(15):128-32.
22. Anonymous. Vectors and diseases. Hazards and risks for travellers: Part 2. *Can Comm Dis Rep* 2001;27(16):139-40.
23. Anonymous. Vectors and diseases. Hazards and risks for travellers: Part 3. *Can Comm Dis Rep* 2001;27(17):146-8.
24. Committee to Advise on Tropical Medicine and Travel (Canada). 2000 Canadian recommendations for the prevention and treatment of malaria among international travellers. *Can Comm Dis Rep* 2000 Mar; 26S2. Available at: http://www.hc-sc.gc.ca/hpb/lcdc/publicat/ccdr/00vol26/26s2/26s2/index.html. Accessed November 27, 2001.
25. Goodyer L. Bite avoidance. *Pharm J* 2000;265:298-304.
26. Centers for Disease Control and Prevention. *Health Information for International Travel 2001-2002*. Atlanta, GA: US Department of Health and Human Services, Public Health Service; 2001. Available at: http://www.cdc.gov/travel/yellowbook.pdf. Accessed January 29, 2002.
27. Kain KC, Shanks D, Keystone JS. Malaria chemoprophylaxis in the age of drug resistance. I. Currently recommended drug regimens. *Clin Infect Dis* 2001;33:226-34.
28. Health Canada, Population and Public Health Branch. *General advice for travellers*. Available at: http://hc-sc.gc.ca/pphb-dgspsp/tmp-pmv/travel/advice_e.html. Accessed October 31, 2001.
29. Dardick KR. General advice and medical kit. *Med Clin N Amer* 1992;76(6):1261-74.
30. Murdoch L. Storage and mixing of insulins – part 1. *New Drugs – Drug News* 1987;5(5):1-2.
31. Ontario College of Pharmacists. Clinical knowledge assessment. *Pharmacy Connection* 2000;Jan/Feb:29.
32. Goodyer L. Medical kits for travellers. *Pharm J* 2001;267:154-8.
33. Ward BJ. Vaccines for travelling minors: The 'shot' heard around the world. *Paediatr Child Health* 2001;6(4):190-3.
34. International Association for Medical Assistance to Travelers. Medical services and the international traveler. Guelph, Ontario: Foundation for the Support of International Medical Training, Inc., 1982.
35. Keystone JS, Kozarsky PE, Freedman DO. Internet and computer-based resources for travel medicine practioners. *Clin Infect Dis* 2001;32(Mar):757-65.
36. Houston S. From Livingstone to ecotourism – what's new in travel medicine. *Can Fam Physician* 2000;46:121-31.
37. Merck Manual. Maintenance of fluid requirements. Available at http://www.merck.com/pubs/mmanual/section19/chapter259/259d.htm. Accessed January 29, 2002
38. United States Enviormental Protection Agency Office of Water. *Current Drinking Water Standards for Contaminants*. Available at: http://www.epa.gov/safewater/mcl.html. Accessed January 29, 2002.
39. Centers for Disease Control Travelers Health. *Risks from food and drink*. Available at: http://www.cdc.gov/travel/foodwatr.htm. Accessed January 29, 2002.
40. Curtis, Rick. Hygiene and water purification. In: *The Backpackers Field Manual: a comprehensive guide to mastering backcountry skills*. New York: Random House Publishing 1998 Rick Curtis, Outdoor Action Program, Princeton University:83.

41. Health Canada Travel Medicine Program. *Travelers Diarrhea and Food and Water Precautions.* Available at: http://www.hc-sc.gc.ca/pphb-dgspsp/tmp-pmv/travel/diarre_e.html. Accessed January 29, 2002.

42. Health Canada. *It's Your Health. Water Treatment Devices.* Available at: http://www.hc-sc.gc.ca/ehp/ehd/catalogue/general/iyh/disinfection_devices.htm. Accessed January 29, 2002.

43. Health Canada. *Drinking Water Away From Home, Emergency or Short Term Water Disinfection.* Available at: http://www.hc-c.gc.ca/ehp/ehd/catalogue/bch_pubs/dw_away.htm Accessed January 29, 2002.

44. American Red Cross. *Water Storage Before Disaster Strikes.* Available at http://www.redcross.org/services/disaster/beprepared/water.html. Accessed January 29, 2002.

45. Reynolds JEF, ed. *Martindale The Extra Pharmacopoeia.* 13th ed. London: The Pharmaceutical Press; 1993:970-1.

Microorganism Abbreviations

Abbreviation	Full Name
Bacteria	
B. forsythus	Bacteroides forsythus
B. fragilis	Bacteroides fragilis
C. jejuni	Campylobacter jejuni
C. pneumoniae	Chlamydia pneumoniae
C. trachomatis	Chlamydia trachomatis
C. difficile	Clostridium difficile
C. diphtheriae	Corynebacterium diphtheriae
E. aerogenes	Enterobacter aerogenes
E. cloacae	Enterobacter cloacae
E. faecalis	Enterococcus faecalis
E. coli	Escherichia coli
F. necrophorum	Fusobacterium necrophorum
F. nucleatum	Fusobacterium nucleatum
G. vaginalis	Gardnerella vaginalis
H. influenzae	Haemophilus influenzae
H. pylori	Helicobacter pylori
K. pneumoniae	Klebsiella pneumoniae
L. acidophilus	Lactobacillus acidophilus
L. vaginalis	Lactobacillus vaginalis
L. pneumophila	Legionella pneumophila
L. monocytogenes	Listeria monocytogenes
M. furfur	Malassezia furfur
M. catarrhalis	Moraxella catarrhalis
M. lacunata	Moraxella lacunata
M. tuberculosis	Mycobacterium tuberculosis
M. pneumoniae	Mycoplasma pneumoniae
N. gonorrhoeae	Neisseria gonorrhoeae
N. gonorrhoeae subsp N. kochii	Neisseria gonorrhoeae subspecies Neisseria kochii
N. meningitidis	Neisseria meningitidis
N. asteroides	Nocardia asteroides

Abbreviation	Full Name
N. asteroides	Nocardia asteroides
N. asteroides	Nocardia asteroides
P. acnes	Propionibacterium acnes
P. gingivalis	Porphyromonas gingivalis
P. intermedia	Prevotella intermedia
P. mirabilis	Proteus mirabilis
P. stuartii	Providencia stuartii
P. aeruginosa	Pseudomonas aeruginosa
S. typhi	Salmonella typhi
S. marcescens	Serratia marcescens
S. aureus	Staphylococcus aureus
S. epidermidis	Staphylococcus epidermidis
S. saprophyticus	Staphylococcus saprophyticus
S. pneumoniae	Streptococcus pneumoniae
S. mutans	Streptococcus mutans
S. pyogenes	Streptococcus pyogenes
S. viridans	Streptococcus viridans
U. urealyticum	Ureaplasma urealyticum
V. cholerae	Vibrio cholerae
Blood Parasites	
P. falciparum	Plasmodium falciparum
P. malariae	Plasmodium malariae
P. ovale	Plasmodium ovale
P. vivax	Plasmodium vivax
Fungi	
C. albicans	Candida albicans
C. glabrata	Candida glabrata
C. neoformans	Cryptococcus neoformans
E. floccosum	Epidermophyton floccosum
T. mentagrophytes	Trichophyton mentagrophytes
T. rubrum	Trichophyton rubrum

Abbreviation	Full Name
Protozoa/Parasites	
C. cayetanesis	*Cyclospora cayetanesis*
C. parvum	*Cryptosporidium parvum*
E. histolytica	*Entamoeba histolytica*
E. vermiculais	*Enterobius vermicularis*
G. lamblia	*Giardia lamblia*
P. carinii	*Pneumocystis carinii*
S. stercoralis	*Strongyloides stercoralis*
T. gondii	*Toxoplasma gondii*
T. vaginalis	*Trichomonas vaginalis*

Abbreviation	Full Name
Viruses	
CMV	Cytomegalovirus
HAV	Hepatitis A virus
HBV	Hepatitis B virus
HCV	Hepatitis C virus
HIV	Human immunodeficiency virus
HPV	Human papillomavirus
HSV	Herpes simplex virus
RSV	Respiratory syncytial virus

Index

patient information 461

prevention 456-57

signs and symptoms 456, 457*t*

treatment 457-59, 458*t*, 459*f*

atopic dermatitis *see also* contact dermatitis; diaper d.; hand d.; stasis d.

associated drugs 482*t*

defined 480

diaper dermatitis 498*t*

etiology 480

monitoring of therapy 494, 494*t*

pathophysiology 479-80

patient assessment 483, 484*f*, 485*t*, 486*t*

patient information 506

signs and symptoms 476*t*

treatment 486, 487*f*, 489*t*-90*t*

atropine sulfate

causing dry mouth 803*t*

exacerbating symptoms of benign prostatic hyperplasia 736*t*

attapulgite

diarrhea 243*t*

auranofin

associated with psoriasis 509*t*

associated with seborrhea 509*t*

causing nausea and vomiting 210*t*

aurothioglucose

associated with psoriasis 509*t*

associated with seborrhea 509*t*

aversion therapy

smoking cessation 104

avulsions *see* cuts and wounds

Ayurveda 829

psoriasis 523

azathioprine

associated with fever 81*t*

caution in breastfeeding 360*t*

azithromycin

causing ototoxicity 184*t*

travelers' diarrhea 247

azole-resistant candidiasis 675-76

B

baby bottles 369-70

bacitracin

acute bacterial conjunctivitis 151

blepharitis 150

burns 633*t*, 637

causing contact dermatitis 481*t*

cuts and wounds 633*t*

hordeolum 146

otitis externa 195*t*

back pain *see* low back pain

backache (pregnancy) 712*t*

bacterial skin infections

furuncles and carbuncles 593-94, 595*f*, 596-97, 597*t*

impetigo 592-93, 594*t*, 596*t*

bacteriostatic soaps

inappropriate for use in acne 536

bad breath *see* halitosis

balanced salt solution

seasonal allergic conjunctivitis 156*t*

bandages *see* dressings

banned/restricted substances 449*t*, 450

barbiturates

associated with constipation 223*t*

associated with depression 59*t*

associated with fever 81*t*

causing erectile dysfunction 723*t*

inappropriate for use in infant colic 281*t*

insomnia 54

barium

associated with constipation 223*t*

barotrauma 183*t*, 185

Barrett's esophagus 257

barrier contraceptives 657-60

barriers

diaper dermatitis 499-500, 501*t*

basal temperature 654, 744, 745*t*

bath boards 813

bath products

dermatitis 489*t*, 491

bath/shower seats 813

bathroom safety products 812-13

bathtub transfer benches 813

bayberry

diarrhea 242

Beano® *see* alpha-galactosidase

beclomethasone, nasal

pregnancy 126

pregnancy and lactation 706

bedrest

low back pain 416, 418*t*

behavior change

action stage 24

contemplation stage 23-24

facilitating 26*t*, 27*t*-28*t*, 29, 34, 39

identifying stages 25

maintenance stage 24

precontemplation stage 23

preparation stage 24

processes of 25, 26*t*

termination stage 24

transtheoretical model of 23, 24*t*

Behcet's disease 782

belching 264-66, 266*t*

belladonna

causing dry mouth 803*t*

orthomolecular therapy 831
oseltamivir
    influenza prophylaxis 135
    influenza treatment 138
osteoarthritis
    clinical features vs rheumatoid arthritis 426, 427*t*
    monitoring of therapy 435*t*
    pathophysiology 426
    patient assessment 426-27, 428*f*
    patient information 438
    signs and symptoms 426, 427*t*
    treatment 427, 429, 429*t*, 430-31*t*, 432-35, 433*t*, 434*f*
osteopathic medicine 831
osteophytes 426
osteoporosis
    associated drugs 406*t*
    defined 405
    monitoring of therapy 412*t*
    pathophysiology 405
    patient assessment 406, 407*f*, 408*f*
    patient information 414
    prevention 406
    risk factors 405, 406*t*, 407*f*
    treatment 351*t* , 406-11, 407*t*, 409*t*
ostomy
    appliances and accessories 301, 304
    changing the appliance 304, 305*f*
    defined 300
    dietary factors 308*t*, 309
    irrigation 305
    lifestyle considerations 309
    medication concerns 309, 310*t*
    patient assessment 301
    problems 306-09
    types 300, 302*f*, 303*f*
otalgia *see* ear disorders, pain
otitis externa
    acute diffuse 192
    acute localized 192
    chronic 192
    eczematous 192
    etiology 192
    monitoring of therapy 196
    necrotizing 192
    pathophysiology 192
    patient assessment 193
    patient information 197
    prevention 195
    seborrheic 510
    treatment 193, 194*t*-95*t*, 195
otitis media
    etiology 183
    signs and symptoms 134*t*, 183, 183*t*
    treatment 184

otorrhea *see* ear disorders, drainage
ototoxicity
    associated drugs 184*t*
ovulation 653, 684, 715, 744, 745*t*
oxazepam
    causing dry mouth 803*t*
oxiconazole
    athlete's foot 458*t*
oxprenolol *see also* beta-blockers
    associated with dermatitis 482*t*
oxybutynin
    causing dry mouth 803*t*
    hyperhidrosis 549
oxygen therapy 816
oxymetazoline
    allergic rhinitis 124*t*
    causing rhinitis medicamentosa 121
    pregnancy and lactation 709*t*
    seasonal allergic conjunctivitis 156*t*
    upper respiratory tract infections 136*t*
oxytocin 359, 360

P

PABA 566*t*
    associated with diaper dermatitis 496*t*
    sunscreen coverage 559*f*
pacifiers 370
pain *see also* abdominal p.; low back p.
    postepisiotomy 710, 714*t*
pancreatitis
    associated with abdominal pain 252*t*, 254
    associated with depression 59*t*
    associated with dyspepsia 256*t*
pantothenic acid
    deficiency 345*t*
    function 345*t*
    recommended nutrient intake 345*t*
    sources 345*t*
papain
    arthropod bites and stings 628*t*
papular acrodermatitis *see* Gianotti-Crosti syndrome
parabens
    associated with diaper dermatitis 496*t*
parabom 692
paraphenylenediamine
    causing contact dermatitis 481*t*
parasitic skin infections
    pediculosis 607-10, 612*t*, 620
    scabies 610-13, 621
Parkinson's disease
    associated with depression 59*t*
paroxetine
    associated with diarrhea 239*t*
    associated with headache 70*t*